Guide to Pediatric Physical Therapy

Guide to Pediatric Physical Therapy

A Clinical Approach

EDITORS

Martha H. Bloyer, PT, DPT
Board-Certified Clinical Specialist in Pediatric Physical Therapy
Assistant Professor
Department of Physical Therapy
Miller School of Medicine
University of Miami
Miami, Florida

Tricia Catalino, PT, DSc
Board-Certified Clinical Specialist in Pediatric Physical Therapy
Professor, Doctor of Physical Therapy Program
Dean, Graduate College of Health Sciences
Hawai'i Pacific University
Honolulu, Hawaii

Eric Shamus, PT, DPT, PhD
Professor
Department of Rehabilitation Sciences
Florida Gulf Coast University
Fort Myers, Florida

Cindy Miles, PT, PhD
Board-Certified Clinical Specialist in Pediatric Physical Therapy
Whitehall, Pennsylvania
Past President, APTA Academy of Pediatric Physical Therapy
Middleton, Wisconsin

McGraw Hill

1 2 3 4 5 6 7 8 9   DSS   29 28 27 26 25 24

ISBN 978-1-264-91709-9
MHID 1-264-91709-0

This book was set in Minion Pro by KnowledgeWorks Global Ltd.
The editors were Michael Weitz and Peter J. Boyle.
The production supervisor was Richard Ruzycka.
Project management was provided by Revathi Viswanathan, KnowledgeWorks Global Ltd.
The interior design was by Mary McKeon.
The cover designer was W2 Design.

Library of Congress Cataloging-in-Publication Data

Names: Bloyer, Martha H., editor. | Catalino, Tricia, editor. | Shamus,
  Eric, editor. | Miles, Cindy, 1954-2023, editor.
Title: Guide to pediatric physical therapy : a clinical approach / editors,
  Martha H. Bloyer, Tricia Catalino, Eric Shamus, Cindy Miles.
Description: New York : McGraw Hill, [2025] | Includes bibliographical
  references and index.
Identifiers: LCCN 2024024905 (print) | LCCN 2024024906 (ebook) | ISBN
  9781264917099 (hardcover) | ISBN 9781264920105 (ebook)
Subjects: MESH: Physical Therapy Modalities | Child | Adolescent
Classification: LCC RM725 (print) | LCC RM725 (ebook) | NLM WB 460 | DDC
  615.8/2—dc23/eng/20240731
LC record available at https://lccn.loc.gov/2024024905
LC ebook record available at https://lccn.loc.gov/2024024906

Contents

Dedications

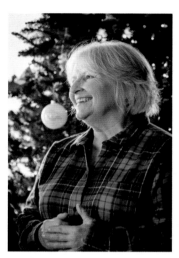

Cindy Miles

Cindy Miles was a mom to two daughters, a grandmother, wife, daughter, supportive friend, adored mentor and teacher, entrepreneur, advocate, and leader. Cindy dedicated her life to pediatric physical therapy, and she was a tireless advocate for all children. She strived every day to make the world a place where every child has the freedom and ability to move, play, and be fit. In her memory, we carry the torch of her mission—to infuse every life with the joy of movement and the boundless possibilities it brings.

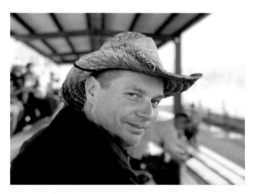

Brent Bloyer

Brent Bloyer's great happiness was his family. He was a wonderful husband, father, son, uncle, and brother-in-law. He took great joy in his children and their accomplishments. Brent was a physical therapist for Miami Dade County Public Schools and provided home-based physical therapy to children, adolescents, and young adults with disabilities. His gift for engaging children and individuals with disabilities made him beloved to many families.

Contributors

Joanna Beachy, MD, PhD
Chief, Newborn Medicine
Baystate Children's Hospital
Professor, Department of Pediatrics
UMass Chan Medical School—Baystate
Springfield, Massachusetts
Chapter 5: Newborn Infants With Medical Fragility

Jason Benincasa, PT, DPT, EP-C
Board-Certified Clinical Specialist in Pediatric
  Physical Therapy
Children's Hospital of Philadelphia
Philadelphia, Pennsylvania
Chapter 6: Pediatric Acute Care

Emily Berry, PT, DPT
Physical Therapist
Benchmark Human Services
Fort Wayne, Indiana
Chapter 6: Pediatric Acute Care

Martha H. Bloyer, PT, DPT
Board-Certified Clinical Specialist in Pediatric Physical Therapy
Assistant Professor
Department of Physical Therapy
Miller School of Medicine
University of Miami
Miami, Florida
*Chapter 7: Cerebral Palsy and Chapter 22: Promoting Successful
  Transition to Adulthood: The Role of Physical Therapy*

Tricia Catalino, PT, DSc
Board-Certified Clinical Specialist in Pediatric Physical Therapy
Professor, Doctor of Physical Therapy Program
Dean, Graduate College of Health Sciences
Hawai'i Pacific University
Honolulu, Hawaii
*Chapter 21: Physical Therapy Practice in Parts C and B of the
  Individuals With Disabilities Education Act*

Susan W. Cecere, PT, MHS
Owner, Sequoia School-Based Therapy Solutions, LLC.
St. Michaels, Maryland
*Chapter 21: Physical Therapy Practice in Parts C and B of the
  Individuals With Disabilities Education Act*

Jason E. Cook, PT, DPT, PhD
Board-Certified Clinical Specialist in Pediatric Physical
  Therapy
Clinical Assistant Professor
Tufts University School of Medicine
Boston, Massachusetts
Chapter 1: Developmental Theory

Megan Geno Dakhlian, PT, DPT
Board-Certified Clinical Specialist in Pediatric Physical Therapy
Manager of Operations—Physical Therapy
Boston Children's Hospital
Boston, Massachusetts
Chapter 9: Neural Tube Defects

Mary Devine, MPH
Senior Director, Emergency Management
Boston Children's Hospital
Boston, Massachusetts
*Chapter 24: Emergency Response of Physical Therapy During a
  Crisis or Pandemic*

Jamie Dyson, PT, DPT
Assistant Clinical Professor
Doctor of Physical Therapy
Graceland University
Independence, Missouri
Chapter 16: Cardiopulmonary Dysfunction in Pediatrics

Elizabeth Ennis, PT, EdD
Senior Academic Program Director – Florida DPT
University of St Augustine for Health Sciences
St Augustine, Florida
Chapter 2: Typical Development

Sarah Fabrizi, OTR/L, PhD
Associate Professor
Occupational Therapy Program
Department of Rehabilitation Sciences
Florida Gulf Coast University
Fort Myers, Florida
Chapter 14: Genetic Disorders

Alicia Fernandez-Fernandez, PT, DPT, PhD
Professor
Physical Therapy Department
Nova Southeastern University
Fort Lauderdale, Florida
*Chapter 8: Neuromuscular Diseases: Muscular Dystrophies and
    Spinal Muscular Atrophy*

Alyssa La Forme Fiss, PT, PhD
Board-Certified Clinical Specialist in Pediatric Physical Therapy
Professor and Director
School of Physical Therapy
Texas Woman's University
Dallas, Texas
Chapter 3: Assessment Tools in Pediatric Physical Therapy

Kendra Gagnon, PT, PhD
Associate Professor
Department of Physical Medicine & Rehabilitation
Johns Hopkins University School of Medicine
Baltimore, Maryland
*Chapter 21: Physical Therapy Practice in Parts C and B of the
    Individuals With Disabilities Education Act*

Roberta Bertie Gatlin, PT, DScPT
Retired Associate Professor Doctor of Physical
    Therapy Program
South College
Knoxville, Tennessee
*Chapter 5: Newborn Infants With Medical Fragility and Chapter 24:
    Emergency Response of Physical Therapy During a Crisis or
    Pandemic*

Jenna Gondelman, PT, DPT
Board-Certified Clinical Specialist in Pediatric Physical Therapy
Physical Therapist, III
Boston Children's Hospital
Boston, Massachusetts
Chapter 6: Pediatric Acute Care

Jonathan Greenwood, PT, MS, MBA, DPT
Board-Certified Clinical Specialist in Pediatric Physical Therapy
Fellow of American College of Health Care Executives
Senior Director of Physical Therapy, Occupational Therapy
    and Rehabilitation Services
Boston Children's Hospital
Boston, Massachusetts
*Chapter 24: Emergency Response of Physical Therapy During a
    Crisis or Pandemic and Chapter 25: The Role of Telehealth in
    Pediatric Physical Therapy*

Dawn James, PT, DPT, DSc
Board-Certified Specialist in Pediatric Physical Therapy
Associate Professor and Program Director
Doctor of Physical Therapy Program
Tarleton State University
Stephenville, Texas
Chapter 2: Typical Development

Lynn Jeffries, PT, DPT, PhD
Board-Certified Clinical Specialist in Pediatric Physical Therapy
Associate Professor
Department of Rehabilitation Sciences
University of Oklahoma Health Sciences Center
Oklahoma City, Oklahoma
*Chapter 2: Typical Development and Chapter 3: Assessment
    Tools in Pediatric Physical Therapy*

Marla Laufer, MD
Board-Certified in General Pediatrics
Board-Certified in Pediatric Hospital Medicine
Senior Instructor
University of Colorado School of Medicine
Denver, Colorado
Chapter 18: Pediatric Wellness and Fitness

Catherine Maher, PT, DPT
Morristown, New Jersey
Chapter 10: Spinal Cord Injury

Kathy Martin, PT, DHSc
Professor
Krannert School of Physical Therapy
University of Indianapolis
Indianapolis, Indiana
Chapter 19: Lower Extremity Orthoses for Children

Rania Massad, PT, DPT
Board-Certified Clinical Specialist in Neurologic Physical
    Therapy
Instructor Physical Therapy
Nova Southeastern University
Davie, Florida
*Chapter 22: Promoting Successful Transition to Adulthood:
    The Role of Physical Therapy*

Teresa Muñecas, PT, DPT, EdD
Assistant Chair and Associate Clinical Professor
Director of Clinical Education
Floirda International University
Miami, Florida
Chapter 7: Cerebral Palsy

Ana Nevares, MA
Assistive Technology & Education Specialist
Regional Coordinator, FAAST Program
University of Miami
Mailman Center for Child Development
Miami, Florida
Chapter 20: The Role of the Physical Therapist in Assistive
Technology Service Delivery

Jennifer Parent-Nichols, DPT, EdD
Board-Certified Pediatric Clinical Specialist in Physical Therapy
Clinical Associate Professor
Associate Program Director
Faculty Director of Student Affairs
Doctor of Physical Therapy Program-Boston
Tufts University School of Medicine
Boston, Massachusetts
Chapter 12: Developmental Coordination Disorder and
Chapter 13: Vestibular Disorders

Mary B. Pengelley, PT, DPT
Assistive Technology Practitioner
Rehab Director of West Palm Beach/Physical Therapist
Progressive Pediatric Therapy, Inc.
West Palm Beach, Florida
Chapter 8: Neuromuscular Diseases: Muscular Dystrophies and
Spinal Muscular Atrophy

Cristina Pujol, MS, CCC-SLP
University of Miami Health System
Miami, Florida
Chapter 20: The Role of the Physical Therapist in Assistive
Technology Service Delivery

Michelle Schladant, PhD, ATP
Board-Certified Assistive Technology Professional
Associate Professor, Pediatrics
University of Miami Miller School of Medicine
Miami, Florida
Chapter 20: The Role of the Physical Therapist in Assistive
Technology Service Delivery

Ron Scott, PT, EdD, JD, LLM, MA (Spanish), MSBA, MSPT
Attorney at Law (Texas)
Faculty Affiliate, DPT Program
University of Montana, Missoula
Content Creator and Instructor
MedBridge Education
Seattle, Washington
Associate Professor and Past Chairperson, Retired
University of Texas Health, San Antonio
Department of Physical Therapy
Current Guest Lecturer, Medical Spanish
Chapter 23: Legal Foundations

Eric Shamus, PT, MS, DPT, PhD, CEEAA, CSCS
Professor
Department of Rehabilitation Sciences
Florida Gulf Coast University
Fort Myers, Florida
Chapter 14: Genetic Disorders; Chapter 15: Juvenile Idiopathic
Arthritis; Chapter 16: Cardiopulmonary Dysfunction in
Pediatrics; Chapter 17: Pediatric Orthopedic and Sports
Injuries; and Chapter 18: Pediatric Wellness and Fitness

Grant Shamus, CPT
Certified Personal Trainer
Exercise Science
Florida Gulf Coast University
Fort Myers, Florida
Chapter 18: Pediatric Wellness and Fitness

Jennifer Shamus, PT, DPT, PhD, COMT, CSCS
Regional Director
Select Physical Therapy
Southeast Florida, Florida
Chapter 15: Juvenile Idiopathic Arthritis and Chapter 17:
Pediatric Orthopedic and Sports Injuries

Rob Sillevis, PT, DPT, PhD
Board-Certified Clinical Specialist in Orthopedic Physical
  Therapy
Fellow in the American Academy of Orthopedic Manual
  Physical Therapists
Associate Professor
Florida Gulf Coast University
Fort Myers, Florida
Chapter 18: Pediatric Wellness and Fitness

Susan Simpkins, PT, EdD
Associate Professor
Department of Physical Therapy
School of Health Professions
UT Southwestern Medical Center
Dallas, Texas
Chapter 4: Movement Systems in Pediatrics

Lori Solo, PT, DPT
Board-Certified Clinical Specialist in Neurologic Physical
  Therapy
Assistant Clinical Professor
Department of Physical Therapy, Movement &
  Rehabilitation Sciences
Northeastern University
Boston, Massachusetts
Chapter 6: Pediatric Acute Care

Jane K. Sweeney, PT, PhD, MS
Board-Certified Clinical Specialist in Pediatric Physical Therapy
Professor and Program Director
Pediatric Science Doctoral Programs and Neonatology
  Fellowship
Rocky Mountain University of Health Professions
Provo, Utah
Chapter 5: Newborn Infants With Medical Fragility

Denise Swensen, PT, DPT
Physical Therapist
Prince George's County Public Schools
Judith P. Hoyer Early Childhood Center
Cheverly, Maryland
*Chapter 21: Physical Therapy Practice in Parts C and B of the
  Individuals With Disabilities Education Act*

Kay Tasso, PT, PhD
Board-Certified Clinical Specialist in Pediatric
  Physical Therapy, Emeritus
Chapter 14: Genetic Disorders

Melissa Moran Tovin, PT, MA, PhD
Board-Certified Clinical Specialist in Pediatric Physical
  Therapy
Associate Professor
Department of Physical Therapy
University of Miami
Miller School of Medicine
Coral Gables, Florida
*Chapter 11: Autism Spectrum Disorder and Chapter 22:
  Promoting Successful Transition to Adulthood: The Role of
  Physical Therapy*

Caroline Ubben, PT, DPT, CSCS
Board-Certified Clinical Specialist in Pediatric Physical Therapy
Pediatric PT Residency Coordinator
Brooks Rehabilitation—Institute of Higher Learning
Jacksonville, Florida
Adjunct Faculty
University of St. Augustine—Health Sciences
St. Augustine, Florida
Chapter 17: Pediatric Orthopedic and Sports Injuries

Sadie Vega-Velasquez, MS, CCC-SLP
Miami, Florida
*Chapter 20: The Role of the Physical Therapist in Assistive
  Technology Service Delivery*

Steven Walczak, PT, DPT
Board-Certified Clinical Specialist in Pediatric Physical
  Therapy
Pediatrics and Brain Injury Program
Brooks Rehabilitation—Institute of Higher Learning
Jacksonville, Florida
Chapter 17: Pediatric Orthopedic and Sports Injuries

Priscilla Weaver, PT, DPT, PhD
Board-Certified Clinical Specialist in Pediatric Physical Therapy
Clinical Professor, Director of Educational Transformation
Northern Arizona University, Department of Physical Therapy
Flagstaff, Arizona
*Chapter 21: Physical Therapy Practice in Parts C and B of the
  Individuals With Disabilities Education Act*

Genevieve Pinto Zipp, PT, EdD
Professor and Program Director PhD in Health Sciences,
  Department of Interprofessional Health Sciences & Health
  Administration, Seton Hall University, School of Health and
  Medical Sciences, HIS Campus Nutley, New Jersey
*Chapter 4: Movement Systems in Pediatrics and Chapter 10:
  Spinal Cord Injury*

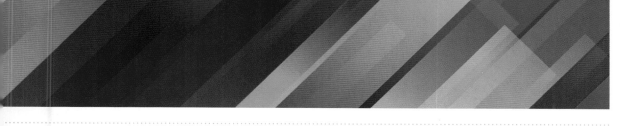

Preface

Guide to Pediatric Physical Therapy: A Clinical Approach provides pedagogy from top experts in the profession to help readers master the practice of physical therapy for kids. Each chapter has multiple cases that help students apply concepts to real-world situations, along with art and illustrations that reinforce what readers have learned. Critical information is presented in tables, which are particularly effective in helping students quickly digest key concepts. With more than 75 collective years teaching pediatric physical therapy, this author team focused on presenting diverse clinical approaches to serve how today's students prefer to learn.

- Chapter summaries are presented to make learning easy and quick.
- 200 illustrations.

- Key tables highlight high-yield information.
- Each case study is followed by open-ended questions for the reader to consider.
- Review questions are written in NPTE Exam format, so students can get early practice in how to handle and solve NPTE questions.

We hope this text will provide everything physical therapists and physical therapy students need to perform safe, effective physical therapy on infants, children, and adolescents.

Developmental Theory

Jason E. Cook, PT, DPT, PhD

LEARNING OBJECTIVES

Upon completion of this chapter, the reader will be able to:

- Understand the historical significance of essential supportive research in the field of human development.
- Apply the developmental theories of dynamic systems theory, neuronal group selection theory, and motor

program theory and schema theory to children with typical and atypical motor development.
- Apply concepts of developmental theories to postural control and gait.

INTRODUCTION

Developmental theory is a scientific attempt to explain how and why humans develop across their life span. A significant amount of human development occurs in the first few years of life as the infant and child learn to move, explore, play, and interact with others. This chapter will introduce some of the most prominent developmental theories and some of the discoveries that help support them. To make sense of the current state in developmental theory, it is important to understand the historical perspectives and discoveries that have helped lead to current understandings. This chapter will begin with a historical perspective of the knowledge about motor development and developmental theory. It will then go over the current principles for understanding the 3 primary developmental theories that explain motor skill acquisition: dynamical systems theory, neuronal group selection theory, and motor programming theory. Cases will be presented to help explain each of these theories to assist in the application of physical therapy clinical practice. Finally, the chapter will discuss an integrative approach of these 3 developmental theories in the skill acquisition of postural control and gait—2 important skills necessary for a child to develop and learn about the world in which they live.

PART I: INTRODUCTION AND HISTORICAL PERSPECTIVES

DEVELOPMENTAL THEORY: A PROGRESSIVE UNDERSTANDING

The science of how and why humans develop is a fascinating journey that has been partly driven by human curiosity and the need to understand why some children struggle with development. Within the past 150 years scientists have advanced their study of the developing infant to gain insight into how humans develop from conception throughout childhood. Around the

mid-19th century, an orthopedic physician, John Little, began to take interest in child development when it was observed that early infant birth asphyxiation led to long-term functional deficits in some children.[1] In the late 19th century, the question of nature versus nurture arose, and Sir Francis Galton began to see the influences that genetics had on the development of characteristics and traits in identical and fraternal twins.[2] Many questions began to arise about how and why humans develop in the way they do. Discoveries led to more questions, which also led to the development of theories that help explain how and why humans develop.

FROM MATURATIONISM TO DEVELOPMENTALISM

Some of our current understandings of human development came from the natural observation of behavior in the developing infant and child. Arnold Gissell, Mary Shirley, and Myrtle McGraw were early 20th-century researchers who documented and recorded infant and childhood movement. They applied these observations to theoretical principles to explain how and why humans develop through changing movement behaviors. Ideas about the importance of reflexes, heredity, and brain maturation were initially explored by these scientists.[3] However, their exploration moved beyond the popular behaviorism models of the time, which did not adequately explain the complex progression found in human development. Arnold Gesell, famous for his support of maturationism, a theory that explains that early development is derived from innate movement patterns and reflexes within the brain itself, helped bring insight to the understanding that heredity as well as predetermined factors influenced motor development.[4] As a physician who was concerned with children with special needs, he contributed significantly to our initial understanding of developmental milestones to assist with diagnosing children who were developmentally delayed.[4] Mary Shirley, a researcher at the Harvard Center for Child Health, wrote in her book, *The First Two Years: A Study* of *Twenty-Five Babies*, about the progression of the developing infant and early child through the stages of gaining independent walking skills.[5] Shirley believed that motor milestones are predetermined and that the developing infant will achieve the skills at a predetermined time.[6]

Myrtle McGraw was able to support the observed ebb and flow of developmental skill progression and the influence that a variety of different lived experiences have on developing human behavior.[7] Her now-famous experiment with a set of twin boys, Jimmy and Johnny, was a highly publicized experiment in the 1930s because of its support of both the nature and nurture models of developmental science.[8,9] Johnny was born hypotonic, leaving him at a developmental disadvantage compared to Jimmy.[10] Johnny was supported through motor training within his first few months, and as this training proceeded, he began to demonstrate advancements over Jimmy. He was able to acquire independent locomotion at the age of 9 months and learned how to roller skate and climb high stools before the age of 2 years.[10] However, by the time the boys reached later childhood, the developmental advancement was not as significant, supporting the idea that nature also has influences, regardless of the advanced motor training that Johnny had received.[9] This argument of whether development is driven by natural influences or a nurturing environment was a big question at this time and drove the maturational versus developmental discussion. There continues to be support that McGraw was at heart a progressive developmentalist.[9,11]

◼ PART II: THEORIES OF SIGNIFICANCE

A lot of what is understood about development today can be explained using 3 primary theories of development: dynamical systems theory, neuronal group selection theory, and motor programming theory/schema theory. These 3 theories are not isolated constructs or ideas but build off of previous theories of reflexive, maturational, and hierarchical theories of human development. These prior theories laid a foundation of knowledge that allows for the building of further understanding of the very complex concept of child development. These theories are primarily viewed in this text as they relate to physical therapy care and motor behavior. Refer to **Table 1-1** for a comparison of the 3 theories. Other theories of cognitivism, behaviorism, psychosocial approaches, and ecological approaches all play an important role in the understanding of child cognitive and psychosocial development; however, they are beyond the scope of this chapter.

DYNAMICAL SYSTEMS THEORY

Dynamical systems theory comes from an integration of multiple fields of study including mathematics, chemistry, physics, biology, and psychology to describe how organisms, including humans, change over time.[12] A.J. Kelso and G. Shöner introduced dynamical systems by recognizing that emerging patterns of movement behavior were not solely associated with hard-wired neural connections but were a dynamic interaction among multiple system that lead to self-organizing patterns.[13,14] Kelso described the development of the brain as being like a river that balances the nature of both flow and turbulence.[13] Within the complex system of motor development, multiple systems interact to make up the projected motor development seen in children.[14]

The structures found within these multiple systems are vast, from internal degrees of freedom, including muscle strength, coordination, and intact neural structures, to external sources of gravity, surface friction, and surface stability, to name only a few external characteristics. These systems work together, self-organizing based on constraints and affordances of the many systems, to produce patterns of movement. This idea of affordance, first described by psychologists J.J. and E.J. Gibson, postulates that internal, perceptual ideas interact with external, environmental factors to influence motor behavior and development.[15,16] The early studies of Johnny and Jimmy helped explain affordances in action. Johnny was exposed to earlier interventions, including the practice of using, struggling with, and ultimately learning to roller skate skillfully by the age of 16 months,[7,17] something that many children today do not learn to master until later in childhood. However, the story of Jimmy learning to skate much later in development, even though exposed to it at the age of 2 years, shows that perception changes over time and that the affordances, even though provided, are factors that interact with other affordances and constraints. In the case of Jimmy, he had established perceptions about the world and became frightened when placed in skates at the age of 2.[7]

TABLE 1-1 • Comparing Theories (key concepts emphasized in bold text)[10-15,17-20,29-34]		
Dynamical Systems Theory	**Neuronal Group Selection Theory**	**Schema and Motor Programming Theory**
• Motor development comes from the **emergence of self-organizing movement patterns**. • **Multiple systems** come together to encourage motor behavior. • Humans have internal **degrees of freedom** like strength, coordination, etc. • Humans interact with **constraints and affordances** that interact with motor patterns and behaviors.	• Incorporates **nature and nurture** together to explain development. • **Primary variability** is observed through movement patterns initiated by cortical development of predetermined neuronal structures. • **Secondary variability** of movement comes from adapting to external and environmental cues.	• Schema are building blocks of learning. • Motor tasks are stored memory, called **general motor programs (GMPs)**. • During the execution of a task, the GMP combines with the changing **parameters** of the task including speed and force. • Some components of a task do not change as the task becomes more skilled. These are called **invariant features** of the task. • Some studies suggest that timing and sequence are invariant features of some tasks.

In a dynamical systems approach, the developing human is a complex integration of multiple systems interacting on both a microscopic and macroscopic level.[14] As the human develops in early life, we see changes in motor behavior. One of the drivers of this change is the dynamic systems interacting, changing, and organizing. A component of dynamical systems theory is the concept that as motor behaviors change from one behavior to another over time, these transitional periods experience states of stability, as the motor behavior is established, and instability, when motor behaviors are changing to progress to a new skill. Those time periods in which the motor behavior is established are referred to as an attractor state.[13,18] As behavior changes from one skill to another, or one level of coordinated task to another, periods of instability are present prior to finding and maintaining the new attractor state. This time period is referred to as a nonequilibrium phase or transition.[19] As the various affordances and constraints of the degrees of freedom change, the movement system of the developing infant and child attempts to self-organize, pushing the motor behavior toward a new developing skill set.

As these new skill sets develop, they are guided by parameters[19] of the environment, variables associated with the given task embedded in the skill set, and the biological constraints that may limit the allowable affordances of the developing child. For instance, when a newborn is placed in standing position on a surface and is slightly leaned forward, this will elicit a stepping action of the leg. However, Thelen et al[20] discovered that this stepping reaction will often diminish, especially in infants who gain more weight early on. When the infants are placed in water to reduce the effects of leg mass, the researchers observed that these stepping reflexes did not disappear, but instead were influenced by bodily constraints of mass and the environmental influences of gravitational forces. In addition, they found that the arousal state was the largest influencer of stepping in neonates.[20] When we consider how human arousal can be influenced by environmental, task-specific, and biological factors associated with the body, we begin to see how these areas can provide an array of constraints and affordances for the developing infant and child.

Progress continues to be made in understanding the changing motor behaviors observed in infancy and childhood. These changes are critically paired with other concepts of cognition, social interaction, social behavior, and play. Through the ideas of dynamical systems theory, childhood development can be viewed as a dynamical process of interacting and self-organizing systems of movement patterns, stability, and variability[14] in motor behavior.

Case 1

Treadmill Training in Infants With Down Syndrome

A family of a 9-month-old boy with a diagnosis of trisomy 21 is being seen by a physical therapist (PT). During the initial evaluation, the PT observes that the child is able to sit for a minimum of 45 seconds without support from the therapist. When the child is not playing with toys, he assumes a propped position, with his arms placed out in front of his body, his shoulders rounded, his trunk in a flexed posture, his pelvis in a posterior tilted position, and his upper cervical region and head extended. When a toy is dangled in front of the child, he is able to reach upward with his arms to get the toy from the PT, and he plays with the toy in sitting without using his arms for balance support. The PT also notices that when the child reaches upward, his spine moves from a flexed posture to a more extended and upright posture and his pelvis moves into a more neutral and upright position.

When the child is placed in supportive standing, the PT observes that he extends both his legs, and his pelvis moves into an anterior pelvic tilt with a protruding abdomen; however, when given encouraging words from his parents, he smiles and extends his hips to assume a more upright standing posture. The parents say that their goal is for their child to walk as close to the age of his peers as is possible. They understand that mobility is linked to learning as the child explores his environment.

The PT explains that research has been performed looking at using treadmill training with infants with Down syndrome to advance the onset of walking.[21-23] Each family performed 8 minutes of supported treadmill walking with their child for 5 days each week and found that walking onset occurred significantly earlier than with the control group that did not participate in treadmill training. The parents agree to watch the therapist show them how their child can walk on a treadmill.

The PT has a special treadmill that begins at 0.1 mph and increases in 0.1-mph increments. The PT sits on a low stool in order to properly support the infant over the treadmill so that the child will walk forward while still facing the PT. While still holding the infant, the PT starts the treadmill at 0.1 mph, and then gently lowers the child's legs onto the slow treadmill. Once the legs touch the treadmill, the PT provides a slight forward lean to the infant's trunk to attempt to initiate stepping reactions. The PT provides encouraging facial expressions and phrases to the child as he begins to take staggered steps on the treadmill.

Questions

1. What affordances were present in this evaluation and treadmill intervention that the child would otherwise not be receiving?
2. What factors are creating a state of nonequilibrium in the infant's stepping by using a treadmill as a tool in this intervention?
3. What factors of affordances and constraints are associated with the environment, the given task, and the body of the infant?

Case 2

Delay in Motor Skill Acquisition

Louise is a 9-month-old girl who has been sent to a pediatric PT because of reports of limited motor development skills. During the parent history, they report that they are concerned their child is not meeting her developmental milestones at the same time as her older 4-year-old sibling did at the same age. The other sibling is observed wearing glasses for vision correction and is playing quietly in the corner of the room. The parents are concerned that the infant may have poor vision like her brother and that this is why the child is delayed. During the physical therapy examination, the therapist notices the following findings:

- The child appears large for her age. The therapist asks about the child's percentiles for height and weight. The parents report that she is in the 80th percentile for height and 95th percentile for weight.
- In the supine position, the child looks around at the surroundings. The child does not attempt to roll or reach for toys that are dangled in front of her, instead looking and smiling at the therapist's face or watching her sibling play in the corner of the room. When the therapist dangles a toy in front of the infant, she watches both the therapist's face and the toy being dangled. She reaches for the toy once, but when her hands come in contact, she stops reaching and returns to watching the sibling play.
- In the prone position, the infant hyperextends in her cervical region. She is limited in her attempts to push through her arms into the floor. Her legs are abducted and externally rotated into a frog-legged position, and she does not attempt to reach for toys.
- The child learned to perform ring sitting in the past month; however, the child does not use her arms for play in this position. Instead, her arms are in a raised, high guard position, where her hands are fisted, elbows are flexed, and shoulders are externally rotated, with mild scapular retraction. She appears mildly unsteady.
- When held up by the PT in standing, the child tucks her legs underneath her and does not push into her legs. While sitting on the floor with the child, the therapist wraps her arms around the torso of the child with one arm, and with the other arm supports her legs into a standing position. The infant appears to catch on and begins to bounce her legs in standing and eventually pushes into knee extension in both of her legs.
- When asked about nutrition, the parents report that the baby is eating a combination of solid foods and infant formula. They report that the child does not perform finger food eating, but instead only wants to be fed by her parents via a spoon.

Questions

1. What activities is the child currently unable to perform that are ideal for functional tasks for an infant at 9 months of age?
2. What degrees of freedom limit this child's ability to perform these functional tasks?
3. As you summarize your answer for question 1, what primary global deficit(s) limit this child's mobility?

NEURONAL GROUP SELECTION THEORY

Neuronal group selection theory (NGST) is a developmental theory that incorporates the understanding of neuroanatomic development with observed changes in early motor behavior. The NGST helps provide an explanation for the "nature versus nurture" debate because, through its theoretical underpinnings, it explains that human development occurs through an amazing integration of both genetic, predetermined neuronal structures of the developing brain and environmental influences.[17] Combined, these 2 elements influence the variation of activity seen in early motor development. NGST categorizes the variability of movement patterns into 2 phases of variability, primary and secondary variability. The primary phase of variability is observed as a repertoire of patterned movements initiated by early cortical development; the secondary phase of variability is observed as complex motor behaviors that are adaptive to external and environmental cues.

Neuronal Group Selection Theory and the Developing Brain

In early postconception development, the cells multiply and differentiate into different structures of ectoderm, endoderm, and mesoderm.[24] Further differentiation forms the developing cells into varying phases of being, from a blastocyst, to an embryo, and finally, by week 8 postmenstrual age, a developing fetus.[24] It is around this time that we begin to see early movements of the developing fetus.[25] These early movements coincide with the developing brain structures.[10] Much of this early process of brain development is predetermined by molecularly driven cues for axonal migration mechanisms.[26] However, as the brain continues to develop, genetically driven mechanisms are countered by environmental influences on brain development. Not only does an interplay between genes and environment affect the brain, but also environmental factors can actually influence gene expression.[27] This concept of evolving co-dominance of genetic and environmental influences is the basis of NGST.[10]

Within NGST, the 2 phases of variability, both primary variability and secondary variability, occur throughout development.[17] Primary variability is evident during even the earliest movements of in utero development, where motor movements have a large amount of variation and patterning.[17,25] It is believed that the primary variability seen in movement occurs from neuronal structure. These movements provide mechanisms in which the developing fetus can experience movement, and the afferent system is primarily a system that allows for the exploration of these experiences without purposeful adaptation to the sensory input.[17] However, once the developing fetus and infant begin to adapt to the sensory, afferent input, we begin to see the transition into secondary variability. It is within the secondary phase of variability that adaptation of movement begins to play an important role in the movement system. The infant begins to feel surfaces as the infant pushes into them through tactile input, and the body begins to respond to visual-perceptual changes and the pulls of gravity using the visual and vestibular systems. Both primary and secondary phases of variability are necessary to develop the infant so the infant can move and develop into a walking, running, and playing human being.[28]

Case 3

NGST and the Impact of Motor Function on a Child Born With Intraventricular Hemorrhage

A 28-year-old mother went into premature labor and gave birth to a premature infant born at 27 weeks of gestational age. A neonatologist was present for the birth of the child and immediately began to care for the newborn in the neonatal intensive care unit (NICU). The newborn was given surfactants shortly after birth to allow for greater lung compliance and was placed on a ventilator. Two days after the child was born, an ultrasound revealed a grade IV intraventricular hemorrhage (IVH). The child stayed in the NICU for 11 weeks and then was discharged to home.

The parents began early intervention physical therapy 3 weeks following the baby's discharge from the NICU. The baby is now 6 months old, or approximately 3 months old when calculated for the adjusted age based on the child being born 13 weeks premature. The PT has observed that as the child progressed with typical development, she kicked with the left leg very frequently; however, she did not kick with the right leg very often. When the child was first seen by the PT, the right leg was fairly inactive; however, over the past month, it appears to have more stiffness and sustained extension when the left leg is kicking. When the PT turns the child's head toward the left side, the infant will sometimes enter into an asymmetrical tonic neck reflex, but at other times, the child is able to bring her hand to her mouth in this position. However, when the therapist turns the child's head toward the right side, her arm will often move into elbow extension, demonstrating an active asymmetrical tonic neck reflex on the right side of her body.

Questions

1. How did the IVH influence primary and secondary variation of movement in this child's motor development?
2. When considering interventions for this child, what would be important characteristics that would support the primary and secondary variations of movement in NGST?

SCHEMA AND MOTOR PROGRAM THEORY

Schema theory and motor program theory have been around for over 40 years as concepts in motor learning and motor control, respectively. They continue to be a strong influence in scientific inquiry and understanding of human movement.[29] Schema theory, when applied to motor activity, is based around the idea that motor learning is a series of situations and motor responses that build upon each other to produce new or refined motor memories and motor behaviors.[30] It comprises 4 continuous events that, when combined and integrated, produce progressive skill development.[30] These 4 steps are as follows: (1) a situation that requires a response resulting in an observable motor behavior and the preunderstanding of sensory stimuli, body position, and factors that presume the motor activity; (2) the action and characteristics that occur with the action including speed and force production; (3) the afferent signaling that provides feedback from the motor behavior; and (4) the success of the motor behavior in the intended goal, otherwise known as the outcome.[30] The last step then provides information to know how future tasks should occur. With repeated practice, the process of motor learning refines the task to the targeted activity.[30]

Schema theory is used to provide insight into how discrete tasks are performed, like throwing a ball; however, it does not solely describe how continuous tasks are controlled, like pedaling or steering a tricycle. This, in part, is because continuous tasks utilize online sensory feedback to allow for corrective responses due to the adequate time allowed for feedback interpretation and action.[29]

It is difficult to separate schema theory from motor program theory because they occur simultaneously during motor development. The basis of motor program theory begins with the idea that motor tasks, called general motor programs (GMPs), are learned and stored within memory. Motor program theory begins to really come to life when we ask questions like "How does a baseball player learn to catch and throw so quickly and accurately?" or "How does a soccer player learn to control the ball when kicking it to another player?" Motor programming theory postulates that some mechanisms of motor control are controlled by GMPs.[29] This occurs in both closed-loop and open-loop versions of feedback mechanisms.[29] In the closed-loop feedback system, the motor task performance is checked against a reference memory of the movement, and any errors made from the reference memory are corrected and stored as a new reference memory.[30] In the open-loop feedback system, a motor task is performed via a GMP, yet in this open-loop system, the GMP is elicited without afferent modulation.[29,30]

Within motor program theory, when a motor behavior is executed, it is composed of both the GMP of the task itself and the parameters of the task, including the speed and the force production applied during the execution of the GMP.[29] When a new GMP is present, many studies support the idea that GMPs are often invariant in temporal, or time-based, sequence.[29,31,32] For instance, there are invariant features when looking at throwing an object overhand including certain grip qualities and the timing sequence of each joint motion, regardless of whether the object is a baseball or a newspaper.[31] One of the factors to consider when performing tasks is that although some components of the task are invariant, there are many parameters that are adjustable to meet the needs of the given task.[31]

When considering how people learn tasks, the old joke of "How do you get to Carnegie Hall?" comes to mind. The answer still rings true today: practice, practice, practice. When considering what leads to the learning of a GMP, a lot of research has looked at 2 specific forms of practice, blocked practice and random practice. Blocked practice is the repeated practice of a skill without breaks or changes in the task, and random practice is the integration of a task among other activities.[33] Studies have supported that random practice helps to establish GMPs but may not be as strong an influence in building skills associated with the parameters of a motor program.[29,34] Therefore, it has been hypothesized that blocked practice can be used as a tool for learning new motor tasks.[31] As the individual works on a given task, repeated use of the GMP reduces the variability observed in the motor program and provides repeated practice to stabilize the performance of the GMP. In addition, research has also supported that randomized practice enhances the parameters of a GMP.[34] Also, varied practice, or practice in which a sequence of different versions of a task is practiced, has also been explained as a method for developing the different parameters of a given task.[31,34,35] It is believed that this is due to the fluctuation in parameters required to carry out the task over a multitude of changing activities within a given time period, thereby requiring adjustments to the parameters of the GMP.

Therefore, it has been hypothesized that random and varied practice can be a method of intervention when trying to learn variation in parameters in motor tasks.

Schema theory and motor program theory help explain how individuals learn and excel at higher-order fundamental movement skills of skipping, hopping, jumping, throwing, and kicking. These theories, when combined with dynamical systems theory and NGST, help provide a greater understanding of how and why motor skills develop in infancy and childhood. As PTs continue to integrate motor theories into practice, there is an awareness that these theories are based on current understanding of movement science. As movement science progresses, it brings with it new understanding that PTs are charged to investigate and utilize for the betterment of the populations they serve.

Case 4

Developmental Coordination Disorder

Matthew is a 7-year-old boy who was referred to physical therapy because of a diagnosis of developmental coordination disorder. He presents with age-appropriate intelligence. He was tested for neurologic disorders associated with poor motor skill and coordination acquisition; however, all tests were negative. When tested using the Movement Assessment Battery for Children (Movement ABCs), his total impairment score, once converted, was below the 5th percentile. In collaboration with a developmental specialist, Matthew was given a diagnosis of developmental coordination disorder because of the impact that his coordination deficit has on his daily function.

Matthew's parents report that he has trouble kicking a ball and having it move forward. Sometimes when he kicks the ball, he misses it; other times when he kicks the ball, he hits it with his foot without much targeted direction of the ball. They report that they are most concerned about his safety because he has been known to fall when walking upstairs and is cautiously slow when negotiating downstairs, always using the rail and primarily using a step-to pattern. He throws a ball by pushing it forward from his chest, unable to reach an intended large target 10 feet away. His parents also report that he struggles with handwriting, stating that it is very difficult to read.

As a part of the treatment, the therapist decides to implement a task-oriented approach to intervention of Neuromotor Task Training (NTT).[36,37] An assessment, including a parent interview, is performed to determine the strengths and weaknesses of each activity with which the child is having difficulties. NTT exercises incorporate a close resemblance to the activity the child is having trouble with. The PT decides to begin by tackling stair negotiation, because Matthew has to walk up and down stairs in his home and school environments. The therapist begins by performing stair activities on a pediatric set of stairs in the clinic with a single handrail. At home, the PT encourages the parents to work on walking up and down the first 4 bottom steps, placing puzzle pieces on the fifth step, and assembling the puzzle at the bottom of the stairs. The goal is for the child to perform this activity multiple times in succession every day for continuous practice of the activity. As the child progresses with the skill, the therapist encourages the child to hold more puzzle pieces in his opposite, non–rail-side hand to limit its usefulness with the handrail. He encourages the family to do this during home practice as well. As the child becomes more comfortable with the task of walking up and down the 4 stairs during practice, the practice is moved to a set of stairs that includes a full flight. The therapist gradually increases the number of steps in the therapy session and in the home practice.

Questions
1. How does the intervention of NTT resemble principles discovered in motor programming theory and schema theory?
2. Sensory feedback is a necessary component associated with coordinated movement. Why didn't the therapist focus on activities that, although not task specific, tap into the sensory system?

◼ PART III: INTEGRATION OF POSTURE AND GAIT IN DEVELOPMENT THEORY

As PTs continue to integrate motor theories into practice, there is the realization that these theories are based on current understanding of movement science. When trying to understand and explain complex motor behavior such as postural control and gait, these developmental theories are often complimentary in their explanation of how and why humans are able to develop these skills necessary for exploration and play.

POSTURAL CONTROL

Postural control is a sophisticated way in which humans learn to move within a gravitational environment. Postural control has been described as awareness of body orientation in which the center of mass is dynamically controlled within a base of support and is used for preparation of movement or as a method for reacting to both internal and external movement-related disturbances.[38] Although maintaining an upright position in a typically developing human requires little forethought, it is, in fact, a complex integration of neuronal, bodily, and environmental factors that work together to make this sophisticated task come to life. However, when one of these factors does not support being upright, this task of postural control can be difficult. By understanding some of the current research in postural control development and how it fits into developmental theory, PTs can utilize this knowledge to analyze and assist their clients in learning to be successful in a world surrounded by a gravitational pull. We can see the attributes of posture development fitting into the perspectives of both the dynamical systems theory and the NGST.

From a dynamical systems perspective, postural control requires multiple systems both internal and external to the body to interact and formulate the developing skill of posture. The developing infant is motivated through auditory and visual sensory stimulation, causing them to learn about the surrounding environment. Perception, motivation, and growing curiosity direct the child to move and explore. Each changing posture will lead the infant to reorganize and find a new, adapted posture, or the infant will regress to the previous postural position as a point of stability.[3] The goal of physical therapy treatment in a dynamic systems framework is to work on skill transformation during time periods and activities of non-equilibrium states.[3] For an infant learning to control posture, a nonequilibrium state may include being in a position in which the child is not stable, yet there is potential for a strategy to be organized to create a new state of stability or state of equilibrium of postural control. During typical development, this new state of equilibrium often leads to the disappearance of a previous state (ie, loss of reflexive behavior) and/or an advancement in developmental motor skills.

Specific characteristics of postural control are also supported by NGST. It has been suggested that the development of postural control has 2 distinguishable levels. The first level utilizes innate motor control mechanisms that activate direction-specific muscle activity during postural sway.[39] It has been observed in 1-month-old infants that the dorsal extensor back muscles are activated when an infant's body is swayed backward, and the ventral anterior flexor muscles are activated when the infant's body is swayed forward.[40] This early observation of postural responses suggests an innate precursor to postural control.[40] These findings about early postural development support the concept of primary variability in NGST, where the infant first develops a repertoire of movement strategies that are innately derived motor activity.[10]

A second level of postural control emerges transitionally as the child develops multisensory responses to postural adjustments to perform the skills of sitting and, ultimately, standing and walking.[39] This second level incorporates a multisensory postural response that integrates input from the somatosensory, vestibular, and visual systems.[39,41] The idea that postural control emerges as an innate motor behavior that evolves into an adjustable motor behavior utilizing sensory feedback supports the concept of secondary variability discussed in NGST.

Postural control does not only develop in sitting. As infants gain experience in standing, they also begin to show signs of developing postural control in the form of anticipatory postural adjustments, or adjustments to postural muscles as the body prepares itself to react to disturbances in the center of mass in relationship to the base of support in standing.[42] Infants first learn to pull up to stand with external support by pulling their body upright in front of a couch or a coffee table around the age of 8 to 9 months.[43] As the child gains more experience in standing, they are afforded the opportunity to repeatedly practice early balance and postural control skills.

Between the ages of 10 and 17 months, there is a significant improvement in standing postural control.[42] As the infant gains experience in standing and walking, they continually utilize posture and balance reactions that lead to enhanced anticipatory postural adjustment with faster reaction time, greater consistency, and greater distal gastrocnemius muscle recruitment.[42] Throughout childhood, there is also an observed decrease in the overall magnitude and frequency of postural sway.[44,45] This progress continues throughout the first 10 years of life as the child masters greater posture and balance control during quiet stance.[44]

As the child develops a greater repertoire of movement strategies, the concept of multiple systems self-organizing and interacting with the brain through multisensory experiences of feedback and feedforward mechanisms takes shape. When considering the relationship of motor program theory and postural control, it is also recognized that postural control must take place and adapt during higher-order skill acquisition of hopping, skipping, jumping, kicking, and throwing a ball.

GAIT

Walking is an amazing skill that is achieved around the 12th month of life. At this point, the infant learns to play, explore, and learn through a bipedal, upright modality of locomotion. So much knowledge has been gained throughout much of the past century to help explain what it takes for human locomotion to occur, and yet so much information is still unknown when considering the questions of how and why humans learn to walk like they do. There are even disputes as to when children reach adult-like gait patterns, with some researcher suggesting by 2 years of age[46,47] and others suggesting 7 to 8 years of age.[46,48] Regardless of our state of knowledge, human locomotion is so much more than a task; it is a means to explore and perceive the world. One thing is for certain: many factors come together over the first year of life in order to produce the human bipedal pattern of locomotion.

Much of the past work performed in looking at infant gait has focused on both the onset of specific gait characteristics[49] and the transition of prone and quadruped skills toward a skill of locomotor behavior.[50,51] This concept is referred to as "functional continuity," where new skills emerge from prior motor skill acquisition.[52] It has been argued that it is through this progressing emergence of higher-order developmental motor skills that children build strength and balance through the practice of body movements during play and exploration. These movements interact with the vestibular, visual, proprioception, and tactile sensory inputs in an environmental and task-specific context.[53] For instance, as discussed in the dynamical systems theoretical model, this continuous interaction among the body, environment, and task begins in the womb and integrates multiple degrees of freedom, constraints, and affordances to build experiences across the prenatal, antenatal, and infant year that lead to the synthesis of a functional repertoire of movement strategies.[53]

Movement in the developing fetus begins around 7.5 to 8 weeks of postmenstrual age, and many of the movements, including those in the arms and legs, consist of distinct movement patterns that are similar to those observed in the newborn infant.[25,54,55] A newborn will perform repetitive kicking motions in the supine position; these movements have been hypothesized to represent a motor program specifically devoted to initiating the necessary motions for gait.[56] In addition, when a newborn infant is held upright in the vertical position, a stepping reflex is observed that appears to be related to the same motor program associated with supine kicking.[57] This stepping reflex will be less observable after the first 2 to 3 months of life as the increasing body weight of the developing infant impacts the mass of the limbs and the infant's decreased strength limits their ability to mobilize the legs.[20] These characteristics associated with newborn stepping have been described as potential precursors to walking; in fact, early treadmill walking that elicits the stepping reflex in newborns has been shown to both increase the response to stepping reactions during this time period in which typical newborn stepping diminishes and also produce an earlier onset to walking by approximately 1 month in the typically developing infant.[58]

Although there appear to be some elements of functional continuity in motor development, as seen in the early reflex stepping and later walking, as well as an association between infant belly crawling and infant creeping skills, not all characteristics of motor activities are directly linked to the progression of other similar motor skills.[52] For instance, functional continuity would suggest that creeping, cruising, and walking are progressively emerging skills; however, some studies have demonstrated that perception of the infant's environment during these tasks is not continuous.[52] A child will negotiate a gap in a handrail during cruising safely yet will not perceive gaps in the floor and will drop into them during cruising. Also, infants will safely negotiate slopes on the floor during cruising, but when first learning to ambulate, will not perceive the slope and will simply fall down the slope when walking. This is an example of functional discontinuity because a skill that was learned during earlier milestones (negotiating gaps and slopes during creeping and cruising) did not carry over into higher-order tasks (walking) that otherwise would appear to be functionally continuous motor skills. One suggestion as to why this occurs is because of the differences in the onset of the emergence of hand versus foot awareness for perceived affordances in the infant's environment.[52] The arms experience a lot of perceptual activities through many prone and grasping activities during the first year when compared to perceptual learning through the legs. This difference could account for the functional discontinuity of negotiating a slope and gap during crawling, cruising, and walking.

As infants move toward the stage of walking independently, it is thought that the primary causes of progression toward this achievement are a growing and evolving strength and postural control in the typically developing infant.[46,53] When a child first learns to walk, they actually walk using a controlled falling action. The new walker will engage in a falling pattern of movement where during initial foot contact, the center of mass of the baby displaces inferiorly. This inferior displacement decreases as the child learns postural control during ambulation.[46] As the child reaches adult-like ambulation, this vertical displacement actually shifts to where the center of mass moves superiorly during initial foot contact.[46] The child uses this motion for weight acceptance as a dynamic mechanism of postural control during gait.

One principle that has emerged over time is that learning to walk incorporates a continuous online process of problem solving for the developing infant.[48] As PTs continue to work toward enhancing life through movement, it will be important for the profession to uphold a standard of reviewing, interpreting, and integrating the discoveries of science and scientific theories of motor development into evidence-based practice.

So much knowledge, however, awaits to be understood. As we make sense of the processes necessary to produce the skill of ambulation, this knowledge will shape the practice of pediatric physical therapy.

CONCLUSION

Many scientists have contributed to our understanding of development and have played an incremental role in how we understand, interpret, and assist children in reaching their fullest potential. The dynamical systems theory, NGST, and motor programming theory help explain how and why children develop as they do. Additionally, these theories can be complementary when trying to explain the complex mechanisms associated with postural control and gait. This knowledge can help the individual therapist explore the needs of the children they serve and help guide them in the process of examination, assessment, and intervention.

STUDY QUESTIONS

1. What are the significant differences between the 3 primary developmental theories discussed in this chapter?

2. When considering development across the first year of life, what significant motor behaviors are observed that reflect characteristics of dynamical systems theory?

3. When considering development across the first year of life, what significant motor behaviors are observed that reflect principles associated with primary and secondary variability in NGST?

4. When considering development through childhood, what significant motor behaviors are observed that reflect principles associated with motor programming theory and schema theory?

5. How does postural control develop during the first 2 years of life?

6. Describe how the 3 primary developmental theories explain how and why children build the skill of independent locomotion.

References

1. Raju TN. Historical perspectives on the etiology of cerebral palsy. *Clin Perinatol.* 2006;33(2):233-250. doi:10.1016/j.clp.2006.03.006.
2. Tredoux G. Francis Galton as differential psychologist. Accessed September 21, 2019. http://galton.org/psychologist/index.html.
3. Kamm K, Thelen E, Jensen JL. A dynamical systems approach to motor development. *Phys Ther.* 1990;70(12):763-775.
4. Dalton TC. Arnold Gesell and the maturation controversy. *Integr Physiol Behav Sci.* 2005;40(4):182-204.
5. Shirley MM. The first two years: a study of twenty-five babies. *Am J Public Health Nations Health.* 1933;23(11):1217-1218.
6. Johnson A. Babes in arms. *Monitor Psychol.* 2011;42(5):24.
7. Hunt JM. Psychological development: early experience. *Annu Rev Psych.* 1979;30(1):103.
8. McGraw M. *Growth: A Study of Jimmy and Johnny.* Appleton Century Company; 1935.

9. Acredolo LP. Beyond heredity and environment: Myrtle McGraw and the maturation controversy. *Syst Res Behav Sci*. 1998;15(2): 152-155.

10. Hadders-Algra M. Variation and variability: key words in human motor development. *Phys Ther*. 2010;90(12):1823-1837. doi:10.2522/ptj.20100006.

11. Thelen E. Motor development as foundation and future of developmental psychology. *Int J Behav Dev*. 2000;24(4):385-397.

12. Davids K, Glazier P, Araújo D, Bartlett R. Movement systems as dynamical systems. *Sports Med*. 2003;33(4):245-260. doi:10.2165/00007256-200333040-00001.

13. Kelso JS, Opstal AV. Dynamic patterns: the self-organization of brain and behavior. *J Cogn Neurosci*. 1996;8(4):385.

14. Schoner G, Kelso J. Dynamic pattern generation in behavioral and neural systems. *Science*. 1988;239(4847):1513-1520.

15. Gibson EJ. Exploratory behavior in the development of perceiving, acting, and the acquiring of knowledge. *Annu Rev Psychol*. 1988;39(1):1-42.

16. Bruineberg J, Rietveld E. Self-organization, free energy minimization, and optimal grip on a field of affordances. *Front Hum Neurosci*. 2014;8:599.

17. Hadders-Algra M. The neuronal group selection theory: a framework to explain variation in normal motor development. *Dev Med Child Neurol*. 2000;42(8):566-572.

18. Metzger MA. Applications of nonlinear dynamical systems theory in developmental psychology: motor and cognitive development. *Nonlinear Dynam Psychol Life Sci*. 1997;1(1):55-68.

19. Kelso JAS, Schöner G. Self-organization of coordinative movement patterns. *Hum Movement Sci*. 1988;7(1):27-46. doi: https://doi.org/10.1016/0167-9457(88)90003-6.

20. Thelen E, Fisher DM, Ridley-Johnson R. The relationship between physical growth and a newborn reflex. *Infant Behav Dev*. 1984;7(4):479-493.

21. Ulrich DA, Lloyd MC, Tiernan CW, Looper JE, Angulo-Barroso RM. Effects of intensity of treadmill training on developmental outcomes and stepping in infants with Down syndrome: a randomized trial. *Phys Ther*. 2008;88(1):114-122.

22. Ulrich DA, Ulrich BD, Angulo-Kinzler RM, Yun J. Treadmill training of infants with Down syndrome: evidence-based developmental outcomes. *Pediatrics*. 2001;108(5):e84.

23. Kınacı-Biber E, Önerge K, Mutlu A. Gait characteristics and effects of early treadmill intervention in infants and toddlers with down syndrome: a systematic review. *Disabil Rehabil*. 2022;44(26):8139-8148.

24. Mitchell B, Sharma R. *Embryology: An Illustrated Colour Text*. Elsevier Health Sciences; 2005.

25. Prechtl HF. *Ultrasound Studies of Human Fetal Behaviour*. Elsevier; 1985.

26. Polleux F. Genetic mechanisms specifying cortical connectivity: let's make some projections together. *Neuron*. 2005;46(3):395-400.

27. Diamond A. The interplay of biology and the environment broadly defined. *Dev Psych*. 2009;45(1):1.

28. Law M, Darrah J. Emerging therapy approaches: an emphasis on function. *J Child Neurol*. 2014;29(8):1101-1107.

29. Schmidt RA. Motor schema theory after 27 years: reflections and implications for a new theory. *Res Q Exerc Sport*. 2003;74(4):366-375.

30. Schmidt RA. A schema theory of discrete motor skill learning. *Psychol Rev*. 1975;82(4):225.

31. Schmidt RA, Wrisberg CA. *Motor Learning and Performance: A Problem-Based Learning Approach*. 3rd ed. Kinetics; 2004.

32. Gentner DR. Timing of skilled motor performance: tests of the proportional duration model. *Psychol Rev*. 1987;94(2):255.

33. Di Tore PA, Schiavo R, D'Isanto T. Physical education, motor control and motor learning: theoretical paradigms and teaching practices from kindergarten to high school. *J Phys Educ Sport*. 2016;16(4):1293.

34. Wright DL, Shea CH. Manipulating generalized motor program difficulty during blocked and random practice does not affect parameter learning. *Res Q Exerc Sport*. 2001;72(1):32-38.

35. Czyż SH, Zvonař M, Pretorius E. The development of generalized motor program in constant and variable practice conditions. *Front Psychol*. 2019;10:2760.

36. Niemeijer AS, Smits-Engelsman BC, Schoemaker MM. Neuromotor task training for children with developmental coordination disorder: a controlled trial. *Dev Med Child Neurol*. 2007;49(6):406-411.

37. Smits-Engelsman BC, Blank R, van der Kaay AC, et al. Efficacy of interventions to improve motor performance in children with developmental coordination disorder: a combined systematic review and meta-analysis. *Dev Med Child Neurol*. 2013;55(3):229-237.

38. Dusing SC, Harbourne RT. Variability in postural control during infancy: implications for development, assessment, and intervention. *Phys Ther*. 2010;90(12):1838-1849.

39. Forssberg H, Hirschfeld H. Postural adjustments in sitting humans following external perturbations: muscle activity and kinematics. *Exp Brain Res*. 1994;97(3):515-527.

40. Hedberg Å, Forssberg H, Hadders-Algra M. Postural adjustments due to external perturbations during sitting in 1-month-old infants: evidence for the innate origin of direction specificity. *Exp Brain Res*. 2004;157(1):10-17.

41. Dusing SC. Postural variability and sensorimotor development in infancy. *Dev Med Child Neurol*. 2016;58:17-21.

42. Witherington DC, Hofsten C, Rosander K, Robinette A, Woollacott MH, Bertenthal BI. The development of anticipatory postural adjustments in infancy. *Infancy*. 2002;3(4):495-517.

43. Woollacott MH, Shumway-Cook A. Changes in posture control across the life span—a systems approach. *Phys Ther*. 1990;70(12): 799-807.

44. Kirshenbaum N, Riach CL, Starkes JL. Non-linear development of postural control and strategy use in young children: a longitudinal study. *Exp Brain Res*. 2001;140(4):420-431.

45. Riach CL, Starkes JL. Velocity of centre of pressure excursions as an indicator of postural control systems in children. *Gait Posture*. 1994;2(3):167-172. doi: https://doi.org/10.1016/0966-6362(94)90004-3.

46. Adolph KE, Vereijken B, Shrout PE. What changes in infant walking and why. *Child Dev*. 2003;74(2):475-497.

47. Burnett CN, Johnson EW. Development of gait in childhood: part II. *Dev Med Child Neurol*. 1971;13(2):207-215.

48. Sutherland DH, Olshen R, Cooper L, Woo SL. The development of mature gait. *J Bone Joint Surg Am*. 1980;62(3):336-353.

49. McGraw MB. Neuromuscular development of the human infant as exemplified in the achievement of erect locomotion. *J Pediatr*. 1940;17(6):747-771. doi: https://doi.org/10.1016/S0022-3476(40)80021-8.

50. Gesell A, Ames LB. The ontogenetic organization of prone behavior in human infancy. *Pedagog Seminary J Genet Psychol*. 1940;56(2):247-263.

51. Berger SE, Adolph KE. Learning and development in infant locomotion. *Prog Brain Res*. 2007;164:237-255.

52. Adolph KE, Berger SE, Leo AJ. Developmental continuity? Crawling, cruising, and walking. *Dev Sci*. 2011;14(2):306-318.

53. Thelen E, Ulrich BD. Hidden skills: a dynamic systems analysis of treadmill stepping during the first year. *Monogr Soc Res Child Dev*. 1991;56(1):1-98.

54. De Vries J, Visser G, Prechtl H. Fetal behaviour in early pregnancy. *Eur J Obstet Gynecol*. 1986;21(5):271-276.

55. De Vries JI, Visser GH, Prechtl HF. The emergence of fetal behaviour. I. Qualitative aspects. *Early Hum Dev*. 1982;7(4):301-322.

56. Thelen E, Bradshaw G, Ward JA. Spontaneous kicking in month-old infants: manifestation of a human central locomotor program. *Behav Neural Biol*. 1981;32(1):45-53.

57. Thelen E, Fisher DM. Newborn stepping: an explanation for a "disappearing" reflex. *Dev Psychol*. 1982;18(5):760.

58. Zelazo PR, Zelazo NA, Kolb S. "Walking" in the newborn. *Science*. 1972;176(4032):314-315.

Typical Development

Lynn Jeffries, PT, DPT, PhD, Elizabeth Ennis, PT, EdD, and Dawn James, PT, DPT, DSc

LEARNING OBJECTIVES

Upon completion of this chapter, the reader will be able to:

- Describe a child's developmental progression across each developmental domain.
- Discuss the interrelatedness of a child's development between developmental domains.
- Describe the influence of environment on a child's development.
- Identify red flags related to the development of a child indicating the need for future evaluation or referral to a pediatrician.

INTRODUCTION

Children's development is complex, and each child develops at their own pace, but typically within the same time frame and along the same trajectory as their peers. Caregivers often ask us to identify if a child is developing typically and, if not, when they will gain a certain skill or why they do not have the same motor skills as other children. Physical therapists must not only understand the typical progression of motor development but also be aware of the multitude of factors that influence the child's development. We must analyze movement and identify the child's challenges to determine if therapy services are needed and, if so, how to facilitate the achievement of the particular skill to assist the child as they participate in their daily activities and routines.

Besides thoroughly understanding the development of movement, therapists must consider the context in which movement is developing. Each child has a multitude of factors that influence their growth. Therapists must be aware of the individual (temperament, cognition, and genetics) and environmental factors that influence the child's development (**Figure 2-1**). Environmental factors are the physical (eg, space and terrain), social (eg, interactions with people), and attitudinal (eg, attitudes of family, community members, and peers toward supporting and encouraging participation) components that can either enhance or limit the child's participation in naturally occurring activities.[1] Also at the environmental level, therapists must consider the child's microsystem (home, family, and siblings), exosystem (day care, school, and extended family), and macrosystem (culture, community, and health care resources) level influences on the child.[2]

Each of these layers affects the child, their behavior, and their family and influences the family's values and beliefs. As physical therapists, we must be aware of these child and environmental factors and their contributions to the child's attainment of movement and development of refined motor control. Additionally, therapists must be aware of the interrelatedness the development of movement has with all areas of child development.

In this chapter, we focus on the development of gross and fine motor skills but provide reference to the child's language, cognitive, adaptive, and social-emotional skills that are all developing at the same time. We recognize that child development is not a linear process and that not all children develop particular skills at the same time. However, achievement of motor skills using an ages and stages format provides physical therapists with a reference to typical expectations. We provide a general overview of in utero movement and then, by ages, provide examples of typical gross and fine motor development. We then address the other areas of child development and highlight some key "red flags" that indicate the need for future evaluation and potentially physical therapy services. In this chapter, we have compiled a summary of skills by developmental domain and age (**Table 2-1**)

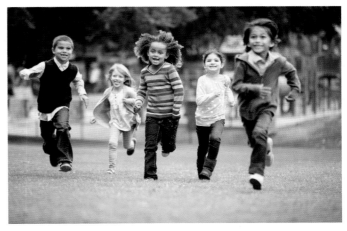

FIGURE 2-1 Therapists must consider the environmental, social, and attitudinal factors that influence a child's development. (Used with permission from Monkey Business Images/Shutterstock.)

TABLE 2-1 · Child Development Chart

	Gross Motor/Mobility	Fine Motor/Upper Extremity	Language	Cognitive	Adaptive	Social-Emotional
0–3 months	Lifts head slightly from prone; when held in sitting, head bobs initially but eventually becomes steady; when held in standing position, takes some weight on legs; turns head from side to side and midline alignment achieved in supported sitting	Opens and closes hands, although they stay primarily closed or clasped together; visually looks at and may swipe at objects; grasp reflex strong initially, but infant begins involuntary release around 1 month	Vocalizes to caregiver's smile and voice; coos; cries to get attention; vocalizes displeasure; responds to changes in speaker's tone, pitch, and volume; attempts to imitate sounds	Can focus on and follow moving objects, including faces; sees all colors; distinguishes pitch and volume of sound; discriminates sweet, sour, bitter, and salty tastes; responds with facial expressions to strong stimuli; begins to anticipate events	Coordinated suck, swallow, breath sequence; sleeps for 4–10 hours; brings hand to mouth	Listens to voices; smiles purposely in response to caregiver's face or voice; respond positively to touch
3–6 months	Raises head to 90 degrees when placed on stomach; initially rolls supine to side lying and eventually prone to supine; static ring sitting when placed; supported standing bears some weight on legs	Extends arms to reach for objects or bring hands to midline; palmar grasp; holds items with both hands; may transfer item from hand to hand	Turns head toward a voice; vocalizes; laughs and babbles; exchanges sounds, facial expressions, or gestures with caregiver; listens to conversations; repeats some vowel and consonant sounds	Recognizes faces; differentiates between different people based on look, sound, or feel; reacts to and imitates facial expressions; responds to familiar sounds; will drop something and watch it fall (beginning problem solving)	Rooting reflex is inhibited; mouths toys; swallows pureed foods	Laughs aloud; excited by food; smiles at self in mirror; pays attention to own name
6–9 months	Segmental rolling; can sit alone steadily and play with a toy; begins moving out of sitting to quadruped and from sitting to prone; rocks on hands and knees; may pull to stand at furniture using arms; belly crawls; raises back into sitting	Reaches with one hand while weight bearing on other forearm; transfers objects between hands; reach and grasp occurs in one continuous movement; radial palmar moving to radial digital grasp; raking small items; controlled release; throws, shakes, and bangs items	Begins repetitive babbling; vocalizes 4 different syllables; has 2-syllable combinations; shouts or vocalizes to gain attention; understands and responds to firm "no"; imitates speech sounds	Responds to name and simple commands; distinguishes between inanimate and animate objects; distinguishes among pictures that show different numbers of items; uses the relative size of an object as a clue to how close or far away it is; object permanence	Moves food around in mouth with tongue; holds own bottle; feeds self a cracker; sleeps through the night	Lively responses and preferences to familiar people; distinguishes friends from strangers; responds actively to language and gestures; expresses several clearly differentiated emotions; desires to be with people; waves goodbye

Age	Gross Motor	Fine Motor	Language	Cognitive	Self-Help	Social/Emotional
9-12 months	Sits without support, rotating to reach and play; pulls to standing using legs more than arms at first then through half kneeling; cruises around furniture; may take independent steps but falls easily; while walking, high hand guard and wide base of support; lowers self with control from standing; hands and knees up stairs if available	Pincer grasp; pokes with index finger; throws objects; turns pages of book by flipping many pages at a time	Says repetitive consonant/vowel sounds like "mama" and "dada"; vocalizes with intent; understands simple demands; understands the names of familiar people and objects; tries to imitate animal sounds	Responds to simple directions and questions with gestures, sounds, and perhaps words; imitates gestures and actions; experiments with objects (eg, seeing how object fits into a container); enjoys looking at picture books	Feeds themselves finger foods; holds cup with 2 hands and drinks with help; holds out arms and legs while being dressed	Actively engages in play such as peek-a-boo and patty-cake; has fear of strangers and separation from primary caregiver; performs for attention
12-18 months	Walks alone; walks backward; carries or pulls small items; squats and recovers; equilibrium reactions are present in standing; seats self in child's chair; initially up stairs on hands and knees, then progresses to walking up and down stairs while holding on	Imitative scribble; palmar-supinate grasp of pencil; precise release of objects; holds 2 cubes in same hand; puts rings on a peg; turns knob; grasps small ball and flings with elbow extension	Uses expressive jargon; talks rather than gestures; understands more than they can say: says 50 meaningful words by the end of this age range; responds correctly when asked "Where?"	Understands and follows simple commands; includes others as recipients of play behaviors; points to 3 body parts; distinguishes between "you" and "me"; recognizes familiar objects in storybooks	Begins to be helpful, such as by helping put things away; brings spoon to mouth; chews food; naps 1-2 times during the day; begins to show discomfort when soiled	Recognizes self in picture or mirror; smiles and makes faces at themselves; initiate their own play experiences; peak of separation distress; expresses negative feelings; shows pride and pleasure in new accomplishments; imitates other children and adult behaviors in play
18-24 months	Begins to run stiffly; creeps backward downstairs or climbs stairs using railing and one hand; seldom falls while walking; able to get into small chairs without help; steps over small barriers	Spontaneous scribble; can build tower of 3-5 cubes; places small items in a bottle; turns 2 or 3 pages at a time; seperates pop-beads	Understands multiword utterances; uses 2 words to express thoughts (eg, "Mommy go"); 50-200+ word vocabulary; identifies pictures when named	Demonstrates invention of new means through mental combinations; finds hidden objects; activates a toy or doll in pretend play	Able to control muscles used to urinate and have a bowel movement, but may not be ready to use toilet; uses spoon and cup to help feed self; removes some clothing items, such as gloves, hats, and socks	Demonstrates less separation distress; begins to show empathetic responses to another's distress; uses words to protest; often imitates; shows affection; listens to story or looks at pictures
2 years old	Runs with better coordination; jumps off low step with one foot, leading up off ground with both feet together; up and down stairs holding on with step-to pattern; kicks a small ball; throws overhand; stands on one foot for 1-2 seconds	Holds crayon with thumb and fingers, not fist; imitates vertical, horizontal, and circular strokes; strings large beads; turns pages one by one; paints with wrist actions; makes dots and lines; rolls, pounds, and squeezes Play-Doh; turns doorknob; stacks 6-7 cubes	Language explosion; strings 3-5 words together (eg, "Me go home"); demands response from others; 300+ word vocabularies; responds to "what" and "where" questions; enjoys listening to stories; recounts events from the day	During pretend play can substitute objects; groups objects by category; relates what they are doing to others; sings song phrases; communicates personal needs; attention span is increasing	Indicates toileting needs, may be ready to begin toilet training; helps to dress and undress themselves	Shows awareness of gender identity; begins to respond verbally to another's distress; includes others in pretend plan; pretends to perform caregiver's routines; begin self-evaluation and develops notions of themselves as good, bad, etc.

(Continued)

TABLE 2-1 • Child Development Chart (Continued)

	Gross Motor/Mobility	Fine Motor/Upper Extremity	Language	Cognitive	Adaptive	Social-Emotional
3 years old	Demonstrates true run, with both feet leaving the ground and reciprocal arm movement; walks up stairs reciprocally; walks down stairs without support marking time; stands on tip toes; can run around obstacles; jumps off step and over 2-inch objects; rides a tricycle; hops on preferred foot and balances on one foot; uses a slide without help	Copies circles; imitates crossed strokes; traces diamond with angles rounded; can catch and throw a ball; stacks up to 9 cubes; imitates building bridges with cubes; puts pegs into holes; manipulates Play-Doh by making balls and snakes; unscrews lids	Follows 2-step commands without forgetting; rereads favorite storybooks using picture to guide story; vocabulary now several hundred words; speaks in sentences of 3 words or more; uses plurals and pronouns; almost all of child's speech should be understandable, even to strangers	Tells simple stories; repeats songs and nursery rhymes; counts up to 5; tells action in pictures; completes multiple-piece puzzles; unable to distinguish from fantasy; often asks questions; comprehends 3 prepositions: onto, under, and inside	May have daytime control over bowel and bladder functions (possibly nighttime control as well); feeds self easily; can dress self, only needing help with shoelaces, buttons, and fasteners in awkward places	Uses physical aggression more than verbal aggression; shows an interest in why and how things work; has difficulty generating alternatives in a conflict situation; will learn aggressive behavior rapidly if initially successful
4 years old	Walks down stairs alternating feet; gallops; stands on tiptoes; rotation of body forward with throwing; catches a ball with arm preparation; hops on one foot without losing balance	Cuts straight line with scissors; cuts out a square; copies cross; uses static tripod grasp; may begin to hold pencil in finger grip; can button small buttons; copies square and cross; throws ball overhand with coordination	Vocabulary of 1000+ words; creates questioning and negative sentences using correct word arrangement; voice well modulated and firm; often reverses letters when writing; understands beside, between, and back; may use words they do not understand	Can follow 3-step commands in correct order; makes opposite analogies; matches and names 4 colors; counts to 15; better able to distinguish reality from fantasy; can identify parts of a whole; can state their whole name and age; shows awareness of past and present; understands size comparisons	Can complete tasks with food without assistance, such as spreading soft butter with a dull knife and pouring from a small pitcher; washes hands unassisted; blows nose when reminded; may still wet bed	Becomes more interested in other children; shares toys, takes turns with assistance, and initiates or joins in play with other children; begins dramatic play, acting out whole scenes; commonly has imaginary playmates; lacks moral concept of right and wrong
5 years old	Can stop and change directions quickly when running; hops 8-10 steps on one foot; one-foot balance with eyes closed; jumps over 6- to 8-inch items; throws ball and hits target at 10 feet; drop kicks a ball; roller skates; rides bike; turns somersaults	Uses dynamic tripod grasp of pencil; copies triangle with sharp edges; draws simple shapes, letters, or numbers; uses safety scissors and cuts on a line continuously	Vocabulary of 2,000+ words; can speak in sentences of 5 or more words; understands passive sentences; may begin to use invented spellings; combines thoughts into one sentence; follows unrelated multiple commands appropriately; understands comparatives such as small, smaller, and smallest	Understands past, present, and future and event sequences; creates classes of items based on a defining characteristic; counts to 20; points to and names many colors; draws a person with detail; draws, names, and describes pictures; knows address; can answer "why" questions	Begins to help with small chores, such as setting the table; brushes teeth and bathes with assistance; dresses self independently	Has a group of friends; still poor at self-control; success depends on removal of temptation or diversion by others; begins to show some understanding of moral reasoning; says "I'm sorry" when they make a mistake; compares themselves to others; develops friendships; shows interest in exploring sexual differences; enjoys imaginative play

Sources: References 3, 16,20,21,69-80.

based on norm-referenced measures. Details related to particular measures can be reviewed in Chapter 3. The developmental expectations presented in Table 2-1 are slightly different than the developmental surveillance milestones on the Centers for Disease Control and Prevention (CDC) website.[3] The CDC milestones were developed based on literature focusing on the age when most (75%) children are expected to demonstrate a particular milestone as compared to the average age when children achieve a milestone.[4] We recognize there can be different developmental age targets based on the resources referenced; however, the table and text in this chapter provide averages and ranges of developmental skill acquisition.

■ NEONATAL MOVEMENT

All movements present in newborns are seen in the fetus by 16 to 18 weeks' gestation; however, movement begins with slight head and lateral trunk bending by 7 to 8 weeks.[5,6] Isolated hand and leg movements begin around 9 weeks, sucking and swallowing is clearly present by 13 to 14 weeks, and finger sucking is present by 15 weeks.[7,8] Fetuses explore their intrauterine environments including their own body, umbilical cord, and uterine wall with their hands and demonstrate identifiable kinematic movement patterns of their hand to mouth by 22 weeks.[9,10] As the fetus develops, they are moving during the first and second trimesters up to 30% of the day.[5] Whole-body rotation and somersaults are present in addition to the refinement of hand, face, and respiratory movements. As the fetus transitions into the third trimester, general gross body movements decrease due to fetal growth reducing the uterine space.[11,12] Refined facial movements, however, increase with more mouthing (jaw opening/closing, swallowing, chewing) and eyelid movement.[8] Fetal breathing movements increase with rhythmic contractions of the diaphragm in coordination with abdominal and intercostal muscle contractions.[10] Sleep and sleep cycles also appear in the third trimester and are considered essential for the development of the sensory and motor systems.[13]

■ GROSS MOTOR DEVELOPMENT

In this section, we explore gross motor development by age ranges and body positions. We recognize the infant and child will not acquire a movement in isolation and that opportunity and environment can support skill acquisition.

0 TO 3 MONTHS

At birth, when positioned prone, the infant is in physiological flexion with particularly strong hip flexion that prevents the pelvis from flattening to the surface. Over the next few months, the physiological flexion decreases, allowing the infant's pelvis to flatten onto the surface. This gradual transition permits the infant to shift their weight caudally, letting them lift their head up to approximately 45 degrees by 3 months (**Figure 2-2**).[14] In this position with the head elevated, the infant's legs are typically abducted and externally rotated at the hips with slight knee flexion. Their weight shifts caudally, letting the infant bring their arms up toward their head, often in an abducted

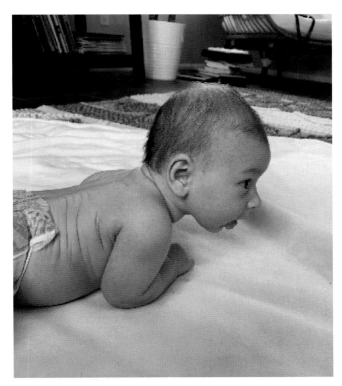

FIGURE 2-2 **Infant in prone with head lifted to approximately 45 degrees.**

position, allowing for the weight-bearing surface to be on the forearms and elbows.

In supine, physiological flexion dominates during the first month, but as the flexion relaxes, reciprocal and symmetrical leg kicking begins. At first, the infant is unable to maintain a symmetrical trunk position, but during the second and third months, the infant develops a symmetrical trunk posture, holding their head in midline while continuing to kick their legs and bring their arms to midline. During a pull to sit, you may not see an initial head lag due to the infant's physiological flexion, but head lag increases over the first month as the infant lacks the cervical muscular control to activate and pull the head, which is quite large in proportion to the body, up into alignment with the body. As the infant gains more active cervical flexor control, their head lag during a pull to sit will decrease.

In sitting, the infant must be supported. The infant does not have head or trunk control and, when positioned in sitting, is in a "C" curved position. Over the next 2 months, the infant begins to gain cervical extension control and early eye movement, and visual attention facilitates this ability. As the infant gains the ability to bring their head into a more upright position, they will still need trunk support to maintain an upright position.

In supported standing, the infant may partially bear weight on their legs and automatically step. This supported standing reflex diminishes by 2 to 3 months due to the increase in body mass.

3 TO 6 MONTHS

In prone, the infant typically achieves 90 degrees of head elevation by 4 months of age. Weight shifting from side to side in prone develops the muscular control equilibrium responses for movement and unweighting of an upper extremity for reaching. During this time, the infant develops control of shoulder retraction and protraction, which facilitates prone pivoting (turning in a circle) as well as crawling.

In supine, by 4 to 5 months, the infant will lead with cervical flexion during a pull to sit movement. The infant should be able to hold a symmetrical head and trunk position, and as more trunk and hip flexor control is developed, the infant will lift their pelvis and bring their feet to their hands and mouth. Early rolling from prone to side lying or supine is frequently accidental as the infant pushes up on their elbows or hands and weight shifts to one side or the other. From supine, as the infant looks to the side or brings their feet to hands, their weight shifts away from midline and gravity assists the infant to roll to the side. Initially, rolling during this phase is nonsegmental, but as the infant continues to be positioned in prone, they quickly learn how to shift their weight and roll eventually into supine.

As the infant gains more trunk control in supine and prone, one can see greater trunk control in sitting. By about 3 months, when held by their hands, the infant can hold their head upright in a vertical position with beginning thoracic extension noted. By 4 to 6 months, if placed with their legs abducted and flexed at the knees and hands propped between their legs, the infant can maintain this propped position as long as they maintain this forward midline position. If they lean too far to the side or sit more upright, without good anterior/posterior trunk co-activation, the infant will topple. Harbourne and Stergiou[15] describe this as stage 1 of sitting development. The infant may

attempt to lift their arm to bat at a toy, but this disrupts the tripod position necessary to maintain stability in this early sitting position. As the infant nears 5 months, stage 2 of sitting develops where the infant has the ability to sit with their arms lifted for short periods of time (1-2 minutes) but cannot maintain the upright unsupported posture to manipulate toys during play.

In supported standing, the infant will again begin to partially accept weight on their legs when held upright around 3 to 4 months of age. The infant's hips are typically externally rotation and abducted, knees are flexed, and feet are pronated. As they near 6 months of age, they will begin to fully bear weight on their legs and even begin to take volitional steps when held upright, with their body weight supported.

6 TO 9 MONTHS

As the infant gains greater control of their trunk, rolling becomes segmental with intra-axial rotation (**Figure 2-3**). By around 6 months, most infants begin rolling from supine to prone leading with either their shoulders/arms or pelvis/legs. As they realize rolling gets them from one place to another, continuous rolling emerges.

In sitting, as the infant gains control of intra-axial rotation, weight shifting, and stabilization of their trunk, they will continually work to erect their trunk into an upright sitting position without hand support. Initially the infant often brings their arms up and to the side in a "high guard" position to facilitate balancing. As upright control improves, the infant will begin to weight shift from side to side, rotate their trunk and head

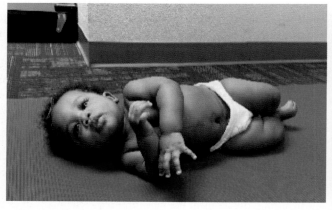
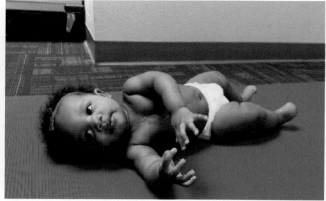
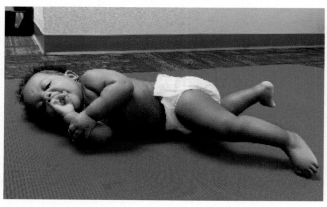
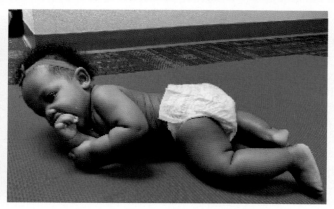

FIGURE 2-3 Rolling progression. Note intra-axial rotation.

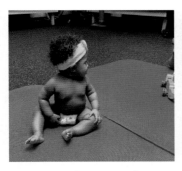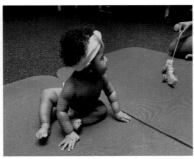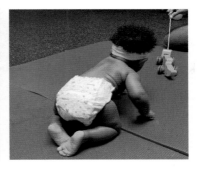

FIGURE 2-4 **Sitting to creeping progression.**

to look around the environment, hold toys in their hands, and dissociate their leg positions. Typically, "ring sitting" upright without hand support is achieved around 6 to 7 months with the ability to successfully manipulate items.[15] And by 9 months, as the infant has gained more control of movement in sitting, as well as rolling and creeping, the infant has the foundational control necessary to transition into and out of sitting from various body positions (prone, supine, side lying). In prone, infants being to pull themselves forward on their belly using their arms with a reciprocal leg movement. This activity is referred to as crawling. As the infant gains trunk and pelvic control, they push up into quadruped with their abdomen lifted off the surface and bodyweight supported on all 4 extremities. Often, they will rock in this hands and knees position in preparation for creeping (crawling on hands and knees with counterrotation of the trunk). Creeping requires hip stability, trunk control with the pelvis in a posterior pelvic tilt position, and the ability to weight shift to one side so the infant can unweight one extremity to allow for reciprocal movement (**Figure 2-4**). On average, infants begin creeping at 8.5 months.[16] One advantage of creeping is the infant can now reach higher surfaces, which will facilitate pulling to stand.

To obtain standing from prone, the infant will try and pull up onto higher surfaces using their arms, and once quadruped is obtained, they will more efficiently reach up and pull up into standing next to stable surfaces as they near 7 to 10 months. As they gain more control of their legs, the infant will actually begin to pull to stand through a half-kneel position, using a leg to help push themselves up into standing as compared to pulling up with just their arms (**Figure 2-5**). When held in standing, the infant will continue to take steps if their hands are supported and will gain more trunk and pelvic control over time. As they near 7 to 9 months, when placed in standing next

to a supportive surface, the infant will independently maintain the position for longer periods of time.

9 TO 12 MONTHS

In prone, creeping continues, but it is not unusual for the infant to vary their movement pattern. Most infants continue to creep in quadruped, but some creep with one foot and one knee, called hitching, or push themselves up into a hands and foot position termed plantigrade creeping. At least 18 different variations of creeping have been documented, and some infants use several types during their development of mobility.[17] If stairs are available, infants may start creeping up stairs. Be aware they may try to go down stairs in a forward descent; therefore, guarding is necessary for safety.

In standing, the infant continues to gain stability and control. During this time frame, the infant will begin to cruise along a solid surface. Cruising is a side-stepping movement while holding onto a surface. Initially in standing, the infant will try and reach for a toy at their side and lean to the point of often falling to the ground. As they learn to weight shift to the opposite leg from the direction they are moving, they can then unweight one leg and step sideways. This weight shifting facilitates pelvis and hip control for standing and eventual walking. While in supported standing, infant's will begin to squat down to pick up toys, which helps develop hip, knee, and ankle stability for walking (**Figure 2-6**). The infant will eventually let go of the stable surface and stand independently around 11 months. Additionally, during this time frame, the infant will take forward steps holding an adult's hands or a push toy.

12 TO 24 MONTHS

In standing, independent forward walking on average begins around 12 months.[16] The toddler's hips are typically externally

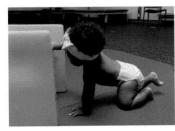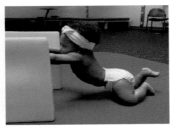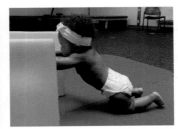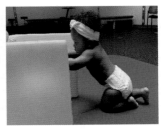

FIGURE 2-5 **Pulling to stand. Note the early reaching, then trunk extension, followed by the infant bringing her legs up under her body to improve the base of support.**

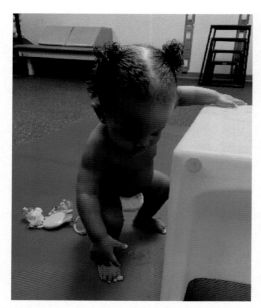

FIGURE 2-6 **Squatting to transition from standing on the floor next to a support surface.**

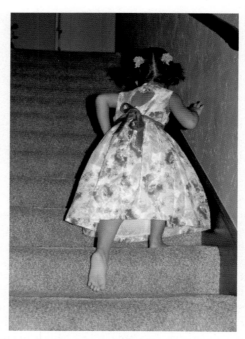

FIGURE 2-7 **Climbing stairs alternating feet.**

rotated, abducted, and flexed, knees are flexed, feet are pronated, and steps are with a flat foot. Initially the toddler's arms are in a high guard position for stability, but as balance and trunk/pelvis control improve, their arms will lower to their sides. Over the next 4 months, the toddler gains greater control in standing and walking but loss of balance is typical. They are able to stop, squat, and return to standing without loss of balance. However, the toddler continues to fall a lot, which is not unusual during this early upright mobile period. The toddler's hips begin to adduct during walking so their feet are under their shoulders, but there is no plantar flexion for push-off. The amount of time in single-leg stance is brief (32% of gait cycle) during early walking, and the toddler's step length is short (~22 cm).[18,19]

By 15 to 18 months, most toddlers will go upstairs holding a rail using a step-to pattern, putting both feet on a step before progressing to the next. They will continue to creep backward down stairs until closer to 2 years old when they will attempt to start going down holding onto a rail and placing both feet on each step in a step-to pattern.

2 TO 4 YEARS

By approximately 2 years of age, a child's step length increases (28 cm at 2 years, 33 cm at 3 years), single-limb stance increases (34% of gait cycle), and arm swing, heel strike, and push off in stance develop.[18,19] The child learns to adapt to their environment, managing slopes, different surfaces, and obstacles with less loss of balance as strength and coordination improve. They are now starting to run, which is really a fast walk. They run with a short, stiff, uneven stride with little to no flight phase.[20] By 3 years old, a mature running pattern with a consistent flight phase is present.

Children 2 to 3 years of age learn to jump down from a step (~2 years old), jump up off the floor with both feet using their arms to help initiate the movement (~3 years old), and jump over objects (between 3 and 5 years old).[20] By 30 months old, most

children are going up stairs alternating their feet while holding a rail, but may still go down using a step-to pattern (**Figure 2-7**).[21]

By 3 to 4 years old, children have gained the strength and balance to hop on one foot, gallop (a step and hop pattern with the same leg leading), jump forward approximately 2 to 3 inches (**Figure 2-8**), walk on a straight line without stepping off, and walk up and down stairs alternating feet. Motor skills continue to refine with speed and coordination increasing. Most children learn to ride a tricycle near their third birthday depending on when the weather allows for outside practice.

5 TO 7 YEARS

Over the next few years, coordination increases to the point the child can hop on a straight line (~5 years old), skip (~5-6 years old), and quickly stop and change directions when running. Most children can ride a bicycle by 5 years old and roller skate if the opportunities for practice exist.

Mature walking is typically present by 7 years of age. The child has a narrow base of support, heel strike, and reciprocal arm swing. They are in single-leg stance on average 38% of the gait cycle, and their step length has increased to 48 cm.[19,20]

8+ YEARS

Gross motor control continues to improve as the child's coordination, balance, and strength develop. Long jump distances increase into the teen years (14-16 years old), as does running speed (11-14 years). Skills continue to develop based on specific sports and practice.

■ MUSCULOSKELETAL ALIGNMENT

Physical therapists must be aware that normal range of motion (ROM) measurements for infants and children are quite variable. Understanding the typical progression of musculoskeletal

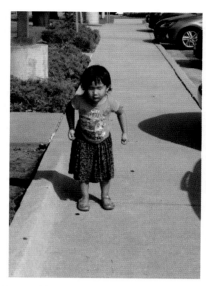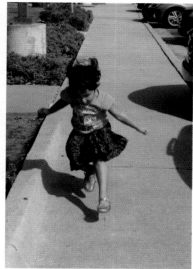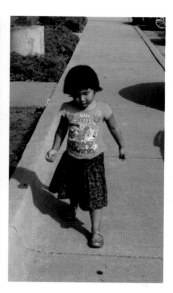

FIGURE 2-8 **Forward jump.**

alignment and having an awareness of asymmetries will assist in the assessment of the child. In this section, we present some generalities of musculoskeletal alignment that help guide the assessment of the child.

SPINAL ALIGNMENT

As presented in the previous section, the infant is born in physiological flexion, which presents as a kyphotic spinal position and posteriorly tilted pelvis. As the infant gains the ability to raise their head in prone and prop on elbows/arms, cervical and lumbar lordosis begins to develop. The quadruped position accentuates the lumbar lordosis.[22] In upright positions of sitting, standing, and walking, the infant's lumbar lordosis continues to increase until adolescence.[23,24] The 1-year-old's pelvis is most anteriorly tilted during standing and walking and decreases to a mature alignment by 3 years of age.

LOWER EXTREMITY ALIGNMENT

Infants are born with a hip flexion contracture due to the intrauterine positioning.[25] This typical contracture diminishes as the infant spends more time in prone and then moves into upright positions. According to Phelps et al,[26] on average, toddlers present with a hip flexion contracture of 3 degrees (standard deviation = 3 degrees) at 24 months.

At birth, hip abduction and external rotation are prominent and decrease as the infant moves into standing. By 2 years of age, external rotation has decreased to an average of 52 degrees and internal rotation has increased to an average of 47 degrees.[25] Knee flexion contractures of approximately 20 to 30 degrees are present at birth and decrease as the infant moves into standing.[25] At birth, the infant's knees are bowlegged (genu varum) and, over the next 18 months, straighten into a neutral alignment.[27,28] The knee angle then progresses toward a knocked knee position (genu valgum) with a peak between 2 and 4 years of approximately 10 to 15 degrees.[27,29] Genu valgum then regresses back toward neutral and stabilizes at approximately 5 degrees of valgus between 6 and 7 years old.[30]

In adolescents and adults, the average knee angle differs slightly depending on gender and race.[31,32]

FOOT ALIGNMENT: ARCH DEVELOPMENT

Newborns have very flexible feet. They are very dorsiflexed due to intrauterine positioning but gain plantar flexion quickly during the first year of life.[28] The primary question asked about a child's foot is "Should it be flat?" Newborns have flat feet due to a thick fat pad and midfoot joint laxity.[33] Midfoot musculature and longitudinal arch are developed as the infant stands, rotates in supported standing, and cruises. The longitudinal arch of the foot should be observable in standing on average by 4 to 5 years.[34] Most believe that even after 5 years of age, intervention is not needed unless the child is having pain or presenting with a neuromuscular or musculoskeletal disorder where the foot alignment could be influencing stability of the pelvis and trunk. However, significant pronation, which allows weight bearing on the medial border of the foot or malleolus, should be evaluated to determine if support is needed.

■ FINE MOTOR DEVELOPMENT

0 TO 6 MONTHS

In the first 6 months of life, infants use their hands to explore the near parts of their environment. Initially, an infant's hands are closed, although they should be able to open their grasp periodically. A firmer grasp exists initially, due to the presence of the palmar grasp reflex, but this decreases over the first few months of life. As the closed fist relaxes, infants will begin to regard their hands, moving their fingers and bringing their hand to their mouth to explore and self-calm.

Around 3 months of age, infants will have enough stability in their shoulder girdle to swipe toward objects they are attempting to obtain, and this is often with both hands at the same time. If they are able to contact the item, grasp is generally raking, with them holding the object on the ulnar side of the hand with the ring and little fingers. Dropping of objects is still involuntary at this age and generally occurs when they see another object of interest.

As shoulder stability improves and upright trunk control increases, infants develop a more controlled unilateral reach and are more likely to obtain an object. Their grasp shifts from a cylindrical grasp to beginning to use their thumb and fingers between 5 and 6 months of age, although a raking grasp is often still used for smaller objects. By 6 months, infants are able to shift objects from one hand to the other and can hold 2 objects at the same time. If the infant has good upright postural control, they may also bang 2 toys together in midline.

6 TO 9 MONTHS

By 6 months, hands should be free to play in sitting, and the infant has a good targeted reach. They are reaching into containers to take things out and are banging toys together and shaking them to explore how they work. Forearm supination is seen early in this age range to allow further exploration of toys and improved accuracy getting food to their mouth. The infant obtains smaller objects using the thumb and several fingers and larger objects using thumb and finger opposition. If a crayon is put in the infant's hand, they use a cylindrical grasp to hold it and might make dots on the paper prior to bringing the crayon to their mouth.

In prone, the infant can weight bear on one forearm and reach with the other, eventually developing the shoulder stability to perform the reach while up on an extended arm. Protective reactions using their arms to the front and sides develop during this age range, and they are beginning to develop the precision to put objects into small areas, like a peg in a board.

9 TO 12 MONTHS

Early in this age range, taking things out of containers is a favorite pastime, either using both hands to remove the items or by lifting the container and dumping it. Toward the end of the age range, precise opposition with fingers is developed to pick up items, and controlled released begins to emerge. Initially, the infant will learn to let go of objects when their hand hits the edge of a container, causing fingers to relax slightly. Eventually, this develops into intentional release into a defined space. Poking with an index finger in a hole develops into pushing a button to make a toy work. Coordinated 2-hand activities, such as holding a book and turning several pages at a time, are practiced during this time. Throwing is also practiced during this age range, although it is more of a fling, without intention or direction.

Depending on practice and availability of activities, putting things into containers also leads to the development of manipulation of objects to put them in specific spaces, like a circle in a puzzle. Generally, by the end of this age range, the infant masters placing easy shapes like circles, whereas shapes with corners take more time.

12 TO 18 MONTHS

After 12 months, depending on experience, a crayon placed in the child's hand will result in a scribble while holding the crayon in their fist (palmer-supinated or cylindrical grasp). Over time, they will attempt to imitate lines and circles but tend to use their whole arm to draw and paint, rather than fine movements of the wrist and hand.

During this time, the child learns to manipulate objects to fit them into precise shapes, like square, triangle, and star; begins to stack larger objects, aligning them so they do not fall; and develops rotational movement of the wrist and hand to turn knobs. The child should still be alternating hands to perform activities and not showing a consistent hand preference at this age.

18 MONTHS TO 2 YEARS

Between 1.5 and 2 years of age, the child is beginning to shift their grasp of a writing implement, scribbling on whatever is available, and starting to stack smaller objects without them falling over. The child is able to turn single pages in a book and orient the book right side up, and can manipulate push-buttons, levers, and knobs. If zippers are started, they can complete the zip up, and they can use both hands to pull pants up.

2 TO 3 YEARS

During the second year, the child transitions their grasp of crayons and pencils to a more mature digital pronated grasp and is accurate at imitation of lines and circles (**Figure 2-9**). Writing and painting become more refined, using wrist movements rather than whole arm movements. After demonstration, the child is able to put beads on a string using both hands doing different components of the task.

Stacking of smaller items improves, and the child is able to stack 6 to 8 small blocks with good alignment to keep them from falling. They are also able to manipulate a doorknob and unscrew the lid on a container. A hand preference could emerge during this time, although it may not be consistent until 5 years of age.

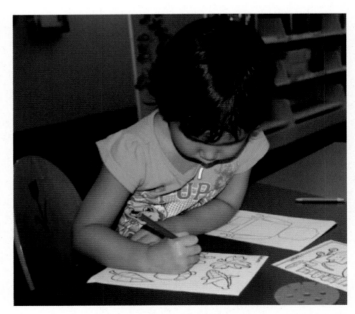

FIGURE 2-9 Coloring with grasp progressing toward a mature static tripod.

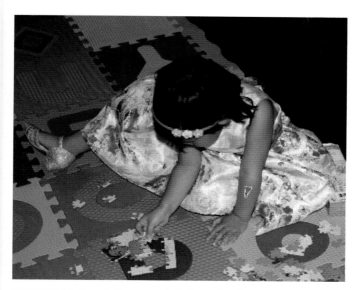

FIGURE 2-10 **Completing a puzzle independently.**

3 TO 4 YEARS

During this period, precision with writing implements improves, and the child is able to trace simple shapes and manipulate substances like Play-Doh, rolling and shaping the dough. They should be working with 20- to 40-piece puzzles (**Figure 2-10**). Throwing becomes a bit more directed at this point, as the child is able to throw within 30 degrees of a target and uses both hands to trap-catch a ball.

4 TO 6 YEARS

During this age range, the child is shifting to a mature tripod grasp during writing and coloring activities and begins to use scissors, initially cutting straight lines and then following more complex pathways. The overhand throw becomes more accurate (**Figure 2-11**), and catching is less of a trap, but the child still uses both hands even though they are away from the body. The child is able to accurately trace shapes with sharp corners and is beginning to print, starting with capital letters. They are able to manipulate buttons, zippers, and laces with practice and completely dress and undress.

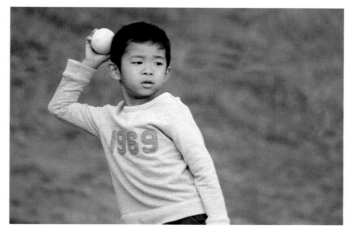

FIGURE 2-11 **Overhand throwing accuracy improves with age.**
(Used with permission from ziggy_mars/Shutterstock.)

■ LANGUAGE DEVELOPMENT

When addressing language development in children, it is important to recognize the 2 main components of language: receptive, or understanding, and expressive, or providing information. Both of these areas should be addressed when evaluating a child's development because a child with a delay will often have more skills in one area than another.

It is also important to recognize contributing factors in the development of language, such as hearing and verbal interaction with others. If either of these factors is limited, there will be an impact on the child's development of communication. There is also a link between the development of movement and the development of language skills. Generally, the first year of life is a movement explosion, whereas the second year has more of a language emphasis. This does not mean skills in those areas only develop during that time; however, the greatest increase in language skills begins in the second year of life.

0 TO 6 MONTHS

Infants recognize caregiver voices early on, having heard the voices while in utero, and will alert to sounds and voices even before they have the ability to turn toward them. They will startle to loud noises, although this should decrease during the first 6 months, and as head control improves, and will look toward and then turn toward sounds to see where they are coming from. Initially infants make social smiles and coos, using cries to make their wants and needs known. Later in the 6 months, a variety of vowel sounds emerge. In the first 3 months, the infant recognizes changes in tone, and between 3 and 6 months, they begin to assign meaning to the different tones of voice. At the end of 6 months, 1 or 2 consonant sounds begin to emerge.

6 TO 12 MONTHS

During the second 6 months of life, the child begins to recognize labels for certain people or objects and will often look toward the person or object named. Occasionally, they will reach for or point to the object named as they approach 1 year. The child will recognize a simple command when it is combined with a gesture and understands "no."

Also during these second 6 months of life, more consonant sounds emerge and the infant begins to use them repetitively. They will also start to play with volume and pitch, getting louder to demonstrate intent. By the end of the first year, the child should have 1 to 2 sounds that they are using consistently to represent a person, object, or action.

12 TO 18 MONTHS

This 6-month period represents the beginning of the language explosion. The child is beginning to string a variety of sounds together (expressive jargon) that sound like a sentence but may or may not have any recognizable words. They are imitating words and developing the use of labels so that by 18 months, the child has up to 50 words that they use consistently.

During this time, the child begins to understand directional words such as "where" and point to objects in their environment that are named. They also begin to develop the ability to point to pictures in a book that are named but do not yet recognize that the ball in the book represents the ball on the floor.

18 TO 24 MONTHS

As the child approaches 2 years of age, they begin to understand the words in requests and do not require a gesture to follow a direction. They will consistently point to a picture in a book when it is named and will follow a simple command but cannot complete a 2-step task. Their vocabulary increases to over 200 words, and the child is beginning to put 2 words together to express their thoughts.

2 TO 3 YEARS

This is the age of the question, as the child demands answers to their questions. Vocabulary increases to over 300 words, and the child is putting 3 to 5 words together, using verbs and pronouns. The child in this year can answer simple questions and enjoys listening to stories, but may also "read" the book themselves, repeating what they have heard on each page.

3 TO 4 YEARS

Children at this age are beginning to follow 2-step related commands without losing track of the purpose and to use plurals and pronouns consistently. While some of the child's speech may have been difficult for strangers to understand previously, by this age, anyone should be able to recognize what the child is intending to say.

4 TO 5 YEARS

At this age, sentences have a much more typical structure for questions and getting their point across. They are imitating intonation and pattern and understand directional words. At this age, children may use words they have overheard without understanding their meaning. They may also try to communicate through writing, but letters could be reversed or in the wrong place. The child can recognize and follow a 2-step command even if the 2 parts are unrelated.

5 YEARS AND OLDER

Communication continues to become more complex as the child is able to tell stories, invent their own spellings of words, and recognize comparative variations such as small, smaller, and smallest.

■ COGNITIVE DEVELOPMENT

Cognitive development is the reasoning and processing that helps a child think about and understand the world around them. Cognitive development includes the construction of thought processes, development of memory and problem solving, and skilled decision-making.[35] For infants and toddlers, it is often difficult to differentiate language and cognitive development, and one should realize they are developing alongside each other. Additionally, therapists should be aware that as children age, we often "know" a child's cognitive ability through their expressive language; therefore, if the child has delayed language expression, we must identify alternate ways of identifying the child's cognitive abilities.

0 TO 6 MONTHS

We know that infants are aware of their surroundings and interested in exploration from the time they are born. They actively gather, sort, and process information, using the data to develop perception and thinking skills. Infant learning is observed by their ability to focus on and follow objects, distinguish sounds, and anticipate events. By 3 months old, infants can recognize faces, imitate facial expressions, and respond to familiar sounds. By 6 months, they can drop an object and demonstrate simple problem solving by watching it fall to the floor and roll away.

6 TO 12 MONTHS

At 6 months, infants begin to imitate sounds, enjoy hearing their own voice, recognize parents, distinguish between animate and inanimate objects, and base distance on the size of an object. They develop object permanence around 7 months old, realizing an object still exists even when they cannot see it. They also figure out that if they drop an object, they can pick it up again. At 4 to 7 months, babies can recognize their names. By 9 months, infants can imitate gestures and actions and begin to test parental responses to their behavior, such as throwing food on the floor. They play pat-a-cake, wave bye-bye, and respond to no-no. They remember their parents' reactions and test them again to see if they get the same reaction.

12 TO 18 MONTHS

Besides their language development, toddlers are associating names with objects; developing attachment to objects, such as a doll or blanket; and experiencing separation anxiety when away from their consistent caregiver. By 18 months of age, toddlers feel a sense of ownership by using the word "my" with certain people or objects and can follow directions that involve 2 different tasks, such as picking up toys and putting them in a box. This demonstrates the learning of concepts, sequences, and words.

18 MONTHS TO 3 YEARS

Between 18 months and 3 years of age, children have reached the "sensorimotor" stage of Piaget's theory of cognitive development that involves rudimentary thought.[36,37] Besides permanence of objects, they understand permanence of people. They strive for independence but do not understand safety. In this age range, the child learns appropriate and inappropriate behavior and understands discipline. The child has a better understanding of emotions, such as love, trust, and fear. They begin to understand some of the ordinary aspects of everyday life, such as shopping for food, going to daycare, and bedtime routines. The child often thrives on this routine because it provides consistency.

3 TO 6 YEARS

At this age, children function in the "preoperational" stage of Piaget's cognitive development theory, meaning they use their imagination and memory skills.[36,37] They are typically self-centered but develop social interaction skills, such as playing and cooperating with other children, but often push boundaries to test their limits. Children are developing an increased attention span, learning to read, and developing structured routines, such as doing household chores.

6 TO 12 YEARS

Children at this age are in the "concrete operations" stage of Piaget's cognitive development theory and should demonstrate logical and coherent actions in thinking and problem solving.[36,37] They understand the concepts of permanence and conservation by learning that volume, weight, and numbers may remain constant despite changes in outward appearance. They build on past experiences, using them to explain why some things happen. Their attention span should increase with age, from being able to focus on a task for about 15 minutes at age 6 to an hour by age 9.

■ ADAPTIVE DEVELOPMENT

Adaptive skills and behaviors are used in a variety of environments during daily life to engage in work and play and are described according to age and cultural standards.[38,39] Adaptive function is generally described in terms of practical, social, and conceptual sills needed to engage in meaningful daily activities including play and schoolwork. Adaptive skills and behaviors include taking care of daily needs related to bathing, dressing, and eating; maintaining interpersonal relationships and following rules; solving problems; and maintaining safety.[21,40]

Hand and finger strength, motor control, sensory processing, communication skills, and the ability to follow directions influence the development of independent self-care skills. Difficulty with self-care skills may be interpreted as limited play skills, immaturity, laziness, or lack of independence. A child who has difficulty with self-care skills may have difficulty using utensils, refuse to eat certain foods, struggle to open food packaging, have toileting accidents, or require adult support to fall asleep. When self-care skills such as toileting and feeding are difficult, children may not be comfortable participating in social activities such as playdates, birthday parties, or sleepovers. This can have a significant impact on self-esteem and participation in leisure and school-related activities.[41,42]

Therapists can support the development of self-care skills by using strategies including breaking down skills into smaller tasks, frequent opportunities for structured skill practice, visual supports, feedback and reinforcement, and role-play activities such as pretending to feed stuffed animals.[40,43-45]

■ SOCIAL-EMOTIONAL SKILLS

Social-emotional skills refer to the experience, expression, and management of emotions and the ability to establish relationships with others. Research suggests "that the neural mechanisms underlying emotion regulation may be the same as those underlying cognitive processes, specifically, higher order cognitive processes such as volitional sustained attention or working memory."[46] Infants experience and express emotions before they are able to manage and explain them to others. For example, infants turn toward and respond to voices, cry to get attention and have their needs met, and smile or vocalize to interact with others. Older children and adults use social-emotional skills in conjunction with cognitive processes to process information and make decisions related to participation in social situations.[44] Development of social-emotional skills contributes to attention, the ability to seek help when needed, and participation in interpersonal relationships.

Major components of social-emotional skills include self-management, self-awareness, social awareness, relationship skills, and responsible decision-making skills. Self-management is the ability to recognize one's own emotions and associate related thoughts and emotions. This can include managing stress, controlling impulses, and motivating oneself to achieve goals. Self-awareness is the ability to label one's emotions and identify their influence on behavior. The development of self-awareness begins in infancy when infants begin to realize that they are separate from others and notice the difference between self-touch and being touched by others. More complex self-awareness skills can be seen when infants begin to recognize themselves in a mirror and begin to identify, label, and manage their own feelings.[47,48] In infancy, children rely on others for soothing and calming. As they age, they are able to ask others for help or ask for a turn with a toy. Social awareness is the ability to understand things from another person's perspective and to empathize with others.[49,50] Social awareness is seen in infants when they react differently to happy or angry voices, attempt to comfort others, or label the emotions of peers. Relationship skills refer to the ability to develop and maintain healthy, meaningful interpersonal relationships. This includes reciprocal communication, turn-taking skills, and conflict resolution and is seen as play skills emerge. Children initially play by themselves, then alongside others in parallel play, and then reciprocally and in turn-taking activities with others. Responsible decision-making is the ability to make thoughtful and constructive decisions about personal behaviors. This can include maintaining one's safety, making ethical decisions, and responding to peer pressure.

Children develop social-emotional skills through interactions with others. Development of these skills can vary due to environmental and cultural issues. Therapists can promote the development of social-emotional skills by modeling words to describe or express emotion, providing interventions that make the child feel safe and secure, promoting self-efficacy, and actively responding to a child's attempts to communicate emotions and feelings.

■ PLAY

Play is how children learn and is essential to their physical, cognitive, social, and emotional growth. Play can be defined as "any spontaneous or organized activity that provides enjoyment, entertainment, amusement or diversion."[51] Unstructured play allows children to initiate their own activities and experiment with open-ended rules helping them learn the difference between plans and outcomes. Play allows children to create and engage in activities individually, with other children, or with adult caregivers, learning rules, social interaction, negotiation, and eventually self-advocacy skills.[52] Play can be solitary and calm or physical and active.

Pellegrini and Smith[53] proposed 3 development stages to describe physical play that includes vigorous physical activity. In the first stage, infants perform what Thelen[54] called "rhythmic stereotypies" or repetitive gross motor activities that do not have a specific purpose but provide movement for the development of body schema. These repetitive behaviors, such as body rocking and leg kicking, peak around 6 months of age, occurring as much as 40% of an hour's activity when the child is awake and playing. Besides the development of body schema, these movement are hypothesized to support the development of strength and endurance in preparation for other motor activities.

The second stage, "exercise play," starts around 12 months of age, peaks in the preschool years, and continues into the elementary years. Exercise play is the never-ending gross motor movement of a child including running, chasing, and climbing. Think of the child who seems to never sit still. They are up and active either by themselves or with others, always moving until they suddenly are sitting still and potentially asleep. The hypothesized function of exercise play is the development of strength and endurance for vigorous activity and the promotion of muscle differentiation.

Finally, "rough-and-tumble" play is the third physical activity play stage that begins with tumbling and wrestling in a social context initially with a caregiver. This physical activity play increases through elementary school and peaks prior to middle school. Rough-and-tumble play can be preparatory for group sports and organized physical activities and can help build social skills related to interacting with peers during group sports events.

One can also view play as a developmental process where children learn how to interact with other children, cooperate, share, and make friends. Parten's 6 stages of play, described in 1932, continue to hold to this day as a description of the process children progress through as they develop play and social skills.[55] These stages are not 100% linear, as you will see children alternate between the play types based on opportunities and influences of other circumstances.[56] **Table 2-2** provides an overview of the play stages. As physical therapists, we must be aware that play is how children learn, and we must understand how to engage a child in play activities.

■ ENVIRONMENTAL INFLUENCES ON DEVELOPMENT

Genetics plays an important role in setting the trajectory for a child's development; however, the environment in which the child develops, from the prenatal period on, affords or hinders the child's opportunities for successful outcomes. For this discussion, we focus on environmental factors that can influence the child after birth, but we acknowledge there are many environmental factors that support a mother's health prior to and

TABLE 2-2 • Parten's 6 Stages of Play[55]	
Stage	**Description**
Unoccupied play (0-12 months)	The infant is making random movements with no clear purpose, but this is play for an infant. Often the infant is just observing.
Solitary (independent) play (0-24 months)	The child plays alone maintaining focus on an activity. They are unaware and uninterested in what others are doing. Make-believe play in older children.
Onlooker play (18-30 months)	The toddler watches others at play but does not engage. The child may interact with others in the environment but does not actually join the play activity.
Parallel play (30 months- 3 years)	The children play side by side with similar toys, often mimicking the actions but not interacting. This type of play is seen as a transitory stage from a socially immature solitary and onlooker type of play to a more socially mature associative and cooperative type of play.[56]
Associative play (3-4 years)	The child plays with a group of children with similar goals, but there is no coordination of the activities with the other children. The children often are interacting with each other, but the activities are not in sync.
Cooperative play (4 year and older)	The children play in a group with an organized goal in mind. The activity is organized, and participants have assigned roles.

during pregnancy and reduce the risk of maternal and fetal complications.[57,58] An environment that provides nurturing care, which is defined as behaviors, attitudes, and knowledge regarding caregiving (eg, health, hygiene, nutrition); stimulation/early learning opportunities (eg, talking, singing, playing); security and safety (eg, routines, protection from harm); and responsive caregiving (eg, early bonding, attachment, trust) provided by the caregivers, supports a child's early development.[59,60] As physical therapists, we may or may not observe each of these components of the environment but should be aware and offer support and resources when indicated.

The environment physical therapists often consider is the child's physical environment. The physical environment includes the physical space, toys, and opportunities for play and exploration in the child's natural environment including the home, extended family's homes, and the childcare environments.[16] As children develop, we consider the physical environment's influence, particularly on gross motor development. For example, do parents place a child on their stomach so they can learn to lift their head up against gravity or is the floor surface slick, making the child's ability to gain traction for creeping more difficult? These considerations continue as the child ages. For example, are there stairs the child can practice on or is the outside play area safe enough to allow tricycle riding and climbing on playground equipment? As therapists, we should be aware of the physical environment but also consider the environment's influence on other areas of development (eg, reading to support language development, offering a cup and spoon to support adaptive development, providing opportunities for parent-child interaction to support attachment and social development). As therapists working with children and their families, we cannot solely focus on motor skills, as we have already shown the interrelatedness of all of the developmental domains.

Therapists should, however, be aware that the family's socioeconomic status (SES) can influence the child's physical environment. Often, homes of those with lower SES are more crowded and provide less cognitive stimulation.[61] Parents have to juggle many stressors and make choices regarding where to place resources. Does their money go to housing and utilities or food and toys? Do they work the extra job or spend more time with their children? Children living in poverty experience less parental nurturing and are exposed to greater life stresses and violence.[62] This continued exposure has demonstrated long-term physiological and brain development consequences that impact attachment and cognition.[63,64] As children living in poverty enter school, many demonstrate lower standardized testing scores on academic achievement tests and poorer grades in school.[65,66] A positive, however, is that maternal nurturing care during the early childhood years can protect early brain development and attenuate the negative effects of a low SES.[63,67] The positive caregiving interactions, which are components of the child's physical environment, have supported positive motor, cognitive, language, and adaptive development.[67,68] As therapists, we should identify ways to support a nurturing physical environment so children have the best developmental opportunities possible.

■ RED FLAGS IN TYPICAL DEVELOPMENT AND REASONS FOR REFERRAL

As a physical therapist, whether you work in pediatrics or not, you will be asked if you think "such and such related to motor development" is a concern. As stated earlier, children meet developmental milestones at varying ages, and we provided what is "typical" within the literature. We also described how environment influences development. However, there is a point when you should recommend a referral for future evaluation. The sections below provide a summary of key development skills that, if a child is not demonstrating, indicate the need for referral. Additionally, if anyone reports that the child is losing skills (regressing), then an immediate referral to the child's pediatrician is warranted.

Birth to 2 months

- Excessively low muscle tone
- Not alerting to sound

3-4 months

- Difficulty nursing
- Unable to grasp objects placed in hands
- Keeping hand fisted
- No eye contact
- No cooing or making sounds

4-6 months

- Not bringing objects to mouth
- Unable to hold head up in prone
- Poor midline head control in supported sitting
- No vowel sounds
- Not batting toward toys

6-8 months

- Not sitting without support
- Not rolling tummy to back and back to tummy
- Not bringing hands to midline
- Not shifting toys from one hand to the other
- Not using thumb and sides of fingers to grasp toys
- Not playing with volume or pitch (varying sounds)
- Not watching toys as they fall to the floor
- Not exploring toys either using their mouth or by shaking and banging

9-10 months

- Not moving around room in some fashion to explore
- Not recognizing their name when called
- Not using several consonant sounds
- Not beginning to string consonant-vowel pairs together (da-da)
- Not using thumb and finger tips to grasp large options
- Not banging 2 toys together
- Not getting into or out of sitting
- Not recognizing "no" and pausing before resuming the activity
- Not showing interest in familiar toys, pets, or people

11-12 months

- Not getting into or out of sitting
- Not creeping in some fashion
- Not pulling toys out of containers
- Not stringing a variety of sounds together
- Not recognizing labels for familiar people
- Not eating mashed table foods

12-18 months

- Not pulling to stand
- Not trying to stand without support
- Not using 1 or 2 words to label objects, people, or actions
- Not putting objects into containers
- Not pushing buttons to make a toy work
- Not interested in what is going on around them
- Not trying to drink out of an open cup that is held for them by an adult

18-24 months

- Not walking independently
- Not using words to indicate wants and needs
- Not marking on paper with pencil or crayon
- Not using up to 200 words by age 2
- Not trying to climb stairs
- Using one hand more than the other (no hand preference until 2-5 years old)

2-3 years old

- Not putting several words together
- Not being able to be understood by familiar people

- Not trying to climb onto furniture or creep up steps
- Not scribbling with a crayon using a more pronated grasp
- Not having the strength to pull pop beads or Legos apart
- Not walking on uneven surfaces
- Not follow a 2-step related command
- Not being able to calm themselves down from a tantrum

4 years old

- Not jumping up, onto, or off using both feet for take-off and landing
- Not navigating obstacles to avoid bumping into things while moving
- Not using pronouns to indicate self or others during speech
- Not recognizing basic colors and shapes
- Not using digital pronated grasp to mark on paper and trace shapes with some reasonable approximation
- Not running with coordination
- Not able to accomplish basic self-dressing tasks (pull on and off)

5 years old

- Not able to walk up and down steps using the rail
- Not able to walk on a line on the floor
- Not able to attempt to write name or several letters
- Not able to string beads using both hands
- Not able to use utensils and open cup effectively
- Not able to follow 2-step unrelated command without cuing
- Not able to ask questions using complete sentences

■ CONCLUSION

A child's development is individualized, but within a typical period and along a typical trajectory. As physical therapists, we must understand the expected sequence within each developmental domain and recognize if the child is progressing similar to their peers or if future evaluations are indicated. We must recognize that the child's environment and family expectations can either support and enhance a child's development or potentially provide barriers to the child's developmental progression. Understanding the interrelatedness of development and the complexity of potential influences on a child is key to supporting children and their families.

STUDY QUESTIONS

1. Describe the progression of prone motor development across an infant's life span.
2. Describe the progression of supine motor development across an infant's life span.
3. Describe the profession of upright motor development across an infant/toddler's life span.
4. A neighbor asks you if their child is developing typically. How would you describe a child's functioning at 3, 6, 9, 12, and 18 months in all areas of development?
5. You started working with a toddler whose parents have limited resources. What strategies could you provide to support development without making them choose between their child's development and living expenses?

References

1. World Health Organization. *The International Classification of Functioning, Disability and Health: An Overview.* WHO; 2001.
2. Brofenbrenner U. Ecology of the family as context for human development: research perspectives. *Dev Psychol.* 1986;22(6):723.
3. Centers for Disease Control and Prevention. CDC's Developmental Milestones website. Accessed February 1, 2022. https://www.cdc.gov/ncbddd/actearly/milestones/.
4. Zubler JM, Wiggins LK, Macia MM, et al. Evidence-informed milestones for developmental surveillance tools. *Pediatrics.* 2022;149(3):e2021052138.
5. de Vries JI, Fong BF. Normal fetal movement: an overview. *Ultrasound Obste Gynecol.* 2006;278:701-711.
6. Prechtl HFR. Fetal behavior. In: Hill A, Volpe JJ, eds. *Fetal Neurology.* Raven Press; 1989:1-106.
7. Blackburn ST. *Maternal, Fetal and Neonatal Physiology: A Clinical Perspective.* 4th ed. Saunders Elsevier; 2012.
8. Kurjak A, Tikvica A, Stanojevic M, et al. The assessment of fetal neurobehavior by three-dimensional and four-dimensional ultrasound. *J Maternal-Fetal Neonatal Med.* 2008;21(10):675-684.
9. Sparling JW, Van Tol J, Chescheir NC. Fetal and neonatal hand movement. *Phys Ther.* 1999;71(1):24-39.
10. Zoia S, Blason L, D'Ottavio G, et al. Evidence of early development of action planning in the human fetus: a kinematic study. *Exp Brain Res.* 2006;176:217-226.
11. Piontelli A. *Development of Normal Fetal Movements.* Springer; 2014.
12. Richardson BS, Harding R, Walker DW. Behavioral states in the fetus: relationship to fetal health and development. In: Creasy RK, Resnik R, Iams JD, Lockwood CJ, Moore TR, Greene MF, eds. *Maternal-Fetal Medicine: Principles and Practice.* 7th ed. Sanders; 2014:155-162.
13. Graven SN, Browne JV. Sleep and brain development: the critical role of sleep in fetal and early neonatal brain development. *Newborn Infant Nur Rev.* 2008;8(4):173-179.
14. Green EM, Mulcahy CM, Pountney TE. An investigation into the development of early postural control. *Dev Med Child Neurol.* 1995;37:437-488.
15. Harbourne TR, Stergiou N. Nonlinear analysis of the development of sitting postural control. *Dev Psychobiol.* 2003;42(4):368-377.
16. World Health Organization Multicentre Growth Reference Study Group. WHO motor development study: windows of achievement for six gross motor developmental milestones. *Acta Paediatrica.* 2006;suppl 450:86-95.
17. Adolph KE, Vereijken B, Denny MA. Learning to crawl. *Child Dev.* 1998;69(5):1299-1312.
18. Sutherland D, Olshen R, Biden E, Wyatt M. The development of a mature gait. *Clin Dev Med.* No. 104/105. Lippincott; 1988.
19. Sutherland D, Olshen R, Cooper L, Woo S. The development of a mature gait. *J Bone Joint Surg.* 1980;62-A(3):336-353.
20. Gallahue DL, Ozmum JC. *Understanding Motor Development: Infants, Children, Adolescents, Adults.* 6th ed. McGraw Hill; 2006.
21. Bayley N. *Bayley Scales of Infant and Toddler Development.* 4th ed. Pearson; 2019.
22. LeVeau BF, Bernhardt DB. Developmental biomechanics. *Phys Ther.* 1984;64(12):1874-1881.
23. Widhe T. Spine, posture, mobility and pain. A longitudinal study from childhood to adolescence. *Eur Spine J.* 2001;10:118-123.
24. Wright JC, Bell D. Lumbosacral joint angles in children. *J Pediatr Orthop.* 1991;11:748-751.

25. Drews JE, Vraciu JK, Pellino G. Range of motion of the joints of the lower extremities of newborns. *Phys Occup Ther Ped.* 1984;4(2):49-62.

26. Phelps E, Smith LJ, Hallum A. Normal ranges of hip motion of infants between nine and 24 months of age. *Dev Med Child Neurol.* 1985;27:785-792.

27. Beeson P. Frontal plane configuration of the knee in children. *Foot.* 1999;9:18-26.

28. Cusick BD. *Progressive Casting and Splinting for Lower Extremity Deformities in Children With Neuromotor Dysfunction.* Therapy Skills Builders; 1990.

29. Hensinger RN, Jones ET. Developmental orthopedics: I: the lower limb. *Dev Med Child Neurol.* 1982;24:95-116.

30. Bleck EE. The showing of children: sham or science. *Dev Med Child Neurol.* 1982;13:188-195.

31. Arazi M, Ogun TC, Memik R. Normal development of the tibiofemoral angle in children: a clinical study of 590 normal subjects from 3-17 years of age. *J Pediatr Orthop.* 2001;21:264-267.

32. Cahuzac JP, Sales de Gauzy D, Vardon J. Development of the clinical tibiofemoral angle in normal adolescents: a study of 427 normal subjects from 10-16 years of age. *J Bone Joint Surg Am Br.* 1995;77:729-732.

33. Staheli LT. *Fundamentals of Pediatric Orthopedics.* Raven Press; 1992.

34. Engel GM, Staheli LT. The natural history of torsion and other factors influencing gait in childhood. *Clin Orthop Relat Res.* 1974;99:12-17.

35. Bowe FG. *Birth to Five: Early Childhood Special Education.* Delmar; 1995.

36. Piaget J. *The Origins of Intelligence in Children.* International University Press; 1952.

37. Parke RD, Gauvain M. *Child Psychology: A Contemporary Viewpoint.* 7th ed. McGraw-Hill; 2009.

38. Grossman HJ. *Classification in Mental Retardation.* American Association on Mental Deficiency; 1993.

39. Chapparo CJ, Hooper E. Self-care at school: perceptions of 6-year-old children. *Am J Occup Ther.* 2005;59(1):67-77.

40. Weaver LL. Effectiveness of work, activities of daily living, education, and sleep interventions for people with autism spectrum disorder: a systematic review. *Am J Occup Ther.* 2015; 69(5):1-11.

41. O'Donnell S, Deitz J, Kartin D, Nalty T, Dawson G. Sensory processing, problem behavior, adaptive behavior, and cognition in preschool children with autism spectrum disorders. *Am J Occup Ther.* 2012;66(5):586-594.

42. Schaaf RC, Benevides T, Mailloux Z, et al. An intervention for sensory difficulties in children with autism: a randomized trial. *J Autism Develop Dis.* 2014;44(7):1493-1506.

43. Jamison TR, Schuttler JO. Overview and preliminary evidence for a social skills and self-care curriculum for adolescent females with autism: the girls night out model. *J Autism Develop Dis.* 2017;47(1):110-125.

44. Campbell PH, Sawyer LB. Supporting learning opportunities in natural settings through participation-based services. *J Early Intervention.* 2007;29(4):287-305.

45. Kellegrew DH. Creating opportunities for occupation: an intervention to promote the self-care independence of young children with special needs. *Am J Occup Ther.* 1998;2(6):457-465.

46. Bell MA, Wolfe CD. Emotion and cognition: an intricately bound developmental process. *Child Dev.* 2004;75(2):366-370.

47. Suddendorf T, Simcock G, Nielsen M. Visual self-recognition in mirrors and live videos: evidence for a developmental asynchrony. *Child Dev.* 2007;22(2):185-196.

48. Suddendorf T, Butler DL. The nature of visual self-recognition. *Trends Cogn Sci.* 2013;17(3):121-127.

49. Markova G, Legerstee M. Contingency, imitation, and affect sharing: foundations of infants' social awareness. *Dev Psychol.* 2006;42(1):132.

50. Uithol S, Paulus M. What do infants understand of others' action? A theoretical account of early social cognition. *Psychol Res.* 2014;78(5):609-622.

51. Parham D. Fazio S. *Play in Occupational Therapy for Children.* 2nd ed. Mosby Elsevier; 2008.

52. Ginsburg KR. The importance of play in promoting health child development and maintaining strong parent-child bonds. *Pediatrics.* 2007;119:182-191.

53. Pellegrini AD, Smith PK. Physical activity play: the nature and function of a neglected aspect of play. *Child Dev.* 1998;69:577-598.

54. Thelen E. Motor development. A new synthesis. *Am Psychol.* 1995;50:79-95.

55. Parten MB. Social participation among preschool children. *J Abnor Soc Psychol.* 1932;27(3):243-269.

56. Hughes F. *Children, Play, and Development.* Sage; 2009.

57. Centers for Disease Control and Prevention. Before Pregnancy website. Accessed February 1, 2019. https://www.cdc.gov/preconception/planning.html.

58. Lu MC. Recommendations for preconception care. *Am Fam Physician.* 2007;6:397-400.

59. Bornstein MH, ed. *Handbook of Parenting.* Psychology Press; 2012.

60. Britto PR, Engle P. Parenting education and support: maximizing the most critical enabling environment. In: Narope TPM, Kaga Y, eds. *Investing Against Evidence: The Global State of Early Childhood Care and Education.* United Nations Educational, Scientific and Cultural Organizations; 2015:157-176.

61. Evans GW. The environment of childhood poverty. *Am Psychol.* 2004;59(2):77-92.

62. Shonkoff JP, Garner AS. The lifelong effect of early childhood adversity and toxic stress. *Pediatrics.* 2012;129:e232-246.

63. Luby JF. Poverty's most insidious damage: the developing brain. *JAMA Pediatr.* 2015;169:810-811.

64. Noble KG, Houston SM, Britto NH, et al. Family income, parental education and brain structure in children and adolescents. *Nat Neurosci.* 2015;18:773-778.

65. Duncan GJ, Brooks-Gunn J. *Consequences of Growing Up Poor.* Russell Sage Foundation; 1997.

66. Haverman R, Wolfe B. The determinants of children's attachments: a review of methods and findings. *J Econ Lit.* 1995;33(3):1829-1278.

67. Holditch-Davis D, Miles MS, Burchinal MR, Goldman BD. Maternal role attainment with medically fragile infants: part 2. Relationship to quality of parenting. *Res Nur Health.* 2011;34:35-48.

68. Treyvaud K, Anderson VA, Howard K, et al. Parenting behavior is associated with the early neurobehavioral development of very preterm children. *Pediatrics.* 2009;123:555-561.

69. Bly L. *Motor Skills Acquisition in the First Year: An Illustrated Guide to Normal Development.* Therapy Skill Builders; 1994.

70. Case-Smith J. Development of childhood Occupations. In: Case-Smith J, O'Brien JC, eds. *Occupational Therapy for Children and Adolescents.* 7th ed. Mosby Elsevier; 2015:65-94.

71. Child Development Institute. Child development website. Accessed February 1, 2022. https://childdevelopmentinfo.com/child-development/#.XFXrVc0nbcs.

72. Edhardt RP. *Developmental Hand Dysfunction: Theory, Assessment, Treatment.* 2nd ed. Pro-Ed, Inc; 1994.

73. Folio MR, Fewell RR. *Peabody Development Motor Scales (PDMS-2)*. Pro-Ed, Inc; 2000.

74. Gesell A, Amatruda CS. *Developmental Diagnosis: Normal and Abnormal Child Development, Clinical Methods and Pediatrics Application*. Haper & Row; 1947.

75. Halverson HM. An experimental study of prehension in infants by means of systematic cinema records. *Genetic Psychol Mono*. 1931;10:107-286.

76. Knobloch H, Pasamanick B. *Gesell and Amatruda's Manual of Development Diagnosis*. 3rd ed. Harper & Row; 1997.

77. Long TM, Battaile B, Toscano K. *Handbook of Pediatric Physical Therapy*. 3rd ed. Wolters Kluwer; 2018.

78. Owen RS. *Language Development: An Introduction*. 10th ed. Pearson; 2020.

79. Rossetti L. *The Rossetti Infant-Toddler Language Scale*. Lingui Systems, Inc; 2005.

80. Schickedanz JA, Schickendanz DI, Forsyth PD, Forsyth GA. *Understanding Children and Adolescents*. 4th ed. Pearson; 2001.

Assessment Tools in Pediatric Physical Therapy

Alyssa La Forme Fiss, PT, PhD, and Lynn Jeffries, PT, DPT, PhD

LEARNING OBJECTIVES

Upon completion of this chapter, the reader will be able to:

- Identify common considerations when selecting an assessment tool.
- Differentiate between discriminative, predictive, and evaluative measures.
- Identify specific types of measures to use for each domain of the International Classification of Functioning, Disability, and Health.
- Interpret the psychometric properties of a given assessment tool.
- Describe common strategies for the administration of assessment tools.
- Interpret the results of common data obtained from assessment tools.

INTRODUCTION

Assessment tools include a wide variety of tests and measures and are commonly used in pediatric physical therapy to document a child's current developmental status, determine eligibility for services, determine prognosis of future delay or impairment, or measure progress over time. Assessment tools allow for the objective gathering of information to guide physical therapist decision-making and service delivery. There are numerous assessment tools available for therapists to use clinically, each with unique properties and purposes. This chapter will detail strategies for selecting and completing appropriate measures in pediatric clinical practice.

SELECTION OF AN ASSESSMENT TOOL

DISCRIMINATIVE, PREDICTIVE, AND EVALUATIVE PURPOSE

Selecting an appropriate assessment tool is an important component of a pediatric physical therapy examination and requires consideration of multiple factors. Selection may begin with a review of the purpose of the test to assist the therapist in narrowing appropriate options for measures by providing important information as to how the test is intended to be used. For example, assessment tools can be categorized as discriminative, predictive, and/or evaluative.[1] A discriminative or norm-referenced measure is a type of assessment that provides information about a child's ability compared to the abilities of other children.[2] Norm-referenced measures are often used to establish a child's current developmental ability as compared to peers or to determine eligibility for services. The Bayley Scales of Infant and Toddler Development–Fourth Edition[3] is an example of a norm-referenced test that examines a child's adaptive behavior, cognition, language, motor skills, and social-emotional skills compared to same-age peers from 1 to 42 months of age and is widely used to determine eligibility for services for children in early intervention programs.[4] Norm-referenced measures are helpful to determine if a child is demonstrating developmental delay.

Predictive measures help to predict or estimate outcomes for a child as they age and can assist with service planning. For example, the Test of Infant Motor Performance (TIMP)[5] may be used as a predictive measure. The TIMP was designed as a measure of functional movement for infants from 32 weeks' gestational age to 4 months postconceptual age and has demonstrated validity at 3 months of age to predict motor performance at 12 months of age,[6] 2 years of age,[7] and preschool age,[8] and from between 34 weeks' postmenstrual age and 16 weeks of age to predict motor development. This ability to predict future performance may assist therapists in determining appropriate service needs for a child at younger ages and to intervene at earlier, opportune times.

An evaluative or criterion-referenced measure assesses a child's abilities compared to an established criterion standard and provides information about the child's performance that is independent of the performance or abilities of other children.[2] Criterion-referenced measures can be used to measure change over time. The Gross Motor Function Measure (GMFM)[9] is an example of an evaluative measure as it was originally designed to detect change in gross motor function over time for children with cerebral palsy. By monitoring change over time, therapists can assess the effectiveness of interventions and monitor the development of the child.

Case 1

Predictive Assessment Example

Alexander is a 5-month-old infant (corrected age, 3 months) who is referred for a physical therapy examination in a local neonatal intensive care unit (NICU) follow-up clinic. Alexander was born at 30 weeks' gestational age, after his mother went into preterm labor, and spent 9 weeks in the NICU. After birth, Alexander was diagnosed with grade 3 intraventricular hemorrhage and received supplemental oxygen. The physical therapist decided to complete the Test of Infant Motor Performance (TIMP) to assess whether Alexander was at high risk for developmental delay. The TIMP is a measure of functional motor ability of newborns and infants from 32 weeks' gestational age up to 4 months of age and includes 28 observed items and 31 elicited items.[3] Research has supported use of the TIMP to predict motor development at 12 months and at preschool age from infant tests at 90 days after term age.[6,8] Alexander's TIMP z-score was −0.6 standard deviations (SDs) below the mean. Based on this result, the therapist predicts that Alexander is likely to demonstrate delays at both 12 months, as measured by scores below the 10th percentile on the Alberta Infant Motor Scales, and at preschool age, as measured by scores less than −2 SDs below the mean on the PDMS-2. These findings suggest that intervention should be initiated to attempt to reduce or prevent these future motor delays.

AGE AND DIAGNOSIS

In addition to the categorization of the test, characteristics of the child being assessed, such as age or diagnosis, may guide the therapist's selection of a measure. Individual measures are frequently designed for use with a defined age group. For example, the Peabody Developmental Motor Scales-2 (PDMS-2)[10] assesses gross and fine motor development for children from birth through age 5 years, whereas the Bruininks-Oseretsky Test of Motor Proficiency, Second Edition (BOT-2)[11] assesses similar domains for children ages 4 through 21 years. Recognizing the intended age range of a measure is important as assessment tools are designed for and validated with children in the identified age range. If the measure is norm-referenced, reference values will not be available for comparison for a child outside of the intended age range, and interpretation of the assessment tool results will not be possible. In addition, use of an assessment tool for children outside of this range may increase the risk of floor or ceiling effects or may make interpretation of the information attained from the measure difficult. Floor effects occur when the items on the measure are too difficult for the child and may occur if a child is too young or lacks the abilities of the intended age range of a measure. Ceiling effects occur when the items on the measure are too easy for the child, resulting in a top score, and may occur if the child is too old or too advanced in skills for the intended measure. Both floor and ceiling effects make the assessment of a child's true abilities more challenging for the therapist.

Measures may also be validated for use with children with specific diagnoses. The GMFM,[9] for example, was initially designed for use with children with cerebral palsy[12] and has subsequently been validated for use with children with Down syndrome,[13] traumatic brain injury,[14] and spinal muscular atrophy.[15] While it is still possible to use the GMFM with children with other diagnoses, therapists should consider that the validity of the measure has not been fully investigated for all diagnoses and results should be interpreted with caution. Therapists must, therefore, determine if the personal characteristics of the child they are assessing are similar enough to the children assessed during validity testing of the measure to have confidence that the measure will appropriately assess the child's abilities.

INTERNATIONAL CLASSIFICATION OF FUNCTIONING, DISABILITY, AND HEALTH

The International Classification of Functioning, Disability, and Health (ICF) is a classification of health and disability and includes dimensions of body function and structure, activity, participation, and contextual factors.[16] The dimension of the ICF the therapist is interested in assessing for a child should be matched to the purpose of the measure to inform assessment selection. Measures are available to assess each dimension of the ICF. **Table 3-1** outlines common assessment tools across the ICF.

Assessment tools may be designed to examine potential impairments of body function and/or structure. Examples of impairment-focused measures include the Pediatric Balance Scale (PBS),[17] the Functional Strength Assessment (FSA),[18] and the Spinal Alignment and Range of Motion Measure (SAROMM).[19] These assessment tools specifically focus on a single body function and provide the therapist with information on impairments that can be monitored over time.

Activity level assessment tools are common in pediatric physical therapy practice and often assess gross motor and/or fine motor functional skills. Examples of activity measures include the previously mentioned GMFM,[9] PDMS-2,[10] and BOT-2.[11] These assessments focus on specific activity level skills as defined by the purpose of the measure. It is important to note, however, that activity level assessments may be norm-referenced and/or criterion-referenced, and consideration of this characteristic is needed when determining which activity level assessment is most appropriate for a given situation.

TABLE 3-1 • Assessment Measures by ICF

Measure	Purpose	Age Range
Participation		
Assessment of Life Habits (LIFE-H)*[42]	To assess the quality of daily activities and social participation of individuals with disabilities	All ages
Canadian Occupational Performance Measure (COPM)*[43]	To detect change in an individual's perception of occupational performance over time	All ages
Children's Assessment of Participation and Enjoyment (CAPE)[20]	To assess how children participate in activities outside of the school environment	6-21 years
Participation and Environment Measure–Children and Youth (PEM-CY)[21]	To examine participation in home, school, and community, including environmental factors for children and youth	5-17 years
School Function Assessment (SFA)*[22]	To assess a student's participation and function within the educational environment	Grades K-6
Activity		
Gross Motor		
Alberta Infant Motor Scales (AIMS)[44]	To identify infants and toddlers with gross motor delay and to evaluate gross motor skill maturation over time	Birth-18 months
Gross Motor Function Measure (GMFM)[9]	To evaluate change in gross motor function in children with cerebral palsy; also validated for children with Down syndrome	5 months-16 years
Test of Gross Motor Development, Third Edition (TGMD-3)[45]	To identify children who have delays in gross motor skills	3-11 years
Test of Infant Motor Performance (TIMP)[5]	To identify infants with risk of poor motor outcome	Premature infants 34 weeks postconceptual age to 4 months
Fine Motor		
Assisting Hand Assessment[46]	To assess how children collaboratively use affected and nonaffected hands in bimanual performance	18 months-12 years
Shriner's Upper Extremity Assessment[47]	To assess upper extremity function in children with hemiplegic cerebral palsy	3-18 years
Melbourne Unilateral Upper Limb Function (MUUL)[48]	To measure the quality of unilateral upper limb movement in children with neurologic conditions	5-15 years
Developmental Screening Tools		
Ages and Stages Questionnaires (ASQ-3)[49]	To assess communication, fine and gross motor, problem solving, and social-emotional skills in young children	1 month-5.5 years
Assessment, Evaluation, and Programming System for Infants and Children (AEPS)–Second Edition[50]	To assess fine motor, gross motor, cognitive, adaptive, social-communication, and social skills in young children	Birth-3 years and 3-6 years
Bayley Infant Neurodevelopmental Screener (BINS)[51]	To assess basic neurologic functions; gross motor, fine motor, oral motor, and verbal skills; receptive functions; and cognitive processes	3-24 months
Hawaii Early Learning Profile (HELP-Strands)[52]	To assess cognitive, language, gross motor, fine motor, social-emotional, and self-help skills	Birth-36 months and 3-6 years
Multiple Domain Assessments		
Activities Scale for Kids (ASK)[53]	To assess personal care, dressing, other skills, locomotion, play, standing skills, and transfers for children with disabilities	5-15 years
Battelle Developmental Inventory, Second Edition (BDI-2)[54]	To assess developmental skills of infants and young children	Birth-8 years
Bayley Scales of Infant Development-4[31]	To identify developmental delay in multiple domains of development	1-42 months

(Continued)

TABLE 3-1 • Assessment Measures by ICF (*Continued*)

Measure	Purpose	Age Range
Brigance Inventory of Early Development, III Edition[55]	To evaluate and monitor progress of perambulatory, gross motor and fine motor skills, prespeech, speech and language, general knowledge, readiness, basic reading, manuscript writing, and basic math skills	Birth-7 years
Bruininks-Oseretsky Test of Motor Proficiency (BOTP-2)[11]	To assess higher-level gross and fine motor skills	4-21 years
Developmental Assessment of Young Children–Second Edition (DAYC-2)[56]	To identify potential developmental delay in cognition, communication, social-emotional development, physical development, and adaptive behavior	Birth-5 years
Functional Independence Measure for Children (WeeFIM)[57]	To measure changes in function over time	6 months-7 years
Harris Infant Motor Test (HINT)[58]	To screen for low- and high-risk infants to categorize infant's level of motor delay	2.5-12.5 months
Merrill-Palmer Scale, Revised[59]	To identify developmental delays and evaluate progress with intervention	1-78 months
Miller Assessment of Preschoolers[60]	To evaluate sensory and motor abilities, cognitive abilities, and combined abilities of preschool-aged children	2 years 9 months-5 years 8 months
Movement Assessment Battery for Children (Movement ABC-2)[61]	To identify impairments in motor function of children with milder movement disorders	3-16 years
Peabody Developmental Motor Scales Second Edition (PDMS-2)[10]	To assess gross motor and/or fine motor skills of young children	1-72 months
Pediatric Evaluation of Disability Inventory (PEDI)[34]	To identify functional delay and examine improvement with intervention	Birth-20 years
Toddler and Infant Motor Evaluation (TIME)[62]	To assess gross and fine motor skills and evaluate motor development over time	4 months-3.5 years
Vineland Adaptive Behavior Scales–Second Edition[63]	To assist in identifying intellectual and developmental disabilities	Birth-90 years
Body Function and Structure		
Coordination		
Selective Control Assessment of the Lower Extremity (SCALE)[64]	To quantify selective voluntary motor control of the lower extremities of children with cerebral palsy	Children
Selective Control Assessment of the Upper Extremity (SCAUE)[65]	To quantify selective voluntary motor control of the upper extremity in children with hemiplegic cerebral palsy	Children
Endurance/Energy		
Early Activity Scale for Endurance (EASE)[35]	To measure endurance for physical activity in young children with cerebral palsy	18 months-12 years
6-Minute Push Test[66]	To assess capacity to self-propel a wheelchair	Any age
6-Minute Walk Test[27]	To assess functional walking capacity	Any age
Standardized Walking Obstacle Course[67]	To determine walking capacity including stability and speed under different conditions	>4 years
Pain		
CRIES Scale (Cries, Require Oxygen, Increased Vital Signs, Expression, Sleep)[68]	To measure postoperative pain	0-4 years
Faces Pain Scale[69]	To measure self-reported pain intensity	4-12 years
FLACC (Faces, Legs, Activity, Crying, Consolability Behavioral Pain Scale)[70]	To assess pain in young children	2 months-7 years

(Continued)

TABLE 3-1 • Assessment Measures by ICF (*Continued*)

Measure	Purpose	Age Range
Postural Control/Balance		
Early Clinical Assessment of Balance (ECAB)[33]	To assess postural control and balance in children with cerebral palsy	18 months-5 years
Movement Assessment of Infants (MAI)[71]	To assess motor development including muscle tone, primitive reflexes, automatic reactions, and volitional movements	Birth-18 months
Pediatric Balance Scale (PBS)[17]	To assess functional balance of children	4-15 years
Pediatric Clinical Test of Sensory Interaction for Balance (P-CTSIB)[72]	To assess the contribution of vestibular, somatosensory, and visual systems to balance	4-9 years
Pediatric Reach Test (Pediatric Functional Reach Test)[73]	To measure balance and postural control in sitting and standing through reaching	2.5-14 years
Segmental Assessment of Trunk Control (SATCO)[74]	To assess discrete levels of trunk control in children with motor and/or cognitive disabilities	Young children
Timed Up and Go–Pediatric[75]	To assess functional ambulatory mobility and monitor change over time	3-12 years
Range of Motion		
Spinal Alignment and Range of Motion Measure (SAROMM)[19]	To evaluate test of spinal alignment and range of motion in children with cerebral palsy	2-18 years
Sensory Processing		
Infant/Toddler Sensory Profile[76]	To assess sensory processing abilities and to profile the effect of sensory processing on functional performance in daily life	Birth-36 months
Sensory Profile-2[77]	To evaluate sensory processing patterns in the context of home, school, and community-based activities	Birth-12 years
Strength		
1-Stroke Push Test–Pediatric[66]	To measuring the distance a wheelchair travels with 1 stroke	6 and older
Functional Strength Assessment[18]	To estimate strength of major muscle groups	18 months-12 years
5-Repetitions Sit to Stand With Children[78]	To measure functional lower limb muscle strength	5-12 years
Environmental Factors		
Infant/Toddler Environment Rating Scale (ITERS-R)[23]	To assess the environment and teacher-child interactions in the school environment	Birth-30 months
Early Childhood Environmental Rating Scales–Third Edition (ECERS-3)[24]	To assess the environment and teacher-child interactions in the school environment	3-5 years
Home Observation for Measurement of the Environment (HOME)[25]	To assess the quality of the home environment including the physical environment and interactions with caregivers	Infant/Toddler: Birth-3 months
Early Childhood: 3-6 years
Middle Childhood: 6-10 years
Personal Factors		
The Revised Dimensions of Mastery Questionnaire[26]	To assess parent perception of a child's persistence and response when presented with a challenge	6 months-5 years
Kidscreen[79]	To assess subjective health and well-being	8-18 years
Pediatric Quality of Life Inventory 4.0 (PEDS QL)[80]	To assess health-related quality of life	2-18 years
Child Health Questionnaire (CHQ)[81]	To measure health-related quality of life	5-18 years

*Measure contain items that assess both participation- and activity-level abilities.

Case 2

Assessing Change Over Time

Sophia is a 3-year-old girl with cerebral palsy classified as Gross Motor Function Classification System (GMFCS) level III. Her therapist is interested in tracking her progress with intervention over time. The therapist completes the GMFM, an activity level assessment of gross motor skills designed for use with children with cerebral palsy.[13] The therapist completed the GMFM at her initial assessment (total score, 41%) and then completed the same measure 1 year later (total score, 45%). The therapist then uses published reference percentiles to determine how this change in motor skills compares to peers with cerebral palsy in GMFCS level III.[41] In this instance, the therapist determines that the child's gross motor skills as measured by the GMFM are progressing below what is expected. This may indicate that the child's plan of care may need to be modified to prevent Sophia from falling further behind her motor skill potential.

Measures of participation aim to assess a child's involvement in life situations in their home, school, and/or community environments. Examples of participation measures include the Children's Assessment of Participation and Enjoyment (CAPE),[20] the Participation and Environment Measure–Children and Youth (PEM-CY),[21] and portions of the School Function Assessment (SFA).[22] The CAPE is a questionnaire designed to assess 5 dimensions of participation of children and youth 6 to 21 years of age in everyday life outside of the school environment.[20] The PEM-CY assesses participation of children 5 to 17 years of age in the home, school, and community settings, as well as environmental factors that may impact participation in each setting.[21] The SFA assesses participation of children in the school setting for children 6 to 12 years of age and includes participation, task supports, and activity performance components.[22] These participation level measures provide important information on how the child engages in everyday life in particular settings, which may help to guide appropriate measure selection.

In addition to the 3 main domains of the ICF, therapists may also be interested in assessing contextual factors, the environmental and/or personal factors that may impact clinical decision-making and intervention effectiveness. Environmental factors include the physical, social, and attitudinal environment in which children live and may influence activity and participation. Often therapists use observation of environments to identify the existing environmental facilitators or barriers; however, environmental assessment measures are available for clinical use. Examples of measures of the environment include the Infant/Toddler Environment Rating Scale (ITERS-R),[23] the Early Childhood Environmental Rating Scales–Third Edition (ECERS-3),[24] and the Home Observation for Measurement of the Environment (HOME),[25] which has both infant/toddler and early childhood measures. The ITERS-R and the ECERS-3 assess the environment and teacher-child interactions in the school environment for infants/toddlers and young children, respectively, with categories such as space and furnishings, personal care routines, language and literacy, learning activities, interaction, and program structure.[23,24] The HOME inventory assesses the quality of the home environment including the physical environment and interactions with caregivers. Multiple versions of the HOME are available depending on the age of the child and include the Infant/Toddler, Early Childhood, and Middle Childhood versions.[25]

Personal factors are aspects of an individual that may have an influence on functioning such as gender, age, race, motivation, interests, or self-determination. Assessment tools that focus on personal factors are less available as these factors include significant variability, and clarity as to the role these factors play in development and function is lacking.[16] Personal factors may play a larger role in helping to select appropriate measures for the therapist to complete. The Revised Dimensions of Mastery Questionnaire (DMQ 18)[26] is an example of a personal factor assessment that examines parent perceptions of a young child's persistence and response when presented with a challenge. By selecting an assessment tool designed to measure a specific ICF domain, the therapist can obtain a more accurate understanding of domain of interest.

CAPACITY, CAPABILITY, AND PERFORMANCE

Therapists must also determine if they are interested in assessing a child's capacity (what the child does in a standardized, controlled environment), capability (what the child can do in their daily environment), or performance (what the child actually does in their daily environment). Capacity, capability, and performance may vary due to personal or other contextual factors. Recognizing this testing characteristic is needed to ensure the therapist is capturing the relevant information of interest. For example, the 6-minute walk test[27] is a self-paced, submaximal walking test, where the distance walked in 6 minutes is measured. This test is frequently used to assess endurance and functional walking capacity. Results from this test, therefore, reflect what the child does under controlled conditions as opposed to what the child actually does in daily life. If this daily activity information is needed, a different test would need to be selected.

GOAL ATTAINMENT SCALING

In some instances, measures to assess an intended area of interest are not available or are not specific enough to meet the needs of the therapist or to capture small changes over time. In these instances, the therapist may consider the use of goal attainment scaling (GAS).[28,29] GAS is an individualized, criterion-referenced measure where behavioral objectives are created for the child at baseline, and ordinal levels of the expected outcome are then determined. Typically, GAS values are assigned to the behavioral objectives or goals as follows:

Value	Predicted Outcome
+2	Much greater than expected outcome
+1	Greater than expected outcome
0	Expected outcome
−1	Less than expected outcome
−2	Much less than expected outcome

After intervention, progress on the GAS can be assessed by calculating the change in the GAS scores. GAS behavioral objectives can be created for all levels of the ICF and are intended to be individualized for a particular child, which allows for broad applicability in clinical practice.

PSYCHOMETRIC PROPERTIES OF ASSESSMENT TOOLS

When selecting an assessment tool, pediatric physical therapists are encouraged to review the measure's reliability, validity, and responsiveness, frequently reported in the assessment manual. *Reliability* refers to the consistency or repeatability of a measure. The intrarater, interrater, and test-retest reliability of a measure each provides information on how consistent scores from an assessment are likely to be. Intrarater reliability refers to the consistency of the results of a measure when it is repeated by the same examiner, whereas interrater reliability refers to the consistency between examiners. Test-retest reliability is a measure of the repeatability of a tool, or the ability of the tool to provide a similar result on repeated testing. Reliability is generally reported by a correlation coefficient ranging from 0 to 1. Portney[30] identifies the need for measures to demonstrate "acceptable" reliability focusing on defining acceptable based on the purpose of the assessment. The following criteria to interpret reliability are proposed:

- 0.00 to 0.50   "poor reliability"
- 0.50 to 0.75   "moderate reliability"
- 0.75 to 0.90   "good reliability"
- 0.90 to 1.00   "excellent reliability"[30]

Therapists are encouraged to select measures that demonstrate good to excellent reliability to help ensure the results obtained on a measure are accurate and consistent.

Validity of an assessment tool refers to how accurately the assessment measures what it is intended to measure. There are several types of validity that can be considered when determining the acceptability of an assessment tool. These types of validity are defined in **Table 3-2**. Therapists should select measures that have been reported to be valid for the construct and the population of interest to ensure accuracy and relevance of assessment results. In addition, attention should be paid to the time frames reported for valid data collection.

OTHER CONSIDERATIONS

Other considerations for selection of an assessment tool may include cost, specialized equipment requirements, or training requirements. Although some pediatric measures are available free of charge, many assessment tools require the purchase of a manual, score forms, and/or specialized equipment. These components of measures can be quite costly, at times over $1000 per assessment. Lack of resources to purchase these measures can limit the clinical feasibility of their use. Conscientious selection of measures that are most applicable to a therapist's current practice and consideration of high-quality tools that are freely available can help to limit the required expense.

Standardized assessments also require training to ensure reliable and accurate data collection. Adequate training in

TABLE 3-2 • Types of Validity

Type of Validity	Definition
Construct validity	The degree to which a test measures what it claims to measure
Convergent validity	The degree to which 2 measures of constructs that should be related are actually related
Divergent validity	The degree to which 2 measures of constructs that should not be related do not have any relationship
Content validity	The degree to which a measure represents all aspects of a given construct
Face validity	The degree to which a measure is viewed as covering the concept it claims to measure
Criterion validity	The degree to which a measure is related to an outcome
Concurrent validity	The degree to which the results of a particular measure correspond to results of a previously established measurement for the same construct
Predictive validity	The degree to which a score on a measure predicts scores on a criterion measure

measure administration is important to ensure efficient and accurate data collection for assessment and intervention planning. Some assessment publishers provide specific training modules therapists can complete to gain competence in administration. For example, the Bayley-4[3] offers independent study training programs, on-site workshops, and prerecorded webinars.[31] In addition, therapists should complete a careful review of the administration manuals and practice administration of test items prior to completing an assessment with a child. The information on the GMFM[9] recommends spending a minimum of 3 hours reviewing the administration manual and an additional 3 hours of practice with the training modules.[32] Therapists can also partner with other therapists to practice test administration, comparing results to establish interrater reliability to ensure they are appropriately and accurately completing assessments. Training may also be required to ensure an understanding of accurate measure interpretation so therapists can appropriately interpret and use the information gained from assessments. Information on appropriate measure interpretation is typically located within the assessment manuals.

Therapists must also consider that developmental delays in one domain of testing may have unintended impacts on the performance of skills and scoring in other domains. For example, consider a child who presents with decreased postural control and delayed gross motor skill acquisition but who can perform age-appropriate fine motor activities. If the child is not well positioned or supported during testing of fine motor activities, the child's score may incorrectly indicate delayed fine motor development as a reflection of the decreased postural control. Careful attention to the child as a whole, and not only to the skill or activity of interest, may help to ensure more accurate and appropriate scoring of assessment tools.

■ ADMINISTRATION OF ASSESSMENT TOOLS

Review of the directions or item administration manual is important prior to completing an assessment tool. These directions will specify the "rules" or requirements of testing such as the number of trials to allow for an individual item, the verbal or visual directions to provide to the child, the specific equipment to use, and the criteria for scoring. For example, the Early Clinical Assessment of Balance (ECAB)[33] allows for 3 trials of each balance item with use of the best attempt for item scoring. The BOT-2 provides specific verbal instructions with large images of each item provided in an item administration easel to provide visual cuing to assist the child in completing the item. As assessment tools are validated following these standardized instructions, it is important to incorporate these guidelines into item administration to ensure validity of the results. Therapists should also determine if the assessment tool allows for parent report for items that are not able to be observed due to lack of appropriate equipment or lack of cooperation from the child. When appropriate, parent report can support greater, more efficient completion of assessment tools.

With clinical experience, therapists often develop various clinical "shortcuts" to improve the efficiency of testing, such as changing the order of item administration to group similar items together. For example, the PDMS-2 has several items that examine the child's ability to stand on one foot with increasing time and stability requirements as the items increase in difficulty. Experienced clinicians may anticipate these increasing requirements and ask the child to maintain the position for as long as possible to score multiple items at once. Additionally, therapists may elect to alter the order of items to begin with items that are generally more tolerated by the child so that the child can gain a level of comfort with the examiner prior to attempting more challenging or more "hands-on" items. For example, therapists may begin with the stationary and locomotor sections of the PDMS-2 and then move to the reflexes section, which includes more direct handling and challenging of protective responses. Finally, if therapists are administering both fine motor and gross motor sections of a measure, it is recommended to start with the fine motor items, as typically the child is seated, prior to moving to more active items like balls skills and gross motor balance and mobility items.

Other strategies that may evolve with clinical experience include the use of observation and preparatory planning. Therapists can observe the child prior to testing to determine assessment tool entry points (the item with which to begin testing) or to score items that are directly observed prior to testing. This observation may help to decrease the number of items that need to be scored directly. Familiarity with the assessment tool also allows the therapist to prepare the space and equipment appropriately to improve the speed and efficiency of item administration and to minimize the need for delays to reset the environment between items.

Coordination with parents and caregivers is vital and is best practiced in family-centered care. Therapists should discuss assessment plans and select appropriate assessment tools based on family concerns and preferences. Assessment tools may include parent report measures to provide direct family input into the assessment process. For example, the Pediatric Evaluation of Disability Inventory (PEDI)[34] may be completed by parent report or by direct observation and includes questions related to the level of caregiver assistance required by the child to complete various activities that may require parental input. Additionally, other assessment tools are fully completed by the parent, such as the Early Activity Scale for Endurance (EASE).[35] The EASE includes 4 questions related to perception of the child's endurance for activity and is intended to be completed by the caregiver. These parent report measures can provide important detail regarding the child's abilities and performance of daily activities that may not be fully captured in a standard, 1-session examination. When possible, it may be helpful to have the family complete these parent report assessments prior to the session to allow the therapist to review the responses with the parents and request any clarifying information. By collaborating with the family, therapists can ensure the family's questions and concerns are addressed and the results of the assessment will provide the needed information for program planning.

■ INTERPRETATION OF ASSESSMENT TOOLS

Norm-referenced tests provide important information that allows comparison of a child's scores to normative values of peers, which is generally a large sample of typically developing children within the age range for which the test is intended. This normative sample should result in scores that follow a bell-shaped curve. Results from norm-referenced tests include raw scores, age equivalents, percentile ranks, developmental quotients, and/or z-scores. Raw scores are the total score or total number of points achieved on a measure or particular section of the measure. Age equivalents represent the mean or median measure score of the normative sample for a given age group. For example, an age equivalent of 4:4 (years:months) would be interpreted to mean the raw score achieved on the measure was equivalent to the average score achieved by children aged 4 years, 4 months in the normative sample. However, use of age equivalents to describe a child's abilities should be considered with caution due to limitations associated with this value. Because age equivalents represent the mean or median score, it can be expected that half of children completing the measure would receive a higher score than their age equivalent and half would receive a lower score.[36] This may lead to a false standard of performances that does not reflect the typical range of performance at a given age.[37] Therapists should, therefore, use care when interpreting age equivalent values and using these values to describe or quantify a child's abilities. Percentile ranks correspond to the percentage of scores in the normative distribution that are equal to or lower than this score. For example, if a child's raw score is calculated to be in the 25th percentile on a particular norm-referenced assessment, this would indicate that the child's score on this assessment is higher than 25% of the normative sample of the measure.

Developmental quotients are a statistic that indicate where the score of an individual child lies in relation to the normative sample mean. They are calculated by taking raw scores and putting them onto a consistent scale with the same standard deviation to allow for comparison to the normative sample. The average or middle distribution developmental quotient on a normative measure would be 100, with 1 standard deviation of scores falling between the developmental quotients of 85 and 115 (68% of the normative sample would have a quotient that falls between 85 and 115). Z-scores represent the number of standard deviations above or below the population mean a particular score falls. For example, a z-score of −1.5 would indicate that a child's score falls 1.5 standard deviations below the population mean on the measure, whereas a z-score of 0.8 would indicate that a child's score falls 0.8 standard deviations above the population mean. Generally, z-scores that fall within −1 to +1 are considered to fall within the typical range of development, as this would represent 1 standard deviation above and below the mean (68% of the normative sample would fall in this range). Based on these results, norm-referenced tests are intended to establish a child's developmental level and are typically used to determine eligibility for services. They should not be used to track progress over time because as children get older, the expectations for skill performance would also be expected to increase, and skill improvement may not be well-reflected in the assessment results.

Case 3

Interpretation of Norm-Referenced Scores

Dimension	Raw Score	Percentile Rank	Age Equivalent	Quotient	Z-Score
Stationary	28	2	7 months		
Locomotor	48	<1	9 months		
Object manipulation	2	5	12 months		
Total		<1		59	−2.73

Interpretation: The child scored 28 points on the stationary section, 48 points on the locomotor section, and 2 points on the object manipulation section of the PDMS-2. The child demonstrates skills better than 2% of same-age peers in stationary skills, less than 1% of same-age peers in locomotor skills, and 5% of same-age peers in object manipulation skills. Overall, this child's gross motor skills are better than less than 1% of same-age peers. The child demonstrates stationary skills similar to the average score of children at 7 months of age; locomotor skills similar to the average score of children 9 months of age; and object manipulation skills similar to the average score of children 12 months of age. The child's developmental quotient of 59 suggests the child's scores are below the average range. A z-score of −2.73 indicates this child presents with a significant developmental delay.

Criterion-referenced tests generally provide raw scores and percentages that can be used to evaluate change over time.

Again, the raw scores reflect the total score attained on the measure. Percentages, not to be confused with percentile rank, represent the percentage of items or points achieved divided by the total possible items or points multiplied by 100. For example, if a child achieves a raw score of 18 points out of a total possible 50 points, the child's percentage would be (18/50) × 100 = 36%. Repeat testing of the measure at a later point in time would allow the therapist to compare results to established reference percentiles to determine if progress has been made on the measure.

In determining how frequently a criterion-referenced measure should be completed, the responsiveness of a measure should be considered. Responsiveness is the ability of a measure to detect change when change has occurred. Responsiveness is often improved when measures are used in younger children and if sufficient time has passed between assessments so that this child has the opportunity to make progress. For example, Vos-Vromans and colleagues[38] noted that both the GMFM and the PEDI are responsive to changes in motor skills over 6 months of intervention and were most responsive for children younger than 4 years of age. Completing measures too frequently may limit the responsiveness of the measure.

Other statistics related to criterion-referenced measures may include minimal detectable change and/or minimal clinically important difference. The minimal detectable change is considered the smallest amount of change that can be detected by a measure beyond measurement error. The minimal detectable change on the PBS has been reported as 1.59.[39] Changes in scores smaller than 1.59 cannot be considered true change and may instead represent measurement error. Minimal clinically important change is defined as the smallest change in the score of a measure that is considered meaningful for patients. These values can provide additional context for the therapist in interpreting scores. For example, Iyer and colleagues[40] report that the minimal clinically important difference on the PEDI is approximately 11 points. This means that from initial to repeat administration, the child's overall PEDI score would need to improve by approximately 11 points for a noticeable difference in functional skills or caregiver assistance to be noted in daily life.

■ CONCLUSION

Assessment tools are an important resource from pediatric physical therapists to document a child's current developmental status, determine eligibility for services, determine prognosis of future delay or impairment, or measure progress over time. Careful consideration of the characteristics of assessment tools and the desired context of assessment facilitate the appropriate selection of assessment tools. Appropriate preparation and administration of measures can produce valuable information to guide services. Therapists are encouraged to understand how to accurately interpret information gained from assessment tools to ensure valid description of the assessment results.

Case 4

Case for Discussion

Donnell is 5-year-old child who presents to physical therapy with concerns about his gross motor skill development. His parents report he academically performs at grade level in school; however, he has difficulty keeping up with his peers during motor play. They describe him as "clumsy and uncoordinated." His teacher has reported concerns with his handwriting skills and controlled manipulation of objects in the classroom. The therapist reviews this information to determine the most appropriate assessment tool to use during the initial evaluation.

For discussion: Identify the potential assessment tools, including benefits and limitations of each tool.

Example answers: Movement ABC-2; Bruininks-Oseretsky Test of Motor Proficiency-2; Peabody Developmental Motor Scales-2; others.

STUDY QUESTIONS

1. Compare and contrast the use of norm-referenced and criterion-referenced measures.

2. Describe specific preparation strategies a therapist could use to facilitate success with standardized testing.

3. Interpret the following scores obtained from a standardized, norm-referenced test for a child aged 3 years and 5 months.
   a. Age equivalent: 36 months
   b. Percentile rank: 30th
   c. Z-score: −0.53

4. A standardized measure reports values for intrarater (intraclass correlation coefficient [ICC] = 0.92) and interrater (ICC = 0.65) reliability. How would the therapist interpret these results for use in clinic?

References

1. Kirshner B, Guyatt G. A methodological framework for assessing health indices. *J Chronic Dis.* 1985;38(1):27-36.

2. Glaser R. Instructional technology and the measurement of learning outcomes: some questions. *Am Psychol.* 1963;18(8):519-521.

3. Bayley N, Aylward G. *Bayley Scales of Infant and Toddler Development.* 4th ed. Pearson; 2019.

4. Aylward GP. Developmental Screening and assessment: what are we thinking? *J Dev Behav Pediatr.* 2009;30(2):169-173.

5. Campbell S. *The Test of Infant Motor Performance. Test User's Manual Version 3.0 for the TIMP Version 5.* Infant Motor Performance Scales, LLC; 2012.

6. Campbell SK, Kolobe TH, Wright BD, Linacre JM. Validity of the Test of Infant Motor Performance for prediction of 6-, 9- and 12-month scores on the Alberta Infant Motor Scale. *Dev Med Child Neurol.* 2002;44(04):263.

7. Madayi A, Shi L, Zhu Y, et al. The Test of Infant Motor Performance (TIMP) in very low birth weight infants and outcome at two years of age. *J Perinatol.* 2021;41(10):2432-2441.

8. Kolobe TH, Bulanda M, Susman L. Predicting motor outcome at preschool age for infants tested at 7, 30, 60, and 90 days after term age using the test of infant motor performance. *Phys Ther.* 2004;84(12):1144-1156.

9. Russell DJ, Rosenbaum PL, Wright M, Avery LM. *Gross Motor Function Measure (GMFM-66 & GMFM-88) User's Manual.* Wiley; 2013.

10. Folio M, Folio R. *Peabody Developmental Motor Scales – Second Edition (PDMS-2): Examiner's Manual.* Pro-Ed; 2000.

11. Bruininks R, Bruininks B. *Bruininks-Oseretsky Test of Motor Proficiency.* 2nd ed. NCS Pearson; 2005.

12. Palisano RJ, Hanna SE, Rosenbaum PL, et al. Validation of a model of gross motor function for children with cerebral palsy. *Phys Ther.* 2000;80(10):974-985.

13. Russell D, Palisano R, Walter S, et al. Evaluating motor function in children with Down syndrome: validity of the GMFM. *Dev Med Child Neurol.* 1998;40(10):693-701.

14. Linder-Lucht M, Othmer V, Walther M, et al. Validation of the gross motor function measure for use in children and adolescents with traumatic brain injuries. *Pediatrics.* 2007;120(4):e880-e886.

15. Nelson L, Owens H, Hynan LS, Iannaccone ST, AmSMART Group. The gross motor function measure is a valid and sensitive outcome measure for spinal muscular atrophy. *Neuromuscul Disord.* 2006;16(6):374-380.

16. World Health Organization. *How to Use the ICF: A Practical Manual for Using the International Classification of Functioning, Disability and Health (ICF). Exposure Draft for Comment.* WHO; 2013.

17. Franjoine MR, Gunther JS, Taylor MJ. Pediatric Balance Scale: a modified version of the Berg Balance Scale for the school-age child with mild to moderate motor impairment: *Pediatr Phys Ther.* 2003;15(2):114-128.

18. Jeffries L, McCoy S, Bartlett D, Chiarello L, Palisano R, Fiss A. Functional strength assessment. Published online 2011. Accessed September 17, 2018. https://canchild.ca/system/tenon/assets/attachments/000/000/.../Muscle_Strength.pdf.

19. Bartlett D, Purdie B. Testing of the spinal alignment and range of motion measure: a discriminative measure of posture and flexibility for children with cerebral palsy. *Dev Med Child Neurol.* 2005;47(11):739.

20. King G, Law M, King S, et al. *Children's Assessment of Participation and Enjoyment (CAPE) and Preferences for Activities of Children (PAC).* Harcourt Assessment Inc; 2004.

21. Coster W, Law M, Bedell G, Khetani M, Cousins M, Teplicky R. Development of the participation and environment measure for children and youth: conceptual basis. *Disabil Rehabil.* 2012;34(3):238-246.

22. Coster W, Deeney T, Haltiwanger J, Haley S. *School Function Assessment.* Psychological Corporation/Therapy Skill Builders; 1998.

23. Harris T, Cryer D, Clifford R. *Infant/Toddler Environmental Rating Scale, Revised Edition, Updated (ITERS-R).* Teachers College Press; 2006.

24. Harris T, Clifford R, Cryer D. *Early Childhood Environmental Rating Scale, Third Edition, Updated (ECERS-3).* Teachers College Press; 2015.

25. Caldwell B, Bradley R. *Home Observation for Measurement of the Environment (HOME)-Revised Edition.* University of Arkansas; 1984.

26. Morgan G, Liao H, Nyitrai A, et al. The Revised Dimensions of Mastery Questionnaire (DMQ 18) for infants and preschool children with and without risks or delays in Hungary, Taiwan and the

US The Revised Dimensions of Mastery Questionnaire (DMQ 18) for infants and preschool children with and without risks or delays in Hungary, Taiwan and the US. *Hungarian Educ Res J.* 2017;(2):48-67.

27. ATS Committee on Proficiency Standards for Clinical Pulmonary Function Laboratories. ATS Statement: Guidelines for the Six-Minute Walk Test. *Am J Repir Crit Care Med.* 2002;166(1):111-117.

28. Kiresuk TJ, Smith A, Cardillo J. *Goal Attainment Scaling.* Psychology Press; 2014.

29. Steenbeek D, Gorter JW, Ketelaar M, Galama K, Lindeman E. Responsiveness of goal attainment scaling in comparison to two standardized measures in outcome evaluation of children with cerebral palsy. *Clin Rehabil.* 2011;25(12):1128-1139.

30. Portney LG. *Foundations of Clinical Research: Applications to Evidence-Based Practice.* 4th ed. F.A. Davis; 2020.

31. Bayley-4 Online Independent Study Training Program®. Published online 2020. Accessed October 18, 2023. https://www.pearsonassessments.com/content/dam/school/global/clinical/us/assets/bayley-4/bayley4-online-training.pdf.

32. CanChild GMFM Team. Gross motor function measure training video. Published online 2022. Accessed January 27, 2022. https://www.canchild.ca/en/shop/33-gross-motor-function-measure-training-video.

33. McCoy SW, Bartlett DJ, Yocum A, et al. Development and validity of the early clinical assessment of balance for young children with cerebral palsy. *Dev Neurorehabil.* 2014;17(6):375-383.

34. Haley S, Andrellos P, Coster W, Haltiwanger J, Ludlow L. *Paediatric Evaluation of Disability Inventory (PEDI): Development, Standardisation and Administration Manual.* New England Medical Centre Hospitals; 1992.

35. Westcott McCoy S, Yocum A, Bartlett DJ, et al. Development of the early activity scale for endurance for children with cerebral palsy. *Pediatr Phys Ther.* 2012;24(3):232-240.

36. Lawrence CW. Assessing the use of age-equivalent scores in clinical management. *Language Speech Hearing Serv Schools.* 1992;23(1):6.

37. Salvia J, Ysseldyke JE, Bolt S. *Assessment in Special and Inclusive Education.* 12th ed. Wadsworth/Cengage Learning; 2013.

38. Vos-Vromans DCWM, Ketelaar M, Gorter JW. Responsiveness of evaluative measures for children with cerebral palsy: the gross motor function measure and the pediatric evaluation of disability inventory. *Disabil Rehabil.* 2005;27(20):1245-1252.

39. Chen CL, Shen IH, Chen CY, Wu CY, Liu WY, Chung CY. Validity, responsiveness, minimal detectable change, and minimal clinically important change of Pediatric Balance Scale in children with cerebral palsy. *Res Dev Disabil.* 2013;34(3):916-922.

40. Iyer LV, Haley SM, Watkins MP, Dumas HM. Establishing minimal clinically important differences for scores on the pediatric evaluation of disability inventory for inpatient rehabilitation. *Phys Ther.* 2003;83(10):888-898.

41. Hanna SE, Bartlett DJ, Rivard LM, Russell DJ. Reference curves for the gross motor function measure: percentiles for clinical description and tracking over time among children with cerebral palsy. *Phys Ther.* 2008;88(5):596-607.

42. Fougeyrollas P, Noreau L, Bergeron H, Cloutier R, Dion SA, St-Michel G. Social consequences of long term impairments and disabilities: conceptual approach and assessment of handicap. *Int J Rehabil Res.* 1998;21(2):127-141.

43. Law M, Baptiste A, Carswell M, Polatajko H, Pollock N. *Canadian Occupational Performance Measure.* 5th ed. CAOT Publications ACE; 2014.

44. Piper M, Darrah J. *Motor Assessment of the Developing Infant.* WB Saunders; 1994.

45. Webster EK, Ulrich DA. Evaluation of the psychometric properties of the Test of Gross Motor Development—Third Edition. *J Motor Learning Dev.* 2017;5(1):45-58.

46. Krumlinde-Sundholm L, Holmefur M, Kottorp A, Eliasson AC. The Assisting Hand Assessment: current evidence of validity, reliability, and responsiveness to change. *Dev Med Child Neurol.* 2007;49(4):259-264.

47. Davids JR, Peace LC, Wagner LV, Gidewall MA, Blackhurst DW, Roberson WM. Validation of the Shriners Hospital for Children Upper Extremity Evaluation (SHUEE) for children with hemiplegic cerebral palsy. *J Bone Joint Surg.* 2006;88(2):326-333.

48. Randall M, Johnson L, Reddihough D. *The Melbourne Assessment of Unilateral Upper Limb Function: Test Administration Manual.* Melbourne Royal Children's Hospital; 1999.

49. Squires J, Bricker DD, Twombly E. *Ages & Stages Questionnaires: A Parent-Completed Child Monitoring System. 3.* 3rd ed. Paul H Brooks; 2009.

50. Bricker D. *Assessment, Evaluation, and Programming System for Infants and Children (AEPS®).* 2nd ed. Paul H Brooks; 2002.

51. Aylward GP. The Bayley Infant Neurodevelopmental Screener (BINS). In: *Bayley-III Clinical Use and Interpretation.* Elsevier; 2010:201-233.

52. Parks S, Celeste M. *Inside HELP: Administrative and Reference Manual for HELP (the Hawaii Early Learning Profile) Birth - 3 Years.* VORT Corp; 2006.

53. Young NL, Williams JI, Yoshida KK, Wright JG. Measurement properties of the activities scale for kids. *J Clin Epidemiol.* 2000;53(2):125-137.

54. Newborg J, Stock J, Wnek L, Guidubaldi J, Svinicki J. *Battelle Developmental Inventory- 2nd Edition.* Riverside Publishing; 2004.

55. Curriculum Associates, Hawker Brownlow Education. *Brigance: Inventory of Early Development III.* Hawker Brownlow Education; 2014.

56. Voress J, Maddox T. *DAYC-2: Developmental Assessment of Young Children.* 2nd ed. PRO-ED; 2013.

57. Msall ME, DiGaudio K, Rogers BT, et al. The Functional Independence Measure for Children (WeeFIM): conceptual basis and pilot use in children with developmental disabilities. *Clin Pediatr.* 1994;33(7):421-430.

58. Harris SR, Megens A, Backman C, Hayes V. Development and standardization of the Harris Infant Neuromotor Test. *Infants Young Children.* 2003;16(2):143-151.

59. Roid G, Sampers J. *Merrill-Palmer-Revised Scales of Development.* Stoelting Company; 2004.

60. Miller L. *The Miller Assessment for Preschoolers Manual (Rev. Ed.).* Psychological Corporation; 1988.

61. Henderson S, Sugden D, Barnett A. *Movement Assessment Battery for Children-2.* Harcourt Assessment; 2007.

62. Mailloux Z. Toddler Infant Motor Evaluation. In: Volkmar FR, ed. *Encyclopedia of Autism Spectrum Disorders.* Springer; 2013.

63. Sparrow S, Cicchetti D, Balla D. *Vineland Adaptive Behavior Scales.* 2nd ed. American Guidance Service; 2005.

64. Fowler EG, Staudt LA, Greenberg MB, Oppenheim WL. Selective Control Assessment of the Lower Extremity (SCALE): development, validation, and interrater reliability of a clinical tool for patients with cerebral palsy. *Dev Med Child Neurol.* 2009;51(8):607-614.

65. Wagner LV, Davids JR, Hardin JW. Selective Control of the Upper Extremity Scale: validation of a clinical assessment tool for

children with hemiplegic cerebral palsy. *Dev Med Child Neurol.* 2016;58(6):612-617.

66. Verschuren O, Ketelaar M, De Groot J, Vila Nova Fá, Takken T. Reproducibility of two functional field exercise tests for children with cerebral palsy who self-propel a manual wheelchair. *Dev Med Child Neurol.* 2013;55(2):185-190.

67. Held SL, Kott KM, Young BL. Standardized Walking Obstacle Course (SWOC): reliability and validity of a new functional measurement tool for children. *Pediatr Phys Ther.* 2006;18(1):23-30.

68. Krechel SW, Bildner J. CRIES: a new neonatal postoperative pain measurement score. Initial testing of validity and reliability. *Pediatr Anesth.* 1995;5(1):53-61.

69. Hicks CL, von Baeyer CL, Spafford PA, van Korlaar I, Goodenough B. The Faces Pain Scale-Revised: toward a common metric in pediatric pain measurement. *Pain.* 2001;93(2):173-183.

70. Merkel SI, Voepel-Lewis T, Shayevitz JR, Malviya S. The FLACC: a behavioral scale for scoring postoperative pain in young children. *Pediatr Nurs.* 1997;23(3):293-297.

71. Chandler L, Andrews M, Swanson MW, Larson A. *Movement Assessment of Infants: A Manual.* Rolling Bay; 1980.

72. Crowe TK, Deitz JC, Richardson PK, Atwater SW. Interrater reliability of the pediatric clinical test of sensory interaction for balance. *Phys Occup Ther Pediatr.* 1991;10(4):1-27.

73. Bartlett D, Birmingham T. Validity and reliability of a pediatric reach test. *Pediatr Phys Ther.* 2003;15(2):84-90.

74. Butler PB, Saavedra S, Sofranac M, Jarvis SE, Woollacott MH. Refinement, reliability, and validity of the segmental assessment of trunk control. *Pediatr Phys Ther.* 2010;22(3):246-257.

75. Williams EN, Carroll SG, Reddihough DS, Phillips BA, Galea MP. Investigation of the timed "up & go" test in children. *Dev Med Child Neurol.* 2005;47(8):518-524.

76. Dunn W, Daniels DB. Initial development of the infant/toddler sensory profile. *J Early Intervent.* 2002;25(1):27-41.

77. Dunn W. *Sensory Profile-2.* Pearson; 2014.

78. Wang TH, Liao HF, Peng YC. Reliability and validity of the five-repetition sit-to-stand test for children with cerebral palsy. *Clin Rehabil.* 2012;26(7):664-671.

79. The European KIDSCREEN Group, Ravens-Sieberer U, Erhart M, et al. Reliability, construct and criterion validity of the KIDSCREEN-10 score: a short measure for children and adolescents' well-being and health-related quality of life. *Qual Life Res.* 2010;19(10):1487-1500.

80. Varni JW, Seid M, Kurtin PS. PedsQL 4.0: reliability and validity of the Pediatric Quality of Life Inventory version 4.0 generic core scales in healthy and patient populations. *Med Care.* 2001;39(8):800-812.

81. Landgraf J, Abetz L, Ware J. *The CHQ User Manual.* The Health Institute, New England Medical Center; 1999.

Movement Systems in Pediatrics

Genevieve Pinto Zipp, PT, EdD, and Susan Simpkins, PT, EdD

LEARNING OBJECTIVE

Upon completion of this chapter, the reader will be able to:

- Describe how movement system diagnosis can decrease the unwanted variability in the management of patients with neuromuscular conditions.
- Explain how movement system diagnosis can minimize the trial-and-error approach to treatment selection.

- Describe how movement system diagnosis can improve communication with other health care professionals.
- Discuss how movement system diagnosis can advance research by enabling creation of homogenous patient groupings.
- Utilize a model for identifying movement system diagnoses in children with neuromuscular conditions.

■ INTRODUCTION

The *movement system* is defined as a collection of interacting systems that move the body or its component parts for purposeful movement (**Figure 4-1A**). The movement system focuses the identity of the physical therapy profession and is at the core of the 2013 American Physical Therapy Association (APTA) House of Delegates professional vision statement: "transforming society by optimizing movement to improve the human experience."* This is a strong vision and one that requires a dedicated effort by all stakeholders to fulfill. An important step in implementing the vision is for physical therapists to embrace their expertise as movement system specialists and leverage their knowledge and skills to optimize an individual's capacity for effective, efficient, and safe movement.

The human movement system represents a group of 6 body systems that function together to support purposeful movement (**Figure 4-1B**). When these individual systems are intact and functioning well, they work cooperatively to move and stabilize body segments, ensure adequate oxygenation and energy to sustain movement, and provide a protective barrier to guard the body against environmental elements. Although these systems serve many more functions than described here, each system provides a unique contribution to human movement. Consequently, each of these systems must be considered to understand why an individual is experiencing movement dysfunction.

Integrating the movement system into clinical practice means clinicians will apply their knowledge of this dynamic system to guide clinical decision-making. The process starts with the development of a comprehensive examination strategy that includes movement observation and analysis. The results of the examination provide the information needed to formulate a movement system diagnosis and prognosis, which include essential steps leading to a plan of care that will target the motor control problems interfering with a child's daily life.

Movement observation and analysis may not be a routine part of every clinician's physical therapy examination. In fact, analysis of movement is not currently included as part of the Patient Management Model from the *Guide to Physical Therapist Practice*. However, movement analysis will be a key element in formulating a movement system diagnosis. Movement analysis involves observing and describing the way a person carries out a task or activity. The information gained from movement analysis is more clinically relevant than a description of a patient's level of independence.[1] Developing a standardized approach to movement analysis and the terminology to describe movement dysfunction is important going forward so clinicians have the tools needed to incorporate this process into their practice. This chapter explores the movement system as a foundation for practice and how knowledge of the movement system can be applied to all aspects of patient management.

■ HISTORICAL PERSPECTIVE SURROUNDING THE MOVEMENT SYSTEM AND ITS VALUE IN HEALTH CARE

An interest in establishing the identity of the physical therapy profession is not new. Over 40 years ago, while delivering the 10th annual Mary McMillian lecture, Helen Hislop stated that we lacked a professional identity and should consider pathokinesiology as the science that anchors physical therapists' practice. While her words were inspiring, there was no meaningful discussion about whether pathokinesiology offered an identity

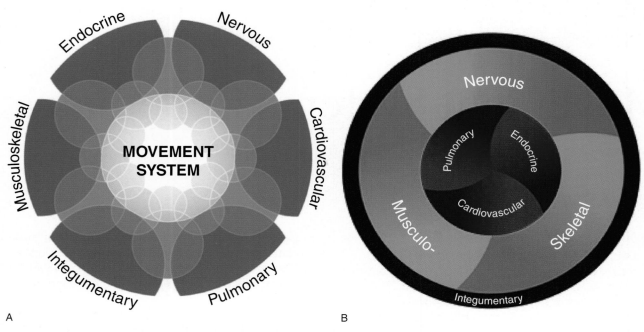

A   B

FIGURE 4-1 Two models depicting interaction of body systems comprising the movement system. **A.** Body systems comprising the movement interact to support movement. **B.** Body systems are nested. The integumentary system provides ongoing external protection as the neurologic and musculoskeletal systems generate movement with the physiological systems at the core to provide energy and oxygenation to support movement.

for the profession. Almost a decade later, the Symposium on Pathokinesiology: Theory, Research, and Practice was held at the 60th Annual Conference of the American Physical Therapy Association (1984) to explore the meaning of the term *pathokinesiology* and its implications as the science of physical therapy.[2] The APTA's House of Delegates did not adopt pathophysiology as our profession's identity; many believed that a focus on abnormal movement was not broad enough to encompass the scope of the profession.

In the early 1990s, a group of physical therapists from academic, research, and clinical backgrounds convened to discuss the movement system and whether movement science was the foundation for practice. The group agreed that both concepts should be developed and incorporated into physical therapist practice.[3] However, there was little movement toward attaining this goal. More than 10 years later, Barbara Norton, PT, PhD, FAPTA, invited a group of therapists to take part in a series of a meetings entitled the Diagnosis Dialogue.[4] The group achieved consensus on support for the movement system as a foundational concept, which extended to the development of movement system diagnoses.

Patricia Scheets, MHS, PT; Shirley Sahrmann, PT, PhD; and Barbara Norton, PT, PhD, published 2 articles that introduced several movement system diagnoses for adults with neuromuscular conditions. The first article was published in 1999, several years before the Diagnosis Dialogues. The diagnostic categories were based on the primary movement system impairments seen in patients with neuromuscular conditions.[5] Notably, each diagnosis was associated with a suggested approach to treatment targeting the specific problems interfering with a patient's purposeful movement. The original diagnostic categories were expanded and revised in 2007[6] and then again in 2014.[7] The diagnostic categories described in

2014 included information specific to children with neuromuscular conditions.

Discussion on the movement system and movement system diagnosis reached a tipping point in 2013 when the House of Delegates adopted a new vision statement that put the movement system front and center as the foundation for physical therapist practice and as the identity of the physical therapy profession. While Vision 2020 and its guiding principles may appear to mark the end of a 40-year journey to find our professional identity, there is still a considerable amount of work ahead to define the diagnostic process before the movement system and movement system diagnoses are integrated into clinical practice, education, and research.

■ INTEGRATION OF MOVEMENT SYSTEMS INTO THE INTERNATIONAL CLASSIFICATION OF FUNCTIONING, DISABILITY, AND HEALTH MODEL

The International Classification of Functioning, Disability, and Health (ICF) is a biopsychosocial model of health that provides a framework and common language for describing health and disability at the level of both individuals and populations.[8] The ICF focuses on how individuals with a health condition function in their everyday life, independent of diagnosis or disease. Function is defined across 3 domains: body structure and function, activity, and participation. Environmental factors such as accessibility are also classified and further defined as facilitators or barriers to function. Personal factors including age, gender, coping style, and social background are noted and serve as a reminder that individual characteristics influence a person's perception of their health condition. APTA endorsed the ICF in 2008 as the profession's model of health.

The 6 systems that form the movement system are listed within the body function and structure domain of the ICF, along with other body systems (**Table 4-1**). The domains of activity and participation include 9 areas of functioning. Given the complexity of the 9 areas of activity and participation, it seems unlikely that disability comes about due to the impairment of just one of the body systems. For example, *mobility* includes tasks such as changing positions, walking in different locations, and moving around using transportation. All of these tasks require mental function (attention, memory, problem solving), sensory function (vision, vestibular), cardiovascular function (blood supply, oxygen exchange), and neuromusculoskeletal function (muscle power, mobility of joints) at the very least. Thus, in many cases, disability is due to impairments in more than one body system. An important role of the physical therapist is to determine through examination how body system impairments affect activity and participation.

The ICF framework describes function, independent of diagnosis or disease. Similarly, a movement system diagnosis describes the problem that interferes with how an individual functions, independent of diagnosis or disease. This means that 2 children with the same diagnosis may experience their condition differently across ICF domains, have different movement system diagnoses, and engage in different types of treatment activities. This is certainly reflective of what we observed in clinical practice. Children with the same medical diagnosis often have very different clinical presentations, which is why the child's medical diagnosis is of limited value in program planning. A medical diagnosis provides the therapist with an expectation of the problems a child *may* have, but the physical therapy examination is what provides information about the child's actual problems and informs development of the plan of care.

The ICF model is well integrated into physical therapists' practice, education, and research. In clinical practice, the ICF can be used to develop an examination strategy to ensure inclusion of tests and measures from all domains. Then, the information gathered during the examination can be organized by domains and contextual factors (see Table 4-1). Once the examination findings are organized in this manner, they are evaluated, which includes weighting, prioritizing, and reorganizing the findings into clusters. From here, the practitioner formulates a hypothesis about the relationship between the child's movement system problems and movement dysfunction. The clinical reasoning process for forming a movement system diagnosis will be much the same as described here, but with the addition of information from clinical observation and movement analysis. Movement analysis allows the practitioner to observe how a child's impairments influence the movement strategies used to execute a functional activity. Watching the child execute different tasks provides information the practitioner needs to identify the specific problems interfering with function. The results of movement analysis and tests and measures considered collectively will aid in forming a movement system diagnosis.

TABLE 4-1 • ICF Domains

Function	Structure
Mental functions	Structure of the nervous system
Sensory functions and pain	The eye, ear, and related structures
Voice and speech functions	Structures involved in voice and speech
Functions of the cardiovascular, hematologic, immunologic, and respiratory systems	Structure of the cardiovascular, immunologic, and respiratory systems
Functions of the digestive, metabolic, and endocrine systems	Structures related to the digestive, metabolic, and endocrine systems
Genitourinary and reproductive functions	Structure related to genitourinary and reproductive systems
Neuromusculoskeletal and movement-related functions	Structure related to movement
Functions of the skin and related structures	Skin and related structures

Activities and Participation
Learning and applying knowledge
General tasks and demands
Communication
Mobility
Self-care
Domestic life
Interpersonal interactions and relationships
Major life areas
Community, social, and civic life

Environmental Factors
Products and technology
Natural environment and human-made changes to environment
Support and relationships
Attitudes
Services, systems, and policies

◼ MOVEMENT SYSTEM OVERVIEW SEEKING PATTERN RECOGNITION USING STANDARDIZED LANGUAGE

Physical therapists, as movement system specialists, design evidenced-based plans of care that effectively and efficiently guide everyone toward meeting their task-specific functional goals in real-world conditions. Before a plan of care is developed, it is imperative that the practitioner understands how the individual's movement problems reflect the interaction of the systems that support human movement, what Guccione et al[9] termed a "behavioral phenomenon in itself." Physical therapists as movement system practitioners have both the knowledge and skills to evaluate, diagnosis, and address how the individual's (learner) dynamic system interacts to solve movement problems given the environmental and task features that constrain the movement. Ongoing changes that emerge naturally across the individual's life span or as a result of injury or disease require continual reexamination and reassessment of the patient-centered, goal-directed plan of care by physical therapists. Using the dynamical systems theory as a framework, we can explore how the interdependent and constantly changing dynamic systems, which evolve over time, as well as the task and environment constraints, which regulate behavioral change, produce purposeful movements. As physical therapists, we acknowledge movement as the primary mediator of human performance regardless of setting or patient population.

The ability to establish a prognosis and predict intervention outcomes is key to creating effective plans of care and establishing the physical therapist's role as a movement specialist. How do physical therapists establish a patient's prognosis and predict outcomes based on interventions employed? One might argue that by seeking to employ a consistent method for establishing pattern recognition of movement system issues and using standardized language across all settings and populations, the profession can then move to a more systematic study of intervention outcomes and thus lead to and support predictions made by physical therapists. Using consistent and meaningful movement system diagnoses can promote clarity specific to what is being observed, communicated, and collaborated with the health care team and lead to the promotion of continuity of care. Establishing movement system diagnoses can enable the characterization of responders and nonresponders when evaluating movement-related intervention effectiveness either in the clinic or in the research environment and can aide in the development of clinical (intervention) prediction rules and ultimately guide clinical decision-making.

Several movement-related classification systems are present in the literature and offer insight to educators, students, and clinicians; however, to date, no specific movement system diagnosis classification system has been supported by APTA.

The Academy of Neurologic Physical Therapy Movement Systems Task Force[1] "recommends that movement system diagnoses for patients with primary neurologic involvement should:

1. be based on a sound, evidence-based theoretical framework,
2. emphasize movement observation and analysis of core standardized tasks as central to the clinical examination and evaluation,
3. represent a unique cluster of movement observations and associated examination findings that can impact a variety of tasks, and
4. provide unique and non-ambiguous labels for each movement system diagnosis."[1]

Acknowledging that no one movement-related classification available today meets all 4 characteristics, the Movement Systems Task Force has proposed a framework for the development of a meaningful movement system diagnosis that can aide physical therapists in their clinical reasoning and decision-making processes. Central to the framework proposed by the task force is a core set of tasks for movement observation regardless of practice setting, patient population, body part, or medical diagnosis. Although not explicitly suggested in the task force white paper, the use of functional tasks within a consistent environmental context supports the dynamical systems theory behavioral phenomenon perspective. The core tasks currently include sitting, standing, sit to stand, stand to sit, walking, step up, step down, reaching, grasping, and manipulating. The task force, recognizing the importance of standardized administration and assessment of these tasks, is working to establish a format for the systematic performance of these standardized core tests. Recognizing that tasks alone do not allow for the integration of all necessary information, the task force proposes infusing Herman's 6-stage movement continuum along with the critical movement-related parameters at each specific stage into the framework to reliably detect movement system problems across a range of tasks (**Figure 4-2**).

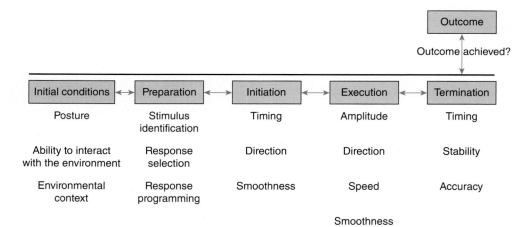

FIGURE 4-2 **Illustration of the sequence of the 5 stages of the Hedman et al temporal model for task analysis, including initial conditions, preparation, initiation, execution, and termination. Key features for each stage are listed.** (Reproduced with permission From Hedman L, Rogers M, and Hanke T. Neurologic Proffessional education: Linking the foundation science of Motor Control With Physical Therapy Interventions for Movement Dysfunction. *J Neurol Phys Ther.* 1996;20(1):9-13.)

To date, the reliability, validity, and clinical utility of the task force's proposed core standardized task framework is unknown. If future testing of the framework supports its reliability and validity, using this observational approach could potentially aide physical therapists' critical thinking skills and ability to hypothesize about how the patient's motor control is affected, why certain movement strategies are or are not employed, and what treatment interventions are best to employ to maximize patient outcomes.

Using both a big data–driven approach and an experience-driven approach will help to identify movement patterns of patient characteristics across different health conditions, inform clinical reasoning, aide in predicting responsiveness to rehabilitation intervention, and direct interventions and outcomes. Practicing physical therapists can assist in moving the discussion regarding movement system diagnoses forward by utilizing the existing 9 movement system diagnoses proposed by Scheets et al[10] and documenting across goal-directed tasks and the patient population's treatment outcomes. This experience-driven practice-based approach to exploring movement system diagnosis will assist in identifying movement system diagnoses that are meaningful, but it will only aide in predicting recovery and guiding treatment if we are diligent in exploring tasks that are functional goal directed and impacted by the learner and environmental constraints. Movement emerges from the interaction among the learner, task, and environmental constraints and thus must be explored in the same manner. Additionally, physical therapists must remember that the diagnostic process is dynamic in nature and must continue throughout treatment, as meaningful movement emerges based on the interaction of an individual's abilities and capabilities and the constraints of the environment at any given moment in time.

Given that movement analysis results from the synthesis of various movement observations, one must acknowledge that while standardized core task testing can support a consistent identification of motor control impairments, observing movement system problems within tasks relevant to the patient under real-world conditions is paramount. Newell discusses 3 types of constraints—organismic, task, and environment—that restrict the movement possibilities. However, through what has been termed a process of "self-organization" among the constraints, a movement resolution emerges into a resultant motor outcome. Based on specifically what the learner brings to the task demands and the environmental constraints, a solution to the movement problem emerges. The movement solution that emerges may or may not be the most ideal or optimal movement solution. Thus, the solution should be seen as the learner's attempt to self-organize the motor outcome with an acceptable degree of error and minimization of metabolic energy expenditure.[11] Finally, through "repetition without repetition" as Bernstein suggests, the self-organized movement evolves into a generalized behavior. Guccione et al[9] suggest "pursing criteria that emphasize the phenomena encompassed in human performance ... through a renewed focus on the interdependencies of the systems that comprise the human body rather than on the structural or physiological systems themselves as the basis for diagnosis by physical therapists."

In 2013, the APTA House of Delegates updated the vision for the profession of physical therapy as follows: to "transform society by optimizing movement to improve the human experience,"[12] with the movement system representing the collection of systems that interact to move the body; thus, physical therapists must explore insightfully how we use the term *movement system diagnoses*. The exploration of movement systems diagnosis must be conducted in the context of a dynamical systems theory where goal-directed movements focus on achieving the "function of the action" and are regulated by the learner, task, and environmental constraints present and observed by the learner. Using similarly recognized, consistent, uniform movement-related terms (movement system diagnosis terminology) to describe similar movements, regardless of pathology, during goal-directed movements, physical therapists can promote clinical reasoning and decision-making processes via promoting the 4 Cs of clarity, communication, collaboration, and continuity in patient-centered care.

The process of linking clusters of clinical presentations to a movement system diagnosis is emerging in the literature, but much work needs to be done. Using movement system diagnoses will enable the physical therapy profession to move further in exploring the efficacy of interventions by studying individuals who share the same cluster of signs and symptoms. This knowledge may promote the introduction of targeted preventive therapeutic interventions. Finally, the promotion of pattern recognition via the implementation of movement system diagnoses can assist in the development of more refined clinical practice guidelines and clinical prediction rules. In 2007, Scheets and colleagues[6] illustrated the use of movement system diagnoses in 3 individuals with a medical diagnosis of stroke (**Table 4-2**). Using impairment tests and movement analysis of functional tasks, Scheets et al[6] systematically observed unique clusters of impairments across the individuals, which resulted in the identification of the following 9 movement system diagnoses: movement pattern coordination deficit, force production deficit, sensory detection deficit, sensory selection and weighting deficit, postural vertical deficit (previously termed *perceptual deficit*), fractionated movement deficit, dysmetria (previously termed *hypermetria*), hypokinesia, and cognitive deficit.

Dysmetria is defined as the "inability to grade forces appropriately for the distance and speed aspects of a task."[7] Rapid movements are generally too large, and slow movements are generally too small. Performance deteriorates with faster speeds, and there is no change with practice. Undershooting or overshooting is present. Abnormal rhythm and incoordination are present during rapidly alternating movements. Wide base of support is present during ambulation and when moving from sit to stand. Repeated stepping when ambulating is observed, along with the potential for excessive swaying at the trunk. Upper extremities are used to stabilize. Dysmetria is generally associated with cerebellar dysfunction.

Force production deficit is defined primarily by weakness in movements. Weakness may be observed in tasks that require

TABLE 4-2 • Movement System Diagnoses

Movement System Diagnosis	Possible Effects on Gait
Movement pattern coordination deficit	Variable foot placement; slow, small steps; may need assistance
Force production deficit	May need assistive device or assistance; may have severe gait deviations such as crouched gait or knee buckling in mid-stance; may not be able to ambulate
Sensory detection deficit	Variable foot placement; may require assistance; gait may improve with vision
Sensory selection and weighting deficit	Deviation from straight path; difficulty with changes in sensory environment
Perceptual deficit	Variable gait impairment; asymmetrical posture
Fractioned movement deficit	Slow, stiff movement; marked gait deviations; may need ankle foot orthosis or assistive device
Hypermetria	Variable foot placement; may need assistance
Hypokinesia	Difficulty initiating gait; variable step length; may need assistance
Cognitive deficit	Unable to modify movement based on instructions; poor memory for movement-related instruction

Adapted from Scheets P, Sahrmann S, Norton B. Diagnosis for physical therapy for patients with neuromuscular conditions. Neurol Rep. 1999;23:158-169; and Scheets P, Sahrmann S, Norton B. Use of movement system diagnoses in the management of patient with neuromuscular conditions. Phys Ther. 2007;87:654-699.

body stability, mobility, controlled mobility, or skill. Limited improvement in performance is observed with practice and may worsen with repeated trials.

Fractionated movement deficit is defined as an inability to fractionate movement and is associated with moderate or greater hyperexcitability. It is always associated with central neurologic deficit. Movements are slow, and the ability to generate force rapidly is lacking. The ability to make rapid reversals in movement is limited.

Hypokinesia is defined as slowness in initiating and executing movement. Slow or lack of preparatory movements is present, thus requiring assistance with movement initiation. Difficulty initiating ambulation, shifting center of mass forward, and maintaining balance on termination are noted.

Movement pattern coordination deficit is defined as the inability to coordinate an intersegmental task because of a deficit in timing and sequencing of one segment in relationship to another. Performance typically improves with practice and instruction. Increased latency in postural movement patterns, inappropriate amplitude of postural adjustments or responses, and increased posterior sway during stance activities are noted.

Postural vertical deficit is defined as inaccurate perception of vertical orientation resulting in postural control deficits and the tendency to resist correction of center of mass alignment. This deficit shifts the center of mass beyond limits of stability to the side or backward without weight acceptance and may have disregard for or neglect involved extremities. It presents with a sensation of "falling" when shifted toward correct vertical alignment.

Sensory detection deficits are defined as the inability to execute intersegmental movement due to lack of joint position sense or multisensory failure affecting joint position sense, vision, and/or the vestibular system. Movements are slow and dyscoordinated, with some improvement noted with visual guidance.

Sensory selection and weighting deficit is defined as the inability to initiate or maintain postural orientation or motor performance as a result of decreased ability to screen for and attend to appropriate sensory inputs. Sensory seeking or sensory avoidance behaviors may be observed. Deviation in line of progression to one or both sides is noted. Increased instability occurs with head turning and turning around. Loss of balance or increased ankle or hip sway occurs upon termination of gait, which worsens with faster movements and may result in dizziness. Increased sway or instability is noted with eyes closed or other changes in sensory conditions. Addressing sensory needs via sensory modifications and practicing stability improve responses.[7]

Cognitive deficit is defined as impaired motor control, which is related to a lack of arousal, attention, or ability to apply meaning to a situation that is appropriate for age.

Scheets et al[10] propose that the 9 movement system diagnoses can be applied across medical diagnosis, age, and intervention setting, thus promoting a possible framework to support the 4 Cs in patient-centered care (clarity, communication, collaboration, and continuity). Others have explored the development of movement system diagnoses specifically in a population of interest such as in children with cerebral palsy, adults with vestibular disorders, and children with developmental coordination disorder; thus, applicability across diagnosis, age, and setting is limited. Presently, the 9 movement system diagnoses proposed by Scheets et al serve as a strong place to start the long journey toward ensuring the utility of movement system diagnoses via validity and reliability testing.

So how can we as students, educators, therapists, and researchers use movement system diagnoses to support the APTA vision and advance the practice of physical therapy? We propose this can be done by continuing to develop and evaluate the viability of the current 9 movement system diagnoses and acknowledging that movement emerges as a response to achieve a goal-directed movement behavior. Movement behavior is the result of complex interactions between many subsystems in the body of the learner, the task demands, and the environment constraints. Given this complexity, dynamic systems theory is an appropriate framework as we seek to analyze how movement behaviors are learned (emerge), change, or are relearned over time and lays a foundation for identifying movement system diagnoses.

TABLE 4-3 • Movement System Diagnosis Documenting System

Task	Movement Pattern Coordination Deficit	Force Production Deficit	Sensory Detection Deficit	Sensory Selection and Weighting Deficit	Postural Vertical Deficit	Fractioned Movement Deficit	Hypermetria	Hypokinesia	Cognitive Deficit	Intervention	Outcome
Example	Action Function • Body stability/ body transport • No object manipulation/ Object manipulation Environmental Context • Regulatory conditions stationary/in motion • No intertrial variability/ intertrial variability										
Level surfaces walking while carrying a bookbag											
Stair ascending in a crowded stairwell											
Stair descending in a crowed stairwell											

47

Additionally, as part of a profession guided by evidence, we must continually immerse ourselves in newly emerging literature, evaluate its efficacy, and integrate when appropriate. Recently, several authors have provided additional insight that can further challenge and guide our assumptions regarding the utilization and implementation of movement system diagnosis. Quinn et al[13] offered recommendations from the Academy of Neurologic Physical Therapy's Movement System Task Force specific to conducting "movement analysis within the context of the movement continuum during 6 core tasks (sitting, sit to stand, standing, walking, step up/down, and reach/grasp/manipulate)" and offered recommendations for variation within a task and the environment Gill-body et al[14] identified 10 unique movement system diagnoses associated with balance dysfunctions based upon a scoping review of the literature. From this review Gill-body et al[14] identified two distinct categories: control strategies for balance and determinants of balance. Control strategies included "steady state postural control, anticipatory postural control, and reactive postural control." Determinants include musculoskeletal system elements, which "contribute to producing and maintaining body orientation and stability during tasks and activities."[14] Exploring these categories as part of our movement analysis can provide additional insight as we move forward in this exploration. McClure et al[15] suggested that "existing movement system models seem inadequate for guiding education, practice, or research. Lack of a clear, broadly applicable model may hamper progress in physical therapists actually adopting this identity." Based on this supposition, McClure et al offered an alternate model used to describe movement. This model addresses the interdependent constructs of motion, force, energy, and control and appreciates and recognizes that all movement is affected by personal factors and occurs within a specific environmental context. In this model, the authors support that a "relevant functional movement task is systematically observed qualitatively while hypotheses are developed to explain abnormal findings."[15] The selection of tests and measures to be completed are then guided by the hypotheses generated from which a movement diagnosis can emerge. Taken together, this process informs the decisions made with regard to intervention strategies employed and further reassessments.

INFUSING KEY ELEMENTS TO PROMOTE CLINICAL UTILITY

The clinical utility of the emerging movement system diagnosis framework is best stated as "unknown." However, as proposed earlier, practicing clinicians can join in the conversation via securing practice-based evidence on the 9 existing movement system diagnoses. For many, the question remains as to where to begin. We suggest refamiliarizing ourselves with some key points discussed previously in this text and throughout the physical therapy community.

First, physical therapists must identify and assess the unique factors contributing to the achievement of a functional goal by an individual. Then, the therapists, in collaboration with the individual (learner), must develop an evidenced-based plan of care that promotes the best match between the individual abilities and resources and the task and environmental demands so that a successful movement can emerge. The goal of the intervention is to match the abilities and resources of the individual to the task and environmental characteristics and progressively challenge the individual while continually reassessing the presence of the movement system diagnosis.

Second, physical therapists must use consistent terminology to identify and assess motor system problems via a specific clustering of impairment level signs and symptoms. Finally, physical therapists must begin the journey to assessing the utility of using movement system diagnoses in practice and embrace both the big data–driven approach and the experience-driven approach. Documentation, that 13-letter word that many see as their enemy, can in turn be our profession's biggest advocate. We propose using a documenting system that captures key elements, including but not limited to information specific to individual, task, and environment characteristics and impairment level signs and systems, when developing a plan of care. **Table 4-3** provides a documenting system that can offer quick but detailed information pertinent to the task, learner, and environment. Once the collective team, including the child, parent, and therapists, determines the appropriate functional tasks that must be assessed, the therapist places the tasks (individually) under the task heading. For each task, the therapist identifies the action function characteristics and the environmental context characteristics and notes them on the document. Once the characteristics have been identified specific to each task, then the therapist, using the 9 existing movement system diagnoses found in the literature, notes which specific movement system diagnoses were observed as being present during the child's execution of each specific task. Based on the therapist's critical review of the child's performance of the tasks and observed movement system diagnoses, an intervention plan is developed and noted on the document. Finally, the document is used to assess the outcome of the plan of care specific to the task-specific individual needs of each child. In Chapter 10, we will again see this documenting system used as a means to organize plan of care information.

CONCLUSION

To support the guiding principles of the 2013 APTA House of Delegates professional vision statement, "transforming society by optimizing movement to improve the human experience,"[12]* physical therapists must insightfully observe and clearly describe the way a person moves when performing a meaningful functional task. Describing how one moves is far more detailed than assigning a label to the patient's level of independence when performing a task. Recognizing that movements emerge based on the individual's unique dynamic interplay of systems, using a movement system diagnosis framework that enables us to identify clusters of impairments, more clearly communicating what we observe, and collaborating across health care professions can support continuity in evidence-based, patient-centered care and our profession's mission statement.[16]

Case 1

For an adult learner, YouTube is a resource available at your fingertips that can be used to enhance your observation skills and apply some of the terms and concepts explored in this chapter. Now that you have completed reading this chapter, find at least 2 YouTube videos of children diagnosed with any of the following medical diagnoses: cerebral palsy, developmental coordination disorder, autism, muscular dystrophy, spinal bifida, or brachial plexus. Find videos of these children engaging in motor tasks, such as walking, stair climbing, creeping, sitting, or playing with toys, or engaging in any age functional task. For each of the video cases that you review, explore the questions below.

In each case:

1. Identify the tasks observed and classify the task based on the action function and environmental context.

2. For those tasks with the same action function/environment context category, do you see a cluster of impairments that could be classified by one of the movement system diagnoses, or do you see the emergence of more than one movement system diagnosis within the same task categories?

Are the movement system diagnoses different between task categories?

3. Are there impairments you identified but could not characterize using one of the 9 movement system diagnoses identified by Scheets et al[6]? If so, what are they?

4. Do you believe the tasks observed were functional and meaningful to the individuals? Were there other tasks that you believe would be key to observe? If so, why?

5. Using best practice, identify the treatment interventions you would employ to promote the best match between the individual abilities and resources and the task and environmental demands so that a successful movement can emerge to successfully execute the task.

6. Did the proposed framework of assessing the task requirements and environmental constraints for each task using similarly recognized, consistent, uniform, movement-related terms (movement system diagnosis terminology) to describe similar movements, regardless of pathology, during goal-directed movements help promote your clinical reasoning and decision-making processes?

STUDY QUESTIONS

1. Establishing the identity of the physical therapy profession took more the 40 years of discussion and debate. All of the following are important milestones on the way to establishing the identity of the physical therapy profession except.

   a. Movement system diagnoses were introduced by Sheets, Sahrmann and Norton in 1999.

   b. Helen Hislop suggests pathokinesiology is the science that anchors our profession.

   c. The 2013 House of Delegates adopts a new vision statement establishes pathokinesiology as the foundation of physical therapists practice.

   d. The Diagnosis Dialogues resulted in agreement that the movement system is foundational to the physical therapy profession.

2. A movement systems diagnosis can be more valuable in developing a child's plan of care than a medical diagnosis because,

   a. Two children with the same medical diagnosis can have different activity limitations.

   b. Movement system diagnoses describes a child's functional movement problems.

   c. Movement system diagnoses integrates well with the ICF framework.

   d. All the above

3. Which statement(s) below underscores the importance of incorporating movement observation and analysis into a comprehensive examination.

   a. Movement analysis enables a practitioner to identify how a child's impairments influence the movement strategies used to carry out a functional activity.

   b. Movement strategies a child demonstrates while executing functional movement tasks can be used to support a movement systems diagnosis.

   c. The cores tasks recommended for movement analysis by the Movement Systems Task Force must be specific to an individual's medical diagnosis in order to standardize the decision-making process across practitioners.

   d. A & B

4. This movement systems diagnosis is described by the inability to initiate or maintain postural orientation or motor performance as a result of decreased ability to screen for and attend to appropriate sensory inputs.

   a. Sensory selection and weighting deficit

   b. Sensory detection deficits

   c. Cognitive deficits

   d. Postural vertical deficit

5. The goal of intervention is to promote the best possible match between the resources of the individual, and the requirements of the task and environmental. Requirements of the task and environment include,

   a. Learner's motivation

   b. Surface conditions

   c. Secondary impairments

   d. Primary impairments

References

1. Hedman LD, Quinn L, Gill-Body K, et al. White paper: movement system diagnoses in neurologic physical therapy. *J Neurol Phys Ther*. 2018;42(2):110-117.
2. Rothstein JM. Pathokinesiology: a name for our times? *Phys Ther*. 1986;66:364-365.
3. Sahrmann SA. The human movement system: our professional identity. *Phys Ther*. 2014;94(7):1034-1042.
4. Scheets PK, Sahrmann SA, Norton BJ. Diagnosis for physical therapy for patients with neuromuscular conditions. *Neurology Report* 1999;23(4):158-169.
5. Norton BJ. Diagnosis dialog: progress report. *Phys Ther*. 2007; 87:1270-1273.
6. Scheets PL, Sahrmann SA, Norton BJ. Use of movement system diagnoses in the management of patients with neuromuscular conditions: a multiple patient case report. *Phys Ther*. 2007; 87(6):654-669.
7. Scheets PK, Bloom NJ, Crowner B, McGee PN, Norton PJ, Sahrmann SA, Stith JS, Strecker SK. Movement system diagnoses neuromuscular conditions description of categories. February 2014. Accessed November 6, 2023. https://cdn-links.lww.com/permalink/jnpt/a/jnpt_39_2_2015_01_28_scheets_jnpt-d-14-00043r2_sdc3.pdf
8. ICF Beginners Guide: Toward a Common Language for Functioning, Disability and Health.
9. January 1, 2002. Accessed November 6, 2023. https://www.who.int/publications/m/item/icf-beginner-s-guide-towards-a-common-language-for-functioning-disability-and-healthGuccione AA, Neville BT, George SZ. Optimization of movement: a dynamical systems approach to movement systems as emergent phenomena. *Phys Ther*. 2019;99(1):3-9.
10. Scheets PL, Sahrmann SA, Norton BJ, Stith JS, Crowner BE. What is backward disequilibrium and how do I treat it? A complex patient case study. *J Neurol Phys Ther*. 2015 Apr;39(2):119-26.
11. Sparrow WA, Newell KM. Metabolic energy expenditure and the regulation of movement economy. *Psychonomic Bulletin & Review*. 1998;5:173-196.
12. American Physical Therapy Association. Physical Therapist Practice and the Movement System. An American Physical Therapy Association White Paper. (2015). Available at: http://www.apta.org/MovementSystem/WhitePaper/. Accessed: November 19, 2017.
13. Quinn L, Riley N, Tyrell CM, et al. A framework for movement analysis of tasks: recommendations from the Academy of Neurologic Physical Therapy's Movement System Task Force. *Phys Ther*. 2021;101(9):pzab154.
14. Gill-Body KM, Hedman LD, Plummer L, et al. Movement system diagnoses for balance dysfunction: recommendations from the Academy of Neurologic Physical Therapy's movement system task force. *Phys Ther*. 2021;101(9):pzab153.
15. McClure P, Tevald M, Zarzycki R, et al. The 4-element movement system model to guide physical therapist education, practice, and movement-related research. *Phys Ther*. 2021;101(3):pzab024.
16. VanSant A. Movement system diagnosis. *J Neurol Phys Ther*. 2017;41:S10-S16.

Newborn Infants With Medical Fragility

Roberta Bertie Gatlin, PT, DScPT, Jane K. Sweeney, PT, PhD, MS, and Joanna Beachy, MD, PhD

LEARNING OBJECTIVES

On completion of this chapter, the reader will be able to:

- Describe the evolution of the neonatal physical therapy subspecialty and origin of neonatology fellowship training for pediatric physical therapists.
- Recognize the high risk of providing neonatal therapy practice without mentored clinical training and the restrictions for student therapists, new graduates, and generalist physical therapists.
- Identify complex medical conditions associated with preterm birth and describe long-term motor and developmental outcomes.

- Determine critical family and cultural factors for inclusion in neonatal physical therapy practice.
- Discuss components of the examination/evaluation and intervention processes used by physical therapists in the neonatal intensive care unit.
- Analyze the neonatal physical therapist role in transition of hospitalized infants to home and coordination of unique outpatient service needs.

INTRODUCTION

This chapter provides an overview of neonatal physical therapy for infants with complex medical conditions requiring neonatal intensive care. Selected neonatal physical therapy examination and intervention procedures are reviewed. Throughout the chapter, themes of collaborative partnership with parents and interdisciplinary team members are emphasized as well as individualization of neonatal developmental care and neuroprotection during neonatal physical therapy procedures. This individualization occurs through judicious selection of procedures depending on the maturation level, medical acuity, physiologic stability, and behavioral tolerance of the infant combined with the subspecialty training and experience levels of the therapist.

NEONATAL PHYSICAL THERAPY SUBSPECIALTY

In the United States, the pediatric subspecialty of neonatal physical therapy emerged in the early to mid-1970s. With increasing survival of infants born prematurely, pediatric physical therapists working in large, regional hospitals and children's hospitals were invited to participate as care team members to address musculoskeletal and developmental needs of this increasing population of hospitalized newborns and infants. In nationwide surveys

of practice in 1980[1] and 1990,[2] examination and intervention for high-risk infants were categorized by pediatric physical therapists as procedures in advanced-level practice requiring advanced-level competencies. The advanced practice perspective was derived from pediatric physical therapists' recognition that unique knowledge and skills for ethical practice in neonatal care units were essential for minimizing risks and adverse reactions from unintended overstimulation and cardiorespiratory consequences (eg, oxygen desaturation, bradycardia, tachypnea) during and after neonatal therapy procedures by well-intentioned therapists with general pediatrics or adult therapy competency.

The first clinical practice guidelines for physical therapists working in neonatal intensive care units were developed in 1989 and 1999 by expert panels representing the American Physical Therapy Association, Section on Pediatric Physical Therapy.[3,4] In subsequent revisions, the advanced practice roles and competencies were expanded,[5] and theoretical and evidence-based practice frameworks[6] were added to the Neonatal Physical Therapy Practice Guidelines. Appropriate physical therapy student observational experiences in neonatal intensive care units were later described and prepared as an addendum to the practice guidelines by Rapport et al.[7]

Postgraduate clinical training models with mentored, individualized neonatal physical therapy preceptorships of varied lengths were created with specialized focus on advanced practice competencies in children's hospitals, university hospitals, and large regional hospitals in the 1980s.[8] The official recognition of neonatology as an advanced practice area in pediatric physical therapy by the American Board of Physical Therapy Residency and Fellowship Education (ABPTRFE) in 2010 was pivotal for the development and accreditation of physical therapy fellowships in neonatology. In 2012, the first neonatology fellowship program for physical therapists was accredited for a university-hospital partnership at Rocky Mountain University of Health Professions and Seattle Children's Hospital and Medical Center. Updated information on accredited neonatology fellowships is available on the ABPTRFE website.[9] National certification in neonatal physical therapy is currently under development through the Academy of Pediatric Physical Therapy, American Physical Therapy Association.

■ THEORETICAL MODELS IN NEONATAL PHYSICAL THERAPY

Four foundational models of service delivery assist the physical therapist in providing services in the neonatal intensive care unit (NICU) and are described in this chapter: (1) the International Classification of Functioning, Disability, and Health[10]; (2) the family-centered care model[11,12]; (3) dynamic systems theory of development; and (4) the Synactive Theory.[13] The 4 models involve complex interactive relationships between a neonate's health and the environmental influences facilitating their ability to function. These models assist the physical therapist in the assessment, development, and implementation of developmental programs for the neonate, family, and NICU health care team.[4,10-13]

INTERNATIONAL CLASSIFICATION OF FUNCTIONING, DISABILITY, AND HEALTH

The International Classification of Functioning, Disability, and Health (ICF) represents interactions among the health condition and various components of the neonate's ability to function.[10] The ICF model represents an interactive, complex relationship between the health and many multifactorial components related to gestational age, health systems, environment, and family dynamics that factor into the neonate's ability to function within the environment. The ICF model offers physical therapists an organizational structure of the neonate's diagnosis(ses), body structure, and functions such as the pathologies, impairments, activity limitations, and difficulties in participatory activities (**Figure 5-1**). The advanced skills of the NICU physical therapist allow the integration of the ICF model for assessment, development of care plans, and implementation of therapeutic interventions while accounting for the multifactorial components that relate to a successful outcome.

FAMILY-CENTERED CARE

The natural bond between the infant and mother takes place immediately after birth. For the infant and mother admitted to the NICU, this important time is disrupted. Families

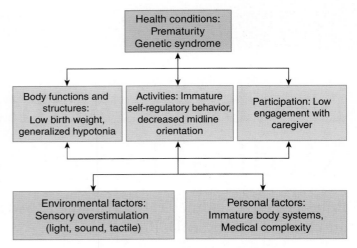

FIGURE 5-1 Modified from The International Classification of Functioning, Disability, and Health (ICF) model. (Adapted from Steiner, Liliane, Huber, Ubelhart, Aeschlimann, Stucki. Use of the ICF model as a clinical problem solving tool in physical therapy and rehabilitation medicine. *Pharm Ther.* 2002;82(11):1098-1107.)

often find the NICU environment to be very intimidating and frightening. Family-centered care (FCC) supports the family's involvement with the infant and assists in decreasing stress levels associated with having a child in the NICU.[11-14] Physical therapists work with the family in helping to recognize their infant's behavioral cues and motor responses. The neonatal therapist may then assist the families with providing interventions in response to their infant's cues. The knowledge the family has about their infant's behavioral cues and how to respond effectively to these cues prior to discharge increases the parents' comfort levels in caring for their child.[14,15] The model and culture of FCC provide an environment that encourages the family to have an active role in the care of the child while in the NICU.

The FCC model is an intervention strategy shown to foster improved outcomes for premature and high-risk infants within the neonatal intensive care environment.[14,15] Nine principles are recognized in the FCC model: (1) respecting the child and family; (2) honoring diversity; (3) recognizing the family's strengths; (4) supporting and facilitating family choices; (5) ensuring flexibility in care procedures; (6) sharing honest and unbiased information; (7) providing support for family needs; (8) collaborating with the family; and (9) empowering the family's strengths.[11,12] Incorporating each principle into the infant's care plan is crucial to neonatal developmental care. The NICU health care team and family should exhibit caring, respectful communication; culturally social and spiritual support; and a flexible, welcoming environment. The FCC model reinforces the importance of preparing the infant and family for transition to home and continued caregiving for the infant.[16]

DYNAMIC SYSTEMS THEORY

The dynamic systems theory (DST) framework recognizes the many interactions that occur among the infant's body systems (ie, ability to move and produce postural control for functional activities), and how the family, home, and community

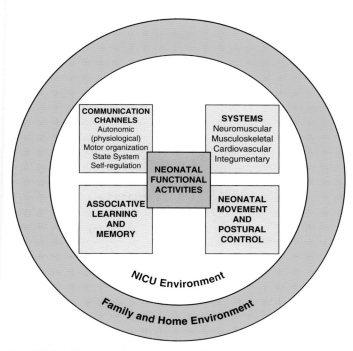

COMMUNICATION
CHANNELS
Autonomic
(physiological)
Motor organization
State System
Self-regulation

SYSTEMS
Neuromuscular
Musculoskeletal
Cardiovascular
Integumentary

NEONATAL
FUNCTIONAL
ACTIVITIES

ASSOCIATIVE
LEARNING
AND
MEMORY

NEONATAL
MOVEMENT
AND
POSTURAL
CONTROL

NICU Environment

Family and Home Environment

FIGURE 5-2 The dynamic systems theory in the neonatal intensive care unit. (Reproduced, with permission, from Sweeney JK, Heriza CB, Blanchard Y, Dusing SC. Neonatal physical therapy. Part II: Practice frameworks and evidence-based practice guidelines. *Pediatr Phys Ther.* 2010;22(1):2-16.)

environments may influence participatory interactions and activities (**Figure 5-2**). The infant's subsystems include body structure, physiology, and behavior. Interactions among the infant's biological makeup, postural control, ability to move and sustain postural control, motor movement patterns, and learned behavioral reactions will influence the ability to perform functional tasks and participate within the infant-family system.[4] The physical therapist must recognize how the infant's postural control and ability to move may directly affect the functioning of physiologic and structural systems.

The DST recognizes the importance of how interventions with the infant and interactions within and around the environment of the infant may produce adverse stress. A change in the environment, such as a loud noise, or a handling technique that moves the infant too quickly may adversely affect the infant and elicit an atypical motor or behavioral response. The DST acknowledges how an interruption of function in one system may be a stressor to the infant and adversely disrupt the ability to maintain stability of other systems. Emphasis in this theory is placed on the contributions of interacting environments in facilitating or constraining the functional performance of the infant. The DST model may assist therapists in considering the many potential positive or negative influences on the infant and how these influences may affect the child's stability.[4,17] All of the theoretical frameworks reviewed in this section support the therapist in designing and implementing an effective neurobehavioral and neurodevelopmental program for the infant and family to facilitate the best outcomes.

SYNACTIVE THEORY OF DEVELOPMENT

Heidelise Als, a developmental psychologist, developed the Synactive Theory of Development to guide the NICU team to understand and interpret the behavior of preterm infants. The Synactive Theory is an example of a dynamic systems theoretical framework. This theory of development is organized into 5 subsystems that may continually activate and influence each other[13] (**Figure 5-3**). The 5 subsystems in the Synactive Theory are organized as a set of interconnected hierarchical behaviors that continually interact with each other.[13,18-21] The least mature subsystem, the autonomic system, oversees the vital functions of the neonate including heart rate, respiratory rate, thermoregulation, and visceral functions. The next subsystem in this hierarchical model is the motor system, responsible for the neonate's postural muscle tone and movement patterns. The third is related to the infant's ability to sustain and transition between various states of alertness, and the fourth subsystem is the infant's ability to maintain attention and engage with a caregiver. The fifth and most mature subsystem is self-regulatory behavior, the ability of the infant to maintain stable and smooth interaction of the other 4 subsystems.

Each subsystem relies on other subsystems' support for intactness and smooth progression. An example of Synactive Theory may be observed when a neonate is medically fragile, functioning in the physiologic subsystem, and attempting to maintain homeostasis of vital functions. As the neonate stabilizes physiologically, they may organize motor activity by presenting with age-appropriate postural muscle tone or actively moving a hand toward the face. As they continue to stabilize, the next subsystem in which they will exhibit behaviors will be their ability to transition smoothly to an alert state, maintain alert behavior, and then transition back into a sleep state. The fourth subsystem is engagement or interaction, often observed prior to discharge when they are able to attend to and interact with the caregiver. The most mature subsystem level is noted when they are able to self-regulate or maintain a balance among the 4 subsystems. These subsystems are important to understand the vulnerability and maturational development of the infant admitted into the NICU.

According to Synactive Theory, infants display communication cues regarding tolerance to stimuli in their environments.[10,17] These cues are considered protective mechanisms that provide the caregiver information regarding the neonate's stress tolerance of an interaction. The cues may be categorized as approach behavioral cues; these behaviors say, "I am ready for interaction" or "I am engaging in this interaction." The infant will present with soft relaxed limbs, quiet and alert state, smooth body movements, or soft, relaxed facial expressions. The infant may exhibit behavioral cues that signify coping or warning behaviors; these behaviors indicate the infant is tolerating the interaction(s) but it is stressful to them. These infants elicit movement patterns of leg bracing, hands to face or mouth, sucking motions, fisting, or attempting to move away from the stimuli. The last category of behaviors an infant may present with are stress cues; these behaviors relay that the infant is not tolerating the stimuli and is experiencing stress that may lead to a change in their homeostasis if continued. These cues must be identified quickly by the caregiver to avoid adverse reactions of the infant, such as losing homeostasis. The behavioral cue may present as a gaze aversion (looking away) and then shift to an avoidance state, such as the

MODEL OF THE SYNACTIVE ORGANIZATION OF BEHAVIORAL DEVELOPMENT

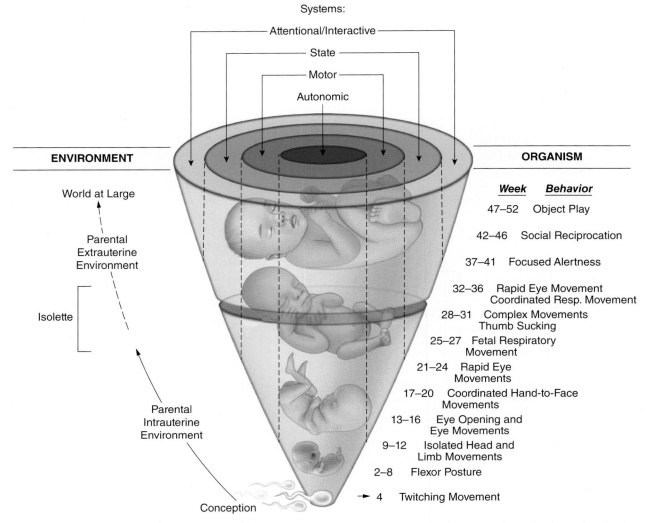

FIGURE 5-3 **The Synactive model of organization of behavioral development by Als.** (Modified with permission from Als. H. Toward a Synactive theory of development: promise for the assessment and support of infant individuality. *Infant Mental Health J.* 1982;3(4):234.)

infant extending the arm with wrist extension and 5-finger salute. Neonatal physical therapists use these cues to guide their interactions with the infant. It is important for the neonatal physical therapist to provide education to assist caregivers in recognizing the infant's individualized behavioral cues. **Table 5-1** presents a list of the behavioral cues that are approach, coping, or stress cues observed by caregivers.

■ NEONATAL INTENSIVE CARE UNIT ENVIRONMENT

In 2012, the American Academy of Pediatrics Committee on Fetus and Newborns defined 4 levels of neonatal care.[22] The levels are designated as basic, specialty, and subspecialty neonatal care (**Table 5-2**).

The neonatal unit is a highly technical environment with many types of equipment that assists in sustaining an infant's life. However, the NICU can cause sensory overstimulation and adversely affect an infant's physiologic stability. For example,

the sound levels, bright lighting, excessive unsupported infant movements, and sensory stimuli that disrupt the neonate's sleep cycles may alter the infant's behavioral states, physiologic stability, and developmental outcomes. The physical therapist can offer suggestions that may eliminate or lessen the impact of neonatal environmental stressors. For example, the neonatal therapist may participate in developing or adapting NICU protocols for reducing sound levels, offering cyclic lighting, promoting postural positioning support to the infant, and initiating feedings based on infant behavioral readiness. The physical therapist providing services in the NICU must be aware of the highly sensitive environment and its crucial role in supporting or challenging neonatal development.

EQUIPMENT

The physical therapist must be familiar with specialized equipment in the NICU (**Figure 5-4**), recognize and

TABLE 5-1 • Self-Regulatory Behavioral Cues

Approach cues	Quiet and alert state
	Soft, relaxed facial expressions
	"Ohh" face
	Cooing
	Relaxed extremities
	Smooth body motions
	Smile
Coping cues	Purposeful shift to a drowsy or light sleep state
	Extremity bracing
	Hand to face
	Sucking motions
	Hand or foot clasping
	Fisting
	Bracing of body to support surface (searching for boundaries)
Stress cues	Gaze aversion
	Grimace/frowning
	"Worry wrinkles"
	Tongue thrusting
	Salute sign
	Stretching or arching away
	Finger splay
	Yawning, burping, or gagging
	Spitting up
	Changes in vital signs homeostasis

understand why certain equipment is being used, and provide input to the team about the infant's response during interventions.

Table 5-3 contains a list of common equipment found in a NICU. Competency-based, mentored training on varied neonatal respiratory and medical equipment is essential for ethical, safe, and effective practice by the physical therapist.

■ NEONATAL MEDICAL CONDITIONS: AN OVERVIEW

Over the past 30 years, many improvements in obstetric care have occurred. These advances include earlier identification of high-risk pregnancies using prenatal ultrasound and noninvasive prenatal screening, medications such as progesterone and betamethasone, and establishment of tertiary care centers for delivery of high-risk infants. Numerous advances in neonatal care have resulted in significantly increased survival of infants born prematurely and at term gestation. Specific innovations are commercial surfactant replacement for lung immaturity, improved ventilator capabilities, noninvasive ventilation leading to decreased pulmonary damage, and medications to improve pulmonary function.

In this section, fetal growth assessment and gestational age assessment at birth are described. Common medical conditions derived from organ system immaturity are reviewed in the context of a premature birth.

GESTATIONAL AGE AND BIRTHWEIGHT

An accurate estimation of gestational age is important for predicting long-term outcomes. Term pregnancy is 40 weeks in duration but spans between 37 and 41 weeks' gestation. Prenatal estimate of gestational age based on the mother's last menses gives an estimated due date and is reliable within 2 weeks. Fetal crown-rump length calculated from ultrasound at less than 14 weeks of gestation is the most reliable assessment of due date with an accuracy of 5 to 7 days. Fetal ultrasound performed later in the second trimester by measuring the biparietal diameter of the head, femur length, and crown-rump length is not as accurate.[23] Gestational age after delivery is usually assessed with the modified Ballard score, which is based on 6 physical and neurologic criteria for neonates at 20 to 44 weeks' gestation.[24] This calculation takes 3 to 5 minutes to complete and accurately estimates gestational age within 2 weeks. The gestational age of the infant is based on the obstetrical dating criteria unless the clinical assessment of the infant deviates more than 2 weeks from the obstetrical calculation. If a fetus has low weight gain in utero, the infant is diagnosed with intrauterine growth restriction. This condition may result in the infant being small for gestational age, which is birth weight less than the 10th percentile for gestational age. Low-birth-weight infants weigh under 2500 g at birth and are usually less than 37 weeks of gestation. Other categories defined by weight are very low birth weight (VLBW; <1500 g) and exceptionally low birth weight (<1000 g).

The organs of infants born prematurely are not fully developed and are highly susceptible to injury that can lead to impaired neurologic functioning and long-term developmental delay. Even infants at term gestation are at increased risk for impairment due to supplemental oxygen requirement, mechanical ventilation, sepsis, multiple noxious stimulation during medical procedures, and decreased infant-parent interactions during hospitalization. Specific organ systems prone to perinatal injury are the brain, eyes, lung, and intestines. Other conditions the infant may experience include in utero drug exposure, birth trauma, and positional deformities.

For infants born under 32 weeks' gestation, intraventricular hemorrhage (IVH) is the most frequent brain injury and can lead to significant neurodevelopmental delays. IVH varies inversely with gestational age and is rarely seen in infants born under 28 weeks' gestation due to the developmental involution of blood vessels in the germinal matrix. Adjacent to the ventricles, the germinal matrix is a highly vascularized capillary network. The germinal matrix is easily ruptured because of the preterm infant's limited ability to maintain cerebral vascular autoregulation. The incidence of IVH (<15% in VLBW infants) has decreased over time due to improved maternal treatment and neonatal respiratory management.[25]

TABLE 5-2 • Levels of Neonatal Care		
Level I	Basic newborn nursery/well-newborn nursery	• Postnatal care and evaluation of the healthy newborn • Neonatal resuscitation at delivery • Stabilization and care for physiologically stable late preterm infants, born between 35 and 36.6 weeks' gestational age (GA) • Stabilization of ill newborns until transfer to a facility at which specialty neonatal care is provided
Level II	Specialty care nursery	Level I capabilities plus: • Resuscitate and stabilize infants with medical needs or preterm infants prior to transfer • Medical intervention to the infant ≥32 weeks' GA and ≥1500 g who has physiologic immaturity or who may be moderately ill with resolution of medical complications within the first 24 hours of life • Provide mechanical ventilation or continuous positive airway pressure for short duration (<24 hours)
Level III	Subspecialty unit/neonatal intensive care unit (NICU)	Level II capabilities plus: • Provide medical intervention for the infant <32 weeks' GA and weighing <1500 g and infants at all GAs and birth weights with critical illness • Offer a full range of respiratory support including conventional mechanical ventilation, continuous positive airway pressure, high-frequency ventilation, and nitric oxide • Provide access to advanced imaging, computed tomography, magnetic resonance imaging, and echocardiography with interpretation for urgency • Support a full range of pediatric medical subspecialists, pediatric surgical specialists, anesthesiologists, and ophthalmologists • Performs surgical procedures • Provides transports to Level IV nursery
Level IV	Regional NICU	Level III capabilities plus: • Surgery for complex surgical diagnoses, ie, CDH Provide access to a full range of pediatric medical subspecialists, pediatric surgical specialists, anesthesiologists, and ophthalmologists • Provide access to specialists for surgical repair of congenital heart anomalies that require cardiopulmonary bypass and/or extracorporeal membrane oxygenation • Provide transport services for Level I, II, and III NICUs • Provide training and educational outreach programs for medical professionals serving the neonatal and high-risk infant population

Source: American Academy of Pediatrics. Policy statement, levels of neonatal care. Pediatrics. 2012;130(3):587-597.

MEDICAL DIAGNOSES

Neurologic

The grades of IVH (grades 1-4) are established by cranial ultrasound within the first 5 days of life. In grade 1 IVH, the hemorrhage is confined to the germinal matrix. If the hemorrhage extends into the ventricle, it is called grade 2 IVH. When

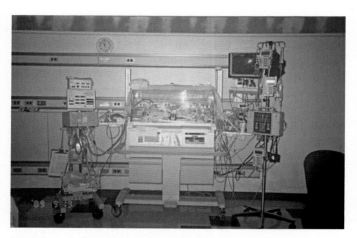

FIGURE 5-4 **Isolette or incubator with infant. To the left of the incubator is the ventilator; to the right is the cardiopulmonary monitor and intravenous poles with various pharmacologic agents, fluids, and nutrition.**

the hemorrhage fills greater than 50% of the ventricle causing ventricular dilatation, it is called grade 3. Grade 4 IVH, or periventricular hemorrhagic infarct (PVHI), is not due to capillary disruption but rather due to venous congestion of veins bordering the lateral ventricles causing destruction of white matter. The PVHI is usually fan-shaped, unilateral, associated with severe IVH, and results in porencephalic cyst generation. Absence of grades 1 and 2 IVH does not ensure normalcy but is not associated with marked developmental delay. Infants with grade 3 IVH and PVHI are at increased risk for developing cerebral palsy, specifically spastic hemiplegia and spastic diplegia.[25] At term gestation, cranial magnetic resonance imaging (MRI) or ultrasound can provide evidence on the extent of cerebral damage from IVH. However, these tests cannot accurately predict neurodevelopmental outcomes because the preterm brain is able to make new connections to ameliorate the impact of hemorrhage and frequently improve neurodevelopmental outcomes (plasticity of the preterm brain).

Posthemorrhagic ventricular dilatation occurs in about 50% of infants with severe IVH (grade 3 or 4), and the majority will develop progressive ventricular enlargement necessitating the need for repeated removal of cerebrospinal fluid (CSF) by spinal tap, subgaleal shunt, or placement of Omaya reservoir. There is no consensus on the optimal management and timing of removal of CSF.[26,27]

TABLE 5-3 • Common Medical Equipment in the Neonatal Intensive Care Unit

Radiant warmer	An open bed for stabilizing an infant's body temperature with an overhead heat source, specialized lighting for examination, and hyperbilirubinemia.
Isolette	An enclosed incubator providing environmental controlled temperature and humidity. Access to the infant is through port holes on each side of the plastic box.
Open crib	Open bassinet bedding without a heat source.
Ventilator:	
IPPV	Intermittent positive pressure ventilation; applies to whole-spectrum ventilation modes that deliver pressure-limited, time-cycled ventilation.
SIMV	Synchronized intermittent mandatory ventilation; similar to IPPV but delivers a predetermined number of breaths per minute (bpm) synchronized with the infant's breaths.
HFOV	High-frequency oscillatory ventilator; employs supraphysiologic ventilation rates and tidal volumes frequently less than dead space.
CPAP-binasal cannula	Continuous positive airway pressure forces high pressures of air into the nasal passages to overcome any obstructions in the airway and stimulate breathing.
Umbilical lines:	
UVC	Umbilical venous catheter is placed into the vein of the umbilical cord allowing access to the central circulation of the newborn. Administration of fluids, nutrition, and medications.
UAC	Umbilical arterial catheter is placed into the artery in the umbilical cord of the newborn. It allows the team to draw blood samples, continuously monitor blood pressure, and perform blood gas sampling.
PICC	Peripherally inserted central catheter is a long slender catheter inserted in a peripheral vein and advanced until termination in a large vein in the chest near the heart. The PICC serves as a central line and may stay in place for weeks, which is less invasive and has decreased complications in neonates who require long-term nutritional and medication needs.
PIV	Peripheral intravenous line is a short-term access through the peripheral vein used to administer fluids, nutrition, or medications.
Monitors:	
Cardiorespiratory Oxygen saturation Transcutaneous CO_2 Near-infrared spectroscopy (NIRS)	Displays heart rate, respiratory rate, and blood pressure with high and low limits. Measures arterial oxygen saturation by using a light sensor. Measures partial pressure of oxygen and carbon dioxide noninvasively using a heated sensor. Noninvasive method to measure tissue (brain, renal, intestinal) oxygen saturation to ensure adequate oxygen delivery.
Amplitude integrated electroencephalogram (aEEG)	Continuous recording of cerebral electrical activity to evaluate presence of seizures and maturation of the brain.
Phototherapy: overhead bili lights	Overhead ultraviolet lights called phototherapy administered to infants with hyperbilirubinemia or jaundice.
Bili blanket	A bilirubin blanket or phototherapy blanket provides an ultraviolet light the infant with jaundice can lie on.
Whole-body cooling blankets	Neonatal whole-body cooling may be utilized with hypoxic-ischemic encephalopathy (HIE). The use of induced hypothermia in postasphyxia has been shown to reduce the incidence of death and disability at 18-22 months of age.
Commercial positioning devices	Positioning aid provides support and maintains a physiologic flexed position for the premature or medically ill infant.
Weighted blankets	A "froggy" or Dandle PAL blankets are smaller plastic pellet-filled positional blankets providing proprioceptive input around the boundaries and/or over the pelvis. Must never be used over the thoracic spine or lungs where the weight may restrict the breathing of the infant.
General pacifier categories	Specialized pacifier designed for the extremely- or very-low-birth-weight premature infant. Specialized pacifier designed for premature infants of low birth weight or typically between 30 and 34 weeks' gestational age.

If the ventricular dilation does not resolve with serial removal of CSF, the infant undergoes placement of a ventriculoperitoneal (V-P) shunt or third ventriculostomy/choroid plexus obliteration. Placement of a V-P shunt is associated with significant complications including sepsis or shunt malfunction requiring shunt revision. These complications further result in increasing compromised neurodevelopmental outcomes.[28]

Periventricular leukomalacia (PVL) is a nonhemorrhagic ischemic injury to the preterm infant's brain due to lack of cerebral blood flow in the "watershed" area usually between the anterior and middle cerebral artery. The PVL lesion presents as cysts adjacent to the ventricles or globally resulting in ventricular enlargement, increased extra-axial fluid, and decreased head growth. The PVL injury can be evident by 3 to 4 weeks after an ischemic insult but may be subtle and not readily evident on cranial ultrasound and should be visualized on cranial MRI.[29] The incidence of PVL increases with decreasing gestational age and is present in less than 10% of VLBW infants.

The cerebellum is involved in coordination, gross and fine motor control, attention, and language development.[30] Frequently, cerebellar damage is associated with IVH indicating similar risk factors. Cerebral damage may impact development in the cerebellum due to neuronal interconnections. In extremely preterm infants, the incidence of cerebellar injury may be as high as 20% and may be clinically silent at birth, but the impact of the injury becomes more evident over time due to the cerebellar involvement in coordination and speech.[28]

Hypoxic-ischemic encephalopathy (HIE) is due to a lack of oxygen around the time of delivery leading to cerebral injury in late preterm (34-36 weeks' gestation) and term infants. About 0.5 to 1 per 1000 births are affected by HIE, resulting in approximately 80% survival with 25% to 30% of the surviving infants showing evidence of significant neurologic damage. The many risk factors for development of HIE include maternal hypotension, placental abruption, placental dysfunction, umbilical cord prolapse, fetal anemia, and infection.[31] There are 3 phases of damage that may occur in HIE. The initial hypoxic insult results in acidosis and neuronal

necrosis. The second phase lasts about 6 hours and involves reperfusion leading to an increase in free radical production and inflammation. The third phase is marked by activation of the apoptotic pathway (programmed cell death) that accounts for the majority of neuronal and glial cell death and worsened morbidity.[25] The damage from HIE is located in the deep structures of the brain such as the basal ganglia, thalamus, and posterior limb of the internal capsule (motor pathways), as well as in the watershed area of the subcortical and parasagittal white matter. This damage can be visualized on MRI using routine T1 and T2 sequences, specific sequences such as diffusion-weighted imaging, apparent diffusion coefficient, and spectroscopy.[32] Clinical or electrographic seizures are present in up to 40% of infants with HIE.

The severity of HIE is based on a clinical scoring system designating mild, moderate, and severe encephalopathy (**Table 5-4**). Mild hypothermia (33.5°C) starting within 6 hours after delivery has become the standard of care of infants at or greater than 35 weeks' gestation with moderate to severe HIE classified by the clinical scoring system.[33] Hypothermia treatment is continued for 72 hours and is more effective in decreasing mortality and morbidity in infants with moderate HIE compared to those with severe HIE.[33] Side effects of mild hypothermia treatment (bradycardia, mild hypotension, thrombocytopenia, and persistent pulmonary hypertension) are transient and usually easily treated medically. Despite hypothermia treatment, only 50% of infants with HIE will have a normal outcome. Due to the location of the injury, infants with HIE demonstrate impaired upper extremity movement and have difficulty in feeding because of bulbar involvement.[33]

Visual

Retinopathy of prematurity (ROP) is a proliferative neovascular disorder of retinal vessels that affects preterm infants and can lead to severe visual impairment (myopia), retinal scarring, retinal detachment, and blindness. Infants with a gestational age under 26 weeks are at the greatest risk for developing ROP. Other risk factors include low birth weight, prolonged assisted ventilation, supplemental oxygen delivery,

TABLE 5-4 • Stages of Encephalopathy				
	Stages of Encephalopathy			
	Normal	**Stage 1 (Mild)**	**Stage 2 (Moderate)**	**Stage 3 (Severe)**
1. Level of consciousness	Alert, responsive	Hyperalert, respond to minimal stimulation	Lethargic	Stupor/coma
2. Spontaneous activity	Changes position	Normal or decreased	Decreased	None
3. Posture	Flexed when quiet	Mild flexion distal	Distal flexion, full extension	Decerebrate
4. Tone	Strong flexor tone	Normal or slightly increased	Hypo- or hypertonia	Flaccid or rigid
5. Reflex: Suck Moro	Strong Complete	Weak or incomplete Intact	Weak Incomplete	Absent Absent
6. Autonomic: Pupils Heart rate Respirations	Normal 100-160 Regular	Mydriasis Tachycardia Hyperventilation	Myosis Bradycardia Periodic breathing	Variable Variable Apnea, assisted

and surgical procedures.[34] Retinal vasculature development originates from the optic disc at 17 weeks' gestation and is completed by approximately 40 weeks' gestation. Preterm infants undergo ophthalmologic retinal examinations starting at 31 weeks' gestation or 4 weeks after birth, and ROP is reported by stage (stage 1-5) and zone (zone 1-3).[35] Infants are followed sequentially until the retinal vessels are mature.[36] The need for treatment (either via laser photocoagulation or injection with anti–vascular endothelial growth factor) is based on location and severity of ROP. Untreated severe ROP can lead to retinal detachment and blindness. Although the incidence of ROP has decreased over time due to tighter control of supplemental oxygen, recent advances in neonatal care have significantly increased the number of VLBW infants who are at the highest risk for developing ROP.

Pulmonary

Hyaline membrane disease or respiratory distress syndrome is frequently present in infants born at or under 35 weeks' gestation and is due to pulmonary surfactant deficiency. Surfactant is composed of a phospholipid and protein layer that helps maintain the structure of terminal airways and alveoli during expiration. Without surfactant, the airways and alveoli collapse, and assisted ventilation, specifically constant distending pressure, is required for respiratory stability. Administration of betamethasone prenatally stimulates surfactant production and is given to mothers starting at 23 weeks' gestation for pregnancies at risk for delivering prematurely. Once delivered, infants with respiratory distress syndrome can be treated with respiratory support and exogenous surfactant to improve pulmonary function. Because the rib cage is compliant, infants with respiratory distress are frequently positioned prone to stabilize the sternum and improve ventilation.[37]

Prolonged assisted ventilation and supplemental oxygen may lead to baro- and volutrauma contributing to bronchopulmonary dysplasia (BPD) or chronic lung disease (CLD). Current definition of moderate BPD is oxygen requirement at 36 weeks' corrected gestational age. Infants with severe BPD require supplemental oxygen and prolonged ventilation and often need tracheostomy for ongoing respiratory insufficiency. Steroids are frequently used to decrease dependence on mechanical ventilation but are associated with impaired neurodevelopmental outcome.[38,39] The severity of BPD is inversely related to gestational age at birth, with the incidence at 33%, 14%, and 6% for infants with birth weight of 751 to 1000 g, 1001 to 1250 g, and 1251 to 1500 g, respectively.[40] Long-term outcomes for infants with CLD are increased incidence of reactive pulmonary disease, asthma, multiple hospitalizations, oral aversion leading to feeding difficulties and delayed speech, and impaired cognitive function.[41,42]

Gastrointestinal

Necrotizing enterocolitis (NEC), the most common intestinal disease of neonates, is an inflammation of the intestine causing feeding intolerance and occasionally intestinal perforation. While the exact etiology is unclear, risk factors for developing NEC include prematurity, congenital heart disease, blood transfusions, rapid enteral feeding advancement, and viral or bacterial infection. The onset of NEC is usually in the first month of life, and it can be treated medically. However, if intestinal perforation or clinical decompensation develops, infants will require surgical intervention. An increased risk for mortality and morbidity occurs in neonates requiring surgical intervention for NEC.[43,44] Common complications of NEC include sepsis, poor growth, cholestasis, "short gut," and stricture formation requiring additional surgeries that further negatively affect neurodevelopment.

Substance Exposure

Maternal medications such as opioids, cocaine, cannabis, and selective serotonin reuptake inhibitors (SSRIs) taken during pregnancy can impact the developing fetal brain depending on the specific drug or combination of drugs and the timing and duration of the medication use. Tolerance occurs when there is continued use of medication, usually opioids, necessitating an increased dose to achieve the same effect. Withdrawal symptoms related to physical dependence on the medication emerge when the drug is abruptly discontinued. Addiction includes tolerance, physical dependence, and psychological craving for the medication.

An increasing concern exists over the expanded use of opioids, either illicit or by prescription, for pain relief. Use of pain relievers, specifically opioids, during pregnancy has increased 5-fold during the past decade.[45] Naturally occurring opioids (morphine and codeine) and synthetic opioids (heroin, methadone, buprenorphine, and fentanyl) can readily cross the placenta and affect the pregnancy by causing premature rupture of membranes, preterm labor, and decreased fetal growth. After delivery, infants are no longer receiving the maternal opioid and begin to demonstrate withdrawal symptoms (neonatal abstinence syndrome [NAS]). Infants will demonstrate a variety of neurologic issues (hyperexcitability, irritability, high-pitched cry, increased muscle tone, tremors, and seizures), gastrointestinal symptoms (frantic sucking, uncoordinated feeding, vomiting, and diarrhea), and autonomic signs (sweating, mottling, hyperthermia, and nasal stuffiness). Symptoms of NAS occur from 2 to 6 days after delivery, depending on the specific opioid. However, severity of withdrawal is not completely related to dose of maternal medication but also depends on genetic differences and other maternal drug use.

The most common scoring tool to determine the need for treatment for NAS is the modified Finnegan scale.[46] Infants exposed to opioids in utero should be placed in a quiet, darkened room; held; swaddled; given a pacifier; and fed on demand. Breastfeeding should be encouraged if the mother is under medical care and without polysubstance use. Once the infant's scores indicate the medical treatment for NAS is necessary, morphine, methadone, or buprenorphine is started. Occasionally the infant will require other medication such as phenobarbital or clonidine. Institution-specific guidelines for assessment and treatment of NAS have greatly decreased the duration of neonatal treatment and length of stay. Even after treatment for NAS is completed, infants exposed to opioids in utero continue to demonstrate hypertonicity, irritability, and delayed fine motor coordination and have an increased risk for sudden infant death syndrome (SIDS).[47,48]

Cocaine is a highly addictive, illicit drug that causes vasoconstriction, which can lead to placental abruption and preterm delivery. Mothers using cocaine tend to use other illicit drugs, drink alcohol, have poor nutrition, and have limited prenatal care. Neonates exposed to cocaine in utero exhibit tremors, hypertonicity, irritability, poor feeding ability, and abnormal sleep patterns. They are at a significantly higher risk of developing SIDS.[49] In addition, in utero cocaine exposure has been linked to abnormalities in executive functioning and an increased incidence of behavioral problems with a need for special education in school-aged children.[50]

Because marijuana (cannabis) has become legal in many states, females will frequently look to cannabis to treat pregnancy-related nausea and vomiting as well as partake in recreational use. As with cocaine, cannabis use is associated with exposure to other illicit drugs, alcohol, and cigarette smoking. An increased incidence of stillbirths, preterm labor, and low birth weight occurs with exposure to cannabis. In addition, in utero marijuana exposure has been linked to increased hyperactivity and impulsivity in children and shorter attention span.[51] The American Academy of Pediatrics discourages the use of marijuana during pregnancy and breastfeeding due to the potential impact on the developing brain.[52]

SSRIs are frequently prescribed during pregnancy because depression can cause serious side effects in both mother and the developing fetus.[53] However, SSRIs readily cross the placenta and can affect fetal brain development, specifically impacting somatosensory processing and the emotional response networks. If maternal use of SSRIs occurs in the third trimester, infants may exhibit symptoms mimicking NAS such as irritable behavior, agitation, tremors, and difficulty sleeping. These symptoms are usually transient and resolve in 2 weeks.[54] The most common clinical sign of in utero SSRI exposure is neonatal feeding difficulty that can persist and prolong length of stay. As with the other maternal medications, it is difficult to predict specific neurodevelopmental outcomes due to the use of multiple medications (prescribed and illicit), timing and duration of all medications, and effect of maternal depression on fetal development.

Birth Trauma

Birth trauma, a relatively infrequent occurrence, can be due to cephalopelvic disproportion, a large for gestational age fetus, or instrumented deliveries (vacuum or forceps). Shoulder dystocia occurs when the fetus's anterior shoulder is caught by the mother's pubic bone after delivery of the head, which can lead to a clavicular fracture or brachial plexus injury (1-5 of 1000 live births).[55] Erb palsy (waiter's tip) is the most common brachial plexus injury affecting the cervical nerves V and VI and causing impaired arm movement. Klumpke palsy (claw hand) affects cervical nerve VIII and thoracic nerve 1 and can be associated with Horner syndrome (eyelid droop and pupillary constriction) and/or diaphragmatic paresis from phrenic nerve involvement. Brachial plexus injury may resolve spontaneously over several months or may require surgical intervention. Care must be given to avoid stretch or compression of the affected shoulder to prevent further discomfort or unintended injury during dressing, lifting, and sleep positioning.

Oligohydramnios (decreased amniotic fluid) or anhydramnios (lack of amniotic fluid) can lead to pulmonary hypoplasia, growth restriction, positional deformities, and joint contractures (arthrogryposis). Low amniotic fluid may be related to premature rupture of membranes, renal disease causing decreased urine production, obstruction of urinary tract (posterior urethral valves), and chromosomal anomalies. Arthrogryposis multiplex congenita is a clinical finding where 2 or more joint contractures are present. This condition can be due to oligohydramnios, neurologic injury leading to decreased movement in utero, genetic abnormalities, or idiopathic causes.

Musculoskeletal

Club foot occurs in 1 in 1000 live births and is composed of 4 specific abnormalities. The foot malalignment may occur in the forefoot (metatarsus adductus), midfoot (high arch or cavus), hindfoot (varus), and or ankle (equinus).[56] The affected foot and calf musculature in club foot are frequently small and atrophic. If conservation treatments of stretching, taping, and/or casting are unsuccessful in correcting the abnormality, surgery is recommended. Positional deformities related to oligohydramnios can usually be passively positioned into normal alignment.

Three main types of acquired skull positional deformities may start in neonatal care units and progress after discharge to the home environment. The 2 most common skull deformities developing in infants born prematurely are dolichocephaly (symmetrical cranial narrowing creating elongated anterior-posterior aspect) and plagiocephaly (asymmetrical unilateral flattening of the occiput with ipsilateral [same side] frontal bossing and anterior displacement of the ipsilateral ear and cheek). Brachycephaly, flattening of the posterior aspect of the head, is more likely to occur in term infants when prolonged head placement in midline may be needed with mechanical ventilation or sedation. These deformities are a result of limited variation in body positioning, incompletely fused sutures, decreased neck tone, and reduced active head movement. The optimal way to treat these deformities is to change position to minimize pressure on the back or side of the head, encourage symmetry in neck motion, and support supervised prone play time.[57] If the positional head deformities are severe and persist, a helmet may be used to realign the cranial bones. Premature closure of suture(s) can cause pronounced head deformity and must be identified and referred early for surgical management. Congenital muscular torticollis, a unilateral shortening or contraction of the sternocleidomastoid muscle, may be evident within the first month of life and may lead to plagiocephaly. Physical therapy with frequent gentle, positional stretching and active strengthening resolves the majority of cases of congenital torticollis, but surgery may be required in selected cases (eg, pseudotumor present or late referral).[58]

■ NEONATAL PHYSICAL THERAPY EXAMINATION

HISTORY/CHART REVIEW

The neonatal examination begins with a comprehensive chart review of the infant's NICU admission and the maternal medical history. The chart review provides the neonatal therapist with the birth history, admission medical diagnosis(ses), gestational age, current medical interventions and medications, and any special procedures and tests results (eg, imaging or genetic testing). After gathering the chart information, the neonatal physical therapist should observe the infant and discuss with the bedside nurse the current respiratory status, nutrition support, intravenous lines, baseline vital signs, and current positioning, as well as the infant's individualized behavioral stress and stability cues. Other pertinent information about the family socioeconomics, home environment, and specific needs or concerns are gathered. After obtaining a thorough chart review, observation and discussion with the bedside nurse provide the neonatal physical therapist critical information to begin the hands-on assessment of the examination, development of an appropriate plan of care, and preparation for discharge readiness.

MEDICAL FRAGILITY

The neonatal physical therapist must continuously evaluate the medical stability of the NICU infant. As physical therapists, we strive to practice under the principle of beneficence ("above all, do no harm" to our patients).[59,60] The therapist must recognize the neonate admitted to the NICU as vulnerable and may present with rapid and unexpected changes in their physiologic stability (**Figure 5-5**). The physiologic stability depends on the medical diagnosis and gestational age. The neonatal physical therapist must have sharp observational skills to identify any behavioral signs that may indicate a compromise in the physiologic stability of the infant.

Infants exhibit self-regulatory behavioral cues that guide the therapists and NICU health care professionals regarding their tolerance to stimuli (see Table 5-1). These behavioral cues are the communication strategies infants use to tell the neonatal care team they are ready for interactions. The approach cues indicate the infants are ready for interaction and intervention

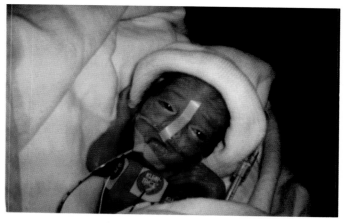
FIGURE 5-6 **Approach cue of relaxed arms and visual engagement.**

(**Figure 5-6**). Coping cues show that babies are handling the intervention but are experiencing some stress (**Figure 5-7**). Adverse stress cues communicate that infants are not handling the intervention and need either a break or rescheduling of the procedure (**Figure 5-8**).

As the neonatal therapist begins the examination process, it is important to collaborate with the bedside nurse to provide intervention during or after the infant's scheduled nursing activity time. This coordinated process ensures the infant receives an uninterrupted period of sleep between interventions. During the collaboration, the therapist and nurse can assist each other in identifying information regarding the stability and behavioral cues of the infant. By providing interventions together, the therapist and nurse offer "cluster care."[61] This care process occurs when the interventions for the infant are clustered together, providing longer undisturbed periods between care activities that may promoting deeper sleep patterns. Working collaboratively with the nursing staff provides a less stressful interaction to the infant.

MEDICALLY STABLE

When examining the medically stable infant, the therapist can have a more hands-on assessment while still letting the

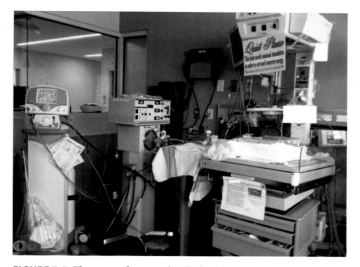
FIGURE 5-5 **The set up for a medically fragile infant under a radiant warmer to provide heat. In the left is the high frequency oscillator ventilator and on the right are pumps for intravenous fluid administration. The quiet please signage indicates medical fragility and overstimulation risk which may lead to loss of homeostasis.**

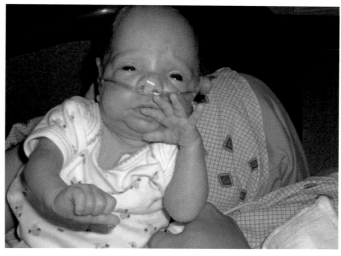
FIGURE 5-7 **Coping cue such as hand to mouth for self-calming.**

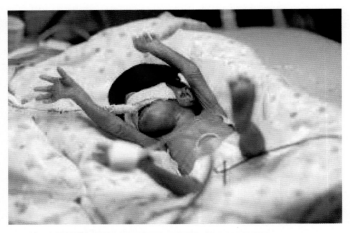

FIGURE 5-8 **Stress cue of stiffly extended extremities.**

infant's behavioral and physiologic stability guide the therapist's pacing. The physical therapist observes the infant's behavioral responses, self-regulatory signs, postural patterns, and motor activities, as well as interactive capabilities and functional activities. Medically stable infants are often progressing with gaining weight, controlling temperature, and learning to feed (bottle and breast methods). Examination of the medically stable infant should occur when the infant is in a calm, awake state. Components of the examination include behavioral states of alertness, review of systems, observation of posture at rest, quality and quantity of active movement patterns, presence of primitive reflexive motor patterns, passive range of motion, sensory processing abilities, habituation patterns to sensory stimuli, tolerance to and self-regulation of environmental stress, and readiness for oral motor examination and/or feeding. The neonatal therapist may also administer special tests and measures (**Table 5-5**).

BEHAVIORAL STATES OF ALERTNESS

During evaluation, the neonate's alertness and transition ability between states of alertness are assessed. Brazelton defined 6 states of behavior for alertness and sleep (**Table 5-6**).[62] Neonates less than 36 weeks' gestational age often do not have the maturity to smoothly transition between these states of alertness. As the neonate matures, the ability to sustain longer periods of alertness and transition between the various states of sleep and alerting should correlate with the feeding schedule. It is important to identify any interventions that may have occurred with the infant prior to the physical therapy examination that may compromise the infant's ability to become or stay alert.[60] This information adds to the therapist's evaluation of the infant's self-regulatory ability.

SYSTEMS REVIEW

The systems review of the infant provides information regarding the maturation and function of the cardiopulmonary, integumentary, musculoskeletal, and neuromuscular systems. Information regarding the current function of each system may be obtained through discussion with nurses and neonatologists and by review of the medical chart. The systems

review includes gathering information about the current baseline status and maturation changes occurring in each of the systems:

- Cardiopulmonary system: Assessment of heart rate, respiratory rate, oxygen saturations, and blood pressure
- Integumentary system: Assessment of risk for skin breakdown, skin condition, pliability (texture), presence of bruising or mottling, skin color, skin integrity, and potential equipment risks to skin
- Musculoskeletal system: Assessment of symmetry, gross active and passive range of motion, gross strength, length, and weight of muscular activity
- Neuromuscular system: General assessment of gross movement patterns and appropriate gestational developmental motor function

The systems review contributes information to the physical therapist in identifying concerns and developing a plan of care that may necessitate a consultation with or referral to health care specialists.

POSITIONING

When examining a preterm infant, the physical therapist assesses the infant's ability to maintain flexion against gravity. The full-term infant typically presents with arms close to midline, shoulders adducted and in neutral internal-external rotation, and elbows flexed and hands near the mouth. The hips are typically flexed with external rotation and abduction, with knees flexed, ankles dorsiflexed, and the head, neck, trunk, and pelvis tucked into flexion. This posture is identified as physiologic flexion (**Figure 5-9**). The younger the gestational age of the infant or the more medically unstable, the less extremity flexion the infant can demonstrate and maintain (**Figure 5-10**).

Positional support is needed and must be individualized. The physical therapist practicing in the NICU must have advanced knowledge of the gestational age progression for each week of development after 23 to 24 weeks, with particular emphasis on developmental changes in the neurologic and musculoskeletal systems and maturation of physiologic flexion.

Positional assessment also includes examination of the infant's cranium shape. The therapist may use the cranial index ratio or a caliper measurement of the widest transverse diameter of the head over the length of the head, or document visual observation of cranial shape and asymmetry. Preterm infants typically do not have sufficient strength for full cervical rotation; therefore, they often spend prolonged periods of time with the head in a side-lying, weight-bearing position. With the weight of the head and the pressure of gravity, the infant's lateral surface of the skull may become bilaterally flattened.[58] This cranial shape is called *dolichocephaly*. Infants in the NICU may develop an asymmetrical cranial shape, such as *plagiocephaly*, or symmetrical posterior flattening termed *brachycephaly*. In 2017, McCarty et al[63] reported that the use of a commercial midliner positioning system in the NICU was associated with decreased dolichocephaly. The NICU therapist examination includes determining the need for

TABLE 5-5 • Standardized Neonatal Assessment Tools

Testing Tool	Authors	Purpose	Age	Time to Administer	Description	Training
Neurological Assessment of Preterm and Full-Term Infants (NAPFI)	Dubowitz V and Dubowitz L	To record and document the functional state of the nervous system or the preterm infant's maturation and recovery from perinatal insult	Preterm and full-term infants	15 minutes	Assessment of behavioral state, neurobehavior, posture, movement, muscle tone, and reflexes with passive manipulation. Emphasis on the patterns of responses. Testing is not quantified or compared with normative age expectations over time.	Requires minimal training and experiences. Items within the area of expertise of developmental therapists.
Neurobehavioral Assessment of the Preterm Infant (NAPI)	Korner AAF and Thom VA	To assess infant maturation, monitor progress, and detect delays in development and any neurologically atypical performance	32-42 weeks' postconceptual age	45 minutes	Assessment of state of alertness, behavior, reflexes, motor patterns, and muscle tone. Many items overlap with other assessments, and infants are assessed during states of rousing, soothing, and alerting.	Training video available with manual. Testing may be used by any professional caring for infants within a neonatal intensive care unit (NICU) environment.
Neonatal Behavioral Assessment Scale (NBAS)	Brazleton TB and Nugent J	To assess the infant's contributions to the interactional process	36-44 weeks' gestational age	30-45 minutes to administer and 15-20 minutes to score	Consists of 28 behavioral items and 18 reflexive items. The sequence of administration is flexible, and the examiner may choose to elicit the infant's best performance for recording of behavior or motor response.	Training requires a reliability administration for scoring. Trainees complete a 4-phase process consisting of self-study, skills assessment, and practice on 25 infants before completing the certification session.
Newborn Behavioral Observation System (NBO)	Nugent JK, Keefer CH, Minear S, Johnson LC, and Blanchard Y	This observational tool is not an examination or assessment but an infant-focused, family-centered tool designed to sensitize parents to their infant's competencies and individuality for promotion of positive infant-parent interactions	Birth through 3 months of life	Dependent on parent observations and their understanding of the behaviors as they pertain to their infant's developmental needs	Consists of 18 neurobehavioral observations, which describe the newborn's capacities and behavioral adaptations.	Training is a 2-day program. Participants are exposed to current research on neurobehavioral development and early parent-child relationships. Then using film and/or live demonstrations, the workshop introduces participants to the kinds of observational strategies necessary to identify newborn behavioral patterns and how to use the NBO as a way of sensitizing parents to the competencies and individuality of their newborn.

(Continued)

TABLE 5-5 · Standardized Neonatal Assessment Tools (*Continued*)

Testing Tool	Authors	Purpose	Age	Time to Administer	Description	Training
Assessment of Preterm Infant Behavior (APIB)	Als H, Lester BM, Tronick EZ, and Brazelton TB	To assess the individual premature infant's behavioral organizational repertoire	Preterm infants	30-45 minutes; scoring may be labor intensive	Focuses on the preterm infant's behavioral and motor responses as in the NBAS. Assesses the preterm infant's physiologic, motoric, and attentional/interactive capabilities, state of alertness, and self-regulation.	Requires extensive training in assessment of preterm infants as well as human development.
NICU Network Neurobehavioral Scale (NNNS)	Lester BM and Tronick EZ	To assess neurologic integrity and behavioral functioning of preterm and high-risk infants	34-46 weeks' postconceptional age	30 minutes	Testing tool draws on NBAS, NAPI, APIB, Neurologic Examination of the Full-Term Newborn Infant, and the Neurological Examination of the Maturity of Newborn Infants. Items are grouped in packages and then presented depending on the infant's state of alertness within that sequence.	Requires certification through a 2- to 5-day training program with certified instruction. Practice and administration of the test are with instruction and in the learner's own clinical environment. Training is dependent on the learner's experience level.
General Movements Assessment (GMA)	Einspieler C, Pretchl HF, Boss AF, Ferrari F, and Cioni G	To assess early signs of brain dysfunction using qualitative measures	36 weeks to 4 months postconceptional age	1 hour for initial videotape and up to 15-30 minutes for follow-up videos plus time for analysis of video recordings	Infants are videotaped, and an observational analysis of the infant's movements are reviewed and scored for variety, fluidity, elegance, and complexity of performance. Video recording and analysis are completed longitudinally.	Two-day training required for basic principles. Practice of 100 video recordings is required to become a skilled observer. Training videos are available and demonstrate qualitative aspects of movement.
Test of Infant Motor Performance (TIMP)	Campbell SK, Girolamo G, Oston E, and Lenke M	To identify motor delay in infants before 4 months of corrected age	34 weeks' gestation to 4 months postterm	15-30 minutes	Consists of 13 observed items focusing on midline alignment, selective control, and quality of movement; 29 elicited items focusing on antigravity postural control elicited by handling typically experienced by the infant.	Workshops or self-study courses provided with online cloud videos for assessment training.
Alberta Infant Motor Scale (AIMS)	Piper M and Darrah J	To identify gross motor delays for newborns through 18 months of age	0-18 months	10-15 minutes	Observational assessment of 58 gross motor postures and transitional patterns in supine, prone, sitting, and standing.	No training required. Recommended for use by professionals with a background in infant motor development.

TABLE 5-6 • Neonatal Behavioral Assessment Scale

State 1	Deep sleep	Eyes closed, regular respirations, no active movements
State 2	Light sleep	Eyes closed, rapid eye movements, small motor movements, no gross body movements
State 3	Drowsy	Eyes open or closed, quiet, diffuse movements but no gross motor movements
State 4	Alert	Eyes open, gross movement, not crying, able to focus on stimulation, taking in information
State 5	Active awake	Eyes open/closed, infant awake/ aroused, fussy but not crying, not taking in information
State 6	Crying	Intense cry

Source: Brazelton TB. Neonatal Behavioral Assessment Scale. Clinics in Developmental Medicine No. 50. Spastics International Medical Publications. J.B. Lippincott Co.; 1973.

supportive boundaries within incubators to promote physiologic flexion posture and the inclusion of varied (including midline) positioning of the head to support skull shaping in the premature infant.

MUSCLE TONE, MOTOR PATTERNS, AND REFLEXES

The motor activity of an infant admitted to the NICU is a crucial part of the physical therapist's examination. Assessment of the preterm infant's resting posture, passive and active muscle tone, and reflexive motor patterns are a few of the components of the neurologic presentation of the infant. The Dubowitz Neurological Examination of the Preterm and Full Term Infant provides the physical therapist with a developmental framework for the assessment of reflexes, muscle tone, and motor patterns in relation to the gestational week of the infant.[64,65] As gestational maturation occurs, primitive reflex patterns emerge, muscle tone and physiologic flexion develop, and active motor patterns

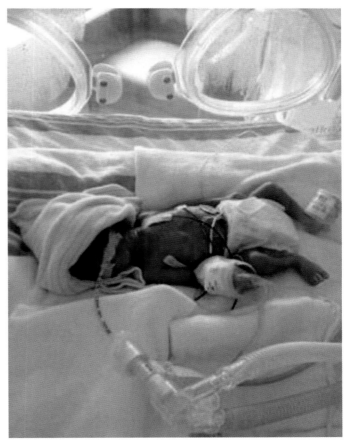

FIGURE 5-10 **Premature infant resting posture with gestational lower tone compared to term-newborn physiological flexion (all extremities).**

become more purposeful.[64,65] Presentation of tone, reflex patterns, and deep tendon reflexes emerge in the lower extremities and then mature in a caudal-cephalic direction. The preterm infant maturing in the extrauterine environment has immature muscle tone and motor activity and is exposed to gravitational forces. These factors predispose the infant to atypical postural and motoric patterns.[17,60,66]

The infant's presentation of muscle tone, posture, and motor patterns is related to physiologic stability. If an infant is struggling to maintain homeostasis, the resting posture and motor activity will be negatively affected, causing the infant to appear hypotonic or lethargic. The infant's tone and motor patterns may be related to the state of alertness and any previous interactions that may have been stressful. When assessing the infant's posture, tone, and movements, the therapist should first observe the infant at rest or in a drowsy state and then progress to a quiet, alert state.

As an infant awakens and transitions to alert state, the physical therapist examines the volitional and nonvolitional movement patterns. Volitional movements, such as hands to mouth, and flexion and extension patterns are assessed for quality and quantity. Volitional movements are documented by the quality and quantity of the movement pattern, which side, and if the movement is a self-regulatory pattern, warning cue, or stress cue. As the infant is actively moving, the appearance of nonvolitional movement may be observed. These are primitive reflex patterns such as the asymmetrical tonic neck reflex

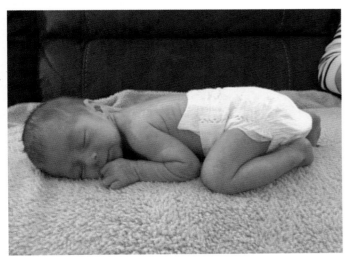

FIGURE 5-9 **Infant in physiologic flexion.**

or rooting reflex. Eliciting a primitive reflex pattern may be too stressful for the premature infant and jeopardize the physiologic stability of the infant. Primitive reflex patterns are best observed when spontaneously produced by the infant and then documented by location and symmetry. Examining muscle tone, motor patterns, and reflex patterns of the premature infant are advanced-level skills regarding administering the procedures and in determining gestational age appropriateness, medical stability, and diagnostic relevance. It is the NICU therapist's role to provide ongoing assessment of the maturational presentation of motor activity in premature infants and recommend referrals for developmental follow-up based on the findings. The motor presentation and maturational development of the infant provide NICU therapists with information regarding discharge recommendations for follow-up programming.

TESTS AND MEASURES

A range of other examination tools are available to the NICU therapist for predictive information about developmental outcomes. These tests and measures offer systematic examination and documentation of infant pain levels and neurobehavioral and neurodevelopmental functioning. The neurobehavioral and neurodevelopmental examination provides objective information to assess an infant's motor function over time, justify the need for developmental intervention, determine intervention outcomes, and identify the need for developmental follow-up and intervention after NICU discharge.[60,67] Tests and measures are available for data collection on pain, neurologic gestational age presentation, and neurobehavioral functioning of the infant.

PAIN ASSESSMENT

An infant's pain level may be identified using multiple tools. The most common scales are the following: Neonatal Infant Pain Scale (NIPS); Neonatal-Pain, Agitation Sedation Scale (N-PASS); Scale of Face, Legs, Activity, Cry, and Consolability (FLACC); and the Crying, Requirement of Oxygen, Increased Vital Signs, Expression, and Sleeplessness (CRIES).[21,60,67-69] For each of the pain scales, documentation includes the infant's facial expression, motor activity, and behavioral state. Assessment of the infant's pain levels prior to, during, and after interventions provides the therapist with information on the infant's ability to tolerate stimuli and function within the environment related to gestational age maturity and medical status.

One tool available to assess the neonate with NAS is the Modified Finnegan scale.[70] This tool provides a comprehensive way to collect objective data on the infant's withdrawal symptoms. The Modified Finnegan is divided into 3 categories of system responsiveness to the opioid withdrawal: (1) central nervous system; (2) metabolic, vasomotor, and respiratory systems; and (3) gastrointestinal and integumentary systems. This tool provides clinicians with objective data about the infant's symptoms of opioid withdrawal.

NEONATAL NEURODEVELOPMENTAL AND NEUROBEHAVIORAL ASSESSMENTS

Assessment tools available for evaluating the preterm infant are individually described in Table 5-5. These tools include

the following: Neurological Assessment of the Preterm and Full-Term Infant (NAPFI); Neurobehavioral Assessment of the Preterm Infant (NAPI); Neonatal Behavioral Assessment Scale (NBAS); Newborn Behavioral Observation System (NBO); Newborn Individualized Developmental Care and Assessment Program (NIDCAP); Assessment of Preterm Infant Behavior (APIB); General Movement Assessment (GMA); Hammersmith Infant Neurological Examination (HINE); and the Test of Infant Motor Performance (TIMP).[21,60,61,67] Training with a mentor is important for the novice NICU therapist to appropriately administer, score, and interpret the results. Administration of the assessments include handling of the infant and determining the infant's ability to tolerate the test administration. If the examination procedures are stressful with marginal tolerance, the results are likely unreliable and require retesting. The neuromotor items (tone, reflexes, and reactions) are often presumed to be benign and yet in a study by Sweeney and Blackburn, they found these neuromotor testing items to be destabilizing in 72 infants.[71] When administering an assessment tool, the therapist must continually evaluate the physiologic and behavioral stability of the infant by observing and respecting the infant's cues and asking, "Is this infant able to tolerate the handling required to complete this assessment?" The physical therapist determines the specific assessment tool as part of the examination, based on the purpose of the examination, medical stability of the infant, and how the information may be used to develop the plan of care and discharge preparation.

In summary, the neonatal examination encompasses an extensive chart review, communication with the NICU team, observational and handling skills of the infant, and administration of assessment tools. The therapists must recognize the stability of the infant, current medical status, postconceptual age, and body systems involvement in relation to diagnoses that may impact the neonatal examination. The physical therapist must synthesize all examination information to determine the strengths, needs, priorities, and developmental expectations of the infant for program development and discharge preparation.

■ NEONATAL PHYSICAL THERAPY INTERVENTION

The advanced practice roles and competencies from the Neonatal Physical Therapy Practice Guidelines provide an important framework for practitioners preparing for NICU clinical practice. Another highly useful guide is an infant care path described by Byrne and Garber.[72] This intervention care path identifies procedures for facilitating a calm state, positioning and handling, movement therapy, and oral motor organization and feeding. Other important neonatal caregiving activities of family education and team collaboration are included in the intervention care path for the NICU. New practitioners are advised to review this care path for both the assessment[73] and intervention[72] components applied to physical therapy in the NICU.

BODY POSITIONING

Consistent, varied body position changes (eg, prone, supine, side lying) are key in supporting body alignment and preventing skull deformity and extremity malalignment. Many positioning aids are available for stabilizing neutral head and trunk alignment and extremity semiflexion while infants remain in incubators. A containment "nest" is commonly constructed with positioning rolls or commercially available neonatal positioner aids to create a cocoon-like environment for the infant inside the incubator. Body swaddling with a blanket inside a containment "nest" facilitated recovery of autonomic and motor stability within 5 minutes of weighing and bathing infants (32-35 weeks of gestation).[74] An important principle in body positioning within "containment boundaries" of a swaddling blanket and "nest" is to provide space for spontaneous movement (**Figure 5-11**). Transition to the supine sleep position on a firm, flat surface in a small crib without positioning aids occurs approximately 2 weeks prior to discharge to prepare infants for a safe sleep environment at home, thereby decreasing risk of SIDS.[75]

Body position after feeding is known to affect gastric emptying and reflux in infants. Infants placed in prone position or in left side-lying position reportedly had decreased reflux.[76] Gastric residual was decreased in the prone and in right side-lying positions,[77] especially when positioned in the first 30 minutes after feeding.[78]

THERAPEUTIC HANDLING

With the current, important emphasis on "brain care" and neuroprotection of preterm infants, the readiness, intensity, sequencing, and duration of neuromotor handling must be guided by each infant's behavioral and physiologic responses and gestational age expectations. Documentation of prehandling physiologic and behavioral baseline status is a critical risk management procedure for determining infant responses. The risk of sensory overload and related physiologic consequences may outweigh potential benefits of sensory and movement experiences. Collaboration with the neonatal nurse is essential to create optimal timing and duration of neuromotor assessment and therapeutic handling, usually 30 minutes before a feeding session.[71]

An aim of therapeutic handling is assisting parents to help infants reach and maintain a quiet, alert behavioral state for maximum visual and auditory interaction. Other aims are facilitating hand-to-mouth movement, spontaneous partial movement of extremities against gravity, and momentary holding of the head in midline.[17]

One handling intervention used by the neonatal physical therapist is facilitated tucking. This therapeutic touch technique by caregivers involves placing their hands over the head and lower body of the infant, offering a constant, moderately deep, touch procedure.

This handling technique may be used to calm an infant or to assist in transition from drowsy to alert behavior. The facilitated tucking procedure may be applied during stressful times such as placement of an intravenous line by nurses. This deep and

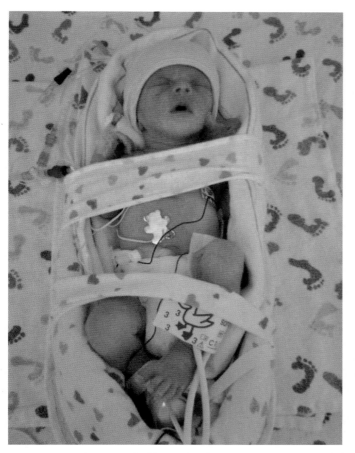 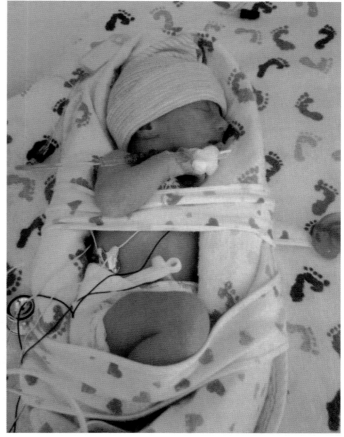

FIGURE 5-11 **Infant nested with positional supports in prone and side lying.**

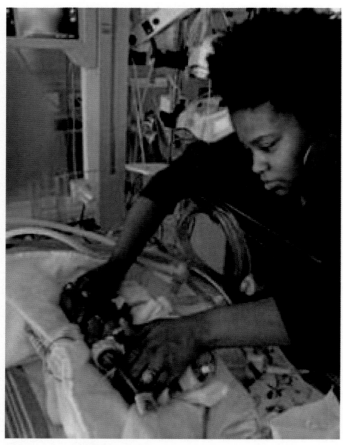

FIGURE 5-12 **Facilitated tucking.**

The epidermis is composed of many layers of stratum corneum, up to 20 layers in full-term infants. Infants born at 24 weeks' gestational age present with only 1 or 2 cellular layers of stratum corneum.[79,80] This lack of epidermal stratum corneum layering decreases the skin integrity. The preterm infant is at a higher risk of an increase in TEWL, which may lead to an increase in evaporation of heat and a state of dehydration. These factors place the infant at risk for skin dehydration, tears, and infections.

The physical therapist plays a role in assessing and treating skin conditions within the NICU. Therapists play a role in monitoring and administering plans of care to decrease skin breakdown due to immobility of the infant and/or equipment needs that may have adverse forces on the skin. Therapists within the NICU must be aware of the advanced areas of skin integrity, skin assessment and wound identification, and application of appropriate wound care products for the premature infant. This practice area is considered an advanced area of practice within the NICU for the physical therapist.

EXTREMITY TAPING AND SPLINTING

The neonatal period is the time of highest plasticity in the infant's musculoskeletal system and therefore the optimal time to address extremity malalignment and positional deformity.[84] Using tape products commonly stocked in the NICU over a foam underwrap layer directly on the infant skin, the neonatal physical therapist with orthopedic expertise can provide expedient management of equinovarus foot deformities (**Figures 5-13** and **5-14**). This management takes advantage of the rapid growth in the newborn infant's skeletal system to

sustained, proprioceptive touch may facilitate a calmness in the infant and reduce excessive motor behavior during the medical intervention. In **Figure 5-12**, the infant's mother is providing facilitated tucking with her medically fragile infant. The handling technique provides the mother with an active role in her infant's care. This intervention increases the mother's ability to bond with her infant as well as participate in the care plan.

NEONATAL SKIN SCIENCE

Neonates present with skin characteristics that assist with adaptation to the extrauterine environment by the presence of an antimicrobial vernix mantle and an epidermis and dermis structured to regulate transepidermal water loss (TEWL) and control the surface pH.[79-83] The premature infant's skin is very thin and immature due to the absence of the stratum corneum layers within the epidermis.

At birth, the skin of a newborn is covered with a white, lipophilic substance that is cheesy in appearance referred to as vernix caseosa. This naturally occurring proteolipid material is produced in late pregnancy. Neonates born at less than 28 weeks' gestational age and less than 1000 grams lack this protective mantle of vernix. The vernix functions to prevent water loss, regulates surface and body temperature, and provides surface protection through immunity. The vernix has an antimicrobial function providing a barrier to acute and subacute infections.[82]

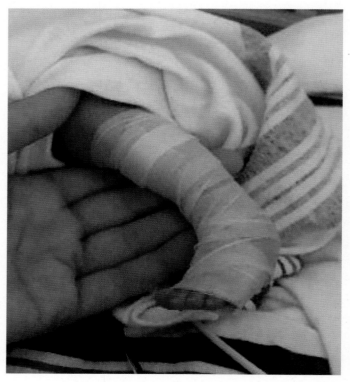

FIGURE 5-13 **Pretaping underwrap foam layer on varus foot and tibia.**

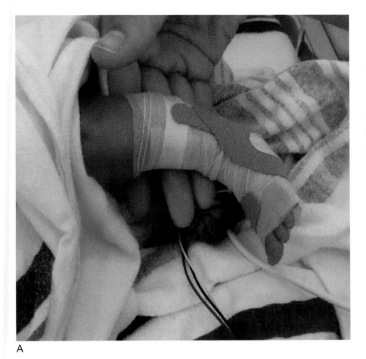
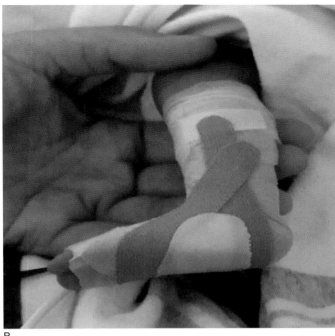

A   B

FIGURE 5-14 **A and B. Lateral stirrup technique for equinovarus foot deformity.**

facilitate correction of deformity when the primary deforming forces are minimized by the taping. Circulatory and dermatologic precautions, physiologic tolerance, behavioral stability, and individualized wearing schedules are emphasized with taping interventions. Infants younger than 32 weeks' corrected age are not considered stable enough for taping procedures. Foot deformity taping in the neonatal period provides initial positional management in preparation for pediatric orthopedist follow-up in the first month after NICU discharge.

Splinting may also be used for promoting postural alignment of an extremity or joint. Products available for splinting often include 1/8-inch-thick polypropylene plastic, moleskin for skin protection, and soft Velcro or a stockinette for securing the splint to an extremity. Gestational age and medical stability must be taken into consideration when determining if a hard splint is indicated for the infant. Splinting may be used to maintain a joint or extremity placed into corrected alignment (**Figures 5-15** and **5-16**). The improved alignment the neonatal physical therapist gently elicits during passive joint movement is the appropriate starting point (alignment) for the splint to support. Because modulated soft tissue stretching is the focus of hard splint application for selected infants in the NICU, daily examination and monitoring are essential for custom fit, alignment, and skin integrity. Scheduled wearing times are created by the patient's needs and influenced by NICU caregiving protocols. The infant's rapid growth may promote realignment quickly but may also increase the risk of skin breakdown.

NEONATAL HYDROTHERAPY

Hydrotherapy for stable neonates was conceptualized and piloted by Sweeney in 1980 for infants with BPD and muscular stiffness (**Figure 5-17**). The therapeutic use of warm water to

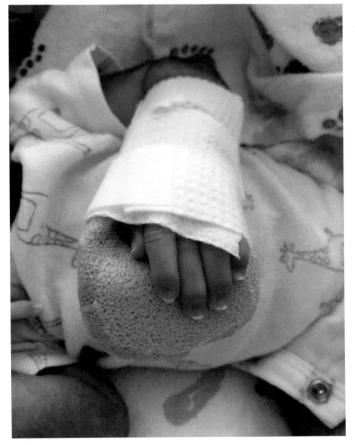

FIGURE 5-15 **Hand splint.**

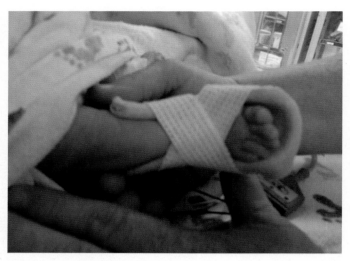

FIGURE 5-16 **Ankle-foot splint.**

facilitate spontaneous movement was also useful for neonates with low muscle tone (Prader-Willi syndrome, trisomy 21/Down syndrome, congenital myopathies, and congenital cardiac defects) and skeletal fragility (osteogenesis imperfecta). Because most infants transition to a quiet, alert behavioral state during the water immersion, a short hydrotherapy session immediately prior to feeding can be strategic in facilitating behavioral readiness for feeding. In a randomized crossover design with 31 preterm infants receiving either hydrotherapy or a rest period before feeding, more efficient feeding (significantly decreased feeding duration) occurred after hydrotherapy. In addition, short-term, increased daily weight gain was present after hydrotherapy.[85]

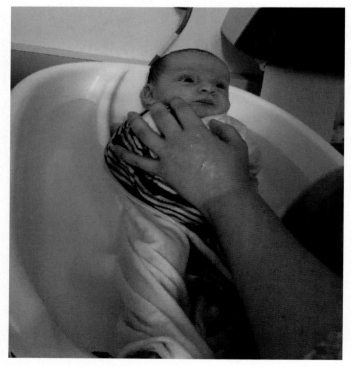

FIGURE 5-17 **Hydrotherapy.**

Hydrotherapy tubs may vary in size, but overhead radiant heat, water temperature to approximately 101°F, and warm receiving towels are recommended to offset hypothermia risk with the procedure. Keeping the infant swaddled before and partially swaddled during the hydrotherapy helps with behavioral and postural stability in the fluid environment. Two caregivers (therapist, nurse, and/or parent) provide head, upper body, and pelvis support for spontaneous and facilitated extremity movement in the buoyant water environment. Agitation of the water, common in athletic hydrotherapy application, is not used with neonates. A floating hot tub thermometer may be useful for continuous monitoring of water temperature. Refer to Sweeney[85] for detailed description of neonatal hydrotherapy procedures.

Risk management considerations for neonatal hydrotherapy involve medical clearance, electronic physiologic monitoring, and calm behavioral state. Resolution of apnea, bradycardia, and temperature instability and discontinued intravenous lines and ventilatory equipment are advised. A portable vital signs monitor can be used with safe immersion of a plastic blood pressure cuff on the distal tibia. Blood pressure and heart rate can be monitored at 2-minute intervals during a 10-minute hydrotherapy session. Range of acceptable vital sign changes during and after hydrotherapy must be determined by the neonatology staff. Pilot data illustrated a 7% increase (mean percent change) from baseline in heart rate and mean arterial pressure during neonatal hydrotherapy.[79] Body swaddling before and during immersion was not implemented and may have modulated the physiologic stress during hydrotherapy.

Behavioral stability is enhanced by immersing the infant with a swaddling blanket and providing a short period of quiet holding without body movement or auditory stimulation to support behavioral adaptation to the warm water. Infants who cry should be removed from the water and comforted with warm towels. The procedure is not therapeutic if infants become destabilized behaviorally or physiologically. Neonatal hydrotherapy research in Brazil indicated improved sleep and behavioral organization[86] and decreased stress (salivary cortisol levels)[87] after 10-minute hydrotherapy sessions with gentle facilitated movement in neonates at 34 to 35 weeks' adjusted age.

Parent participation in swaddled bathing and in swaddled neonatal hydrotherapy can contribute to skill and confidence in bathing activities in the home environment. Because of the multisensory tactile, temperature, and movement stimulation during routine infant bathing, preterm infants are predisposed to sensory overload and behavioral agitation responses. For this reason, early involvement of parents with bathing activities and hydrotherapy can create positive, successful experiences instead of power struggle and sensory overload during infant bathing.

ORAL MOTOR AND FEEDING THERAPY

In advanced practice, the neonatal physical therapist's role incorporates knowledge and competency in oral motor examination and infant feeding.[5] This competency involves assessment of physiologic and behavioral stability and neuromaturation expectations for prefeeding nonnutritive oral stimulation and feeding readiness. Knowledge of varied feeding equipment includes bottle types, nipple flow rates, specialized devices (eg, cleft palate feeding systems), and lactation support aids. Continuous collaboration occurs with lactation consultants, nurses, neonatal dietitians, and neonatologists on feeding procedures, feeding advancement, parent education, and parent competency in infant feeding.

Two oral-motor and feeding assessment instruments commonly used in the NICU are the Neonatal Oral-Motor Assessment Scale (NOMAS)[88] and the Early Feeding Skills (EFS) Assessment for preterm infants.[89,90] The NOMAS is used to examine rate, rhythmicity, jaw excursion, tongue configuration, and tongue movement (timing, direction, and range). Without evaluation of breathing pattern, work of breathing or respiratory exertion, and physiologic variables during feeding, this assessment has limited use in the NICU except for low-risk, healthy neonates.

In contrast, the EFS Assessment can be implemented for a wide range of infants in the NICU. This 36-item observational tool measures oral feeding readiness, feeding skill, and feeding recovery. It includes examination of physiologic and behavioral stability, behavioral feeding readiness cues, oral-motor coordination and endurance, coordination of breathing and swallowing, and postfeeding alertness, energy level, and physiologic state.

To guide neonatal team members and parents in observing infant behavior to direct the feeding process, the Supporting Oral Feeding in Fragile Infants (SOFFI) method has been an important contribution to neonatal feeding practices.[91] The SOFFI method offers a decision-making algorithm for bottle feeding to guide pacing (pausing, restarting, and stopping) of the feeding rather than focusing on volume consumed. The individualized starting and stopping of feedings by caregivers is determined by the infant's physiologic and behavioral responses. Fewer therapy referrals and less trunk arching, gagging, and vomiting with meals were reported in 3- to 5-month corrected-age preterm and term infants when the SOFFI method was used compared to typical NICU feeding methods emphasizing feeding volumes.[92]

Oral motor assessment and feeding trials should not be attempted by physical therapists untrained in current preterm infant feeding approaches and in managing the respiratory and general physiologic monitoring components of neonatal feeding. These competencies are developed in a mentored training program with interdisciplinary feeding experts, infants of varied acuity levels and gestational ages, and parents from diverse cultures.

SKIN-TO-SKIN HOLDING

FCC has been instrumental in offering therapeutic interventions to foster the bonding experience. Skin-to-skin holding or kangaroo care supports the infant-parent bond.[20] The practice of skin-to-skin holding involves placing the infant onto the mother or other designated caregiver's chest and allowing undisrupted prolonged periods of bonding (**Figure 5-18**). The infant is placed prone on the chest, and the parent holds the infant in a flexed posture, with 1 or 2 heated blankets placed

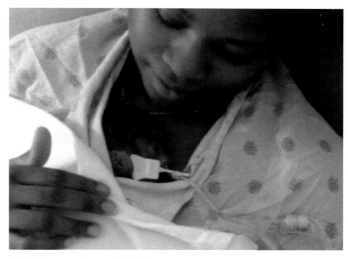

FIGURE 5-18 Skin-to-skin holding.

over the infant. Implementation of skin-to-skin holding may be dependent on the gestational age and medical stability of the infant. Evidence has shown that infants offered skin-to-skin holding demonstrated improved thermoregulation, respirations, and oxygenation; decreased apneic and bradycardic events; improved self-regulatory patterns; and overall decrease in hospital stay.[93,94] Skin-to-skin positioning facilitates milk production and improved breast feeding.[93,94] Another benefit of skin-to-skin holding is the family awareness of the infant's physiologic, behavioral, and motor responses. Parents offered skin-to-skin holding during their infant's NICU admission were reported to be more sensitive to the infant's behavioral cues and felt more prepared to take care of the infant following discharge.[94] The physical therapist can foster skin-to-skin holding in the NICU by discussing benefits with the family and health care team and assisting in monitoring infant neck and body alignment while held.

NEONATAL TEAM ROUNDS

Participation in rounds is another way for the parent to be involved with their infant's plan of care. As part of the developmental care and FCC model, the medical team should invite the family to participate in daily or weekly rounds. Technological advances allow a choice of this bedside rounding including opportunities for the mother and family to utilize telecommunication, especially for the infant transported to another NICU. The bedside rounding is a critical time when the family may learn about their child's medical and developmental progress and prepare for a discharge timeline. Many articles report that parents who have participated in the care of their infant have shown decreased depression rates and improved confidence levels in caring for their infant.[95]

SIBLING SUPPORT

The importance of quality educational programming is important to help ease the stress of the family. The birth of a premature infant is highly stressful and traumatic for the family, specifically the siblings. The NICU sibling often experiences changes within their behavior, such as regression in behaviors, developmental milestones, and communication. The family's daily schedule and the availability of the parents are often disrupted when an infant is admitted to the NICU. Most NICUs offer structured support programming for families, specifically the parents; however, very few offer organized support for siblings. A component of the FCC model is to include the whole family, and yet many NICUs do not allow siblings to visit due to infection risk. In 2016, Sutaria[96] reported in a poster presentation titled "Brothers and Sisters of Infants in the NICUs: Meta-Synthesis" that siblings often experience increased distress and anxiety, regressive behaviors, and a misunderstanding of the medical needs regarding the new sibling. The meta-synthesis reviewed both interventions and qualitative studies that demonstrated the importance and effectiveness of sibling supportive programming in reducing negative behaviors exhibited by the sibling. The challenge is that many NICUs do not address the siblings. As physical therapists, we can play an important role in providing supportive programming to assist in the siblings' understanding and coping with the infant in the NICU.

PALLIATIVE CARE

Physical therapists may have the opportunity to support parents and newborn infants with a life-limiting genetic or medical condition (**Figure 5-19**). With an emphasis on "comfort care," physical therapists can assist parents with creating individualized body positioning strategies and adapting infant equipment (eg, swing, infant seat, bathtub) and bed space to design a calm, comfortable caregiving environment during the hospital stay.

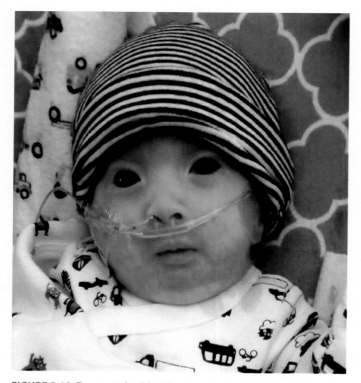

FIGURE 5-19 **Two-month-old with trisomy 18, nasal oxygen, and nasogastric tube for home palliative care.**

Problem-solving assistance on equipment and physical management for short-term caregiving in the home environment can support the parents' goal of taking the baby home, even for a week or month. Working with a palliative care team and grieving families, neonatal therapists have an opportunity to develop and expand qualities of empathy and nonjudgement and contribute to comfort and acceptance rather than striving for developmental advancement.

Neonatal therapists should not miss the opportunity to participate with the palliative care team and nurses in bereavement follow-up care to the family after the baby's death. This follow-up may consist of attending a memorial service, sending a sympathy note with a remembrance of a special attribute of the infant, and contacting the family a year later on the baby's birthday. Bereavement support activities and grief management for NICU team members including neonatal physical therapists are critical for preventing compassion fatigue and for processing the palliative care experience.[97]

TRANSITIONING TO HOME

The happiest time of an NICU family is discharge day. Communication regarding discharge preparation is vital to the family with a child admitted to the NICU. This communication should begin on the admission day by the NICU team assisting the family in understanding and preparing for their infant's individualized care needs. Offering the family diverse opportunities for engagement in their child's daily care needs and providing educational information regarding diagnoses and expectations have shown to improve family stress levels during and after discharge.[98-100] The physical therapist can contribute valuable information regarding the infant's postural needs and motor activities, provide parent education and interactions, and assess the infant for future needs. The physical therapist is able to gather information about the infant's developmental maturation throughout the NICU admission and assess future rehabilitative needs. Information presented to the family by the physical therapist regarding concerns of developmental prognoses assists the family in understanding future concerns and may decrease feelings of anxiety. Various educational methods may be used to assist in the education of parents; examples include combinations of demonstrations, videos, and written materials.

UNIQUE OUTPATIENT SERVICE NEEDS OF NICU GRADUATES

A range of outcomes have been reported in prematurely born infants, including muscle tone changes, developmental delays, and behavioral concerns.[101-105] Appropriate discharge planning and referrals may be directed to interdisciplinary developmental follow-up clinics, federally funded early intervention programs, or direct physical therapy outpatient services. The infant admitted to the NICU may qualify for state or federally funded programs, such as Social Security Administration programs, Medicaid, and/or early intervention programming through the Individuals With Disabilities Education Act (IDEA). Specific diagnoses and/or referral criteria are required for state and federally funded early intervention programming.[101] In most

NICUs, a perinatal social worker assists the family with obtaining authorization for referrals to any agency prior to discharge. The physical therapist provides information regarding the need for direct therapy services for infants at high risk for neurodevelopmental and/or musculoskeletal conditions.

Some NICUs may be associated with a neonatal follow-up clinic. These clinics may offer an interdisciplinary approach to assessing the NICU graduate. The NICU follow-up health care team often includes a developmental pediatrician and/or neonatologist, nutritionist, social worker, physical therapist, occupational therapist and/or speech-language pathologist, child psychologist, and other specialists in child development. Neonatal follow-up clinics often gather outcome data for the NICU team. This information assists the team in developing, altering, and changing current interventions based on the outcomes of the NICU graduate. The NICU follow-up programs may also determine the need for developmental intervention, either individualized therapy services or state-funded early intervention programming. Infants spending prolonged time in a NICU environment are at high risk for developmental delays or disabilities.

Physical therapists bring a unique strength to NICU follow-up programming by providing expertise in movement analysis, musculoskeletal alignment, and developmental expectations consistent with gestational age. These advanced skills assist the NICU team in identifying developmental concerns and referral needs. The therapist offers specialized understanding of movement patterns and the identification of motor changes over time that may indicate the need for further intervention. The referral for direct, individualized services may be recommended for physical, occupational, and/or speech-language services immediately following discharge. Clinical conditions that warrant a referral for direct rehabilitative services may be those diagnoses that present with a documented high risk for developmental concerns, such as a suspected acute brain injury, an abnormal cranial ultrasound, atypical systems examination, or any diagnosis with an associated risk of brain dysfunction or skeletal deformity.[104] The objective of discharge preparation is to provide the family with information regarding their infant's current musculoskeletal, neurodevelopmental, and neurobehavioral functioning, thereby reinforcing the importance of the referral to direct rehabilitative services.

■ OUTCOMES IN THE PREMATURE HIGH-RISK POPULATION

Prematurity is reported as a significant cause of infant morbidity and mortality; however, over the past 20 years, a steady decrease has occurred in the premature death rate.[102-105] Improvement is directly related to advanced resuscitation and pharmacologic agents, such as surfactant replacement therapy and supplemental oxygenation and ventilation.[106] As the gestational age is pushed younger and younger, the preterm infants born at 22 to 23 weeks' gestation continue to present with neurodevelopmental and neurobehavioral concerns.

As discussed, survival of extremely preterm infants has dramatically increased over time, resulting in an increased number of surviving infants with long-term neurodevelopmental delay.

Some of the disease processes have an identified impairment. Infants with IVH and PVL may exhibit spastic hemiplegia or diplegia and cerebral palsy,[25] infants with HIE can have feeding and speech impairments due to bulbar involvement,[106] infants with detached retinas are blind due to ROP,[35] and infants with chronic lung disease have a marked increased risk for asthma, limited pulmonary reserve, and cognitive deficits.[42] Because infants are exposed to many different events after they are born, such as noxious stimuli, pain, disrupted sleep/wake cycles, too much or too little stimulation, parental deprivation, and medications, it is difficult to identify which specific disease processes and environmental factors lead to abnormal brain development and neurodevelopmental delays. Therefore, long-term neurodevelopmental outcomes are likely related to a compilation of all prenatal, perinatal, and neonatal insults and deprivations.

The Bayley Scales of Infant Development (BSID) are the most frequently used assessments for long-term neurodevelopmental outcomes, usually at around 2 years of age. This scale was first published in 1969, revised in 1993 (BSID-II), and again revised in 2006 (BSID-III). This assessment tool evaluates infants from 1 month to 42 months and is administered by sub-specialist pediatric professionals. The postmenstrual age (gestational age at birth plus chronological age) is used for preterm infants to account for prematurity until the infant is between 2 and 3 years old. The BSID-II has 4 subscales (cognitive, language, gross motor, and fine motor), whereas the BSID-III has 6 subscales (expressive and receptive language, cognitive, gross and fine motor development, and social-emotional development). A concern is reported that the BSID-III overestimates the developmental status and underestimates the incidence of developmental delay.[107] When children born prematurely are evaluated at school age, a variety of other assessments tools are used to evaluate language skills, mathematical ability, more complex tasks, and higher executive functioning.

Outcomes of extremely preterm infants assessed at 18 to 30 months of age with the BSID have been published from many countries with relatively consistent findings.[28,108-111] Approximately 50% of infants born at or under 27 weeks' gestation and surviving to 2 years had neurodevelopmental or motor impairment. Significant language delays were present in less than 20% of this population, and cognitive difficulties were found in a little over 10%. Motor impairments were identified in 15%, with 7% of the infants diagnosed with cerebral palsy. Infants born at 27 to 31 weeks' gestation were more likely to survive to 2 years with minimal deficits (15%), whereas only 2% of term infants displayed neurodevelopmental impairments.[115] At school age, less than 40% of children born at under 27 weeks' gestation had a normal IQ, with the average IQ score more than 15 points below that of children born at term.[112] In addition, one-third of these infants at school age had cognitive delay in working memory, verbal comprehension, processing speed, and reasoning, whereas two-thirds of the infants were found to be functioning within normal range. In a cohort of surviving children born under 27 weeks' gestation tested at both 2 and 6 years of age, two-thirds had only mild or no delay. Approximately a quarter of the children demonstrated improvement in cognitive outcome, whereas one-third of the children had worse outcomes, probably related to emphasis on higher skills such as executive functioning.[109,112]

Children with younger gestational ages at birth had increased risk for moderate to severe disability over time. Although neurodevelopmental testing at a corrected age of 2 years identifies children at risk for developmental delay, ongoing assessments are needed as these children approach school age for referral and enrollment in pediatric therapy and school assistance to maximize development.

■ CONCLUSION

The NICU is an environment with striking evolutionary changes and ongoing medical and technological advances. In addition, the expanded knowledge and understanding of physiologic systems of infants born as early as 23 weeks' gestation have transformed the range and effectiveness of interventions implemented by neonatal teams for fragile infants. The physical therapist must have advanced knowledge of the equipment, environment, and medical approaches provided for the care of these extremely vulnerable babies and their families. Providing collaborative care with the family has contributed positively to the neurobehavioral and neurodevelopmental outcomes of the infant and family. Physical therapists have an important role in promoting developmentally appropriate interventions, offering carefully modulated, physiologically supportive therapeutic interventions and facilitating an environment where families are actively involved in their infants' care in preparation for the long-awaited discharge to home. Neonatal physical therapists are privileged to participate in rewarding, pivotal experiences collaborating with parents to support and maximize dramatic developmental changes as the infants stabilize, grow, and thrive.

Case 1

An infant is born at 29.2 weeks' gestational age and weighing 850 g at the local women and children's hospital in a suburban community. She is currently on an overhead warmer bed in a humidified environment and receiving cardiopulmonary monitoring, supplemental high-flow oxygen, and phototherapy. She has an umbilical line for fluids and pharmacologic therapies as well as an oral gastric tube for breastmilk feedings. Her parents are at the bedside participating in discussion of their daughter's medical plan of care.

1. The hospital neonatal intensive care unit (NICU) would most likely have which level of NICU designation?
   a. Level IA
   b. Level IIA
   c. Level IIB
   d. Level IIIB

2. The family participating at the bedside in their daughter's medical plan of care would represent which of the following care models?
   a. Medical model
   b. Patient- and family-centered care (PFCC)
   c. Early intervention model
   d. Individuals With Disability Educational Act (IDEA)

Case 2

An infant is born at 29.2 weeks' gestational age and weighing 850 g at the local women and children's hospital in a suburban community. She is currently on an overhead warmer bed in a humidified environment. She is receiving supplemental high-flow oxygen after one dose of beractant. She is positioned in the supine position or positioned supine with eyes closed and a grimace facial expression. Her postural activity presents with trunk arching, left upper extremity shoulder flexion, elbow extension, and the hand displayed in a "stop" sign presentation. Her oxygenation saturation drops to 80% during this motor behavior. The bedside nurse increases her supplemental oxygen from 21% FiO_2 to 30% FiO_2 with an increase in the infant's oxygenation saturation increasing to 95%.

1. Which neonatal state classification is this infant exhibiting?
   a. State 3/drowsy
   b. State 1/deep sleep
   c. State 5/active awake state
   d. State 6/agitated

Case 3

An infant boy is born to a 34-year-old G2P2 mother with pregnancy-induced hypertension (PIH) and signs and symptoms of preeclampsia. Mother had consistent prenatal care. The infant was born by emergent cesarean section at 30 weeks' gestation weighing 1000 g (2 lb, 2 oz). The infant's Apgar scores were 6 at 1 minute of age and 7 at 5 minutes of age. He is currently 7 days old and in an incubator within a temperature-controlled environment. He is on cardiopulmonary monitoring and requires continuous positive airway pressure (CPAP) and supplemental oxygen of 4 L/min at 32% FiO_2. His cranial ultrasound showed bilateral Grade III intraventricular hemorrhage (IVH). He is positioned in supine with eyes closed, head rotated to the right, and both upper and lower extremities abducted and externally rotated away from his body. His vital signs are stable.

1. What are *all* the facts in the above case scenario's history that a therapist would include in their rehabilitation evaluation's medical history?
   a. Infant's gestational age, birth weight, Apgar scores, and the mother's age and maternal (mother's) prenatal diagnoses
   b. Infant's gestational age, birth weight, Apgar scores, current medical diagnoses, and respiratory support
   c. Infant's gestational age, mother's age, prenatal medical diagnoses, and type of birth
   d. Infant's gestational age, birth weight, Apgar score, day of life of infant, medical diagnoses, and current respiratory support, as well as the mother's age and maternal prenatal diagnoses

Case 4

An infant boy is born at 35 weeks' gestational age and weighing 1500 g (3 lb, 3 oz). He is age 21 days of life and is in an open crib. He is on cardiopulmonary monitoring and (CPAP) of 5 mL water and supplemental oxygen at 32%. He is swaddled in a blanket and positioned in side lying with eyes open and both upper and lower extremities tucked into flexion at midline. He has positional supports nesting him cephalocaudally into facilitated tucked position. He is rooting and mouthing on his hands. His vital signs have been stable, and his Neonatal Infant Pain Scale score is 2/7. Small movements of both upper and lower extremities are noted within the swaddling blanket. You are preparing this infant for an intervention of oral (bottle) feeding.

1. In this case scenario, the therapist would want to document what type of information about the infant prior to, during, and after the intervention?

   a. Document the positioning posture and any positional supports the infant requires, the infant's pain level, heart rate (HR), respiratory rate (RR), oxygen saturation (SaO_2), alert state(s), motor patterns, and behavioral cues.

   b. Document the positioning posture and any positional supports the infant requires.

   c. Document the vital signs of the infant: HR, RR, and SaO_2 only.

   d. Document the infant's pain level, HR, RR, SaO_2, alert state(s), motor patterns, and behavioral cues.

STUDY QUESTIONS

1. In the Synactive Theory of Development, which is the correct maturational order of the hierarchical set of behaviors seen in neonates?

   a. Physiological, Motor, Alertness, Interaction, Self-Regulation

   b. Alertness, Physiological, Motor, Interaction, Self-Regulation

   c. Alertness, Physiological, Interaction, Motor, Self-Regulation

   d. Physiological, Alertness, Motor, Interaction, Self-Regulation

2. Infants born preterm may be designated by which of the following terms?

   a. Gender, ethnicity, and medical stability

   b. Gestational age, birth weight and size

   c. Gestational age, gender, and ethnicity

   d. Gender, ethnicity, and birth weight

3. An infant born between 34 and 37 weeks' gestational age may be referred to as premature; however, the best descriptive term for this GA is which of the following?

   a. Small for gestational age (SGA)

   b. Late preterm infant (LPI)

   c. Appropriate for gestational age (AGA)

   d. Low birth weight (LBW)

4. Which behavioral cues may an infant present with to relay to the caregiver "I am ready for intervention"?

   a. Finger splay, salute sign

   b. Fisting or clasping hands and feet

   c. Gaze aversion and shifting to drowsy state

   d. Smooth body motions and quiet alert state

5. A physical therapy interaction with an infant in the NICU should be timed with the bedside nursing care of that infant. This is referred to as what type of care?

   a. Individualized patient care

   b. Cluster care

   c. Family centered care

   d. Cue based care

6. The following characteristics are expected in examination of infants with Neonatal Opiate Withdrawal Syndrome EXCEPT

   a. Irritability

   b. Lethargy

   c. Tremulousness

   d. Inconsolability

7. The positioning intervention of body swaddling with a blanket is expected to inhibit which of the following in the baby with opiate withdrawal?

   a. Extremity flexor tone

   b. Conscious attention to a task or object

   c. Hand-to-mouth movement

   d. Smooth coordinated movements

8. Which clinical tool was developed to score and document symptoms of Neonatal Abstinence Syndrome ?

   a. Brazelton Neonatal Behavioral Assessment Scale

   b. Test of Infant Motor Performance

   c. Modified Finnegan Scale

   d. Hammersmith Neonatal Neurological Examination

9. Which positional foot deformity is common in neonates and responsive to extremity taping in the NICU after reaching corrected gestational age of 32 weeks?

   a. Pes planus

   b. Equino varus

   c. Equino valgus

   d. Rocker bottom foot

10. Which of the following adverse effects is the LEAST likely to occur in neonates receiving hydrotherapy in the NICU?

    a. Epidermal infection

    b. Hypothermia

    c. Fatigue

    d. Increased blood pressure

References

1. Heriza C, Lunnen K, Fischer, J, Harris M. Pediatric practice in physical therapy: a survey. *Phys Ther.* 1983;63:948-956.
2. Sweeney JK, Heriza C, Markowitz R. The changing profile of pediatric physical therapy: a ten year analysis of clinical practice. *Pediatr Phys Ther.* 1994;6(3):113-118.
3. Scull S, Diets J. Competencies for the physical therapist in the neonatal intensive care unit (NICU). *Pediatr Phys Ther.* 1989;1:11-14.
4. Sweeney JK, Heriza CB, Reilly MA, Smith C, Van Sant AF. Practice guidelines for the physical therapist in the neonatal intensive care unit (NICU). *Pediatr Phys Ther.* 1999;11:119-132.
5. Sweeney JK, Heriza CB, Blanchard Y. Neonatal physical therapy. Part I: clinical competencies and neonatal intensive care unit clinical training models. *Pediatr Phys Ther.* 2009;21:296-307.
6. Sweeney JK, Heriza CB, Blanchard Y, Dusing SC. Neonatal physical therapy. Part II: practice frameworks and evidence-based practice guidelines. *Pediatr Phys Ther.* 2010;22:3-16.
7. Rapport MJ, Sweeney JK, Dannemiller L, Heriza CB. Student experiences in the neonatal intensive care unit: addendum to neonatal physical therapy competencies and clinical training models. *Pediatr Phys Ther.* 2010;22:439-440.
8. Sweeney JK, Chandler LS. Neonatal physical therapy: medical risks and professional education. *Infant Young Child.* 1990;2(3):59-68.
9. American Board of Physical Therapy Residency and Fellowship Education. Accessed March 25, 2019. www.abptrfe.org/home.aspx.
10. Steiner WA, Liliane R, Huber E, Uebelhart D, Aeschlimann A, Stucki G. Use of the ICF model as a clinical problem-solving tool in physical therapy and rehabilitation medicine. *Phys Ther.* 2002;82(11):1098-1107.
11. Malusky SK. A concept analysis of family-centered care in the NICU. *Neonatal Netw.* 2005;24(6):25-32.
12. Institute for Patient and Family Centered Care. Principles of the FCC model. Accessed January 2018. www.ipfcc.org.
13. Als H. Toward a Synactive Theory of development: promise for the assessment and support of infant individuality. *Infant Ment Health J.* 1982;3(4):229-243
14. White Z, Gilstrap C, Hull J. "Me against the world": parental uncertainty management at home following neonatal intensive care unit discharge. *J Fam Commun.* 2017;17(2):105-116.
15. Hagen IH, Iversen VC, Nesset E, et al. Parental satisfaction with neonatal intensive care units: a quantitative cross-sectional study. *BMC Health Services Res.* 2019;19:37.
16. Cleveland LM. Parenting in the neonatal intensive care unit. *J Obstet Gynecol Neonatal Nurs.* 2008;37(6):666-691.
17. Sweeney JK, Gutierrez T, Beachy JC. Neonates and parents: neurodevelopmental perspectives in the NICU and follow-up. In: Umphred D, Lazaro RT, Roller ML, Burton GU, eds. *Umphred's Neurological Rehabilitation.* 6th ed. Mosby/Elsevier; 2013:271-316.
18. Als H. A Synactive model of neonatal behavioral organization: framework for the assessment and support of the neurobehavioral development of the premature infant and his parents in the environment of the neonatal intensive care unit. *Phys Occup Ther Pediatr.* 1986;6(3-4):3-55.
19. Als H, Lawhon G, Duffy FH, McAnulty GB, Gibes-Grossman R, Blickman JG. Individualized developmental care for the very low birthweight infant: medical and neurofunctional effects. *JAMA.* 1994;272(11):853-858.
20. Als H, Gikerson L. Developmental supportive care in the neonatal intensive care unit: zero to three. *Curr Opin Pediatr.* 1995;15(6):1-10.
21. Als H, Butler S, Kosta S, McAnulty G. The assessment of preterm infants' behavior (APIB): furthering the understanding and measurement of neurodevelopmental competence in preterm and full-term infants. *Ment Retard Dev D R.* 2005;11(1):94-102.
22. American Academy of Pediatrics. Policy statement, levels of neonatal care. *Pediatrics.* 2012;130(3):587-597.
23. Committee on Obstetric Practice, American Institute of Ultrasound in Medicine, and the Society for Maternal-Fetal Medicine. Committee Opinion No 700: Methods for Estimating the Due Date. *Obstet Gynecol.* 2017;129:e150-e154.
24. Ballard JL, Khoury JC, Wedig K, et al. New Ballard Score, expanded to include extremely premature infants. *J Pediatr.* 1991;119:417-423.
25. Volpe JJ. Intracranial hemorrhage: germinal matrix-intraventricular hemorrhage of the preterm infant. In: Volpe JJ, Inder TE, Darras BT, et al, eds. *Neurology of the Neonate.* Elsevier; 2017:591-698.
26. Bassan H. Intracranial hemorrhage in the preterm infant: understanding it, preventing it. *Clin Perinatol.* 2009;36:737-762.
27. Srinivasakumar P, Limbrick D, Munro R, et al. Posthemorrhagic ventricular dilatation-impact on early neurodevelopmental outcome. *Am J Perinatol.* 2013;30:207-214.
28. Adams-Chapman I, Hansen NI, Stoll BJ, et al. Neurodevelopmental outcome of extremely low birth weight infants with posthemorrhagic hydrocephalus requiring shunt insertion. *Pediatrics.* 2008;121:1167-1177.
29. Woodward LJ, Anderson PJ, Austin NC, et al. Neonatal MRI to predict neurodevelopmental outcomes in preterm infants. *N Engl J Med.* 2006;355:685-694.
30. Limperopoulos C, Bassan H, Gauvreau K, et al. Does cerebellar injury in premature infants contribute to the high prevalence of long-term cognitive, learning, and behavioral disability in survivors? *Pediatrics.* 2007;120:584-593.
31. American College of Obstetricians and Gynecologists. *Neonatal Encephalopathy and Cerebral Palsy: Defining the Pathogenesis and Pathophysiology.* American College of Obstetricians and Gynecologists; 2003:1-8.
32. Chau V, Poskitt KJ, Miller SP. Advanced neuroimaging techniques for the term newborn with encephalopathy. *Pediatr Neurol.* 2009;40:181-188.
33. Shankaran S, Pappas A, McDonald SA, et al. Childhood outcomes after hypothermia for neonatal encephalopathy. *N Engl J Med.* 2012;366:2085-2092.
34. Torr C, Yoder B, Beachy J. Assessing the surgical experience to identify risk factors associated with severe retinopathy of prematurity and laser intervention. *Neonatology.* 2018;114:230-234.
35. Wheatley CM, Dickinson JL, Mackey DA, et al. Retinopathy of prematurity: recent advances in our understanding. *Br J Ophthalmol.* 2002;86:696-700.
36. Fierson WM. American Academy of Pediatrics Section on Ophthalmology, American Academy of Ophthalmology, American Association for Pediatric Ophthalmology, Strabismus, American Association of Certified Ophthalmology. Screening examination of premature infants for retinopathy of prematurity. *Pediatrics.* 2013;131:189-195.
37. Whisett JA, Pryhuber GS, Wert S. Acute respiratory disorders. In: MacDonald MG, ed. *Avery's Neonatology: Pathophysiology and Management of the Newborn.* Wolters Kluwer; 2016:397-415.
38. Doyle LW, Ehrenkranz RA, Halliday HL. Early (< 8 days) postnatal corticosteroids for preventing chronic lung disease in preterm infants. *Cochrane Database Syst Rev.* 2014;CD001146.

39. Doyle LW, Ehrenkranz RA, Halliday HL. Late (> 7 days) post-natal corticosteroids for chronic lung disease in preterm infants. *Cochrane Database Syst Rev.* 2014;CD001145.

40. Renault A, Patkai J, Dassieu G, et al. Hydrocortisone use in ven-tilated extremely preterm infants decreased bronchopulmonary dysplasia with no effects on neurodevelopment after two years. *Acta Paediatr.* 2016;105:1047-1055.

41. Adams-Chapman I, Heyne RJ, DeMauro SB, et al. Neurodevel-opmental impairment among extremely preterm infants in the neonatal research network. *Pediatrics.* 2018;141:e20173091.

42. Donn SM. Bronchopulmonary dysplasia: myths of pharmaco-logic management. *Semin Fetal Neonatal Med.* 2017;22:354-358.

43. Hintz SR, Kendrick DE, Stoll BJ, et al. Neurodevelopmental and growth outcomes of extremely low birth weight infants after necrotizing enterocolitis. *Pediatrics.* 2005;115:696-703.

44. Rees CM, Pierro A, Eaton S. Neurodevelopmental outcomes of neonates with medically and surgically treated necrotiz-ing enterocolitis. *Arch Dis Child Fetal Neonatal Ed.* 2007;92: F193-198.

45. Wiles JR, Isemann B, Ward LP, et al. Current management of neonatal abstinence syndrome secondary to intrauterine opioid exposure. *J Pediatr.* 2014;165:440-446.

46. Finnegan LP, Kron RE, Connaughton JF, et al. Assessment and treatment of abstinence in the infant of the drug-dependent mother. *Int J Clin Pharmacol Biopharm.* 1975;12:19-32.

47. Ornoy A, Michailevskaya V, Lukashov I, et al. The developmen-tal outcome of children born to heroin-dependent mothers, raised at home or adopted. *Child Abuse Negl.* 1996;20:385-396.

48. Ornoy A, Segal J, Bar-Hamburger R, Greenbaum C. Develop-mental outcome of school-age children born to mothers with heroin dependency: importance of environmental factors. *Dev Med Child Neurol.* 2001;43:668-675.

49. Young SL, Vosper HJ, Phillips SA. Cocaine: its effects on maternal and child health. *Pharmacotherapy.* 1992;12:2-17.

50. Frank DA, Bresnahan K, Zuckerman BS. Maternal cocaine use: impact on child health and development. *Curr Probl Pediatr.* 1996;26:57-70.

51. Grant KS, Petroff R, Isoherranen N, et al. Cannabis use during pregnancy: pharmacokinetics and effects on child development. *Pharmacol Ther.* 2018;182:133-151.

52. Ryan SA, Ammerman SD, O'Connor ME, et al. Marijuana use during pregnancy and breastfeeding: implications for neonatal and childhood outcomes. *Pediatrics.* 2018;142:e20181889.

53. Marcus SM, Flynn HA, Blow F, Barry K. A screening study of antidepressant treatment rates and mood symptoms in preg-nancy. *Arch Womens Mental Health.* 2005;8:25-27.

54. Moses-Kolko EL, Bogen D, Perel J, Bregar A, et al. Neonatal signs after late in utero exposure to serotonin reuptake inhibi-tors: literature review and implications for clinical applications. *JAMA.* 2005;293:2372-2383.

55. Andersen J, Watt J, Olson J, Van Aerde J. Perinatal brachial plexus palsy. *Paediatr Child Health.* 2006;11:93-100.

56. Balasankar G, Luximon A, Al-Jumaily A. Current conservative management and classification of club foot: a review. *J Pediatr Rehabil Med.* 2016;9:257-264.

57. American Academy of Pediatrics Task Force on Sudden Infant Death Syndrome. The changing concept of sudden infant death syndrome: diagnostic coding shifts, controversies regarding the sleeping environment, and new variables to consider in reducing risk. *Pediatrics.* 2005;116:1245-1255.

58. Do TT. Congenital muscular torticollis: current concepts and review of treatment. *Curr Opin Pediatr.* 2006;18:26-29.

59. Harris MH, Welch R. Physical therapy in the neonatal intensive care unit. In: Connolly BH, Montgomery PC, eds. *Therapeutic Exercise for Children With Developmental Disabilities.* 3rd ed. Slack Incorporated; 2005:157-188.

60. Versaw-Barnes D, Wood A. The infant at high risk for develop-mental delay. In: Tecklin JS, ed. *Pediatric Physical Therapy.* 5th ed. Lippincott Williams & Wilkins; 2015:103-186.

61. Dusing SC, Murray T, Stern M. Parent preferences for motor development education in the neonatal intensive care unit. *Pediatr Phys Ther.* 2008;20(4):363-368.

62. Brazelton TB. *Neonatal Behavioral Assessment Scale. Clinics in Developmental Medicine No. 50. Spastics International Medical Publications.* J.B. Lippincott Co.; 1973.

63. McCarty DB, O'Donnell S, Goldstein RF, Smith PB, Fisher K, Malcolm WF. Use of a midliner positioning system for preven-tion of dolichocephaly in preterm infants. *Pediatr Phys Ther.* 2018;30(2):126-134.

64. Dargassies SS. *Neurological Development in the Full-Term and Premature Neonate.* Experta Medica; 1977.

65. Prechtl H, Beintema D. *The Neurological Examination of the Newborn Infant. Clinics in Developmental Medicine.* 12th ed. Heinemann Educational Books; 1964.

66. Nwabara O, Rogers C, Inder T, Pineda R. Early therapy services following neonatal intensive care unit discharge. *Phys Occup Ther Pediatr.* 2007;37(4):414-424.

67. McManus B, Blanchard Y, Dusing S. The neonatal intensive care unit. In: Palisano RJ, Orlin M, Schreiber J, eds. *Campbell's Physical Therapy for Children.* 5th ed. Elsevier; 2017:672-702.

68. Hillman BA, Tabrizi MN, Gauda EB, Carson KA, Aucott SW. The neonatal pain, agitation and sedation scale and the bed-side nurse's assessment of neonates. *J Perinatol.* 2015;35(2): 128-131.

69. O'Neal K, Olds D. Differences in pediatric pain management by unit types. *J Nurs Scholarsh.* 2016;48(4):378-386.

70. Maguire D, Cline GJ, Parnell L, Tai CY. Validation of the Finnegan neonatal abstinence syndrome tool-short form. *Adv Neonatal Care.* 2013;13(6):430-437.

71. Sweeney JK, Blackburn ST. Neonatal physiological and behav-ioral stress during neurological assessment. *J Perinatol Neonat Nur.* 2013;27(3):242-252.

72. Byrne E, Garber J. Physical therapy intervention in the neonatal intensive care unit. *Phys Occup Ther Pediatr.* 2013;33(1):75-110.

73. Byrne E, Campbell SK. Physical therapy observation and assess-ment in the neonatal intensive care unit. *Phys Occup Ther Pedi-atr.* 2013;33(1):39-74.

74. Bembich S, Fiani G, Strajn T, Sanesi C, Demarini S, Sanson G. Longitudinal responses to weighing and bathing procedures in preterm infants. *J Perinatol Neonatal Nurs.* 2017;31(1):67-74.

75. AAP Task Force on Sudden Infant Death Syndrome. SIDS and other sleep-related infant deaths: updated 2016 recommendations for a safe infant sleeping environment. *Pediatrics.* 2016;138(5): e20162938.

76. Ewer AK, James ME, Tobin JM. Prone and left lateral position-ing reduce gastro-oesophageal reflux in preterm infants. *Arch Dis Child Fetal Neonatal Ed.* 1999;81(3):F201-205.

77. Sangers H, de Jong PM, Mulder SE, et al. Outcomes of gastric residuals whilst feeding preterm infants in various body posi-tions. *J Neonatal Nurs.* 2013;19(6):337-341.

78. Chen SS, Tzeng YL, Gau BS, Kuo PC, Chen JY. Effects of prone and supine positioning on gastric residuals in preterm infants: a time series with cross-over study. *Int J Nurs Stud.* 2013;50(11): 1459-1467.

79. Baker SF, Smith BJ, Donohue PK, Gleason CA. Skin care management practices for premature infants. *J Perinatol.* 1999;19:426-431.

80. Blume-Peytavi U, Hauser M, Stamatas GN, et al. Skin care practices for newborns and infants: review of the clinical evidence for best practices. *Pediatr Dermatol.* 2012;28(3):241-254.

81. Afsar FS. Physiological skin conditions of preterm and term neonates. *Clin Exp Dermatol.* 2009;35:346-350.

82. Lund CH, Osborne JW, Kuller J, et al. Neonatal skin care: clinical outcomes of the AWHONN/NANN Evidence-Based Clinical Practice Guideline. Association of Women's Health, Obstetric and Neonatal Nurses and the National Association of Neonatal Nurses. *J Obstet Gynecol Neonatal Nurs.* 2001;30:41-51.

83. Sweeney JK. Neonatal hydrotherapy: an adjunct to developmental intervention in an intensive care nursery setting. *Phys Occup Ther Pediatr.* 1983;3:39-52.

84. Hensinger RN, Jones ET. *Neonatal Orthopedics.* Grune & Stratton; 1981.

85. Sweeney JK. Feeding proficiency in preterm neonates following hydrotherapy in the NICU setting. *Pediatr Phys Ther.* 2003;15(1):63.

86. Vignochi C, Teixeira PP, Nader SS. Effect of aquatic physical therapy on pain and state of sleep and wakefulness among stable preterm newborns in neonatal intensive care units. *Rev Bras Fisioter.* 2010;14:214-220.

87. De Oliveria Tobinaga W, de Lima Marinho C, Barros Abelenda VL, et al. Short-term effects of hydrokinesiotherapy in hospitalized preterm newborns. *Rehabil Res Pract.* 2016;1-8.

88. Braun MA, Palmer MM. A pilot study of oral-motor dysfunction in "at-risk" infants. *Phys Occup Ther Pediatr.* 1985;5:13.

89. Thoyre SM, Shaker CS, Pridham KF. The early feeding skills assessment for preterm infants. *Neonatal Netw.* 2005;24:7-16.

90. Thoyre S, Pados B, Shaker C, Park J, Fuller K. Psychometric properties of the early feeding skills (EFS) assessment tool. *Adv Neonatal Care.* 2018;18(5):E13-E23.

91. Ross ES, Philbin KM. SOFFI: an evidence-based method for quality bottle feedings of preterm, ill, and fragile infants. *J Perinatol Neonatal Nurs.* 2011;25:349-359.

92. Horner S, Simonelli AM, Schmidt H, et al. Setting the stage for successful oral feeding: the impact of implementing the SOFFI feeding program with medically fragile NICU infants. *J Perinatol Neonatal Nurs.* 2014;28(1):59-68.

93. Anderson G. Kangaroo care and breastfeeding for preterm infants. *Breastfeeding Abstr.* 1989;9(20):7.

94. Nunes CR, Campos LG, Lucena AM, et al. Relationship between the use of kangaroo position on preterm babies and mother-child interaction upon discharge. *Rev Paul Pediatr.* 2017;35(2):136-143.

95. Maghaireh DF, Abdullah KL, Chan CM, et al. Systematic review of qualitative studies exploring parental experience in the neonatal intensive care unit. *J Clin Nurs.* 2016;10(19-20):2745-2756.

96. Sutaria P. Brothers and sisters of infants in the neonatal intensive care units: meta-synthesis. *Am J Occup Ther.* 2016;70(suppl 1):7011505133p1.

97. National Association for Neonatal Nurses. Palliative and end-of-life care for newborns and infants. Position statement #3063. February 2015. Accessed April 7, 2019. www.nann.org/aboutposition-statements.

98. O'Brien K, Robson K, Bracht M, et al. Effectiveness of family integrated care in neonatal intensive care units on infant and parent outcomes: a multicenter, multinational, cluster-randomized controlled trial. *Lancet Child Adolesc Health.* 2018;2(4):245-254.

99. Lakshmanan A, Agni M, Lieu T, et al. The impact of preterm birth <37 weeks on parents and families: a cross-sectional study in the 2 years after discharge from the neonatal intensive care unit. *Health Qual Life Out.* 2017;15:38.

100. Dusing SC, Murray T, Stern M. Parent preferences for motor development education in the neonatal intensive care unit. *Pediatr Phys Ther.* 2008;20(4):363-368.

101. Centers for Disease Control and Prevention. What is "early intervention"? Accessed October 18, 2023. https://www.cdc.gov/ncbddd/actearly/parents/states.html#textlinks

102. Glass HC, Costarino AT, Stayer SA, Brett C, Cladis F, Davis PJ. Outcomes for extremely premature infants. *Anesth Analg.* 2015;120(6):1337-1351.

103. Nwabara O, Rogers C, Inder T, Pineda R. Early therapy services following neonatal intensive care unit discharge. *Phys Occup Ther Pediatr.* 2007;37(4):414-424.

104. O'Shea TM, Allred EN, Kuban KC, et al. Intraventricular hemorrhage and developmental outcomes at 24 months of age in extremely preterm infants. *J Child Neurol.* 2012;27(1):22-29.

105. Glass H, Costarino AT, Stayer SA, et al. Outcomes of extremely premature infants. *Anesth Analg.* 2015;120(6):1337-1351.

106. Volpe JJ. Hypoxic ischemic encephalopathy: neuropathology and pathogenesis. In: Volpe JJ, Inder TE, Darras BT, et al, eds. *Neurology of the Neonate.* Elsevier; 2017:232-590.

107. Anderson PJ, De Luca CR, Hutchinson E, Roberts G, Doyle LW, Victorian Infant Collaborative Group. Underestimation of developmental delay by the new Bayley-III Scale. *Arch Pediatr Adolesc Med.* 2010;164:352-356.

108. Pierrat V, Marchand-Martin L, Arnaud C, et al. Neurodevelopmental outcome at 2 years for preterm children born at 22 to 34 weeks' gestation in France in 2011: EPIPAGE-2 cohort study. *BMJ.* 2017;358:j3448.

109. Serenius F, Ewald U, Farooqi A, et al. Neurodevelopmental outcomes among extremely preterm infants 6.5 years after active perinatal care in Sweden. *JAMA Pediatr.* 2016;170:954-963.

110. Synnes A, Luu TM, Moddemann D, et al. Determinants of developmental outcomes in a very preterm Canadian cohort. *Arch Dis Child Fetal Neonatal Ed.* 2017;102:F235-F234.

111. Glass HC, Costarino AT, Stayer SA, Brett C, Cladis F, Davis PJ. Outcomes for extremely premature infants. *Anesth Analg.* 2015;120(6):1337-1351.

112. Serenius F, Kallen K, Blennow M, et al. Neurodevelopmental outcome in extremely preterm infants at 2.5 years after active perinatal care in Sweden. *JAMA.* 2013;309:1810-1820.

Pediatric Acute Care

Jason Benincasa, PT, DPT, EP-C, Emily Berry, PT, DPT,
Jenna Gondelman, PT, DPT, and Lori Solo, PT, DPT

LEARNING OBJECTIVES

Upon completion of this chapter, the reader will be able to:

- Identify the role of physical therapy in the pediatric acute care setting.
- Identify and understand the unique challenges, both medical and physical, presented in the acute care setting.
- Identify elements required for a complete functional history or prior level of function (PLOF).
- Identify important objective information required to determine appropriate discharge environment.
- Identify common precautions and how they may affect the physical therapist's plan of care.

- Identify the clinical presentation of the most common diagnoses encountered in the inpatient pediatric setting.
- Identify appropriate evaluative tests and measures for the most common diagnoses found in the inpatient setting.
- Identify and support with clinical reasoning a variety of therapeutic interventions appropriate for the inpatient setting.
- Identify appropriate measurable goals for the inpatient setting.

■ INTRODUCTION

In the year 2019, there were 5.2 million pediatric hospital admissions reported, with the majority (76.2%) being newborns and infants under the age of one year.[1]

This number includes medical as well as surgical admissions. Respiratory conditions were the primary reason for admissions in children younger than 10 years while mental disorders were the leading reason for admissions for children older than 10 years.[1] These children present with a wide variety of acuity levels—some stable and others having experienced severe trauma or are at high risk of experiencing rapid decompensation.[2] Acuity refers to the level of complexity of health problems that a patient poses and the level of care that the patient requires to address these complexities. Each hospital uses a system they have developed to determine acuity. The number of patients in the hospital and their acuity levels are used to determine medical staffing patterns for each shift.

Given the variety of diagnoses encountered in the acute care setting, the practice of physical therapy can be challenging, but it remains of great importance to the recovery and improved function of a patient. Physical therapy must take place within the confines of the comprehensive care a child in the hospital is receiving. This requires scheduling around competing medical tests and interventions, medication administration, and caregivers are availability for training. The physical therapist (PT) has a responsibility to be familiar with a wide variety of medical diagnoses and interventions. Patients can have changing clinical presentations related to emerging deficits from disease progression or physiologic instability. The acute care PT must be attuned to changes in patient status that may be indicative of a medical emergency or a significant event that affects overall function.

It is in the acute care hospital that many families and patients may first encounter the profession of physical therapy. PTs are an integral part of the inpatient medical team, and their contributions are an important component of a child's medical care. The data collected during an acute care PT evaluation may be used by other medical professions to guide a child's medical course, determine best treatments, educate families, and ultimately determine the best discharge environment for our patients.

MEET THE STAFF: MEMBERS OF THE MULTIDISCIPLINARY TEAM

Within the hospital, there is a primary team of medical providers who serve as the coordinators of a patient's care. Based on the unique needs of the patient, additional staff members may also be consulted. In the inpatient setting, consultative services include physical therapy but can also consist of additional medical teams that are devoted to a specific body system or medical subspecialty. The consult services, together with the primary medical team, the patient, the patient's family, and bedside nurses, provide a multidisciplinary team approach to patient care.

TABLE 6-1 • Members of the Multidisciplinary Team	
Discipline	**Collaboration With Physical Therapy**
Occupational therapy	Provide therapy sessions focused on fine motor function and ADLs. Cotreat with PT to address bed mobility transfers and balance through functional activities.
Speech therapy	Address communication and cognitive issues during changes in position and gross motor tasks. Collaborate to provide suggestions for gross motor–related phrases and symbols to be added to a patient's augmentative communication device or daily schedule. Perform cotreatments with PT as able.
Respiratory therapy	Assist during physical therapy sessions to transition and manage supplemental oxygen supports.
Psychology	Assist with the development of a patient behavior plan to maximize the effectiveness of a session. Cotreatments to help manage patient behaviors and improve compliance to PT-directed tasks.
Child life specialist	Assist with providing structure to a child's daily schedule and encourage PT-related activities outside of sessions. Cotreatments to assist with motivating a patient and improve participation within a session.
Social work	Collaborate to connect a family with PT-related resources in the community. Assist with attaining equipment that may not be covered by insurance.
Case management	Collaborate with PT to determine what durable medical equipment a patient may need for discharge. Schedule home-based PT services. Make a referral for inpatient rehabilitation and schedule transport at discharge as needed.

Abbreviations: ADLs, activities of daily living; PT, physical therapy.

Teaching hospitals are associated with academic programs and participate in the education and training of providers. These hospitals support a commitment to on-site teaching, with various levels of trainees present for the process. The medical team of physicians is arranged as a hierarchy and can include an attending, fellow, resident, intern, and medical student. In a teaching hospital, children and families may encounter large medical teams rounding at their bedside. It is therefore important to understand and identify all of the members in order to provide consistent communication and education. For more information regarding additional members of the multidisciplinary team, please see **Table 6-1**.

CHART REVIEW AND PATIENT AND FAMILY HISTORY

After receiving a physical therapy consult, it is the responsibility of the PT to complete a thorough chart review. In the inpatient setting, a patient is likely presenting with an acute medical condition and/or recovering from a medical or surgical procedure. As a result, there is great importance in understanding how the patient's course of treatment, medications, lab values, and prior medical history have the potential to affect their presentation.

When completing a chart review, the PT should first confirm the details of the physician's orders, which will indicate the patient's diagnosis and the reason for the consult. Next, any pertinent precautions and activity orders should be reviewed. Precautions can include weight-bearing restrictions, range of motion restrictions, recommendations for positioning, and ranges for safe lab values and vital signs. Activity orders can often include a patient's precautions as well as recommendations for activity a patient is cleared to perform, ranging from restricted bedrest to activity as tolerated. The medical chart also provides documentation of vital signs, medications, and lab values that may affect the PT session. The presence of lines and tubes is also documented and should be considered prior to the examination. Understanding the precautions associated with specific lines and tubes and maintaining their integrity during

mobilization is essential. See **Tables 6-2** and **6-3** for normal pediatric lab values. **Tables 6-4**, **6-5**, and **6-6** outline normal pediatric vital signs.

If available, diagnostic imaging, such as radiographs and magnetic resonance imaging (MRI) scans, should also be viewed. This review is important because a patient's physiologic presentation on imaging can potentially affect their presentation during an examination. Finally, reviewing medical notes as well as examinations from fellow members of the multidisciplinary team allows a PT to determine an anticipated medical course of treatment and other aspects of a patient's presentation that may not be addressed by physical therapy. These notes may also indicate important pieces of information regarding a patient's past medical history, history of present illness, social history, and anticipated discharge plan. This may include baseline deficits in strength or cognition or specific documentation regarding functional skills.

TABLE 6-2 • Normal Pediatric Lab Values[3]			
Age	**Hematocrit (%)**	**Hemoglobin (g/dL)**	**Red Blood Cell Count (× 10⁶/μL)**
0-30 days	44-70	15.0-22.0	4.1-6.7
1 month	32-42	10.5-14.0	3.0-5.4
2-6 months	29-41	9.5-13.5	2.7-4.5
7 months-2 years	33-39	10.5-14.0	3.7-5.3
3-6 years	34-40	11.5-14.5	3.9-5.3
7-12 years	35-45	11.5-15.5	4.0-5.2
13-18 years/female	36-45	12.0-16.0	4.1-5.1
13-18 years/male	37-49	13.0-16.0	4.5-5.3
≥19 years/female	36-46	12.0-16.0	4.0-5.4
≥19 years/male	41-53	13.5-17.5	4.7-6.0

Platelet count 150,000-450,000/μL.

TABLE 6-3 • Normal Pediatric White Blood Cell Count[3]

Age	White Blood Cell Count (× 10³/μL)
0-30 days	9.1-34.0
1 month	5.0-19.5
2-11 months	6.0-17.5
1-6 years	5.0-14.5
7-12 years	5.0-14.5
13-18 years	4.5-13.5
≥19 years	4.5-11.0

Reproduced with permission from Gregory GA, Andropoulos DB. Gregory's Pediatric Anesthesia, With Wiley Desktop Edition. John Wiley & Sons; 2012.

TABLE 6-4 • Age-Based Heart Rate Norms[4]

Age	Awake Rate (bpm)	Asleep Rate (bpm)
Neonate	100-205	90-160
Infant	100-180	90-160
Toddler	98-140	80-120
Preschooler	80-120	65-100
School-age child	75-118	58-90
Adolescent	60-100	50-90

TABLE 6-5 • Respiratory Rate Norms[4]

Age	Rate (breaths/min)
Infant	30-53
Toddler	22-37
Preschooler	20-28
School-age child	18-25
Adolescent	12-20

TABLE 6-6 • Blood Pressure Norms[4]

Age	Systolic Pressure (mm Hg)	Diastolic Pressure (mm Hg)	Mean Arterial Pressure (mm Hg)
Birth (12 hours, <1000 g)	39-59	16-36	28-42
Birth (12 hours, 3000 g)	60-76	31-45	48-57
Neonate (96 hours)	67-84	35-53	45-60
Infant (1-12 months)	72-104	37-56	50-62
Toddler (1-2 years)	86-106	42-63	49-62
Preschooler (3-5 years)	89-112	46-72	58-69
School-age child (6-7 years)	97-115	57-76	66-72
Preadolescent (10-12 years)	102-120	61-80	71-79
Adolescent (13-15 years)	110-131	64-83	73-84

Following a complete chart review and communication with the multidisciplinary team as needed, a PT will move forward with the completion of the initial evaluation. As with all other physical therapy settings, the patient and family interview is a vital portion of the evaluation process. The interview should be family centered and include input directly from the patient when appropriate. The context of each family and patient experience needs to be taken into consideration when planning the physical therapy examination. Some patients receiving physical therapy in the acute care setting have a long-standing relationship with the hospital environment, whereas others are unfamiliar with hospitals and are experiencing the emotions of an unexpected admission related to a new diagnosis or a traumatic event. This may affect the time required for patients and families to process new information and education.

An important topic to discuss with the family is the patient's prior level of function including prior participation in physical therapy. This information will guide the physical therapy plan of care. Understanding how much assistance a patient needs at baseline as well as available caregiver support after discharge will provide insight on the amount of family training that will be needed during this hospitalization. Caregivers may already be comfortable assisting a patient or may require further training should the patient demonstrate a change in function. Information related to a patient's home setup and personal equipment should also be obtained. Environmental factors such as the presence of stairs, type of shower, and room size to accommodate equipment are important to obtain. Finally, it is beneficial to identify interests, hobbies, or items that are motivating to the patient. This information can help guide conversations with a patient to build rapport and decrease anxiety while also improving a patient's willingness to participate in activities. Identifying what is important to the patient and making it applicable within the inpatient setting can help create an overall successful plan of care.

EXAMINATION AND EVALUATION

Once orders have been verified and a thorough chart review and family history have been obtained, the PT can begin the examination and evaluation. A patient's ability to participate in standardized tests and functional assessment as part of the examination is largely dependent on the child's age and cognitive function as well as level of pain. The evaluation synthesizes this information in order to identify disorders of movement and how the disorder may cause an activity limitation or participation restriction. Once the evaluation is complete, the PT will establish goals and a plan of care appropriate to a child's current medical issues and functional needs in order to assist with a safe and prepared discharge.

Information can be gathered about range of motion, muscle strength, sensation, coordination, balance, and functional level in nearly any child, keeping special considerations such as age and medical status in mind. For example, an 8-year-old previously healthy child with a new diagnosis of leukemia would be expected to have the ability to participate in a standardized manual muscle test to measure strength. A 2-year-old child with the same diagnosis would not be expected to have the cognitive skills to participate in a standardized manual muscle test. The therapist must be creative in order to obtain pertinent and accurate information about this young child's strength. The therapist may ask the child to give them a "high five," moving the child's hand to a variety of positions and asking the child to use each upper extremity. In reporting this on the evaluation form, the therapist might state the following: "A standard manual muscle test is unable to be given secondary to the child's age, but the child demonstrates the ability to raise bilateral upper extremities against gravity to give a high five in all directions including across midline." When considering medical status, it is important to consider the patient's acuity level and medical diagnosis. For example, a patient who is on the intensive care unit (ICU) may not tolerate the same examination techniques as a stable patient admitted to the oncology floor for a course of chemotherapy.

Throughout the remainder of this chapter, special considerations will be discussed in more detail for each diagnostic grouping.

Standardized Tests and Measures

The use of standardized tests and measures during the initial PT evaluation establishes a quantifiable baseline to enable measurable goals to be set. Reassessment using the same standardized tests and measures allows the therapist to measure the patient's progress using the same measuring tool each time. A wide variety of tests and measures are available for the pediatric patient. In accordance with the International Classification of Functioning, Disability, and Health (ICF) model, standardized tests and measures are available to assess body function and structure, activity, and participation. When selecting the appropriate standardized test and measure, the therapist must consider the patient's age and diagnosis, the cognitive and functional level of the patient, and the impairment or functional skill that is most applicable to the patient's diagnosis and clinical presentation. The pediatric section of the American Physical Therapy Association (APTA) has references for standardized tests that have been validated in the pediatric population.

Given the time constraints of the acute care setting and the acuity of the patients, long standardized tests are often not realistic or valuable. Often this patient population is treated for a short length of time, and therefore, significant changes in score and the opportunity to retest would not always be expected. An acute care PT will typically utilize a combination of standardized tests, screenings, and observational assessment during the initial examination. This combination allows the therapist to collect data surrounding impairment level tests and the patient's current level of independence with functional mobility. For patients who have an expected longer length of stay, standardized developmental tests are appropriate to measure the patient's progression through the developmental sequence. **Table 6-7** provides examples of commonly used standardized tests that are appropriate for the pediatric population in the acute care setting. These tests were selected with consideration of time taken to administer, difficulty level of the tasks, and appropriateness for the pediatric population.

PLAN OF CARE

Following a physical therapy examination and evaluation, a plan of care will be established. The PT will need to anticipate the trajectory of the hospital course and how this has impacted or will impact a child's function compared to their baseline. This will allow appropriate goals to be established and clinically appropriate recommendations to be provided. The proposed plan of care should include measurable goals, a patient's rehab potential, frequency and duration of PT services, and discharge recommendations.

Measurable Goals

In the pediatric acute care setting, short-term goals are typically achievable in 2 weeks or less, whereas long-term goals are more often achieved in 4 weeks or more. All goals should be written in SMART format (specific, measurable, attainable, realistic, timely). For children whose discharge is dependent on mobility, goals are typically focused on functional skills and caregiver education to ensure a safe discharge. For children with anticipated prolonged hospitalization, goals should focus on preventing the development of impairments or loss of functional skills. For young children, goals would focus on progression through the developmental sequence. Physical therapy goals should be patient-centered and are often generated along with patient and caregiver input.

Discharge Planning

Discharge recommendations should be made for each patient in the acute care setting. Children recommended for inpatient rehabilitation are those seen frequently or intensively in the hospital settings with potential for continued daily progress. These children may present with significant deficits that prevent safe discharge to home, requiring acute rehabilitation to continue to progress toward a home discharge. Long-term care is most appropriate for children receiving physical therapy on a consultative basis in the acute care setting with anticipated long-term physical therapy or medical needs. Home care physical therapy is most appropriate for children and adolescents who require a home safety evaluation or ongoing functional mobility training in which they are unable to leave their home until such training is complete. Early intervention is state-funded physical therapy in the home or community for children from birth to 3 years old. Finally, outpatient physical therapy is recommended for children with occasional to frequent physical therapy needs who are able to access a community clinic.

Factors such as age, cognition, psychosocial barriers, and baseline and current level of functioning will impact and guide discharge planning. Discharge recommendations should be made on evaluation but are often assessed and modified throughout a child's hospital course. For example, a 12-year-old child who had a stroke with significant impairments, activity limitations, and participation restrictions on evaluation will likely be referred to acute rehabilitation. However, as their hospital course progresses, they may have achieved a level of mobility for which a home discharge is now appropriate with outpatient PT follow-up. A patient with the same medical diagnosis but who

TABLE 6-7 • Standardized Tests and Measures[5]		
Body Structure/Function	**Standardized Test/Measure**	**Screening or Observation**
Cardiopulmonary	Heart rate Blood pressure Borg scale Rate of perceived exertion (RPE) Oxygen saturation	Skin color of face Breathing patterns Use of accessory muscles
Coordination	SCALE test of coordination Clinical measure of motor and postural skills	Finger-nose-finger Finger to nose Rapid alternating movements Heel to shin
Pain	Wong-Baker Faces Pain Scale Individualized Numeric Rating Scale (INRS) Face, Legs, Activity, Cry, and Consolability (FLACC) Scale Visual analog scale	Observe for splinting Observe facial expression Observe change in heart rate
Endurance	6-minute walk test 30-second walk test	Observe a young child's skill level decompensating or look for signs of fatigue such as change in mood
Strength/muscle power	Manual muscle testing Dynamometer	Observation of active control of movement
Somatosensation	Pediatric–Modified Total Neuropathy Score	Light touch, proprioception, deep pressure, kinesthesia, vibratory sense, monofilament testing
Posture and balance	Pediatric Balance Scale Movement Assessment of Infants Romberg test Pediatric Berg Balance Scale	Tandem stance and tandem gait
Oculomotor skills		Observation of: Saccadic movements Convergence and divergence Ability to follow a target through visual fields
Arousal/cognition	Pediatric Confusion Assessment Method for the ICU Cornell Assessment for Pediatric Delirium	Orientation Delayed recall Response to stimuli
Activity		
Gait	Dynamic Gait Index Timed Up and Go Functional Mobility Assessment	Observational gait analysis
Gross motor	Alberta Infant Motor Scale Gross Motor Function Measure Gross Motor Performance Measure	Observation of movement against gravity Observation of developmental skill level
Fine motor control	9-Hole Peg Test	Finger opposition

Abbreviations: ICU, intensive care unit; SCALE, selective control assessment of the lower extremity.

is 13 months old and was non-ambulatory prior to the stroke may not be recommended to transition to inpatient rehab at any point in the hospitalization. In these circumstances, consistent communication with the medical team and case management is essential.

Although patients are often followed by other rehabilitation or ancillary services, it may be important for the inpatient PT to facilitate a referral for additional outpatient services. If patients are noted to have impairments that contribute to decreased independence with activities of daily living (ADLs) or fine motor tasks, they may require a referral for outpatient

occupational therapy. Patients may also require outpatient follow-up from a speech-language pathologist if they demonstrate impairments in their speech and/or cognition. This may be the case after an acute neurologic event or following respiratory decline requiring intubation.

Equipment Needs

If it is determined that a patient is safe to be discharged to their home environment, it is important to identify any new pieces of durable medical equipment (DME) that are necessary to overcome any identified environmental barriers.

Patients who have weight-bearing precautions postoperatively will require an assistive device for ambulation such as axillary crutches or a rolling walker. Patients with postoperative mobility impairments may also have difficulty accessing their bathrooms either because of their precautions or simply due to their home setup. They may therefore require a commode that can be placed at the bedside or over a toilet to aid with ease of toilet transfers. They may also benefit from a shower seat in order to increase safety while showering, particularly if they are not able to fully bear weight through one leg. These patients may also require a wheelchair for long-distance mobility or use at school. Because school hallways are busy and may put a patient at a higher risk for falling, it is often recommended that patients using an assistive device for ambulation have a wheelchair for use at school.

Patients who have custom equipment may require separate rental equipment or adaptations to their personal equipment. For example, a patient who typically sits in a custom manual wheelchair with standard leg rests may require a wider rental wheelchair with elevating leg rests to accommodate casting or orthotic support if they have had a hip surgery. Rental wheelchairs can come equipped with elevating leg rests, seatbelts, or reclining back supports. However, rental wheelchairs do not provide a 4-point harness or approved tie downs for transport. It is important to be clear with patients and families regarding these limitations of rental wheelchairs in order to assess if the patient is able to sit safely and be transported throughout the community following discharge. Some patients may require modifications to their custom equipment due to the nature of their hospitalization, such as following a spinal fusion for scoliosis. It is important to assess what modifications can be made in the hospital and what requires consultation with an equipment vendor. In some cases, specialized car seats can be obtained to accommodate children requiring additional support or maintenance of postsurgical precautions. In instances when a patient cannot be safely transported in a car, an ambulance transport home may be necessary.

Patients whose diagnosis is not orthopedic in nature may also require DME for discharge. These patients include anyone who is medically ready for discharge and can return safely to their homes but who has not returned to their baseline level of functional mobility. These patients may require assistive devices for ambulation due to weakness, impaired balance, or decreased endurance. They may also require a rental wheelchair or commode chair for these same reasons.

Although some equipment, such as axillary crutches, may be provided directly from the hospital, other equipment will need to be ordered. This will require knowledge of a patient's insurance benefits as well as communication with DME companies. Each hospital is different with regard to how equipment is ordered. If the case management department typically orders DME for a patient, it is important to remain in close contact with that team in order to ensure that equipment is delivered in a timely manner or that active problem solving can occur in the event of an insurance denial. It could also be the PT's role to order equipment. Regardless of who is responsible for completing this task, it is important to initiate the process as soon as needs are identified.

■ DIAGNOSTIC GROUPINGS

Inpatient units are typically compartmentalized by common diagnoses or by common level of acuity. Levels of acuity in the hospital escalate from general floor to intermediate-care or step-down units and ICUs. PTs are trained to evaluate and treat patients throughout all inpatient units, as well as the emergency department and operating room when clinically indicated.

GENERAL PEDIATRIC UNIT

Introduction

Many children admitted to the hospital do not require a specialized medical team. These children are cared for by a general pediatric physician team. Diagnoses on this unit include but are not limited to respiratory illnesses, gastrointestinal disorders, musculoskeletal dysfunction, and endocrine/metabolic disorders.[6] Length of stay for these patients can vary greatly from observation over a few days to several months. If a child falls below their functional baseline or is at risk for development delay, physical therapy may be required.

It is also important to note that not every child admitted to the hospital will need physical therapy. The initial focus of the admission will be to address the presenting medical issues. A screening is a way to identify children who require a full PT evaluation and those who do not. The mechanisms used for conducting screenings are set through policies and procedures of each institution and may include participation in multidisciplinary rounds.

Role of the PT on a General Medicine Floor

Developmental Play

Infants may be hospitalized to treat routine illnesses unable to be managed at home, for staged medical procedures such as hernia repairs and abdominal surgeries, and for various respiratory illnesses. The pediatric PT is often consulted for suggestions on how to foster motor development opportunities in the confines of the hospital setting. Treatment activities focus on manual facilitation of gross motor skills through developmental play outside of the crib environment. Education is also vital for carryover of developmental activities. Handouts posted at the bedside and provided to caregivers will maximize communication and continuity of care regarding activities and positioning programs.

Functional Mobility

This population includes both typically developing children as well as those who have a baseline developmental delay. PT intervention would focus on the acquisition of any skills lost in the setting of the hospital admission. Prolonged bed rest related to acute hospitalization may result in decreased independence with functional mobility. This may include quality of movement during transitions and gait as well as higher-level activities such as standing balance and coordination. For younger patients, this is addressed through a combination of functional tasks and play activities, whereas older children may be able to participate in formal therapeutic exercise programs.

Children may also be admitted to the hospital with impairments related to an infection, soft tissue injury, or hematologic process such as sickle cell disease. In these instances, PT interventions will focus on restoring range of motion at the affected joint(s) and assisting with return to independent functional mobility. In some cases, an assistive device may be required to support safe ambulation until patients return to their baseline.

Respiratory Illness

According to Witt et al,[6] respiratory conditions account for 22% of all nonneonatal hospital stays. In many hospitals, respiratory therapists provide airway clearance techniques, but PTs are also trained in and often provide postural drainage and manual chest physical therapy. In addition, the PT can assist in positional modifications to achieve upright posture, which facilitates improved pulmonary function. For infants, this can be achieved through the use of soft positioning rolls, infant seats, or caregiver handling. For toddlers and older children, adaptive seating and positioning devices such as tumble form seats, pediatric cardiac chairs, or custom wheelchairs and strollers can provide opportunities for upright positioning. **Figure 6-1** is an example of upright positioning in a tumble form seat for a child requiring bilevel positive airway pressure for respiratory compromise. The acute care PT may also provide opportunities

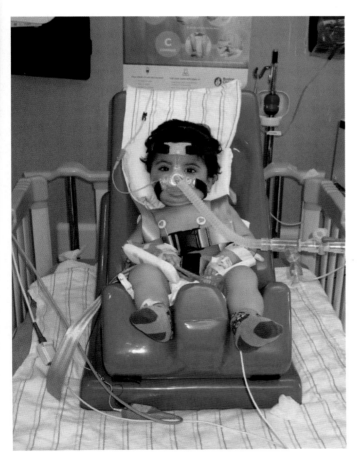

FIGURE 6-1 **Upright positioning in a Tumble Form seat for a child requiring bilevel positive airway pressure for respiratory compromise.**

for aerobic exercise to facilitate airway clearance as well as improved cardiopulmonary health.

Examination and Plan of Care

Taking into account the patient's age, cognition, baseline function, and reason for hospitalization, a full examination includes impairment level testing and identification of activity limitations through standardized testing or functional observation. When selecting appropriate tests and measures, a patient's anticipated length of stay should be taken into consideration. Standardized assessments, such as those noted in the introductory section of this chapter, should be considered for patients whose length of stay may be prolonged, as they can provide information regarding meaningful change. In contrast, observational assessments will provide more relevant information for short admissions. Length of stay will also provide information regarding what interventions will be most beneficial when establishing the patient's plan of care. For example, if a patient will likely be discharged within 1 to 2 weeks, minimal impact will be made on impairments such as strength and gross motor skill development that require long-term PT treatment for measurable change.

Goals

The following are some examples of appropriate goals for patients on the general pediatric unit based on acuity, age, and developmental stage.

Scenario 1: A 6-month-old child with Down syndrome is admitted for placement of a gastrostomy tube followed by extended admission to maximize weight gain and feeding volume. The child is noted to have poor tolerance to handling.

Short-Term Goals (to be met in 2 weeks)

1. Caregiver(s) will be independent with facilitating daily motor activities as instructed by PT and confirmed per parent or nursing report.
2. Patient will remain calm and alert with Face, Legs, Activity, Cry, and Consolability (FLACC) scale score ≤3 for 15 minutes of motor play.

Long-Term Goals (to be met in 4-6 weeks)

1. Patient will tolerate modified prone on forearms, lifting head to 45 degrees and holding for 30 seconds with stable vital signs.
2. Infant will prop sit unassisted for 30 seconds.

Scenario 2: An 8-year-old child with right plantar foot infection requires irrigation and debridement procedures and intravenous antibiotic treatment. Patient is to remain non–weight bearing on right lower extremity. Anticipated length of stay is 5 days.

Short-Term Goals = Long-Term Goals (to be met by discharge)

1. Patient will transfer sit to/from stand with supervision using least restrictive assistive device.
2. Patient will ambulate 50 feet on a level surface with least restrictive assistive device and contact guard assist.
3. Patient will negotiate 5 steps with 1 rail and 1 axillary crutch, with contact guard assist.

Scenario 3: A 15-year-old girl with cerebral palsy, Gross Motor Function Classification System level IV, is admitted with a diagnosis of acute pneumonia, presenting with desaturations requiring supplemental oxygen, cough, fever, and lethargy. Expected length of stay is 2 weeks or less.

Short-Term Goals = Long-Term Goals (to be met in 2 weeks)

1. Patient will return to baseline respiratory status indicated by clear breath sounds and oxygen saturation of greater than 92% on room air.
2. Caregiver will demonstrate safe and independent performance of manual chest physical therapy.
3. Patient will tolerate semi-upright sitting in personal wheelchair up to 2 hours, maintaining oxygen saturation of greater than 92% per report.

INTENSIVE CARE UNIT

Introduction

Approximately 250,000 children are admitted to a pediatric ICU each year in the United States.[7,8] The focus of care in a pediatric ICU is on resuscitation, stabilization, management of critical disease process, and reversal of organ failure.[7,9] Mortality rates of children admitted to the pediatric ICU have decreased significantly in the past 3 decades.[10,12] However, as mortality rates have declined, the population in pediatric ICUs has become more complex. Recent research has found that 53% of critically ill children had underlying chronic, complex illnesses.[12] There has also been an increase in ICU-acquired morbidities.[13,14] Recent literature suggests that pediatric survivors of critical illness experience significant physical, psychosocial, and cognitive morbidities, leading to delayed recovery, functional impairments, and reduced quality of life.[13] Furthermore, ICU-acquired weakness is being increasingly recognized as a significant clinical problem in children.[15] Research has shown that patients who are mechanically ventilated or immobile for greater than 7 days are at increased risk for deconditioning and muscle atrophy.[16] As such, PTs play a vital role in addressing impairments and restoring function in hospitalized children with critical illness.

Children admitted to a pediatric ICU vary in chronological age, developmental stage, and medical complexity. Children may be admitted to the ICU for management of medical diagnoses or following surgical procedures. This may also include respiratory failure, multisystem organ failure, congenital heart disease, neurologic monitoring following an event or surgery involving the brain or spinal cord, organ transplant, and trauma.[7] As mentioned previously, a general hospital may have just one pediatric ICU, whereas a children's hospital may have several ICUs. Each ICU may be categorized by a certain population or department. Examples of ICUs found in a children's hospital are the medical ICU (MICU), surgical ICU (SICU), neonatal ICU (NICU), and cardiac ICU (CICU).

ICU Team

When a child is admitted to the ICU, their primary care team is the critical care team and is composed of physicians specialized in critical care or anesthesia. Depending on the patient's diagnosis, there may be other consulting teams of specialty physicians working together with the critical care team to provide care for the patient in the ICU. For example, the therapist may receive a consult for a child admitted to the ICU who had an orthopedic procedure requiring respiratory support postoperatively. Their primary team is the critical care team, with orthopedics as a consulting team. Furthermore, this same patient may have an underlying diagnosis such as type 1 diabetes for which endocrinology is also a consulting team. For the PT in the ICU setting, communication typically occurs with the primary care team regarding orders, hemodynamic parameters, and additional precautions for mobilization. The critical care team will communicate with consulting teams to determine the most appropriate approach for medical management and rehabilitation of the child in the ICU.

Environment of Care

Knowledge of the environment is essential to prepare for examination and treatment in the ICU. The therapist in the ICU should be able to identify all lines and tubes; understand precautions for mobilizing patients with certain lines, tubes, or ventilatory support; understand normal pediatric vital signs; and recognize pharmacologic therapies and implications for physical therapy.

When preparing for mobility in an ICU setting, the therapist must prepare the environment to ensure the safety of the patient and the integrity of lines, tubes, and devices. The therapist should first visualize all lines and tubes connected to the patient prior to mobilizing. In general, the therapist should consider moving all lines/tubes to the same side of the bed in which the patient will be mobilizing from to ensure the integrity of these lines will not be compromised during mobility. This may include moving an intravenous (IV) pole or Foley catheter or obtaining a portable monitor. In certain circumstances, nursing or respiratory therapy assistance may be necessary to help prepare the environment and mobilize the patient safely.

Figure 6-2 illustrates placement of a ventilator and multiple IV poles for a patient mobilized to a chair.

Advanced Life Support Measures

A critically ill patient may require advanced life support measures. PTs may be involved with these patients to optimize positioning, maintain joint range of motion, provide appropriate education to caregivers and staff, and in some cases, assist with mobilization out of bed. Therefore, it is important to note these devices and their medical use. **Table 6-8** summarizes advanced life support devices, their use in the critically ill population, and PT considerations.

Respiratory Support

Children in the ICU often require oxygen or ventilatory airway support. Ventilatory support can be delivered invasively or noninvasively. **Table 6-9** describes the different methods of oxygen or ventilatory support used.[22-24]

Common Medications

There are many pharmacologic interventions used throughout the hospital setting, some of which require close hemodynamic monitoring in an ICU. Medication classes commonly used in

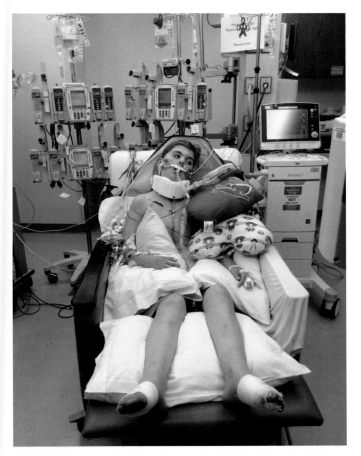

FIGURE 6-2 **Placement of a ventilator and multiple intravenous line poles for a patient mobilized to a chair.**

the ICU are vasopressors, inotropes, sedatives and paralytics, and pain medications.

Inotropes such as dopamine, dobutamine, and milrinone are used in the cardiac ICU to increase contractility of the heart and therefore improve cardiac output. These medications are typically used for children with severe heart failure or following cardiac surgery. Conversely, vasopressors work to increase vasoconstriction. Both inotropes and vasopressors can be used to increase blood pressure, thereby increasing organ perfusion in the critically ill patient. Common types of vasopressors used in the pediatric setting are epinephrine, norepinephrine, and phenylephrine.[25,26] Use of both inotropes and vasopressors requires ICU level of care for close hemodynamic monitoring.

Sedatives are commonly used in the pediatric ICU to suppress the central nervous system and induce sleep. Common pharmacologic agents for sedation include midazolam, propofol, clonidine, dexmedetomidine, and barbiturates such as phenobarbital. Certain opioids such as fentanyl, morphine, and hydromorphone can also have sedative properties.[27-30]

There are times when a patient may need to be medically paralyzed to prevent movement due to safety or medical instability such as following the placement of a new tracheostomy tube. In these instances, paralytics are used. It is important to note that paralytics only eliminate muscle activity and do not have sedative or analgesic properties. As such, they are often used in combination with other medications during procedures such as intubation or insertion of central lines. Common muscle relaxants or neuromuscular blockades used in pediatrics include succinylcholine, pancuronium, vecuronium, and other nondepolarizing agents of the -curium drug class.[30]

TABLE 6-8 • Advanced Life Support Devices		
Device	**Definition and Purpose**	**Physical Therapy Considerations**
Extracorporeal membrane oxygenation (ECMO)	Machine used to pump and oxygenate a patient's blood outside the body, similar to heart-lung bypass machine. Used for patients with heart or lung failure as a bridge to further treatment such as ventricular assist devices or heart or lung transplantation.[17]	• Consult for positioning or range of motion • Early mobilization on ambulatory ECMO circuit • Risk for neurologic insult with external device
Ventricular assist device (VAD)	Implantable mechanical device that helps pump blood from the ventricles to the rest of the body. Can be placed in either or both ventricles, but most commonly used in the left ventricle and referred to as left ventricular assist device (LVAD). Used for patients with heart failure as long-term management or while awaiting heart transplantation.[18,19]	• Early mobilization • Patient and caregiver education • Risk for neurologic insult with external device • Long-term anticoagulation
EXCOR Berlin Heart (**Figure 6-3**)	A paracorporeal ventricular assist device specific for infants and children with heart failure. Can be used as a bridge to transplant or a bridge to recovery.[20]	• Early mobilization and developmental care ○ Risk for kinking of cannulas during developmental activity • Caregiver education • Risk for neurologic insult • Long-term anticoagulation
Continuous renal replacement therapy (CRRT)	Slow, continuous removal of waste and water via hemodialysis machine and central dialysis catheter. Used in critically ill patients to prevent hemodynamic fluctuations associated with rapid intermittent hemodialysis.[21]	• Early mobilization ○ Care for mobility with femoral catheterization

TABLE 6-9 • Respiratory Support[22-24]

Respiratory Support	Definition and Purpose
Noninvasive	
Oxygen delivery systems 1. Low flow 2. Reservoir systems 3. High flow	1. Nasal cannula inserted in the nares for rapid oxygen delivery of <1 L/min up to 8 L/min. 2. Oxygen delivered via facemask or cannula with reservoir incorporating mechanism for gathering and storing oxygen. 3. High concentration of oxygen or high flow rate of oxygen delivered via mask or high-flow nasal cannula (HFNC). Able to achieve flow rates 10-60 L/min with fraction of inspired oxygen (FiO_2) of 21%-100%.
Continuous positive airway pressure (CPAP)	Mild airway pressure delivered continuously during inhalation and exhalation via mask fitted over nose and/or mouth connected to machine, used to keep airway open during ventilation. In infants, HFNC may be used instead of CPAP to provide positive end-expiratory pressure (PEEP) with or without the addition of supplementary FiO_2.
Bilevel positive airway pressure (BiPAP)	Airway pressure delivered at varying levels during inhalation and exhalation via mask fitted over nose and/or mouth connected to machine. Used to keep airway open during ventilation. A higher pressure is provided during inhalation than during exhalation in contrast to CPAP.
Invasive	
Endotracheal intubation	Flexible tube passed through the nose or mouth and into the trachea. Connected to ventilator to maintain open airway, provide oxygen, support breathing, and protect the lungs in critically ill patients.
Tracheostomy	Surgically created hole (stoma) in the trachea. Used for conditions requiring long-term ventilation or when airway is blocked. Can be connected to ventilator to provide pressure support to lungs or tracheostomy collar for delivery of oxygen.

Children in the ICU often require medications for pain following trauma or surgical procedures. For mild pain, nonopioid analgesics may be used such as acetaminophen, nonsteroidal anti-inflammatory drugs (NSAIDs), and tramadol. Morphine, hydromorphone, and fentanyl are all opioids used to treat more severe pain. These can be delivered intravenously for rapid action. For pain medications administered enterally, opioids such as hydrocodone and oxycodone can be used.[31,32]

Certain medications used in the acute care and ICU settings may impact the evaluation or treatment of a patient. Several medications can cause muscle wasting, motor impairments, osteopenia, and delirium, all of which are further exacerbated by immobilization. Additionally, patients may be weaning off of sedatives or analgesics and exhibiting symptoms of withdrawal including agitation, anxiety, muscle tension, diaphoresis, tachypnea, and tachycardia. Recognizing these medications and understanding their use will help prepare you for managing patients in the acute care setting. **Table 6-10** outlines PT considerations for medication classes commonly used in the ICU setting.

Setting Up a Room and Patient Preparation

Management of a patient in the ICU takes careful planning and coordination. Communication with nursing is essential to determine appropriate timing of PT intervention recognizing certain medication effects, respiratory status, and potential support and collaboration with respiratory therapy. Prior to mobilizing a patient out of bed, it is imperative the therapist work with the bedside nurse to set up the room in order to safely mobilize the patient and maintain integrity of lines and tubes. This may include rearranging the hospital room to accommodate placement of a chair in the room. Additionally, IV poles, ventilators, urinary catheters, and hemodynamic

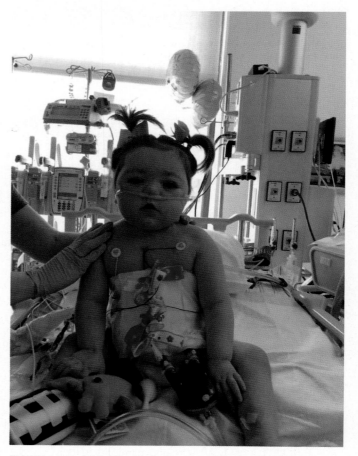

FIGURE 6-3 A child with a Berlin Heart participating in a sitting balance activity.

TABLE 6-10 • Common Medications in Pediatric Intensive Care Unit

Medication Class	Examples	Physical Therapy (PT) Considerations
Inotropes and vasopressors	Inotropes: dopamine, dobutamine, milrinone Vasopressors: epinephrine, norepinephrine, phenylephrine	• Monitoring of blood pressure during mobility • Need for continuous hemodynamic monitoring • Decreased activity tolerance and endurance
Sedatives	Midazolam, propofol, clonidine, dexmedetomidine, phenobarbital	• Level of arousal • Ability to participate in PT examination/intervention • Decreased motor function • Fall risk
Paralytics	Succinylcholine, pancuronium, vecuronium	• Impaired motor function
Pain medications	Fentanyl, morphine, hydromorphone, hydrocodone, oxycodone Nonsteroidal anti-inflammatory drugs (NSAIDs), acetaminophen	• Sedation effects • Opioid-induced delirium • Impact on gastrointestinal system • Respiratory depression • Dizziness/orthostasis • Timing of PT interventions

monitoring systems should be moved to the same side of the bed to which the patient will be mobilizing prior to initiating mobility. The therapist should take care to ensure they are positioned in a manner to physically assist the patient while not compromising lines or tubes. Often, assistance from the bedside nurse is required for management of lines and tubes during PT intervention. Similarly, when mobilizing a patient on cardiorespiratory supports such as continuous positive airway pressure (CPAP) or extracorporeal membrane oxygenation (ECMO), a respiratory therapist or ECMO specialist will need to be present for assistance and management of equipment during PT intervention. In addition to room setup, the therapist should ensure the patient is prepared for safe mobility. This includes donning of nonslip footwear, application of gait belt, and bracing when applicable. Once the patient and environment are prepared, the therapist can complete their assessment or intervention.

Special Considerations

Prior to and during intervention in the ICU setting, several things should be considered. First, it is necessary to understand the acuity of the patient and current medical status. The therapist should be able to identify if the child is hemodynamically stable enough to initiate mobility and recognize how mobility may impact hemodynamic stability. Careful planning for possibilities where mobility may compromise medical stability or where medical diagnosis or medications may compromise the patient's physiologic response to mobility or safety is imperative.[33] The therapist must understand how precautions and activity restrictions may impact treatment. Consider infectious diseases or immunocompromise that prevents the patient from leaving their hospital room or the need for medical staff to don protective equipment. Sternal precautions should be considered for all children who have undergone median sternotomy. Weight bearing and other orthopedic precautions will additionally impact the ability to safely mobilize a patient in the ICU.

Vital sign precautions should be considered prior to and during mobilization, and the therapist should be prepared to

react appropriately should the patient have a rapid change in vital signs that prohibits progression of mobility.[33] **Table 6-11** outlines "rest and reassess" criteria for changes during mobilization of patients in the ICU. If the patient experiences changes outlined from baseline vital signs or behaviors, the therapist should be prompted to reassess whether continued mobilization is safe.

In an ICU setting, therapists should consider the patient's level of alertness and implications for therapeutic interventions. Several pharmacologic agents in the ICU can impact a patient's level of alertness and therefore their ability to participate in physical therapy. For children heavily sedated, PT intervention may consist of positioning to maintain skin integrity, passive range of motion or bracing to maintain joint flexibility, and caregiver education. Additionally, children may be lethargic and able to participate in limited mobility initially. Furthermore, ICU delirium may impact PT intervention.

TABLE 6-11 • Rest and Reassess Criteria[9]

Change in heart rate 20%
Change in blood pressure 20%
Change in respiratory rate 20%
Decrease in oxygen saturation 15%
Increase in fraction of inspired oxygen 20%
Increase in end-tidal carbon dioxide 20%
Ventilator/CPAP/BiPAP asynchrony
Respiratory distress
New arrhythmia
Hemodynamic concerns
Change in mental status
Concern for airway device, vascular access, or external ventricular drain integrity
Behavior interfering with safe activity

Modified with permission from Wieczorek B, Ascenzi J, Kim Y, et al. PICU Up!: Impact of a Quality Improvement Intervention to Promote Early Mobilization in Critically Ill Children. Pediatr Crit Care Med. 2016;17(12):e559-e566. Abbreviations: BiPAP, bilevel positive airway pressure; CPAP, continuous positive airway pressure.

ICU-Acquired Delirium

Delirium has been well defined and studied in the adult population, with recent research defining delirium in pediatrics.[34] Delirium is defined by the *Diagnostic and Statistical Manual of Mental Disorders* as "an acute disturbance in level of consciousness, attention, cognition, and perception that develops over a short period of time and can have fluctuations."[35,36] Recent reports have found that pediatric delirium has a prevalence rate between 12% and 65% in pediatric medical, surgical, and cardiac ICUs.[37] According to Patel et al,[37] "delirium in children is marked by changes in psychomotor activity, ranging from delayed responsiveness to constant, agitated movements. Emotional lability is also common, evidenced by inconsolability or, alternatively, inappropriate calmness. Some pediatric patients (particularly adolescents) experience auditory and visual hallucinations." Changes in sleep patterns may also be present. **Table 6-12** categorizes risk factors for development of delirium into 2 categories, predisposing and precipitating risk factors.[37]

Preliminary studies on pediatric delirium suggest a link to short-term morbidity, including increased duration of mechanical ventilation. Several studies have shown that pediatric delirium is associated with increased length of hospital stay, higher resource utilization, and increased health care costs.[34,37]

There are 2 bedside tools used to diagnose pediatric delirium: the Pediatric Confusion Assessment Method for the ICU (pCAM-ICU or psCAM-ICU for preschool-age children) and the Cornell Assessment for Pediatric Delirium (CAPD). Both assessments have been proven to be valid and reliable for detection of delirium in critically ill children. Each assessment should take minutes to complete and requires that the child is arousable to verbal stimulation. The pCAM-ICU and psCAM-ICU are point-in-time screens designed to detect delirium present at the time of screening. They yield an objective result of delirium as present or absent.[37,38] The CAPD is a longitudinal screen used over the course of a nursing shift. It is validated in both developmentally typical and developmentally delayed children 0 to 21 years of age. A score of 9 or higher yields a diagnosis of delirium. Furthermore, it can be trended over time to assess trajectory and response to interventions.[35,37] As a PT in the ICU setting, you should be familiar with each assessment tool and may at times perform the pCAM-ICU/psCAM-ICU to determine the presence of delirium in your patients.[39]

PTs often play a vital role in the prevention and management of ICU delirium. PTs should adhere to clustered care to assist in promoting good sleep hygiene, as reduction or disruption in sleep can interfere with physiologic processes and lead to delirium. Additionally, therapists can help reduce light and noise in the ICU setting that can contribute to delirium. Perhaps most importantly, PTs often provide cognitive stimulation and early mobilization to prevent or manage ICU delirium.[34,37,38]

Early Mobilization

Early mobilization in general is defined as clinically safe and developmentally appropriate rehabilitation exercises of varying degrees initiated within the first 48 to 72 hours of ICU admission.[13] In a 2018 systematic review, mobilization was described in 4 of 11 individual studies as graduated, developmentally appropriate, active, and/or strengthening exercises. The same studies categorized range of motion, stretching, and positioning as nonmobility interventions. Other studies included developmental play as mobility and use of interactive video games and/or in-bed cycling to facilitate mobility. All 11 studies included in this systematic review report that mobilization was feasible in a pediatric ICU.[40]

Several contraindications to early mobility exist, including cardiorespiratory instability, intracranial hypertension, and spinal instability.[40] Additionally, barriers such as patient sedation, cooperation, and health care or family apprehension may limit the ability to promote early mobilization in the ICU setting.[7,40,41] Although the literature is limited on the effect of early mobilization on the pediatric patient in the ICU setting, early research suggests decreased duration of mechanical ventilation, decreased ICU length of stay, decreased mortality rate, and decreased risk of ICU-acquired morbidities.[7] Although literature is limited, early mobility in the pediatric ICU continues to gain momentum. It is appropriate for the entry-level PT to be aware of current literature and health care trends as this may impact their practice.

Examination and Plan of Care

Evaluation and intervention for a critically ill child will vary depending on level of acuity. Careful consideration of precautions, hemodynamic parameters, and level of arousal will guide selection of tests and measures to complete the assessment. For children able to participate in the assessment, impairment level testing and standardized assessments should be completed with consideration and modification based on developmental stage and cognitive ability. The following sections will discuss appropriate tests and measures for certain diagnostic groupings, all of which may be encountered in an ICU setting. Many critically ill children may not tolerate a complete evaluation, and often, impairments are assessed creatively or through functional or developmental activity. Some standardized assessments may not be appropriate because lines, tubes, and respiratory support will impact performance or patient safety. Furthermore, patient tolerance, respiratory status, and hemodynamics may impact the ability to complete a formal examination or standardized assessment.

Goals and treatment of the pediatric patient in the ICU will also vary based on level of alertness. For children under sedation or with decreased responsiveness to stimulation, maintaining joint range of motion, skin integrity, and arousal is typically the focus. Joint range of motion can be provided to children of all ages and should be provided with care for lines and tubes. Often, caregiver education on appropriate range

TABLE 6-12 • Risk Factors for Delirium[37]	
Predisposing Risk Factors	**Precipitating Risk Factors**
Age <2 years	Anticholinergic medications
Developmental delay	Benzodiazepines
High severity of illness	Cardiac bypass surgery
Mechanical ventilation	Immobilization
Low albumin	Prolonged ICU length of stay
Preexisting medical condition	Use of restraints

Reproduced with permission from Patel AK, Bell MJ, Traube C. Delirium in Pediatric Critical Care. Pediatr Clin North Am. 2017;64(5):1117-1132.

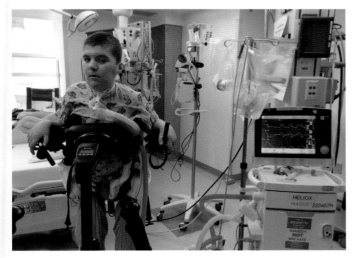

FIGURE 6-4 **A patient requiring ventilator support standing in a body weight supported gait trainer.**

of motion is provided to ensure carryover between therapy sessions. Positioning is imperative to maintaining skin integrity. For adolescents, pillows, rolls, and positioning aids can assist with maintaining skin integrity. For infants and toddlers, several commercial products are available to assist with positioning. These children are typically seen 1 to 2 times per week to monitor changes in range of motion and arousal. Once medications have been weaned and the child is able to participate, the frequency of physical therapy is most often increased based on their presentation, according to guidelines mentioned earlier. Developmentally appropriate mobility will be the focus of PT intervention for children with the ability to participate. There are various products to assist in mobilizing patients in an ICU setting including, but not limited to, mechanical lifts, ceiling lifts, transfer sheets, tilt tables, sit to standers, ambulation aides, and portable medical equipment such as ventilators and monitors. **Figures 6-4** and **6-5** illustrate early mobility activities for children in an ICU setting on respiratory support.

The following are some examples of appropriate goals for the infant or child in the ICU based on acuity, age, and developmental stage. It is important to note that as children are transitioned out of the ICU, the goals may continue to be appropriate or may need to be revised to reflect progress or change in medical status.

Scenario 1: A 3-week-old infant is admitted to the neonatal ICU with bronchopulmonary dysplasia. The patient is currently intubated, sedated, and paralyzed.

Short-Term Goal (to met be in 2 weeks)

1. Patient will tolerate appropriate positioning devices to maintain skin integrity and promote physiologic flexion without FLACC scale score of greater than 2.

Long-Term Goal (to remain appropriate while sedated and/or paralyzed)

1. Patient will tolerate range of motion to all joints in all planes of motion without change in heart rate of greater than 20 bpm while sedated and/or paralyzed.

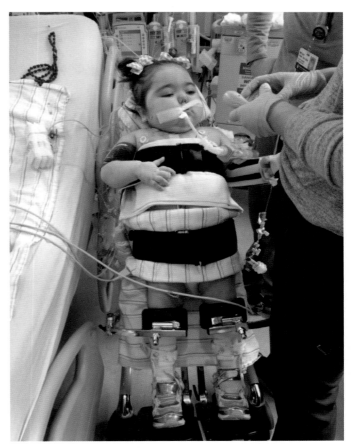

FIGURE 6-5 **A child who is intubated participating in a standing activity in a supine stander.**

Scenario 2: A 10-month-old child is 2 weeks status post lung transplantation and is currently on 0.5 L of oxygen via nasal cannula, awake, and interactive.

Short-Term Goals (to be met in 2 weeks)

1. Patient will tolerate 30 minutes of developmental stimulation or sequencing without cardiorespiratory compromise, evidenced by change in heart rate of no greater than 20 bpm or respiratory rate of no greater than 20 breaths/min.
2. Patient will roll to alternate side lying with no more than minimal assistance via facilitation through pelvis.
3. Patient will maintain supported sit for 5 minutes with no more than contact guard assistance.

Long-Term Goals (to be met in 4-6 weeks)

1. Patient will transition from sit to quadruped with moderate or less assistance.
2. Patient will pull to stand with no more than minimal assistance.

Scenario 3: A 17-year-old child status post motor vehicle accident who sustained multiple extremity fractures and traumatic brain injury is currently intubated on fraction of inspired oxygen (FiO_2) 40% and weaning sedation with decreased arousal.

Short-Term Goals (to be met in 2 weeks)

1. Patient will have appropriate positioning device to encourage upright positioning to maintain skin integrity and tolerate for 30 minutes without cardiorespiratory compromise evidenced by significant change in vital signs.
2. Patient will follow 3 of 5 simple 1-step motor commands with no greater than 10-second delay.
3. Patient will tolerate positioning to alternate side lying without change in vital signs and without signs of pain.

Scenario 4: A 10-year-old child with complex pneumonia required 1 week of intubation. The patient is now extubated to 4 L of oxygen. The patient is awake and participatory with deconditioning from prolonged immobility.

Short-Term Goals (to be met in 2 weeks)

1. Patient will complete transition from supine to sit with no more than minimal assistance.
2. Patient will transition from bed to chair via stand step transfer with no more than minimal assistance.
3. Patient will ambulate 50 feet with least restrictive assistive device and no more than minimal assistance maintaining hemodynamic stability.
4. Patient will ambulate 50 feet with least restrictive assistive device and require no more than minimal assistance maintaining oxygen saturation (SpO_2) >95% on 4 L oxygen via nasal cannula.

As children progress through their ICU course, goals will be continually updated. For children who have an acute decline in status, certain goals may be placed on hold, while new goals are created. Similarly, for a child with a quick recovery, goals may be met quicker than expected, necessitating the creation of new goals. Furthermore, frequency of PT services may also change throughout a child's ICU course, based on medical stability, response and tolerance to PT intervention, and progress toward goals.

ORTHOPEDICS

Introduction

In the pediatric acute care setting, PTs will encounter a variety of orthopedic conditions. These conditions vary from planned surgical procedures to unplanned events such as traumatic fractures or sports-related injuries. Similar to other units of the hospital, the PT's primary roles while working with patients with orthopedic conditions are to ensure that the patient is able to safely mobilize during the recovery process and assist the family with discharge planning and training. In this section, basic principles related to common pediatric orthopedic conditions and how they may appear in the acute care setting will be presented. Key aspects related to an orthopedic evaluation as well as unique concepts related to patient progression and discharge planning will additionally be discussed. These basic principles can be applied to the treatment of patients with a variety of acute orthopedic diagnoses, including those not discussed in this section.

Trauma

Traumas are among the leading causes of death in children, and for patients who experience polytraumas, 63% have associated orthopedic injuries.[42] The most common orthopedic fractures include femur (21.7%), tibia/fibula (21.5%), humerus (17%), and radius/ulna (14.7%).[42]

Following a hip fracture, early reduction of the injury becomes important in order to restore blood flow to the area in the event vasculature becomes compressed by the fracture.[43] If blood flow is not restored, a patient is at increased risk for osteonecrosis, which is the most common complication following hip fractures.[43] This risk is further increased if the fracture has been found to be displaced.[43] Additional complications can include nonunion, premature physeal closure, leg-length discrepancy, coxa vara, coxa valga, and coxa magna.[44]

Pediatric femoral shaft fractures are among the most common type of fractures that require hospitalization.[45] The most common causes of these fractures are falls from a height or road traffic accidents (90%), but a smaller number of cases (10%) are the result of low-energy mechanisms such as a fall from standing or a twisting motion.[45,46] Classification of femoral shaft fractures is based on a descriptive process: configuration (transverse, spiral, oblique), comminution, and open or closed.[45] Management of femoral shaft fractures is often guided in large part by the patient's age.[45] Patients with a fracture who are younger than 6 years are typically managed nonoperatively due to the excellent remodeling potential of the bones. Conservative options include use of a Pavlik harness (works best for infants up to 6 months), traction, and hip spica casts.[45] For older children, there are several factors that impact fracture management and often without a clear consensus.[45] Surgical options include external fixations, plating, and the use of intramedullary nails (flexible or rigid nails). External fixation is often used in children when there is an associated soft tissue injury, head injury, polytrauma, or identification of a pathologic fracture.[45] Complications with external fixation procedures include pin site infections (up to 72% of patients) and secondary fractures (1%-22% of patients).[45]

Functional mobility following femur fracture is largely determined by the patient's age and stability of the reduction. Children less than 6 years old may not be cleared to weight bear and could be restricted to bed-to-chair transfers only within a spica cast (**Figure 6-6**).[43] Immobilization within the cast will often remain in place for 6 to 8 weeks.[43] Children older than 6 years may be cleared for ambulation with weight-bearing restrictions based on the stability of the femur reduction and possible internal fixation.[43] After 6 to 8 weeks, children will often undergo updated radiographic imaging to confirm healing.[43] As cleared by the physician, the patient will begin progressive weight bearing with physical therapy and a return to full activities in 3 to 4 months.[43] If applicable, screw removal is recommended 4 to 6 months following complete reunion of the fracture site.

With tibial fractures, options for management include nonoperative approaches as well as surgical techniques such as open reduction and internal fixation (ORIF) and external fixation.[47] Often the severity of the fracture displacement as well as the degree of soft tissue damage will dictate the approach used.[48]

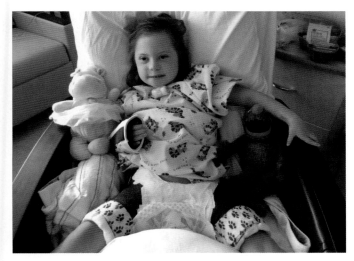

FIGURE 6-6   A child following a femur fracture and SPICA cast placement.

ORIF allows for anatomic restoration of the bone with plates and screws but does so by dissecting the surrounding soft tissue (**Figure 6-7**).[47] External fixation allows for an indirect fixation but with less soft tissue damage.[47] External fixation is accomplished using Taylor spatial frames, Illizarov circular frames, and Monticelli-Spinelli circular fixators.[48] As with femur fractures, there is an increased risk of superficial infections at the pin sites with external fixations; however, there is a higher rate of the need for hardware removal due to deep infection complications for patients undergoing an ORIF.[47]

Spinal injuries account for 1% to 10% of traumatic injuries in children, with cervical followed by lumbar and then thoracic injuries as the most common.[42] Although vertebral and pelvic

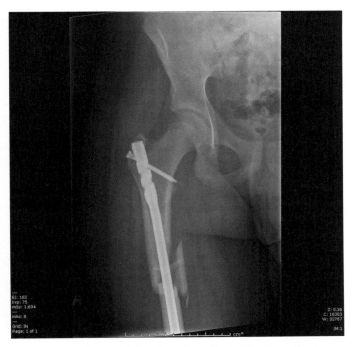

FIGURE 6-7   Radiographic imaging of a patient with a femur fracture following an open reduction and internal fixation (ORIF) procedure.

fractures only account for 5.2% and 4% of fractures, respectively, they are associated with the highest rates of mortality.[42] Depending on the severity of the injury, a patient may be treated conservatively through measures such as bed rest or the use of a spinal orthosis for immobilization.[42] If surgical management is warranted, procedures may include decompression of the spine through fusion and/or instrumentation; however, these interventions account for only 18% to 26% of patients.[42]

With all fractures, PTs should be aware of signs of compartment syndrome, which is defined by Loubani et al[42] as excessive swelling and pressure that occurs in a fascial compartment and results in the compression of nerves and vessels. In adults, signs and symptoms of compartment syndrome include paresthesia, paralysis, pallor, pulselessness, and pain with passive range of motion.[42] These findings often occur late in the pediatric population and instead may present as anxiety, agitation, and an increased need for pain medication.[42]

Hip Conditions

Impairments of the hip joint vary from those associated with neuromuscular conditions that affect muscle tone and subsequent joint development to congenital abnormalities of the hip joint. In each case, the surgical approach is unique and aimed to improve not only the mechanics of the hip joint but also the overall function and quality of life of the patient.

Neuromuscular Disorders

One of the most common neuromuscular disorders that result in secondary effects to the hip joint is cerebral palsy (CP). Patients with CP often experience complications at the hip joint as a result of spastic muscles placing abnormal forces across the hip joint as well as decreased or absent weight-bearing activites.[49] These abnormal forces ultimately impact the formation of the femur and acetabulum in the growing child, resulting in the formation of hip dysplasia, femoral anteversion, coxa valga, and/or posterolateral and superior migration of the femoral head from the acetabulum (**Figure 6-8**).[49] Ultimately, the combination of the atypical hip development as well as the abnormal muscular forces can lead to hip subluxations and dislocations.[49]

Long-standing hip subluxation or dislocation can also result in the development of femoral head deformities and degenerative disease due to the impingement of the femoral head on the acetabular rim.[50] Spastic hip dislocation and subluxation affects 7% of independent ambulators with CP and up to 60% to 90% of nonwalking patients with severe spastic quadriplegia.[51] Patients with hips that go untreated may begin to experience difficulties with perineal care, impaired sitting balance, difficulty tolerating standing activities, and development of a pelvic obliquity that leads to scoliosis.[49,51]

Conservative treatment to address hip dysplasia and subluxations/dislocations includes hip adductor stretching, abduction bracing, and botulinum toxin injections. When conservative treatment fails, soft tissue releases and reconstructive bony procedures involving the proximal femur and/or acetabulum may be required.[49] The goal of a soft tissue procedure is to slow the progression of the dislocation, but it does not correct it.[50] This allows for additional time until the patient is old enough to undergo reconstructive bony surgery.[50] Surgical techniques

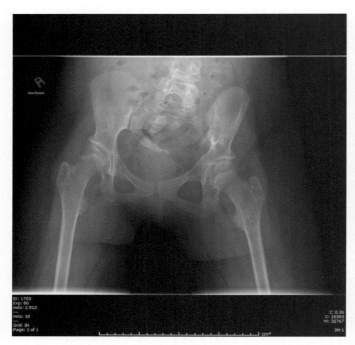

FIGURE 6-8 Radiographic imaging of a patient with hip dysplasia and coxa valga secondary to a neuromuscular condition.

directed at the hip joint include a proximal femoral varus derotational osteotomy (VDRO) alone or in conjunction with an open hip reduction or pelvic osteotomy (**Figure 6-9**).[49] If hip dysplasia becomes severe with concurrent femoral head deformity, the likelihood of a successful joint reconstruction is low. As a result, salvage procedures are performed.[50] The ultimate goal of all treatments is to create a reduced, stable, mobile, and pain-free hip.[49]

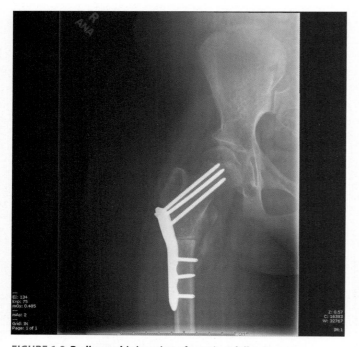

FIGURE 6-9 Radiographic imaging of a patient following a varus derotational osteotomy (VDRO).

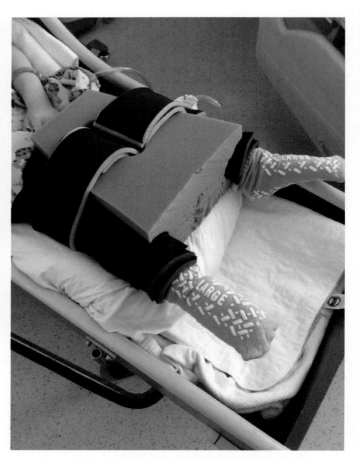

FIGURE 6-10 Positioning of a patient's lower extremities using an abduction pillow and knee immobilizers following a varus derotational osteotomy (VDRO).

Postoperatively, patients are often placed in a spica cast, A-frame cast, or abduction wedge for 4 to 6 weeks.[49] **Figure 6-10** shows a patient who is positioned in an abduction wedge and knee immobilizers to help maintain good hip and lower extremity alignment during the recovery process. During this time, patients may require additional assistance from caregivers to perform self-care and basic functional tasks as well as rely on the use of a rental wheelchair to accommodate for the new lower extremity supports. Once the casts are removed, outpatient physical therapy can be initiated. Weight bearing can begin once there is radiographic evidence of healing.[49]

Congenital Abnormalities

Patients without a neuromuscular disorder may also present with abnormal development of the hip, resulting in a diagnosis of developmental dysplasia of the hip (DDH).[51] DDH occurs when the femur develops incongruently in the acetabulum, which may lead patients to begin to develop pain and functional limitations.[52,53] The deformity may also result in the instability of the joint with an overload of the acetabular rim, leading to labral and cartilage damage.[52] There has also been a correlation found between DDH and osteoarthritis (OA), with 20% to 40% of patients with OA also having DDH.[52] Acetabular dysplasia can be surgically addressed through a periacetabular osteotomy (PAO), which aims to reorient the acetabulum in an ideal

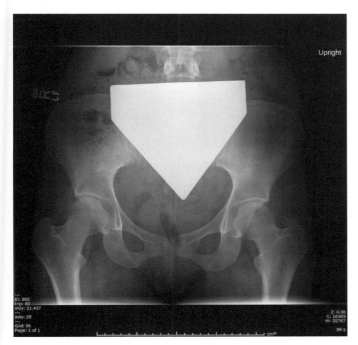

FIGURE 6-11 Radiographic imaging of a patient with hip dysplasia prior to a periacetabular osteotomy (PAO).

position to improve load distributions across the joint.[53] **Figures 6-11** and **6-12** are radiographic examples of a patient before and after a PAO procedure. Although postoperative protocols vary by each institution, the primary goal is to begin patient mobilization as soon as possible.[52] Physical therapy interventions for this population include exercises to initiate active and passive range of motion as well as mobility training that includes bed mobility, transfers, and ambulation with the least

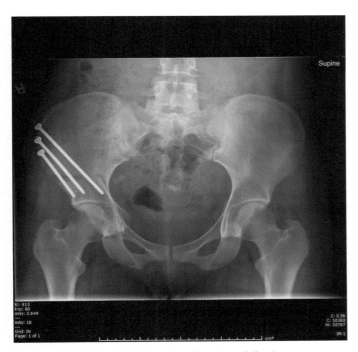

FIGURE 6-12 Radiographic imaging of a patient following a periacetabular osteotomy (PAO).

restrictive assistive device. The PT also educates the patient and caregivers on maintenance of appropriate weight-bearing and range of motion restrictions per facility protocol. Six to eight weeks postoperatively, a patient will meet with the surgeon for a follow-up with repeat imaging.[53] If adequate healing has been achieved, the patient may begin to assume full weight bearing and complete muscular strengthening.[53] Flexion strength can take up to 6 months to return, and complete bony union will take several months.[53]

Additional common hip disorders in pediatric patients include slipped capital femoral epiphysis (SCFE) and Legg-Calvé-Perthes disease. According to Peck,[54] slipped femoral epiphysis (SCFE) is defined as the posterior and inferior slippage of the proximal femoral epiphysis on the metaphysis (femoral neck), which occurs through the epiphyseal plate (growth plate). It is one of the most common disorders in adolescents and occurs typically in patients ages 8 to 15 years old.[54] Patients typically present with a limp and complain of associated pain in the hip, groin, thigh, and knee.[54] A SCFE is categorized as stable or unstable, with the level of stability determined by a patient's ability to ambulate with or without crutches.[54] The condition is more common in boys than girls and has been found to be associated with obesity, growth spurts, and endocrine disorders.[54] Common treatment of a SCFE is in situ fixation with the use of a single screw.[54] During the recovery process, patients may be limited with the amount of weight they may be able to place through the operative leg and thus require training on the use of an assistive device. Ultimately once the growth plate has been found to be closed, a patient will be cleared to return to athletics, including high-impact and contact sports.[54] If left untreated or diagnosis is prolonged, a patient may experience avascular necrosis of the femoral head, degenerative OA, and/or acute loss of cartilage (chondrolysis).[54]

Legg-Calvé-Perthes disease is a childhood hip condition that results in the idiopathic loss of blood supply to the capital femoral epiphysis, resulting in osteonecrosis and chondronecrosis that leads to deformity of the femoral head and degenerative OA later in life.[55] The clinical age of onset usually occurs between 4 and 8 years old, with the diagnosis being 5 times more common in males versus females.[55] Although a specific etiology is not clear, common thought is that the condition is the result of both genetic and environmental factors, such as hyperactivity or mechanical overload.[55] The aim of treatment is to minimize adverse effects on the shape of the femoral head and thus decrease the risk of the development of degenerative arthritis later in life.[56] Nonoperative treatment includes prescription of the use of an abduction orthosis or recommendation that the patient avoids placement of weight through the affected lower extremity and ambulates with the use of an assistive device.[55] Operative management typically includes pelvic osteotomies to provide optimal containment of the femoral head within the acetabulum to maintain the shape as revascularization occurs.[55] For patients younger than 5 years old, nonoperative treatment is typically recommended.[56] Overall prognosis is improved when patients are diagnosed and treated at 8 years of age or younger.[56] As with the previously mentioned hip surgeries, a PT's role will be to provide functional mobility training within the patient's precautions as well as initiate an exercise program to progress a patient's strength and range of motion during the recovery process.

Knee Conditions

Orthopedic conditions that involve the knee joint often occur as a result of acute injuries or abnormal growth patterns that impact baseline joint mechanics. Diagnoses that are commonly treated in the acute care setting include patellofemoral instability, anterior cruciate ligament (ACL) injuries, and excessive genu valgum or varus deformities.

Patellofemoral problems are considered to be among the most frequent causes of knee pain in children, with an incidence rate for children 10 to 18 years old of 29 per 100,000.[57] The pain and limitations that arise from patellofemoral issues are the result of abnormal patellar tracking often with lateral displacement and/or a lateral tilt of the patella.[57] Risk factors for patellar instability include trochlear dysplasia, patella alta, a lateralized tibial tubercle with increased tibial tuberosity–trochlear groove distance, knee joint laxity, femoral groove dysplasia, or lateral patellar tilt.[57] Treatment for patellofemoral issues includes off-loading knee braces and stretching and strengthening, particularly of the vastus medialis oblique (VMO) and rectus femoris.[57] Surgical management includes repairs and reconstruction to the medial patellofemoral ligament (MPFL) and VMO following frequent dislocations. Studies examining MPFL reconstructions have found that the rate of recurrent instability was low (3%) and return to sport was high (86%).[58]

ACL injuries typically occur as a result of a pivot mechanism with the knee partially flexed and the foot planted on the ground or as hyperextension of the knee with a valgus or a rotational force.[59] Because of the mechanism of injury, tearing the ACL is a common injury in contact sports or sports that involve quick changes in directions.[59] Screening for an ACL injury by the medical team upon presentation of a knee injury is important, as there is an incidence of ACL tears in 47% of preadolescents and 65% of adolescents who present with an acute hemarthrosis.[59]

Nonoperative management of ACL injuries may include positioning in a hinged knee brace, partial weight bearing for 6 to 8 weeks, progressive ACL rehabilitation, and activity restrictions from sports.[60] Nonoperative management of ACL injuries were found to have the greatest success in children and adolescents who experienced tears less than half the thickness of the ACL, those with a negative pivot shift test, and those with a skeletal age younger than 14 years.[59,60]

Surgical management for reconstruction of the ACL has increased nearly for children under 20 years old over the years.[60] Indications for surgery include the patient's inability to participate in sports, instability that affects ADLs, associated meniscal tear or chondral lesion, and/or multiple torn ligaments.[59] Surgical management often begin with preoperative physical therapy including reduction of pain and swelling, normalization of gait mechanics, and quadriceps and hamstring strengthening.[59] Surgical techniques prior to skeletal maturity may include the use of the iliotibial band as part of the reconstruction, which has the advantage of avoiding impact to the physes through fixation to the outer portion of the bone.[59]

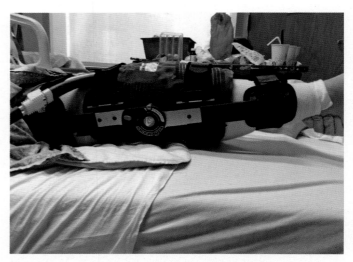

FIGURE 6-13 **Example of a hinged knee brace to assist with maintaining post operative precautions.**

Alternatively, patients may undergo transphyseal ACL reconstruction with hamstring autograft.[59]

Following surgery for both patellofemoral and ACL reconstruction/repairs, patients will often be placed in a knee brace (**Figure 6-13**) that limits knee flexion in order to avoid stress to the patella or graft site and ambulate with limited weight bearing through the affected lower extremity. Acute postoperative training is provided by physical therapy for the use of assistive devices and mobilization with the recommended precautions. There is also a focus on engaging the quadriceps and introducing range of motion within the postoperative precautions.

Finally, children may present with angular deformities of the knees in the coronal plane, resulting in excessive genu valgus or genu valgum.[61] Patients who are obese or present with neuromuscular disorders that alter the muscular force at the knee joint are at further risk for these persistent angular deformities or growth plate disturbances from fractures.[62] Often, these deviations will spontaneously correct during a typically developing child's growth period; however, there are times in which they persist further into adolescence.[61] In these instances, surgical interventions may be used in order to avoid degeneration of cartilage, changes in the orientation of soft tissue, and the ultimate negative impact on functional mobility.[61] A common surgical approach known as hemiepiphysiodesis is often used. This technique aims to halt the growth of one side of the physis, thus changing the angular orientation of the knee and gradually correcting the deformity.[61] The technique can result in permanent or temporary slowing of growth through the use of staples, screws, and tension bands.[61]

Scoliosis

According to El-hawary and Chukwunyerenwa,[63] scoliosis is defined as a 3-dimensional structural deformity that includes a curvature in the anterior-posterior plane, angulation in the sagittal plane, and rotation in the transverse plane (**Figure 6-14**). There are 3 categories of scoliosis, which are based on the way in which the curve develops: idiopathic, congenital, and neuromuscular.

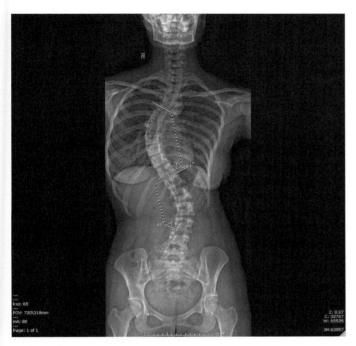

FIGURE 6-14   Radiographic imaging of a patient with scoliosis.

Idiopathic scoliosis is the most common cause of scoliosis, accounting for 80% of cases in children, and includes curves that are greater than 10 degrees.[63] Idiopathic scoliosis is further classified based on the age of onset: infantile (0-3 years), juvenile (3-10 years), and adolescent (>10 years).[63] Infantile onset accounts for less than 1% of cases, most of which ultimately resolve spontaneously.[63,64] Juvenile-onset scoliosis accounts for 12% to 21% of idiopathic scoliosis cases, exhibits a slight female predominance, and presents as a right thoracic curve primarily.[63] In general, the most common type of idiopathic scoliosis is adolescent onset.[63] The risk of progression of the curve depends on the skeletal maturity, sex, and curve magnitude of the patient.[63] The more skeletally immature the patient, the more likely there will be a curve progression.[63]

Congenital scoliosis is the result of malformations of the spine present at birth.[63] These malformations can include a failure of formation of a vertebral body, failure of segmentation between two vertebrae, or a combination of both.[63] Of the patients with a diagnosis of congenital scoliosis, 61% have an associated anomaly in other organ systems or the curve may be a part of a syndrome.[63]

Finally, neuromuscular scoliosis is a curve in the spine that is the result of neurologic or muscular disorders.[63] Patients with a neuromuscular scoliosis lack the muscular support around the spinal column, resulting in a deformity of the spine due to the effects of gravity and posturing.[63] Conditions associated with neuromuscular scoliosis include CP, muscular dystrophies, myelomeningocele, and spinal muscular atrophy.[63]

Treatment Options for Scoliosis

For patients with scoliosis, there are a range of treatment options based on the magnitude of the curve. For curves less than 25 degrees, physicians may choose to simply monitor

the progression with close follow-up appointments every 3 to 6 months in conjunction with outpatient physical therapy.[63] Bracing is recommended for patients with curves of 25 to 45 degrees, with a goal to ultimately prevent progression below the surgical level until skeletal maturity is reached.[63] For patients with neuromuscular scoliosis, nonsurgical management includes wheelchair modifications such a custom-molded seatback or bracing.[63] Bracing to address neuromuscular scoliosis, however, tends to be less effective than in idiopathic scoliosis but can delay the need for surgery if indicated.[63]

Surgical management of scoliosis is recommended for curves of 50 degrees or greater; however, other factors are also considered such as age, curve progression (categorized as a progression of 5 degrees between serial imaging) and related symptoms.[63,64] Any compromise in pulmonary function may warrant surgery despite the magnitude of the curve.[64] Surgery typically includes correction of the spinal curve with fusion through instrumentation and bone grafting (**Figure 6-15**).[63] The goal of surgery is to halt curve progression while improving spinal balance and alignment.[63] For patients who are still skeletally immature, growth-friendly surgeries are performed and include spine or rib-based distractions that are secured to the proximal and distal ends of the curve and grown every 6 months.[63] New techniques that include the use of magnetically controlled growing rods have additionally been performed and forego the need for ongoing invasive surgery.[63] The goal of these surgeries is to allow for appropriate spinal growth, prevent further curve progression, and allow for adequate pulmonary development. In addition, for patients with severe spinal deformities, halo-gravity traction may be used prior to a spinal fusion surgery. Halo-gravity traction (**Figures 6-16** and **6-17**) allows for a preoperative partial correction of the spinal

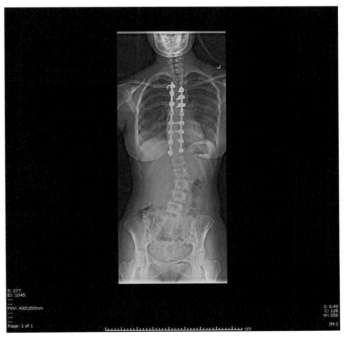

FIGURE 6-15   Radiographic imaging of a patient following a posterior spinal fusion.

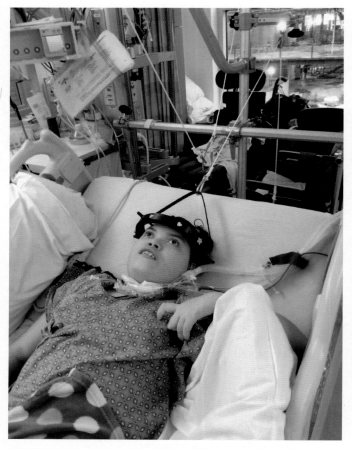

FIGURE 6-16 **A patient resting in bed with halo-gravity traction.**

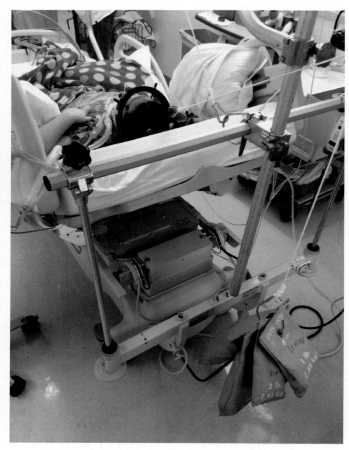

FIGURE 6-17 **Additional view of the halo-gravity traction setup.**

curve, which leads to an improvement in a patient's pulmonary function and tolerance to surgery as well as the need for a less aggressive surgical correction.[65]

For patients with neuromuscular scoliosis who undergo a spinal fusion, there is often a high rate of postoperative complications.[66] Studies have shown that patients with a pre-operative curve greater than 60 degrees with a nonambulatory status have a risk of developing at least one complication.[66] These complications include pulmonary complications (22.7%-28.2%), implant complications (12.5%-12.7%), infections (4.0%-10.9%), neurologic complications (1.8%-3.0%), cardiac complications (1.8%), and wound dehiscence (1.6%).[66,67] Patients with neuromuscular disorders additionally tend to experience the greatest blood loss and require a transfusion either during surgery or postoperatively.[66]

Following a patient's procedure for either a spinal fusion or placement of growing rods, physical therapy will often be consulted to address a patient's mobility needs. Patients are instructed to follow "spinal precautions" as a means to improve their comfort following surgery. These precautions often include limiting hip and trunk flexion past 90 degrees, avoiding lifting heavy objects, and minimizing twisting through the spine. A PT will instruct the patients on appropriate ways to complete bed mobility via log rolling as well as to perform transitions and transfers to adhere to

the spinal precautions. With respect to ambulation, patients will often be limited by pain and decreased endurance. They may report feeling "stiff" along their spine and subsequently demonstrate associated gait deviations. Patients will often have Jackson-Pratt drains placed at the surgical site as well as Foley catheters during the immediate postoperative period. As always, a PT should consider these lines prior to having a patient mobilize out of bed.

Patients undergoing spinal procedures who may have been dependent for transfers and use a wheelchair as their primary means of mobility prior to the surgery will have different PT needs postoperatively. Caregivers will need to complete training on appropriate ways to assist a patient with bed mobility that adhere to spinal precautions. They will additionally need practice on proper lifting techniques while performing transfers, as the methods performed preoperatively may no longer be possible given the patient's precautions and decreased spinal and pelvic mobility. If the patient uses a lift system to perform transfers, clearance to resume use of the lift will need to be obtained from the orthopedic team. With respect to the patient's wheelchair, adjustments to grow the chair will often be required given the patient's newly corrected posture. If a patient previously used a molded seat back, a new back will need to be ordered. Given the patient's postoperative discomfort, a gradual progression and tolerance to sitting in their wheelchair per the patient's baseline will be needed in the days following surgery.

Pain Control

Acute pain is defined as pain of a short duration (hours to days) and is typically associated with trauma, illness, or surgery.[32] For patients presenting to physical therapy with orthopedic complications or recovering from orthopedic surgery, it is particularly important to ensure that pain is adequately controlled. Scheduling a physical therapy session during optimal pain control will not only maximize a patient's comfort during movement but also improve the overall level of participation and learning that occurs. Often a patient's level of pain will fluctuate based on the activities performed.[32] As a result, it is important for a PT to provide feedback to a patient's nurse as well as the medical team if a patient's progression during sessions is limited due to poor pain control. Many hospitals have a dedicated pain management team, whose primary role is to establish and adjust a patient's pain management regime as needed. In the pediatric population, pain can be measured and monitored through the use of scales that quantify pain such as the Wong-Baker Faces Pain Scale or the visual analog scale.[32] Ultimately, adequate pain control is a vital component of a patient's recovery process because it helps to maximize the ability to mobilize, improves patient satisfaction, and reduces stress.[68]

In pediatric patients, there are a variety of measures to assist with managing pain, including medications and local anesthetics. Medication may be administered orally or through a peripheral IV including the use of a patient-controlled analgesia (PCA).[32] A PCA has been shown to be effective at controlling pain in children older than 6 years old.[32] For patients younger than 6 years old or with physical disabilities or cognitive impairments, the medical team may use continuous IV infusions.[32] These infusions allow for a steady state of medication levels in the blood without wide fluctuations.[32] Additional medication may be required during episodes of breakthrough pain. Among nonopioid analgesics, acetaminophen is one of the most common medications prescribed to patients.[32] The duration of the effects of pain medication and how often it can be provided to a patient vary by drug. As a result, it is important to discuss the medication regimen with the nurse to determine the most optimal time to schedule a PT session.

NSAIDs are also used with children as young as 3 to 12 months old but can be associated with gastrointestinal disturbances and renal damage and can impact a patient's hemostasis.[32,69] Benzodiazepines (eg, diazepam) can be used to control the inflammation of muscles following surgery, which can lead to spasms and pain.[32] Medications classified as opioids include some of the most powerful drugs available for pain relief and include codeine, hydrocodone, and oxycodone.[69] Unfortunately, common side effects of opioid use can include itching, nausea, and sedation, which can ultimately hinder a patient's participation during PT sessions.[32] Side effects from pain medication should also be conveyed to the medical team to further help establish a medication balance for full participation.

In addition to medications, local anesthetics may be used during surgeries to temporarily block signals along nerve fibers.[32] Epidural catheters are placed directly into the spine for continuous administration of local anesthetics and/or opioids.[32] Side effects include nausea, dizziness, hypotension, motor weakness, respiratory depression, and potential development of an epidural hematoma.[69] Peripheral nerve blocks include placement of a local anesthetic at a peripheral nerve to block pain signals to the central nervous system.[32] These nerve blocks can be used as a single injection or a catheter for continuous injections.[32] The use of the blocks helps to minimize the use of opioids, avoiding adverse side effects as well as aiding in postoperative return of gastrointestinal function.[69] It is important to remember, however, that although these local anesthetics assist with pain management, they also can mask potential postoperative complications such as compartment syndrome, as well as negatively impact a patient's balance and lower extremity stability during weight-bearing tasks.[32] For instance, a patient with a local anesthetic may experience decreased sensation and subsequently impaired motor control while standing, resulting in an increased risk of knee buckling. As a result, patients should be closely monitored and guarded during gait training.

Orthopedic Examination and Evaluation

As previously reported, once a PT receives a consult order for an inpatient physical therapy evaluation and treatment, a thorough chart review is completed along with the acknowledgement of pertinent precautions and activity guidelines. With orthopedic conditions, these precautions and guidelines will be an important aspect of the examination and will ultimately guide activity progression, DME recommendations, and discharge planning.

Gaining an understanding of a patient's weight-bearing precautions will allow a PT to begin to evaluate the most appropriate assistive device that will yield the greatest level of safety and independence within the home environment. All key aspects of the patient and family interview previously reviewed should be included as part of the initial evaluation. With orthopedic cases, a patient may have previous experience and comfort in using an assistive device, either during a previous injury or as part of a baseline level of function. This experience will in turn affect the level of training that will be required for a safe discharge. In addition, a patient's age and level of cognition will also influence which specific assistive device, if any, is recommended during the recovery process.

As part of the initial examination, a baseline strength and range of motion assessment should be performed. Manual muscle testing at both the upper and lower extremities can be used to quantify the patient's strength; however, special care and decision-making should be taken when determining the appropriateness of applying resistance at joints that recently underwent a surgical procedure. Modified strength testing can be performed at the affected joints through use of observation and palpation of isometric muscle contractions. Furthermore, based on the patient's postoperative presentation, pain, lethargy, and/or nausea may limit a patient's ability to participate in formal manual muscle testing. In these instances, a gross assessment of a patient's strength can be gained as the patient begins to participate in functional activities. With respect to range of motion, a PT should perform an active and passive screen of the upper extremities, spine, and lower extremities, assessing for limitations that may affect a patient's presentation and function during the recovery process. A patient may additionally begin to perform active assisted range of motion at the affected joints to begin the process of postoperative joint range of motion and surrounding muscle activation. A sensory and proprioception screen should be performed to assess not only for potential complications from surgery but also effects of local anesthetics. Any identified impairments have the potential to influence balance, skin integrity, and overall function during recovery. The patient's current level of pain should also be objectively obtained through the most appropriate means (eg, Wong-Baker Faces Pain Scale, FLACC scale, numeric rating scale) to begin tracking the patient's baseline pain, the impact of activity on pain, and the effectiveness of a patient's pain medication regimen. Finally, monitoring a patient's vital signs throughout the examination can further guide a progression of activities. Patients may experience episodes of hypotension when first transferring out of bed following surgery, warranting close monitoring. Please refer to earlier in this chapter for a reference of normal values for pediatric vitals. For patients who are nonverbal or with cognitive delays, autonomic responses, such as an increase in respiratory rate or heart rate, as well as the Individualized Numeric Rating Scale, can be used to monitor pain responses.

From a functional perspective, the PT should then begin to examine a patient's ability to perform bed mobility tasks, transfers, ambulation, and stair negotiation (if needed). Early mobilization following any orthopedic procedure is an important part of the recovery process as it promotes movement of joints and muscle activation, leading to improved function. As a reminder, it is important to consider a patient's baseline level of function and cognition when formulating an expected prognosis and appropriate goals to ensure a safe discharge. Following an orthopedic procedure, patients need to learn to perform movements with new joint alignments (eg, status post spinal fusion), precautions, and/or brace and cast support. As a result, PTs play a vital role in educating patients and their families on a safe and appropriate way to move postoperatively. This training is important as patients may require increased support from equipment or caregivers from their typical baseline level of function. Caregiver support may include guarding for safety and/or hands-on assistance, such as in the case of a patient following PAO who has postoperative weakness and range of motion restrictions and therefore requires assistance to maneuver their operative leg during bed mobility. The PT is also a valuable resource to provide recommendations for physical activities and exercises, if applicable, the patient can perform as part of a daily routine upon discharge. These guidelines will help to ensure a patient appropriately recovers and maximizes their ability to function during this process.

The following is a list of sample goals for a variety of patient ages and orthopedic procedures. Due to the generally short admission time frame for patients who undergo orthopedic procedures, short-term goals often equate to long-term goals. Goals should be created and based on the expected presentation in order for a patient to be deemed safe to function in their respective discharge environment. Ideally, once these goals are met, a patient can be considered appropriate to discharge home from a physical therapy perspective once they are medically cleared.

Scenario 1: A 3-year-old child status post femur fracture with spica application.

Short-Term Goals (to be met in 3 sessions)

1. Patient's caregivers will be independent with performing dependent cradle transfers bed to/from wheelchair.
2. Patient's caregivers will be independent with assisting the patient with all bed mobility with proper body mechanics.
3. Patient's caregivers will be independent with all PT-provided activity and positioning recommendations.

Scenario 2: A 16-year-old patient with ACL tear now status post ACL reconstruction of the left knee.

Short-Term Goals (to be met in 5 days)

1. Patient will complete all bed mobility with assist from a caregiver to only support the left lower extremity as needed.
2. Patient will complete all transfers via sit to/from stand with least restrictive device and no more than close supervision from caregivers.
3. Patient will ambulate at least 50 feet with least restrictive device and no more than close supervision from caregivers.
4. Patient will negotiate a flight of stairs with single rail support and least restrictive device with no more than contact guard assistance.
5. Patient will be independent with maintaining weight-bearing precautions during all functional mobility.

Scenario 3: A 14-year-old child with past medical history of idiopathic scoliosis who is now status post posterior spinal fusion of T12-L5.

Short-Term Goals (to be met in 1 week)

1. Patient will complete all bed mobility independently.
2. Patient will complete all transfers via sit to/from stand independently.
3. Patient will ambulate at least 200 feet with no more than close supervision.
4. Patient will negotiate a flight of stairs with single rail support and no more than contact guard assistance.
5. Patient will accurately recall all spinal precautions without the need for assistance.

ONCOLOGY

Introduction

In the United States, approximately 1 in 400 children under 15 years of age and 1 in 300 children under 20 years of age will be diagnosed with cancer. Cancer is also the second leading cause of death in children 5 to 14 years of age. Despite this fact, the 5-year survival rate for childhood cancer is approximately 80%, and more than half (70%) of survivors are at least 20 years old. It is also notable that, in general, children and adolescents who survive 5 years after their primary diagnosis have a high probability of subsequent survival for at least the next 10 years.[70] The most common types of cancers as well as survival rates vary by age, sex, and race/ethnicity. It is the role of the pediatric acute care PT to address impairments caused by medical interventions, disease process, and hospital course related to a patient's oncologic diagnosis.

Cancer diagnoses are generally categorized by the area in which the cancers grow including the brain and nervous system, blood and lymphatic systems, and musculoskeletal system. They are further categorized by origin and/or cell type. The most common types of childhood cancer will be described in this section.

Common Pediatric Cancers

Cancers of the Brain and Central Nervous System

Although brain and nervous system cancers are not the most commonly diagnosed cancers in the pediatric population, they are the leading cause of mortality related to childhood cancer.[71] These types of cancerous tumors are named for the type of cell they originated from and/or the location within the nervous system. There are different grades of tumors, graded for how fast they are growing and how likely they are to invade neighboring tissue.

According to the American Cancer Society, grade I and II cancers are slow growing or benign and are less likely to grow into nearby tissue, whereas grade III and IV cancers grow quickly or are metastatic and are more likely to grow into nearby tissue.

In children over 1 year old, over two-thirds of intracranial tumors arise from the posterior fossa of the cranium, which includes the cerebellum and brain stem. This grouping of tumors is referred to as posterior fossa tumors. The most commonly diagnosed intracranial tumors are pilocytic astrocytoma, medulloblastoma, ependymoma, and brain stem glioma.[72]

Glioma Family Glioma is a general term used to describe cancer that arises from the glial cells of the brain. Gliomas are the most common type of brain tumor in children and adolescents.[73,74]

Types of glioma include:

1. **Astrocytomas:** Astrocytoma, anaplastic astrocytoma, and glioblastoma
2. **Ependymomas:** Anaplastic ependymoma, myxopapillary ependymoma, and subependymoma
3. **Oligodendrogliomas:** Oligodendroglioma, anaplastic oligodendroglioma, and anaplastic oligoastrocytoma.[73]

Astrocytoma Cerebellar astrocytomas are the most frequently occurring posterior fossa tumors in children, accounting for up to 35% of these lesions.[75] Cerebellar pilocytic astrocytomas are generally resectable without the need for additional therapy. Those arising from the brain stem, however, are often not completely resectable and require chemotherapy.[72] Anaplastic astrocytoma and glioblastoma are rare and aggressive grade III and IV astrocytomas.

Ependymoma Ependymomas are rare tumors originating from the ependymal cells that line the ventricular system of the brain, the central canal of the spinal cord. They account for 6% to 12% of all intracranial tumors in children and up to 50% of the intracranial tumors in children under 5 years of age.[76] Ninety percent of the childhood intracranial ependymomas are found in the posterior fossa.[76] Because of the aggressive nature of these tumors, they are often treated with surgery (resection) and followed with radiation and/or chemotherapy.[76] Relapse in the pediatric population is high, and the best known prognostic indicator for survival is success of surgical resection.

Oligoastrocytoma This is a mixed glioma made up of cells from oligodendroglioma and diffuse astrocytoma. They can be low grade (World Health Organization [WHO] grade II) or high grade (WHO grade III).[77] Oligoastrocytomas account for less than 20% of the intracranial tumors and are rare among the pediatric population, most often presenting in the temporal lobe.[78] Fifty percent of patients ultimately diagnosed with oligoastrocytoma present with new-onset seizures.[78]

Presenting symptoms of gliomas depend on the area of the brain in which they arise but often include headache or nausea and vomiting.[79] Vision changes are likely apparent in an optic glioma. Treatment depends on the type, grade, and location of the tumor but often includes surgical resection possibly followed by radiation therapy or chemotherapy.

Medulloblastoma Also called grade IV primitive neuroectodermal tumors, medulloblastomas are relatively fast-growing tumors of the posterior fossa. They often arise in the cerebellar vermis and extend into the fourth ventricle. Patients may present with progressive symptoms of cerebellar dysfunction and increased intracranial pressure (ICP) over a period of weeks to months. Patients may also present with cranial nerve involvement.[80] The survival rate for these tumors has improved in recent years, but because of the aggressive nature of the treatment options, the survivors are often left with sequelae that include neurologic, endocrinologic, and communication issues and the inability to interact socially.[81] Patients under the age of 3 often do not receive radiation therapy due to the high risk of neurocognitive impairment.[80]

Neuroblastoma Neuroblastomas are also considered central nervous system tumors because they arise from neural crest cells, but the tumors themselves can be found in many areas of the body, most commonly the abdomen, given the migratory nature of the cells. Neuroblastomas account for 10% of pediatric cancer diagnoses but 15% of pediatric cancer deaths.[82] This is likely due to the low survival rate of patients with high-risk neuroblastoma. In contrast, patients with low-risk neuroblastomas have a 90% survival rate. Treatment for neuroblastomas, similar to that for medulloblastomas and gliomas, is determined by risk categorization: low, intermediate, or high. Low- and intermediate-risk patients are often treated with surgical resection alone, whereas high-risk patients require aggressive multimodal treatment.[82]

Posterior Fossa Syndrome Posterior fossa syndrome (PFS) is a term used for a group of symptoms that are sometimes present in children following the removal of a posterior fossa tumor. It is unclear why some children experience this syndrome and others do not. The symptoms can become evident 24 to 107 hours postsurgically. The symptoms include aphasia, dysphasia, mutism or other speech disturbances, decreased motor output of a single or multiple limbs, emotional lability, and cranial nerve palsy. These symptoms can take weeks or months to resolve. Many children continue to struggle with these symptoms years after the tumor removal.[83]

Cancers of the Blood and Lymphatic System

The 2 most common categories of blood and lymphatic cancers in children and adolescents are leukemia and lymphoma. Leukemias begin in the bone marrow, often in the white blood cells, whereas lymphomas develop in the lymphatic system.[84]

Leukemias are the most common cancers diagnosed in children. There are many types of leukemias, the most common being acute lymphocytic leukemia (ALL) and acute myelogenous leukemia (AML). ALL, which accounts for approximately 25% of total childhood cancer diagnoses, begins in the lymphocytes.[85] It can be further differentiated by the specific type of lymphocyte, with B-cell being more common than T-cell leukemia.[85] AML begins in myeloid cells, which typically grow to form nonlymphocyte white blood cells, red blood cells, and platelets. Children with leukemias typically present with fatigue, weakness, signs of chronic infection such as fever secondary to low white blood cell counts, easy bruising or bleeding secondary to low platelet counts, bone and/or joint pain, and/or weight loss.[86] Initial treatment for both AML and ALL involves multiple cycles of chemotherapy.[87] Some patients also undergo stem cell transplant or chimeric antigen receptor T-cell (CAR-T) therapy, which will both be discussed in further detail later in this section. Survival rates over the past 10 years have significantly improved secondary to continued advances in treatment.[85]

Lymphomas are the third most common type of cancer diagnosed in the pediatric population. The 2 most common types of lymphomas are classified as Hodgkin lymphoma (HL) and non-Hodgkin lymphoma (NHL), although these can be further subcategorized as well. The defining characteristic of HL is the presence of Reed-Sternberg cells.[88] Patients typically present with painless adenopathy (swelling of lymph nodes), often in the cervical or supraclavicular areas.[89] There are multiple subtypes of NHL, differentiated by the grade and histology of the tumors. The majority of NHLs in children are high grade.[90] NHL is more common in children under the age of 15, after which HL becomes more common. The survival rate of each has improved in the past 30 years, with that of HL being greater than 97% in patients under 20 years of age and that of NHL being greater than 88% in the same age range.[70] The treatment for both HL and NHL includes chemotherapy and/or radiation therapy pending the specific subtype and grade.

Cancers of the Musculoskeletal System

Cancers that develop from connective tissues are classified under the general term of sarcoma. There are several subtypes of sarcoma, which are named for the tissue and cell types affected. Primary cancers that start in the bone are relatively rare, making up less than 1% of all cancer diagnoses.[91] A patient may also present with metastatic bone tumors; however, these

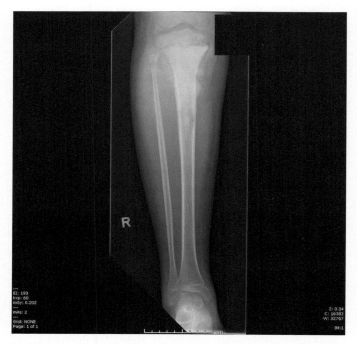

FIGURE 6-18 Radiographic imaging of a tumor surrounding the tibia.

are made up of cells from the primary cancer. Osteosarcoma and Ewing sarcoma are seen rarely in adults and are more common in children, adolescents, and young adults.

Osteosarcoma is the most common type of sarcoma seen in the pediatric population. Osteosarcoma occurs most frequently in the metaphysis of long bones, specifically the distal femur (43%), proximal tibia (23%), or humerus (10%).[92] **Figures 6-18** and **6-19** show significant tumor burden of the

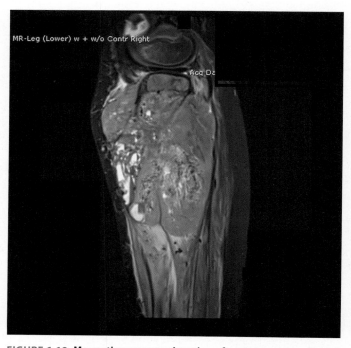

FIGURE 6-19 Magnetic resonance imaging of a tumor surrounding the tibia.

tibia and surrounding soft tissue structures via x-ray and MRI, respectively. Ewing sarcoma is the second most common primary bone cancer in the pediatric population. Unlike osteosarcoma, Ewing sarcoma is most commonly found in the pelvis, chest, and middle of the long bones.[93] Patients typically present with swelling of the affected area and pain that is significant enough to wake them from sleep.[94] Rhabdomyosarcoma (RMS) begins in the cells that make up skeletal muscles. It is the most common soft tissue sarcoma of childhood.[95] Because there are so many areas of skeletal muscle in the body, presenting symptoms of RMS are varied.[96] Treatment for all of these types of sarcoma typically includes chemotherapy both prior to and following surgical resection.

Other Solid Tumors

There are several types of solid tumor that occur outside of the musculoskeletal system in children. These include Wilms tumor and hepatoblastoma. Wilms tumor is the most common malignant tumor of the kidney, diagnosed in children at an average age of 30 to 33 months.[97] Treatment for Wilms tumor involves surgical resection, possibly followed by chemotherapy, with a survival rate of approximately 90%.[97] Hepatoblastoma is the most common malignant hepatic tumor diagnosed in the pediatric population. Treatment includes chemotherapy in addition to surgical resection, although 40% of hepatoblastomas are unresectable and require liver transplant.[98]

Medical Treatment Options

There are many types of cancer treatments. Often, patients will require a combination of several treatment techniques. This section will discuss the techniques used frequently for treatment of cancer in the pediatric population, although more exist.

Chemotherapy

Chemotherapy refers to the use of medication to treat cancer. As noted earlier, chemotherapy is a common technique for treating most types of cancer. Patients typically undergo multiple cycles of chemotherapy, although the specific treatment regimen depends on the type and stage of cancer. The 3 possible goals of chemotherapy are to cure the cancer, control the cancer, or provide palliative control such as pain relief.[99] Chemotherapeutic agents are used to disrupt the growth and spread of cancer cells; however, because they are used systemically, they are unable to distinguish between normal and cancerous cells, causing the death of normal cells as well.[99] Thus, there are many side effects of chemotherapy. **Table 6-13** includes several common chemotherapy agents, and their commonly associated side effects.

Because of the nonspecific nature of chemotherapy agents, one major risk of treatment is infection. Leukemias and chemotherapy agents both cause neutropenia, or diminished number of healthy white cells that make up the immune system. This increases a patient's risk of developing and fighting an infection. Patients who are neutropenic should not be in proximity to any person or patient who could pass an infection. This may involve being placed on "contact precautions" or "reverse precautions"

while in hospital and requiring all providers to wear a gown and gloves when entering the patient's room. This would also limit that patient to their hospital room. Although this is an important precaution in order to maintain the patient's safety, it also limits the ability to participate in functional activities, particularly given that many hospital rooms are quite small. This may require education with regard to beneficial activities that can be performed in the patient's room that will facilitate physical activity.

Some chemotherapy agents may cause chemotherapy-induced peripheral neuropathy (CIPN). There are multiple areas of the neuron that can be affected by chemotherapy agents, leading to CIPN. Although the incidence of CIPN has not been well studied in children as of yet, up to one-third of adult patients with cancer treated with multiple chemotherapy agents are diagnosed with CIPN.[100] The most common symptoms of CIPN include sensory loss in a stocking glove distribution of the hands and feet; this may include loss of light tough, proprioception, and/or vibration, as well as distal muscle weakness. Many patients also report neuropathic pain, which may impact their ability to tolerate weight-bearing activities and/or socks or other clothing.[101] With regard to impairments and activity limitations, these symptoms are likely to impact balance, gait, and coordination, which will significantly impact the patient's functional mobility and safety. Many patients experience foot drop, which often manifests itself by patients appearing to trip over their feet due to a lack of foot clearance during the swing phase of gait. Patients who are too young to verbalize their subjective symptoms may demonstrate a resistance to bearing weight through their legs either due to discomfort or the feeling of instability. Because many pediatric patients are admitted for some, if not all, of their chemotherapy treatments, they may begin to show symptoms during their admission. It is important that a PT perform a comprehensive sensory, strength, and functional evaluation if any of these signs or symptoms are reported by the patient, family, or medical team. Physical therapy treatment may include strengthening, balance activities, and desensitization. Although many cases of CIPN resolve once the chemotherapy treatment has stopped,[101] there is limited information regarding the lasting symptoms of CIPN. Therefore, long-term recommendations may be required, such as bracing or the use of an assistive device in the event of persistent foot drop and gait impairments.

Radiation

Radiation therapy uses high-energy particles to disrupt the DNA of cancer cells, causing cell death.[102] Unlike chemotherapy, most radiation therapy is local. Although it may affect nearby healthy cells, there are typically fewer systemic side effects than are caused by chemotherapy. Some side effects may still be significant, such as potential neurocognitive effects of radiation to the brain, particularly in young children. The acute care PT should be aware of whether radiation is a part of a patient's treatment plan. From an administrative perspective, radiation will require the patient to leave the floor for treatment. It is also important to be cognizant of possible side effects, which typically involve the direct area being treated but may also impact

TABLE 6-13 • Common Chemotherapy Agents and Adverse Effects[99]

Drug Class	Common Agent(s)	Adverse Effects	Considerations for PT
Alkaylating agents	Cyclophosphamide Cisplatin Busulfan Thiotepa	Myelosuppression Mucositis Nausea/vomiting Neurotoxicity Alopecia Pulmonary fibrosis Infertility Secondary malignancies	Risk of bleeding with falls, resistance exercise, etc due to myelosuppression Changes in neurological symptoms General tolerance to activity due to nausea/vomiting Respiratory insufficiency during activity
Topoisomerase II inhibitors	Doxorubicin	Myelosuppression Cardiotoxicity Nausea/vomiting Alopecia Vesicant (causes skin blisters) Secondary malignancies (rare but associated with poor prognosis)	Risk of bleeding with falls, resistance exercise, etc due to myelosuppression Cardiovascular response to activity
Antimicrotubular agents	Vincristine (VCR)	Neurotoxicities/Peripheral neuropathies • Loss of deep tendon reflexes • Distal sensory changes • Distal motor changes Myelosuppression	Risk of bleeding with falls, resistance exercise, etc due to myelosuppression Neuropathic pain and fall risk related to neuropathy
Antimetabolites	Methotrexate (MTX) Cytarabine Mercaptopurine Nelarabine	Mucositis Hepatotoxicity Nephrotoxicity Nausea/vomiting/GI symptoms Myelosuppression Immunosupression Elevated liver enzymes Generalized aches/pains Peripheral neuropathies Neurotoxcity Veno-occlusive disease Skin reactions	Risk of bleeding with falls, resistance exercise, etc due to myelosuppression Infection risk Neurological symptoms: headache, dizziness, nystagmus Fall risk

the patient's ability to participate in PT session. For example, if a patient is receiving radiation to the abdomen, side effects may include nausea and/or vomiting, which will limit a patient's tolerance to activity.

Stem Cell Transplant

Hematopoietic stem cells are located in the bone marrow and develop into blood cells. Stem cell transplants allow a patient to receive aggressive chemotherapy that would otherwise destroy their bone marrow or, in some types of leukemia, provide the opportunity for transplanted cells to attack the patient's cancer (known as graft-versus-cancer effect).[103] Stem cell transplants are most commonly used in the treatment of leukemias and lymphomas but are also used in the treatment of some other cancers such as neuroblastoma.[104] Transplants are most successful when the patient is in remission but may also be used if the patient is at high risk or if the patient has relapsed after previous successful treatment. The transplant

may also be referred to as a bone marrow transplant, but the difference is only in the process for retrieval of the transplanted cells; cells can come from the donor's bone marrow or peripheral blood.

The 2 primary types of stem cell transplants are autologous and allogenic. In the case of an autologous stem cell transplant, the cells belong to the patient and are harvested during a period of remission. This type of transplant is used to restore the patient's ability to make their own blood cells after the bone marrow has been destroyed by chemotherapy, such as used for neuroblastoma. It does not provide the graft-versus-cancer effect, which can occur following allogenic stem cell transplant. In the case of an allogenic stem cell transplant, cells are harvested from a donor, ideally a relative.[105]

The process for a stem cell transplant has several steps. First, the patient is admitted to the hospital for high-dose chemotherapy, possibly in conjunction with total-body irradiation therapy.[105] This process is called "conditioning" and is used to completely destroy the bone marrow (and hopefully cancerous cells if they are present). The patient then receives their stem cells through an IV infusion. Over approximately 2 to 4 weeks, if the transplant is successful, the patient will go through "engraftment," during which the body begins to produce its own blood cells.[105] During this time, the patient is especially immunocompromised and is isolated from the outside population given the high risk that any infection could pose. In the hospital, these patients remain in a separate wing from all other patients, and after discharge, they remain isolated for a prolonged period of time in order to allow the immune system to fully recover. It is therefore important that the PT treating in this area of the hospital be aware of their own health. No person—hospital employee or patient guest—should enter the stem cell transplant wing if they are experiencing any symptoms of illness at all, even those of the common cold, which might not otherwise limit the PT's ability to work. These isolation precautions also continue following discharge from the acute care hospital, and any discharge PT recommendations should take this fact into account. For example, a patient may benefit from continued PT services on an outpatient basis; however, because of the post-transplant precautions, the patient cannot be treated in an outpatient clinic and home PT services should be arranged.

It is also important to consider the systemic effects of hematopoietic stem cell transplantation (HSCT) beyond those of the conditioning regimen. Mucositis of the mouth and/or intestine is the most common early side effect of HSCT and causes pain as well as possible nausea, cramping, and diarrhea.[106] As the acute care PT, it is necessary to identify if and when a patient will tolerate participation despite these symptoms and when sessions will need to be postponed. This requires regular communication with nursing staff, patients, and families as well as coordination with pain control.

The other primary risk factor following HSCT is graft-versus-host disease (GVHD), which can occur either spontaneously or as an immune response to an allogenic transplant.[106] GVHD may occur in one of several body systems including the gastrointestinal system, liver, lungs, and skin.[107] GVHD can be recalcitrant to treatment and, when chronic, is one of the highest risk factors for mortality.[107] It is possible for GVHD to arise after the patient's initial hospitalization and thus require readmission for treatment. It is therefore important for the acute care PT to identify if these patients, who may require prolonged admission, will require additional PT intervention while in the hospital.

Studies have shown that exercise has a positive effect on both physical measures and health-related quality of life in patients undergoing cancer treatment.[108-110] With specific relation to HSCT, the most benefits have been observed at hospital discharge for patients who participated in exercise during hospitalization.[110] This is an especially important consideration for the acute care PT, as it indicates that education and intervention regarding regular exercise throughout a patient's hospitalization have the opportunity to mitigate several of the negative sequelae of cancer treatment. Given that patients are admitted to the hospital several days prior to HSCT for conditioning, there is often ample time to initiate physical therapy activities before patients begin to experience the effects of engraftment.[111]

CAR-T

CAR-T therapy is a new treatment used for patients with B-cell leukemias and lymphomas that are refractory to treatment or have relapsed multiple times.[112] It is a form of immune therapy that uses the patient's own cells to target malignant cells.[113] Patients who are admitted for CAR-T therapy may benefit from a PT evaluation or consultation if they have baseline PT needs, although the therapy itself does not typically result in specific deficits in body structure and function. It is important for the acute care PT to be aware, however, of the risk of cytokine release syndrome (CRS), which is an acute toxicity caused by CAR-T infusion.[112] CRS can often be treated with medication, but at its most toxic, it can lead to cardiac dysfunction and neurologic toxicity, among other life-threatening symptoms, which could require PT treatment once the patient becomes medically stable.[114]

Surgery

When the goal of a surgical approach to treatment of a solid tumor is curative, complete resection is necessary. This is the goal for many solid tumors. In some cases, tumors may not require complete resection, such as a low-grade glioma, which is slow growing and may cause limited symptoms. In these cases, a biopsy may be sufficient to provide diagnostic information but no direct treatment.[115] In other cases, the goal may be curative; however, complete resection may not be possible. This may occur if the tumor is encapsulating a primary vessel or is too large to completely resect without damaging surrounding structures. In this event, partial resection is performed. In the event of metastatic tumors in the lung, a wedge resection is performed.

Surgical decision-making for musculoskeletal tumors is based on tumor location, size, and age of patient. Patient and family input is critical with regard to decision-making because there are multiple options, all with differing functional outcomes and aesthetic changes. For tumors that occur in the extremities, the typical standard of care involves tumor resection while sparing the limb, using prosthetic devices or allografts within the long bone.[116] In the event that there is inadequate remaining healthy tissue in order to preserve the limb, a complete amputation is performed. **Figures 6-20** and **6-21** show a patient status post above-the-knee amputation secondary to osteosarcoma. A rotationplasty may also be considered in cases where the tumor occurs in the distal femur and/or proximal tibia. To provide an anatomic knee joint, rather than an above-knee amputation, the distal tibia including the foot and ankle joint are rotated 180 degrees and surgically attached to the distal femur. The muscles of the ankle are also attached such that the plantar flexors now act as knee extensors and dorsiflexors act as knee flexors. While this avoids a 2-joint prosthetic device, it does have aesthetic consequences that need to be considered. Although limb salvage procedures have a higher risk of complications such as nonunion of the endoprosthetic device, they are associated with improved functional outcomes and 5-year survival rates.[117,118]

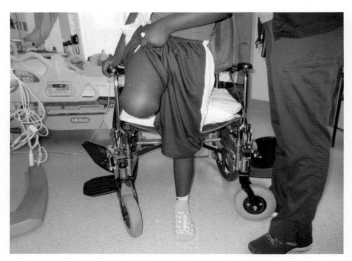

FIGURE 6-20 A patient following an above-the-knee amputation as treatment for an osteosarcoma.

For patients with musculoskeletal tumors who are immediately postoperative, the role of the acute care PT is much like that for any other orthopedic surgery. Patients and families will require education and training regarding functional mobility including bed mobility and transfers as well as ambulation and stair climbing as cleared by the surgeon. The acute care PT is also involved in discharge planning, including identifying equipment or ongoing PT needs. It is also important to remember that, as noted earlier, many patients with a musculoskeletal tumor also receive chemotherapy following their surgical resection. Patients may be admitted to the hospital during this time period for a number of reasons related to their treatment such as neutropenia or infection. These patients may require inpatient physical therapy for progression of their outpatient physical therapy—in the event of a prolonged hospitalization—or due to an acute change in their strength or function. It is important to remember that they may continue to have

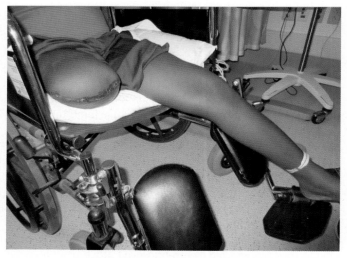

FIGURE 6-21 Additional view of the patient's surgical site following an above-the-knee amputation for treatment of an osteosarcoma.

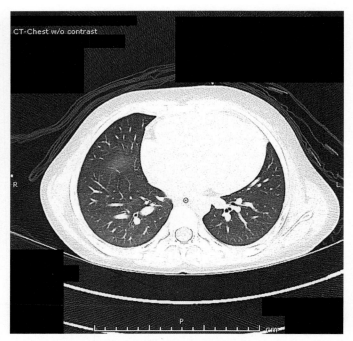

FIGURE 6-22 Computed tomography imaging that shows lung nodules for a patient with an osteosarcoma.

weight-bearing or range of motion precautions at this time. If these restrictions are not clear or are unknown by the patients' inpatient medical team, it is important to have communication with the primary surgeon. These patients may also return to the hospital for biopsy or resection of a pulmonary metastasis. For patients who typically ambulate using axillary crutches for mobility, it is necessary to assess if this is still tolerated or if they require a change of assistive device to a walker or Lofstrand crutches. **Figure 6-22** shows lung nodules seen on chest computed tomography in a patient with osteosarcoma.

Special Considerations

Multiple studies have shown that children diagnosed with cancer demonstrate impaired aerobic capacity and muscle strength when compared with their healthy peers.[108] There are likely many contributing factors leading to these impairments including lower levels of physical activity caused by side effects from chemotherapy or cancer-related fatigue (CRF). It is therefore important to encourage daily out of bed activity early in treatment in order to prevent such impairments. This is particularly important in the acute care setting, where patients are outside of their home environment and have fewer opportunities or possibly decreased motivation to participate in such activities. Caregiver education is especially critical at this time in order to discuss the balance of providing rest and choice as appropriate with necessary regular functional activities.

It is also important to consider a patient's laboratory values that apply to a patient's red blood cells. Low platelet count, or thrombocytopenia, is a vital lab value to monitor due to its high incidence and serious consequences. Patients become thrombocytopenic due to the nature of either their cancer or cancer treatment. When patients are thrombocytopenic, they have a higher risk of bleeding. Normal platelet values vary by age and gender; however, as noted earlier in this chapter, the minimum normal value is never less than 140,000. With a platelet count of 50,000, surgical procedures (eg, lumbar punctures, which may be required as part of cancer treatment or assessment) are more likely to be complicated by bleeding.[119] With a platelet count of 10,000, a patient is at a higher risk of spontaneous bleeding.[119] This is also important for the acute care PT because physical resistance, such as manual muscle testing or resistive exercises, may also increase patients' risks of bleeding. Many hospitals therefore have guidelines for exercise and activity based on platelet counts. Patients who are actively bleeding due to thrombocytopenia or who are at a high risk of bleeding, based on a threshold established by the hospital and individual patients, will likely receive a transfusion of platelets, and this should be considered when scheduling PT sessions.[120]

Cancer related fatigue (CRF) is defined as "distressing, persistent, subjective sense of physical, emotional, and/or cognitive tiredness or exhaustion related to cancer or cancer treatment that is not proportional to recent activity and interferes with usual functioning."[121] CRF is common in patients of all ages, including children, but is most common (up to 90%) in patients receiving chemotherapy.[122] It can exist at any point from diagnosis through and following treatment and has been reported as the most distressing symptom of cancer.[123] Fatigue itself can be a barrier to participation in physical activity; however, it has been determined that exercise is a successful intervention for improving CRF.[109,124] It is therefore important for the PT to provide education regarding participation in exercise as well as the intervention itself. The acute care PT has a particularly unique opportunity to provide this education for patients who may be at the beginning of their treatment courses. Many studies have demonstrated that regular exercise for a total of 30 minutes at a time has been effective at decreasing CRF.[109] For older patients who are able to perform formal exercise, a program can be developed. Younger children, however, will benefit from incorporation of therapeutic activities into their ADLs and play such as scavenger hunts to encourage participation in a walking program or placement of toys at varied levels to facilitate active lower extremity strengthening. Parental education and understanding of preferred activities will be important. Patients who are hesitant to participate may benefit from collaboration with the child life specialist in order to establish a daily schedule and/or reward system.

Physical Therapy Examination and Evaluation

As described earlier, a thorough chart review is a vital component of any evaluation. Identifying a patient's primary diagnosis, sequelae, and past medical history will help to direct the physical examination. Additionally, any pertinent precautions and activity guidelines should be documented. For example, is it anticipated based on the patient's medical plan that laboratory values, such as platelet count, will be decreased? If so, it may be important to modify the planned strength assessment. Knowledge of the medical plan is also valuable in identifying risk factors for future impairments, such as those related to

CIPN. As previously discussed, weight-bearing precautions for patients who have undergone surgical resection of a lower extremity tumor should be appropriately documented and taken into account during evaluation. A conversation with the bedside nurse will then provide valuable insight regarding if the patient will be leaving the unit for treatment or if the patient is fatigued or in pain following or during a particular medical treatment in order to appropriately schedule the PT evaluation.

Based on the chart review and history from the patient and family, the PT can determine appropriate tests and measures to perform. A strength assessment, either against gravity or resistance pending platelet counts, should always be performed. Particular attention should be paid to the foot and ankle muscles if it is identified that the patient is at risk for CIPN. Similarly, an in-depth balance assessment, including progression to single limb stance with eyes both open and closed as appropriate, should be performed if this is the case. The Pediatric–Modified Total Neuropathy Score (Ped-mTNS) is a valid and reliable measure of CIPN in children.[125] It uses a combination of subjective and objective measures of neuropathy including sensation (light touch, proprioception), reflexes, and strength to determine if a patient has a neuropathy.[126] A patient's tolerance to activity should also be assessed. In the acute care setting, this is often evaluated during functional activities such as ADLs and ambulation, but a standardized test such as the 6-minute walk test could also be used. For younger children who are not able to participate in standardized testing, focus will remain on ADLs, tolerance to play in sitting versus standing as appropriate based on age, and parental report.

Plan of Care

As with all diagnoses, the PT plan of care, including frequency and duration of treatment, will depend on patient presentation and goals of care. A patient's functional status and likelihood of making progress also need to be considered. For example, a patient who is admitted following surgical resection of a musculoskeletal tumor will likely have a short hospital stay and need to receive physical therapy once to twice daily given that there will be progress made between each session. Goals will pertain to safety, functional mobility, and discharge planning. In contrast, a patient who is admitted for the duration of an HSCT or chemotherapy course may not present with significant impairments upon evaluation; however, this patient remains at high risk for deconditioning based on the anticipated hospital course and medical treatment. The physical therapy frequency will likely be much lower than that for the previous patient, perhaps weekly or biweekly. Sessions may be more consultative in nature, with the PT providing education and activities for the patient and family to complete independently. If patients do not have notable impairments upon admission, they will benefit from education regarding an exercise program that can be completed independently throughout their hospital stay with monitoring and progression from the PT as appropriate. Goals will involve endurance, strength, and balance. For infants and toddlers, treatment and goals will focus on progression of age-appropriate developmental skills. If patients and families are able to demonstrate independence with a home program and do not require regular monitoring or progression of activities, the patient may be discharged from the acute physical therapy service. In this case, patients and families should be educated on red flags, such as decreased tolerance to standing, gait impairments such as tripping or falls, or decreased activity tolerance, which would indicate that the PT should be reengaged.

The following are some examples of appropriate goals for patients on the oncology floor based on acuity, age, and developmental stage.

Scenario 1: A 17-year-old female admitted for HSCT evaluated prior to start of treatment who presents without specific impairments.

Short-Term Goals (to be met within 2 weeks)

1. Patient will verbalize compliance with home exercise program 5 out of 7 days of the week.
2. Patient will verbalize compliance with out-of-bed activities for ≥3 hours daily.

Long-Term Goals (to be met within 4-6 weeks)

1. Patient will tolerate 20 minutes of dynamic standing activity without signs or symptoms of fatigue.
2. Patient will ambulate >1000 feet independently without gait deviations or rest break.

Scenario 2: A 9-year-old male with ALL admitted for chemotherapy presents with evidence of bilateral lower extremity peripheral neuropathy.

Short-Term Goals (to be met within 2 weeks)

1. Patient will tolerate having hospital socks donned for ≥1 hour with pain ≤2/10 via Numeric Rating Scale.
2. Patient will ambulate ≥100 feet with least restrictive assistive device and minimal assistance.

Long-Term Goals (to be met within 4 weeks)

1. Patient will ambulate ≥300 feet with least restrictive assistive device and supervision from caregiver.
2. Patient will demonstrate fair or greater strength of ankle dorsiflexors bilaterally.
3. Patient will maintain Rhomberg stance for ≥10 seconds with eyes open.
4. Patient will maintain Rhomberg stance for ≥10 seconds with eyes closed.

Scenario 3: A 4-year-old male status post surgical resection of brain stem glioma.

Short-Term Goals (to be met by discharge [within 1 week])

1. Patient will tandem walk for 10 feet with supervision and without loss of balance.
2. Patient will perform all bed mobility independently.
3. Patient will perform transfers via stand step with supervision from caregiver.
4. Patient will ambulate ≥350 feet with supervision from caregiver and no loss of balance.
5. Patient will ascend/descend 1 flight of stairs with close supervision from caregiver.

Long-term goals were not established due to short anticipated length of stay.

NEUROLOGY

Introduction

A neurologic disorder refers to any injury, disease process, or residual sequelae involving the central or peripheral nervous system.[127] These deficits may be a result of a congenital anomaly, a traumatic birth, an acute insult to the central nervous system such as a bleed, or a progressive disorder.[127] With advances in medical technology, more children are surviving, but with survival, there may also be the presence of deficits of motor control, sensation, cognition, and ability to function as an independent member of society.[127] There are a multitude of neurologic disorders that are not within the scope of this chapter. There are also diagnoses that affect both the adult and pediatric populations that will be addressed as separate chapter topics outside the acute care setting. These include spinal cord injury, traumatic brain injury, Guillain-Barré syndrome, and other systemic diseases that may have neurologic sequelae. This section discusses both rare and common disorders that are pediatric specific in nature.

Intercranial Hemorrhage and Disorders of CNS Vascularization

An intracranial hemorrhage (ICH) is defined as bleeding within the intracranial vault or brain including the surrounding meningeal spaces.[128] These types of bleeds, also referred to as cerebrovascular accidents, can be a result of a trauma, malformation, or fragility of the venous-arterial system. Hemorrhagic stroke accounts for between 39% and 54% of all childhood stroke.[129] An ICH is identified by the part of the brain in which it takes place: subdural hemorrhage, subarachnoid hemorrhage, intraparenchymal hemorrhage, and intraventricular hemorrhage.

Often, these hemorrhages are not addressed surgically.[130-133] In the very young infant or neonate, medical intervention consists of early identification and management of sequelae, including seizures, elevated intracranial pressure, abnormal tone and spasticity, apnea, and respiratory distress.[131,132] In the older pediatric population, hemorrhage resulting in increased intracranial edema and pressure may require a decompressive craniotomy.[129] **Table 6-14** lists the types of ICHs and on their locations and risk factors.

Arteriovenous Malformation

Arteriovenous malformation (AVM) is a congenital malformation resembling a tangle of the arteries and veins that are fed by a large artery and drained by a large vein. AVMs can occur anywhere in the body but are most often found in the brain.[134] These can cause an ICH, especially in the young individual or the pediatric patient.[135] The larger vessels of an AVM have a higher blood flow and have fewer capillaries or are void of smaller capillaries.[136] Because of this, there is shunting or decrease in blood supplied to the tissue around the AVM itself.[136,137] Over time, the decrease in blood flow to brain tissue can lead to cerebral wasting. In a patient with both AVM and aneurysms, there is a risk for hypoxic brain injury as well as in increased incidence of stroke caused by bleeding. Some of the most common symptoms of the presence of an AVM are hemorrhage or seizure.[137]

TABLE 6-14 • Types of Intracranial Hemorrhage

Type of Hemorrhage	Location	Risk Factors
Subgaleal	Between the galeal aponeurosis and the periosteum (just outside the skull)	Prematurity Vacuum- or forceps-assisted delivery Coagulopathy
Subdural (SDH)	Between the dura mater and the arachnoid mater (within the skull, outside the brain)	Prematurity Vacuum- or forceps-assisted delivery Coagulopathy
Subarachnoid (SAH)	Below the arachnoid mater (on the surface of the brain)	Prematurity Vacuum- or forceps-assisted delivery Coagulopathy
Interventricular (IVH)	Originates in the germinal matrix (adjacent to the ventricles)	Prematurity Chorioamnionitis Hypotension Acidosis Respiratory distress Bicarbonate therapy Coagulopathy

Treatments of cerebral AVM are both surgical and non-surgical. Smaller asymptomatic AVMs (eg, those discovered incidentally during a scan for an unrelated issue) may simply be monitored. An AVM that is considered at high risk of hemorrhage, is symptomatic, or has already bled may be managed through resection, stereotactic radiotherapy, and endovascular embolization.[129] Surgical intervention is the treatment of choice if an AVM has ruptured.[129]

Cavernous Malformation

Cavernous malformations are malformations made up of tiny venules and capillaries that are tangled together. Unlike an AVM, there are no large feeder vessels involved. These malformations are most often familial and are associated with a genetic abnormality passed from parent to child. Most cavernomas are monitored through serial imaging and patient report of number and severity of symptoms.[138] When the symptoms become refractory (unable to be controlled with medication) or if a bleed occurs, surgery will be considered.[138] It is after a bleed that PTs encounter patients with cavernous malformations.

Physical therapy interventions for cerebral hemorrhage, no matter what the cause, are largely dependent on the area of the brain in which the hemorrhage occurred, age of the patient, and extent of the neurologic damage.[129] Motor deficits are the most common sequelae of childhood cerebral hemorrhage.[129] In many cases, this weakness is accompanied by abnormal tone (usually hypertonicity and, in some cases, spasticity).[129] Children who have experienced a hemorrhagic stroke may also present with cognitive disorders, decreased sensation, dysphagia, and seizures. The severity of the disability following stroke is largely dependent on the location and the presence of additional preexisting diagnoses. If the bleed occurs at Broca's

area, one would expect an aphasia, whereas if the bleed occurs in the motor cortex, one would expect a hemiparesis. Because of the wide variability of presentations following a cerebral hemorrhage, the physical therapy plan of care is dependent on the objective findings of the assessment and evaluation. It is the job of the PT to address the neurologic sequelae from the bleed and provide experiences that encourage recovery and normal development. In the case of the infant, therapy would be focused on experiences to encourage them to move through the developmental sequence. In the case of the older pediatric patient, the therapy experience should use principles of neuroplasticity to provide experiences that encourage neurologic reeducation and recovery of motor function and motor skills. As with all physical therapy treatments, caregiver education and training and discharge planning are included in the PT plan of care.

Moyamoya Syndrome

Moyamoya syndrome is characterized by a progressive stenosis at the apices of the internal carotid arteries. As this occurs, there is simultaneous growth of collateral vascularization at the base of the skull. The collaterals appear on angiography as a "puff of smoke;" or *moyamoya* in Japanese. This syndrome was first documented in 1957 by Takeuchi and Shimizu who reported a case of "hypoplasia of the bilateral internal carotid arteries," but was first named as moyamoya in 1969 by Suzuki and Takaku.[139-141] An AVM or aneurysm in the area of the moyamoya are also commonly diagnosed.[139,142,143]

Children who are ultimately diagnosed with moyamoya often present with headache, irritability, or symptoms of transient ischemic attack (episodic aphasia, sensory changes, or hemiparesis). These symptoms often follow an episode of intense crying or physical exertion where hypoventilation took place. There are also a certain number of children, both young and old, who will present after having had a bleed associated with as-yet undiagnosed moyamoya.[139] The severity of disability due to moyamoya is variable. If a child is diagnosed prior to a major stroke, the overall prognosis is good even when the moyamoya is severe in its progression.[139] PTs often become involved with this patient population at the time of diagnosis and as part of the posttreatment team.

Treatments for this population include aspirin or other blood thinners with close monitoring of the disease progression, calcium channel blockers to decrease headache symptoms, and surgical interventions aimed at increasing or restoring blood flow to the hypoperfused areas of the cortex.[139]

Physical therapy intervention for this population is largely dependent on whether the malformation was discovered prior to a neurologic event or discovered after a rupture and bleed. If the malformation was discovered without a neurologic event, physical therapy is largely focused on a postoperative examination of functional mobility. This type of evaluation includes screens and tests for impairments such as strength and sensation but focuses on current functional mobility, ability to perform bed mobility, household ambulation, and stairs if needed. Education would be inclusive of guarding techniques, energy conservation for the initial postoperative days due to fragility of the vasculature, and signs and symptoms for which the caregivers should contact a physician. The education of the family would include information related to changes in the patient's mental status, new motor deficits, or, for the young child, inconsolability. It is also recommended that the child avoid playing in an inverted position and anything that would significantly increase the blood pressure and put undue stress on the vessels at the surgical site. Often, patients with this diagnosis do not require additional follow-up physical therapy after being discharged from the hospital.

If moyamoya syndrome is discovered following a neurologic event, the physical therapy evaluation and plan of care would involve identification of impairment-level deficits (eg, strength, tone, sensory changes) and impairments affecting function (balance and gait abnormalities). Physical therapy focus would be on neurorecovery of gross motor skills for older children and continued progression through the developmental sequence for younger children. The plan of care would be directed toward deficits, with therapeutic interventions focusing on addressing impairments, improving mobility, and educating caregivers. In the case where moyamoya has been discovered as a result of a bleed, additional physical therapy in an inpatient rehabilitation facility, the home setting, or the outpatient clinic is often required.

Chiari Malformation

A Chiari malformation, first described by Arnold Chiari early in the 19th century, is characterized by the overcrowding of the contents in the hindbrain that results in a prolapse through the foramen magnum.[144] Despite this abnormal shift in the hindbrain, Chiari malformation is fairly common.[144] Often, this herniation results in progressive neurologic symptoms. The structures that can be affected by a Chiari malformation include the cerebellar tonsils, medulla, fourth ventricle, and pons. Chiari malformations are divided into 4 distinct groupings. The groupings are divided according to the structures involved and the distance of the herniation of these structures through the foramen magnum.[145]

Chiari I malformation: Characterized by the downward herniation of the cerebellar tonsils below the foramen magnum (the distance of the protrusion required to be classified as a true Chiari is variable from >3 cm to >5 cm throughout the research).[144-146] Often, no symptoms are present and Chiari I malformations are identified during imaging for unrelated symptoms. Some children with Chiari I malformations can present with a variety of symptoms such as head or neck ache, dizziness, decreased strength of the upper extremities, or symptoms associated with secondary hydrocephalus.[144,145]

Chiari II malformation: Characterized by cerebellum and brain stem tissue prolapse into the foramen magnum. It is often accompanied by a myelomeningocele, tethered cord, or other spinal dysraphism (congenital anomaly of the spinal cord).[147]

Chiari III and IV malformations: Rare and often result in death or severe neurologic devastation. Chiari III malformations are characterized by the cerebellum, brain stem, occipital lobe, and fourth ventricle prolapsing through the foramen

magnum.[145,148] These malformations are so rare and have such poor prognosis that there is very little literature found for medical intervention and follow-up rehabilitation.[148]

Treatment for Chiari malformation is surgical correction through decompression. This often includes a laminectomy of one or more of the cervical vertebrae.

Physical therapy interventions for Chiari I and II malformations include treatment techniques focusing on the neurologic sequelae such as tone management, developmental stimulation, and neurologic recovery associated with hydrocephalus and neurologic damage associated with prolapse of the hindbrain contents. Patients are also taught range of motion activities to address the stiff neck that often accompanies a laminectomy.

Hydrocephalus

Hydrocephalus is defined by Pople[149] as "an excessive accumulation of cerebrospinal fluid (CSF) within the head caused by a disturbance of formation, flow or absorption." "CSF is circulated along the ventricular system into the subarachnoid space and then absorbed into the venous system within the arachnoid granulations that line the convexity of the brain. An equilibrium normally exists between its production and absorption."[150] Disruption of this equilibrium can lead to hydrocephalus.[150] There are 2 types of hydrocephalus: communicating and noncommunicating.

Communicating hydrocephalus refers to hydrocephalus where the CSF is able to leave the ventricular system and enter the subarachnoid space. Normal CSF flow is obstructed outside of the ventricular system. This increase in CSF volume results in increased ICP.[149,151] *Noncommunicating hydrocephalus* refers to hydrocephalus where the CSF is unable to leave the ventricular system and the access of CSF in that system creates increased ICP.[149,151]

An increase in ICP can result in transient changes in neurologic status such as altered speech, balance issues, facial droop, vomiting, headache (most often in the morning), and gait ataxias. Sensation and strength remain intact.[151] There are a variety of causes for both forms of hydrocephalus; they include, but are not limited to, congenital malformations, tumors or cysts obstructing flow, intraventricular hematoma, and cerebellar infarct, to name a few.[152]

Treatment for hydrocephalus is to normalize the CSF flow, thus decreasing the ICP and resolving the neurologic symptoms associated with that elevated ICP. The cause of the obstructed ventricular pathways can at times determine the course of treatment. For example, if a hydrocephalus is caused by a posterior fossa tumor, the removal of the tumor may relieve the hydrocephalus. If the hydrocephalus is thought to be temporary, as in the case of edema caused by trauma or surgery, a temporary external ventricular drain may be inserted.[150] This is a way of temporarily managing increased ICP. When hydrocephalus is unable to be corrected through removal of a physical barrier within the CSF pathways or through a temporary drain (external ventricular drain), there are 2 commonly used options to address the hydrocephalus: surgically inserting a shunting system or surgically performing an endoscopic third ventriculocisternostomy (ETV).[151] Often, the ETV is performed in conjunction with a choroid plexus cauterization. This is where a hole is made at the bottom of the third ventricle to allow for CSF to drain into the basal cistern and there is a burning of the tissue that produces CSF. The ETV provides the CSF a pathway around the obstruction, whereas the choroid plexus cauterization decreases the amount of CSF fluid produced.[153]

Encephalitis and Meningitis

Meningitis is inflammation of the meninges of the brain and can lead to encephalitis, an infection of the brain itself. The inflammation can be caused by a virus, a bacteria, or an autoimmune process.[154-156] Encephalitis affects people of all ages but is found more often in the pediatric, immunocompromised, and elderly populations.[154,155] Often, viral meningitis causes severe flulike symptoms or no symptoms at all.[154] Autoimmune and bacterial meningitis, however, often present with days or weeks of fluctuation in memory and cognitive skills.[156,157] It can result in neurologic sequelae including cognitive deficits, motor sensory deficits, behavioral issues, and amnesia.[156,157] Patients with autoimmune encephalitis may present with abnormal movement patterns, altered mental status, or seizure activity. Dystonic, ataxic, or choreic movements are a more common presenting symptom in the pediatric population than in the older populations.[157] Medical treatment for autoimmune and bacterial encephalitis is focused on decreasing or minimizing the damaging inflammation caused by the bacteria or autoimmune process. It may include high-dose steroids and/or IV immunoglobulin (IVIG).[156,157] Due to its multiple anti-inflammatory and immunomodulatory properties, IVIG is used successfully in a wide range of autoimmune and inflammatory conditions.[156]

Because patients with encephalitis and meningitis will vary in symptom presentation according to the severity of the infection and the response to treatment, the physical therapy plan of care will focus on the impairment-level deficits and their impact on functional mobility. In the acute care setting, the PT evaluation will assist the medical team in determining the discharge location. Some patients may require acute inpatient rehabilitation, and others will be discharged to home with minimal residual deficits.

Myelitis

Acute Flaccid Myelitis

Acute flaccid myelitis (AFM) is described by the Centers for Disease Control and Prevention (CDC) as a sudden onset of flaccid paralysis of one or more limbs with loss of deep tendon reflexes.[158] In the past, this grouping of symptoms was referred to as "poliomyelitis" or "polio-like syndrome."[159] During the years 2012 to 2015, there was a significant increase in the reports of these symptoms being reported in the United States, leading to tracking and classification as AFM.[160] This diagnosis requires confirmation with MRI demonstrating lesions of gray matter in the anterior horn of the spinal cord.[158,159] Because the anterior horn of the spinal cord contains the cell bodies of the neurons controlling the skeletal muscles, lesions in this area result in the paralysis noted with AFM. There is epidemiologic evidence to suggest this acute neurologic decompensation is linked to the enterovirus D-68.[160] The mechanism of how and why in some cases the enterovirus D-68 virus transitions from an upper respiratory illness to a neurodegenerative illness remains unclear.

Below are the signs and symptoms of AFM that may be found on physical therapy evaluation.[159,160]

- Proximal weakness greater than distal weakness (may be asymmetric)
- May have cranial nerve involvement
- Loss of reflexes
- Hypotonia or flaccid muscles
- Sensory involvement without clear sensory level

Some children may demonstrate motor recovery and some may have improved function, but most or all have significant residual deficits 1 year after the original infectious episode and most have what is believed to be permanent motor deficits.[160]

Acute Transverse Myelitis

According to Varina and colleagues, acute transverse myelitis (ATM) is a potentially devastating clinical syndrome affecting the spinal cord that is characterized by acute onset of motor, sensory, and autonomic dysfunction.[161,162] According to the National Institute of Neurological Disorders and Stroke, there are 1400 new cases of ATM diagnosed in the United States every year. One of the tenets of ATM is a clear spinal level for sensory disturbance. This level can be used to establish a plateau or nadir in the disease progression and to chart or track recovery. In some cases, ATM is the first episode of a more aggressive demyelinating disease such as acute demyelinating encephalomyelitis or neuromyelitis, and in older children and young adults, it can transition into multiple sclerosis.[162] Because ATM is a diagnosis of exclusion, the Transverse Myelitis Consortium Working Group has proposed a list of criteria of inclusion to assist in the diagnosis of ATM. Below are the signs and symptoms of ATM that would be found on a thorough physical therapy evaluation.[162] These symptoms would be expected to reportedly have increased over several hours or days.

A history of or presence of low back pain is often present. Bilateral weakness of the lower extremities may be present but is often asymmetrical. Depending on the location of the spinal cord lesion, upper extremity involvement may also be present. There is often bowel and bladder involvement. A clear sensory level should be present but may be difficult to assess in younger children given their ability/inability to participate in objective testing.

It is reported that pain is the first symptom to show improvement before motor symptoms, with the remaining sensory systems" being the last to show improvement.[162] The devastation caused by ATM is variable but severe. Long-term studies show that 10% to 20% of patients do not recover bladder function or the ability to ambulate.[163] Up to 50% report ongoing sensory disturbances.[163] Some studies show there is a prolonged period between onset of symptoms and diagnosis for children under 3 years of age.[163] Children of this age group also present with longer spinal segment involvement and lack of white blood cells in the CSF.[163] Mortality is associated with respiratory issues caused by involvement at higher spinal levels.[163]

Because PT would most likely be consulted to work with children presenting with weakness and sensory changes, it is important for the PT to be familiar with the signs and symptoms of AFM and ATM. Therapy would focus on motor recovery, optimizing functional mobility, and determination of discharge environment.

Traumatic Brain Injury

Traumatic brain injury (TBI) is a neurologic injury that can have devastating physical, emotional, and financial sequelae.[164] Over 57 million people worldwide are living with neurologic deficits as a result of TBI.[164] Approximately 1.7 million Americans sustain a TBI each year, and 52,000 will die from the injury.[164] The severity of a brain injury of this type can range from a concussive injury to a trauma that results in a vegetative/minimally responsive state or coma.

Concussion

Recent media coverage of concussions in athletes has brought a focus on concussions caused by the impact of contact sports.[165] According to Kimbler et al,[164] "TBI is more prevalent than breast cancer, AIDS, multiple sclerosis, and spinal cord injury combined; however, these data reflect only the number of neurotrauma patients seeking emergency medical treatment." Because not all people who sustain a concussion seek medical intervention, the prevalence could be significantly higher. A concussion is a pathophysiologic disruption of the brain caused by blunt force trauma.[166] A concussion is characterized by the presence of altered mental status, memory loss, headache, photophobia, and attention issues in the absence of a gross anatomic lesion.[166] These symptoms may last for several hours or, in some cases, several months.

Treatment for Patients With Concussion In the inpatient setting, it is often the job of the PT to evaluate balance and mobility for safe discharge home, to address oculomotor dysfunction with the appropriate exercises, to screen for vestibular dysfunction, and to assess cranial nerve function. The PT should also educate the patient and family on how to appropriately return to learning as well as return to sports. It is important to consider the demands of the school setting. It presents challenges of memory and cognition, as well as bright lights and increased sensory input. Because there are no outward signs of the injury, it is sometimes difficult for friends and educators to understand the deficits of the child. The concussed brain should be allowed to rest with minimal stimulation, including screen time, until the child can experience stimulation without return of any symptoms.

Guidelines for "return to learn" continue to change as research moves forward. As a result, it is recommended that the patient and family refer to the CDC guidelines for return to learning.

Because many concussed adolescents are athletes, there have been policies formulated as guidelines for schools in how to safely return athletes to the field following a concussion. Many towns are implementing preseason sideline or computerized tests to obtain baseline cognitive and physical skill levels. These data are then used as a comparison as a retest to determine readiness to return to sports. States that institute formal pans require they be followed by coaching staff when returning a player to the field.

The CDC suggested return to play steps are as follows[167]:

- **Step 1: Back to regular activities:** Athlete is back to their regular activities (eg, school).
- **Step 2: Light aerobic activity:** Begin with light aerobic exercise only to increase an athlete's heart rate. This means about 5 to 10 minutes on an exercise bike, walking, or light jogging. There should be no weightlifting at this point.
- **Step 3: Moderate activity:** Continue with activities to increase an athlete's heart rate with body or head movement. This includes moderate jogging, brief running, moderate-intensity stationary biking, and moderate-intensity weightlifting (less time and/or less weight from their typical routine).
- **Step 4: Heavy, noncontact activity:** Add heavy noncontact physical activity, such as sprinting/running, high-intensity stationary biking, regular weightlifting routine, or noncontact sport-specific drills (in 3 planes of movement).
- **Step 5: Practice and full contact:** Young athlete may return to practice and full contact (if appropriate for the sport) in controlled practice.
- **Step 6: Competition:** Young athlete may return to competition.

The athlete must tolerate the activity at each level without experiencing additional symptoms before they are allowed to progress to the next step. If symptoms occur, it is a sign the athlete was not ready to place that level of demand on their body. In this situation, the athlete should return to the previous level for 1 to 3 days before attempting to advance to the next level.

There are some people who sustain one or more concussions who continue to experience concussion symptoms long after the expected recovery time has passed. This population is referred to as having postconcussive syndrome. The therapeutic and medical needs of this group are largely handled on an outpatient basis. Please refer to the sports injury section of this book for additional details surrounding outpatient treatment of children and adolescents with concussions requiring outpatient therapy.

Moderate to severe TBI is a complex injury causing a cascade of physiologic responses leading to life-altering physical and cognitive sequelae. The details of moderate and severe TBI are beyond the scope of the inpatient pediatric section of this book. Please refer to the section on TBI for details of the medical and physical challenges faced by this patient population.

Functional Neurologic Symptom Disorder

Functional neurologic symptom disorder (FNSD; formerly known as conversion disorder) refers to presentation of neurologic symptoms in the absence of an organic basis. That is to say, there are no structural deficits in the patient's neurologic systems.[168-170] Patients with a functional neurologic disorder can present with blindness, hemiparesis, muscle weakness, jerky movement patterns, tremor, syncope, or any other neurologically based symptomatology. These symptoms are present in the absence of positive neurologic testing or imaging. Diagnostic tests such as electroencephalogram and imaging are negative despite the sometimes severe clinical presentation. There are no diagnostic tests that rule in FNSD, and it is a diagnosis of exclusion. This diagnosis is often described as a problem with "the software not the hardware."[171] Individuals with conversion or functional neurologic disorder are not faking their symptoms; the symptoms are real, but they stem from psychological need rather than a medical condition.[170]

PTs are often involved in assisting with the diagnosis of functional disorder. The PT evaluation can be valuable in providing the medical team with additional information to appropriately make a diagnosis of FNSD. The physical therapy evaluation is carried out in its usual manner. The therapist would perform impairment-level testing such as strength and somatosensation as well as a functional evaluation to assess the level to which the patient's impairments have affected functional mobility. Throughout the evaluation, the therapist will observe for signs and symptoms of neurologic disorder. The classic symptoms of FNSD are inconsistencies in results when manual muscle testing (MMT) and sensation as these tests are repeated.[172,173] There may also be evidence of sensory testing that does not follow any anatomic patterns. The overall functional presentation is often not in agreement with the muscle testing. In repeated testing the PT would note manual muscle testing grades that do not correlate with the patients functional abilities and/or sensory impairments that do not follow anatomic patterns.[172,173] For example, the therapist may ask the patient to lift their lower extremity against gravity or participate in a MMT, and they demonstrate an inability to do this. Later in the session, often during a functional activity, the patient will demonstrate the ability to move that lower extremity with minimal difficulty. Other signs may include jerky, exaggerated movements; unexplained tremors; bizarre gait patterns; and simultaneous contraction of agonist and antagonist muscles.[172,173] A common motor complaint is astasia-abasia, which is an unsteadiness of gait presenting with unusual incoordination, especially in walking or standing still.[172,173] There are specific screening tests that therapists can conduct that may help differentiate between a functional disorder and a disorder that is organic in nature. The following are tests and screens that may help the therapist differentiate between an organic disorder and a functional disorder.

When tremor is present in suspected FNSD, there are ways to challenge that tremor and gather further evidence of the possibility of an FNSD. For example, a tremor with an organic base will not vary in amplitude and rhythm with distraction. If the tremor varies or stops when the patient is distracted, functional disorder should be suspected.[172] This can be formally assessed with an entrainment test. The clinician asks the patient to tap an uninvolved limb at a different frequency than the tremor of the involved limb. If the frequency of the tremor of the involved limb changes (usually to match the tempo of the uninvolved limb), this is evidence in support of a functional disorder.[172,173]

Observational gait analysis can also be valuable when considering the diagnosis of FNSD. If the patient's gait does not follow typical movement pattern disorders, varies throughout the treatment, or changes/normalizes with distraction, FNSD would be suspected. Patients with a diagnosis of FNSD demonstrate large truncal and extremity movements but are able to control their balance.[172-174] They often will grab onto walls or chairs or "fall" into bed but will avoid a complete fall or injury.[174] Often, the patient will grab onto furniture or people in the environment but will maintain their balance when unassisted.[168,175]

A hip adduction test is a test where the patient is asked to adduct the uninvolved hip against resistance given by the PT. While the therapist resists adduction on the uninvolved side, there will be an isometric contraction of the involved side. This may indicate FNSD.[176]

Treatment of a functional neurologic disorder requires a team of medical personnel and must include psychology, as it is a psychological diagnosis. It consists of standard physical therapy procedures such as motor retraining and functional part-to-whole training. Education regarding the disorder and expectation of recovery is an essential element of the physical therapy process and paramount to recovery.

Special Considerations

External Ventricular Drain

A variety of neurologic disease processes and neurologic trauma can result in an increase in ICP. This represents a medical emergency that requires monitoring of ICP and diversion of CSF. One way to relieve the pressure is to insert an external ventricular drain (EVD).[150] An EVD is a catheter usually placed within the right frontal lobe (to avoid speech centers in the majority of patients). The spinal fluid drains through the catheter to a collection bag. It drains through a combination of the patient's anatomy, ICP, and gravity in relation to the placement of the collection bag. As such, the collection bag must be "leveled" with an anatomic landmark determined by the surgeon. This landmark is often the tragus of the ear as this coincides with the skull base. Because the relationship between the ventricles of the brain and the position of the collection bag is integral in the success of the drain and the accuracy of the ICP monitor, the drain must be clamped and releveled with all movements of the patient. This includes bed mobility and all transfers. Moving a patient with an open EVD can result in large-volume dumping of CSF from the collection bag to the patient's brain or from the patient's brain into the collection bag. This causes a sudden change of ICP, which could go undetected and untreated.[150]

Shunting Hydrocephalus

According to the Hydrocephalus Foundation, "an implanted shunt diverts CSF from the ventricles within the brain or the subarachnoid spaces around the brain and spinal cord to another body region where it will be absorbed."[177] This catheter is named for where it originates and to where it diverts the CSF. For example, a ventriculoperitoneal (VP) shunt begins in the cerebral ventricle and ends in the peritoneal cavity, and a ventriculoatrial (VA) shunt begins in the cerebral ventricle and ends in the atrium of the heart. The complications associated with shunting include infection, shunt failure, epilepsy, and cognitive and neurologic deficits.[151] The long-term outcomes of these interventions are uncertain and vary greatly within the

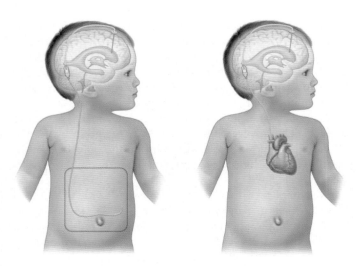

FIGURE 6-23 View of the route throughout the body of a ventriculoperitoneal (VP) (pictured left) and ventriculoartrial (VA) (pictured right) shunt.

published documentation.[151] **Figure 6-23** shows the course of a VP (left) and VA (right) shunt.

Endoscopic Third Ventriculostomy

ETV is considered as a treatment of choice for obstructive hydrocephalus.[151,152] It is a technique where an opening is put in the floor of the third ventricle of the brain.[152] This allows for the excess CSF to drain directly to the basal cistern, also known as the interpeduncular cistern (part of the natural CSF pathway system), bypassing the obstruction.

Examination and Plan of Care

As with all PT examinations, a thorough chart review and interview of the patient and/or their caregivers is necessary. When identifying appropriate impairment-level testing, one must consider the patient's physical and cognitive abilities both at baseline and with the acute medical issue. For example, if the patient has abnormal tone of left upper and lower extremities at baseline, they may struggle to isolate single muscles to participate in standardized MMT. In this case, the therapist should have a plan for alternate means to assess the patient's functional strength. This can be achieved through functional tasks such as having the patient squat to retrieve an object from the floor to assess functional quad control (both eccentrically and concentrically). Through the same task, the therapist can observe weight bearing on the right and left, balance, motor planning, gross coordination (eg, tremor, overshoot), and functional range of motion. Depending on where the object to be retrieved is placed, the therapist may also be able to observe the patient's ability to perform and recover from internal perturbations. When using function to assess impairments, the therapist must document appropriately. To use the example above, the therapist may document the following:

> *Patient unable to isolate muscle strength for the left upper extremity/left lower extremity (LUE/LLE) secondary to abnormal tone. He demonstrates sufficient strength and motor control of bilateral lower extremity (BLE) to perform*

a full squat without upper extremity (UE) support to retrieve a light object form the floor. He demonstrates the ability to reach with LUE out of his base of support in the squatted position and return to midline without assist. There is an intentional tremor noted when reaching for desired object with LUE and there is greater weightbearing (WB'ing) on the RLE as compared to left throughout the activity.

The Gait Cycle

Because many patients who have had a neurologic insult or neurologic surgery have gait disturbances, it is imperative to have a deep understanding of the gait cycle. To train the proper muscles during recovery, one must provide the appropriate training. For example, if a patient demonstrates knee hyperextension in stance phase and the therapist does not understand that this can be due to poor eccentric hamstring control or adaptive shortening of or increased tone in the plantar flexors, they could waste valuable time on functional quad training that may not remedy the issue.[178]

When compiling a treatment plan for the neurologically involved patient, it is important to keep in mind the principles of neuroplasticity and specificity of training as well as considering the functional and cognitive level of each individual patient. The role of the acute care physical therapy plan of care is to provide experiences and challenges that encourage normalized movement patterns and promote neuroplastic recovery. This is not a setting in which adaptive compensation should yet be considered.

Using Principles of Neuroplasticity

Research supports the findings that spontaneous recovery occurs for weeks and possibly months following a neurologic injury and that behavioral experience is the most important factor in encouraging brain plasticity.[179] Through carefully planned rehabilitative experiences, the PT must provide the appropriate environmental challenges and experiences at the appropriate time in recovery to support and nurture brain recovery using known neuroplastic principals. To affect the most widespread neuroplastic changes, the therapist must provide experiences that are meaningful to the patient, repetitive and functional in nature, and foster normal movement patterns.[179]

Specificity Training

Specificity of training refers to the principal of training a specific skill by repeatedly performing that specific skill under a variety of conditions.[180] This means that, just as you would not train a soccer player to improve the accuracy of kicking by having them dribble the ball, you would not expect a person's gait pattern to improve static balance activities. This principle of training is imperative for motor recovery following a neurologic event. Research using functional MRI shows that slow repetitive practice of a skill first presents on functional MRI as changes in the motor cortex consistent with the setting up of "task-specific motor routines."[180] While the motor cortex is setting these routines, the patient's skill level may not yet be showing improvement. Although functional gains may not be evident at the onset of training, neuroplastic changes in the motor cortex may be occurring that will become evident in skill acquisition and improvement at a later date.[180]

The following are examples of goals that may be appropriate for the neurologically involved patient in the inpatient setting:

Scenario 1: A 5-week-old infant with multiple subdural hematomas is now medically stable and remains hospitalized for feeding issues.

Short-Term Goals (to be met in 2 weeks)

1. The baby will tolerate >20 minutes of developmental stimulation with 3 rest breaks with ≤2 signs of stress.
2. The baby will demonstrate spontaneous antigravity movements of all 4 extremities.
3. The baby will demonstrate the ability to bring hand to mouth, both right and left, when in the side-lying position.
4. In supine, the baby will demonstrate reciprocal kicking when both soles of feet are stimulated with light touch.

Long-Term goals (to be met in 4 weeks)

1. The baby will tolerate >30 minutes of developmental stimulation including 3 position changes with stable vital signs.
2. The baby will demonstrate the ability to bring hand to mouth, both right and left, when in the side-lying position.
3. In supine, the baby will demonstrate spontaneous reciprocal kicking.

Scenario 2: A 10-year-old previously healthy male is status post ruptured AVM with resultant left hemiparesis.

Short-Term Goals (to be met in 2 weeks)

1. The patient will perform supine to sit rolling through right side lying with minimal assist to roll and moderate assist to move side lying to sit.
2. The patient will demonstrate the ability to maintain upright midline posture sitting at the edge of bed with both lower extremities supported, without upper extremity or posterior support for >4 minutes.
3. The patient will perform a stand step transfer from bed to chair to the right with minimal assist of 1.

■ CONCLUSION

The acute care therapist relies on a wide spectrum of clinical reasoning skills to improve the medical and mobility needs of children throughout the hospital. Given the wide range of diagnoses encountered, inpatient pediatric physical therapy is a dynamic and exciting area of practice. There is ample opportunity to develop skills in a variety of practice areas including but not limited to general medicine, ICU, orthopedics, oncology, and neurology. The acute care setting also has a high demand for patient, family, and staff education. The therapist who is most successful in the acute care setting is highly flexible, thrives on complex problem solving, and is a skilled communicator.

Case 1

Patient is a typically developing 16-year-old male who was struck by a car while crossing the street. He sustained a right femur fracture as well as multiple abrasions. He is postoperative day (POD) 1 from open reduction internal fixation of the right femur. He is non–weight bearing and cleared for range of motion as tolerated on his right lower extremity postoperatively.

1. What assistive device do you anticipate will be best for progression of ambulation?
   A. Rolling walker
   B. Axillary crutches
   C. Lofstrand crutches
   D. Patient will be unable to progress to ambulation and should complete transfers only with assistance from a caregiver

2. What is the least important question to ask as part of the patient/family interview in planning for discharge home?
   A. Who will be present at home to provide support?
   B. What is the home setup?
   C. What are the patient's allergies to medication?
   D. What are the patient's extracurricular activities?

3. Based on the patient's precautions, which activity would not be appropriate to recommend as part of a home exercise program?
   A. Quadriceps isometric exercises
   B. Mini squats with bilateral upper extremity support
   C. Long arc quads while seated at the side of the bed
   D. Active assisted range of motion at the hip and knee with caregiver assist

Case 2

The patient is a 5-year-old girl with past medical history significant for end-stage renal disease who was independent with ambulation and is now POD5 status post left kidney transplant. She is referred to physical therapy for evaluation while on the surgical intensive care unit due to concern for deconditioning postoperatively. She presents with the following lines/tubes: Jackson-Pratt (JP) drain, arterial line (right wrist), nasogastric tube to suction, 2 peripheral intravenous lines (PIVs; left upper extremity and left lower extremity), and Foley catheter.

1. In preparation for mobilizing the patient out of bed, what would be the most important thing to consider with regard to lines or tubes?
   A. Ensuring PIV has been capped
   B. Making sure the patient has hospital socks donned
   C. Ensuring all lines and tubes are on the same side of the bed as the chair
   D. Making sure the Foley catheter and JP drains are empty

2. You successfully transfer the patient to a chair. After 2 minutes, her blood pressure drops from 110/65 to 83/50 mm Hg. How do you proceed?
   A. Rest and reassess
   B. Notify the medical team immediately
   C. Transfer the patient back to bed
   D. Give her a drink of water

3. You return for your physical therapy session on POD8. The patient presents ring sitting independently in bed. Her arterial line and left foot PIV have been removed. What are your mobility goals for this session?
   A. Sitting on edge of bed
   B. Dependent transfer to chair
   C. Single leg stance activities
   D. Walking in hallway with assistance

Case 3

The patient is an 11-year-old previously healthy boy who presented to his primary care physician (PCP) with complaints of headache for 3 weeks and recent vomiting in the morning. PCP referred the patient to your hospital for further workup, and a medulloblastoma in the area of the cerebellum was discovered. He presents to physical therapy after 6 weeks of chemotherapy and is POD1 from a debulking surgery during which neurologic damage occurred.

1. What is the most immediate and relevant history information you would want to know given the information you currently have?
   A. Prior level of function (PLOF)
   B. Home setup
   C. Any support in school
   D. Activities outside of school
2. Given the location of the tumor and your knowledge of neuroanatomy, what impairment-level deficits would you expect to find?
   A. Disturbance of proprioception, light touch, temperature and/or pain
   B. 2-point discrimination and graphesthesia
   C. Disturbance of language
   D. Ataxic or discoordinated movements
3. Taking into consideration the 6 weeks of chemotherapy preoperatively, what potential areas would you expect to be most affected?
   A. Light touch sensation, hearing, and endurance
   B. Vision, strength, and endurance
   C. Strength, endurance, and perception of hot and cold
   D. Vision, endurance, and resting heart rate
4. Following your evaluation, you find the child has ≥3/5 for all manual muscle testing (MMT) grades and has decreased proprioception at the left ankle and great toe. He is able to perform bed mobility with increased time, he can move from sit to stand with contact guard, and he requires minimal assist of 1 to ambulate. During gait, he has difficulty with left foot placement, has a shortened stance phase on the left, and requires increased support when changing directions. You suggest he use a straight cane or a Lofstrand crutch when walking alone to increase his safety. What standardized test would be most appropriate for this patient and why?
   A. 6 Minute Walk Test
   B. Pediatric Berg Balance Scale
   C. 30 second Sit to Stand Test
   D. Functional Reach Test

References

1. Weiss AJ, Liang L, Martin K. Overview of Hospital Stays in the United States, 2019. HCUP Statistical Brief #299. November 2022. Agency for Healthcare Research and Quality. Accessed November 4, 2023. https://hcup-us.ahrq.gov/reports/statbriefs/sb299-Hospital-Stays-Children-2019.jsp.
2. Russ CM, Agus M. Triage of intermediate-care patients in pediatric hospitals. *Hosp Pediatr.* 2015;5(10):542-547.
3. Gregory GA, Andropoulos DB. *Gregory's Pediatric Anesthesia.* Wiley Desktop Edition. John Wiley & Sons; 2012.
4. American Heart Association. *Advanced Cardiovascular Life Support, Provider Manual.* American Heart Association Incorporated; 2015.
5. Practice Committee of Academy of Pediatric Physical Therapy. List of Pediatric Assessment Tools Categorized by ICF Model. APTA website. Accessed July 27, 2019. https://pediatricapta.org.
6. Witt W, Weiss A, Elixhauser A. Overview of Hospital Stays for Children in the United States, 2012. HCUP Statistical Brief #187. December 2014. Accessed October 23, 2023. https://hcup-us.ahrq.gov/reports/statbriefs/sb187-Hospital-Stays-Children-2012.jsp.
7. Wieczorek B, Burke C, Al-harbi A, Kudchadkar SR. Early mobilization in the pediatric intensive care unit: a systematic review. *J Pediatr Intensive Care.* 2015;2015:129-170.
8. Randolph AG, Gonzales CA, Cortellini L, Yeh TS. Growth of pediatric intensive care units in the United States from 1995 to 2001. *J Pediatr.* 2004;144(6):792-798.
9. Wieczorek B, Ascenzi J, Kim Y, et al. PICU Up!: Impact of a quality improvement intervention to promote early mobilization in critically ill children. *Pediatr Crit Care Med.* 2016;17(12): e559-e566.
10. Rennick JE, Childerhose JE. Redefining success in the PICU: new patient populations shift targets of care. *Pediatrics.* 2015;135(2):e289-291.
11. Namachivayam P, Shann F, Shekerdemian L, et al. Three decades of pediatric intensive care: who was admitted, what happened in intensive care, and what happened afterward. *Pediatr Crit Care Med.* 2010;11(5):549-555.
12. Edwards JD, Houtrow AJ, Vasilevskis EE, et al. Chronic conditions among children admitted to U.S. pediatric intensive care units: their prevalence and impact on risk for mortality and prolonged length of stay. *Crit Care Med.* 2012;40(7):2196-2203.
13. Walker TC, Kudchadkar SR. Early mobilization in the pediatric intensive care unit. *Transl Pediatr.* 2018;7(4):308-313.
14. Pinto NP, Rhinesmith EW, Kim TY, Ladner PH, Pollack MM. Long-term function after pediatric critical illness: results from the survivor outcomes study. *Pediatr Crit Care Med.* 2017;18(3): e122-e130.
15. Kukreti V, Shamim M, Khilnani P. Intensive care unit acquired weakness in children: critical illness polyneuropathy and myopathy. *Indian J Crit Care Med.* 2014;18(2):95-101.
16. Parchem K, Peck A, Tales K. A multidisciplinary approach to equipment use in pediatric patient mobilization. *Crit Care Nurs Q.* 2018;41(3):330-339.
17. Garcia AV, Jeyaraju M, Ladd MR, et al. Survey of the American Pediatric Surgical Association on cannulation practices in pediatric ECMO. *J Pediatr Surg.* 2018;53(9):1843-1848.
18. Adachi I, Burki S, Fraser CD. Current status of pediatric ventricular assist device support. *Semin Thorac Cardiovasc Surg Pediatr Card Surg Annu.* 2017;20:2-8.
19. Burki S, Adachi I. Pediatric ventricular assist devices: current challenges and future prospects. *Vasc Health Risk Manag.* 2017; 13:177-185.

20. Hetzer R, Kaufmann F, Delmo Walter EM. Paediatric mechanical circulatory support with Berlin Heart EXCOR: development and outcome of a 23-year experience. *Eur J Cardiothorac Surg.* 2016;50(2):203-210.

21. Cho MH, Kang HG. Acute kidney injury and continuous renal replacement therapy in children; what pediatricians need to know. *Korean J Pediatr.* 2018;61(11):339-347.

22. Schibler A, Franklin D. Respiratory support for children in the emergency department. *J Paediatr Child Health.* 2016;52(2):192-196.

23. Shelly MP, Nightingale P. ABC of intensive care: respiratory support. *BMJ.* 1999;318(7199):1674-1677.

24. Watters KF. Tracheostomy in infants and children. *Respir Care.* 2017;62(6):799-825.

25. Joynt C, Cheung PY. Cardiovascular supportive therapies for neonates with asphyxia: a literature review of pre-clinical and clinical studies. *Front Pediatr.* 2018;6:363.

26. Maconochie IK, De Caen AR, Aickin R, et al. Part 6: Pediatric basic life support and pediatric advanced life support: 2015 International Consensus on Cardiopulmonary Resuscitation and Emergency Cardiovascular Care Science with Treatment Recommendations. *Resuscitation.* 2015;95:e147-168.

27. Beckman EJ. Analgesia and sedation in hospitalized children. In: *Pediatric Self-Assessment Program. Vol 3. Sedation and Analgesia.* American College of Clinical Pharmacy; 2017:7-30.

28. Benedetti GM, Silverstein FS, Rau SM, Lester SG, Benedetti MH, Shellhaas RA. Sedation and analgesia influence electroencephalography monitoring in pediatric neurocritical care. *Pediatr Neurol.* 2018;87:57-64.

29. Kudchadkar SR, Yaster M, Punjabi NM. Sedation, sleep promotion, and delirium screening practices in the care of mechanically ventilated children: a wake-up call for the pediatric critical care community. *Crit Care Med.* 2014;42(7):1592-1600.

30. Zuppa AF, Curley MAQ. Sedation analgesia and neuromuscular blockade in pediatric critical care: overview and current landscape. *Pediatr Clin North Am.* 2017;64(5):1103-1116.

31. Hauer J, Houtrow AJ. Pain assessment and treatment in children with significant impairment of the central nervous system. *Pediatrics.* 2017;139(6):e20171002.

32. Nowicki PD, Vanderhave KL, Gibbons K, et al. Perioperative pain control in pediatric patients undergoing orthopaedic surgery. *J Am Acad Orthop Surg.* 2012;20(12):755-765.

33. Greenwood K, Stewart E, Milton E, Hake M, Mitchell L, Sanders B. *Core Competencies for Entry-Level Practice in Acute Care Physical Therapy.* Academy of Acute Care Physical Therapy; 2015.

34. Traube C, Silver G, Gerber LM, et al. Delirium and mortality in critically ill children: epidemiology and outcomes of pediatric delirium. *Crit Care Med.* 2017;45(5):891-898.

35. Franken A, Sebbens D, Mensik J. Pediatric delirium: early identification of barriers to optimize success of screening and prevention. *J Pediatr Health Care.* 2019;33(3):228-233.

36. American Psychiatric Association. *Diagnostic and Statistical Manual of Mental Disorders, Fifth Edition.* American Psychiatric Association; 2013.

37. Patel AK, Bell MJ, Traube C. Delirium in pediatric critical care. *Pediatr Clin North Am.* 2017;64(5):1117-1132.

38. Martínez F, Donoso AM, Marquez C, Labarca E. Implementing a multicomponent intervention to prevent delirium among critically ill patients. *Crit Care Nurse.* 2017;37(6):36-46.

39. Madden K, Burns MM, Tasker RC. Differentiating delirium from sedative/hypnotic-related iatrogenic withdrawal syndrome: lack of specificity in pediatric critical care assessment tools. *Pediatr Crit Care Med.* 2017;18(6):580-588.

40. Cuello-Garcia CA, Mai SHC, Simpson R, Al-harbi S, Choong K. Early mobilization in critically ill children: a systematic review. *J Pediatr.* 2018;203:25-33.e6.

41. Choong K, Foster G, Fraser DD, et al. Acute rehabilitation practices in critically ill children: a multicenter study. *Pediatr Crit Care Med.* 2014;15(6):e270-e279.

42. Loubani E, Bartley D, Forward K. Orthopedic injuries in pediatric trauma. *Curr Pediatr Rev.* 2018;14(1):52-58.

43. Boardman MJ, Herman MJ, Buck B, Pizzutillo PD. Hip fractures in children. *J Am Acad Orthop Surg.* 2009;17(3):162-173.

44. Kuo FC, Kuo SJ, Ko JY, Wong T. Complications of hip fractures in children. *Chang Gung Med J.* 2011;34(5):512-519.

45. John R, Sharma S, Raj GN, et al. Current concepts in paediatric femoral shaft fractures. *Open Orthop J.* 2017;11:353-368.

46. Dial BL, Lark RK. Pediatric proximal femur fractures. *J Orthop.* 2018;15(2):529-535.

47. Meng YC, Zhou XH. External fixation versus open reduction and internal fixation for tibial pilon fractures: a meta-analysis based on observational studies. *Chin J Traumatol.* 2016;19(5):278-282.

48. Yang Z, Yuan ZZ, Ma JX, Ma XL. Long-term efficacy of open reduction and internal fixation versus external fixation for unstable distal radius fractures: a meta-analysis. *Zhonghua Yi Xue Za Zhi.* 2017;97(41):3269-3272.

49. Huh K, Rethlefsen SA, Wren TA, Kay RM. Surgical management of hip subluxation and dislocation in children with cerebral palsy: isolated VDRO or combined surgery? *J Pediatr Orthop.* 2011;31(8):858-863.

50. Givon U. Management of the spastic hip in cerebral palsy. *Curr Opin Pediatr.* 2017;29(1):65-69.

51. Reidy K, Heidt C, Dierauer S, Huber H. A balanced approach for stable hips in children with cerebral palsy: a combination of moderate VDRO and pelvic osteotomy. *J Child Orthop.* 2016;10(4):281-288.

52. Pascual-Garrido C, Harris MD, Clohisy JC. Innovations in joint preservation procedures for the dysplastic hip: "the periacetabular osteotomy." *J Arthroplasty.* 2017;32(9S):S32-S37.

53. Kamath AF. Bernese periacetabular osteotomy for hip dysplasia: surgical technique and indications. *World J Orthop.* 2016;7(5):280-286.

54. Peck D. Slipped capital femoral epiphysis: diagnosis and management. *Am Fam Physician.* 2010;82(3):258-262.

55. Ibrahim T, Little DG. The pathogenesis and treatment of Legg-Calvé-Perthes disease. *JBJS Rev.* 2016;4(7):e4.

56. Shah H. Perthes disease: evaluation and management. *Orthop Clin North Am.* 2014;45(1):87-97.

57. Antinolfi P, Bartoli M, Placella G, et al. Acute patellofemoral instability in children and adolescents. *Joints.* 2016;4(1):47-51.

58. Gao B, Dwivedi S, Fabricant PD, Cruz AI. Patterns in outcomes reporting of operatively managed pediatric patellofemoral instability: a systematic review and meta-analysis. *Am J Sports Med.* 2019;47(6):1516-1524.

59. Trivedi V, Mishra P, Verma D. Pediatric ACL injuries: a review of current concepts. *Open Orthop J.* 2017;11:378-388.

60. Fabricant PD, Kocher MS. Anterior cruciate ligament injuries in children and adolescents. *Orthop Clin North Am.* 2016;47(4):777-788.

61. Martínez G, Drago S, Avilés C, Ibañez A, Hodgson F, Ramírez C. Distal femoral hemiepiphysiodesis using screw and nonabsorbable filament for the treatment of idiopathic genu valgum. Preliminary results of 12 knees. *Orthop Traumatol Surg Res.* 2017;103(2):269-273.

62. Zajonz D, Schumann E, Wojan M, et al. Treatment of genu valgum in children by means of temporary hemiepiphysiodesis using eight-plates: short-term findings. *BMC Musculoskelet Disord.* 2017;18(1):456.

63. El-hawary R, Chukwunyerenwa C. Update on evaluation and treatment of scoliosis. *Pediatr Clin North Am.* 2014;61(6):1223-1241.

64. Kim HJ, Blanco JS, Widmann RF. Update on the management of idiopathic scoliosis. *Curr Opin Pediatr.* 2009;21(1):55-64.

65. Yang C, Wang H, Zheng Z, et al. Halo-gravity traction in the treatment of severe spinal deformity: a systematic review and meta-analysis. *Eur Spine J.* 2017;26(7):1810-1816.

66. Brooks JT, Sponseller PD. What's new in the management of neuromuscular scoliosis. *J Pediatr Orthop.* 2016;36(6):627-633.

67. Rumalla K, Yarbrough CK, Pugely AJ, Koester L, Dorward IG. Spinal fusion for pediatric neuromuscular scoliosis: national trends, complications, and in-hospital outcomes. *J Neurosurg Spine.* 2016;25(4):500-508.

68. Sheffer BW, Kelly DM, Rhodes LN, Sawyer JR. Perioperative pain management in pediatric spine surgery. *Orthop Clin North Am.* 2017;48(4):481-486.

69. Frizzell KH, Cavanaugh PK, Herman MJ. Pediatric perioperative pain management. *Orthop Clin North Am.* 2017;48(4): 467-480.

70. Ward E, DeSantis C, Robbins A, Kohler B, Jemal A. Childhood and adolescent cancer statistics, 2014. Childhood and adolescent cancer statistics, 2014. *CA Cancer J Clin.* 2014;64(2):83-103.

71. Withrow DR, Berrington de Gonzalez A, Lam CJ, Warren KE, Shiels MS. Trends in pediatric central nervous system tumor incidence in the United States, 1998-2013. *Cancer Epidemiol Biomarkers Prev.* 2019;28(3):522-530.

72. Anquilina K. Posterior fossa tumours in children: part 1. *Adv Clin Neurosci Rehabil.* 2013;13(4):24-28.

73. Sturm D, Bender S, Jones DT, et al. Paediatric and adult glioblastoma: multiform (epi)genomic culprits emerge. *Nat Rev Cancer.* 2014;14(2):92-107.

74. Bauchet L, Rigau V, Mathieu-Daudé H, et al. Clinical epidemiology for childhood primary central nervous system tumors. *J Neurooncol.* 2009;92(1):87-98.

75. Davis FG, Mccarthy BJ. Epidemiology of brain tumors. *Curr Opin Neurol.* 2000;13(6):635-640.

76. Kilday JP, Rahman R, Dyer S, et al. Pediatric ependymoma: biological perspectives. *Mol Cancer Res.* 2009;7:765-786.

77. Gandhi P, Khare R, Niraj K, Garg N, Sorte SK, Gulwani H. Unique case of oligoastrocytoma with recurrence and grade progression: exhibiting differential expression of high mobility group-A1 and human telomerase reverse transcriptase. *World J Clin Cases.* 2016;4(9):296-301.

78. Lau CS, Mahendraraj K, Chamberlain RS. Oligodendrogliomas in pediatric and adult patients: an outcome-based study from the Surveillance, Epidemiology, and End Result database. *Cancer Manag Res.* 2017;9:159-166.

79. Wilne SH, Ferris RC, Nathwani A, Kennedy CR. The presenting features of brain tumours: a review of 200 cases. *Arch Dis Child.* 2006;91(6):502-506.

80. Millard NE, De Braganca KC. Medulloblastoma. *J Child Neurol.* 2016;31(12):1341-1353.

81. Northcott PA, Korshunov A, Witt H, et al. Medulloblastoma comprises four distinct molecular variants. *J Clin Oncol.* 2011;29(11):1408-1414.

82. Whittle SB, Smith V, Doherty E, Zhao S, Mccarty S, Zage PE. Overview and recent advances in the treatment of neuroblastoma. *Expert Rev Anticancer Ther.* 2017;17(4):369-386.

83. Kirk EA, Howard VC, Scott CA. Description of posterior fossa syndrome in children after posterior fossa brain tumor surgery. *J Pediatr Oncol Nurs.* 1995;12(4):181-187.

84. Swerdlow SH, Campo E, Harris NL, et al, eds. *WHO Classification of Tumours of Haematopoietic and Lymphoid Tissues.* Revised 4th ed. International Agency for Research on Cancer (IARC); 2017.

85. Bhojwani D, Yang JJ, Pui CH. Biology of childhood acute lymphoblastic leukemia. *Pediatr Clin North Am.* 2015;62(1):47-60.

86. Clarke RT, Van den Bruel A, Bankhead C, Mitchell CD, Phillips B, Thompson MJ. Clinical presentation of childhood leukaemia: a systematic review and meta-analysis. *Arch Dis Child.* 2016;101(10):894-901.

87. Gaynon PS, Angiolillo AL, Carroll WL, et al. Long-term results of the children's cancer group studies for childhood acute lymphoblastic leukemia 1983-2002: a Children's Oncology Group report. *Leukemia.* 2010;24(2):285-297.

88. Bräuninger A, Schmitz R, Bechtel D, Renné C, Hansmann ML, Küppers R. Molecular biology of Hodgkin's and Reed/Sternberg cells in Hodgkin's lymphoma. *Int J Cancer.* 2006;118(8): 1853-1861.

89. Nachman JB, Sposto R, Herzog P, et al. Randomized comparison of low-dose involved-field radiotherapy and no radiotherapy for children with Hodgkin's disease who achieve a complete response to chemotherapy. *J Clin Oncol.* 2002;20(18):3765-3771.

90. Allen CE, Kelly KM, Bollard CM. Pediatric lymphomas and histiocytic disorders of childhood. *Pediatr Clin North Am.* 2015;62(1):139-165.

91. Gurney JG, Swensen AR, Bulterys M. Malignant bone tumors. In: Ries LA, Smith MAS, Gurney JG, et al, eds. *Cancer Incidence and Survival Among Children and Adolescents: United States SEER Program 1975-1995.* National Cancer Institute; 1999:99.

92. Isakoff MS, Bielack SS, Meltzer P, Gorlick R. Osteosarcoma: current treatment and a collaborative pathway to success. *J Clin Oncol.* 2015;33(27):3029-3035.

93. Applebaum MA, Worch J, Matthay KK, et al. Clinical features and outcomes in patients with extraskeletal Ewing sarcoma. *Cancer.* 2011;117(13):3027-3032.

94. Widhe B, Widhe T. Initial symptoms and clinical features in osteosarcoma and Ewing sarcoma. *J Bone Joint Surg Am.* 2000;82(5):667-674.

95. Shern JF, Yohe ME, Khan J. Pediatric rhabdomyosarcoma. *Crit Rev Oncog.* 2015;20(3-4):227-243.

96. Maurer HM, Beltangady M, Gehan EA, et al. The Intergroup Rhabdomyosarcoma Study-I. A final report. *Cancer.* 1988;61(2): 209-220.

97. Al-Hussain T, Ali A, Akhtar M. Wilms tumor: an update. *Adv Anat Pathol.* 2014;21(3):166-173.

98. Sharma D, Subbarao G, Saxena R. Hepatoblastoma. *Semin Diagn Pathol.* 2017;34(2):192-200.

99. Amjad MT, Chidharla A, Kasi A. Cancer Chemotherapy (https://www.ncbi.nlm.nih.gov/books/NBK564367/). 2022 Mar 3.

100. Staff NP, Grisold A, Grisold W, Windebank AJ. Chemotherapy-induced peripheral neuropathy: a current review. *Ann Neurol.* 2017;81(6):772-781.

101. Moore RJ, Groninger H. Chemotherapy-induced peripheral neuropathy in pediatric cancer patients. *Cureus.* 2013;5(6):e124.

102. Revell SH. *Relationship Between Chromosome Damage and Cell Death.* AR Liss; 1983:113.

103. Ishaqi M, Afzal S, Dupuis A, et al. Important role for absolute lymphocyte count in predicting risk of relapse in pediatric acute lymphoblastic leukemia post allogeneic hematopoietic stem cell transplantation. *Pediatr Blood Cancer.* 2006;108(11):3669.

104. Matthay KK, Villablanca JG, Seeger RC, et al. Treatment of high-risk neuroblastoma with intensive chemotherapy, radiotherapy, autologous bone marrow transplantation, and 13-cis-retinoic acid. Children's Cancer Group. *N Engl J Med*. 1999; 341(16): 1165-1173.

105. Peters C, Schrappe M, Von stackelberg A, et al. Stem-cell transplantation in children with acute lymphoblastic leukemia: a prospective international multicenter trial comparing sibling donors with matched unrelated donors—the ALL-SCT-BFM-2003 trial. *J Clin Oncol*. 2015;33(11):1265-1274.

106. Copelan EA. Hematopoietic stem-cell transplantation. *N Engl J Med*. 2006;354(17):1813-1826.

107. Pidala J. Graft-vs-host disease following allogenic hematopoietic cell transplant. *Cancer Control*. 2011;18(4):268-276.

108. Braam KI, Van der Torre P, Takken T, Veening MA, Van Dulmen-Den Broeder E, Kaspers GJ. Physical exercise training interventions for children and young adults during and after treatment for childhood cancer. *Cochrane Database Syst Rev*. 2016;3:CD008796.

109. Simioni C, Zauli G, Martelli AM, et al. Physical training interventions for children and teenagers affected by acute lymphoblastic leukemia and related treatment impairments. *Oncotarget*. 2018;9(24):17199-17209.

110. Van Haren IE, Timmerman H, Potting CM, Blijlevens NM, Staal JB, Nijhuis-Van Der Sanden MW. Physical exercise for patients undergoing hematopoietic stem cell transplantation: systematic review and meta-analyses of randomized controlled trials. *Phys Ther*. 2013;93(4):514-528.

111. Van Haren IEPM, Staal JB, Potting CM, et al. Physical exercise prior to hematopoietic stem cell transplantation: a feasibility study. *Physiother Theory Pract*. 2018;34(10):747-756.

112. Schuster SJ, Svoboda J, Chong EA, et al. Chimeric antigen receptor T cells in refractory B-cell lymphomas. *N Engl J Med*. 2017;377(26):2545-2554.

113. Salter AI, Pont MJ, Riddell SR. Chimeric antigen receptor-modified T cells: CD19 and the road beyond. *Blood*. 2018; 131(24):2621-2629.

114. Lee DW, Gardner R, Porter DL, et al. Current concepts in the diagnosis and management of cytokine release syndrome. *Blood*. 2014;124(2):188-195.

115. Veeravagu A, Jiang B, Ludwig C, Chang SD, Black KL, Patil CG. Biopsy versus resection for the management of low-grade gliomas. *Cochrane Database Syst Rev*. 2013;4:CD009319.

116. Grimer RJ, Taminiau AM, Cannon SR. Surgical outcomes in osteosarcoma. *J Bone Joint Surg Br*. 2002;84(3):395-400.

117. Li X, Zhang Y, Wan S, et al. A comparative study between limb-salvage and amputation for treating osteosarcoma. *J Bone Oncol*. 2016;5(1):15-21.

118. Han G, Bi WZ, Xu M, Jia JP, Wang Y. Amputation versus limb-salvage surgery in patients with osteosarcoma: a meta-analysis. *World J Surg*. 2016;40(8):2016-2027.

119. Kuter D. Managing thrombocytopenia associated with cancer chemotherapy. *Oncology (Williston Park)*. 2015;29(4): 282-294.

120. Bercovitz RS, Josephson CD. Thrombocytopenia and bleeding in pediatric oncology patients. *Hematology Am Soc Hematol Educ Program*. 2012;2012:499-505.

121. Berger AM, Mooney K, Alvarez-perez A, et al. Cancer-Related Fatigue, Version 2.2015. *J Natl Compr Canc Netw*. 2015;13(8): 1012-1039.

122. Silva MC, Lopes LC, Nascimento LC, Lima RA. Fatigue in children and adolescents with cancer from the perspective of health professionals. *Rev Lat Am Enfermagem*. 2016;24:e2784.

123. Ryan JL, Carroll JK, Ryan EP, Mustian KM, Fiscella K, Morrow GR. Mechanisms of cancer-related fatigue. *Oncologist*. 2007;12(suppl 1):22-34.

124. Kangas M, Bovbjerg DH, Montgomery GH. Cancer-related fatigue: a systematic and meta-analytic review of non-pharmacological therapies for cancer patients. *Psychol Bull*. 2008; 134(5):700-741.

125. Gilchrist LS, Tanner L. The pediatric-modified total neuropathy score: a reliable and valid measure of chemotherapy-induced peripheral neuropathy in children with non-CNS cancers. *Support Care Cancer*. 2013;21(3):847-856.

126. Gilchrist LS, Marais L, Tanner L. Comparison of two chemotherapy-induced peripheral neuropathy measurement approaches in children. *Support Care Cancer*. 2014;22(2):359-366.

127. Berry JG, Poduri A, Bonkowsky JL, et al. Trends in resource utilization by children with neurological impairment in the United States inpatient health care system: a repeat cross-sectional study. *PLoS Med*. 2012;9(1):e1001158.

128. Caceres JA, Goldstein JN. Intracranial hemorrhage. *Emerg Med Clin North Am*. 2012;30(3):771-794.

129. Lo WD. Childhood hemorrhagic stroke: an important but understudied problem. *J Child Neurol*. 2011;26(9):1174-1185.

130. Whitby EH, Griffiths PD, Rutter S, et al. Frequency and natural history of subdural haemorrhages in babies and relation to obstetric factors. *Lancet*. 2004;363(9412):846-851.

131. Brouwer AJ, Groenendaal F, Koopman C, Nievelstein RJ, Han SK, De Vries LS. Intracranial hemorrhage in full-term newborns: a hospital-based cohort study. *Neuroradiology*. 2010; 52(6):567-576.

132. Shah NA, Wusthoff CJ. Intracranial hemorrhage in the neonate. *Neonatal Netw*. 2016;35(2):67-71.

133. Intrapiromkul J, Northington F, Huisman TA, Izbudak I, Meoded A, Tekes A. Accuracy of head ultrasound for the detection of intracranial hemorrhage in preterm neonates: comparison with brain MRI and susceptibility-weighted imaging. *J Neuroradiol*. 2013;40(2):81-88.

134. Geibprasert S, Pongpech S, Jiarakongmun P, Shroff MM, Armstrong DC, Krings T. Radiologic assessment of brain arteriovenous malformations: what clinicians need to know. *Radiographics*. 2010;30(2):483-501.

135. Da Costa L, Wallace MC, Ter Brugge KG, O'Kelly C, Willinsky RA, Tymianski M. The natural history and predictive features of hemorrhage from brain arteriovenous malformations. *Stroke*. 2009;40(1):100-105.

136. Li G, Han K, Yang H, Huang H, Yang H, Zhu D. Risk factors of intracranial hemorrhage after brain AVM interventional therapy and its effects on prognosis. *Int J Clin Exp Med*. 2015;8(7): 11014-11019.

137. Ajiboye N, Chalouhi N, Starke RM, Zanaty M, Bell R. Cerebral arteriovenous malformations: evaluation and management. *Sci World J*. 2014;2014:649036.

138. Nundia L, Marsh R. Hemorrhagic progression of cavernous angiomas: a review. *Neurosci Commun*. 2017;3:e1519.

139. Smith ER, Scott RM. Surgical management of moyamoya syndrome. *Skull Base*. 2005;15(1):15-26.

140. Takeuchi K, Shimizu K. Hypoplasia of the bilateral internal carotid arteries. *Brain Nerve*. 1957;9:37-43.

141. Suzuki J, Takaku A. Cerebrovascular "moyamoya" disease. Disease showing abnormal net-like vessels in base of brain. *Arch Neurol*. 1969;20(3):288-299.

142. Jha V, Behari S, Jaiswal AK, Bhaisora KS, Shende YP, Phadke RV. The "focus on aneurysm" principle: classification and surgical principles of management of concurrent arterial aneurysm with

arteriovenous malformation causing intracranial hemorrhage. *Asian J Neurosurg.* 2016;11(3):240-254.

143. Marks MP, Lane B, Steinberg GK, Chang PJ. Hemorrhage in intracerebral arteriovenous malformations: angiographic determinants. *Radiology.* 1990;176(3):807-813.

144. Klein R, Hopewell CA, Oien M. Chiari malformation type I: a neuropsychological case study. *Mil Med.* 2014;179(6):e712-e718.

145. Urbizu A, Toma C, Poca MA, et al. Chiari malformation type I: a case-control association study of 58 developmental genes. *PLoS ONE.* 2013;8(2):e57241.

146. Andica C, Soetikno RD. Chiari malformation type III: case report and review of the literature. *Radiol Case Rep.* 2013;8(3):831.

147. Geerdink N, Van der Vliet T, Rotteveel JJ, Feuth T, Roeleveld N, Mullaart RA. Essential features of Chiari II malformation in MR imaging: an interobserver reliability study—part 1. *Childs Nerv Syst.* 2012;28(7):977-985.

148. Jeong DH, Kim CH, Kim MO, Chung H, Kim TH, Jung HY. Arnold-Chiari malformation type III with meningoencephalocele: a case report. *Ann Rehabil Med.* 2014;38(3):401-404.

149. Pople IK. Hydrocephalus and shunts: what the neurologist should know. *J Neurol Neurosurg Psychiatry.* 2002;73(suppl 1):i17-22.

150. Muralidharan R. External ventricular drains: management and complications. *Surg Neurol Int.* 2015;6(suppl 6):S271-274.

151. Vinchon M, Rekate H, Kulkarni AV. Pediatric hydrocephalus outcomes: a review. *Fluids Barriers CNS.* 2012;9(1):18.

152. Van Beijnum J, Hanlo PW, Fischer K, et al. Laser-assisted endoscopic third ventriculostomy: long-term results in a series of 202 patients. *Neurosurgery.* 2008;62(2):437-443.

153. Demerdash A, Rocque BG, Johnston J, et al. Endoscopic third ventriculostomy: a historical review. *Br J Neurosurg.* 2017; 31(1):28-32.

154. Granerod J, Crowcroft NS. The epidemiology of acute encephalitis. *Neuropsychol Rehabil.* 2007;17(4-5):406-428.

155. Christie S, Chan V, Mollayeva T, Colantonio A. Rehabilitation interventions in children and adults with infectious encephalitis: a systematic review protocol. *BMJ Open.* 2016;6(3):e010754.

156. Moorthi S, Schneider WN, Dombovy ML. Rehabilitation outcomes in encephalitis: a retrospective study 1990-1997. *Brain Inj.* 1999;13(2):139-146.

157. Hartung HP, Mouthon L, Ahmed R, Jordan S, Laupland KB, Jolles S. Clinical applications of intravenous immunoglobulins (IVIg): beyond immunodeficiencies and neurology. *Clin Exp Immunol.* 2009;158(suppl 1):23-33.

158. Mckay SL, Lee AD, Lopez AS, et al. Increase in acute flaccid myelitis - United States, 2018. *MMWR Morb Mortal Wkly Rep.* 2018;67(45):1273-1275.

159. Messacar K, Asturias EJ, Hixon AM, et al. Enterovirus D68 and acute flaccid myelitis: evaluating the evidence for causality. *Lancet Infect Dis.* 2018;18(8):e239-e247.

160. Messacar K, Schreiner TL, Van Haren K, et al. Acute flaccid myelitis: a clinical review of US cases 2012-2015. *Ann Neurol.* 2016;80(3):326-338.

161. Wolf VL, Lupo PJ, Lotze TE. Pediatric acute transverse myelitis overview and differential diagnosis. *J Child Neurol.* 2012;27(11):1426-1436.

162. Absoud M, Greenberg BM, Lim M, Lotze T, Thomas T, Deiva K. Pediatric transverse myelitis. *Neurology.* 2016;87(9 suppl 2):S46-52.

163. Pidcock FS, Krishnan C, Crawford TO, Salorio CF, Trovato M, Kerr DA. Acute transverse myelitis in childhood: center-based analysis of 47 cases. *Neurology.* 2007;68:1474-1480.

164. Kimbler DE, Murphy M, Dhandapani KM. Concussion and the adolescent athlete. *J Neurosci Nurs.* 2011;43(6):286-290.

165. Zhang AL, Sing DC, Rugg CM, Feeley BT, Senter C. The rise of concussions in the adolescent population. *Orthop J Sports Med.* 2016;4(8):2325967116662458.

166. Signoretti S, Lazzarino G, Tavazzi B, Vagnozzi R. The pathophysiology of concussion. *PM R.* 2011;3(10 suppl 2):S359-368.

167. Tator CH. Concussions and their consequences: current diagnosis, management and prevention. *CMAJ.* 2013;185(11):975-979.

168. Keane JR. Hysterical gait disorders: 60 cases. *Neurology.* 1989;39(4):586-589.

169. Heruti RJ, Reznik J, Adunski A, Levy A, Weingarden H, Ohry A. Conversion motor paralysis disorder: analysis of 34 consecutive referrals. *Spinal Cord.* 2002;40(7):335-340.

170. Ness D. Physical therapy management for conversion disorder: case series. *J Neurol Phys Ther.* 2007;31(1):30-39.

171. Evens A, Vendetta L, Krebs K, Herath P. Medically unexplained neurologic symptoms: a primer for physicians who make the initial encounter. *Am J Med.* 2015;128(10):1059-1064.

172. Roper LS, Saifee TA, Parees I, Rickards H, Edwards MJ. How to use the entrainment test in the diagnosis of functional tremor. *Pract Neurol.* 2013;13(6):396-398.

173. Roper LS, Rickards H. The entrainment test in tremor assessment: influence of historical factors and clinical methodology. *J Neurol Neurosurg Psychiatry.* 2013;84:e1.

174. Parobek VM. Distinguishing conversion disorder from neurologic impairment. *J Neurosci Nurs.* 1997;29(2):128-134.

175. Heruti RJ, Reznik J, Adunski A, Levy A, Weingarden H, Ohry A. Conversion motor paralysis disorder: analysis of 34 consecutive referrals. *Spinal Cord.* 2002;40(7):335-340.

176. Mehndiratta MM, Kumar M, Nayak R, Gatg H, Pandey S. Hoover's sign. *Clin Rel Neurol.* 2014;60(3):297-299.

177. Groat J, Neumiller J. Review of the treatment and management of hydrocephalus. *US Pharm.* 2013;38(3):HS8-HS11.

178. Moseley A, Wales A, Herbert R, Schurr K, Moore S. Observation and analysis of hemiplegic gait: stance phase. *Aust J Physiother.* 1993;39(4):259-267.

179. Nudo RJ. Recovery after brain injury: mechanisms and principles. *Front Hum Neurosci.* 2013;7:887.

180. Karni A, Meyer G, Rey-Hipolito C, et al. The acquisition of skilled motor performance: fast and slow experience-driven changes in primary motor cortex. *Proc Natl Acad Sci USA.* 1998; 95(3):861-868.

Cerebral Palsy

Martha H. Bloyer, PT, DPT, and Teresa Muñecas, PT, DPT, EdD

LEARNING OBJECTIVES

Upon completion of this chapter, the reader will be able to:

- Define cerebral palsy (CP) and differentiate between the various classifications.
- Integrate information regarding pathophysiology, diagnostic criteria, and potential differential and associated diagnoses of CP.
- Identify appropriate screening and diagnostic tools used to determine motor function classification.

- Apply evidenced-based interventions and management strategies in developing a plan of care for individuals with the diagnosis of CP.
- Discuss the prognosis for individuals with CP and identify appropriate referrals and available community resources.

■ INTRODUCTION

CEREBRAL PALSY DEFINITION

Cerebral palsy (CP) refers to a group of clinical presentations due to an insult or pathogenic event in the developing and immature brain, resulting in motor deficiency affecting movement and posture, with nonprogression of the initial condition or insult.[1-3] According to Graham et al,[4] the stage of brain maturation during which the pathogenetic events occur defines the type and site of lesions, as well as the specific response to insult resulting in activity limitations and participation restrictions.[2,4] The motor disorders of CP are often accompanied by disturbances of sensation, perception, cognition, communication, and behavior; epilepsy; and secondary musculoskeletal problems.[3]

The purpose of this chapter is to use the International Classification of Functioning, Disability, and Health (ICF) framework to provide evidenced-based decision-making and management of the movement disorders in individuals diagnosed with CP. The role of the physical therapist and physical therapist assistant, as part of the interdisciplinary team, will be discussed, and case examples will be used to guide and instruct the reader to critically think and develop skills in order to formulate evidence-informed diagnosis, prognosis, and selection and implementation of interventions.

PREVALENCE AND RISK FACTORS

The pooled prevalence of CP is 2.11 per 1000 live births, despite improved survival of at-risk preterm infants, as reported by Oskoui et al.[5] Estimates using young children as the denominator are somewhat higher, ranging from 3.1 to 4.4 per 1000.[6] Among population-based studies of CP, males have been found to have a higher prevalence of CP than females, with sex ratios ranging from 1.1:1 to 1.5:1.[7] A higher prevalence in black non-Hispanic children compared with white non-Hispanic children has been reported.[7] There is an increasing body of evidence pointing to strong genetic influences on the occurrence of CP of up to 14%, and a multifactorial inheritance pattern is suggested.[8-10] Potential risk factors associated with the development of CP are shown in **Figure 7-1** and can be associated with maternal or infant factors.[4,11,12]

PHYSIOLOGIC AND TOPOGRAPHIC CLASSIFICATION OF CEREBRAL PALSY

CP can be divided into 2 main *physiologic* groups, the *pyramidal* (a term used to refer to cases in which spasticity is prominent) and the *extrapyramidal types* (term used to refer to cases in which chorea, athetosis, dystonia, and ataxia are prominent). Refer to **Table 7-1**. Extrapyramidal CP has 4-limb involvement, with the upper extremities typically being functionally more involved than the lower extremities. A combination of these tone patterns in the same patient is common, creating potential difficulty in finding the proper diagnostic terminology.[6]

In addition, the *topographic* classification (**Figure 7-2**) is restricted to the *spastic* group for practical purposes. There are concerns with the reliability of the topographic and physiologic classifications, as they do not consider functional abilities.[6]

MOTOR SYNDROMES OR TYPE: CLASSIFICATION OF CEREBRAL PALSY

Spastic CP is the most common type of CP, affecting approximately 70% to 80% of the children identified with CP.[13] Those with spastic CP have increased muscle tone (hypertonicity), or

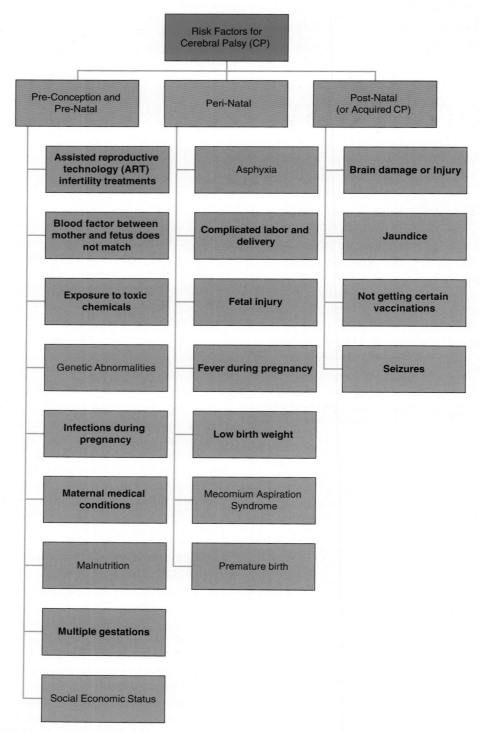

FIGURE 7-1 **Potential risk factors for cerebral palsy.** (https://www.ninds.nih.gov/health-information/disorders/cerebral-palsy#toc-who-is-more-likely-to-get-cerebral-palsy-)

resistance to passive movements. Spasticity has been defined as "a motor disorder, characterized by a velocity-dependent increase in tonic stretch reflexes (muscle tone) with exaggerated tendon jerks, resulting from hyper-excitability of the stretch reflex as one component of the upper motor neuron syndrome."[14] Spasticity can be measured and graded using the Modified Ashworth Scale (MAS).[15] Further explanation and

use of the MAS can be found in the examination section of this chapter.

Spastic CP is usually described by what parts of the body are affected, as follows:[16,17]

- **Spastic diplegia:** Muscle hypertonicity is mainly in the legs, with the arms less affected or not affected at all. Individuals with spastic diplegia may have difficulty walking because

TABLE 7-1 • Physiologic and Topographic Classification of Cerebral Palsy[4,6]			
Physiologic Classification	**Muscle Tone/Motor Type**	**Limb Involvement**	**Injury**
Pyramidal type	Spasticity is prominent	Varies	Within the pyramidal tract
Extrapyramidal types	Chorea, athetosis, dystonia, ataxia	4 limbs	Basal ganglia, thalamus, and cerebellum
Topographic Classification (subgroups of spastic CP)			
Monoplegia	1 limb is affected and more often the lower limb		
Diplegia	Bilateral lower extremity involvement > upper extremity involvement		
Hemiplegia	Unilateral upper and lower extremity involvement		
Triplegia	Involvement of 3 extremities (typically both lower extremities and 1 upper extremity)		
Double hemiplegia	4-extremity involvement with more severe spasticity of the upper extremities		
Quadriplegia/tetraplegia	Severe 4-extremity involvement		

tight hip and leg muscles cause their legs to pull together, turn inward, and/or cross at the knees, resulting in crouched or scissoring gait patterns.

- **Spastic hemiplegia:** This type of CP affects only one side of the person's body; usually the arm is more affected than the leg.
- **Spastic quadriplegia:** Spastic quadriplegia is the most severe form of spastic CP and affects all 4 limbs, the trunk, and the face. Individuals with spastic quadriplegia usually present with severe motor impairments, resulting in inability to walk, and often have other developmental disabilities such as intellectual disability; seizures; or problems with vision, hearing, or speech.

Dyskinetic CP includes athetoid, choreoathetoid, and dystonic cerebral palsies.[16,18] Individuals with dyskinetic CP have problems controlling the movements of their hands, arms, feet, and legs, making it difficult to perform activities such as sitting or walking independently. The movements are uncontrollable and can be slow and writhing or rapid and jerky. Sometimes the face and tongue are affected, and the individual has a hard time sucking, swallowing, and talking. Those with dyskinetic CP present with muscle tone that can change (varying from hypertonia to hypotonia) not only from day to day, but even during a single day.[18]

Ataxic CP is the least frequent type of CP.[16] Individuals with ataxic CP have problems with balance and coordination. They may present with unsteady shaky movements leading to difficulties with walking steadily and controlled. They may have a hard time with quick movements or movements that require greater graded control, like writing or picking up a glass filled with water. They may also present with difficulty in timing the movements of their hands or arms when they reach for something, resulting in clumsiness due to the overcorrection of inaccurate movements. For example, when the individual reaches for an object, they may overshoot and miss the intended target.[13]

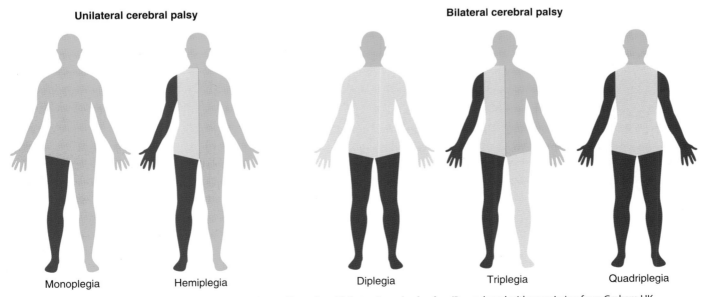

FIGURE 7-2 Topographical description in cerebral palsy: unilateral and bilateral cerebral palsy. (Reproduced with permission from Graham HK, Rosenbaum P, Paneth N, et al. Cerebral palsy. Nature Reviews Disease Primers. 2016;2(1):15082.)

Mixed CP is the term used in cases where no one type dominates and the individual may have symptoms of more than one type of CP. The most common type of mixed CP is spastic-dyskinetic CP. However, it is stated in recent literature that the term *mixed CP* should not be used without elaboration and description of the component motor disorders.[4]

Although typically used, topographic and physiologic classifications do not aid therapy selection and interventions. Because brain dysfunction has diffuse manifestations in childhood, each child must be evaluated thoroughly for associated impairments in areas such as learning and cognition, vision, behavior, epilepsy, and secondary neuromuscular abnormalities. It is not possible to direct clinical assessments simply based on correlations between topography and associated dysfunctions.[6]

ADDITIONAL CLASSIFICATION SYSTEMS

Additional attempts to classify CP have included *etiologic* and *neuropathologic*.[6] *Etiologic* classifications have aimed at preventive strategies; however, to date, a system has not been fully developed. *Neuropathologic* classifications attempt to reflect, highlight, and relate brain structure to brain function. With the advent of advanced neuroimaging, such as computed tomography (CT) and magnetic resonance imaging (MRI), 2 important *associations* have been described: (1) periventricular leukomalacia (white matter damage with prematurity)[3,11] and (2) basal ganglia injury with term asphyxia.[11] Although advances in neuroimaging techniques continues to be realized, neuroimaging has not demonstrated the ability to *consistently* demonstrate a relationship between structure and function.

Supplemental classifications include syndromes such as bilirubin encephalopathy, which presents as choreoathetoid CP, vertical gaze palsy, dental enamel dysplasia, and sensorineural hearing loss. It has a predictable clinical course, with extensor spells during the first few months, followed by hypotonia, then choreoathetosis, and finally dystonia during adolescence.[6]

Classification of CP from an *epidemiologic* perspective led to many international surveillance systems such as the Surveillance of Cerebral Palsy in Europe (SCPE).[6,17,18] In addition, surveillance systems began using formalized methods to assess function in addition to impairment, and the Gross Motor Function Measure (GMFM) was developed for clinical use.[6,19,20] The GMFM is an assessment tool designed and evaluated to measure changes in gross motor function over time or with intervention in children with CP. There are 2 versions of the GMFM: the original GMFM-88 and the shortened GMFM-66. It addresses gross motor activities in the following 5 dimensions:

A: Lying and rolling
B: Sitting
C: Crawling and kneeling
D: Standing
E: Walking, running, and jumping

Additional information regarding the GMFM-88 or GMFM-66 can be found at the following website: https://canchild.ca/en/resources/44-gross-motor-function-measure-gmfm.

Based on the concepts of disability and functional limitations, today, the trend in clinical practice is to classify individuals with CP by functional independence. Reflecting this trend, several classifications systems have been developed (**Table 7-2**).[21,22]

The Gross Motor Function Classification System–Expanded and Revised

The Gross Motor Function Classification System–Expanded and Revised (GMFCS-E&R) describes self-initiated movement in children before the second birthday through 18 years of age with emphasis on sitting, walking, and wheeled mobility. It is a 5-level classification with clinically meaningful distinctions among the levels. Distinction levels are based on functional limitations and the need for handheld mobility devices (eg, walkers, crutches, or canes) or wheeled mobility (see https://cparf.org/what-is-cerebral-palsy/severity-of-cerebral-palsy/gross-motor-function-classification-system-gmfcs/).[22-26]

TABLE 7-2 • Functional Classification Systems		
Classification System	**Website**	**English Version Website**
Gross Motor Function Classification System–Expanded and Revised (GMFCS-E&R)[22-24,26]	https://canchild.ca/en/resources/42-gross-motor-function-classification-system-expanded-revised-gmfcs-e-r[24]	https://canchild.ca/system/tenon/assets/attachments/000/000/058/original/GMFCS-ER_English.pdf[25]
Manual Ability Classification System (MACS)[27]	https://www.macs.nu/index.php[28]	http://www.macs.nu/files/MACS_English_2010.pdf[29]
Bimanual Fine Motor Function (BFMF)[30]	https://eu-rd-platform.jrc.ec.europa.eu/scpe/data-collection/reference-documents_en[31]	https://eu-rd-platform.jrc.ec.europa.eu/sites/default/files/Bimanual-Fine-Motor-Function-2.0.pdf[31]
Communication Function Classification System (CFCS)[32]	http://cfcs.us/[33]	http://cfcs.us/wp-content/uploads/2018/11/CFCS_English_CP.pdf[34]
Eating and Drinking Ability Classification System (EDACS)[35]	https://www.sussexcommunity.nhs.uk/get-involved/research/chailey-research/eating-drinking-classification.htm[36]	https://www.sussexcommunity.nhs.uk/get-involved/research/chailey-research/edacs-request[37]

https://www.cpqcc.org/sites/default/files/GMFCS-ER.pdf

Similar scales for fine motor, communication, and eating abilities have been developed: the Manual Ability Classification System (MACS), the Bimanual Fine Motor Function (BFMF) scales, the Communication Function Classification System (CFCS), and the Eating and Drinking Ability Classification System (EDACS).[21]

The Manual Ability Classification System

MACS has been developed to classify how children with CP age 4 to 18 years use their hands when handling objects in daily activities. The developers of the MACS, consisting of a multidisciplinary team, stated that they wanted to highlight the importance of hand use in children and that there was no previous valid and reliable way to classify hand function. (See https://www.macs.nu/why-macs.php.)

It has also been noted by Eliasson et al, that the high but not perfect correlation between MACS and GMFCS indicates that the MACS is built on a different construct to GMFCS. In only half of the children was there exact agreement between MACS and GMFCS levels. This suggests that gross and fine motor function in children with CP "do not neatly run in parallel," and can and should be independently classified separately.[27]

The Bimanual Fine Motor Function

The BFMF scale classifies fine motor function in children with CP age 3 to 18 years. The BFMF describes 5 levels of fine motor function and covers the entire spectrum of limitations in fine motor function that may be found among children with various CP subtypes.[30]

The Communication Function Classification System

The CFCS for individuals with CP is used to classify the everyday communication performance of an individual greater than 4 years of age into 1 of 5 levels.[32]

The Eating and Drinking Ability Classification System

The EDACS describes the functional eating and drinking abilities of children with CP aged 3 to 17 years using 5 distinct levels. The developers of the EDACS reported that there was no previous way to systematically describe how eating and drinking ability was affected in individuals with CP. This system is distinct from available detailed clinical assessments for mealtime management and offers a means for parents and professionals to communicate effectively these specific abilities.[38] The EDACS refers to key features of safety (aspiration and choking) and efficiency (amount of food lost and time taken to eat). The EDACS also provides a 3-level ordinal rating scale to describe the degree of assistance required (independent, requires assistance, or totally dependent).[35]

■ EXAMINATION AND EVALUATION

Each individual with CP must be evaluated for an array of neuromotor impairments and associated conditions, including deficits in vision, hearing, speech, cognition, and academic achievement. A thorough systems review should be included as part of the examination. Although the focus of this section is related to the physical therapist's examination of neuromotor impairments, a team approach and referral to appropriate professionals is warranted to address the following associated conditions:

- Visual impairments and disorders of ocular motility are common in 28% of children with CP. There is an increased presence of strabismus, amblyopia, nystagmus, optic atrophy, and refractive errors.
- Hearing impairment occurs in approximately 12% of children with CP. This occurs more commonly if the etiology of CP is related to very low birth weight, kernicterus, neonatal meningitis, or severe hypoxic-ischemic insults.
- Epilepsy is common in children with CP, and 35% to 62% of children develop epilepsy. Children with spastic quadriplegia (50%-94%) or hemiplegia (30%) have a higher incidence of epilepsy than patients with diplegia or ataxic CP (16%-27%).
- Speech is affected in CP due to bilateral corticobulbar and oral motor dysfunctions. Receptive and expressive language deficits are common and are linked with the level of cognitive involvement. Articulation disorders and impaired speech are present in 38% of children with CP. Oral motor problems with feeding difficulties and swallowing dysfunction can also result in nutritional problems affecting physical growth.
- Abnormalities of proprioception and tactile sensations are common in children with CP.
- Psychiatric disorders such as anxiety, depression, conduct disorders, and hyperkinesis and inattention were seen in 61% of 6- to 10-year-old children with hemiplegic CP.[18,39]

Specialized clinicians in each field should address the associated diagnoses. Physical therapists should identify limitations in associated diagnosis and refer to the specialized clinician. Communication and education of parents and/or caregivers is a priority. Physical therapy assessment of infants, children, and youth with CP should be adapted to meet the needs of the child and family based on their age and the setting in which the assessment is conducted and should occur to ensure realistic goal setting, provide a baseline for therapy, and evaluate therapy programs.

HISTORY

As with any physical therapy examination, in addition to demographic information (eg, name, age, sex, caregiver/guardian), a full thorough history should be gathered. The history can include, but may not be limited to, the sample questions listed in **Table 7-3**.

INTERNATIONAL CLASSIFICATION OF FUNCTIONING, DISABILITY, AND HEALTH CORE SETS FOR CEREBRAL PALSY

The ICF model provides the framework in examining a child or adolescent with a medical of diagnosis CP. The Children and Youth with Disability in Society (CYDiS) research unit at the University of British Columbia in Canada, the ICF Research Branch, and the Classification, Terminology, and Standards Team at the World Health Organization have teamed up to tackle the issue of the lack of appropriate instruments that assess the effects of CP on everyday life and the lack of guidelines on how to measure and evaluate specific interventions. Together, they developed the first version of the ICF Core Sets for children and youth with CP.[40,41]

TABLE 7-3 • Sample Background and History Questions

Pregnancy and birth	Duration of pregnancy: _____ (weeks) Type of delivery: _____ Birth weight: _____ Birth length: _____ inches Baby discharged from hospital at: _____ (days/weeks) after birth Did the mother experience any problems/complications during pregnancy and/or labor? ☐ Yes ☐ No If "Yes," please describe:
Medical and surgical	Has your child had any medical problem(s) and/or received any previous diagnoses? ☐ Yes ☐ No If "Yes," please describe: Has your child had any procedure(s)/hospitalization(s)? ☐ Yes ☐ No If "Yes," please describe:
Medication or supplements	Has your child ever taken or is your child currently taking any prescribed medications? ☐ Yes ☐ No If "Yes," please describe: Has your child ever taken or is your child currently taking over-the-counter medication, including vitamins and/or nutritional supplements? ☐ Yes ☐ No If "Yes," please describe:
Previous evaluations and therapies	Has your child had any previous evaluations? ☐ Yes ☐ No If "Yes," please describe: Has your child received any treatments or therapies? ☐ Yes ☐ No If "Yes," please describe:
Child/family goals with physical therapy services	What specific gross motor concerns do you have? What are your goals with physical therapy services provided?

The Core Sets can be downloaded at the following website: https://www.icf-research-branch.org/icf-core-sets/category/8-neurologicalconditions.[42]

SELECTED TESTS AND MEASURES FOR INFANTS, CHILDREN, AND YOUTH WITH CEREBRAL PALSY

The physical therapist (PT) can play a significant role as part of an interdisciplinary team for early diagnosis of CP. Most children with CP are historically diagnosed around 12 to 24 months of age.[43] The examination of the infant, child, or adolescent with CP should include the following components using the ICF model: body structure and function, activity limitations, and participation restrictions to include environmental and personal factors.

Early Diagnosis Examination

Early diagnosis of CP is now possible with full workups that include the PT as part of the evaluation of neonates born prematurely. Providing an early diagnosis can lead to timely access to services and appropriate interventions. **Figure 7-3** provides an early diagnosis algorithm for diagnosing CP. In conjunction with other team members' examinations, the PT can perform a neurologic examination using the standardized Hammersmith Infant Neurological Evaluation (HINE). The HINE can be used for *identifying the risk* of CP in infants between 2 and 24 months of age. The HINE contains cutoff scores that can help in identifying infants at risk for CP and provides additional information on the severity level.[44] Additionally, as part of the motor assessment of *quality* of movements, the PT can utilize Prechtl's General Movement Assessment (GMA) to observe spontaneous movements in infants lying in supine from the preterm period to 20 weeks postterm. GMA is considered the most accurate clinical tool to *predict* CP before the age of 5 months.[45-48] The PT can also assess volitional movement of the infant by using the parent questionnaire, the Developmental Assessment of Young Children (DAYC), for infants 6 to 12 months of age. The DAYC has been found to be a good predictive tool for infants greater than 5 months of age.[49]

Examination: Body Structure and Function

A thorough examination of body structure and function should be completed when examining an individual diagnosed with CP. Over time, the imbalance of muscle strength and tone causes muscle weakness and atrophy, as well as soft tissue contracture and eventual joint deformity.[49] The *most common* primary and secondary neuromuscular impairments seen in children with CP will be discussed.

- **Tone**
  Tone can manifest as hypotonicity, hypertonicity, or normal resting tension.
  - In children presenting with spasticity (hypertonicity), as previously mentioned, the **Modified Ashworth Scale (MAS)** can be used can be used as a clinical measure for grading muscle tone and is a nominal-level measure of resistance to passive movement (**Table 7-4**). In the literature, it has been found to have improved reliability when assessing the upper extremities as compared to the lower extremities.[15,51,52]
  - The **Modified Tardieu Scale (MTS)** assesses resistance to passive movement at both slow (V1) and fast (V3) speeds. V2 represents the speed of limb movement due to gravity (**Table 7-5**).[52,53] Using a goniometer, the clinician compares the angle of full slow speed (V1) passive range of movement (R2) and the angle of resistance first felt during fast speed (V3) passive movements (R1) to identify the physiologic and neurologic mechanisms affecting resistance to passive movements, respectively. Refer to **Figure 7-4** for angle reference suggested positions for elbow flexors, ankle dorsiflexors, and knee flexors.[54]
    - R1 angle of resistance first felt during fast passive movements
    - R2 angle of full, slow passive range of movement[55]

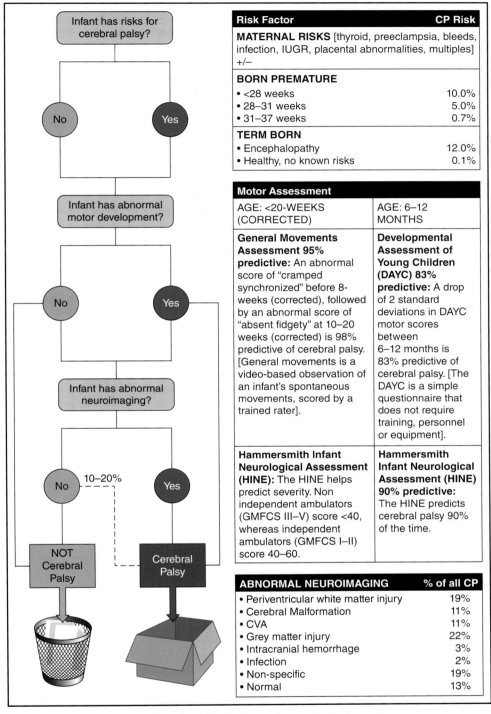

Infant has risks for cerebral palsy?

No   Yes

Infant has abnormal motor development?

No   Yes

Infant has abnormal neuroimaging?

No   10–20%   Yes

NOT Cerebral Palsy   Cerebral Palsy

Risk Factor	CP Risk
MATERNAL RISKS [thyroid, preeclampsia, bleeds, infection, IUGR, placental abnormalities, multiples] +/–	
BORN PREMATURE	
• <28 weeks	10.0%
• 28–31 weeks	5.0%
• 31–37 weeks	0.7%
TERM BORN	
• Encephalopathy	12.0%
• Healthy, no known risks	0.1%

Motor Assessment	
AGE: <20-WEEKS (CORRECTED)	AGE: 6–12 MONTHS
General Movements Assessment 95% predictive: An abnormal score of "cramped synchronized" before 8-weeks (corrected), followed by an abnormal score of "absent fidgety" at 10–20 weeks (corrected) is 98% predictive of cerebral palsy. [General movements is a video-based observation of an infant's spontaneous movements, scored by a trained rater].	**Developmental Assessment of Young Children (DAYC) 83% predictive:** A drop of 2 standard deviations in DAYC motor scores between 6–12 months is 83% predictive of cerebral palsy. [The DAYC is a simple questionnaire that does not require training, personnel or equipment].
Hammersmith Infant Neurological Assessment (HINE): The HINE helps predict severity. Non independent ambulators (GMFCS III–V) score <40, whereas independent ambulators (GMFCS I–II) score 40–60.	**Hammersmith Infant Neurological Assessment (HINE) 90% predictive:** The HINE predicts cerebral palsy 90% of the time.

ABNORMAL NEUROIMAGING	% of all CP
• Periventricular white matter injury	19%
• Cerebral Malformation	11%
• CVA	11%
• Grey matter injury	22%
• Intracranial hemorrhage	3%
• Infection	2%
• Non-specific	19%
• Normal	13%

1. Evidence-based decision-making algorithm for diagnosing cerebral palsy early.

FIGURE 7-3 Early diagnosis algorithm for diagnosing cerebral palsy. (Reproduced with permission from Novak I. Evidence-based diagnosis, health care, and rehabilitation for children with cerebral palsy. *J Child Neurol.* 2014;29[8]:1141-1156.)

- **Muscular strength**

The ability to produce sufficient force to create a strong and controlled muscular contraction is decreased in individuals with CP and is well documented in the literature.[41,43,50,55,56] Depending on the child's age or their ability to follow multiple-step commands, testing muscular strength and performance in young children can be challenging. Traditional manual muscle testing (MMT), isometric muscle strength testing using a handheld dynamometry,[57] and isokinetic muscle testing using an isokinetic dynamometer can be used in determining muscular strength and performance in children with CP. Movement analysis in antigravity

TABLE 7-4 • Modified Ashworth Scale[15]
0 No increase in muscle tone
1 Slight increase in muscle tone, manifested by a catch and release or by minimal resistance at the end of the range of motion when the affected part(s) is (are) moved in flexion or extension
1+ Slight increase in muscle tone, manifested by a catch followed by minimal resistance through the remainder of the range of motion but the affected part(s) is (are) easily moved
2 More marked increase in muscle tone through most of the range of movement, but the affected part(s) is (are) easily moved
3 Considerable increases in muscle tone; passive movement difficult
4 Affected part(s) is (are) rigid in flexion or extension

TABLE 7-5 • Tardieu Scale[56]	
Grading is always performed at the same time of the day, in a constant position of the body for a given limb. Other joints, particularly the neck, must also remain in a constant position throughout the test and between tests. For each muscle group, reaction to stretch is rated at a specified stretch velocity with 2 parameters, X and Y.	
Velocity of stretch	V1: As slow as possible (minimizing stretch reflex) V2: Speed of the limb segment falling under gravity V3: As fast as possible (faster than the rate of the natural drop of the limb segment under gravity) V1 is used to measure the passive range of motion (PROM). V2 or V3 is used to rate spasticity.
Quality of muscle reaction (X)	0: No resistance throughout the course of the passive movement 1: Slight resistance throughout the course of the passive movement, with no clear catch at a precise angle 2: Clear catch at a precise angle, interrupting the passive movement, followed by release 3: Fatigable clonus (<10 seconds when maintaining pressure) occurring at a precise angle 4: Infatigable clonus (>10 seconds when maintaining pressure) occurring at a precise angle
Angle of muscle reaction (Y)	Measured relative to the position of minimal stretch of the muscle (corresponding to angle 0) for all joints except the hip, where it is relative to the resting anatomic position

Reproduced with permission from Fosang AL, Galea MP, McCoy AT, Reddihough DS, Story I. Measures of muscle and joint performance in the lower limb of children with cerebral palsy. Developmental Medicine & Child Neurology. 2003;45(10):664-670.

positions can be used to describe activities where decreased muscular strength may present as an impairment; for example, when a child performs an abdominal crunch or "sit-up," is a head lag present? When other causes have been ruled out, the head lag may be due to poor strength of the sternocleidomastoids (<3 on a traditional MMT).

- Functional tests, such as the 30-Second Sit-to-Stand Test (30sSTST), can also be used in determining strength and physical performance. The 30sSTST is a measurement of functional lower limb muscle strength and performance with a high test-retest reliability. 30sSTST measures the number of repetitions for a sit-to-stand task within a 30-second period. The individual should sit on a chair without a backrest or armrest with feet flat on the ground and hips and knees flexed at 90 and 105 degrees, respectively, to the best of their abilities. In addition, the individual may use an assistive device if necessary. The individual is instructed to repetitively move from the sitting to standing position as many times as they can within a 30-second period without using arms for support.[58]
- **Range of motion**
  - Passive range of motion (PROM) and active range of motion (AROM) can be measured using a goniometer.[49] The PT can also compare the angle of full slow (V1) passive range of movement (R2) and the angle of resistance first felt during fast (V3) passive movements (R1) to identify the physiologic and neurologic mechanisms affecting resistance to passive movements, respectively.[55]
- **Exercise capacity**
  - 6-Minute Walk Test (6MWT) can be used to quantify functional exercise capacity. The individual walks at a self-selected comfortable velocity and is instructed to cover as much ground as possible in 6 minutes. The distance walked (6-minute walk distance) is recorded. The individual can use a walking assistive device and is allowed to rest, if necessary, during the walking session.[59]
  - 10-Meter Shuttle Run Tests (SRT-I and SRT-II). The SRT-I was developed for children at GMFCS level I, and the SRT-II was developed for children at GMFCS level II. The SRT-I starts at 5 km/h, and the SRT II starts

at 2 km/h. The SRT measures aerobic power in children with CP. The SRT requires children to walk or run between 2 markers delineating the respective course of 10 m, at a set incremental speed determined by a prerecorded signal, which can be played on an electronic device. As the test proceeds, the interval between each successive beep reduces, forcing the child to increase speed over the course of the test, until it is impossible to keep in sync with the recording.[60]

- **Perceived exertion**
  - Children's OMNI Scale of Perceived Exertion (OMNI Scale) can be used to determine a child's perceived exertion during activities, such as walking and running. The OMNI Scale has a developmentally indexed category format that contains both pictorial and verbal descriptors positioned along a comparatively narrow numerical response range of 0 to 10 perceived exertion (**Figure 7-5**).[61,62]

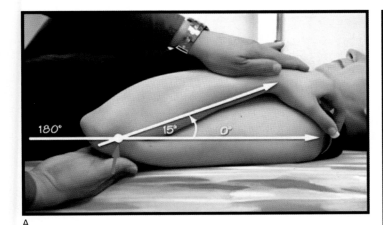

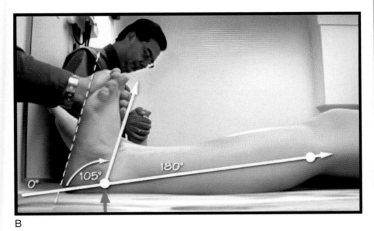

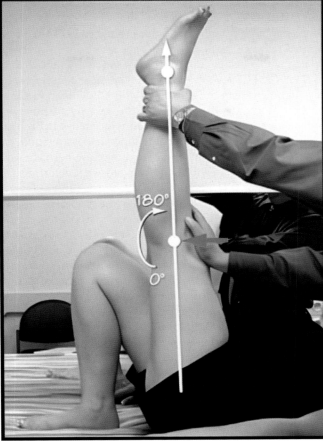

FIGURE 7-4 Angles used in the Tardieu Scale for the elbow flexors (A), ankle plantar flexors (B), and knee flexors (C). Zero is the theoretical position of minimal stretch of the muscle to be assessed. (Reproduced from Gracies J-M, Burke K, Clegg NJ, et al. Reliability of the Tardieu Scale for assessing spasticity in children with cerebral palsy. *Arch Phys Med Rehabil.* 2010;91[3]:421-428. doi:10.1016/j.apmr.2009.11.017.)

PAIN

Pain in children with CP is common, and if it persists greater than 3 months and takes a longer than expected time to heal, it is defined as *chronic pain*. Chronic pain in individuals with CP and other conditions can be caused by gastrointestinal dysfunctions, musculoskeletal complications, therapeutic procedures, and other universal causes including trauma, infection, and common childhood pain. Chronic pain can have significant consequences, leading to activity limitations and participation restrictions, and therefore should be identified and measured. The following are tools that can be used to assess chronic pain accurately in individuals with CP with or without intellectual disabilities.[63]

- Body Diagram
- Bath Adolescent Pain Questionnaire (BAPQ)
- Child Activity Limitations Interview (CALI)
- Wong-Baker Faces Pain Rating Scale Noncommunicating Children's Pain Checklist–Revised (NCCPC-R)
- Pediatric Pain Interference Scale (PPIS)
- Pediatric Pain Questionnaire (PPQ)
- Pediatric Pain Profile (PPP)

SPINAL ALIGNMENT

Children with severe CP often present with more musculoskeletal problems than those with mild CP, and their musculoskeletal structures often deteriorate with advancing age.

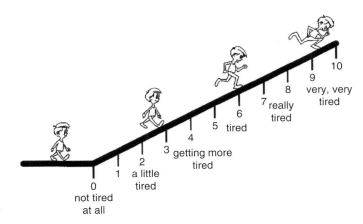

FIGURE 7-5 Children's OMNI Scale of perceived exertion for walking/running. (Reproduced with permission from Robertson RJ, Goss FL, Boer NF, et al. Children's OMNI Scale of perceived exertion: mixed gender and race validation. *Med Sci Sports Exerc.* 2000;32(2):452-458.)

Tightness of spastic muscles, joint contractures, and spinal malalignment are common and significant CP-related problems in children. In addition, spinal malalignment and limited range of motion (ROM) have also been strongly correlated with a decline in gross motor function and correlated to their GMFCS level.[64] Scoliosis is the most common spinal malalignment seen in individuals with CP, with an incidence of 25% or greater depending on the severity of functional independence.[65,66] Scoliosis has been associated with problems in sitting, pressure ulcers, cardiopulmonary dysfunction, gastrointestinal dysfunction, and pain. It has also been shown to be associated with pelvic obliquity, windswept deformity, and hip dislocation.[67] The presence of a scoliosis can be classified according to the criteria defined by the Scoliosis Research Society and a Cobb angle of greater than 10 degrees, and its severity is established using the Cobb angle, with a severe curve being greater than 40 degrees. If the Cobb angle is greater than 40 degrees, it may warrant the need for surgical intervention.[64] Therefore, it is important to identify, assess, and monitor the presence of a progressive scoliosis early as the result of spinal surgery is related to the curve magnitude. The CPUP (Uppföljningsprogram för personer med cerebral pares) has been a Swedish CP surveillance program for over 2 decades. The CPUP classification of scoliosis is as follows:[68]

- No scoliosis
- Mild scoliosis: Discreet curve visible only on thorough examination in forward bending
- Moderate scoliosis: Obvious curve in both upright and forward bending
- Severe scoliosis: Pronounced curve preventing upright position without external support

The following describes physical therapy assessments for the presence and monitoring of scoliosis.

- Forward bend test: A commonly used screening tool for *adolescent idiopathic scoliosis* is the forward bending test that measures asymmetrical rib prominence.
- Scoliometer reliably measures the angle of trunk rotation due to rib prominence or "rib hump," and it is a commonly used tool to screen for *adolescent idiopathic scoliosis*.[69] The cutoff value that warrants a radiographic referral in adolescent idiopathic scoliosis varies but 7 degrees or greater has been suggested (**Figure 7-6**).
- These 2 measures to assess and monitor scoliosis progression in idiopathic scoliosis have also been found to have excellent interrater reliability in children with CP.[68] In addition, a scoliometer can be used in individuals who are unable to stand, and therefore, the scoliosis is measured when the individual is seated and bends forward.
- In sitting position, a scoliometer can be placed in forward bending at the top of the thoracic spine, with the 0 (zero) mark over the spinous process, and slowly moved down the spine noting the highest degree of truncal rotation. A higher degree of truncal rotation indicates worse inclination.[68]
- The Spinal Alignment and Range of Motion Measure (SAROMM) allows clinicians to determine whether a

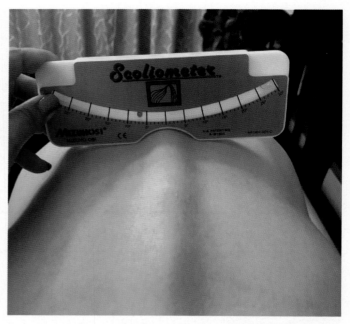

FIGURE 7-6 **Scoliometer reading: angle of trunk rotation of 7 degrees.**

change in SAROMM score represents a clinically meaningful change. The SAROMM has fair to good intrarater and interrater reliability and construct validity and is a discriminative tool for children and adolescents with CP aged 2 to 18 years. SAROMM may be simpler to apply and a more meaningful indicator of whether or not a child has normal alignment and ROM.[70]

Examination: Activity Limitations

Neuromotor impairments in body structure and function commonly seen in individuals with CP may lead to limitations in their ability to perform activities in the same manner as their aged-match peers. As previously described, the GMFM can be used to measure changes in gross motor function over time or as a result of interventions. The following are examples of selected tests and measures that can address activity limitations in individuals with CP, such as walking ability, reaching, and ascending/descending stairs.

- The 10-Meter Walk Test (10mWT) has a high test-retest reliability and is correlated with gross motor functions for individuals with CP. The test is conducted on a 14-m walkway that includes 2 m at the start and end points to allow for acceleration and deceleration. Before the test, the examiner instructs the individual to walk at their usual speed. The time it takes to walk the 10-m path is recorded.[58,71]
- The Timed Up and Go Test (TUGT) and the Modified Timed Up and Go (TUG) are measures used to assess functional dynamic balance that have good test-retest reliability. They are quick and practical methods of testing balance in basic mobility maneuvers. The TUGT is based on a functional task of rising from a height-adjustable chair or bench without backrest or armrests, walking 3 m, turning, and returning to the chair. The individual should be seated with feet flat on the floor in such a way that hip and knee remain in 90 degrees of flexion to the best of their abilities. Patients

can use orthotics or their assistive device to complete the activity. In the Modified TUG, a target is placed at the end of the 3 m, and the individual is asked to touch the target (eg, a star on the wall) and return to the chair or bench. The Modified TUG version has been found to have *less abstract instruction,* which can limit a child's performance. The time in seconds required to complete the task is recorded. The time in seconds is recorded from the "go" until the individual sits down in the chair.[58,72]

- The Functional Reach Test (FRT) is a clinical measure of balance that has excellent reliability. FRT measures the distance between the length of the flexed shoulder to 90 degrees and a maximal forward reach in the standing position (using the third metacarpal head as the measuring landmark of the distanced reached). The individual is instructed to stand close to a wall, but not touching the wall, with the dominant side arm position set at the zero mark of the stick, which is placed on a measuring stick against the wall at the height of the individuals' acromion. The individual is asked to reach as far as they can forward without taking a step.[58]

- The Timed Stair Test measures the ability to walk up and down stairs, a task that is commonly difficult for individuals with CP. The Timed Stair Test is based on items 84 and 87 of the GMFM. The test requires participants to walk up and down 3 steps of standard size (17.5 cm) as quickly as possible, using rails if required. The time taken to complete the task is measured using a stopwatch. The Timed Stair Test is a simple measure of functional mobility that can be easily completed in a variety of settings and can be used for testing and potentially documenting improvement of children with CP in their functional mobility and balance abilities.[57]

- Walking ability: Gait analysis using observational or video instrumented assessments is recommended to identify abnormal movement patterns and variations of gait kinematics and walking ability.[73] Key gait parameters/characteristics, views assessed, and definitions are described in **Table 7-6**.

The most common gait deviation for children with CP is stiff knee in swing, followed by crouched gait, excessive hip flexion, in-toeing, and equinovarus.[74] These gait deviations increase the energy cost of walking, which is twice that of typically developing children.[73] Within the school setting, it is reported that walking is the largest hindrance in children with CP, followed by vision, dexterity, and speech impairments.[75]

Among children with CP, it has been reported that 58.2% to 58.9% of children walk independently, 7.8% to 11.3% use a handheld assistive device, and 30.6% to 33.3% have limited or no walking. It has also been reported that nearly all children with unilateral spastic CP (96.6%) walk independently compared with less than half of those with spastic CP (45.5%).[76,77]

- The Functional Mobility Scale (FMS) (version 2) has been constructed to classify functional mobility in children 4 to 18 years, taking into account a range of assistive devices a child might use over 3 distances: 5 m (in and around the home), 50 m (in and around school/preschool), and 500 m (in the community). Further information about the FMS and the instrument can be found at the following website: https://www.sralab.org/rehabilitation-measures/functional-mobility-scale.[78,79]

Participation Restrictions

The ICF defines participation as involvement in life situations, and it is captured across 9 domains including self-care, interpersonal relationships, schooling, and employment. Participation

TABLE 7-6 • Gait Parameters and Characteristics

Gait Characteristic	View	Operational Definition
Genu recurvatum (%)	Lateral	The percentage of steps in which >0 degrees of knee extension was observed during stance phase.
Heel strike (%)	Lateral	The percentage of steps in which initial contact was made with only the posterior one-third of the foot.
Hip extension (degrees)	Lateral	The maximum angle of hip extension from neutral achieved in stance phase of gait. The axis is placed at the greater trochanter, whereas the proximal vector is placed along the midaxillary line of the trunk, and the distal vector is placed in line with lateral midline of the femur, using the femoral condyle as a reference point.
Stiff knee in swing (%)	Lateral	The percentage of steps taken in which a progression from knee flexion to extension is observed during the swing phase of gait.
Neutral foot placement (%)	Frontal	Percentage of steps in which the plantar surface of the first digit and metatarsal phalangeal joint make contact with the ground during midstance phase of gait.
Scissoring (%)	Frontal	The percentage of steps in which the stance foot is visually blocked by the swing foot from anterior to posterior view at any point within the gait cycle.
Toe-in (%)	Frontal	The percentage of steps in which the lateral calcaneus is visible in the stance phase.
Mean step length (cm)	Marker on floor	Distance from heel strike contact point to the next heel strike contact point on the ipsilateral leg. Contact points are marked on walking surface then measured in centimeters. A mean is calculated from a minimum of 10 steps.
Mean gait velocity	Lateral	The time (in seconds) to ambulate 10 m with the walker. A mean of 3 trials in which the subject ambulated at least 10 m without stopping is calculated per rater. The mean of the 2 raters is then calculated.

Refer to https://www.cpqcc.org/sites/default/files/GMFCS-ER.pdf. Adapted from Fergus A. A novel mobility device to improve walking for a child with cerebral palsy. Pediatr Phys Ther. 2017;29(4):E1-E7.

is consistently reduced in children with CP compared with the general population and in proportion to the severity and number of impairments.[18] Furthermore, the participation interactions are influenced by the context in which an individual lives, and the ICF recognizes 2 further constructs: environmental and personal factors. It is important to address participation restrictions as part of the physical therapy examination of individuals with CP.

- The Children's Participation and Enjoyment (CAPE) and the Preferences for Activities of Children (PAC) are companion self-report or interview assisted measures of children's participation in recreation and leisure activities outside of school activities. The CAPE is a 55-item questionnaire designed to examine how children and young adults (ages 6 -21y) participate in everyday activities outside of the school setting. It provides information related to; diversity (number of activities done), intensity (frequency of participation measured as a function of the number of possible activities within a category), enjoyment of activities and additional information about the context in which they participate in these activities. The PAC provides the individuals' preferences for involvement in each activity. The authors report there is a relationship between gross motor capacity and daily-life mobility in children with CP, and using the user-friendly CAPE and PAC allows for a holistic understanding of their participation patterns.[80]
- Assessment of Life Habits (LIFE-H) for children: The LIFE-H for children, with versions for parental report of children age 0 to 4 years and 5 to 13 years, was designed and validated to assess the social participation of children with disabilities.[80]

For an additional list of commonly used assessments to address participation restrictions, refer to Chapter 3.

Environmental Construct

Environmental factors such as physical barriers, attitudes, or social policies can act as either supports or barriers to activity and participation for disabled children. Therefore, it necessary to understand and measure these environmental factors that influence activity and participation for children with disabilities.

The 10-item Craig Hospital Inventory of Environmental Factors (CHIEF) for Children–Parent Version is an acceptable, easy-to-complete, and reliable measure of perceived environmental barriers for disabled children 2 to 12 years of age.[81]

Personal Factors

Personal factors such as age, gender, values, and lifestyle can influence an individual with a disability in participating with their peers. Therefore, it is necessary to address subjective dimensions such as well-being and quality of life (QOL).[82] QOL is also defined as a person's feelings of well-being across many domains, including physical, social, emotional, and spiritual aspects of life.[83]

The Pediatric Quality of Life Inventory (PedsQL), version 3.0, Cerebral Palsy Module is used to measure specific health-related QOL for individuals with CP. PedsQL can discriminate QOL between typically developing children and children with CP age 2 to 18 years.[82]

TABLE 7-7 • Summary of Examination
Examination

• Musculoskeletal assessment
  ◦ Range of motion (ROM) limitations (contracture)
  ◦ Muscle weakness
  ◦ Posture
  ◦ Alignment
    • Between segments and with reference to gravity

• Neuromuscular assessment
  ◦ Muscle tone
  ◦ Muscle extensibility
  ◦ Loss of selective motor control
  ◦ Pain
  ◦ Balance and postural control
  ◦ Alignment
    • Between segments and with reference to gravity

• Gait assessment
  ◦ Know the walking characteristics that are age appropriate for children
  ◦ Observational and instrumented gait analyses
    • Visual description and/or other noninstrumented measure
    • Instrumented measure
    • Kinematics or joint rotations
    • Kinetics or forces
    • Muscle activation (electromyography confirms underlying muscular causes—activation and sequence of activation)
• Measure of functional walking ability
• Measure of aerobic capacity and energy expenditure

• Functional skills assessment
• Orthoses assessment and prescription
• Adaptive equipment, positioning equipment, and assistive devices

In summary, a detailed examination needs to be considered when examining a child or adolescent with CP (**Table 7-7**). This includes assessments of orthoses, adaptive equipment, and assistive devices. Refer to those specific chapters for additional information.

■ INTERVENTIONS

A team approach in a format of multidisciplinary, interdisciplinary, or transdisciplinary care is considered best practice when working with children with complex needs. Extra attention should be focused on times of transition with early forward planning being essential for positive outcomes across various practice settings. Refer to Chapter 22 for further information regarding life span transition.

Physical therapy interventions should be aimed at addressing limitations identified and can strengthen muscles, improve coordination, improve balance, and increase flexibility. Stretching, exercises, adaptive equipment, and other activities are used in physical therapy to achieve these goals and give children greater independence, physical function, and ultimately more mobility. Bailes et al[84] support the incorporation of frequently used evidence-based interventions of neuromuscular motor control, functional strengthening, caregiver education, ankle-foot orthoses, treadmill training, and fit of adaptive equipment. These and other selected physical interventions will be described.

CAREGIVER EDUCATION

PTs must educate the child's primary caregiver on various components involved with medical and rehabilitative care of the child. Caregivers can be educated via home exercise programs, neuromuscular rehabilitation evidence-based practice rationale, and home safety awareness. In addition, education of other related services, such as occupational therapy, speech therapy, or other health care services, should be provided.[85]

STRETCHING

Although there is conflicting evidence regarding stretching techniques for children with CP, the 3 main stretching interventions include casting and serial casting (casts that are changed at regular intervals), application of orthoses or a specific positioning program, and a manual stretch program.[86]

- **Casting:** Casting is indicated when soft tissue contracture is interfering with function or causing potential biomechanical misalignment. It only provides a short-term stretch and is usually required to be repeated at regular intervals and has been shown to be effective following botulinum toxin injections. Casting imposes a continuous stretch on a group of muscles, leading to an increase in muscle fiber length due to an increase in the number of sarcomeres. However, a cast should never be left on for more than 5 to 7 days as there is evidence to support the loss of sarcomeres if a joint is left immobilized in a cast for too long and longer casting periods do not necessarily translate to greater gains in ROM.[87] Casting is not indicated for long-term contractures or when there are bony changes at a joint.
- **Orthoses and splinting:** The main purposes of orthoses or splints are to maintain ROM and assist with function. An orthosis is usually applied at the tolerable end of joint range. Functional orthoses generally position joints in a biomechanically advantageous position to either enable or improve function. Examples may include ankle-foot orthoses (AFOs; a variety of AFOs are available with varying purposes), wrist extension orthoses, and wrist and thumb orthoses. Positional orthoses aim to maintain corrected anatomic alignment of the joint and maintain ROM around that joint. Some AFOs have been shown to improve postural stability and decrease loss of balance.[88] Refer to Chapter 19 for additional information.
- **Manual stretching:** Manual stretch can be self-administered or applied manually by therapists.[89] It involves the mechanical elongation of soft tissues for varying periods of time. The evidence is not consistent regarding the parameters for stretching intervention and varies considerably. Some evidence has demonstrated its effectiveness on PROM and spasticity.[41] The number of repetitions for passive stretching ranged from 1 to 10 (median, 4), and the length of time to hold the stretch varied from 15 to 90 seconds (median, 30 seconds). Parameters for active stretching ranged from 1 to 10 repetitions (median, 4) and 15 to 90 seconds duration (median, 21 seconds).[90]

EXERCISE

Children diagnosed with CP demonstrate reduced physical activity and increased sedentary behavior compared to sex-matched controls without CP. Frequency, intensity, duration, and type of physical activity and exercise for individuals with CP recommendations include a frequency of 5 days/week of moderate exercise or 3 days/week of vigorous exercise for 20 to 60 minutes of continuous and rhythmic exercises that involve major muscle groups. It is suggested that exercise prescription should include an intensity between 60% and 95% of peak heart rate or between 40% and 80% of the heart rate reserve. A warm-up and cool-down should be added to reduce musculoskeletal injury. For individuals with CP who are very deconditioned, it is recommended to start with 1 to 2 sessions per week and progress gradually as adaptations occur. Clinicians must become aware of the importance of exercise among high-risk populations, such as CP, and also use the best evidenced-based practice in designing an individualized exercise program.[91,92]

- **Neuromuscular Motor Control:** Neuromuscular electrical stimulation (NMES) is electrical stimulation to specific muscles either in a stationary position or during a specific task (functional electrical stimulation) to increase strength and function.[93] Evidence has shown that NMES can increase muscle fiber diameter, muscle size, and muscle strength in children with CP.[94] According to Yan and Vasser,[94] "NMES also reduces spasticity by decreasing stretch reflex sensitivity and can indirectly improve selective motor control by applying it during specific movement phases such as wrist extension during reach and grasp when the elbow is flexed, or during knee extension at the end of the swing phase of gait when the hip is flexed."
- **Functional strengthening:** Task-specific strengthening exercises and activities with appropriate hand placement to help facilitate movement have been shown to improve overall motor control, mobility, and independence of the child.[84]

MEDICAL AND SURGICAL INTERVENTIONS

Botulinum Toxin Type A

Botulinum toxin type A (BTX-A) is a neurotoxin that is injected into the muscle and affects the neuromuscular synapses by inhibiting the release of acetylcholine. This causes spasticity reduction in a safe and selective way. Studies have demonstrated the benefits of intramuscular BTX-A injections for the management of spasticity in children with CP. The effect, however, is reversible, and the period of clinically useful relaxation is usually 12 to 16 weeks. During the effective period, positive effects have been noted by improved ROM, spasticity reduction, pain reduction, and improved gait pattern in individuals with CP. These positive effects translate to improvements in nursing care and sitting and walking abilities. It is suggested that the maximum dosage delivered is 23 MU/kg bodyweight, limited to no more than 400 units per limb, within an overall maximum dose of 1200 MU per session. Sessions can include multilevel treatments. Additionally, the total dosage is defined by standardized dosages per muscle group. The dose injected in one muscle is dependent on the muscle volume, the amount of spasticity, and the degree of involvement of the muscle in the pathologic gait pattern. Ultimately, the duration of the effect of a BTX-A treatment is mainly determined by the pre- and postinjection care, consisting of intensive physical therapy, orthotic management, and casting.[94,95]

Selective Dorsal Rhizotomy

Selective dorsal rhizotomy (SDR) is a neurosurgical procedure aimed at reducing spasticity and has been performed mainly in children diagnosed with bilateral spastic CP. The most common area for the operation is at the lumbosacral level to reduce spasticity in the lower limbs and includes surgical interruption of the afferent input of the monosynaptic stretch reflex. During the SDR procedure, the dorsal root is divided into separate rootlets and only a portion of these are transected, leaving the others intact, thereby preserving certain sensory and sphincter function. SDR is an irreversible procedure that can also negatively influence motor function; therefore, strict patient selection criteria are essential. It has been noted that the SDR-related reduction in spasticity may reveal underlying muscle weakness, and this might lead to a worsening gait performance in patients lacking sufficient antigravity strength.

After an SDR procedure, it is recommended that physical therapy sessions start immediately. During the first few days postoperatively, therapy consists of PROM exercises of the lower limb joints and strengthening of the hip abductors and extensors, knee extensors, and ankle dorsiflexors. Progression to standing, weight bearing, and gait training standing (if possible) with a rigid AFO in 0 degrees of dorsiflexion with a floor reaction orthosis to stimulate knee extension during walking is encouraged. An intensive therapy frequency is recommended with an emphasis on strength training and practicing normal patterns of movement, standing, and walking.[96,97]

Additional Interventions

- **Functional taping:** This method supports joint function by exerting an effect on muscle function, improving proprioception by normalization of muscle tone, correction of inappropriate position, and stimulating effect on skin receptors.[98]
- **Equine-assisted therapy and hippotherapy:** Equine-assisted therapy uses a horse's movement, which has an individual and variable gait, tempo, rhythm, repetition, and cadence. Improvements in trunk control and balance have been noted in children with CP due to the physical adjustments to maintain proper alignment on the horse. Current evidence supports equine-assisted therapies, especially hippotherapy, and therapeutic horse riding as having positive effects on balance and gross motor function in children with CP, although current literature and evidence are limited.[86] Equine-assisted therapies should be considered as therapeutic tools for children initiating ambulation or to promote stability during gait.[99]
- **Treadmill training:** Treadmill training, even though the research varies, has been shown to be a common intervention to promote gait in children with CP. Findings indicate that treadmill intervention may increase motor skill attainment in children with CP.[100]
- **Adaptive equipment:** Adaptive equipment options include orthoses; gait assistive devices; and positioning equipment for standing, sitting, feeding, and activities of daily living. The specific needs of the child and caregiver must be considered. **Figures 7-7** to **7-12** depict evidence-based and promising interventions for individuals with CP by topography.[43]

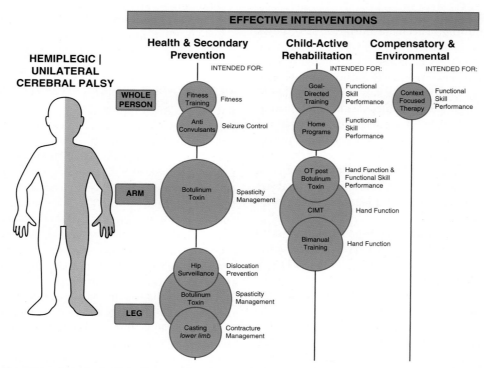

FIGURE 7-7 Hemiplegic/unilateral cerebral palsy effective interventions. (Novak I, Evidence-Based Diagnosis, Health Care, and Rehabilitation for Children With Cerebral Palsy. (29(8):1141-1156, Copyright © 2014 by SAGE publication). Reprinted by permission of SAGE publications.)

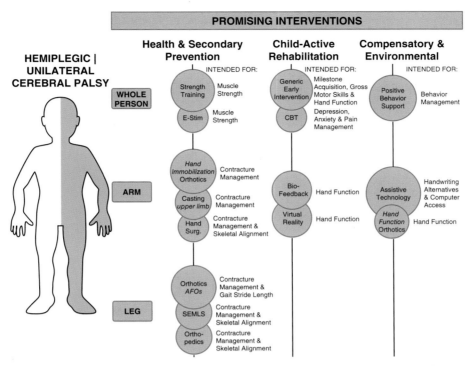

FIGURE 7-8 Hemiplegic/unilateral cerebral palsy promising interventions. (Novak I, Evidence-Based Diagnosis, Health Care, and Rehabilitation for Children With Cerebral Palsy. (29(8):1141-1156, Copyright © 2014 by SAGE publication). Reprinted by permission of SAGE publications.)

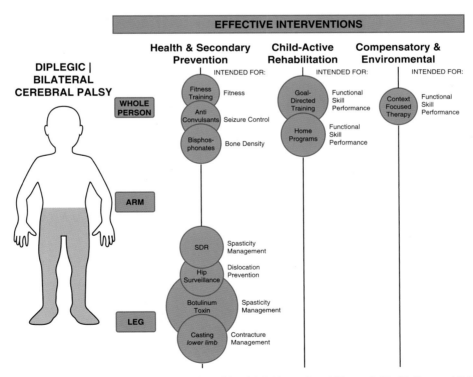

FIGURE 7-9 Diplegic/bilateral cerebral palsy effective interventions. (Novak I, Evidence-Based Diagnosis, Health Care, and Rehabilitation for Children With Cerebral Palsy. (29(8):1141-1156, Copyright © 2014 by SAGE publication). Reprinted by permission of SAGE publications.)

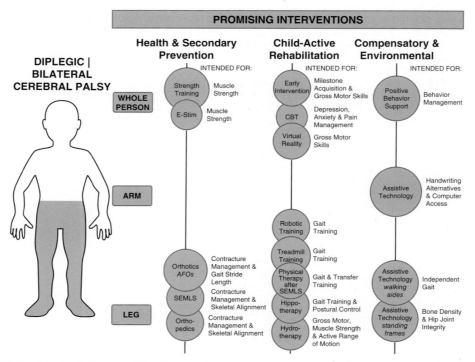

FIGURE 7-10 Diplegic/bilateral cerebral palsy promising interventions. (Novak I, Evidence-Based Diagnosis, Health Care, and Rehabilitation for Children With Cerebral Palsy. (29(8):1141-1156, Copyright © 2014 by SAGE publication). Reprinted by permission of SAGE publications.)

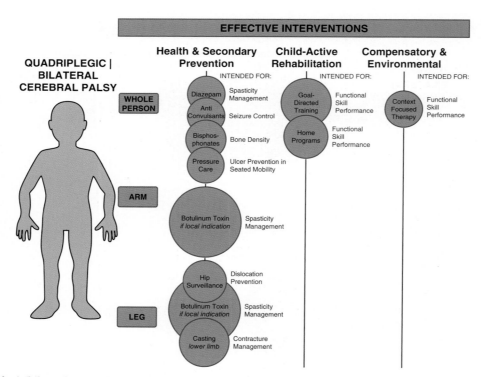

FIGURE 7-11 Quadriplegic/bilateral cerebral palsy effective interventions. (Novak I, Evidence-Based Diagnosis, Health Care, and Rehabilitation for Children With Cerebral Palsy. (29(8):1141-1156, Copyright © 2014 by SAGE publication). Reprinted by permission of SAGE publications.)

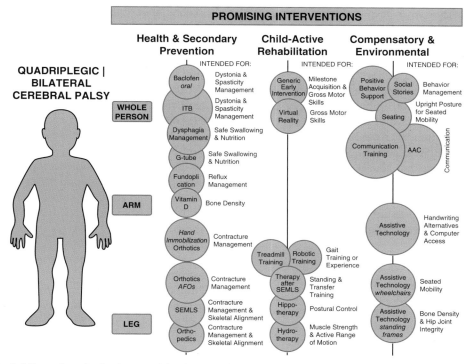

FIGURE 7-12 **Quadriplegic/bilateral cerebral palsy promising interventions.** (Novak I, Evidence-Based Diagnosis, Health Care, and Rehabilitation for Children With Cerebral Palsy. (29(8):1141-1156, Copyright © 2014 by SAGE publication). Reprinted by permission of SAGE publications.)

■ GOALS

Goals should be developed to promote independence, with safety as a priority. Goals for the *pediatric* patient will require ongoing revisions throughout various treatment sessions and may need to be attained over the course of 6 months to a year. Developing clear, measurable, and realistic goals is necessary for the patient's success and compliance for caregivers. Assessing the quality of movement throughout treatment sessions is crucial to limit further musculoskeletal impairments and/or dysfunction. Developing goals for patients with CP will require input from various sources. Input from parents, caregivers, and the child will provide the priority needs for the child overall. One framework that can be used to develop goals is Goal Attainment Scaling (GAS).

GAS can be used across multiple practice settings, GMFCS levels, and age ranges. GAS is an individualized criterion-referenced approach to documenting changes over time. It is a 5-point goal scale that is developed via interview with the client, family, and caregivers. Graded levels of possible goal attainment with descriptions of anticipated outcome are described for each goal. Goals are scaled from least favorable to most favorable outcome, with an expected outcome level in the middle. GAS has been found to be useful for progress monitoring and documentation of outcomes.[101,102]

If the patient achieves a better-than-expected outcome, this is scored at +1 (somewhat better) or +2 (much better). If the patient achieves the expected level, this is scored at 0. If the patient achieves a worse-than-expected outcome, this is scored at −1 (somewhat worse) or −2 (much worse). For more information regarding the GAS, see the following website: https://www.sralab.org/rehabilitation-measures/goal-attainment-scale.[103]

■ CONCLUSION

In summary, an accurate and thorough physical therapy examination is necessary to ensure the selection and provision of treatment interventions that are evidenced-based tools and techniques in order to improve overall function, promote independent mobility, and provide patient and caregiver education for individuals with CP. In a study by Rozkalne and Bertule,[104] it was shown that determining accurate prognosis among children with CP is difficult and individual patient variables must be taken into consideration. Following the ICF for Children and Youth (ICF-CY) can help guide and develop appropriate goals, outcome measures, and effectiveness of treatment intervention. The ICF-CY describes a conceptual framework to report a variety of health information (diagnosis and functioning) and thereby delivers a common language and terminology to describe the child's problems in relation to functions and anatomic properties, activity limitations, and participation restrictions.[41]

Case 1

Background Information/Past Medical History

Andrea is 3 years and 2 months old and was diagnosed with spastic diplegic CP, GMFCS level III. She has been referred for an outpatient physical therapy evaluation. Concerns and goals for therapy expressed by her parents are to improve Andrea's ability to walk and get around independently.

Andrea's parents report she was diagnosed with CP at the age of 1, after the pediatrician was concerned that she was still unable to sit independently or transition between positions independently. Her parents report that her medical history includes having had a seizure when she was 3 months old. Since then, she has been on a daily dose of carbamazepine with no seizures reported within the past year. No additional medications or allergies are reported. Parents also report that Andrea only eats pureed thickened foods and milk with cereal. She requires assistance with dressing and toileting. She sleeps well at night. As per Andrea's parents, she began ambulating for 5 to 10 feet about 1 year ago, at the age of 2, with 2 hands held.

Andrea recently started attending a pre-K program at her local public school and has an Individualized Education Plan (IEP) for accommodations and personalized education goals. Main gross motor concerns identified by the IEP team are access to the school environment safely; she exhibits loss of balance and decreased safety awareness. In addition, Andrea presents with limited expressive and receptive language and mild cognitive involvement.

Examination
Observation/Systems Review
Andrea is in the 25% percentile for both weight and height for her age. She is able to understand simple commands and expresses herself with sounds and limited gestures. Andrea has no reported cardiac and gastrointestinal concerns identified. Integumentary system is intact.

Andrea is motivated to play and explore her environment. Andrea did not have any issues working with the therapist and transitioning between therapist-led activities. Andrea does exhibit impulsive behaviors and decreased safety awareness negotiating the environment.

Outcome Measures
- Results from the GMFM-66: total score of 44
- FMS: rating 1 for 5 m

Neuromuscular/Gross Motor
Upon assessment, the following impairments are present:
- Tone
  - Spasticity is noted in bilateral lower extremities throughout the available ROM in hip flexors (MAS = 1 bilaterally) and knee flexors (MAS 1+ bilaterally).
  - Mild low tone throughout trunk musculature is noted.
- ROM
  - Passive hip extension of 0 degrees noted bilaterally
  - Biomechanical assessment reveals internal and external rotation within normal limits of bother lower extremities
  - Hamstring length
    - Left: R1 = 35 degrees, R2 = 52 degrees
    - Right: R1 = 45 degrees, R2 = 56 degrees
  - Minus 8 degrees of active knee extension on left
  - Minus 5 degrees of active knee extension on right
  - Ankle active plantar flexion (PF) 50 degrees bilaterally
  - Ankle passive dorsiflexion (DF) approximately 5 degrees bilaterally
  - No notable limitations in AROM within bilateral upper extremities
  - Limited active trunk rotation noted during sitting and walking activities
- Posture/spinal alignment
  - Neck hyperextension noted when working in prone and shoulder elevation when prone on elbows
  - In floor tailor sitting, mild spinal curvature noted with rounded shoulders
  - No evidence of scoliosis noted
- Strength
  - Functional testing shows evidence of decreased strength in trunk musculature (abdominals, trunk extensors, gluteals, hip abductors). She is unable to maintain a chin tuck during pull from supine to sit. She is unable to transition from the floor to standing without upper extremity support or without pulling up on a table. She is able to assume tall kneeling, however, and maintains the position using a wide base of support for support, demonstrating decreased hip abductor strength. She is able to perform sit to stand from a bench with upper extremity support and supervision.
- Sensation
  - No sensation deficits noted to light touch in bilateral lower extremities
  - Proprioception appears to be impaired with decreased awareness of body in space
- Balance
  - She is able to stand unsupported for 40 seconds.
  - She is unable to perform a single leg stance on either lower extremity.
  - Floor sitting dynamic balance is good with wide base of support noted when reaching for an object.
- Reflexes/reactions
  - Andrea presents with obligatory asymmetric tonic neck reflex to the right (tested in quadruped).
  - Associated reactions into flexion synergy of both upper extremities are observed during challenging activities that require extra effort on her part.
  - In supine, a supine tonic labyrinthine reflex with extension bias is noted, although she is able to bring arms down or to midline when instructed.
  - Postural reactions in standing are delayed in all directions, with greatest delay noted when perturbations are given toward the right side. She demonstrates appropriate upper extremity protective reactions forward and sideways when perturbations are provided in tall kneeling. However, she has delayed responses in standing resulting in near falls (needs physical assistance to prevent a fall).
- Gait and endurance
  - Andrea can take approximately 10 steps independently with a high guard posturing of upper extremities.
  - She is able to ambulate for 25 ft with one handheld assistance on level surfaces and requires moderate bilateral handheld assistance when ambulating on uneven surface.
  - She is learning to use a posterior walker but requires moderate assistance for steering and safety.
  - She requires moderate assistance to negotiate stairs; she ascends and descends with nonreciprocal pattern and use of 2 handrails for 3 steps.
  - Hips and knees are flexed during stance phase of gait.
  - She exhibits a wide base of support, lower center of mass, and limited heel strike present (right greater than left).

Her upper extremities are in a high guard position during ambulation on level surfaces.
- Orthotics: She uses bilateral articulated AFOs.
• Equipment
- She has a parent/caregiver-propelled custom stroller for long distances.
- No other equipment is reported.
• Movement system diagnosis[105]
- Fractionated movement deficit
- Decreased force production

Refer to Chapter 4 for more information regarding movement systems.

Additional quality of life measures should be provided to Andrea's parents.

For Andrea, a typical outcome measure will include the GMFM-66. The Rasch model that underlies the GMFM-66 also estimates the difficulty of the items, so that a child's total ability score can be easily related to the probability of attaining common motor milestones. Total possible scores range from 0 to 100.[106,107] Initial scores should be documented and reassessed every 3 months to determine appropriate treatment clinical decision. Refer to **Figure 7-13** for gross motor development curves.

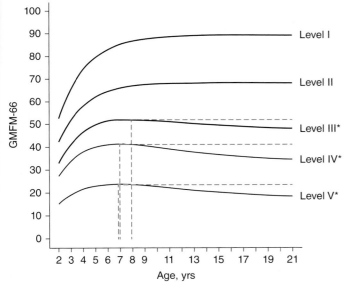

FIGURE 7-13 Gross motor development curves representing average development predicted by the Gross Motor Classification System. The diamonds on the vertical axis identify 4 items of the 66-item Gross Motor Function Measure (GMFM-66) that predict when children are expected to have a 50% chance of completing that item successfully. The GMFM-66 item 21 (diamond A) assesses whether a child can lift and maintain their head in a vertical position with trunk support by a therapist while sitting, item 24 (diamond B) assesses whether a child can maintain a sitting position on a mat without support from their arms for 3 seconds, item 69 (diamond C) measures a child's ability to walk forward 10 steps without support, and item 87 (diamond D) assesses the task of walking down 4 steps by alternating feet with arms free. (Reproduced with permission from Hanna SE et al. Stability and decline in gross motor function among children and youth with cerebral palsy aged 2 to 21 years. *Dev Med Child Neurol.* 2009;51(4):295-302.)

As previously stated, common treatment techniques to address impaired mobility in children with CP include, but are not limited to, stretching, soft tissue mobilization, balance training, strength training, endurance and physical fitness training, and weight-bearing activities. For Andrea, outpatient treatment sessions will be recommended at 3 times per week for 45-minute sessions, taking into consideration age and ability to tolerate sessions. Initial sessions will assess Andrea's compensatory movement patterns and determine priority needs for function and educating caregivers. Incorporating strengthening, balance, and muscle elongation activities within functional play is crucial to promote engagement in sessions and maintain patient-centered treatment.

As treatments continue, sessions should be increasingly challenging, increasing the level of difficulty by advancing through the neurodevelopmental sequence. For instance, as Andrea progresses, stairs and ambulating on grass or unsteady surfaces should be incorporated in treatment sessions to challenge the central nervous system and righting reactions and increase muscle strength and overall endurance. Monitoring of orthotics and other equipment needs should also be considered throughout her episode of care.

Case 2

Background Information/Past Medical History
Ben is an 11-year-1-month-old boy currently enrolled in an inclusive 5th-grade classroom at his local public school with additional support services identified on his Individualized Education Plan (IEP). He presents at GMFCS level IV. He has been referred to physical therapy at an outpatient clinic.

Concerns and goals expressed by his parents are Ben's recent growth spurt, decreased physical activity, and concerns regarding physical readiness and transition to middle school in the upcoming year.

Ben was diagnosed at 2 years of age with spastic quadriplegic cerebral palsy. Ben's mom's pregnancy was unremarkable, and there were no complications during delivery. Ben suffered a seizure at 1 month of age, resulting in placement of a ventriculoperitoneal (VP) shunt and hospitalization for 3 weeks. Since then, he has not had any further episodes of seizures and has never had the shunt revised. Ben has been receiving physical, occupational, and speech therapy for episodes of care since he was 2 months of age. Parents report that Ben has received BTX-A injections in bilateral hamstrings and adductors of lower extremity to minimize tone and promote appropriate graded muscle control.

Examination
Observations/Systems Review
Ben is at the 85% percentile for both weight and height. Integumentary system is intact. Ben is able to communicate verbally, but it is slow and laborious. He exhibits shortness of breath during speaking beyond simple sentences and with excitement, but no immediate cardiac concerns are noted. Ben's parents express concerns with constipation secondary to Ben being sedentary for the majority of the day.

Ben is social and enjoys communicating with peers, teachers, and therapists. He transitions well between activities and is motivated to participate but is easily distracted to avoid higher-level activities. In addition, he gets frustrated when tasks increase in difficulty or require increased musculoskeletal effort.

No prescribed medications or allergies are reported. Ben takes a daily multivitamin.

Outcome Measure
• Result from the GMFM-88: total score of 36%

Neuromuscular/Gross Motor Assessment
Upon assessment, the following impairments are present:
• Tone
  - Spasticity is noted in all 4 extremities: MAS 1+ throughout available upper extremity ROM and MAS 2 throughout available lower extremity ROM.
  - Low tone throughout trunk musculature is noted.
• ROM
  - Limited trunk rotation noted during sitting and static standing activities
  - No notable limitation in passive ROM within bilateral upper extremities
  - Active assistive (AA)/AROM shoulder flexion 120 degrees bilaterally
  - AA/AROM shoulder abduction 110 degrees bilaterally
  - Hamstring length
    • Right R1 = 40 degrees, R2 = 56 degrees
    • Left R1 = 45 degrees; R2 = 58 degrees
  - PROM hip extension = minus 15 degrees bilaterally
  - Active knee extension on right = minus 20 degrees
  - Active knee extension on left = minus 15 degrees
  - PROM ankle DF on right = minus 5 degrees
  - PROM ankle DF on left = to neutral
  - PROM ankle PF bilaterally = 55 degrees
• Strength
  - Functional testing shows evidence of decreased strength in trunk musculature (abdominals, trunk extensors, gluteal and hip abductors).
  - He is able to roll from supine to prone and back, but he is unable to transition into sitting without maximum assistance due to increased muscle tone during active movements.
  - He requires moderate to maximum assistance to transition from sit to stand with bilateral handheld assistance.
  - He is unable to write and exhibits poor finger dexterity but is able to exhibit fair upper extremity gross motor movements.
  - He requires moderate to maximum assistance to work in midline on bilateral upper extremity tasks.
• Posture/spinal alignment
  - In unsupported floor sitting with legs partially extended, Ben presents with rounded back and posterior pelvic tilt.
  - No evidence of structural/fixed scoliosis is noted upon observation.
• Sensation
  - No sensation deficits are noted with light touch.
• Balance
  - He can maintain static standing holding on to a support surface with upper extremities or bilateral hands held; however, full erect upright is not achieved.

  - In addition, tight bilateral hip flexors and bilateral hamstrings are noted in static standing with trunk support at maximum assistance.
  - Sitting static balance with legs in ring sitting is fair.
• Reflexes/reactions
  - Increased startle reflex is noted throughout the day (ie, when an alarm sounds).
  - Positive asymmetric tonic neck reflex, more significant to the right than left, is noted in sitting and during higher-effort, upper-body activities.
  - Delayed postural reactions are noted in all directions when seated.
• Gait and endurance
  - Ben is able to walk with a gait trainer–assisted mobility equipment for about 50 ft without showing signs of fatigue and minimal assistance for steering and lower extremity placement. Scissoring gait is noted throughout the swing phase of gait and requires moderate to maximum assistance to correct as distance increases.
  - OMNI Scale: Ben reported/pointed at the #7 after gait assessment.
  - To get around the school and large public areas, Ben uses a parent/caregiver-propelled custom manual wheelchair to transition between classes and within the lunch area, supermarket, and malls.
• Standing equipment
  - Ben uses a sit-to-stand system during the school day to help promote weight bearing and joint approximation throughout lower extremities, strengthening, trunk support, and overall digestion. The sit-to-stand system provides trunk support, thigh support, and knee blocks to maintain proper alignment.
  - Ben can tolerate approximately 45 minutes of standing in the assistive device. The sit to stand system is elevated to approximately 75 degrees of standing (as measured on the angle dial indicator).
• Orthotics
  - Bilateral total-contact AFOs

Movement System Diagnosis
• Fractionated movement deficit
• Decreased force production
Refer to Chapter 4 for more information regarding movement systems.

Additional quality of life measures should be provided to both Ben and his parents.

Based on the examination, Ben presents with the following impairments: limited independent ambulation secondary to muscle tone deficits, decreased A/PROM in both lower extremities, impaired posture, and decreased strength, balance, and endurance. Based on Ben's age and current functional level, it is recommended that he receive episodes of care that address changes in motor performance, especially during growth spurts. It is crucial that all providers aiding in his care collaborate regularly in order to maximize clinical outcomes. The interdisciplinary team may include the physical therapist, occupation therapist, speech-language pathologist, teacher, neurologist, social worker, and any personnel directly involved in his care.

As previously mentioned, treatment sessions should include various techniques, such as stretching, soft tissue mobilization, balance training, strength training, endurance and physical fitness training, weight bearing, and gait training activities. The sessions should be increasingly challenging and increase in level of difficulty. Taking into consideration Ben's age and priorities, developmental progression of activities does not need to be emphasized; emphasis in sessions should instead be on incorporating various positions (sitting, quadruped, tall or half kneeling, standing) that will help increase stability and strength and improve postural reactions, balance, and overall functional movement.

Nonetheless, it is important to maintain all available ROM and functional movement, while minimizing contractures and pulmonary and gastrointestinal complications while working on improving overall strength, balance, and independence in activities of daily living. Improved performance among adolescents with CP is more likely to occur in specific activities as a result of instruction and practice, accommodations, assistive technology, environmental modifications, or some combination of these factors.[108] Therefore, it is crucial to focus on overall neurodevelopmental improvements and overall independence based on the patient's age and functional priorities.

For PTs, clinical implications are based on the assumption that providing adolescents the opportunity to participate actively in decision-making is important for the planning for the transition into adulthood. Therapists are encouraged to problem solve with adolescents and their families on how adolescents can be more self-sufficient and assume more responsibility despite limitations in physical capability.[108] The PT, in conjunction with an occupational therapist and other related service providers, must consider adaptive equipment, assistive technology, and support personnel in order to promote functional independence. Refer to Chapter 22 regarding life span transition to adulthood,

Case 3

Background Information/Past Medical History

Tyler is a 6-year-6-month-old boy referred for a physical therapy evaluation in his home environment. He is in a regular education kindergarten classroom at a private school. He does not receive any support services while at school. He lives in a 2-story home with both parents and has 2 siblings: a 12-year-old sister and a twin brother.

Tyler was born via cesarean section. No complications are reported by his mother during her pregnancy or after delivery.

His past medical history includes delays in all activities, which were identified early on as an infant, as compared to his twin brother. He was diagnosed with CP with right-side hemiplegia at the age of 2 and has been receiving occupational and physical therapy services since he was an infant.

Tyler has no reported speech, hearing, or vision problems. He presents at GMFCS level I. No medications or allergies are reported. He sleeps well and eats a well-balanced meal.

Concerns expressed by his parents are Tyler's decreased ability to perform activities with good posture and control and decreased ability to participate in activities with the family, such as riding a tricycle/bicycle. In addition, his parents are concerned about his current leg length discrepancy and that he maintains his right heel off the floor during all activities. Goals that Tyler and his parents would like for him to achieve are to improve his age-appropriate overall development (eg, ride a bicycle or scooter during family outings) and to encourage increased use of right extremities to improve his posture and assist with minimizing leg length discrepancy.

Examination

Observations/Systems Review

Tyler is very social, follows multiple-step directions, maintains joint attention, and enjoys dancing and painting.

Integumentary system: blanchable erythema noted on right navicular after AFO removed

Cardiorespiratory system: Resting heart rate = 88 bpm, blood pressure at rest = 90/60 mm Hg

Outcome Measure

GMFM-88 total score = 81.6%

Neuromuscular/Gross Motor Assessment

- Tone
  - Left upper extremity (UE) and lower extremity (LE) present with normal tone
  - Right UE and LE present with spasticity
    - MAS = wrist/finger flexors 2 and 2 elbow flexors
    - MAS = hamstrings 1
    - MAS = gastrocnemius/soleus 2
- ROM
  - Left UE and LE present with full AROM
  - Right UE PROM:
    - Shoulder flexion and abduction have functional full range
      - Scapular winging and abduction noted with movements; decreased scapulohumeral dissociation
    - Elbow flexion = full ROM
    - Elbow extension = minus 5 degrees
    - Full forearm supination and pronation limited
    - Wrist is held in flexion, PROM in extension approximately 45 degrees
    - Fingers flexed and thumb adducted; can open actively but unable to obtain full finger extension
  - Right LE
    - Knee AROM functional full range achieved
    - Hip PROM prone
      - Internal rotation (IR) = 40 degrees
      - External rotation (ER) = 10 degrees
    - Ankle
      - Passive dorsiflexion (DF) to neutral
      - Passive plantarflexion (PF) to 45 degrees
- Strength
  - Left UE and LE have good strength
  - Right UE
    - Shoulder flexors: fair antigravity strength
    - Shoulder abductors: fair antigravity strength
    - Hand strength/grip: can grasp and release

- Right LE
  - Hip flexor strength: good
  - Hip abductor strength: fair
  - Knee extensor strength: fair
  - Knee flexor strength: fair minus
  - Ankle/foot: increased tone limits MMT
    - Tendency to invert and PF foot during active movements
- Fair minus abdominal strength as he is unable to complete a "sit-up" activity with good control
- He is able to sustain prone (V-up) extension for approximately 5 seconds
• Sensation
- Normal to light touch in all 4 extremities
• Pain
- Right ankle with DF, using Wong-Baker Faces Pain Rating Scale = 4/10 = hurts a little more
• Posture/spinal alignment
- Presents with asymmetrical alignment of the spine with a right scoliosis of 13 degrees using scoliometer at the mid-thoracic area
- Presents with an elevated right shoulder, scapular winging, and left cervical spine lateral tilt
- Posture in tailor sitting is fair with rounded shoulders and posterior pelvic tilt
- Presents with a leg length discrepancy measured in supine from umbilicus to medial malleoli, left = 55.5 cm and right = 54 cm
- Thigh-foot angle (measured in prone) is <5 degrees on right side and approximately 8 degrees on left
- In standing, with a right total contact posterior stop AFO on and with a one-quarter-inch shoe heelpost insert, his LE alignment is improved and popliteal lines are equal
• Balance
- Static standing balance: single leg stance: left >30 seconds, right <1 second
- Static and dynamic sitting balance are good
• Reflexes/reactions
- Positive plantar grasp noted on right side
- Presence of obligatory symmetrical tonic neck reflex noted in quadruped position; flexion bias of UE with cervical flexion
- Optical and head righting reactions are normal
- Protective reactions are delayed on right side in all directions and in all positions
- Associated reactions are present in right UE and LE and increase with effortful activities
• Gait and endurance
- Tyler is able to ambulate on all terrain, grass, gravel, and cement with and without his AFO; however, he presents with various compensations during movement, as follows:
  - Right foot/ankle is PF with weight bearing at end of toes and no heel strike present and maintains knee in full extension throughout the gait cycle without AFO.
  - With AFO (as described above) and one-quarter-inch heelpost in shoe, he is able to place foot flat during gait.
- He is able to go up a flight of stairs (15 steps) independently in a reciprocal pattern and down stairs leading with left LE in a nonreciprocal pattern.
- He is unable to ride a bicycle or a Razor scooter board independently.
- He is able to kick a rolling ball with right LE while standing on left LE.
• Orthotics
- Wears a right total-contact posterior stop AFO with a one-quarter-inch shoe heelpost insert
- Uses a pedantic wrist splint with thumb abduction during the day
- Has a night splint for stretching and improving DF; not used consistently
• Activities of Daily living
- Tyler requires assistance in donning/doffing socks, shoes, orthotic, shirts, and pants with buttons.
- He is able to feed himself using left UE.
- He drinks from a regular cup using left UE.

Movement System Diagnosis
• Fractionated movement deficit
• Decreased force production
Refer to Chapter 4 for more information regarding movement systems.

Additional quality of life measures should be provided to both Tyler and his parents.

Based on Tyler's examination, he presents with decreased quality of movements and relies on compensatory strategies for activities. In addition, he is unable to perform activities and tasks equivalent to his aged-matched peers (and twin brother). Positive contextual factors include his willingness to participate in all activities, ability to comply with tasks, eagerness to learn and try new activities, and supportive family.

Based on the examination, Tyler presents with the following impairments: right UE and LE strength deficits and decreased full AROM. Additional impairments include decreased standing dynamic balance, decreased motor control resulting in decreased quality of movement during transitions and gait, inability to run efficiently, poor jumping skills, and dependence in self-care activities. He presents with delays in gross motor activities that limit his independence and participation in all environments (school, home, and community). It is important to note that although Tyler's GMFM total score is 81% and he is able to complete activities, the quality and efficiency of movements are impaired. He is at risk for progressive musculoskeletal deformities given his right hemiplegia and significant use of his left dominant side. It is recommended that Tyler receive episodic physical therapy services at home or an outpatient clinic to address impairments, activity limitations, and participation restrictions within his home and community environments. In addition, the therapist should provide ongoing consultation regarding a home exercise program and orthotic needs and address and monitor his scoliosis, leg length discrepancy, and overall gross and fine motor development. Consultation with his teachers can also be provided in order to have continuity of performance and practice with activities throughout his school day, such as using an alternating reciprocal pattern when going up and down stairs, encouraging use of both hands when carrying books or tray at school, and recommendations for physical education participation.

References

1. Bax M, Goldstein M, Rosenbaum P, et al. Proposed definition and classification of cerebral palsy, April 2005. *Dev Med Child Neurol.* 2005;47(8):571-576. doi:10.1017/S001216220500112X

2. Morris C. Definition and classification of cerebral palsy: a historical perspective. *Dev Med Child Neurol.* 2007;49:3-7. doi:10.1111/j.1469-8749.2007.tb12609.x

3. Rosenbaum P, Paneth N, Leviton A, et al. The definition and classification of cerebral palsy. *Dev Med Child Neurol.* 2007;49(Suppl 109):8-14. doi:10.1111/j.1469-8749.2007.00201.x

4. Graham HK, Rosenbaum P, Paneth N, et al. Cerebral palsy. *Nat Rev Dis Primers.* 2016;2(1):15082. doi:10.1038/nrdp.2015.82

5. Oskoui M, Coutinho F, Dykeman J, Jetté N, Pringsheim T. An update on the prevalence of cerebral palsy: a systematic review and meta-analysis. *Dev Med Child Neurol.* 2013;55(6):509-519. doi:10.1111/dmcn.12080

6. Pakula A, Van Naarden Braun K, Yeargin-Allsopp M. Cerebral palsy: classification and epidemiology. *Phys Med Rehabil Clin North Am.* 2009;20(3):425-452.

7. Yeargin-Allsopp M, Braun KVN, Doernberg NS, Benedict RE, Kirby RS, Durkin MS. Prevalence of cerebral palsy in 8-year-old children in three areas of the United States in 2002: a multi-site collaboration. *Pediatrics.* 2008;121(3):547-554. doi:10.1542/peds.2007-1270

8. Schaefer GB. Genetics considerations in cerebral palsy. *Semin Pediatr Neurol.* 2008;15(1):21-26. doi:10.1016/j.spen.2008.01.004

9. Novak I, Morgan C, Adde L, *et al.* Early, accurate diagnosis and early intervention in cerebral palsy: advances in diagnosis and treatment. *JAMA Pediatr.* 2017;171(9):897-907. doi:10.1001/jamapediatrics.2017.1689

10. Centers for Disease Control and Prevention. Data and Statistics for Cerebral Palsy. Accessed September 9, 2022. https://www.cdc.gov/ncbddd/cp/data.html.

11. Drougia A, Giapros V, Krallis N, et al. Incidence and risk factors for cerebral palsy in infants with perinatal problems: a 15-year review. *Early Hum Dev.* 2007;83(8):541-547. doi:10.1016/j.earlhumdev.2006.10.004

12. Sadowska M, Sarecka-Hujar B, Kopyta I. Cerebral palsy: current opinions on definition, epidemiology, risk factors, classification and treatment options. *Neuropsychiatr Dis Treat.* 2020;16:1505-1518. https://doi.org/10.2147/NDT.S235165

13. Cerebral Palsy Alliance Research Foundation. Types of cerebral palsy. Accessed September 10, 2022. https://cparf.org/what-is-cerebral-palsy/types-of-cerebral-palsy/?gclid=EAIaIQobChM-IqIGT1-335wIVi5-zCh2NuA1rEAAYASAAEgJimfD_BwE

14. Lance J. What is spasticity? *Lancet.* 1990;335(8689):606-606. doi:10.1016/0140-6736(90)90389-M

15. Bohannon RW, Smith MB. Interrater reliability of a modified Ashworth scale of muscle spasticity. *Phys Ther.* 1987;67(2):206-207. doi:10.1093/ptj/67.2.206

16. National Institutes of Health. What are the types of cerebral palsy? Accessed September 10, 2022. https://www.nichd.nih.gov/health/topics/cerebral-palsy/conditioninfo/type.

17. Cans C. Surveillance of cerebral palsy in Europe: a collaboration of cerebral palsy surveys and registers. *Dev Med Child Neurol.* 2000;42(12):816-824. doi:10.1017/S0012162200001511

18. Colver A, Fairhurst C, Pharoah PO. Cerebral palsy. *Lancet.* 2014;383(9924):1240-1249. doi:10.1016/S0140-6736(13)61835-8

19. Russell DJ, Rosenbaum PL, Cadman DT, Gowland C, Hardy S, Jarvis S. The gross motor function measure: a means to evaluate the effects of physical therapy. *Dev Med Child Neurol.* 1989;31(3):341-352. doi:10.1111/j.1469-8749.1989.tb04003.x

20. Can Child. Resources. Gross Motor Function Measure (GMFM). Accessed September 10, 2022. https://canchild.ca/en/resources/44-gross-motor-function-measure-gmfm

21. Compagnone E, Maniglio J, Camposeo S, et al. Functional classifications for cerebral palsy: correlations between the Gross Motor Function Classification System (GMFCS), the Manual Ability Classification System (MACS) and the Communication Function Classification System (CFCS). *Res Dev Disabil.* 2014;35(11):2651-2657. doi:10.1016/j.ridd.2014.07.005

22. Palisano R, Rosenbaum P, Walter S, Russell D, Wood E, Galuppi B. Development and reliability of a system to classify gross motor function in children with cerebral palsy. *Dev Med Child Neurol.* 1997;39(4):214-223. doi:10.1111/j.1469-8749.1997.tb07414.x

23. Palisano RJ, Rosenbaum P, Bartlett D, Livingston MH. Content validity of the expanded and revised gross motor function classification system. *Dev Med Child Neurol.* 2008;50(10):744-750. doi:10.1111/j.1469-8749.2008.03089.x

24. Can Child. Resources. Gross Motor Function Classification System–Expanded & Revised (GMFCS-E&R). Accessed September 10, 2022. https://canchild.ca/en/resources/42-gross-motor-function-classification-system-expanded-revised-gmfcs-e-r.

25. Can Child. GMFCS–E&R. Gross Motor Function Classification System Expanded and Revised. Accessed September 10, 2022. https://canchild.ca/system/tenon/assets/attachments/000/000/058/original/GMFCS-ER_English.pdf.

26. Palisano R, Rosenbaum P, Bartlett D, Livingston M. *GMFCS-E&R. Gross Motor Function Classification System Expanded and Revised.* Canchild Centre for Childhood Disability Research, McMaster University; Institute for Applied Health Sciences McMaster University; 2007:b15.

27. Eliasson A-C, Krumlinde-Sundholm L, Rösblad B, et al. The Manual Ability Classification System (MACS) for children with cerebral palsy: scale development and evidence of validity and reliability. *Dev Med Child Neurol.* 2006;48(7):549-554. doi:10.1017/S0012162206001162

28. MACS. Manual Ability Classification System for children with cerebral palsy 1-18 years. Accessed September 10, 2022. https://www.macs.nu/index.php.

29. MCAS. Manual Ability Classification System for children with cerebral palsy 4-18 years. Accessed September 10, 2022. http://www.macs.nu/files/MACS_English_2010.pdf.

30. Elvrum AK, Andersen GL, Himmelmann K, et al. Bimanual Fine Motor Function (BFMF) classification in children with cerebral palsy: aspects of construct and content validity. *Phys Occup Ther Pediatr.* 2016;36(1):1-16. doi:10.3109/01942638.2014.975314

31. Bimanual Fine Motor Function Version 2.0. 2016. Accessed September 10, 2022. https://eu-rd-platform.jrc.ec.europa.eu/sites/default/files/Bimanual-Fine-Motor-Function-2.0.pdf.

32. Hidecker MJ, Paneth N, Rosenbaum PL, et al. Developing and validating the Communication Function Classification System for individuals with cerebral palsy. *Dev Med Child Neurol.* 2011;53(8):704-710. doi:10.1111/j.1469-8749.2011.03996.x

33. CFCS. Communication Function Classification Systems website. Accessed September 10, 2022. http://cfcs.us/.

34. Communication Function Classification System (CFCS). Accessed September 10, 2022. http://cfcs.us/wp-content/uploads/2018/11/CFCS_English_CP.pdf.

35. Tschirren L, Bauer S, Hanser C, Marsico P, Sellers D, Hedel HJA. The Eating and Drinking Ability Classification System: concurrent validity and reliability in children with cerebral palsy. *Dev Med Child Neurol.* 2018;60(6):611-617. doi:10.1111/dmcn.13751

36. National Health Service Sussex Community. Eating and Drinking Ability Classification System for Individuals with Cerebral Palsy (EDACS). Accessed September 10, 2022. https://www.sussexcommunity.nhs.uk/get-involved/research/chailey-research/eating-drinking-classification.htm.

37. The Eating and Drinking Ability Classification System (EDACS). Accessed September 10, 2022. https://www.sussexcommunity.nhs.uk/get-involved/research/chailey-research/edacs-request.

38. Sellers D, Mandy A, Pennington L, Hankins M, Morris C. Development and reliability of a system to classify the eating and drinking ability of people with cerebral palsy. *Dev Med Child Neurol.* 2014;56:245-251. https://doi.org/10.1111/dmcn.12352

39. Sankar C, Mundkur N. Cerebral palsy-definition, classification, etiology and early diagnosis. *Indian J Pediatr.* 2005;72(10):865-868. doi:10.1007/BF02731117

40. World Health Organization. International Classification of Functioning, Disability and Health: Children and Youth Version: ICF-CY. Accessed September 10, 2022. https://apps.who.int/iris/handle/10665/43737

41. Franki I, Desloovere K, De Cat J, et al. The evidence-base for basic physical therapy techniques targeting lower limb function in children with cerebral palsy: a systematic review using the International Classification of Functioning, Disability and Health as a conceptual framework. *J Rehabil Med.* 2012;44(5):385-395. doi:10.2340/16501977-0983

42. ICF Research Branch. Neurological conditions website. Accessed September 20, 2022. https://www.icf-research-branch.org/icf-core-sets/category/8-neurologicalconditions

43. Novak I. Evidence-based diagnosis, health care, and rehabilitation for children with cerebral palsy. *J Child Neurol.* 2014;29(8):1141-1156. doi:10.1177/0883073814535503

44. Romeo DM, Ricci D, Brogna C, Mercuri E. Use of the Hammersmith Infant Neurological Examination in infants with cerebral palsy: a critical review of the literature. *Dev Med Child Neurol.* 2016;58(3):240-245. doi:10.1111/dmcn.12876

45. Gmmash AS, Effgen SK. Early intervention therapy services for infants with or at risk for cerebral palsy. *Pediatr Phys Ther.* 2019;31(3):242-249. doi:10.1097/PEP.0000000000000619

46. Einspieler C, Bos AF, Libertus ME, Marschik PB. The general movement assessment helps us to identify preterm infants at risk for cognitive dysfunction. *Front Psychol.* 2016;7:406. doi:10.3389/fpsyg.2016.00406

47. Mcintyre S, Morgan C, Walker K, Novak I. Cerebral palsy: don't delay. *Dev Disabil Res Rev.* 2011;17(2):114-129. doi:10.1002/ddrr.1106

48. Wang Y, Zhu P, Yang Z, Gu G. Establishing an early identification score system for cerebral palsy based on detailed assessment of general movements. *J Int Med Res.* 2020;48(4):300060520902579. doi:10.1177/0300060520902579

49. Novak I, Morgan C, Adde L, et al. Early, accurate diagnosis and early intervention in cerebral palsy: advances in diagnosis and treatment. *JAMA Pediatr.* 2017;171(9):897-907. doi:10.1001/jamapediatrics.2017.1689

50. Andersson C, Grooten W, Hellsten M, Kaping K, Mattsson E. Adults with cerebral palsy: walking ability after progressive strength training. *Dev Med Child Neurol.* 2003;45(4):220-228. doi:10.1017/S0012162203000446

51. Mutlu A, Livanelioglu A, Gunel MK. Reliability of Ashworth and Modified Ashworth scales in children with spastic cerebral palsy. *BMC Musculoskelet Disord.* 2008;9(1):44. doi:10.1186/1471-2474-9-44

52. Waninge A, Rook RA, Dijkhuizen A, Gielen E, van Der Schans CP. Feasibility, test–retest reliability, and interrater reliability of the Modified Ashworth Scale and Modified Tardieu Scale in persons with profound intellectual and multiple disabilities. *Res Dev Disabil.* 2011;32(2):613-620. doi:10.1016/j.ridd.2010.12.013

53. Mackey AH, Walt SE, Lobb G, Stott NS. Intraobserver reliability of the modified Tardieu scale in the upper limb of children with hemiplegia. *Dev Med Child Neurol.* 2004;46(4):267-272. doi:10.1111/j.1469-8749.2004.tb00481.x

54. Gracies J-M, Burke K, Clegg NJ, et al. Reliability of the Tardieu Scale for assessing spasticity in children with cerebral palsy. *Arch Phys Med Rehabil.* 2010;91(3):421-428. doi:10.1016/j.apmr.2009.11.017

55. Ben-Shabat E, Palit M, Fini NA, Brooks CT, Winter A, Holland AE. Intra- and interrater reliability of the Modified Tardieu Scale for the assessment of lower limb spasticity in adults with neurologic injuries. *Arch Phys Med Rehabil.* 2013;94(12):2494-2501. doi:10.1016/j.apmr.2013.06.026

56. Fosang AL, Galea MP, McCoy AT, Reddihough DS, Story I. Measures of muscle and joint performance in the lower limb of children with cerebral palsy. *Dev Med Child Neurol.* 2003;45(10):664-670. doi:10.1017/S0012162203001245

57. Dodd KJ, Taylor NF, Graham HK. A randomized clinical trial of strength training in young people with cerebral palsy. *Dev Med Child Neurol.* 2003;45(10):652-657. doi:10.1017/S0012162203001221

58. Peungsuwan P, Parasin P, Siriratratiwat W, Prasertnu J, Yamauchi J. Effects of combined exercise training on functional performance in children with cerebral palsy: a randomized-controlled study. *Pediatr Phys Ther.* 2017;29(1):39-46. doi:10.1097/PEP.0000000000000338

59. Ulrich S, Hildenbrand FF, Treder U, et al. Reference values for the 6-minute walk test in healthy children and adolescents in Switzerland. *BMC Pulm Med.* 2013;13(1):49. doi:10.1186/1471-2466-13-49

60. Verschuren O, Takken T, Ketelaar M, Gorter, JW, Helders PJM. Reliability and validity of data for 2 newly developed shuttle run tests in children with cerebral palsy. *Phys Ther.* 2006;86(8):1107-1117. doi:10.1093/ptj/86.8.1107

61. Utter AC, Robertson RJ, Nieman DC, Kang J. Children's OMNI scale of perceived exertion: walking/running evaluation. *Med Sci Sports Exerc.* 2002;34(1):139-144.

62. Robertson RJ, Goss FL, Boer NF, et al. Children's OMNI scale of perceived exertion: mixed gender and race validation. *Med Sci Sports Exerc.* 2000;32:452-458.

63. Kingsnorth S, Orava T, Provvidenza C, et al. Chronic pain assessment tools for cerebral palsy: a systematic review. *Pediatrics.* 2015;136(4):E947-E960. doi:10.1542/peds.2015-0273

64. Bertoncelli CM, Solla F, Loughenbury PR, Tsirikos AI, Bertoncelli D, Rampal V. Risk factors for developing scoliosis in cerebral palsy: a cross-sectional descriptive study. *J Child Neurol.* 2017;32(7):657-662. doi:10.1177/0883073817701047

65. Littleton SR, Heriza CB, Mullens PA, Moerchen V, Bjornson K. Effects of positioning on respiratory measures in individuals with cerebral palsy and severe scoliosis. *Pediatr Phys Ther.* 2011;23(2):159-169. doi:10.1097/PEP.0b013e318218e306

66. Abousamra OT, Sullivan BF, Samdani AJ, et al. Three methods of pelvic fixation for scoliosis in children with cerebral palsy: differences at 5-year follow-up. *Spine.* 2019;44(1):E19-E25. doi:10.1097/BRS.0000000000002761

67. Persson-Bunke MW, Hägglund G, Lauge-Pedersen H, Ma P, Westbom L. Scoliosis in a total population of children with cerebral palsy. *Spine.* 2012;37(12):E708-E713. doi:10.1097/BRS.0b013e318246a962

68. Persson-Bunke M, Czuba T, Hägglund G, et al. Psychometric evaluation of spinal assessment methods to screen for scoliosis in children and adolescents with cerebral palsy. *BMC Musculoskelet Disord.* 2015;16:351. https://doi.org/10.1186/s12891-015-0801-1

69. Tyrakowski M, Czaprowski D, Szczodry M, Siemionow K. Cobb angle measurements on digital radiographs using Bunnell scoliometer: validation of the method. *J Back Musculoskelet Rehabil.* 2017;30(4):667-673. doi:10.3233/BMR-150338

70. Chen C-L, Wu KPH, Liu W-Y, Cheng H-YK, Shen I-H, Lin K-C. Validity and clinimetric properties of the Spinal Alignment and Range of Motion Measure in children with cerebral palsy. *Dev Med Child Neurol.* 2013;55(8):745-750. doi:10.1111/dmcn.12153

71. Thompson P, Beath T, Bell J, et al. Test–retest reliability of the 10-metre fast walk test and 6-minute walk test in ambulatory school-aged children with cerebral palsy. *Dev Med Child Neurol.* 2008;50(5):370-376. doi:10.1111/j.1469-8749.2008.02048.x

72. Dhote S, Khatri P, Ganvir S. Reliability of "Modified Timed Up and Go" test in children with cerebral palsy. *J Pediatr Neurosci.* 2012;7(2):96-100. doi:10.4103/1817-1745.102564

73. Fergus A. A novel mobility device to improve walking for a child with cerebral palsy. *Pediatr Phys Ther.* 2017;29(4):E1-E7. doi:10.1097/pep.0000000000000451

74. Wren TAL, Rethlefsen SP, Kay RM. Prevalence of specific gait abnormalities in children with CP: influence of CP subtype, age, and previous surgery. *J Pediatr Orthop.* 2005;25(1): 79-83.

75. Kennes J, Rosenbaum P, Hanna SE, et al. Health status of school-aged children with CP: information from a population-based sample. *Dev Med Child Neurol.* 2002;44(4):240-247.

76. Christensen D, Van NB, Doernberg NS, et al. Prevalence of cerebral palsy, co-occurring autism spectrum disorders, and motor functioning: autism and developmental disabilities monitoring network, USA, 2008. *Dev Med Child Neurol.* 2014;56(1):59-65. doi:10.1111/dmcn.12268

77. Centers for Disease Control and Prevention. Data and statistics for cerebral palsy. Accessed September 19, 2022. https://www.cdc.gov/ncbddd/cp/data.html.

78. Ryan S, Ability Lab. Functional Mobility Scale. Accessed September 19, 2022. https://www.sralab.org/rehabilitation-measures/functional-mobility-scale.

79. Functional Mobility Scale. Accessed September 19, 2022. https://www.schn.health.nsw.gov.au/files/attachments/the_functional_mobility_scale_version_2.pdf.

80. Bjornson KF, Zhou C, Stevenson R, Christakis DA. Capacity to participation in cerebral palsy: evidence of an indirect path via performance. *Arch Phys Med Rehabil.* 2013;94(12):2365-2372. doi:10.1016/j.apmr.2013.06.020

81. McCauley G, Rosenbaum R, Law K. Assessment of environmental factors in disabled children 2-12 years: development and reliability of the Craig Hospital Inventory of Environmental Factors (CHIEF) for Children–Parent Version. *Child Care Health Dev.* 2013;39(3):337-344. doi:10.1111/j.1365-2214.2012.01388.x

82. Mcdougall J, Wright V, Rosenbaum P. The ICF model of functioning and disability: incorporating quality of life and human development. *Dev Neurorehabil.* 2010;13(3):204-211. doi:10.3109/17518421003620525

83. Carlon S, Shields N, Yong K, Gilmore R, Sakzewski L, Boyd R. A systematic review of the psychometric properties of quality of life measures for school aged children with cerebral palsy. *BMC Pediatr.* 2010;10:81. doi:10.1186/1471-2431-10-81

84. Bailes AF, Greve K, Long J, et al. Describing the delivery of evidence-based physical therapy intervention to individuals with cerebral palsy. *Pediatr Phys Ther.* 2021;33(2):65-72. doi:10.1097/pep.0000000000000783

85. Demont A, Gedda M, Lager C, et al. Evidence-based, implementable motor rehabilitation guidelines for individuals with cerebral palsy. *Neurology.* 2022;99(7):283-297. doi:10.1212/wnl.0000000000200936

86. NSW Health. *Management of Cerebral Palsy in Children: A Guide for Allied Health Professionals.* 2018. Accessed September 20, 2022. http://www1.health.nsw.gov.au/pds/Pages/doc.aspx?dn=GL2018_006.

87. Pohl M, Rückriem S, Mehrholz J, Ritschel C, Strik H, Pause MR. Effectiveness of serial casting in patients with severe cerebral spasticity: a comparison study. *Arch Phys Med Rehabil.* 2002;83(6):784-790.

88. Leonard R, Sweeney J, Damiano D, Bjornson K, Ries J. Effects of orthoses on standing postural control and muscle activity in children with cerebral palsy. *Pediatr Phys Ther.* 2021;33(3): 129-135. doi:10.1097/pep.0000000000000802

89. Harvey LA, Katalinic OM, Herbert RD, Moseley AM, Lannin NA, Schurr K. Stretch for the treatment and prevention of contractures. *Cochrane Database Syst Rev.* 2017;1(1):CD007455. doi:10.1002/14651858.CD007455.pub3

90. Wiart L, Darrah J, Kembhavi G. Stretching with children with cerebral palsy: what do we know and where are we going? *Pediatr Phys Ther.* 2008;20(2):173-178. doi:10.1097/PEP.0b013e3181728a8c

91. Verschuren O, Takken T. 10-metre shuttle run test. *J Physiother.* 2010;56(2):136. doi:10.1016/s1836-9553(10)70046-1

92. Verschuren O, Takken T. Aerobic capacity in children and adolescents with cerebral palsy. *Res Dev Disabil.* 2010;31(6): 1352-1357. doi:10.1016/j.ridd.2010.07.005

93. Yan D, Vassar R. Neuromuscular electrical stimulation for motor recovery in pediatric neurological conditions: a scoping review. *Dev Med Child Neurol.* 2021;63(12):1394-1401. doi:10.1111/dmcn.14974

94. Vles GF, de Louw AJA, Speth LA, et al. Visual analogue scale to score the effects of botulinum toxin A treatment in children with cerebral palsy in daily clinical practice. *Eur J Paediatr Neurol.* 2008;12(3):231-238. doi:10.1016/j.ejpn.2007.08.002

95. Molenaers G, Fagard K, Campenhout A, Desloovere K. Botulinum toxin A treatment of the lower extremities in children with cerebral palsy. *J Child Orthopaed.* 2013;7(5):383-387. doi:10.1007/s11832-013-0511-x

96. Grunt S, Fieggen AG, Vermeulen RJ, Becher JG, Langerak NG. Selection criteria for selective dorsal rhizotomy in children with spastic cerebral palsy: a systematic review of the literature. *Dev Med Child Neurol.* 2014;56(4):302-312. doi:10.1111/dmcn.12277

97. Oudenhoven LM, van Der Krogt MM, Romei M, et al. Factors associated with long-term improvement of gait after selective dorsal rhizotomy. *Arch Phys Med Rehabil.* 2019;100(3):474-480. doi:10.1016/j.apmr.2018.06.016

98. Souza Neves da Costa C, Simioni Rodrigues F, Mustafe Leal F, Cicuto Ferreira Rocha NA. Pilot study: investigating the effects of Kinesio Taping® on functional activities in children with cerebral palsy. *Dev Neurorehabil.* 2013;16:121-128. doi:10.3109/17518423.2012.727106

99. Heussen N, Häusler M. Equine-assisted therapies for children with cerebral palsy: a meta-analysis. *Pediatrics.* 2022;150(1): e2021055229. doi:10.1542/peds.2021-055229

100. Valentín-Gudiol M, Mattern-Baxter K, Girabent-Farrés M, Bagur-Calafat C, Hadders-Algra M, Angulo-Barroso RM. Treadmill interventions in children under six years of age at risk of neuromotor delay. *Cochrane Database Syst Rev.* 2017;7(7): CD009242. doi:10.1002/14651858.cd009242.pub3

101. Roach AT, Elliott SN. Goal attainment scaling: an efficient and effective approach to monitoring student progress. *TEACHING Exceptional Children.* 2005;37(4):8-17. doi:10.1177/004005990503700401

102. Chiarello LA, Effgen SK, Jeffries LW, McCoy S, Bush H. Student outcomes of school-based physical therapy as measured by goal attainment scaling. *Pediatr Phys Ther.* 2016;28(3):277-284. doi:10.1097/PEP.0000000000000268

103. Shirley Ryan Ability Lab. Accessed September 20, 2022. https://www.sralab.org/rehabilitation-measures/goal-attainment-scale.

104. Rozkalne Z, Bertule D. Measurement of activities and participation for children with cerebral palsy: a systematic review. *SHS Web Conferences.* 2014;10. doi:10.1051/shsconf/20141000038

105. Scheets PL, Sahrmann SA, Norton BJ. Use of movement systems diagnoses in the management of patients with neuromuscular conditions: a multiple case report. *Phys Ther.* 2007; 87(6):654-669.

106. Hanna SE, Bartlett DJ, Rivard LM, Russell DJ. Reference curves for the Gross Motor Function Measure: percentiles for clinical description and tracking over time among children with cerebral palsy. *Phys Ther.* 2008;88(5):596-607. doi:10.2522/ptj.20070314

107. Avery LM, Russell DJ, Raina P, et al. Rasch analysis of the Gross Motor Function Measure: validating the assumptions of the Rasch model to create an interval measure. *Arch Phys Med Rehabil.* 2003;84:697-705.

108. Palisano R, Copeland W, Galuppi B. Performance of physical activities by adolescents with cerebral palsy. *Phys Ther.* 2007; 87(1):77-87.

8

Neuromuscular Diseases: Muscular Dystrophies and Spinal Muscular Atrophy

Alicia Fernandez-Fernandez, PT, DPT, PhD, and Mary B. Pengelley, PT, DPT

LEARNING OBJECTIVES

Upon completion of this chapter, the reader will be able to:

- Describe the expected clinical presentation, natural history, and medical management of different types of muscular dystrophy or spinal muscular atrophy (SMA).
- List appropriate tests and measures for children with muscular dystrophy or SMA.

- Describe potential physical therapy interventions in children with muscular dystrophy or SMA.
- Provide a rationale for the use of specific interventions based on the child's impairments, functional limitations, and participation restrictions.
- Discuss the role of assistive and adaptive technology in the management of children with muscular dystrophy or SMA.

INTRODUCTION

The spectrum of neuromuscular diseases can affect any of the components of the motor unit, including the motor neuron, peripheral nerves, neuromuscular junction, and muscle. In these diseases, dysfunction of the motor unit results in loss of strength, range of motion, and functional abilities. In the past few decades, knowledge of the specific genetic causes of several neuromuscular diseases has greatly increased, which has enhanced the ability to correctly diagnose these patients and create informed prognoses. This information has opened the door to not only a better understanding of disease pathophysiology and presentation but also earlier diagnosis, new preventative approaches, targeted therapies, and improved personalized care. Physical therapy is an essential component of patient management, with the aim of preserving available functional abilities for as long as possible at each life stage, preventing complications, and maximizing quality of life within the context of disease progression.

This chapter provides an overview of neuromuscular diseases in children, with a focus on Duchenne muscular dystrophy and spinal muscular atrophy (SMA). The clinical presentation of these diseases will be reviewed, along with medical management and selected physical therapy tests and measures across

the spectrum of the International Classification of Functioning, Disability, and Health (ICF). Current evidence-based physical therapy management strategies will be discussed within the context of child development. Case studies will be presented to illustrate management across the life span, as well as a family-centered perspective.

MUSCULAR DYSTROPHIES

CLASSIFICATION AND KEY FEATURES

Muscular dystrophies are a diverse collection of inherited disorders that affect the muscle component of the motor unit and can be classified in several ways including age of onset, rate of progression, genotype, and other factors. **Table 8-1** lists the most common muscular dystrophies in pediatrics, affecting children in infancy, childhood and/or adolescence.[1]

The hallmark of muscular dystrophies is that progressive muscle dysfunction results in insidious weakness accompanied by secondary impairments such as contractures, postural changes, pathologic biomechanics, decreased endurance, difficulties with functional tasks, and impaired motor development when the onset occurs during childhood or infancy. Although the primary effect is on the musculoskeletal system, other systems are often also impacted, including, among others, the

> **Key Concept**
>
> Muscular dystrophies present with progressive muscle dysfunction, weakness, postural/biomechanical changes, and functional impairments. They affect multiple body systems, and early diagnosis is crucial for medical and therapeutic management.

cardiovascular system, the respiratory system, the gastrointestinal system, and the central nervous system.[2,3] Improvements in the understanding of the genetic etiology of these diseases has enhanced the ability to correctly diagnose patients, which is crucial for informing the family about prognosis and for making appropriate decisions regarding patient management.[4] For some of the muscular dystrophies, such as Duchenne muscular dystrophy, mutation-specific drugs have also been approved or are in clinical trials or in development. This means that genetic mapping is also important in order to determine if a patient can benefit from any available therapies based on their specific genetic mutation.[4]

DUCHENNE MUSCULAR DYSTROPHY

The dystrophinopathies, which include Duchenne muscular dystrophy (DMD), Becker muscular dystrophy (BMD) and DMD-associated cardiomyopathy (DCM),[5] all present with some type of mutation in the DMD gene located in the short arm of the X chromosome. Therefore, these diseases affect boys, whereas females are typically asymptomatic carriers, although a very small percentage of females may be symptomatic carriers.[6,7] Genetic mutations such as deletions, duplications, and point mutations can affect the DMD gene that encodes dystrophin. Depending on the type of mutation, dystrophin may be present but in smaller amounts or with impaired

function (e.g., in BMD), whereas in DMD, dystrophin will be completely absent or dysfunctional.[8] DMD is the most common of the childhood muscular dystrophies, with an incidence of approximately 1 in 3800 to 6300 male births and a prevalence of 15.9 cases per 100,000 male live births in the United States.[3,9] DMD was first described in the mid-1800s and is characterized by mutations that result in no functional dystrophin production.[10,11] Dystrophin is naturally present in skeletal and cardiac muscle but also in other tissues such as the brain and the retina.[6,12] In muscle, dystrophin associates with other proteins known as dystrophin-associated glycoproteins to form the dystrophin-associated protein complex (DAPC), which has important roles in the integrity of muscle fibers.[13] The DAPC is involved in anchoring actin to the extracellular matrix, which allows for stabilization of the sarcolemma during muscle contraction and for appropriate force transmission, and also plays a role in cell signaling, calcium homeostasis, and the nitric oxide pathways.[14]

The absence of functional dystrophin, or a complete lack of dystrophin, disrupt the function of the DAPC and eliminates the link between actin and the extracellular membrane, resulting in sarcolemma instability that is worsened by repeated contractions. Additionally, the microenvironment of the muscle fiber changes with increases in cell membrane permeability, abnormal influx of calcium into the muscle fiber, increased levels of intracellular reactive oxygen species, and decreased activity of nitric oxide synthase, which affects vasodilation pathways during exertion.[15] As a result, there is cumulative microscopic damage to the muscle fiber with a chronic inflammatory response that furthers tissue injury and eventually results in fibrosis, fat infiltration, muscle degeneration, atrophy, loss of contractile function, and progressive weakness (**Figure 8-1**).[11,15-17]

Cardiac muscle is also affected by the absence of dystrophin, resulting in cardiomyopathy.[18] This effect, together with the involvement of respiratory muscles, translates into impaired

TABLE 8-1 • Some Types of Muscular Dystrophies With Onset by Adolescence and Their Main Characteristics[1]	
Type of Muscular Dystrophy	**Characteristics**
Congenital	Very early onset in first few months of life, different forms and different progression depending on genetic profile, presents with hypotonia, weakness, contractures; Fukuyama form can affect brain function
Duchenne	X-linked, lack of dystrophin, onset in early childhood, rapidly progressive proximal to distal weakness and atrophy, loss of ambulation, eventual cardiorespiratory failure
Becker	X-linked, insufficient dystrophin, later onset than Duchenne with longer life span and better prognosis, "milder form"
Emery-Dreifuss	Can be X-linked, autosomal dominant, or autosomal recessive; affects the joints, muscles, and heart; childhood symptoms are often focused on joints and muscles, with heart symptoms developing in adulthood
Facioscapulohumeral	Autosomal dominant; large spectrum of severity from very mild to completely disabling; affects face, scapula, and upper extremities but can extend beyond those; slow progression; age of onset varies but typically in adolescence
Limb-girdle	Many different types (eg, limb-girdle muscular dystrophy [LGMD] 1A, LGMD2I), autosomal recessive or dominant, onset varies from child to adult, most common is proximal weakness starting in hips and progressing
Myotonic	Autosomal dominant, onset can be in late adolescence but most commonly over age of 20, weakness with myotonia and delay in muscle relaxation time

Note. This list is not exhaustive, and many of these classifications include several subtypes. Other classifications are possible depending on the criterion used to create the groups, such as mode of inheritance, age of onset, functional impact, prognosis, and others.

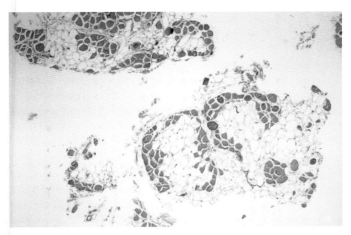

FIGURE 8-1 **Cross-section of dystrophic versus healthy muscle tissue, demonstrating extensive fat infiltration.** (From CDC/Dr. Edwin P. Ewing, Jr.)

cardiorespiratory function and decreased endurance, and death typically occurs due to compromise of cardiorespiratory function in the late stages of the disease. Additionally, neurodevelopmental issues including delayed speech, developmental delay, behavioral problems, learning disabilities, attention-hyperactivity disorder, and autism spectrum disorder have been reported in boys with DMD.[19-21]

Diagnosis

Diagnosis of DMD had classically been based on clinical observation and muscle biopsy. Today, new tools are available to aid in diagnosis and monitoring, including genetic testing, metabolite testing, magnetic resonance imaging (MRI), and ultrasound. An early diagnosis is important in order to promptly initiate interventions and prevent or delay complications,[22] and the possibility of newborn screening is gaining interest.[9] The literature suggests that starting steroid treatment before age 4 can improve long-term outcomes such as increasing the time that the child is able to remain ambulatory and delaying the onset of severe cardiorespiratory involvement.[23]

One-third of mutations in DMD are spontaneous mutations.[24] In the absence of known family history, clinical observation remains the most common initial step for diagnosis, which is typically made at a mean age of 4 to 5 years.[25,26] In England, it has been reported that the mean delay from parental concern to obtaining an accurate diagnosis for

children with DMD is 1.6 years,[25] and the average is similar in a United States report from the Muscular Dystrophy Surveillance, Tracking, and Research Network (MD STARnet), which found a mean delay of 2.5 years from concerns to diagnosis.[26] This highlights how crucial it is for pediatricians, physical therapists, and other clinicians who may have direct access to the patient to be aware of red flags that might indicate the presence of DMD. The typical presentation of a young child with DMD includes delayed motor milestones, decreased antigravity control, delayed walking,[27] frequent falls, calf hypertrophy, Gower's sign upon standing from the floor (**Figure 8-2**), and potential regression in functional abilities such as negotiating stairs.[24] Parents or caregivers may recognize that the child has "become clumsy" or does not seem to be able to keep up with peers as they did before, and this leads to a consult where clinical red flags are identified. **Table 8-2** illustrates the most common signs and symptoms that a clinician would observe in a young child with DMD.[3]

Blood tests can aid in the diagnosis of DMD because they can detect the presence of biomarkers such as creatine kinase. Because creatine kinase exists primarily in muscle, the presence of high levels of creatine kinase in serum is indicative of muscle injury. Highly elevated creatine kinase levels, with values over 5000 IU/L compared to the normal range (<200 IU/L) and without a history of major trauma or infections, are considered a potential biomarker for DMD in children and should lead to further testing for dystrophinopathies.[24,28,29] Additionally, recent research suggests that as many as 44 serum metabolites that are significantly elevated or decreased in patients with DMD may have the potential to be used as diagnostic biomarkers, including arginine, creatine, creatinine, androgen derivatives, and other proteins as well as several unknown compounds.[30,31] In a natural history study that investigated some of these biomarkers, the authors also reported that the creatine/creatinine ratio in DMD increased as the disease progressed, compared with healthy controls where it decreased with age.[30] Serum biomarkers thus show potential promise for diagnostic and monitoring purposes (e.g., evaluating treatment effects) in patients with DMD.[32]

Genetic testing, with DNA obtained from sources such as serum, saliva, urine, skin, or muscle, provides definitive confirmation of the diagnosis of DMD. Establishment of the precise mutation that is present in a patient can inform management

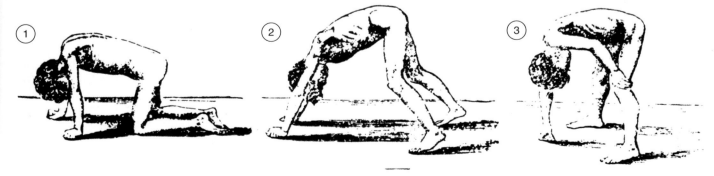

FIGURE 8-2 **Gower's sign upon transitioning to stand.** (From Gowers WR. *Pseudo-Hypertrophic Muscular Paralysis: A Clinical Lecture.* J. & A. Churchill; 1879.)

TABLE 8-2 • Clinical Signs and Symptoms of Duchenne Muscular Dystrophy That Would Indicate Need for Diagnostic Referral

Motor	Nonmotor
• Pseudohypertrophy, particularly in calves or quadriceps	issues in the following domains:
• Decreased muscle tone	• Cognitive
• Muscle pain or cramping	• Behavior
• Gait deviations, including toe walking	• Learning
• Decreased endurance	• Attention
• Regression in motor skills in a child that was previously on target	• Growth
• Difficulty negotiating stairs, running, climbing, or jumping, or general difficulty with antigravity control	• Speech
• Difficulty with transitions from floor, Gower's sign (**Figure 8-2**), head lag in pull to sit	
• Frequent falls, reports of "clumsiness" or inability to keep up with peers	

Adapted from Birnkrant DJ, Bushby K, Bann CM, et al. Diagnosis and management of Duchenne muscular dystrophy, part 1: diagnosis, and neuromuscular, rehabilitation, endocrine, and gastrointestinal and nutritional management. Lancet Neurol. 2018;17(3):251-267.

because targeted therapies may be available for specific mutations, and some genotypes can be related to rate of progression and specific clinical markers such as age at loss of ambulation.[33] Additionally, disease progression may be affected by other genes, with reports that specific single-nucleotide polymorphisms (SNPs) in the *LTBP4* gene and the *SPP1* gene may modulate DMD progression and potentially delay loss of ambulation in these children. The *LTBP4* gene regulates fibrosis signaling processes, and the *SPP1* gene regulates inflammation, so different genotypes in these 2 genes can result in slower or quicker progression of DMD based on the activity of inflammation and fibrosis pathways. Research continues to evolve in this area in order to confirm whether these SNPs, identified as disease modifiers, can inform prognosis and management.[34-37]

The use of imaging techniques in DMD has recently been reported for diagnostic and monitoring purposes. Several groups describe the use of ultrasound to detect areas of muscle damage and differentiate between healthy and DMD muscle or to monitor the progression of the disease by quantifying muscle thickness or using edge detection, and this is a developing area of diagnostics in DMD.[38-40] Jansen et al[38] report that the presence of dystrophic changes is related to ambulatory status, functional grading, muscle strength, and motor ability, and Zaidman et al[41] found that quantitative ultrasound was able to detect differences between children with DMD and healthy controls earlier than some functional tests such as the supine-to-stand and 6-minute walk tests. Therefore, quantitative ultrasound shows promise as an adjuvant to other diagnostic and monitoring techniques.[40]

Another imaging technique that has demonstrated sensitivity to DMD progression is MRI, accompanied by quantitative magnetic resonance spectroscopy (MRS), which can measure composition of muscle tissue, such as the fraction of fat. In a study of 136 children with DMD, Barnard et al[42] found that T2-weighted MRI combined with MRS showed significant correlation to functional measures such as the 10-minute walk/run, climb 4 stairs, supine-to-stand, and 6-minute walk tests. This correlation was particularly strong for data from the vastus lateralis looking at muscle morphology and fat fraction, where fat fraction increased as DMD progressed. The authors were able to establish a quantitative threshold for fat fraction (0.40) that was associated with loss of ambulation.[42] Willcocks et al[43] were able to detect subclinical disease progression in DMD over long time periods (1-2 years) as well as short time periods (3-6 months) using T2-weighted MRI and MRS. In the short time period study, the researchers were able to detect significant changes in fat fraction before significant changes in functional clinical measures, with the vastus lateralis and biceps femoris showing the most changes.[43,44] Arpan et al[45] observed reduction in muscle inflammation, damage, and fat infiltration in T2 MRI and MRS over a period of 1 year for boys who were treated with corticosteroids versus those who were not. Other authors have also been able to identify fat replacement of muscle over time using T1-weighted imaging.[46] These findings open up the possibility that MRI and MRS can be used to detect preclinical changes in boys with DMD, as well as to monitor disease progression and the effects of treatment.

Natural History and Medical Management

The natural history of DMD has changed significantly over the past few decades with advances in medical management, including the use of mechanical ventilation and glucocorticoids, which have resulted in prolonged life spans (from old teens into the late twenties or early thirties). These interventions have also allowed improvements or extensions in functional ability, such as ambulatory status until older ages.[47,48] The Cooperative International Neuromuscular Research Group (CINRG) ran a large, prospective, multicenter, natural history study, the CINRG Duchenne Natural History Study (DNHS), which enrolled over 400 boys and young adults between 2006 and 2015 and resulted in an improved understanding of the natural history of the disease and how it has shifted overtime, as well as provided valuable information on strength and mobility, cardiovascular function, clinical care, behavior, community participation, and quality of life.[49-51] Nowadays, there is the potential for further positive shifts with the advent of dystrophin-specific therapeutics that are currently in their initial market stages.

The latest version of the standards of care for DMD, published in 3 parts in 2018,[2,3,52] reflected this shift in timeline with the addition of a section on care during transition to adulthood. The standards of care also reflect a more contemporary understanding of the importance of early diagnosis and therapy and of the interdisciplinary nature of optimal patient management. The standards divide care into 3 major stages with some subdivisions: preclinical or at diagnosis, ambulatory (including early and late), and nonambulatory (including early and late). Recommendations are made for all areas of care at each stage and spanning the different stages (**Figure 8-3**).

Glucocorticoids, a class of corticosteroids, are well established in the treatment of the child with DMD. Evidence

	Stage 1: At diagnosis	Stage 2: Early ambulatory	Stage 3: Late ambulatory	Stage 4: Early non-ambulatory	Stage 5: Late non-ambulatory
Neuromuscular management	Lead the multidisciplinary clinic, advise on new therapies; provide patient and family support, education, and genetic counselling				
	Ensure immunisation schedule is complete	Assess function, strength, and range of movement at least every 6 months to define stage of disease			
	Discuss use of glucocorticosteroids	Initiate and manage use of glucocorticosteroids			
	Refer female carriers to cardiologist				Help navigate end-of-life care
Rehabilitation management	Provide comprehensive multidisciplinary assessments, including standardised assessments, at least every 6 months				
	Provide direct treatment by physical and occupational therapists, and speech-language pathologist, based on assessments and individualised to the patient				
	Assist in prevention of contracture or deformity, overexertion, and falls; promote energy conservation and appropriate exercise or activity; provide orthoses, equipment, and learning support		Continue all previous measures; provide mobility devices, seating, supported standing devices, and assistive technology; assist in pain and fracture prevention or management; advocate for funding, access, participation, and self-actualisation into adulthood		
Endocrine management	Measure standing height every 6 months				
	Assess non-standing growth every 6 months				
		Assess pubertal status every 6 months starting by age 9 years			
		Provide family education and stress dose steroid prescription if on glucocorticosteroids			
Gastrointestinal and nutritional management	Include assessment by registered dietitian nutritionist at clinic visits (every 6 months): initiate obesity prevention strategies; monitor for overweight and underweight, especially during critical transition periods				
	Provide annual assessments of serum 25-hydroxyvitamin D and calcium intake				
		Assess swallowing dysfunction, constipation, gastro-oesophageal reflux disease, and gastroparesis every 6 months			
		Initiate annual discussion of gastrostomy tube as part of usual care			
Respiratory management		Provide spirometry teaching and sleep studies as needed (low risk of problems)		Assess respiratory function at least every 6 months	
	Ensure immunisations are up to date: pneumococcal vaccines and yearly inactivated influenza vaccine				
				Initiate use of lung volume recruitment	
				Begin assisted cough and nocturnal ventilation	
					Add daytime ventilation
Cardiac management	Consult cardiologist assess with electrocardiogram and echocardiogram* or cardiac MRI†	Assess cardiac function annually, initiate ACE inhibitors or angiotensin receptor blockers by age 10 years	Assess cardiac function at least annually, more often if symptoms or abnormal imaging are present; monitor for rhythm abnormalities		
			Use standard heart failure interventions with deterioration of function		
Bone health management		Assess with lateral spine x-rays (patients on glucocorticosteroids: every 1–2 years; patients not on glucocorticosteroids: every 2–3 years)			
		Refer to bone health expert at the earliest sign of fracture (Genant grade 1 or higher vertebral fracture or first long-bone fracture)			
Orthopaedic management	Assess range of motion at least every 6 months				
		Monitor for scoliosis annually		Monitor for scoliosis every 6 months	
	Refer for orthopedic surgery if needed (rarely necessary)	Refer for surgery on foot and achilles tendon to improve gait in selected situations		Consider intervention for foot position for wheelchair positioning; initiate intervention with posterior spinal fusion in defined situations	
Psychosocial management	Assess mental health of patient and family at every clinic visit and provide ongoing support				
	Provide neuropsychological evaluation/interventions for learning, emotional, and behavioural problems				
		Assess educational needs and available resources (individualised education programme, 504 plan); assess vocational support needs for adults			
		Promote age-appropriate independence and social development			
Transitions	Engage in optimistic discussions about the future, expecting life into adulthood	Foster goal setting and future expectations for adult life; assess readiness for transition (by age 12 years)	Initiate transition planning for health care, education, employment, and adult living (by age 13–14 years); monitor progress at least annually; enlist care coordinator or social worker for guidance and monitoring		
			Provide transition support and anticipatory guidance about health changes		

FIGURE 8-3 **Summary of medical and rehabilitative management of Duchenne muscular dystrophy.** (Reproduced with permission from Birnkrant DJ, Bushby K, Bann CM, et al. Diagnosis and management of Duchenne muscular dystrophy, part 1: diagnosis, and neuromuscular, rehabilitation, endocrine, and gastrointestinal and nutritional management. *Lancet Neurol.* 2018;17(3):251-267.)

supports their early initiation after diagnosis, before physical decline begins, as well as their continuation after loss of ambulation, along with physical therapy.[3] Long-term use of glucocorticoids results in slower progression of muscle degeneration and damage, with prolonged functional use of lower extremities (ambulation extended by an average of 1.2-3.9 years depending on the steroid used), upper extremities, and respiratory muscles.[3,53,54] Corticosteroid treatment has also been shown to result in reduced muscle tissue inflammation and fat infiltration.[45] When possible, treatment is initiated preclinically with prednisolone or deflazacort (Emflaza®, a daily oral regimen of corticosteroid produg, Food and Drug Administration [FDA] approved in 2017).[55] Corticosteroid treatment requires careful monitoring for side effects and for dose efficacy (impact on functional status).[3] There are still benefits to initiating steroid regimens later on, even in patients who are already nonambulatory.[54] More research is needed to standardize care and more clearly delineate optimal dosage for each patient, as well as determine how to weigh the potential benefits of some steroids over others in terms of their efficacy versus their side effects, such as weight gain, osteopenia, insulin resistance, or decreased growth among others.[53,56-59]

In recent years, there has been an increase in research and development of novel drug therapies for DMD. Many drugs are being investigated as of 2022 in different areas including antifibrotic, anti-inflammatory, drugs affecting mitochondrial function, and gene therapies, among others.[60] The reader can refer to the ClinicalTrials.gov website (http://clinicaltrials.gov) for updated information on current clinical trials using these diverse approaches. Of particular interest are gene-based therapies, which attempt to directly address the genetic defects that affect dystrophin production and some of which have reached market. Because these defects are varied and there are different subgroups of children with DMD depending on the exact type of genetic mutation that is involved, these treatments are typically only applicable to certain subpopulations of individuals with DMD. As a result, some therapies have been brought to market based on relatively small samples. For instance, in 2016, the FDA granted accelerated approval for eteplirsen (Exondys 51), a drug that promotes dystrophin production by excision of exon 51 when it is defective (a mutation present in about 14% of DMD patients). Skipping over the defect allows for the reading frame to still be translated. Eteplirsen does not "cure" DMD, but there is some evidence that this drug is able to induce the expression of dystrophin in a shorter but functional form.[61,62] In 2019, the FDA also approved golodirsen (Vyondys 53), which uses a similar approach, but for patients with a mutation amenable to exon 53 skipping (about 7% of children with DMD).[63,64] Other recently approved treatments include the exon 53–skipping antisense oligonucleotide viltolarsen (Viltepso®), which was FDA approved in 2020, and ataluren (Translarna®), which is currently only approved in Europe and can be used in nonsense DMD mutations.[55]

Two important considerations that present a challenge for clinical applicability of some of these drugs are access to treatment (e.g., eteplirsen currently costs several hundred thousand dollars per year) and the fact that approval was based on small sample sizes and limited data, with the need to obtain stronger evidence regarding their impact on function. Several larger and longer-term clinical trials are ongoing.

Management Across the Life Span

The 2018 clinical guidelines describe 3 distinct functional stages to frame intervention: preclinical or at diagnosis, ambulatory, and nonambulatory, with the latter 2 stages subdivided into early and late periods. Each stage is specifically defined by clinical milestones or predicted functional losses, and specific management needs vary as the stages progress. The focus is on individualized treatment plans that address current problems, but due to the progressive nature of DMD, it is also necessary to actively predict and anticipate future functional losses to properly plan and adapt upcoming care. Appropriate objective tests and measures are critical to determining rate of progression, planning, and providing customized care that includes appropriate caregiver education. Physical therapy should start as soon as the child is diagnosed, and baseline measures of range of motion (ROM), strength, and functional ability should be obtained at the initial visit and reassessed periodically thereafter, with new measures added as necessary. Current guidelines recommend reassessments every 6 months.[2]

Weakness is the main impairment, and it progresses proximal to distal starting with antigravity muscle groups such as the hip extensors or the neck flexors, with more involvement of the lower extremities than the upper extremities in initial stages. As weakness increases, postural changes due to compensations begin to emerge, and contractures start to develop in unopposed muscle groups or muscles that are trying to compensate to preserve function. In standing, there is a progressive posterior weight shift in an attempt to provide a biomechanical advantage to weak hip extensors by driving the ground reaction force vector behind the hip joint. This results in a characteristic lordotic stance that increases with time, as can be observed in **Figure 8-4**. Increased lateral trunk sway (swaddling) is typically observed during gait due to hip abductor weakness, along with reduced arm swing, decreased step length, and wide base of support due to tensor fascia lata contractures. Toe walking typically emerges as an attempt to compensate for hip extension deficits, along with increasing ankle dorsiflexor weakness, and eventually leads to plantar flexor contractures. As the quadriceps gets weaker and antigravity knee extension becomes more challenging, compensatory displacement of the line of gravity is even more marked due to the need for maintaining the ground reaction force vector behind the hip and in front of the knee at the same time. Plantar flexion compensation also increases at this stage in an attempt to assist knee extension.

As weakness progresses, functional ability declines and sequential milestones characterized by loss of function will occur. In the presymptomatic stage, a child may only demonstrate qualitative changes in functional ability, such as partial Gower's sign, or initial difficulty with some functional tasks that require antigravity control, such as transitions, squatting, or negotiating stairs, but will still be able to complete these tasks. As time passes and the child is in the

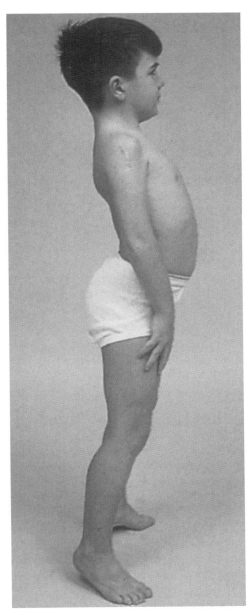

FIGURE 8-4 Lordotic stance in child with Duchenne muscular dystrophy. Notice the increase in lumbar lordosis, posterior weight shift to promote antigravity control of the hip, and increased anterior pelvic tilt due to hip flexor tightness. (Reproduced with permission from Hauser SL, Josephson SA, *Harrison's Neurology in Clinical Medicine*, 4e, New York: McGraw Hill; 2017.)

living (ADLs) including transfers, dressing, grooming, bathing or feeding. Accordingly, functional loss milestones in this stage include loss of ability to reach overhead, loss of bed mobility, loss of manual dexterity to utilize equipment, and loss of ability to perform different ADLs that require independent upper extremity use (e.g., grooming or feeding). In this stage, cardiorespiratory involvement also increases and can result in the need for cough assist, ventilation, or other support measures.

> ### Key Concept
>
> Physical therapy assessments in Duchenne's muscular dystrophy should encompass strength, range of motion, gait, and various detailed aspects of functional ability to enable clinicians to monitor change over time and proactively manage care.

Understanding the natural progression of DMD frames the physical therapy assessments, interventions, and expected outcomes at each stage. Important assessment components across the life span that should be followed over time include ROM (measured using goniometry), strength (measured using manual muscle testing and dynamometry), gait and posture, balance, respiratory function (spirometry, chest wall excursion, ability to cough and clear secretions), aerobic capacity and endurance, functional ability, and participation at home and school. **Table 8-3** summarizes the most commonly used assessments of functional ability for children with DMD. Patient-reported outcome measures are also crucial to obtain more information about the patient's clinical picture. From a clinical point of view, self-report scales to measure pain, fatigue, or perceived exertion are important components of the assessment of the child with DMD. In terms of quality of life and participation, some of the tools that can be used include the Pediatric Outcomes Data Collection Instrument, the Pediatric Evaluation of Disability Inventory, the Pediatric Functional Independence Measure, the School Function Assessment, the Pediatric Quality of Life Inventory, and the Activities-Specific Scale for Kids, among others.[65]

Periodic reassessment can help inform management because the North Star Ambulatory Assessment, timed function tests, 6-minute walk test, and Motor Function Measure have all been shown to be predictive of disease progression, as discussed in Table 8-3. Also, both knee extensor strength and plantar flexor strength are moderately correlated with functional outcomes, with loss of strength resulting in decreased function, although strength loss is not the only factor impacting function.[76] Periodic assessment information is crucial because it can provide rationale for change in medication or treatment based on functional status, support preventative care, and direct the need for equipment such as mobility equipment, transfer equipment, home modifications, or school accommodations. The current guidelines recommend that assessments are repeated at least every 6 months.[3]

ambulatory stage, critical loss milestones will occur including loss of standing from the floor, loss of ability to negotiate stairs, loss of sit to stand, and ultimately loss of ambulation. Predicting loss of ambulation is crucial to plan for needed adaptations, assistive and mobility equipment, and home modifications.

Once in the nonambulatory stage, the focus of compensatory biomechanics shifts to stability in sitting and assisting and maintaining upper extremity function. Weakness and contractures will develop and significantly affect the upper extremities at this stage, thus impacting all activities of daily

TABLE 8-3 • Functional Assessments in Duchenne Muscular Dystrophy

Functional Assessments	Details
North Star Ambulatory Assessment (NSAA)[66-68]	Functional assessment for preclinical or ambulatory stages. Includes 17 items, graded by quality and ability to perform with or without compensation. Functional items include stand, walk, sit to stand, single leg stance (left and right), climb box step (left and right), descend box step (left and right), lift head in supine, floor to sit, rise from floor, stand on heels, jump, hop (left and right), run 10 m. Maximum score is 34. A revised version has been developed for early use as young as 3 years old. The NSAA was derived from the Hammersmith Functional Motor Scale Expanded (HFMSE).[69]
Timed functional tests[68,70]	10-m walk test (over 12 seconds predicts loss of ambulation within 12 months), supine to stand (over 30 seconds predicts loss of ambulation within 12 months), climb 4 stairs (over 8 seconds predicts loss of ambulation within 12 months), Timed Up and Go (TUG), single limb stance. The TUG is a useful tool as it includes not only walking but also functional sit/stand components.
6-Minute walk test (6MWT)[68,71]	Functional assessment of endurance. Measures how far the child can walk in 6 minutes. Clinically significant change is 20-30 m.
Motor Function Measure (MFM)[72]	Functional assessment with 32 items in 3 subsections: standing and transfers, axial and proximal motor capacity, and distal motor capacity. Predictive threshold for loss of ambulation in 12 months: total score 70% and standing and transfers subscore 40%.
Vignos functional scale for lower extremities[73]	Functional 1-10 scale, from 1 = walks and climbs stairs without assistance to 10 = in bed, cannot do activities of daily living (ADLs) without assistance.
Brooke functional scale for upper extremities[73]	Functional 1-6 scale, from 1 = abducts arms in full circle overhead to 6 = no hand to mouth and no use of hands.
Egen Klassifikation (EK) scale[74,75]	For use in the nonambulatory stage, functional scale focused on ADLs that also includes coughing ability. 17 items scored by interview and observation. Available in several languages.

Note. This table is nonexhaustive but highlights the most commonly used instruments in this population. Also included are known predictor thresholds for loss of ambulation.

While we should not expect improvement during the course of care with these patients, preservation of function does significantly improve quality of life, and management should be organized around prevention, proactive care, and anticipation of future changes. All therapeutic interventions should be adapted to the child's unique needs, as disease progression depends on a variety of aspects including not only genetic variations but also medical management (e.g., use of steroids) and environmental factors. When providing therapeutic instruction and presenting goal-oriented tasks, it is important to consider that research has shown that boys with DMD may have significant impairments in executive aspects of cognition, such as multitasking, problem solving, and working memory, which is needed to plan and direct behavior,[77] even in the absence of diagnosed intellectual disability.

The focus of therapy in the initial preclinical stage is prevention of contractures, promotion of appropriate activities, and monitoring of disease progression. It is critically important to begin to document ROM, muscle strength, gait and posture, and functional scores to provide a baseline for future reference. The main role of the physical therapist is to educate the family on disease progression, activities to avoid, and consistent stretching exercises. It is important to avoid overuse and fatigue, focusing instead on submaximal activity to avoid muscle damage,[78] while allowing and encouraging age-appropriate functional activities, including aquatic activities.[79] Resistive exercises and eccentric activities should not be used as therapy or recommended to the family due to the potential for increased damage.[80] When possible, it is desirable to coordinate with the physical education teacher at the child's school to

ensure that activities can be adapted to the child's needs while they still get the physical and social peer-interaction benefits of exercise. Stretching protocols can be incorporated into the child's daily routine at home and school, with a recommended frequency of up to 6 times per week,[3] and should be active when possible. In the initial stages, target muscle groups for stretching would include the gastrocnemius-soleus and the tensor fascia lata, with progressive addition of other muscle groups such as hamstrings, hip flexors, or foot evertors. For instance, an incline standing board can be used for plantar flexion stretches, long sitting for hamstring stretches, and prone positioning for hip flexor stretching. At this stage, it is also important to discuss the initiation of night bracing to support the effects of active stretching, as a combined approach has been shown to be more effective and lengthen the period of independent walking.[81,82] The use of ankle-foot orthoses (AFOs) for stretching at night is best tolerated if it starts at a young age with a preventative focus.[3] Increased plantar flexion contractures demonstrate a correlation with decreased functional scores in assessments such as the NSAA,[83] highlighting the importance of early and proactive management.

In the early to late ambulatory stage, as biomechanical changes and compensations become apparent, it is important to continue with a consistent stretching protocol that progressively incorporates additional muscle groups as necessary, as well as with appropriate physical activity that will help slow down loss of function and endurance. The child should carry on utilizing night braces to complement active stretching or start using night braces at this time if they had not previously. Energy conservation techniques and fall prevention strategies should be discussed with the family as well, as posture and gait changes will increase in this stage, thus generating increased exertion and difficulties with dynamic postural adjustment. Assessment of the school, home, and community environments is important to determine appropriate safe activities and potential need for assistive equipment. Knee-ankle-foot orthoses (KAFOs) may be used to support ambulation. In general, the use of AFOs for ambulation is not desirable because they tend to create increased knee flexor moments, which are hard for a weakened quadriceps to counteract. At this time, long-term considerations such as use of mobility equipment for long distances should be discussed.

In the late ambulatory stage, tightness and biomechanical changes will have increased to the point where ambulation becomes progressively challenged. Transfers and functional antigravity use of the lower extremities become more difficult, and tightness starts to develop in the upper extremities as well. Maintaining a consistent stretching protocol becomes even more important in this stage, including both active stretching and night bracing, which should now both include the upper extremity. For some children, serial casting may be an alternative to improve ROM,[84] and other children may have surgery at this stage (e.g., tenotomies) to prolong ambulation. Prolonged ambulation has important benefits including a reduction in the severity of scoliosis[85] and prevention of cardiorespiratory, musculoskeletal, gastrointestinal, integumentary, and psychological complications. However, surgical intervention does not always provide good outcomes because eliminating the contracture sometimes takes away some of the child's compensatory strategies, which may actually result in decreased functional ability. Thus, the recommendation is to use surgery in children who have severe contractures but still strong ambulation.[86] Physical therapy involvement in the postoperative stage is crucial to promote recovery and return to functional gait.

While still in the ambulatory stage, physical activity can continue but may have to be adapted to limit fatigue and exertion, for instance, in an aquatic environment. Energy conservation techniques are important as cardiorespiratory function starts to show signs of impairment. Upper extremity exercises are also important at this stage, and ergometry has been shown to preserve upper extremity function better than ROM exercises alone.[87] Respiratory function should also be closely assessed, and the family can be instructed in breathing exercises, assisted coughing, chest percussion, or bronchial drainage. The physical therapist can obtain valuable information regarding respiratory function from formal pulmonary function testing, which is typically performed at regular intervals by the medical team at this stage.[2] Finally, one of the most important aspects of management in the late ambulatory period is planning for alternative mobility equipment and environmental adaptations; for instance, the purchase of a wheelchair, modifications to the home and school environment, or future transportation needs (e.g., adaptations to the family car). The rate of progression can dictate the most logical choice of mobility device and the equipment needed. Predictors of loss of ambulation can help delineate an appropriate timeline to start considering these issues,

and it is crucial to be proactive, as it may take a long time and some financial planning and coordination to make the proper arrangements. Appropriate accessories for pressure relief, spinal support, or adaptive control systems should be considered at this time as well.

In the early nonambulatory stage, one of the most important aspects of therapy is training the child and family on wheelchair use, safety, and transfers. Although cessation of ambulation can sometimes bring a feeling of disappointment, it is important to highlight the benefits of using a wheelchair, including more access to the environment, less exertion and fatigue, ability to cover longer distances, and improved ability to participate, compared to the end of the previous stage where ambulation had become laborious. The child and the family should be trained in safe transfer techniques, and equipment may need to be ordered for ergonomically safe transfers in the home environment. ROM exercises and bracing should continue with an emphasis on both upper and lower extremities, as should physical activity such as aquatic exercises, ergometer use, or activities while using the wheelchair. Shoulder depressors and triceps are essential muscles to maintain active due to their role in transfers. As previously mentioned, coordination with the child's physical education teacher can be a crucial means of maintaining activity and inclusion during this important transition. Standing programs during nonactive time can also be initiated to obtain some of the benefits of weight bearing. Pain is usually of biomechanical origin and can be alleviated with positional changes. Respiratory interventions to promote breathing and drainage should be continued. Research has shown that assessments such as motor strength and Pediatric Evaluation of Disability Inventory (PEDI) mobility scores can be reliably assessed in sitting regardless of ambulatory status, so they can continue to be used to inform clinical decision-making and optimize care during this stage.[88]

In the late nonambulatory stage, respiratory function declines quickly and will most likely require the use of ventilation and cough assist machines. Progressive weakness and increased contractures also result in greater dependence on caregivers and decreased ability to perform ADLs. It is important to train caregivers in proper body mechanics and in the use of hydraulic lifts or other transfer mechanisms. Decreased mobility and long-term use of glucocorticoids often results in high rates of obesity among individuals with DMD in the nonambulatory stage, highlighting the need for caregiver education in safe transfers. For the individual, the emphasis on stretching and appropriate physical activity still continues, along with a renewed emphasis on respiratory therapy and training in pulmonary clearing techniques and breathing exercises. Assistive technology, such as environmental control devices or power chair voice or head controls, may be useful at this stage.

Eventually, respiratory insufficiency or cardiomyopathy will bring the patient into the final stages of life. But it is important to understand that although there is no cure for DMD and life expectancy is short, incredible advances have been made in the management of DMD and in improving life expectancy and quality of life. Passamano et al,[89] who followed life expectancy in cohorts born from the 1960s to the 2010s, found that with early glucocorticoids and use of assistive ventilation, life

TABLE 8-4 • ICF Considerations for Noah's Case	
Child's name and age	Noah, age 4 years
Health condition	• Duchenne muscular dystrophy • Pulmonary complications: pneumonia, respiratory syncytial virus infection, bronchiolitis • Premature birth
Body function and structures	• Muscle weakness • Multiple bouts of respiratory illness • Feeding difficulties: food aversions/limited preferences
Activity limitations	• Difficulty with developmentally appropriate gross motor skills such as running, climbing, squatting, kicking • Unable to navigate uneven surfaces/stairs • Difficulty with eating regular diet
Participation restrictions	• Difficulty with community mobility and unable to walk for long distances such as outings • Unable to participate in playground activities with peers at daycare • Requires special foods for meals at daycare
Environmental factors	• Facilitators: Proactive medical and therapeutic interventions (aquatic therapy, night splints, pulmonary care, medications), daycare supportive, family proactive and aware • Barriers: daycare not adapted
Personal factors	• Facilitators: early diagnosis • Barriers: sensory sensitivities and corresponding behavioral protests

expectancy for individuals with DMD has increased in the past few decades from 17 years 9 months to 27 years 9 months and that function was also prolonged several years; the authors conclude that "DMD should be now considered an adulthood disease as well … and more public health interventions are needed to support these patients and their families as they pass from childhood into adult age."

> ### Key Concept
> More individuals with Duchenne's muscular dystrophy are now reaching adult age and encountering issues with continuity of care. Pediatric therapists should plan in collaboration with the patient, family, and care team to ensure successful transitions.

The general principles we have discussed for the management of children and adolescents with DMD also apply to other muscular dystrophies, with specific consideration of their unique presentation, rate of progression, and primary clinical characteristics. A focus on preserving function, maintaining ROM and strength, promoting submaximal physical activity, and maximizing participation through the use of assistive and adaptive equipment is also applicable in these cases, with individualized care based on functional ability and prognosis.

Case 1

Noah

Noah was diagnosed with DMD before the age of 2. He had a family history of DMD and a complicated medical history during his infancy, including premature birth, tongue and lip tie, multiple pneumonias, respiratory syncytial virus (RSV) and bronchiolitis

from age 4 to 17 months, pressure equalizer tubes at 17 months, and a febrile seizure during respiratory illness. He was given cough assist and a high-frequency vibrating vest to help with pulmonary health and was brought in for therapy evaluations at 23 months of age due to recent difficulty with swallowing. At that time, he was walking with a wide base of support and could squat to play and recover but could not run. He had normal passive ROM but began wearing night stretching splints. He also began participating in weekly aquatic therapy to improve pulmonary health, while maintaining strength through activities in a reduced gravity environment to prevent breakdown of muscle fibers. At age 3, he began taking deflazacort, using a 10-day-on/10-day-off regimen, coenzyme Q10, calcium, vitamin D, and probiotics. At age 4, he stopped attending aquatic therapy due to mother's work schedule but was noted to have some hypertrophy of the gastrocnemius muscles. He was tested using the Expanded Hammersmith Functional Motor Scale and scored 20%. He was then fitted with new night stretching splints as well as foot orthoses to support his medial arches, as he had begun bearing weight with bilateral calcaneal valgus due to decreased ROM of the heel cords. **Table 8-4** shows ICF considerations for Noah's case. See also **Figure 8-5**.

Case Question

Why do you think Noah's therapist recommended starting the use of night splints at such an early age, even though his passive ROM was still normal?

Case 2

James

James came into the physical therapy outpatient clinic at age 13 for evaluation and recommendations for equipment needs and home programming. He was diagnosed at age 5 with DMD and had recently been hospitalized for cardiac arrhythmia. At

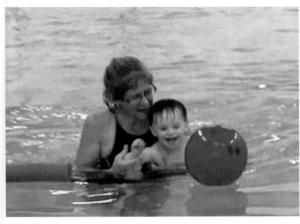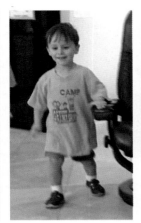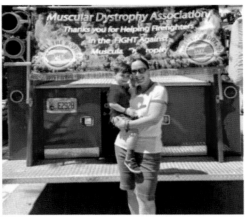

FIGURE 8-5 From left to right: Noah in his aquatic therapy session, Noah walking with proper medial arch support, and Noah and his mother at a Muscular Dystrophy Association event.

the evaluation visit, James had 20-degree hip and knee flexion contractures and 15-degree plantar flexion contractures. He could transfer to and from the floor using a Gower's maneuver and was able to independently ambulate at home and for short distances at school using a wide-based toe-toe gait with excessive lumbar lordosis. He used a manual wheelchair as his primary means of mobility at school and reported that his manual wheelchair was fitted with power assist wheels to reduce upper extremity effort, but James did not like it and said it worked like a "bucking bronco." He was given bilateral heel wedges in his shoes and bilateral knee immobilizers, and the family was shown how to perform myofascial release to stretch hamstrings and gastrocnemius muscles. It was recommended that James be fitted with a power wheelchair with seat elevator. He was only seen for 3 months to help the family develop an appropriate

home program and obtain needed equipment. Two years later, his therapist met the family at a social event and James was happily maneuvering among the crowd with his power chair, raised to eye level with others. His family reported that he had started high school that year, and they had gotten reports from the teachers that he was often late to class. They were concerned that the crowded hallways may have been an issue for him to access his classes on time, but when they asked James, he told them it was because all the kids wanted to "high-five" him as he rolled through the halls. **Table 8-5** shows ICF considerations for James's case. See also **Figure 8-6**.

Case Question

Why do you think a power wheelchair with seat elevator option was recommended for James?

TABLE 8-5 • ICF Considerations for James's Case	
Child's name and age	James, age 13 years
Health condition	• Duchenne muscular dystrophy (DMD) • Cardiomyopathy
Body function and structures	• Muscle weakness • Joint contractures • Cardiac arrhythmias • Respiratory muscle dysfunction
Activity limitations	• Difficulty with independent mobility: walking, manual wheelchair • Difficulty with bathing and self-care routines
Participation restrictions	• Decreasing ability to self-propel wheelchair in community/school settings • Difficulty with keeping up with peers: school, social outings • Unable to participate in athletic activities with peers • Unable to participate in household duties such as meal prep, cleaning, etc.
Environmental factors	• Facilitators: computers/technology, school supports (Individualized Education Plan, paraprofessional assistance, additional time for class change), home modifications (ramps, bathchair), proactive family, social acceptance and peer support • Barriers: manual wheelchair (unable to use in community/school); insurance/funding limitations for power wheelchair, therapy, etc.
Personal factors	• Facilitators: self-awareness and positive attitude about DMD • Barriers: limited knowledge of adaptive modifications (heel wedges/orthoses) and power wheelchair options (seat elevator, smaller power base, custom seating)

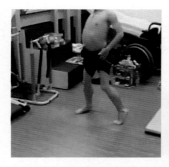
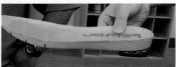
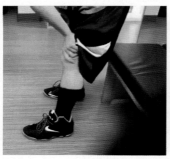
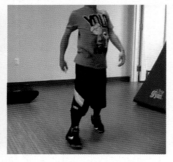

FIGURE 8-6 From left to right: James toe walks with a wide base of support and excessive lordosis when barefoot. Bilateral heel wedges and consistent stretching result in improved gait pattern, although some compensations persist.

Case 3

Matthew

Matthew was first seen upon request of the local wheelchair supplier who had been servicing Matthew's wheelchair for years. Matthew was going to turn 40 years old in 2 weeks and had a diagnosis of DMD, along with an extensive medical history as follows.

Medical/Surgical History for Matthew

1. Left lateral skull fracture, age 2
2. Diagnosed with DMD via muscle biopsy, age 5
3. Achilles tendon lengthening, age 10
4. Buckled compression fracture left humerus, age 10
5. Wheelchair dependent, age 10
6. Spinal stabilization with Luki-Harrington rod, age 13
7. Respiratory failure, age 25
8. Pneumothorax left upper lobe, age 25
9. Tracheostomy and ventilator dependent, age 25
10. Gastrostomy tube placed then removed after swallow study with tracheostomy, age 25
11. Infusaport placement right subclavian, age 25
12. Pneumonia left lower lobe, age 28
13. Cardiomegaly, age 33
14. Appendicitis/appendectomy, age 38

Matthew's medications include an albuterol inhaler, heparin, and furosemide.

Matthew had recently been having difficulty tolerating the planar custom seating system in his power wheelchair, which he operated using a sip and puff control interface. The chair was over 10 years old, and the seat was over 5 years old. Matthew was fully dependent for all transfers and ADLs and used a ventilator full time, but he was a very bright and articulate young man, who easily described his needs for wheelchair modifications and what had been successfully used in the past. A new custom-molded seating system and power wheelchair with power tilt and recline was ordered and fitted. Approximately a year later, Matthew was seen again and was noted to have difficulty with the sip and puff interface and had gained weight and thus was not fitting comfortably in his custom-molded seating. He wanted to try a track ball or mini joystick to control the chair but also noted that he was using a touchscreen on his phone. While seated in the chair, Matthew's lumbar lordosis was increased, and he was not actually sitting against the seat back. When given manual support to the abdomen, he was much more comfortable and was able to fit into the seat back. Modifications were made to his current wheelchair for a touch pad interface, abdominal binder, and custom-molded upper extremity supports on the wheelchair for his fingers to be appropriately positioned and supported for control while driving. **Table 8-6** shows ICF considerations for Matthew's case. See also **Figure 8-7**.

Case Activity: Investigate!

Look up the different types of adaptive wheelchair controls online, like the sip and puff system, touchpad interface, or joystick controls. What factors would you have to consider in deciding which option is best?

Answers will vary depending on your search. There are many options out there! ROM, strength, motor control, cognitive level, dexterity, and cost factors, among others, may impact the choice.

■ SPINAL MUSCULAR ATROPHY

ETIOLOGY, CLASSIFICATION, KEY FEATURES, AND DIAGNOSIS

SMA is a disease in which degeneration of α-motor neurons in the lower spinal cord leads to progressive muscle weakness and atrophy. The death of these motor neurons is related to lack of survival motor neuron (SMN), a protein encoded by the *SMN1* and *SMN2* genes. In healthy individuals, *SMN1* is the gene in charge of producing functional SMN protein, whereas the *SMN2* gene produces only partially functional SMN protein. Most forms of SMA are caused by mutations in *SMN1*, so production of partially functional SMN protein by the neighboring *SMN2* gene will take precedence and will modulate the prognosis and severity of the disease.[1,90] Despite its name, SMN protein is not exclusive to the nervous system and actually fulfills a variety of roles in many different cell tissues. SMN is involved in cellular homeostatic pathways, mRNA trafficking and local translation, cytoskeletal dynamics, endocytosis, and bioenergetic pathways, among other processes.[91] SMA can affect the muscles that act in walking, sitting, upper extremity movement, head control, breathing, and swallowing.

> ### Key Concept
>
> SMA not only affects trunk and extremity function, but can also impact muscles involved in head control, breathing, and swallowing.

TABLE 8-6 • ICF Considerations for Matthew's Case

Name and age	Matthew, age 40 years
Health condition	• Duchenne muscular dystrophy (DMD) • Tracheostomy/ventilator dependent • Cardiomegaly • History of multiple fractures
Body function and structures	• Muscle weakness/flaccidity • Cardiopulmonary dysfunction • Osteoporosis • Scoliosis • Joint contractures • Increased weight gain
Activity limitations	• Difficulty with all gross motor–related functions: positioning, transfers, mobility • Difficulty with all self-care activities • Unable to change positions, transfer, or manage activities of daily living
Participation restrictions	• Unable to independently use power wheelchair in the community with current sip and puff controls • Unable to participate in activities/outings without attendant
Environmental factors	• Facilitators: appropriate medical care, adaptive technology for computer use, alternative controls for power wheelchair, adaptive equipment for home (bathchair, bed, patient lift, ventilator), supportive family • Barriers: aging parents who are primary caretakers, needs new power wheelchair, custom-molded seating, and new alternative controls using mini joystick and touch pad
Personal factors	• Facilitators: proactive in own care and decision-making, well-informed and knowledgeable about DMD, positive outlook regarding his condition • Barriers: distance from siblings and other family members for support

Classically, SMA types were defined by the age of disease onset and the achievement of motor milestones, as described in **Table 8-7**.

In 2007, standard-of-care guidelines for SMA were published,[92] with the most recent update developed in 2017 and released in 2018. The latest standard-of-care guidelines for SMA highlight the importance of early identification, anticipatory guidance, proactive care, and interdisciplinary care.[90,93] The guidelines recommend that clinical suspicion of SMA warrants referral for genetic testing because testing is highly sensitive and specific. Mutations of the *SMN1* gene confirm the diagnosis of SMA, and the number of copies of *SMN2* determines the prognosis.[90] Additional testing components may include compound motor action potential (CMAP) and nerve conduction velocity (NCV); CMAP would be diminished,[94] whereas NCV would be normal.

The clinical findings listed in **Table 8-8** are red flags that would indicate the need for diagnostic referral to a neurologist for suspicion of SMA.

MEDICAL MANAGEMENT

Historically, the management of patients with SMA was guided by the type of SMA determined during initial diagnosis (SMA type I, II, or III). However, there has been a recent major shift in management strategies, particularly since the publication of the latest revision of the SMA clinical guidelines. Nowadays, management is focused on current functional ability (nonsitters, sitters, or walkers) rather than on disease classification. This results in a more customized, patient-centered approach that recognizes the uniqueness of each child and the potential for

varied outcomes, rather than the previously more rigid framework that prejudged each child's future abilities based on a diagnostic label. This has become particularly important in the age of therapeutic drug innovations for SMA. Although some of these therapies are still in the early stages of clinical application, so far there have been striking differences in functional outcomes for most children who have received the treatment versus those who do not (or those who started the treatment later in life), regardless of having the same diagnostic classification (see Kaden and Kenna's case study later in this chapter). An additional development in the management of SMA has been the move toward early diagnosis, with some regions of the world implementing standardized newborn screening. The United States added SMA to the Recommended Uniform Screening Panel (RUSP) in 2018.[1]

> **Key Concept**
>
> Management of SMA has become more customized to individual patient functional needs rather than being solely based on disease classification. Advances in pharmacological interventions have blurred the lines between SMA types and have created an even bigger need for tailored approaches.

Management of children with SMA involves orthopedic care, pulmonary care, rehabilitative care, nutritional and gastrointestinal care, and care of other organs. One of the main areas of concern in orthopedic care is scoliosis, which

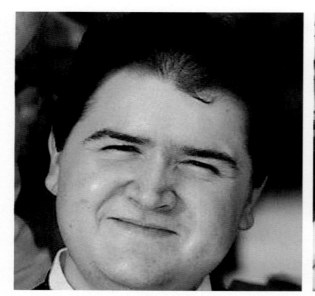
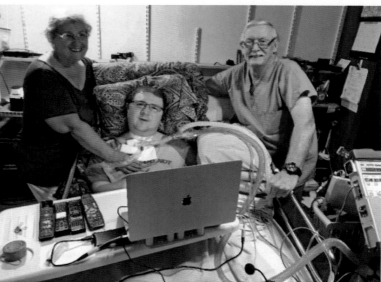
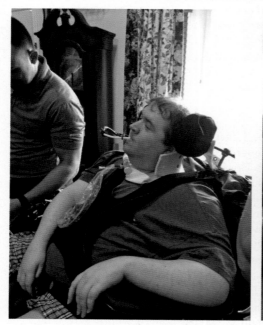
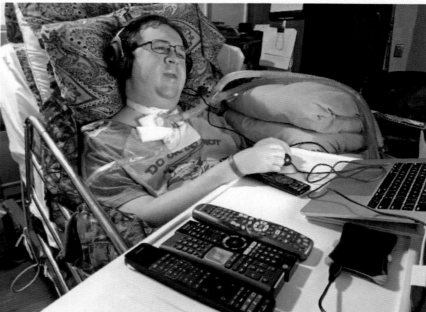

FIGURE 8-7 **Matthew receives supportive ventilation. He uses different adaptive controls to operate his chair and his computer.**

TABLE 8-7 • Types of Spinal Muscular Atrophy (SMA) in Children[1]	
SMA Type	**Characteristics**
Type I (Werdnig-Hoffmann)	Onset before 6 months of age, head lag, difficulty with antigravity movement in supine and prone, oral motor weakness, limited respiratory function, life expectancy around 2 years
Type II	Onset between 6 months and 1 year, not pulling to stand in first year of life, progressive weakness, fasciculations and fine tremors, delay in motor skills particularly quadruped and prone, can sit but not walk, often survive to adulthood (~70%) but may require ventilation
Type III (Kugelberg-Welander)	Onset after age 1, achieve independent ambulation but may eventually lose it, prognosis worse with earlier onset, progressive weakness, fasciculations, decreased deep tendon reflexes

Note. Note that other forms of SMA exist, such as type IV (onset in adulthood) and type X-linked (similar to type I SMA but with a different inheritance pattern and severe joint involvement), among others. The 3 types listed in the table are the most common and are autosomal recessive.

TABLE 8-8 • Clinical Red Flags for Spinal Muscular Atrophy[92,95]

- Hypotonia
- Baby who does not bear weight on legs when suspended by armpits
- Lack of head control by age 1-2 months, or head control not improving
- Lack of righting response: body acting on body
- Progressive symmetric proximal weakness, lower extremities more affected than upper extremities
- Weakness of the intercostal muscles with paradoxical breathing; diaphragm relatively spared
- Decreased deep tendon reflexes
- Regression of motor skills

is managed with orthoses or with surgery in curves greater than 50 degrees and after age 4. Surgery may involve growing rods or spinal fusion depending on skeletal maturity.[96] One of the most recent advances in surgical considerations is the potential for creation of a window for future intrathecal access to deliver medication. Pulmonary care includes clinical assessment of inspiratory and expiratory weakness and chest wall abnormalities, functional pulmonary testing, assessment and treatment of sleep-disordered breathing, and promotion of effective airway clearance. Again, the approach is proactive, with use of noninvasive positive-pressure ventilation prior to signs of respiratory failure. Individuals with SMA are particularly susceptible to respiratory infection, aspiration, and impaired airway clearance. Nutritional and gastrointestinal care includes assessment and treatment of swallowing dysfunction and dysphagia, weight management, monitoring intake of fluids and nutrients with special emphasis on vitamin D and calcium to promote bone health, and in some cases, placement of a feeding tube. Finally, the guidelines also emphasize the importance of parent education on the diagnosis, treatment options, and prognosis. Studies have shown, particularly in the case of severe SMA, that parent education and resources for decision-making and advocacy need to be improved and expanded.[97]

Research into medications to treat SMA has included both SMN-dependent and SMN-independent approaches. SMN-dependent strategies try to increase the available amount of functional SMN protein by either modifying the splicing of *SMN2* RNA (with the goal of producing functional SMN protein) or replacing the faulty *SMN1* gene (using viral vector–based gene therapy). SMN-independent strategies aim to reduce symptoms by enhancing muscle activation. Several molecules, some SMN-dependent approaches and some SMN-independent, are currently in clinical trials. In December 2016, the splicing modifier nusinersen (Spinraza®) became the first approved treatment for SMA.[98] Nusinersen is an antisense oligonucleotide that targets *SMN2*, resulting in an increase in functional production of SMN protein. It is administered by intrathecal injection and was approved after showing great promise in several clinical trials (CS3A, ENDEAR, CHERISH, and NURTURE),[99] with improvement

of motor function for pediatric patients with type II and type III SMA and improved survival in pediatric patients with type I SMA.[98,100,101] Although nusinersen does not technically "make the patient change SMA type," it does change the phenotype and clinical progression of SMA, so patients who may not have been expected to sit or walk are able to do so. Starting the treatment at an earlier age seems to have a larger impact on function,[99,102] when comparing children who otherwise had similar trajectories. Like many other genetic therapies, one of the main disadvantages of nusinersen is its high cost.[98] A more recent alternative to nusinersen is risdiplam (Evrysdi®), which was approved by the FDA in 2020 and can be administered orally.[103] Both treatments require long-term administration, but other emerging treatments can be administered in a single dose, such as onasemnogene abeparvovec-xioi (Zongelsma®), which was approved by the FDA in 2019 and is an adeno-associated virus vector–based gene therapy.[55] Cost, however, continues to be a barrier.[104]

Nutritional supplementation has also been proposed as a treatment approach for SMA, including the administration of valproic acid and L-carnitine, but clinical trials have not demonstrated any significant functional effect.[105-107]

SPINAL MUSCULAR ATROPHY PHYSICAL THERAPY MANAGEMENT ACROSS THE LIFE SPAN

The characteristic features of SMA are progressive muscle weakness and loss of motor function.[108] The progression trajectories, however, are different depending on the age of onset because some patients in the ambulatory group may gain function over time but eventually decline.[109] Also, the existence of new medications is changing the phenotype of the patients who come to physical therapy clinics. These patients may actually start gaining skills, which is something that was previously not possible. Functionally, patients are classified as nonsitters, sitters, or walkers.[90] The goal of physical therapy is to promote optimal motor function and independence, while minimizing contractures. ROM, positioning, exercises, orthoses, developmental milestones, weight-bearing activities for bone health, and caregiver education are crucial components of the overall approach to rehabilitation of children with SMA. An important general precaution when treating patients with SMA is their increased incidence of hip dislocation,[110] which must be considered in therapeutic planning.

> **Key Concept**
>
> Physical therapy management of children with SMA focuses on functional independence, developmentally appropriate activities, positional support, maintaining functional range of motion and strength, and education.

As with other neuromuscular diseases, it is crucial to establish an assessment baseline, which is then periodically updated. **Table 8-9** summarizes the most commonly used assessments

TABLE 8-9 • Functional Assessments in Spinal Muscular Atrophy (SMA)

Functional Assessment	Details
Hammersmith Functional Motor Scale–Expanded (HFMSE)[99,111-113] and Revised Hammersmith Scale (RHS)[114]	Key outcome measure in SMA clinical trials. Gives objective information on motor ability and clinical progression for individuals with type II and type III SMA. Quick, easy to use, reproducible and reliable, and validated in SMA. Correlates with respiratory and motor strength. Items assessed include the ability to roll, sit independently, or walk. Maximum score is 66 points. Has floor and ceiling effects so may need to be combined with other measures below. A revised version of the scale, the RHS, has been developed to address some of the psychometric issues with the expanded scale. It was published in 2017 and consists of 36 items and 2 timed tests.
Children's Hospital of Philadelphia Infant Test for Neuromuscular Disorder scale (CHOP INTEND)[115]	16-item scale (0-64 points) designed specifically to capture motor function in infants with SMA type I. Items include spontaneous movement (upper and lower extremities), hand grip, head in midline with visual stimulation, hip adductors, rolling elicited from legs and from arms, shoulder and elbow combined motions, knee extension, hip flexion and foot dorsiflexion, head control, elbow flexion, neck flexion, head and neck extension, and spinal incurvation.
6-Minute walk test (6MWT)[99,116,117]	Functional assessment of endurance. Measures how far child can walk in 6 minutes. Can be safely performed in ambulatory patients with SMA. Correlates with established outcome measures and is sensitive to fatigue-related changes.
Revised Upper Limb Scale (RULM)[99]	20-item instrument to assess activities of daily living in patients with SMA through items involving shoulder, elbow, wrist, and hand function such as bringing hands from lap to table, picking up small items, pushing buttons, and bringing hands above shoulders.
Functional Composite Score[118]	A composite of the scores from the HFMSE, RULM, and 6MWT, where HFMSE and RULM are expressed as a percentage of the maximum score and 6MWT as percentage of predicted normal distance.
Motor Function Measure (MFM)[119]	Functional assessment with 32 items in 3 subsections: standing and transfers, axial and proximal motor capacity, and distal motor capacity.
Timed functional tests[120]	10-m walk test, supine to stand (children with SMA may also demonstrate a Gower's maneuver upon standing from the floor), climb 4 stairs, Timed Up and Go (TUG), single limb stance. The TUG is a useful tool as it includes not only walking but also functional sit/stand components.
Egen Klassifikation (EK) scale[74,75]	For use with children who are not ambulatory. Functional scale focused on activities of daily living, which also includes coughing ability. 17 items scored by interview and observation. Available in several languages.
Hammersmith Infant Neurological Examination (HINE)[121]	For infants from 2 months to 2 years. Includes 3 sections: (1) neurologic examination assessing cranial nerve function, posture, movements, tone, reflexes, and reactions; (2) developmental milestones (head control, sitting, voluntary grasp, ability to kick, rolling, crawling, standing, and walking); and (3) behavioral assessment (state of consciousness, emotional state, social orientation).

Note. This table is not exhaustive but highlights the most commonly used instruments in this population.

of functional ability for children with SMA. The recommendation from the standard SMA care guidelines is that functional assessments should be repeated at 6-month intervals.[90] Therapists should perform baseline and periodic assessment of function, ROM, strength, posture, balance, respiratory function (spirometry, chest wall excursion, ability to cough and clear secretions), aerobic capacity and endurance, functional ability, and participation at home and school.

Participation can be measured, similarly as for other pediatric neuromuscular disorders, using the Pediatric Outcomes Data Collection Instrument, the Pediatric Evaluation of Disability Inventory, the Pediatric Functional Independence Measure, the School Function Assessment, the Pediatric Quality of Life Inventory, and the Activities-Specific Scale for Kids, among others. Increased participation and quality of life are meaningful outcomes that should guide intervention over time.

Physical therapy is a fundamental component of interdisciplinary care in SMA.[122] Therapeutic interventions in children with SMA must consider current function and prognosis and emphasize optimization of functional outcomes. Joint contractures and malalignment have been particularly associated with

reduced functional ability,[123] so maintaining ROM and proper alignment are important in all types of SMA, along with a customized functional developmental progression and the promotion of functional mobility through appropriate use of assistive technology. Orthoses to promote proper positioning and facilitate function are also a relevant component of care.[124]

In nonsitters, therapy will focus on stretching, positioning, achievable developmental milestones, and chest physical therapy. Stretching and positioning may include active and passing stretching along with use of orthoses such as knee immobilizers, KAFOs, thoracolumbosacral orthoses (TLSOs; such as the one shown in **Figure 8-8**), and standers. Recommended minimal frequency for stretching, ROM, and orthosis wear is about 5 times per week.[90] Seating systems must be properly designed to provide alignment, support, and proper positioning, and adaptive equipment may be recommended to assist upper extremity function in supported sitting. Developmental progressions will focus on appropriate milestones such as head and trunk control, floor mobility and presitting functional progressions, weight shifting, dynamic balance, and weight bearing as able, including the use of standers as appropriate. Aquatic

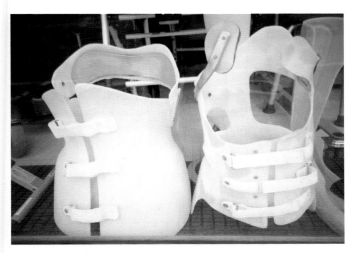

FIGURE 8-8 **Back brace used for Scoliosis correction.** (Used with permission from Luis Diaz Devesa/Getty Images.)

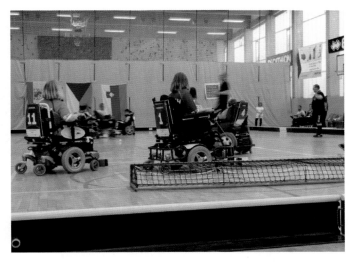

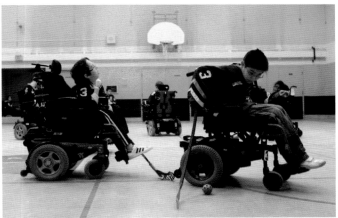

FIGURE 8-9 **(A) Czech Republic, PRAGUE - OCTOBER 11 2019: Powerchair hockey IPCH Qualification Tournament 2019. (B) Wheel chair hockey.** ((A) Used with permission from Gre jak/Alamy Stock Photo. (B) Used with permission from Tara Walton/Getty Images.)

therapy may be feasible with proper support and supervision.[90] Chest physical therapy to enhance clearance and improve breathing may include breathing exercises, percussion, cough training, and postural drainage.

For children who are sitters, in addition to the techniques mentioned for nonsitters, additional functional mobility tasks and transitional skills can be emphasized. Reciprocal gait orthoses and KAFOs can be used to promote therapeutic ambulation,[90] and some stronger children may be able to use manual wheelchairs, but powered wheelchairs will be the primary means of functional mobility. Power mobility should be introduced very early on, before the age of 2 (see Lenix's case study in this chapter).[90,125] Prevention of contractures and appropriate positioning continue to be key components of therapy, with active-assisted stretching and use of orthoses. Serial casting may be an adjuvant approach to maintaining ROM. Standing frames can also be used in this population to obtain the benefits of weight bearing, with frequency and duration recommendations of 5 to 7 times per week for at least 60 minutes at a time.[90] Standing programs must be designed with the entire family and care team in mind and considering child status and development, family goals and priorities, and available resources.[126] Scoliosis prevention is a key concern,[127] so custom seating systems are important, and thoracic orthoses are often prescribed to assist function and trunk control. Exercise to increase endurance and strength should be promoted while avoiding fatigue. Aquatic exercise, hippotherapy, or adaptive sports (**Figure 8-9**) may be appropriate depending on the child.[128,129]

For children who are ambulatory, aerobic exercise that promotes endurance, strength, and balance is recommended 3 to 5 days a week for 30 minutes each day.[90] Fatigue is a common characteristic of SMA, even for children who are ambulatory.[109] Thus, the exercise plan should be designed so that it avoids fatigue or overexertion but still has training benefits. Concentric and eccentric exercise can be used, and research has shown that progressive resistance training exercise programs can be feasible and safe in this population.[130] Aquatic therapy may also be used.[131] Maintaining ROM through stretching and orthoses

should also be part of the plan of care as appropriate. Manual wheelchairs or wheelchairs with power assist may be indicated (**Figure 8-10**), as well as power mobility for long distances if the child has limited endurance.

Case 4

Kaden and Kenna, Brother and Sister

Kaden had his initial physical therapy evaluation at 7 months of age, within days of being evaluated by a neurologist who suspected SMA but had not diagnosed it yet. He was assessed with the Alberta Infant Motor Scale (AIMS), with motor skills noted between 0 and 5th percentile. Kaden had no head lifting in prone or rolling, could maintain tripod sitting with rounded spine, could not bear weight on his legs at all, had significantly decreased strength in all proximal muscle groups, and demonstrated better active motion in hands and ankles. Physical therapy goals were established to provide supportive seating and stander, orthoses, and improved head/trunk alignment with supports. Within a few weeks, Kaden had a formal diagnosis of SMA type II. By 13 months of age, his family had initiated

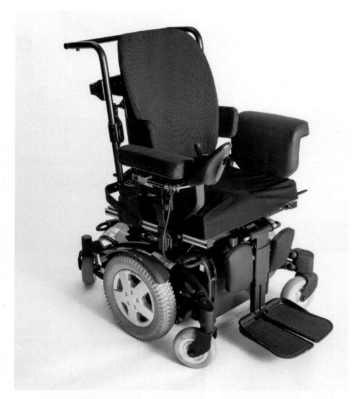

FIGURE 8-10 Empty electric wheel chair. (Used with permission from Risal Khan/Shutterstock.)

support through CureSMA, via online sources. They began supplementing with Tolerex, an elemental free form amino acid formula combined with continued breast feeding; enrolled him in aquatic therapy; and purchased a Panthera ultra-lightweight manual wheelchair (weighs only 5 lb), which Kaden was able to

self-propel. Kaden was fitted with a soft trunk orthosis, AFOs, and a mobile prone stander. By this time, although Kaden was able to sit without upper extremity support, he needed supervision due to lack of protective or righting responses. His AIMS score had progressed from a 3-month-old level to 4-month-old level. By 19 months of age, Kaden could roll over his left side and, if positioned, could push a ride-on toy backward with his feet for short distances with support to trunk for balance. He was fitted with hip-knee-ankle-foot orthoses for improved alignment of his lower extremities, as he was beginning to develop knee flexion contractures, and to allow him the opportunity to play in standing at a low table.

At 2 years 6 months, Kaden was hospitalized and had a nasogastric tube placed for 6 weeks, followed by gastrostomy tube placement to supplement oral feeding and maintain hydration. He began using a cough assist and nebulizer treatments on a regular basis. His little sister Kenna was born when he was 2 years 9 months of age. She was diagnosed at birth with the same genome for SMA as Kaden. Both children were enrolled in the Spinraza (nusinersen) trials as soon as FDA approval was given 2 weeks after Kenna was born. The siblings have been receiving intrathecal nusinersen injections every 4 months. When Kaden was evaluated recently at 4 years of age, it was noted that he had made some improvements in gross motor skills and strength and was able to pivot in sitting, tall kneel with minimal assistance at a supporting surface, perform pelvic bridge with feet supported, reach for toys outside of his base of support in sitting, maintain bench sitting with upper extremities extended overhead, and take 5 steps in his KidWalk gait trainer. **Table 8-10** lists ICF considerations for Kaden's case.

Kenna has never received physical therapy services. She independently sat, crawled, and walked within normal limits for her age. She is 19 months of age in the picture shown in **Figure 8-11**.

TABLE 8-10 • ICF Considerations for Kaden's Case	
Child's name and age	Kaden, age 4
Health condition	• Spinal muscular atrophy (SMA) type II • Gastrostomy tube
Body function and structures	• Muscle weakness • Respiratory dysfunction/history of pneumonia
Activity limitations	• Difficulty with standing/walking/mobility skills • Difficulty with self-help skills • Difficulty with safe swallowing thin liquids • Difficulty with clearing secretions/coughing • Unable to complete self-care activities
Participation restrictions	• Unable to independently transfer or participate in age-appropriate motor activities with peers such as walking, using playground equipment, etc. • Unable to attend daycare
Environmental factors	• Facilitators: participated in clinical trials/currently treated with nusinersen, ongoing therapy supports, adaptive equipment (power wheelchair, stander, orthotics/thoracolumbosacral orthosis, bathchair), proactive and well-informed family, SMA support groups • Barriers: 3 hours from medical center for nusinersen treatment (and needs to return every 4 months), home needs modification for safety and independence
Personal factors	• Facilitators: bright and happy personality, younger sister to play with • Barriers: distance from extended family for support

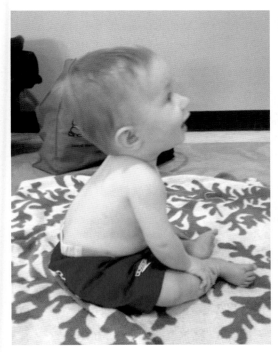 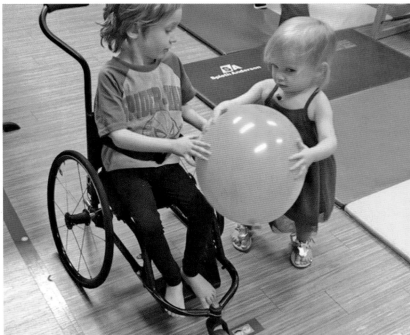

FIGURE 8-11 **Left: Kaden at 7 months of age. Notice decreased trunk tone, rounded spine, and hand use to provide support in sitting. Right: Kaden and Kenna play together.**

Case Activity

Reflect on how Kaden's prognosis has changed over the years. What would be some of the next developmental activities he may be able to work on?

Case 5

Lenix

Lenix was referred through early intervention for evaluation at the child daycare he attended at 9 months of age. At that time, Lenix had been receiving outpatient therapy at a local hospital for 2 months due to motor delays. The evaluation at the daycare revealed that Lenix lacked head control in prone and was unable to lift and turn his head. He exhibited no lower extremity movement off the mat in supine but moved ankles and feet. He was very social and responsive and enjoyed tactile stimulation throughout trunk and extremities. He exhibited a very weak cough, decreased deep tendon reflexes, and tongue fasciculations. The physical therapy evaluation from the outpatient clinic was available for review and was very thorough in describing similar findings in motor skills and strength. However, the hospital documentation included a recommendation to wait 1 to 2 months before referring to a neurologist if improvement was not seen. During the initial early intervention physical therapy evaluation at the daycare, the therapist discussed her findings with the parent and her concerns about the recommendation to wait for improvement. The therapist felt it was important to call the pediatrician to recommend referral to a neurologist as soon as possible, rather than waiting. The therapist also called the family support coordinator for early intervention later to discuss concerns and request additional support.

Lenix was seen the following week by a neurologist for bloodwork and testing. Two weeks later, at the follow-up neurology appointment, his mother was given a diagnosis of SMA type I and was told Lenix would not live past 1 year of age. Four weeks after the diagnosis, Lenix was hospitalized for pneumonia and remained hospitalized for 6 weeks. He was discharged home with nebulizer treatments daily every 4 hours plus oral albuterol. Therapy goals were established to educate family and daycare staff regarding SMA and the need to maintain respiratory health, provide external support in upright sitting, and facilitate participation in daycare and home setting routines. Lenix remained healthy and had no further hospitalizations throughout his time at the daycare. He was a bright and social child, and at 15 months, Lenix was successfully able to maneuver a power wheelchair during a trial. The vendor allowed his family to practice with Lenix using the loaner power wheelchair at home until he was ready for his own wheelchair at 2 years of age. Lenix remained successfully integrated in the regular daycare classrooms for infants and toddlers, with the support of a special positioning chair and with protective supports while sitting on the floor during playtime. Lenix was not able to take the power wheelchair to school, as it would be a safety concern with other toddlers not understanding it was not just another toy, but he used it at home to drive in his house, around the neighborhood, and to go to the park.

Unfortunately, when he turned 3 years old, the daycare staff told Lenix's family that they could not continue to keep him in their program because the children his age were no longer having their diapers changed and were expected to participate in more tabletop activities. The daycare loved Lenix, but they did not feel they had the right equipment for him to be safely and

TABLE 8-11 • ICF Considerations for Lenix's Case

Child's name and age	Lenix, age 3
Health conditions	• Spinal muscular atrophy type I • Pneumonia
Body function and structures	• Muscle weakness • Scoliosis • Pulmonary dysfunction
Activity limitations	• Difficulty with all transfers, positioning, mobility, self-care • Difficulty with positioning, mobility, and toileting • Difficulty with clearing secretions
Participation restrictions	• Unable to use toilet, playground, and change positions at daycare • Unable to participate in motor activities with peers
Environmental factors	• Facilitators: attended same daycare since birth, well-loved by all daycare providers, age-appropriate peers and educational services at daycare, ramp into home, Early Steps therapy services since age 7 months, loving and supportive family • Barriers: daycare not adapted, needed special chair and toilet to progress to 3-year-old class, more exposure to common childhood illness in daycare
Personal factors	• Facilitators: very bright and happy, recent little brother added to family • Barriers: family received limited medical support and information

appropriately positioned and were worried he or his teachers might get hurt. This was devastating news for the family, who loved the daycare and had a new 3-month-old baby at the same daycare. Through a local charity, his therapist helped the family obtain an adaptive toilet system and a hydraulic high-low activity chair to be used at school, and the daycare agreed that Lenix could stay. The therapist trained the staff and teachers to transfer and position Lenix safely. Lenix was toilet trained shortly after he received the adaptive toilet. His teachers noted that when they tested him at age 3, Lenix scored at a 5-year-old level for verbal skills, and they called him the "teacher's assistant." Much of the therapist's role for Lenix involved providing training and adaptive equipment to allow him to remain with his peers at the daycare. The local charity that purchased the adaptive toilet and classroom chair for Lenix invited his family to be guests at their annual fundraiser. Lenix charmed the crowd with his precocious personality and eagerness to pull the raffle tickets during the event. Sadly, a few months later, after a serious pneumonia and a short hospitalization, Lenix died very unexpectedly at the age of 3 years, 4 months. **Table 8-11** lists ICF considerations for Lenix's case. See also **Figure 8-12**.

Case Activity

Reflect on how physical therapists can be advocates for early and accurate diagnosis, as well as promote inclusion for children with neuromuscular disorders. Find examples in the case of how the therapist was able to act as an advocate.

Case 6

AJ

AJ has Spinal Muscular Atrophy (SMA) and has been using a wheelchair since he was two. **Table 8-12** *shows ICF considerations for AJ's case. He has been adamant about not letting his disease define him, and despite only having limited functional*

use of his hands as an adult, he has charted his course as a professional graphic designer by leveraging the use of technology to allow him to create digital art. He graduated with a BFA from Digital Media Arts College and currently works as a designer, specializing in digital illustration techniques, branding, and other print design products.

His webpage is http://ajbrockman.com/, and you can see samples of his digital art at http://www.singlehandedstudio.com. Some publicly available videos highlighting his story and accomplishments include "Painting with one finger: The story of AJ Brockman" (https://vimeo.com/35548780), "AJ Brockman: Anything is possible" (https://www.youtube.com/watch?v=1oP9LWcvTt8), and "Digital Media Arts College Student Spotlight: AJ Brockman" (https://www.youtube.com/watch?v=MyoWmP_JQL0)

■ OTHER PEDIATRIC NEUROMUSCULAR DISEASES

As we mentioned at the beginning of the chapter, there are numerous pediatric neuromuscular diseases, as this is a broad label that can include disorders of the anterior motor neuron (e.g., SMA), the peripheral nerve (e.g., Charcot-Marie-Tooth disease), the neuromuscular junction (eg, congenital myasthenic syndrome), and the muscle (myopathies and muscular dystrophies such as DMD). It is impossible to cover them all in a single chapter, but in this section, we provide a brief overview of congenital myopathies and a case example of a patient with congenital myopathy with neuropathy.

Congenital myopathies (CMs) are genetic muscle disorders that involve abnormal myofiber structure as well as, in some cases, abnormal protein accumulation in the sarcoplasm. There are several different types of CMs depending on their underlying etiology and pathophysiology. The most common CMs are core myopathies, nemaline myopathy, and centronuclear myopathy, although there is a spectrum of CMs.[1,132] A lot remains

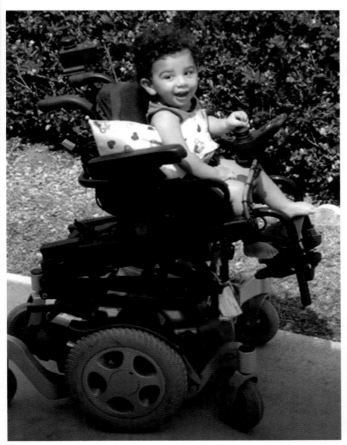 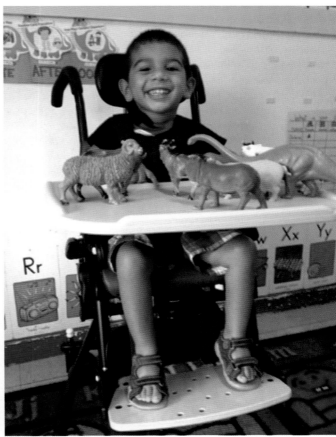

FIGURE 8-12 Left: Lenix using a power chair at age 15 months. Right: Lenix in his adaptive classroom chair.

TABLE 8-12 • ICF Considerations for AJ's Case	
Name and age	AJ, age 30
Health condition	• Spinal muscular atrophy type II • Tracheostomy
Body function and structures	• Muscle weakness • Musculoskeletal deformity/scoliosis • Pulmonary dysfunction
Activity limitations	• Difficulty with transfers, self-help, positioning • Difficulty with clearing secretions
Participation restrictions	• Unable to move independently in home and community without power wheelchair • Unable to hold paintbrush as an artist
Environmental factors	• Facilitators: educational opportunities in high school/college to earn bachelor of fine arts, owns art studio, co-owns art gallery/brewhouse, consistent medical support, access to technology (drives power chair with chin control, paints digitally with 2 fingers) • Barriers: need for personal attendant for all self-care and positioning needs
Personal factors	• Facilitators: bright and motivated, recognizes own talent, willingness and awareness of alternative methods for producing art, living his own dream • Barriers: limited motor skills for all activities

to be explored in terms of the pathophysiology of these myopathies, but recent research suggest that there are common abnormalities in excitation-contraction coupling.[132] These diseases present with hypotonia, weakness, reduced endurance, and pain, but unlike children with congenital muscular dystrophy, weakness is less progressive or even static and there is usually no central nervous system involvement.[133-135] Common orthopedic problems include congenital dislocations of the hip and scoliosis; respiratory complications are also common.[135]

As with many other neuromuscular diseases, muscle weakness and asymmetrical muscle forces can give rise to joint contractures. Minimizing loss of ROM should be an important part of care and can be achieved with stretching, orthoses, and serial casting. Patients may present with exercise-induced myalgias, so exercise must be carefully tailored to each patient, and the therapist should emphasize energy conservation, activity modification, and the use of mobility devices such as walkers, scooters, and wheelchairs as necessary.[135] Environmental modifications such as ramps, lifts, or rails can enhance safety and increase participation at school. Customized exercise programs to increase endurance and maintain strength are recommended 2 to 3 times per week and should be focused on concentric work.[135] Children who have mobility difficulties will benefit from adaptive sports as well as the use of standers to promote bone, gastrointestinal, respiratory, and cardiovascular health.

Case 7

A Parent Perspective, Siblings Alora and Mason: Congenital Myopathy/Axonal Neuropathy *SPTBN4* Genetic Mutation

Mom's story is as follows: (written by mom when Alora was almost 3 years old):

Alora was born in the Bahamas, 6 lbs 2 oz and nothing was ever mentioned about anything being wrong with her. She was tiny, as she did lose weight those first couple days and dropped to 5 lbs 8 oz. She moved her arms and legs around (looking back and now after paying attention to other newborns, she did not have the normal movements of her arms and legs, they did not move a lot), and her neck was very weak, but we thought it was because she was so small and figured she would catch up. Alora had a very weak suck and never actually drank more than 4-5 oz at one time (at about 4 months old). She mostly drank small amounts (2-3 oz) often as she got tired from working so hard to drink her formula. She made eye contact on time, smiled on time, and even rolled once or twice…. We really started to notice when she was about two months old that she had no neck strength and that she was very difficult to hold. Her joints were loose. And this was only because we were around another baby of the same age, and we couldn't believe the difference. We called the pediatrician in Florida (no pediatrician in Abaco), and she said to give her more tummy time. We tried, and she was just barely lifting her head and getting it up and holding for a few seconds. We brought her to Florida when she was around four months old. The pediatrician told us she was extremely floppy, and we needed to get into a neurologist right away. At this time, Alora was able to lift her arms and legs against gravity a fair amount of time when she was lying on her back or in a supported sitting position. We met the neurologist that week and he told us she was on the moderate to severe end for being floppy. He immediately thought SMA but also did some metabolic tests along with some other genetic tests. And he told us to get her into therapy as soon as possible. He also sent us for a heart ultrasound and an EKG to check her out as he said he wanted to be sure that the heart muscle wasn't affected as well. All tests he performed were either normal or negative.

When she was 6 months old, she became sick with RSV and was hospitalized. While in hospital, they also did a video swallow study to confirm that she didn't get pneumonia from aspirating. She passed the video swallow. The negative results for the SMA test came in while she was in hospital and Dr. Liu called the lab to have them agree to test her again, because he was convinced she had SMA after seeing her again in the hospital. They agreed to re-test, but she was negative, again. We went to Miami Children's Hospital to see a geneticist when she was around 10 months old. The doctor wanted us to see an eye doctor because her pupils were different sizes and to also have a brain MRI. We went to the eye doctor, who said that the structure of her eye was fine and she was able to see, only that one eye innervates different than the other. She does not have crossed eyes or anything, but still has different sized pupils. The brain MRI was also normal. The geneticist couldn't really give us anything else to test for as she felt like the neurologist had covered

what she would do. She said we would have to wait and see if any other symptoms appeared unrelated to the hypotonia (like seizures) and see how she developed. We continued in therapy, without much improvement, sadly. Even today, when she is almost 3 years old, therapy still consists of the same things we were doing when she was 6 months old. Working on head control, rolling, and reaching.

I got pregnant with Mason (unplanned) when Alora was a year and a half old in the fall of 2013. We called the doctors and asked if there was anything else we can test for or anything we can do to reveal anything about our developing baby. They of course could not offer any help, only that there would be possibly a 25% chance of the same condition, as he believed it was a recessive disease. At 9 weeks, we tested for chromosome abnormalities, such as Down syndrome and other prenatal diagnostic testing that is routinely available and everything was negative. We decided that we couldn't terminate. Meanwhile Alora was not gaining any weight. It was getting harder for her to eat and swallow. She was unable to drink water or juice and it was taking so long for her to drink from a bottle that she was getting so tired in the process. She was unable to drink from a straw or a sippy cup. The amount of fluid overwhelmed her. The doctors recommended a G-tube with fundoplication to prevent aspiration. She had a test done that revealed she was having some reflux (can't remember what it was—maybe an upper GI). We had already tried adding Duocal to her pureed foods, but she was still falling off the weight charts. In April of 2014 (she had just turned 2 y), we decided to do the G-tube and fundo, and since she would be under anesthesia, we went ahead and did a muscle biopsy. The muscle biopsy did not reveal anything.

Surgery went well, and within a week of her G-tube she already looked better—hydrated and her skin color was so great. She started gaining weight too. She did start rejecting food within a week though. We were told it was probably due to the fundoplication. We still give her foods to taste but she gags after a few tastes.

Alora right now is 100% tube fed. She is unable to hold her head up (she can lift her head but unfortunately it goes straight back). She is unable to sit unassisted, and unable to weight bear on her arms, so she is unable to push up to steady herself and only moves her legs when she is stretching or excited. Her leg movements have decreased over time, in our opinion. The therapists have previously said to us that it could be because she has gotten heavier, but who knows now. She was able to bring her knees up (she doesn't now) and was able to lift her feet and straighten out her legs but now only does this rarely, as mentioned above, when stretching or excited. She still moves her arms around but has never really been able to reach out or hold anything with intention too well. The little she was able to as a baby quickly became harder for her. Any movement against gravity is very hard and very little. When laying on her back she can move her head from side to side and does move her arms. She can roll from her side to her back and with help she can get from her back to her side. She cannot roll from her tummy position. Her chest has a sunk in appearance (pectus excavatum)

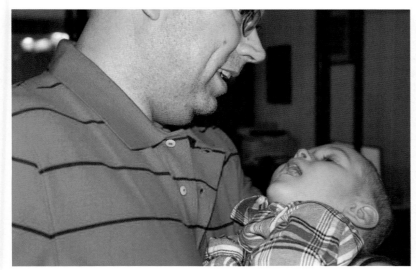
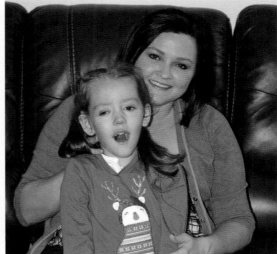

FIGURE 8-13 **Mason (left) and Alora (right).**

due to the lack of muscle tone. She also does not speak, and we are unsure of what she comprehends. We know what TV and toys she likes or dislikes by either smiling/laughing or crying/ whining/complaining. She does recognize people she knows and also takes notice of strangers. She particularly does not like anyone in scrubs.

This family had a history of other relatives with undiagnosed myopathies. Mason was born when Alora was 2 years old but sadly passed away 3 months before his third birthday when Alora was 4 years old (**Figure 8-13**). He was hospitalized at 5 months of age for pneumonia and had a gastrostomy tube with fundoplication placed at that time. Mason remained at home and healthy until both he and Alora contracted RSV, requiring hospitalization in the pediatric intensive care unit for 2 weeks before final respiratory failure. Mason was physically very similar to his sister, with significant muscle weakness, lack of active movement, and normal brain MRI. He loved *Jake and the Never Land Pirates*, loved when his daddy talked silly, and cried when strangers walked into the room. Both children were diagnosed with their own unique genetic disorder following extensive genetic testing and final diagnosis in Texas, identified as the *SPTBN4* genetic mutation. Spectrin is an actin crosslinking and molecular scaffold protein that links the plasma membrane to the actin cytoskeleton and functions in the determination of cell shape, arrangement of transmembrane proteins, and organization of organelles. It is composed of 2 antiparallel dimers of alpha and beta subunits. This gene is one member of a family of beta-spectrin genes. The encoded protein localizes to the nuclear matrix, promyelocytic leukemia nuclear bodies, and cytoplasmic vesicles.

At age 6, Alora has a daily routine of home-based respiratory care, 24-hour postural care, and ROM. She has begun using bilevel positive airway pressure, oxygen as needed, as well as cough assist, vibration vest, and suctioning with nasal cannula and oral cannula. The family has always said they do not want a tracheostomy but recently have begun to consider it. Alora uses the Tobii Eye Gaze communication device and enjoys *Mickey Mouse Clubhouse*, reading books, and playing make-believe with hand-over-hand assistance. Alora is happy and greets familiar people or family with a smile and vocalizes at times with effort to gain attention. Positioning equipment includes nighttime postural supports, a supine stander, tilt and reclining wheelchair with custom seating, contoured supportive seat for relaxation, trunk orthosis, and AFOs, with a variety of pillows, pads, and cushions used as needed to support and align her body optimally and comfortably. **Table 8-13** presents ICF considerations for Alora's case.

Case Activity

Research at least 2 other types of neuromuscular disorders that were not discussed explicitly in this chapter. What is the clinical presentation, prognosis, and therapeutic management for each of them?

■ CONCLUSION

Neuromuscular disorders encompass a large spectrum of diseases, and it is important for the therapist to stay informed of the latest developments in this field. Many of the management principles that we have discussed for DMD and SMA apply to other neuromuscular diagnoses as well, including therapeutic exercise that reduces weakness and increases endurance while avoiding fatigue and tissue damage; ROM exercises, stretching, and orthotic management to promote proper alignment, joint function, posture, and mobility; respiratory care to promote secretion clearance and breathing effectiveness; adaptive and assistive equipment to optimize function and participation in the home, school, and community; and child and caregiver education for self-care and independence. The future of patient management will undoubtedly be shaped by exciting developments emerging from the numerous clinical trials that are investigating therapeutic approaches for many of these diseases.

TABLE 8-13 • ICF Considerations for Alora's Case

Child's name and age	Alora, age 6
Health condition	• Congenital myopathy/axonal neuropathy, *SPTBN4* genetic mutation • Pulmonary complications: pneumonia, respiratory syncytial virus infection • Gastrostomy tube with fundoplication
Body function and structures	• Muscle weakness/hypotonia/atrophy • Multiple bouts of respiratory illness • Feeding difficulties with failure to thrive • Muscle contractures • Scoliosis • Right hip dysplasia
Activity limitations	• Unable to turn in bed • Unable to sit up or stand without maximum support • Unable to use hands for functional activities • Unable to speak • Unable to eat orally
Participation restrictions	• Unable to participate in school, outings >1 hour due to fatigue or play with peers/sibling • Unable to communicate verbally with peers
Environmental factors	• Facilitators: proactive therapeutic interventions including aquatic therapy; trunk, hand, and foot orthoses; positioning equipment; and augmentative and alternative communication eye gaze device. Successful home-based medical care including gastrostomy tube feedings, pulmonary care with suctioning, bilevel positive airway pressure, vibration vest, cough assist, medications, and full-time nursing. Family and nurses are very responsive to needs. • Barriers: peers have difficulty interpreting nonverbal communication.
Personal factors	• Facilitators: able to communicate needs to family and nurses with nonverbal communication • Barriers: unable to self-occupy except with TV/iPad videos

STUDY QUESTIONS

Muscular Dystrophy

1. Often children with a diagnosis of DMD do not need ongoing weekly physical therapy. Why do you think that is the case? What might be some reasons to provide skilled physical therapy interventions and at what frequency?

   a. Considerations: What factors contribute to muscle fiber breakdown, progressive weakness, muscle contractures, and bony deformity? (Resistive exercise, aggressive stretching, impact activities, inactivity, limited position changes, steroids.) What are the parents already doing with their child, and what are their goals? (Most families become very well informed about DMD after receiving the diagnosis through organizations such as the Muscular Dystrophy Association.)

   b. Initial physical therapy may involve caregiver instruction regarding stretching, use of night splints, standing programs, respiratory health, nutrition, and appropriate physical activity such as aquatic therapy/swimming lessons. What are some of the benefits of aquatic activity for children with DMD? (Cardiopulmonary health, strengthening in open chain, reduced resistance, gravity-reduced environment, ROM.)

   c. Episodic care becomes very important during growth spurts, changes in physical activity, when adaptive equipment is needed or needs modifications, or following hospitalizations, surgical interventions, or lengthy illnesses.

2. Often children diagnosed with DMD will need adaptive equipment. What are some things that can help them retain their independence? When and why would you recommend the following devices?

   a. Night stretching AFOs: Needed to maintain heel cord length, may begin as a toddler before significant limitations of passive ROM and to increase family awareness of changes in ROM. May be solid or articulated with toe straps to create dorsiflexor stretch. Usually need to be replaced every year due to growth.

   b. Stander: Needed to maintain heel cord, hip flexor, and knee flexor length; may begin as soon as child demonstrates increased sitting time during elementary school years; best if tied into daily functional routine (e.g., during meals, homework). Prone stander better tolerated than supine; however, as child becomes too large for transfers, a hydraulic sit-to-stand model such as the Easy Stand is easier for caregivers.

(Continued)

c. Wheelchair: manual or power? Family input in the decision-making is important. Consider growth, current physical skills/strength, rate of progression of DMD so far, environment, transportation, functional independence, and social needs. A manual chair is lightweight and will promote upper body strength and pulmonary function but will require adequate strength and endurance for self-propelling longer distances such as at school or in the community. A power wheelchair can have many options that are very helpful for middle to high school students, such as the seat elevator to access cabinets, closets, and counters at home, and have improved ability to navigate through crowded school hallways safely.

3. As children age into adulthood, home modifications, adaptive equipment, and surgical interventions may be needed to assist with care, including the following:

a. Alternative access mode to drive power wheelchairs and use environmental controls help accommodate progressive muscle weakness; plan ahead when ordering.

b. Home modifications may include ramps or level entrances, wider doors for power wheelchairs, roll-in showers for safer, easier transfers and bathing assistance, modified vans with ramps/lifts for transportation of power wheelchair, hospital beds, and spacious rooms to accommodate respiratory supports and additional home care assistants.

c. Adaptive equipment needed may include patient lift systems, such as overhead track lifts and/or portable patient lifts. Track lifts are usually preferred to portable lifts due to space but may not be covered by insurance.

d. A commode/shower transfer chair will allow patient to use the toilet and then be moved into shower on the same chair, with roll-in level entry shower.

e. Respiratory supports are used as needed, including oxygen, ventilator, continuous positive airway pressure, bilevel positive airway pressure, vibration vests, cough assist, and suction machines. Inspiratory muscle training may assist with maintaining pulmonary health, but specific methodology for this type of training has not been well defined, and gains in strength and endurance may not be significant.[136]

f. Surgical interventions may include tendon releases and internal spinal fixation to allow optimal positioning. Tracheostomies, gastrostomy tubes for feeding, and peripherally inserted central catheters (PICC lines) may help to maintain general health and ease of care.

Spinal Muscular Atrophy

1. For children with a diagnosis of SMA types I and II, what rationale can you provide to justify the need for skilled physical therapy intervention and at what frequency?

a. Considerations: What are your physical findings on exam and using standardized testing? Caregivers will have access to well-developed online resources and may have already been seen by specialty centers that have begun treating with nusinersen, so they may have already become well informed about the diagnosis/prognosis, and the patient may have already been fitted with orthoses and adaptive seating, standers, and so on. Therapist's role will be to continue instruction and education, monitoring orthoses and adaptive equipment for appropriate fit, monitoring respiratory function, and adapting developmentally appropriate activities.

b. Children receiving nusinersen injections currently are demonstrating slow improvements in strength and may need ongoing regular services to continue to progress and modify home and school programs. Consider aquatic programs for improving motor function in gravity-reduced environment, as well as building respiratory capacity

c. Children who have not been receiving nusinersen may need more intensive therapy initially, then continued services at decreased frequency to monitor home program, modify equipment for growth, instruct nursing staff, and adapt activities as child ages.

2. Often children diagnosed with SMA need adaptive equipment, but they may be connected to a larger community of families with SMA through larger support organizations. This community often shares outgrown equipment or sell equipment at a reduced cost, such as very small, very lightweight manual wheelchairs or larger power wheelchair sized small enough for toddlers. As a therapist, you may need to help families understand how to use equipment throughout the day to prevent contractures, allow functional control, maintain safety, maintain musculoskeletal alignment, and so on. When and why would you recommend caregivers have their child use the following devices?

a. Trunk orthoses, knee immobilizers, and AFOs: Trunk orthoses for daytime but may interfere with child's ability to self-propel manual wheelchair by inhibiting forward/backward weight shift. Knee immobilizers to prevent knee flexion contractures may be used while long sitting in play, for supported standing, or in stander. AFOs can be worn most of the day to maintain ankle-foot alignment, but they may

(Continued)

interfere with the child's ability to take steps while supported in gait trainer. As the distal muscles tend to be stronger than proximal muscles, the child may compensate for weak hip and knee extension by using ankle plantar flexors for extra push off.

b. Bath/shower chair: Transitioning from infant bath seats to larger bath/shower chair, need to assess family needs, bathroom setup, and so on. Bath chairs are elevated and do not allow the child to play down in the water; however, as the child grows heavier, it is important to maintain safety during bathing and transfers.

c. Stander: Needed to maintain hip integrity and bone integrity, improve bowel function, and improve respiratory function. Prone standers are usually more comfortable and better tolerated. A mobile prone stander allows the child to independently self-propel large wheelchair-style wheels while in the stander, versus being stationary.

Other Neuromuscular Diseases

1. For children with an unknown diagnosis of a neuromuscular disorder, what rationale can you provide to justify the need for skilled physical therapy intervention and at what frequency?

   a. Considerations: What are your physical findings on exam and using standardized testing? For caregivers, there are not going to be the usual online websites to go to because they do not have a diagnosis; there will likely be a lot of questions and need for support. Caregivers will have to rely on the therapist for instruction and education, providing explanation and rationale for implementing stretching; use of orthoses and adaptive equipment for bathing, seating, standing, and so on; respiratory care and monitoring respiratory function; feeding and appropriate nutrition; and adaptive developmentally appropriate activity.

   b. Children may need more intensive therapy initially, then continued services at decreased frequency to monitor home programs, modify equipment for growth, instruct nursing staff, and adapt activities as children age.

2. Often children diagnosed with neuromuscular disorders need adaptive equipment. What are some devices that can help them retain their independence? When and why would you recommend the following devices?

   a. Trunk orthoses, hand splints, and AFOs: Needed to maintain alignment, prevent deformity and limitations of passive ROM, allow improved positioning for feeding, and so on.

   b. Bath chair: Transitioning from infant tubs to larger bath/shower chair, need to assess family needs, bathroom setup, and so on.

   c. Stander: Needed to maintain hip integrity and bone integrity, improve bowel function, and improve respiratory function.

   d. Wheelchair: Manual or power? Family input in the decision-making is important. Consider growth, current physical skills/strength, rate of progression of the disorder so far, environment, transportation, and functional and social skills needs. Stroller-type chair may be needed initially as family begins to transition from infant strollers; eventually wheelchair with custom seating with tilt-in-space option may be needed.

   e. Supine positioning supports for symmetry to decrease progression of deformity in spine, hips, and other areas.

References

1. Rathore G, Kang PB. Pediatric neuromuscular diseases. *Pediatr Neurol.* 2023;149:1-14.
2. Birnkrant DJ, Bushby K, Bann CM, et al. Diagnosis and management of Duchenne muscular dystrophy, part 2: respiratory, cardiac, bone health, and orthopaedic management. *Lancet Neurol.* 2018;17(4):347-361.
3. Birnkrant DJ, Bushby K, Bann CM, et al. Diagnosis and management of Duchenne muscular dystrophy, part 1: diagnosis, and neuromuscular, rehabilitation, endocrine, and gastrointestinal and nutritional management. *Lancet Neurol.* 2018;17(3):251-267.
4. Aartsma-Rus A, Ginjaar IB, Bushby K. The importance of genetic diagnosis for Duchenne muscular dystrophy. *J Med Genet.* 2016;53(3):145-151.
5. Darras BT, Urion DK, Ghosh PS. Dystrophinopathies. September 2000 [Updated Jan 20, 2022]. In: Adam MP, Ardinger HH, Pagon RA, et al., ed. *GeneReviews®* [Internet]. University of Washington, Seattle; 1993-2022. Accessed July 1, 2022. https://www.ncbi.nlm.nih.gov/books/NBK1119/.
6. Muntoni F, Torelli S, Ferlini A. Dystrophin and mutations: one gene, several proteins, multiple phenotypes. *Lancet Neurol.* 2003;2(12):731-740.
7. Nozoe KT, Akamine RT, Mazzotti DR, et al. Phenotypic contrasts of Duchenne muscular dystrophy in women: two case reports. *Sleep Sci.* 2016;9(3):129-133.
8. Flanigan KM. Duchenne and Becker muscular dystrophies. *Neurol Clin.* 2014;32(3):671-688, viii.
9. Mendell JR, Shilling C, Leslie ND, et al. Evidence-based path to newborn screening for Duchenne muscular dystrophy. *Ann Neurol.* 2012;71(3):304-313.
10. Biggar WD, Klamut HJ, Demacio PC, Stevens DJ, Ray PN. Duchenne muscular dystrophy: current knowledge, treatment, and future prospects. *Clin Orthop Relat Res.* 2002(401):88-106.

11. Barnabei MS, Martindale JM, Townsend D, Metzger JM. Exercise and muscular dystrophy: implications and analysis of effects on musculoskeletal and cardiovascular systems. *Compr Physiol*. 2011;1(3):1353-1363.

12. Anderson JL, Head SI, Rae C, Morley JW. Brain function in Duchenne muscular dystrophy. *Brain*. 2002;125(Pt 1):4-13.

13. Ervasti JM. Dystrophin, its interactions with other proteins, and implications for muscular dystrophy. *Biochim Biophys Acta*. 2007;1772(2):108-117.

14. Ehmsen J, Poon E, Davies K. The dystrophin-associated protein complex. *J Cell Sci*. 2002;115(Pt 14):2801-2803.

15. Allen DG, Whitehead NP, Froehner SC. Absence of dystrophin disrupts skeletal muscle signaling: roles of Ca2+, reactive oxygen species, and nitric oxide in the development of muscular dystrophy. *Physiol Rev*. 2016;96(1):253-305.

16. Byrne E, Kornberg AJ, Kapsa R. Duchenne muscular dystrophy: hopes for the sesquicentenary. *Med J Aust*. 2003;179(9):463-464.

17. Morgenroth VH, Hache LP, Clemens PR. Insights into bone health in Duchenne muscular dystrophy. *Bonekey Rep*. 2012; 1:9.

18. Kamdar F, Garry DJ. Dystrophin-deficient cardiomyopathy. *J Am Coll Cardiol*. 2016;67(21):2533-2546.

19. Thangarajh M, Spurney CF, Gordish-Dressman H, et al. Neurodevelopmental needs in young boys with Duchenne muscular dystrophy (DMD): observations from the Cooperative International Neuromuscular Research Group (CINRG) DMD Natural History Study (DNHS). *PLoS Curr*. 2018;10:ecurrents. md.4cdeb6970e54034db54032bc54033dfa54054b54034d54987.

20. Vicari S, Piccini G, Mercuri E, et al. Implicit learning deficit in children with Duchenne muscular dystrophy: evidence for a cerebellar cognitive impairment? *PLoS One*. 2018;13(1): e0191164.

21. Snow WM, Anderson JE, Jakobson LS. Neuropsychological and neurobehavioral functioning in Duchenne muscular dystrophy: a review. *Neurosci Biobehav Rev*. 2013;37(5):743-752.

22. Quinlivan R. Early diagnosis of Duchenne muscular dystrophy is essential to improve long term outcomes. *Arch Dis Child*. 2014;99(12):1061.

23. Merlini L, Gennari M, Malaspina E, et al. Early corticosteroid treatment in 4 Duchenne muscular dystrophy patients: 14-year follow-up. *Muscle Nerve*. 2012;45(6):796-802.

24. Verma S, Anziska Y, Cracco J. Review of Duchenne muscular dystrophy (DMD) for the pediatricians in the community. *Clin Pediatr (Phila)*. 2010;49(11):1011-1017.

25. van Ruiten HJ, Straub V, Bushby K, Guglieri M. Improving recognition of Duchenne muscular dystrophy: a retrospective case note review. *Arch Dis Child*. 2014;99(12):1074-1077.

26. Ciafaloni E, Fox DJ, Pandya S, et al. Delayed diagnosis in Duchenne muscular dystrophy: data from the Muscular Dystrophy Surveillance, Tracking, and Research Network (MD STARnet). *J Pediatr*. 2009;155(3):380-385.

27. Gissy JJ, Johnson T, Fox DJ, et al. Delayed onset of ambulation in boys with Duchenne muscular dystrophy: potential use as an endpoint in clinical trials. *Neuromuscul Disord*. 2017; 27(10):905-910.

28. Brandsema JF, Darras BT. Dystrophinopathies. *Semin Neurol*. 2015;35(4):369-384.

29. Sun SC, Peng YS, He JB. [Changes of serum creatine kinase levels in children with Duchenne muscular dystrophy]. *Zhongguo Dang Dai Er Ke Za Zhi*. 2008;10(1):35-37.

30. Boca SM, Nishida M, Harris M, et al. Discovery of metabolic biomarkers for duchenne muscular dystrophy within a natural history study. *PLoS One*. 2016;11(4):e0153461.

31. Hathout Y, Brody E, Clemens PR, et al. Large-scale serum protein biomarker discovery in Duchenne muscular dystrophy. *Proc Natl Acad Sci U S A*. 2015;112(23):7153-7158.

32. Hathout Y, Seol H, Han MH, Zhang A, Brown KJ, Hoffman EP. Clinical utility of serum biomarkers in Duchenne muscular dystrophy. *Clin Proteomics*. 2016;13:9.

33. Bello L, Morgenroth LP, Gordish-Dressman H, et al. DMD genotypes and loss of ambulation in the CINRG Duchenne Natural History Study. *Neurology*. 2016;87(4):401-409.

34. Bello L, Piva L, Barp A, et al. Importance of SPP1 genotype as a covariate in clinical trials in Duchenne muscular dystrophy. *Neurology*. 2012;79(2):159-162.

35. Pegoraro E, Hoffman EP, Piva L, et al. SPP1 genotype is a determinant of disease severity in Duchenne muscular dystrophy. *Neurology*. 2011;76(3):219-226.

36. Barp A, Bello L, Politano L, et al. Genetic modifiers of Duchenne muscular dystrophy and dilated cardiomyopathy. *PLoS One*. 2015;10(10):e0141240.

37. Flanigan KM, Ceco E, Lamar KM, et al. LTBP4 genotype predicts age of ambulatory loss in Duchenne muscular dystrophy. *Ann Neurol*. 2013;73(4):481-488.

38. Jansen M, van Alfen N, Nijhuis van der Sanden MW, van Dijk JP, Pillen S, de Groot IJ. Quantitative muscle ultrasound is a promising longitudinal follow-up tool in Duchenne muscular dystrophy. *Neuromuscul Disord*. 2012;22(4):306-317.

39. Koppaka S, Shklyar I, Rutkove SB, et al. Quantitative ultrasound assessment of Duchenne muscular dystrophy using edge detection analysis. *J Ultrasound Med*. 2016;35(9):1889-1897.

40. Mah JK, van Alfen N. Neuromuscular ultrasound: clinical applications and diagnostic values. *Can J Neurol Sci*. 2018;45(6): 605-619.

41. Zaidman CM, Wu JS, Kapur K, et al. Quantitative muscle ultrasound detects disease progression in Duchenne muscular dystrophy. *Ann Neurol*. 2017;81(5):633-640.

42. Barnard AM, Willcocks RJ, Finanger EL, et al. Skeletal muscle magnetic resonance biomarkers correlate with function and sentinel events in Duchenne muscular dystrophy. *PLoS One*. 2018;13(3):e0194283.

43. Willcocks RJ, Arpan IA, Forbes SC, et al. Longitudinal measurements of MRI-T2 in boys with Duchenne muscular dystrophy: effects of age and disease progression. *Neuromuscul Disord*. 2014;24(5):393-401.

44. Willcocks RJ, Rooney WD, Triplett WT, et al. Multicenter prospective longitudinal study of magnetic resonance biomarkers in a large Duchenne muscular dystrophy cohort. *Ann Neurol*. 2016;79(4):535-547.

45. Arpan I, Willcocks RJ, Forbes SC, et al. Examination of effects of corticosteroids on skeletal muscles of boys with DMD using MRI and MRS. *Neurology*. 2014;83(11):974-980.

46. Hollingsworth KG, Garrood P, Eagle M, Bushby K, Straub V. Magnetic resonance imaging in Duchenne muscular dystrophy: longitudinal assessment of natural history over 18 months. *Muscle Nerve*. 2013;48(4):586-588.

47. Bushby K, Connor E. Clinical outcome measures for trials in Duchenne muscular dystrophy: report from International Working Group meetings. *Clin Investig (Lond)*. 2011;1(9):1217-1235.

48. van den Bergen JC, Ginjaar HB, van Essen AJ, et al. Forty-five years of Duchenne muscular dystrophy in the Netherlands. *J Neuromuscul Dis*. 2014;1(1):99-109.

49. McDonald CM, Henricson EK, Abresch RT, et al. The cooperative international neuromuscular research group Duchenne natural history study—a longitudinal investigation in the era of glucocorticoid therapy: design of protocol and the methods used. *Muscle Nerve*. 2013;48(1):32-54.

50. Parent Project DMD. Published 2020. Accessed July 21, 2022. https://www.parentprojectmd.org/aiovg_videos/cinrg-expanded-duchenne-natural-history-study-ednhs/.

51. Cooperative International Neuromuscular Research Group. Accessed April 30, 2019. https://cinrgresearch.org/.

52. Birnkrant DJ, Bushby K, Bann CM, et al. Diagnosis and management of Duchenne muscular dystrophy, part 3: primary care, emergency management, psychosocial care, and transitions of care across the lifespan. *Lancet Neurol.* 2018;17(5):445-455.

53. Bello L, Gordish-Dressman H, Morgenroth LP, et al. Prednisone/prednisolone and deflazacort regimens in the CINRG Duchenne Natural History Study. *Neurology.* 2015;85(12): 1048-1055.

54. Pane M, Fanelli L, Mazzone ES, et al. Benefits of glucocorticoids in non-ambulant boys/men with Duchenne muscular dystrophy: a multicentric longitudinal study using the performance of upper limb test. *Neuromuscul Disord.* 2015;25(10):749-753.

55. Abreu NJ, Waldrop MA. Overview of gene therapy in spinal muscular atrophy and Duchenne muscular dystrophy. *Pediatr Pulmonol.* 2021;56(4):710-720.

56. Connolly AM, Zaidman CM, Golumbek PT, et al. Twice-weekly glucocorticosteroids in infants and young boys with Duchenne muscular dystrophy. *Muscle Nerve.* 2019;59(6):650-657.

57. Griggs RC, Herr BE, Reha A, et al. Corticosteroids in Duchenne muscular dystrophy: major variations in practice. *Muscle Nerve.* 2013;48(1):27-31.

58. Guglieri M, Bushby K, McDermott MP, et al. Developing standardized corticosteroid treatment for Duchenne muscular dystrophy. *Contemp Clin Trials.* 2017;58:34-39.

59. Joseph S, Wang C, Bushby K, et al. Fractures and linear growth in a nationwide cohort of boys with Duchenne muscular dystrophy with and without glucocorticoid treatment: results from the UK NorthStar Database. *JAMA Neurol.* 2019;76(6):701-709.

60. Yao S, Chen Z, Yu Y, et al. Current pharmacological strategies for Duchenne muscular dystrophy. *Front Cell Dev Biol.* 2021;9: 689533.

61. Lim KRQ, Maruyama R, Yokota T. Eteplirsen in the treatment of Duchenne muscular dystrophy. *Drug Design Dev Ther.* 2017;11: 533-545.

62. Charleston JS, Schnell FJ, Dworzak J, et al. Eteplirsen treatment for Duchenne muscular dystrophy: exon skipping and dystrophin production. *Neurology.* 2018;90(24):e2146-e2154.

63. Frank DE, Schnell FJ, Akana C, et al. Increased dystrophin production with golodirsen in patients with Duchenne muscular dystrophy. *Neurology.* 2020;94(21):e2270-e2282.

64. Heo YA. Golodirsen: first approval. *Drugs.* 2020;80(3):329-333.

65. Case LE, Apkon SD, Eagle M, et al. Rehabilitation management of the patient with Duchenne muscular dystrophy. *Pediatrics.* 2018;142(Suppl 2):S17-S33.

66. Ricotti V, Ridout DA, Pane M, et al. The NorthStar Ambulatory Assessment in Duchenne muscular dystrophy: considerations for the design of clinical trials. *J Neurol Neurosurg Psychiatry.* 2016;87(2):149-155.

67. Mercuri E, Coratti G, Messina S, et al. Revised North Star Ambulatory Assessment for Young Boys with Duchenne muscular dystrophy. *PLoS One.* 2016;11(8):e0160195.

68. Mazzone E, Martinelli D, Berardinelli A, et al. North Star Ambulatory Assessment, 6-minute walk test and timed items in ambulant boys with Duchenne muscular dystrophy. *Neuromuscul Disord.* 2010;20(11):712-716.

69. Connolly AM, Florence JM, Cradock MM, et al. Motor and cognitive assessment of infants and young boys with Duchenne muscular dystrophy: results from the Muscular Dystrophy Association DMD Clinical Research Network. *Neuromuscul Disord.* 2013;23(7):529-539.

70. Arora H, Willcocks RJ, Lott DJ, et al. Longitudinal timed function tests in Duchenne muscular dystrophy: imaging DMD cohort natural history. *Muscle Nerve.* 2018;58(5):631-638.

71. McDonald CM, Henricson EK, Abresch RT, et al. The 6-minute walk test and other clinical endpoints in Duchenne muscular dystrophy: reliability, concurrent validity, and minimal clinically important differences from a multicenter study. *Muscle Nerve.* 2013;48(3):357-368.

72. Vuillerot C, Girardot F, Payan C, et al. Monitoring changes and predicting loss of ambulation in Duchenne muscular dystrophy with the Motor Function Measure. *Dev Med Child Neurol.* 2010;52(1):60-65.

73. Lue YJ, Lin RF, Chen SS, Lu YM. Measurement of the functional status of patients with different types of muscular dystrophy. *Kaohsiung J Med Sci.* 2009;25(6):325-333.

74. Fagoaga J, Girabent-Farres M, Bagur-Calafat C, Steffensen BF. [Evolution of functional capacity, assessed with the Egen Klassifikation scale, in the Spanish population with spinal muscular atrophy or Duchenne muscular dystrophy. A three year longitudinal study]. *Rev Neurol.* 2015;61(8):344-348.

75. Steffensen B, Hyde S, Lyager S, Mattsson E. Validity of the EK scale: a functional assessment of non-ambulatory individuals with Duchenne muscular dystrophy or spinal muscular atrophy. *Physiother Res Int.* 2001;6(3):119-134.

76. Batra A, Harrington A, Lott DJ, et al. Two-year longitudinal changes in lower limb strength and its relation to loss in function in a large cohort of patients with Duchenne muscular dystrophy. *Am J Phys Med Rehabil.* 2018;97(10):734-740.

77. Battini R, Chieffo D, Bulgheroni S, et al. Cognitive profile in Duchenne muscular dystrophy boys without intellectual disability: the role of executive functions. *Neuromuscul Disord.* 2018; 28(2):122-128.

78. Hughes KJ, Rodriguez A, Flatt KM, et al. Physical exertion exacerbates decline in the musculature of an animal model of Duchenne muscular dystrophy. *Proc Natl Acad Sci USA.* 2019; 116(9):3508-3517.

79. Heutinck L, Kampen NV, Jansen M, Groot IJ. Physical activity in boys with Duchenne muscular dystrophy is lower and less demanding compared to healthy boys. *J Child Neurol.* 2017; 32(5): 450-457.

80. Jansen M, de Groot IJ, van Alfen N, Geurts A. Physical training in boys with Duchenne muscular dystrophy: the protocol of the No Use is Disuse study. *BMC Pediatr.* 2010;10:55.

81. Hyde SA, Lytrup I, Glent S, et al. A randomized comparative study of two methods for controlling Tendo Achilles contracture in Duchenne muscular dystrophy. *Neuromuscul Disord.* 2000;10(4-5):257-263.

82. Hyde SA, Scott OM, Goddard CM, Dubowitz V. Prolongation of ambulation in Duchenne muscular dystrophy by appropriate orthoses. *Physiotherapy.* 1982;68(4):105-108.

83. Kiefer M, Bonarrigo K, Quatman-Yates C, Fowler A, Horn PS, Wong BL. Progression of ankle plantarflexion contractures and functional decline in Duchenne muscular dystrophy: implications for physical therapy management. *Pediatr Phys Ther.* 2019; 31(1):61-66.

84. Main M, Mercuri E, Haliloglu G, Baker R, Kinali M, Muntoni F. Serial casting of the ankles in Duchenne muscular dystrophy: can it be an alternative to surgery? *Neuromuscul Disord.* 2007;17(3):227-230.

85. Kinali M, Main M, Eliahoo J, et al. Predictive factors for the development of scoliosis in Duchenne muscular dystrophy. *Eur J Paediatr Neurol.* 2007;11(3):160-166.

86. Apkon SD, Alman B, Birnkrant DJ, et al. Orthopedic and surgical management of the patient with Duchenne muscular dystrophy. *Pediatrics.* 2018;142(Suppl 2):S82-S89.

87. Alemdaroglu I, Karaduman A, Yilmaz OT, Topaloglu H. Different types of upper extremity exercise training in Duchenne muscular dystrophy: effects on functional performance, strength, endurance, and ambulation. *Muscle Nerve.* 2015;51(5):697-705.

88. Kern R, Carvell K, Gupta A, Verma S. Seated outcome measures in children with Duchenne muscular dystrophy. *Pediatr Phys Ther.* 2022;34(3):375-380.

89. Passamano L, Taglia A, Palladino A, et al. Improvement of survival in Duchenne muscular dystrophy: retrospective analysis of 835 patients. *Acta Myol.* 2012;31(2):121-125.

90. Mercuri E, Finkel RS, Muntoni F, et al. Diagnosis and management of spinal muscular atrophy: part 1: recommendations for diagnosis, rehabilitation, orthopedic and nutritional care. *Neuromuscul Disord.* 2018;28(2):103-115.

91. Chaytow H, Huang YT, Gillingwater TH, Faller KME. The role of survival motor neuron protein (SMN) in protein homeostasis. *Cell Mol Life Sci.* 2018;75(21):3877-3894.

92. Wang CH, Finkel RS, Bertini ES, et al. Consensus statement for standard of care in spinal muscular atrophy. *J Child Neurol.* 2007;22(8):1027-1049.

93. Finkel RS, Mercuri E, Meyer OH, et al. Diagnosis and management of spinal muscular atrophy: part 2: pulmonary and acute care; medications, supplements and immunizations; other organ systems; and ethics. *Neuromuscul Disord.* 2018;28(3):197-207.

94. Kaufmann P, McDermott MP, Darras BT, et al. Observational study of spinal muscular atrophy type 2 and 3: functional outcomes over 1 year. *Arch Neurol.* 2011;68(6):779-786.

95. American Physical Therapy Association. Published 2021. Accessed December 15, 2021. Fact sheet: spinal muscular atrophy. https://pediatricapta.org/includes/fact-sheets/pdfs/FactSheet_SpinalMuscularAtrophy_2021.pdf?v=1.

96. Catteruccia M, Vuillerot C, Vaugier I, et al. Orthopedic management of scoliosis by Garches brace and spinal fusion in SMA type 2 children. *J Neuromuscul Dis.* 2015;2(4):453-462.

97. Beernaert K, Lovgren M, Jeppesen J, et al. Parents' experiences of information and decision making in the care of their child with severe spinal muscular atrophy: a population survey. *J Child Neurol.* 2019:883073818822900.

98. Michelson D, Ciafaloni E, Ashwal S, et al. Evidence in focus: nusinersen use in spinal muscular atrophy: report of the Guideline Development, Dissemination, and Implementation Subcommittee of the American Academy of Neurology. *Neurology.* 2018;91(20):923-933.

99. Chiriboga CA. Nusinersen for the treatment of spinal muscular atrophy. *Expert Rev Neurother.* 2017;17(10):955-962.

100. Finkel RS, Mercuri E, Darras BT, et al. Nusinersen versus sham control in infantile-onset spinal muscular atrophy. *N Engl J Med.* 2017;377(18):1723-1732.

101. Mercuri E, Darras BT, Chiriboga CA, et al. Nusinersen versus sham control in later-onset spinal muscular atrophy. *N Engl J Med.* 2018;378(7):625-635.

102. Dangouloff T, Servais L. Clinical evidence supporting early treatment of patients with spinal muscular atrophy: current perspectives. *Ther Clin Risk Manag.* 2019;15:1153-1161.

103. Ratni H, Ebeling M, Baird J, et al. Discovery of risdiplam, a selective survival of motor neuron-2 (SMN2) gene splicing modifier for the treatment of spinal muscular atrophy (SMA). *J Med Chem.* 2018;61(15):6501-6517.

104. Mahajan R. Onasemnogene abeparvovec for spinal muscular atrophy: the costlier drug ever. *Int J Appl Basic Med Res.* 2019;9(3):127-128.

105. Swoboda KJ, Scott CB, Crawford TO, et al. SMA CARNI-VAL trial part I: double-blind, randomized, placebo-controlled trial of L-carnitine and valproic acid in spinal muscular atrophy. *PLoS One.* 2010;5(8):e12140.

106. Kissel JT, Scott CB, Reyna SP, et al. SMA CARNIVAL trial part II: a prospective, single-armed trial of L-carnitine and valproic acid in ambulatory children with spinal muscular atrophy. *PLoS One.* 2011;6(7):e21296.

107. Kissel JT, Elsheikh B, King WM, et al. SMA valiant trial: a prospective, double-blind, placebo-controlled trial of valproic acid in ambulatory adults with spinal muscular atrophy. *Muscle Nerve.* 2014;49(2):187-192.

108. Wadman RI, Wijngaarde CA, Stam M, et al. Muscle strength and motor function throughout life in a cross-sectional cohort of 180 patients with spinal muscular atrophy types 1c-4. *Eur J Neurol.* 2018;25(3):512-518.

109. Montes J, McDermott MP, Mirek E, et al. Ambulatory function in spinal muscular atrophy: age-related patterns of progression. *PLoS One.* 2018;13(6):e0199657.

110. Sporer SM, Smith BG. Hip dislocation in patients with spinal muscular atrophy. *J Pediatr Orthop.* 2003;23(1):10-14.

111. Main M, Kairon H, Mercuri E, Muntoni F. The Hammersmith functional motor scale for children with spinal muscular atrophy: a scale to test ability and monitor progress in children with limited ambulation. *Eur J Paediatr Neurol.* 2003;7(4):155-159.

112. Pera MC, Coratti G, Forcina N, et al. Content validity and clinical meaningfulness of the HFMSE in spinal muscular atrophy. *BMC Neurol.* 2017;17(1):39.

113. Krosschell KJ, Scott CB, Maczulski JA, et al. Reliability of the Modified Hammersmith Functional Motor Scale in young children with spinal muscular atrophy. *Muscle Nerve.* 2011; 44(2): 246-251.

114. Ramsey D, Scoto M, Mayhew A, et al. Revised Hammersmith Scale for spinal muscular atrophy: a SMA specific clinical outcome assessment tool. *PLoS One.* 2017;12(2):e0172346.

115. De Sanctis R, Pane M, Coratti G, et al. Clinical phenotypes and trajectories of disease progression in type 1 spinal muscular atrophy. *Neuromuscul Disord.* 2018;28(1):24-28.

116. Montes J, McDermott MP, Martens WB, et al. Six-minute walk test demonstrates motor fatigue in spinal muscular atrophy. *Neurology.* 2010;74(10):833-838.

117. Mazzone E, Bianco F, Main M, et al. Six minute walk test in type III spinal muscular atrophy: a 12 month longitudinal study. *Neuromuscul Disord.* 2013;23(8):624-628.

118. Montes J, Glanzman AM, Mazzone ES, et al. Spinal muscular atrophy functional composite score: a functional measure in spinal muscular atrophy. *Muscle Nerve.* 2015;52(6):942-947.

119. Vuillerot C, Payan C, Iwaz J, Ecochard R, Berard C, MFM Spinal Muscular Atrophy Study Group. Responsiveness of the motor function measure in patients with spinal muscular atrophy. *Arch Phys Med Rehabil.* 2013;94(8):1555-1561.

120. Dunaway S, Montes J, Garber CE, et al. Performance of the timed "up & go" test in spinal muscular atrophy. *Muscle Nerve.* 2014;50(2):273-277.

121. Haataja L, Mercuri E, Regev R, et al. Optimality score for the neurologic examination of the infant at 12 and 18 months of age. *J Pediatr.* 1999;135(2 Pt 1):153-161.

122. Dunaway S, Montes J, McDermott MP, et al. Physical therapy services received by individuals with spinal muscular atrophy (SMA). *J Pediatr Rehabil Med.* 2016;9(1):35-44.

123. Salazar R, Montes J, Dunaway Young S, et al. Quantitative evaluation of lower extremity joint contractures in spinal muscular atrophy: implications for motor function. *Pediatr Phys Ther.* 2018;30(3):209-215.

124. Fujak A, Kopschina C, Forst R, Mueller LA, Forst J. Use of orthoses and orthopaedic technical devices in proximal spinal muscular atrophy. Results of survey in 194 SMA patients. *Disabil Rehabil Assist Technol.* 2011;6(4):305-311.

125. Dunaway S, Montes J, O'Hagen J, Sproule DM, Vivo DC, Kaufmann P. Independent mobility after early introduction of a power wheelchair in spinal muscular atrophy. *J Child Neurol.* 2013;28(5):576-582.

126. Townsend EL, Simeone SD, Krosschell KJ, Zhang RZ, Swoboda KJ. Stander use in spinal muscular atrophy: results from a large natural history database. *Pediatr Phys Ther.* 2020;32(3):235-241.

127. Arnold WD, Kassar D, Kissel JT. Spinal muscular atrophy: diagnosis and management in a new therapeutic era. *Muscle Nerve.* 2015;51(2):157-167.

128. Cunha MC, Oliveira AS, Labronici RH, Gabbai AA. Spinal muscular atrophy type II (intermediary) and III (Kugelberg-Welander). Evolution of 50 patients with physiotherapy and hydrotherapy in a swimming pool. *Arq Neuropsiquiatr.* 1996;54(3):402-406.

129. Lemke D, Rothwell E, Newcomb TM, Swoboda KJ. Perceptions of equine-assisted activities and therapies by parents and children with spinal muscular atrophy. *Pediatr Phys Ther.* 2014; 26(2):237-244.

130. Lewelt A, Krosschell KJ, Stoddard GJ, et al. Resistance strength training exercise in children with spinal muscular atrophy. *Muscle Nerve.* 2015;52(4):559-567.

131. Salem Y, Gropack SJ. Aquatic therapy for a child with type III spinal muscular atrophy: a case report. *Phys Occup Ther Pediatr.* 2010;30(4):313-324.

132. Nance JR, Dowling JJ, Gibbs EM, Bonnemann CG. Congenital myopathies: an update. *Curr Neurol Neurosci Rep.* 2012;12(2): 165-174.

133. Harmelink M. Differentiating congenital myopathy from congenital muscular dystrophy. *Clin Perinatol.* 2020;47(1): 197-209.

134. Butterfield RJ. Congenital muscular dystrophy and congenital myopathy. *Continuum (Minneap Minn).* 2019;25(6): 1640-1661.

135. Wang CH, Dowling JJ, North K, et al. Consensus statement on standard of care for congenital myopathies. *J Child Neurol.* 2012;27(3):363-382.

136. Williamson E, Pederson N, Rawson H, Daniel T. The effect of inspiratory muscle training on Duchenne muscular dystrophy: a meta-analysis. *Pediatr Phys Ther.* 2019;31(4):323-330.

9

Neural Tube Defects

Megan Geno Dakhlian, PT, DPT

Upon completion of this chapter, the reader will be able to:

■ Understand the etiology, incidence, and prevalence of spina bifida.

■ Understand the medical and surgical management of spina bifida throughout the life span and identify key factors that prompt referral to medical provider.

■ Understand neurologic, cognitive, musculoskeletal, and urologic problems associated with spina bifida.

■ Understand the role of the physical therapist throughout the life span for an individual with spina bifida.

■ Identify components of physical therapy evaluation and prioritize aspects of the evaluation based on age, setting, and medical status.

■ Understand anticipated functional outcomes and prognosis based on neurologic levels and identify factors that may have an impact on prognosis.

■ Recommend appropriate orthoses, assistive devices, and adaptive equipment for individuals with myelomeningocele based on level of lesion.

■ INTRODUCTION

Spina bifida is a complex, congenital condition associated with abnormalities of the brain and spinal cord with neurologic, cognitive, musculoskeletal, and urologic involvement. With improvements in prenatal screening, management of hydrocephalus, bowel and bladder function, and surgical techniques, people with spina bifida can live well into adulthood.[1] Comprehensive multidisciplinary care has also led to improved health and quality of life for individuals with spina bifida. Multidisciplinary care may include, but is not limited to, medical providers, therapists, and mental health professionals. See **Table 9-1** for members who may be a part of a multidisciplinary team. It is

essential for the physical therapist to have an understanding of the multisystem involvement associated with spina bifida to provide comprehensive care. The body systems are interrelated, and changes in clinical presentation may be indicative of a change in medical status. It is beneficial for the physical therapist to have knowledge of the patient's baseline level of function in order to identify any changes and potential need for referral to other medical providers. Understanding anticipated functional levels can guide treatment interventions to optimize participation in purposeful life activities. There is a shift from primarily managing medical conditions to focusing on long-term outcomes and quality of life for individuals with spina bifida.[2-7] The physical therapist can support prevention of secondary impairments and promote independent participation in physical activities for a healthy lifestyle and improved quality of life.[2,8]

■ NEURAL TUBE DEFECTS

A neural tube defect (NTD) occurs when there is a failure of the neural tube to close or a disruption in neurulation of the spinal placode during fetal development. Neurulation occurs within the first 28 days of gestation.[4,9-11] The neural tube will eventually form the brain, spinal cord, and spinal column. Failure to close can occur anywhere along the neural canal, leading to abnormal development of the brain or spinal cord.[4,9,10] The most common NTD is myelomeningocele, or spina bifida, which has lifelong complications (**Table 9-2**).[4,5,9,12-15] Spina bifida, which is the most commonly occurring NTD, will be the preferred term used and the primary focus of this chapter.[11]

TABLE 9-1 • Multidisciplinary Team Members

Neurosurgeon	Physical therapist
Neurologist	Occupational therapist
Orthopedic/orthopedic surgeon	Neuropsychologist
Physiatrist	Psychologist
Urologist	Nutritionist
Pediatrician/complex care provider	Social worker
Endocrinologist	Nurse
Gastroenterologist	Coordinated care provider
Nephrologist	

TABLE 9-2 • Neural Tube Defect Definitions

Neural Tube Defect	Closed (Occulta)/ Open (Aperta) Lesion	Definition	Key Clinical Features	Other
Spina bifida occulta	Occulta	One or more vertebral arches in spinal column form incompletely	Often asymptomatic	May be benign lesion, have hairy patch, skin tag, or hemangioma
Meningocele	Occulta	One or more vertebral arches in the spinal column are incomplete; cyst formation containing meninges and cerebrospinal fluid (CSF)	No associated brain involvement; may or may not have peripheral nervous system involvement	May or may not be associated with paralysis
Lipomyelomeningocele or lipomeningocele	Occulta	Meningocele with addition of lipoma	No associated brain involvement; may or may not have peripheral nervous system involvement	Can be associated with paralysis; risk of neurologic changes with spinal cord tethering
Myelomeningocele or spina bifida	Aperta	One or more vertebral arches in the spinal column are incomplete; sac containing spinal cord, nerve roots, meninges, and CSF formed outside the body	Central nervous system involvement (hydrocephalus, Chiari II malformation); bowel and bladder involvement; sensory impairments; motor paralysis	Anatomic and neurologic levels may differ; may have asymmetrical involvement
Encephalocele	Aperta	Protrusion of the brain, CSF, and meninges through a bony defect in the skull	Involvement correlated with location of lesion	Mixed prognosis
Anencephaly	Aperta	Failure of anterior end of the neural tube to close; exposure of malformed brain from the skull	Absence of forebrain	Poor neurologic prognosis

NTDs can be open (aperta) or closed (occulta) lesions.[9] Individuals with closed NTDs generally have less neurologic impact than those with open NTDs.[13] Spina bifida occulta is found in up to 10% to 20% of the healthy population. Spina bifida occulta occurs when there is a failed closure along one or more of the posterior elements of the vertebral column with a normal spinal cord.[9] It typically is not associated with neurologic impairments and can often go undetected. Skin abnormalities may be noted at birth, such as a hairy patch, hemangioma, or discoloration of the skin or a skin tag.[16]

A closed or skin-covered NTD associated with a protrusion from the distal end of an intact spinal cord is classified as either a meningocele or a lipomyelomeningocele. These are most commonly found in the lumbosacral region and may or may not be associated with neurologic impairments.[9] With a meningocele, there is a bony defect of the spinal column with a protrusion or cyst containing meninges and cerebrospinal fluid (CSF) but the spinal cord remains intact.[4,17] A lipoma contains a superficial fatty mass with fibrous tissue that extends caudally along the spinal cord.[4,7] Neurologic involvement varies with lipomyelomeningocele, depending on the involvement with the spinal roots.[9] Lipomas can be associated with tethering of the spinal cord, which can have progressive and potentially permanent neurologic damage.[7,9] Tethered spinal cords are discussed later in this chapter.

Spina bifida occurs when there is a failed fusion of the dorsal aspect of the neural tube during neurulation, leading to a failed formation of the posterior vertebral arches along the spinal column and resulting in an open NTD.[4,7,13,18,19] The posterior elements of the spinal column at the level of the lesion do not form typically, and there is abnormal formation of the spinal cord with impaired innervation distally.[4] The lesion is open with a membranous sac that contains the spinal cord, nerve roots, meninges, and CSF.[17] This lesion can occur anywhere from the thoracic to the sacral aspect of the spinal cord (**Figure 9-1**). Spina bifida is often classified by the anatomic location of the lesion or the motor level of paralysis. It is beneficial to know both the anatomic level of lesion and the motor level for classification and identification of anticipated outcomes. Spina bifida is associated with multisystem involvement and can have a wide variety of impairments, including neurologic changes, sensory loss, and motor paralysis that leads to musculoskeletal deformity and bowel and bladder involvement.[9,14,18,20-22] Severity is often associated with the level of the lesion, where higher-level lesions are associated with more neurologic involvement and paralysis.

An encephalocele is a protrusion of the brain, CSF, and meninges through a bony defect in the skull. This typically occurs in the occipital area of the brain but can also be seen

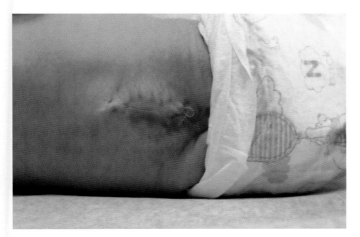

FIGURE 9-1 Picture of infant with spina bifida after closure.

in the frontal portion of the brain. An anencephaly is a failure of the anterior end of the neural tube to close, resulting in exposure of a malformed brain at birth.[6] There is an absence of forebrain and is typically associated with profound neurologic deficits with a poor prognosis.[13] Prognosis is related to the site of the NTD, the amount of exposed neural tissues, and presence of other coexisting malformations.[6]

RISK FACTORS

The cause of spinal bifida is likely multifactorial, including genetic and environmental factors.[11] Genetic risk factors include a prior pregnancy or family member with an NTD as well as race or ethnicity.[4] A prior pregnancy with an NTD increases the risk of subsequent pregnancies with NTDs by 2% to 3%. A woman with spina bifida has a 5% increased risk of having a child with spina bifida.[4,6] Hispanic/Latino race or ethnicity has a higher prevalence of spina bifida.[11] Maternal risk factors include dependence on insulin during gestation, diabetes mellitus, and obesity. Environmental risk factors include maternal exposure to high temperatures during early pregnancy (high fever or frequent hot tub use), use of valproic acid (an antiseizure medication), and paternal exposure to Agent Orange (chemical agent commonly used during the Vietnam War).[4,9,19,22]

Deficiencies in folic acid can lead to an increased incidence of NTDs.[11] In 1992, the US Public Health Service recommended that all women of childbearing age who are capable of becoming pregnant should consume at least 4 mg of folic acid daily. The addition of regular folic acid can decrease the risk of having a pregnancy with an NTD by up to 70% to 75%.[4,6,9,17,19,22] This led to a mandate by the Food and Drug Administration (FDA) to fortify enriched grain products, such as pastas and cereals, with folic acid. The recommendations for folic acid consumption have led to a decrease in the overall birth rate of children with spina bifida in developed countries, but the rate remains higher in developing countries.[14] The birth rate of infants with spina bifida is variable around the world and is currently 0.5 to 1.0 per 1000 live births in the United States.[4,10,13,14,23,24] Other reports have shown the worldwide incidence as 3.4 to 4.6 per 10,000 live births.[19,22,25]

PRENATAL CARE

Advancements in prenatal care, screening, and diagnostic tools have drastically changed the care for children with spina bifida and improved quality of life.[4] High-resolution ultrasound can identify an open NTD during routine prenatal care in up to 90% to 95% of cases around 18 to 20 weeks' gestation.[4,13,22] Magnetic resonance imaging (MRI) can identify the presence of brain and spine malformations, such as the presence of a Chiari II malformation or hydrocephalus, which will be discussed later in this chapter.[4] Amniotic α-fetoprotein (AFP) is a protein that leaks into amniotic fluid with open NTDs. The maternal serum AFP can be detected through routine blood screening between 15 and 20 weeks' gestation.[4,9,22]

Prenatal counseling can occur through high-risk or advanced fetal care programs to support family education and planning. Vaginal deliveries have been shown to increase the risk of rupturing the neural sac, which can lead to further impairment or infection.[4] Cesarean sections are generally planned and coordinated with an identified neurosurgeon who can surgically close the defect within the first 24 to 48 hours after delivery.[4,6,19] Postoperative management is focused on early closure of the defect, preventing infection, management of hydrocephalus, and minimizing musculoskeletal deformity.[8,19]

Research has shown progressive damage to the central and peripheral nervous systems based on serial ultrasound images of fetuses with spina bifida, suggesting worsening hydrocephalus and lower extremity function as pregnancy progressed.[6,15,17] This led to the hypothesis that the final neurologic deficit results from a failure of the neural tube to close and the exposure to the intrauterine environment.[6,15,19,22,26] Performing prenatal surgery on a fetus with spina bifida prior to 26 weeks' gestation could minimize neurologic impairment, preserve function, and improve outcomes for children with spina bifida.[15,26]

The Management of Myelomeningocele Study (MOMS) was funded by the National Institute of Child Health and Human Development and directly compared children with spina bifida who underwent prenatal versus postnatal surgery.[9,15,26-28] Prenatal surgery occurred around 25 weeks' gestation, and then a planned cesarean section was performed closer to term. Those in the postnatal repair group had a scheduled cesarian section at 37 weeks.[15,26,27,29]

The study was terminated in 2010 prior to reaching the goal sample size of 200 women due to maternal safety concerns with increased risk of spontaneous placenta or membrane rupture leading to premature delivery.[15,19,22,26-29] More than one-third of mothers in the prenatal repair group presented at the time of delivery with wound dehiscence or very thin uterus.[27] Fetal safety concerns included increased risk of premature birth. The average gestational age at birth for the prenatal group was 34.1 weeks with 13% being born prior to 30 weeks' gestation. This is compared to the postnatal repair group with an average age of gestation at delivery of 37.3 weeks. There was a higher association with effects of prematurity, such as respiratory distress syndrome, in the prenatal group.[15,27]

Outcomes that were measured in MOMS included the presence of hindbrain herniation, the need for a ventriculoperitoneal (VP) shunt at 12 months, the composite score on the motor index of the Bayley's Scale of Infant Development (BSID) at 30 months, and the functional level associated with the anatomic level of the lesion.[9,15,17,27,29,30] The prenatal repair group showed decreased hindbrain herniation with decreased need for a shunt due to hydrocephalus. The rate of actual shunt placement was 40% for the prenatal group compared to 82% for the postnatal group.[15,22,27-30] The presence of no hindbrain herniation was 35% for the prenatal group and 4% for the postnatal group. The prenatal group also showed improved outcomes in motor function compared to the postnatal group based on the BSID.[6,15,22,27-30] Children in the prenatal group were more likely to function at least 2 neurologic levels better than anticipated based on anatomic level of lesion and were more likely to walk independently.[15,22,28,30] Prenatal surgery did not decrease the need for clean intermittent catheterization at 30 months.[1,28-30] Prenatal surgery shows some benefits in neurologic outcomes, but the risk to fetal and maternal morbidity must be considered.[1,15,26] Further technological advancements with fetal surgical techniques may improve outcomes and lower the maternal and fetal risks of prenatal surgery.[19,22,28,30]

▪ PROBLEMS ASSOCIATED WITH SPINA BIFIDA

MUSCLE WEAKNESS

Most children with spina bifida have muscle weakness or motor paralysis due to the abnormal formation of spinal nerve roots impacting muscle innervation that may be asymmetrical. Thorough strength examinations can identify level of motor innervation and provide information about anticipated functional outcomes as well as potential future deformities. It can help guide physical therapy recommendations and interventions throughout an individual's life. Potential impacts on accurately determining motor level include age, cognitive status, and motivation.[31] For the purpose of this text, the following definitions will be used when discussing motor levels associated with spina bifida: thoracic level (any thoracic level); high lumbar (L1-L2), mid lumbar (L3), or low lumbar level (L4-L5); or sacral level (S1 and below)[9,20,31-33] (**Table 9-3**). Muscle grades are based on standard manual muscle testing (**Table 9-4**).

SENSORY IMPAIRMENTS

Sensory innervation may also be impacted in individuals with spina bifida. As with motor involvement, this can have asymmetrical involvement and differ based on motor level innervation.[9] Sensory impairments can include light touch, pain, and proprioceptive sensory receptors. Musculoskeletal deformities and weakness with impaired mobility may create abnormal pressure or shearing forces across fragile skin. This contributes to the risk of skin injury, especially in areas that are insensate. Nociceptor pain responses may be impaired, which inhibits protective responses and contributes to other injuries, such as fractures or burns.

NEUROLOGIC AND NEUROSURGICAL CONCERNS

Chiari II Malformation

A Chiari II malformation is a complex brain malformation associated with spina bifida.[4,15] This malformation involves a

TABLE 9-3 • Motor Levels Associated With Spina Bifida

Motor Level	Associated Muscle Involvement
Thoracic	No motor activation below the umbilicus
	May have weak abdominals or paraspinals
High lumbar (L1/L2)	Good to normal iliopsoas, hip adductors
	Weak or absent quadriceps
Mid lumbar (L3)	Normal iliopsoas
	Fair or greater quadriceps
Low lumbar (L4/L5)	Normal iliopsoas
	Normal quadriceps
	Fair or greater anterior tibialis
	Poor or greater hamstrings
	Poor to absent gluteal
	Poor to absent gastrocnemius-soleus
Sacral	Normal iliopsoas
	Normal quadriceps
	Normal anterior tibialis
	Normal hamstring
	Poor to normal gluteus medius and maximus
	Poor to normal gastrocnemius-soleus

dysgenesis of the corpus callosum, downward rotation of the cerebellum toward the foramen magnum, development of a small posterior fossa, and elongation of the fourth ventricle.[6,9,10,15,22] Nearly all children with spina bifida have a Chiari II malformation, but not all children will require intervention.[6,22,28,33] Compression on the brain stem, cranial nerves, and cerebellum can lead to upper motor neuron symptoms and lower cranial nerve dysfunction.[4,9,28] Acute changes in Chiari II symptoms can be life-threatening and require immediate medical attention.[4] Respiratory impairment and swallowing dysfunction related to

TABLE 9-4 • Manual Muscle Strength Grades

Grade	Description	Muscle Action
0	Absent	No contracture
1	Trace	Slight twitch/contraction of muscle without movement
2−	Poor minus	Moves partial range in gravity-minimized plane
2	Poor	Moves full range in gravity-minimized plane
2+	Poor plus	Moves against resistance in gravity-minimized plan
3−	Fair minus	Moves partial range against gravity
3	Fair	Moves full range against gravity
3+	Fair plus	Moves against slight resistance against gravity
4	Good	Moves against moderate resistance against gravity
5	Normal	Moves against maximal resistance against gravity, cannot break contraction

TABLE 9-5 • Symptoms of Chiari II Malformation	
Infant	**Child/Young Adult**
Respiratory impairment/stridor/apnea	Respiratory impairment/stridor/apnea
Emesis	Emesis
Swallowing dysfunction	Swallowing dysfunction
Vocal cord paresis	Vocal cord paresis
Upper extremity paresis or increase in tone	Upper extremity paresis
Arching of neck	Neck pain
Weak or absent cry	Headache
Failure to thrive	

brain stem dysfunction with a Chiari II malformation remain the leading causes of early death in children with spina bifida.[6] Clinical signs of a symptomatic Chiari II malformation include neck pain, headache, apnea, stridor, vocal cord paralysis, difficulty with swallowing or feeding, upper extremity weakness, and paralysis. In infants, symptoms may also include a weak or absent cry, arching of the neck, or apnea with or without color changes (**Table 9-5**).[4,6,9,22] Progressive or symptomatic Chiari II malformations may require surgical intervention and warrant a referral to the neurosurgeon.

Hydrocephalus

Hydrocephalus is an abnormal collection of CSF within the ventricular system of the brain and is present in as many as 90% of people with spina bifida.[10,25,33,34]. Hydrocephalus is associated with a Chiari II malformation.[4,9,25,33] Hydrocephalus is often identified by accumulation of CSF fluid within the third or fourth ventricles, also known as ventriculomegaly. Prolonged ventriculomegaly can lead to abnormal shape and structure of the ventricles.[35] Increased intracranial pressure (ICP) can lead to symptoms associated with hydrocephalus, which vary with age and severity[4,36] (**Table 9-6**).[4] As with a Chiari II malformation, acute neurologic changes warrant a referral to a neurosurgeon.

Hydrocephalus can be managed with the surgical placement of a VP shunt.[4,15,25,28] A shunt controls CSF pressure and ventricular volumes, which can limit progressive hydrocephalus. The shunt is a tube with a 1-way valve that is inserted into the

TABLE 9-6 • Symptoms of Hydrocephalus	
Infant	**Child/Young Adult**
Rapid increase in head circumference	Headache
Bulging anterior fontanelle	Emesis
Irritability	Visual changes
Emesis	Stridor
Feeding or swallowing difficulty	Apnea
Gastroesophageal reflux	Upper extremity weakness
Stridor	
Apnea	
Arching of neck	
Increase in upper extremity tone	

enlarged ventricle and allows for the flow of CSF out of the brain and downward to the end of the tube. Approximately 80% to 90% of children with spina bifida have a shunt to manage hydrocephalus.[6,10,28,35,36] A shunt may be placed immediately after birth when the initial closure occurs. Alternatively, an increasing number of institutions are monitoring the infant's clinical presentation and waiting to intervene if symptoms arise.[4,6,33,36]

The use of VP shunts has drastically improved the life expectancy for children with spina bifida; however, VP shunts have challenges and risk.[6,25] Shunt malfunction or shunt infection pose serious risks for children with spina bifida.[4,25] A shunt malfunction occurs when there is an occlusion in the shunt tubing or the tubing becomes disconnected. Signs of shunt malfunction are associated with increases in ICP.[4] Refer to Table 9-6 for symptoms. This requires immediate referral to a medical provider. Early management of the malfunction can help prevent further morbidity or potential death.[6,34] Surgery is often required to repair or replace the malfunctioning shunt, and upward of 50% of children with spina bifida with a VP shunt will require surgical revision at least once.[6,33-35] Some may require several shunt revisions throughout their life.[6,34] Multiple shunt revisions can have a negative impact on cognition and quality of life.[6]

An alternative treatment approach to management of hydrocephalus associated with spina bifida is endoscopic third ventriculostomy (ETV), which is often performed in conjunction with a choroid plexus cauterization (CPC).[25,28,30,34] The ETV procedure involves burrowing a small hole through the base of the third ventricle to provide an alternative route for flow of CSF. The CPC cauterizes the choroid plexus, which is responsible for the production of CSF. The use of an ETV/CPC procedure has decreased the rate of shunt dependence in children with spina bifida; however, it may not prevent the need for shunt later in life.[34,36] The combination of ETV/CPC has been shown to be more effective compared to ETV alone for managing hydrocephalus in children with spina bifida, especially in the first year of life.[25,28] Studies have shown similar neurocognitive outcomes for children when comparing a VP shunt versus ETV/CPC for treating hydrocephalus.[36]

Syringomyelia or Hydromyelia

Syringomyelia and hydromyelia are a dilation within the central canal of the spinal cord that results in an elongated cavity or syrinx that is filled with CSF. Symptoms, which may be dependent on location, include neck pain, changes in upper motor neuron function, new or worsening spasticity, ataxia, upper extremity weakness, or rapid progression of a spinal curve or scoliosis.[9] As with hydrocephalus, syringomyelia or hydromyelia should be monitored closely and any changes warrant a referral to a specialist.

Tethered Cord

A tethered spinal cord occurs when the terminal nerve roots of the spinal cord "get stuck" or tethered, creating a stretching on those nerve roots and resulting in neurologic deterioration.[6,28,37] Neurologic changes associated with tethered cord are common.[4] Symptoms associated with tethered cord include loss of strength, increased or new-onset spasticity, back or leg

TABLE 9-7 • Symptoms of Tethered Cord
Lower extremity weakness
Increase in lower extremity tone
Changes in bowel or bladder function
Back or leg pain
Rapid progression of spinal curve/new-onset scoliosis
Progressive foot deformity
Changes in gait

pain, changes in bowel or bladder function, rapid progression of spinal curve, progressive foot deformities, or changes in gait (**Table 9-7**).[4,6,7,9,37]

MRI may be used to diagnose a tethered cord but should be compared with prior images for progression as all children with spina bifida will appear to have a tethered cord on spinal MRI.[9] Clinical examination may help to identify neurologic changes. Urodynamics are also a useful and reliable diagnostic tool to assess for tethered spinal cord by identifying changes with parasympathetic and sympathetic nerve function.[9]

A tethered spinal cord is managed surgically by releasing nerve roots with the goal of halting progression of neurologic changes.[7] Any clinical signs concerning for a tethered cord should be referred to the neurosurgeon. A majority (at least 78%) of people with spina bifida undergo at least one tethered cord release in their life while some may have multiple surgical releases.[37] Based on review of the National Spina Bifida Registry, rates of tethered cord (measured by need for tethered cord release) increased in a linear relationship from birth to 13 years of age and then decreased between 14 and 21 years of age. There is not an association between tethered cord release rate and neurologic level; however, it was more common in those considered to be community ambulators.[37]

COGNITION AND NEUROPSYCHOLOGICAL CONSIDERATIONS

There are a wide range of cognitive levels and learning abilities in people with spina bifida. Intellectual prognosis is often is associated with complications related to hydrocephalus, shunt dependence, and other anomalies of the central nervous system.[4,6,7,13] Lower levels of cognition can affect an individual's ability to achieve their anticipated level of function and participate in self-care or activities of daily living (ADLs), which can affect quality of life.[5,7,8] Increased number of shunt revisions is also associated with poorer cognitive functioning.[38] Individuals often have challenges with executive functions such as abstract reasoning, visual-perceptual abilities, visual motor integration, problem solving, and writing and math skills.[9,10,38] A referral to occupational therapy may be beneficial for visual-perceptual training and strengthening.[38]

Cognitive challenges may become more apparent during school and can impact school performance. Children with spina bifida may meet the criteria for attention-deficit/hyperactivity disorder (ADHD) due to challenges with attention, organization, and executive functioning skills.[9,10] Behaviors seen may include distractibility, difficulty focusing, and inappropriate

social interactions.[10] Neuropsychological testing is beneficial in identifying cognitive processing styles and providing recommendations for academic supports and learning needs.[4]

MUSCULOSKELETAL INVOLVEMENT

Muscle Imbalances and Deformities

Muscle weakness is associated with abnormal innervation to the muscles. Muscle imbalances occur when one side of the joint experiences muscle forces greater than the opposing side. Muscle imbalances present in children with spina bifida can result in a variety of bone or joint deformities, which can be congenital or acquired. Congenital deformities are present at birth and associated with abnormal or impaired movement patterns in utero, as well as abnormal development of bones and joints. Acquired deformities develop over time from a combination of muscle imbalances, static positioning, effects of gravity, and abnormal weight-bearing forces.[4] The presence of deformities can have a significant impact on an individual's level of functional mobility, limit ability to use orthotics, and increase the risk of skin breakdown.[39,40]

Early physical therapy, orthopedics, or physiatrist involvement can help to optimize functional outcomes by working to counterbalance or minimize the impact of muscle imbalances.[6] Orthoses can provide stability to improve function or prevent the development of acquired deformities. Surgical intervention is considered when a bony deformity further limits an individual's anticipated level of mobility. Any rapid progression of a deformity should be considered if there is an underlying neurologic concern and warrants referral to the medical team.[39]

Hip Deformities

Hip deformities may be congenital or acquired and are related to muscle imbalances, prolonged positioning, and abnormal weight-bearing forces. Hip flexion contractures are common and related to the innervation levels to musculature surrounding the hip joint. The hip flexors (iliopsoas and sartorius) are innervated primarily by L1-L2 nerve roots, whereas the hip extensors (primarily gluteus maximus) are innervated from an L5-S2 level.[9] This creates a muscle imbalance where the hip can actively flex but has absent or weak extension to counter this force, leading to a hip flexion contracture. This can be further compromised by an individual's impaired level of mobility and spending more time in a seated position. The presence of a hip flexion contracture can greatly impact a child's ability to get into an upright or standing position and result in a compensatory lordosis through the lumbar spine.[41,42] It may also have an impact on ambulation.[43] Orthoses and adaptive equipment can accommodate some degree of contracture but severe contractures can impact a child's ability to be in an upright position.[41-43]

Due to the potential impact on mobility, hip flexion contractures should be managed early with stretching and positioning programs. Surgical correction can involve either soft tissue releases or correction of the bony alignment. Soft tissue procedures involve lengthening the sartorius, iliopsoas, or rectus femoris muscles and can be most successful with contractures around 30 to 40 degrees. Correction through the bone can change the alignment of the femur on the pelvis. Surgical correction of hip flexion contractures can improve motion, but there is the risk of the contracture returning due to the persistent muscle imbalance and prolonged positioning in a seated position.[41,43] Stretching the hip flexors should remain a focus throughout the lifetime due to the high risk of contracture development.

Hip dysplasia and subluxation are other common deformities of the hip. Hip dysplasia is present in nearly 50% of children with spina bifida, and many have evidence of subluxation or dislocation at birth.[9,39,44] This is related to the muscle imbalances around the hip, with more active hip flexion and adduction compared to hip extension and abduction.[3] The innervation of the hip flexors and hip adductors is from a higher lumbar level (L1-L2), whereas the counterbalancing force of hip extensors and abductors is innervated from L4 to S1. This muscle imbalance can impact the development of the acetabulum and the femoral head/neck angle.[3] Hip subluxation occurs when there is contact of femoral head against the acetabulum with joint instability, whereas dislocation occurs when the femoral head is not located within the acetabular socket or the femoral head is not covered by the acetabular socket.[45] Subluxation can be progressive as the child begins to weight bear without the presence of counterbalancing hip abduction or extension strength.[3,44]

The management of hip dysplasia and dislocations is complex, and approaches vary from institution to institution.[40,42] It is imperative to have involvement with an orthopedic surgeon to monitor hip integrity and consider treatment options. Hip subluxation or dislocations are often not painful in individuals with spina bifida and may not have an impact on ability to achieve ambulation. Many individual with unilateral and bilateral dislocations have been able to achieve an ambulatory status.[3,40,43,44] Long-term ambulatory outcomes have not been associated with hip status and are more closely associated with neurologic levels and hip range of motion.[46] Studies have shown that contracture is more of a limiting factor to ambulation than subluxation.[39] Therefore, most would agree to address hip flexion contractures due to the negative impact on ambulatory potential.[43]

Surgically managing hip dysplasia or dislocation is complex with more variability with outcomes. Surgery may be more likely to be considered if there is a potential to improve function, but there is a high incidence of complications associated with surgical intervention.[44] Surgical management to realign the hip poses challenges because it can create a more rigid hip and has a risk of re-subluxing due to the ongoing presence of muscle imbalances. It has been reported that up to 40% to 50% of children may re-dislocate after surgical location and nearly a third have stiffness reported postoperatively.[3,44] An increased incidence of pain has been shown postoperatively, whereas less than 10% of people report pain preoperatively.[3] Additional postoperative complications may include infection, fracture, and avascular necrosis.[40] Some children may have poorer outcomes with decreased ambulatory ability, especially if there is decreased hip range of motion.[3,44] Postoperative immobilization

is required, followed by physical therapy for progressive range of motion and strengthening.[42]

Knee Deformities

Knee deformities may be congenital or acquired and are related to muscle imbalances, prolonged positioning, and abnormal weight-bearing forces. The most prevalent is a knee flexion contracture and can occur in individuals who primarily rely on a wheelchair for means of mobility. Knee flexion contractures may also be present in ambulatory individuals with impaired gastrocnemius-soleus function. Children with weak gastrocnemius-soleus (L5-S3) muscles, especially with the presence of anterior tibialis (L3-L5) strength, are prone to a crouch gait pattern. The gastrocnemius-soleus not only has a function of push-off in terminal stance but also eccentrically controls anterior translation of the tibia through mid-stance. In the presence of a weak or absent gastrocnemius-soleus muscle, there is limited control of forward translation of the tibia in stance and a resultant crouch pattern. A crouch gait pattern, or persistent knee flexion through stance, is commonly seen with individuals with low lumbar and sacral level lesions. The individual will rely on quadriceps strength to prevent knee buckle, which can lead to fatigue.[20] The greater the degree of contracture, the more fatiguing this can be, and it will limit an individual's ambulatory potential with increased energy expenditure. Just as with hip flexion contractures, knee flexion contractures should be managed early and aggressively with stretching programs in order to optimize a child's opportunity to participate in upright mobility activities (**Figures 9-2 and 9-3**). Orthoses should also be considered in order to minimize or control the anterior translation of the tibia. Orthotic options are discussed later in this text.

Knee extension contractures can occur with an imbalance of strong quadriceps in the presence of weak or absent hamstrings, creating an extensor moment. Knee extension contractures affect an individual's ability to obtain a seated position. This can also occur in ambulatory children and lead to patellar alta, knee pain, and patellar overuse syndromes. Knee extension

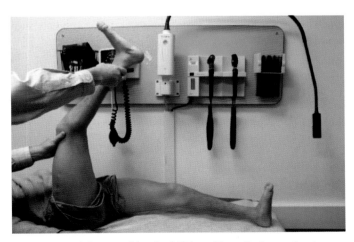

FIGURE 9-2 Adolescent with spina bifida and knee flexion contracture. Individual is supine with popliteal angle indicating knee flexion contracture.

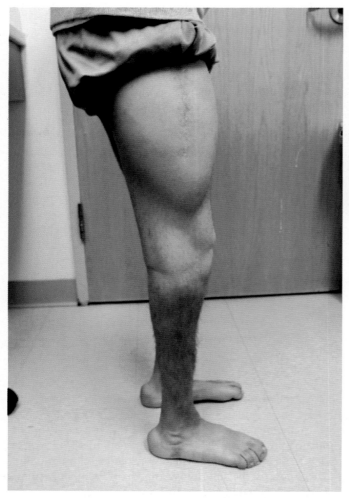

FIGURE 9-3 **Adolescent with spina bifida in standing with knee flexion contractures and foot deformities.**

contractures may contribute to genu recurvatum, or knee hyperextension, during stance or gait.

Knee valgus or knee varus deformities can lead to increased medial or lateral forces through the knee joint, respectively. This can lead to ligamentous laxity and have an impact on the integrity of the joint, especially for those who ambulate into adulthood.

Common Deformities of the Foot

There are many foot deformities or combinations of foot deformities seen with spina bifida. These occur due to asymmetrical muscle forces pulling through the small bones of the foot creating flexible or fixed deformities. A flexible deformity passively corrects to a plantigrade position, whereas a fixed deformity may have a more rigid alignment.

Congenital foot deformities occur due to asymmetrical muscle forces and positioning in utero. One of the most common congenital foot deformities is a club foot, which includes a combination of equinovarus, forefoot adduction, and supination (**Figures 9-4** and **9-5**). Other congenital foot deformities may include calcaneovalgus, cavovarus, or a vertical talus.[9] A vertical talus limits the available range of dorsiflexion through

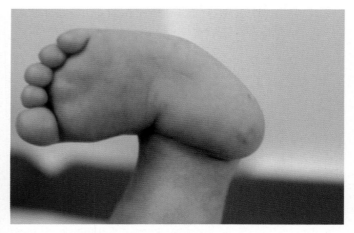

FIGURE 9-4 **Infant with club foot deformity.**

the talonavicular joint. Congenital foot deformities should be addressed early with range of motion/stretching, splinting, or casting. Soft tissue releases may need to be performed as well for persistent deformities.

An acquired foot deformity can result from imbalanced muscle forces and unsupported weight bearing, often seen in children with lower lumbar and sacral levels of spina bifida. These may include equinus contractures, dorsiflexion contractures, calcaneal varus or valgus contractures, or a cavus foot. A calcaneal deformity may occur with over activation of the anterior tibialis tendon with increased calcaneal weight-bearing forces.[39] A cavus foot deformity frequently occurs with activation of the extensor hallucis longus (EHL) over the anterior tibialis to perform dorsiflexion. Over time, this can lead to development of an exaggerated and rigid arch or cavus foot deformity. A valgus foot deformity often occurs from a combination of planovalgus and pronation of the forefoot due to poor motor control (**Figure 9-6**).[47]

Whether congenital or acquired, the goal is to achieve a plantigrade position of the foot to support weight bearing in the upright position. This positioning is ideal for weight bearing and to minimize abnormal joint reaction forces through the foot and upward through the lower extremity and spine. It will

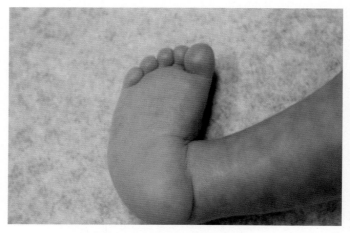

FIGURE 9-5 **Infant with club foot deformity in supine.**

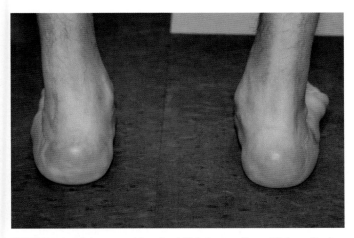

FIGURE 9-6 Adolescent with spina bifida in standing with knee flexion contractures and foot deformities.

also decrease the risk of injury from abnormal weight-bearing forces, especially injury to the skin.[9,47] Orthotics can support the foot and maintain the plantigrade position for weight bearing. Rigid foot deformities can lead to difficulty with fit of orthoses and contribute to skin breakdown.[39]

Treatment may include splinting/serial casting, soft tissue release, or bony correction of the foot deformity through various surgical techniques.[39] As with any surgical intervention, careful consideration of the child's level of function and the risks and benefits associated with surgical correction should be considered.[47] A rapid change in a foot deformity could be related to spinal cord tethering and may require further neurologic evaluation.

Spine Deformities

Scoliosis is defined as a lateral curve in the spine greater than 10 to 20 degrees.[48,49] Spinal curves associated with spina bifida are complex and may be congenital, acquired, or a combination and pose unique challenges for treatment.[39] Congenital scoliosis is related to bony deformities of the vertebrae and may be present in up to 38% of children with spina bifida, most commonly in those with thoracic level lesions.[9,49] Neuromuscular scoliosis is related to muscle imbalances, abnormal skin covering of the back, displacement of neural elements, and abnormal bony spinal structures. These may be associated with a pelvic obliquity or leg length discrepancy.[49] The incidence of acquired spinal curves varies from 50% to 88%, with higher prevalence in individuals with high lumbar or thoracic level lesions.[6,48-51] Spinal curves are often progressive, especially during periods of growth, although it is difficult define the rate of spinal progression in this population.[49-51] Spinal curves may also be associated with an underlying neurologic cause such as a tethered spinal cord or hydromyelia.[49] Rapid progression of a spinal curve can be indicative of a tethered spinal cord, especially in the presence of other neurologic changes, such as changes in bowel or bladder status. This would also warrant evaluation by a neurosurgeon.

The presence of a spinal deformity can have an impact on seating, postural stability, and organ systems, such as pulmonary or gastrointestinal function.[48,49] Impacts on trunk stability

may impede the ability to participate in functional activities and ADLs, especially when there is increased reliance on the upper extremities or external supports for maintaining upright sitting.[49-51] There is also increased risk of skin injury with lack of sensation over bony prominences or due to abnormal sitting pressures created from pelvic obliquities.[48] Back pain may also be associated with neuromuscular scoliosis, further impacting function.[49]

Treatment options vary based on the child's functional level and age. Physical therapy can address postural strength and balance with stretching and strengthening programs. The physical therapist may also consider external supports with seating to accommodate spinal deformities and distributing pressure areas for prevention of skin injury. Spinal orthoses may also be considered to provide additional postural stability and support for children with more flexible curves and promote participation with functional activities. This is most commonly achieved with the use of a thoracolumbosacral orthosis. Any bracing program should be considerate of bony prominences and insensate areas due to the risk for skin breakdown when wearing a rigid orthosis.[49]

Posterior spinal fusion is a surgical procedure that includes fixating hardware along the posterior aspect of the spinal column in order to correct or minimize the curve. The goal of surgical intervention is to better balance the spine while optimizing the patient's quality of life.[49] It is important to consider the impacts on functional mobility when considering spinal fusion and provide opportunity for collaborative discussion between the surgeon and physical therapist. Surgical fixation to the sacrum limits mobility through the lumbar spine.[49] An individual who relies on mobility through the lumbar spine for ambulation may experience a negative impact on their ability to ambulate after surgical fusion.[50] Some reports have shown that children have had more difficulty with ambulation after spinal fusion.[49,50] As with any surgical intervention, the goal should be to prevent further curvature of the spine and optimize quality of life by improving sitting balance or posture, improving pulmonary or gastrointestinal function, decreasing pain, and potentially increasing function.[50,51]

Advances in growth-sparing techniques have been used when surgical intervention is indicated prior to an individual reaching bone maturity. These options include growing rods, vertical expandable prosthetic titanium ribs (VEPTR), or MAGEC growing rods. These allow for growth of the spine but require routine lengthening to the device. A more definitive fusion will be required once skeletal maturity is reached.

Kyphosis or lordosis is a curvature of the spinal curve in the sagittal plane.[49] A kyphosis may be present in the thoracic (excessive kyphosis) or lumbar region of the spine. Kyphosis may also occur with scoliosis, also known as a kyphoscoliosis. Kyphosis may pose a high risk for skin breakdown, especially in individuals who primarily use a wheelchair as their form of mobility. Seating devices should distribute pressure over bony prominences and areas at risk for injury. A lordosis is most commonly seen in the lumbar region of the spine and considered a deformity when the lordosis is greater than 65 degrees.[3] Lordosis may be associated with hip flexion contractures and may be a compensatory posture to achieve a more upright position of the trunk.

NEUROGENIC BOWEL AND BLADDER

Children with spina bifida have parasympathetic and sympathetic nerve impairment that impacts bowel and bladder function.[7,9] Nearly all children with spina bifida will have a neurogenic bladder, with over 90% having dysfunctional voiding.[7] This can result in urinary incontinence, urinary retention, frequent urinary tract infections, or urinary reflux back toward the kidneys (vesicoureteral reflux). Problems associated with neurogenic bladder can lead to significant medical problems, including impacts on renal function.[6]

In neurogenic bladder associated with spina bifida, there is a discoordination or dyssynergy between the contraction and relaxation of the detrusor and sphincter muscles that can contribute to incontinence (leaking of urine) or incomplete emptying of the bladder.[1,7,9,22] Incontinence can occur due to weakness or inability of the pelvic floor to maintain a state of contraction for support or due to the bladder being overactive and contracting to squeeze urine out. Urinary continence is important for social acceptance, prevention of upper urinary tract issues, and prevention of skin integrity issues.[6] Medical issues associated with neurogenic bladder include vesicoureteral reflux, hydronephrosis, renal scarring, bacteriuria, and pyelonephritis.[4,9] Hydronephrosis can lead to renal failure, which can be life-threatening. Renal failure used to be one of the leading causes of death in adults with spina bifida but has since decreased with improved management of bladder function.

Children with spina bifida should have close monitoring of bladder function by a urologist.[7] Urodynamics evaluate muscle and bladder function.[4] This can provide objective measurements of the bladder dynamics and monitor for any neurologic changes associated with bladder function.[1]

Most children will have a bladder management program that starts shortly after birth, and compliance with this program can prevent future complications and preserve the health of the bladder and kidneys.[6] Bladder programs will often include a combination of anticholinergic medications and clean intermittent catheterization (CIC). The addition of CIC has significantly decreased the risk of renal disease in this population.[4,8] Anticholinergic medications help to inhibit detrusor contraction and increase storage capacity.[9] If managed with medications and CIC, 70% to 90% of children achieve some level of continence.[6,9]

Surgical procedures may be performed to promote continence or renal health.[1] A bladder augmentation increases the size or support of the bladder wall.[6,9] A Mitrofanoff procedure uses the appendix to connect the augmented bladder to or near the umbilicus to create a continent stoma to allow for ease of access with CIC.[9] This procedure increases independence and compliance with ADLs, especially for individuals who rely on a wheelchair or have difficulty with fine motor control.

Neurogenic bowel associated with spina bifida includes fecal incontinence or constipation.[7] Fecal incontinence can occur with a lack of pelvic floor or sphincter muscle control.[22,52] Children with spina bifida may have slow motility secondary to decreased parasympathetic activation with decreased colonic movement, leading to constipation.[4,9,52] Bowel dysfunction can have a significant impact on quality of life for individuals with spina bifida.[52] Secondary complications related to bowel dysfunction include urinary incontinence, urinary tract infections, shunt malfunction, risk of skin breakdown, and decreased participation in activities and employment.[52] Once a child reaches the age of toilet training (approximately 3-5 years old), a bowel program should be considered.[9] Bowel programs tailored to meet individual needs have been shown to be most successful.[52] This may include diet modifications, medications, or other means to promote elimination such as enema or suppository use.[4,9] Bowel programs may require prolonged sitting on the toilet or a commode to expel stool.[4] Seating posture and alignment are important considerations due to the risk of skin injury with prolonged sitting in one position. An optimal posture with hip flexion of greater than 90 degrees and the feet resting flat on a surface allows for lengthening of the puborectalis muscle to promote defecation. Surgical procedures include a Malone continent enema (MACE) procedure, which creates an antegrade continence stoma to allow for ease of access to an alternative site to use an enema.[4,9] Achieving bowel continence can have physical and psychological benefits.[7]

OTHER CONSIDERATIONS

Skin Integrity

Many individuals with spina bifida have a high risk of developing issues with skin integrity, especially with higher-level lesions.[3,4,9] According to the National Spina Bifida Registry, in a 2020 study, 26% of individuals had a history of pressure injuries and 19% reported a skin injury within the last year.[53] There is an increased risk of pressure ulcer associated with level of lesion, wheelchair use, urinary incontinence, presence of a shunt, and orthopedic or recent surgery.[11,53] Deformities may create areas of bony prominences with abnormal pressure areas, increasing risk of skin breakdown. This is further compromised by diminished sensation or skin integrity issues. Prolonged sitting contributes to pressure ulcers in this population.[5] Shearing injuries may also occur with abnormal movement or friction over an area with poor sensation or abnormal skin coverage. Burn injuries may occur with poor protective responses.[4] Skin injuries may take weeks to months to heal or be complicated by infection, which can lead to prolonged hospitalization or immobilization. The majority of hospitalizations for adults with spina bifida are related to skin injuries.[5]

Guidelines recommend maximizing skin health while minimizing skin integrity disruption as well as increasing awareness for risk of injury.[53] Education is key to prevention of injuries and secondary complications.[9] Successful skin injury prevention requires daily skin checks, pressure relief throughout the day, regular physician follow-up, proper nutrition, management of bowel and bladder continence, and appropriate seating and positioning. Improving self-management skills and providing individualized education may help to prevent secondary complications associated with skin injury.[5]

Fracture Risk

There is an increased risk of fracture due to low bone density as well as abnormal forces that may be imposed across the bone with muscle imbalances.[4,54,55] Bone mineral density has been shown to be lower in children with spina bifida as compared to age-matched peers.[54] Fractures are common in individuals with spina bifida with an incidence as high as 30%.[54,55] There is a higher association of fractures in individuals who are nonambulatory. Increased mobilization, participation in sports, and increased bone density have a positive correlation with decreased fracture rates.[55] Fractures of the lower extremities may go undetected due to inability to feel pain.[54,55] Careful examination and evaluation should include consideration for potential fracture in an extremity that is red, warm, or swollen.[4,55]

Latex Allergies

There is increased concern for latex allergy in individuals with spina bifida. The etiology is not clear, although it may be related to frequent exposure in home, school, and community environments.[56] There have been several reports of severe anaphylactic responses or death related to exposure to latex in individuals with spina bifida.[4,56] Some people may experience mild systemic responses, such as skin reactions/irritations, rashes, development of hives, skin color changes, or reports of itchy eyes, whereas others may develop wheezing, coughing, nausea, or vomiting.[56] Due to the severity and frequency of allergic responses, it is recommended that all people with spina bifida avoid exposure to latex. Many schools and health care environments are latex-free environments. Guidelines recommend education about latex-containing products, especially items used for medical care, daily activities, or within the community.[56] Adults with spina bifida benefit from ongoing education and support to identify latex products within the work environment as well as consideration of latex-free contraceptives if sexually active.[56]

Weight Management

Obesity is another common comorbidity among people with spina bifida. This is related to decreased mobility with decreased caloric expenditure. Increased body habitus size can further impede mobility or activity.[9] Studies have shown reduced physical activity levels in children and adolescents with spina bifida compared to peers, further contributing to risk of obesity.[2] Education about dietary habits and activity participation can promote participation in home, school, and community activities. Participation in training programs and physical fitness activities has a positive correlation with physical fitness in individuals with spina bifida. Incorporating the individual's and family's priorities will increase success in participation. It can also be beneficial to identify potential perceived barriers to participation for the individual. Factors that may have an impact on physical activity and participation include bowel and bladder continence, level of fitness, ability to complete skills associated with activity, and medical status. Environmental factors may include social supports, the use of assistive devices for mobility, and adequate knowledge and accessibility of adaptive programs.[2]

■ THE PHYSICAL THERAPY EXAMINATION

The physical therapy examination should be comprehensive to address the multiple systems that are associated with spina bifida. This includes examination of joint range of motion, strength, posture, sensation developmental reflexes, motor development, and developmental skills. Using validated and objective assessment tools, the physical therapist can identify an individual's motor level and impairments to provide a basis for intervention by establishing the goals and plan of care. The physical therapist can determine baseline level of function that can help predict anticipated level of function and identify areas of potential deformity or risk of injury. Whenever possible, the physical therapist should work in collaboration with a multidisciplinary team (Table 9-1) to address all aspects of the patient's care and optimize health and quality of life.

Sequential and regular evaluations can help detect any potential changes in a person's condition and indicate a need for a referral to a medical provider.[57] The frequency of formal examinations will depend on the setting, age, and medical status of the individual. Examinations should be more frequent in infancy and childhood and may occur less frequently or annually through adolescence and adulthood.

POSTURAL ASSESSMENT

Postural assessments should be completed in various positions, with and without the effects of gravity, to accurately assess how posture may affect the individual's positioning and ability to participate in functional activities. Postural deformities can be related to motor asymmetries, structural deformities, or muscle tone. Deformities may be considered rigid or flexible. The physical therapist should identify potential deformities and recommend adaptive equipment or orthoses to minimize the detrimental impact on function. Impacts on seating, respiratory function, mobility, and skin integrity should be considered. New onset or progression of a postural deformity may be indicative of a change requiring referral to orthopedics or neurosurgery. For example, a leg length discrepancy may be identified with postural assessments. A real leg length discrepancy occurs when one or both of the long bones of the lower leg are shorter than the contralateral side. An apparent leg length discrepancy may indicate a dislocated hip, pelvic obliquity, scoliosis, or a deformity of the long bone. A rapidly progressing spinal curve or foot deformity may be concerning for neurologic changes related to a tethered cord.

RANGE OF MOTION ASSESSMENT

The development of a joint contracture occurs due to muscle imbalances associated with spina bifida. Range of motion assessments are completed with standardized measurements whenever possible as per the American Academy of Orthopedic Surgeons.[8] Goniometric measurements should be taken in standardized positions and by identifying bony landmarks whenever possible. Any deviation from standardized measurements due to positional restrictions or deformities should be documented for consistency and reproducibility.

Range of motion should be compared to what is considered normal for age-matched peers. Neonates and infants typical present with physiologic flexed positioning and do not have full hip extension, knee extension, ankle plantar flexion, or elbow extension. Maintaining range of motion through the hip, knee, and ankle joints can have a positive impact on functional outcomes and should be a key focus with physical therapy interventions.

STRENGTH ASSESSMENT

Accurate strength assessments help to identify the child's motor level and predict functional outcomes. This can guide interventions and orthopedic management.[31,58] Include upper extremity strength assessments, even for children with lower lumbar or sacral involvement. Asymmetry may be present, and each limb should be examined fully. Establishing a baseline of strength can help identify potential deformities, as well as any neurologic changes that may indicate need for a referral to a neurosurgeon.[31]

The Medical Research Council recommends using a numerical grading scale of 0 through 5 for strength for manual muscle testing in standardized testing positions whenever possible (Table 9-4 and **Figure 9-7**).[17,31,58-61] As with range of motion, modifications should be documented. The physical therapist should isolate and palpate the muscle as best as possible to accurately assign a strength grade. Most authors consider a muscle group to be present or innervated if it is graded as fair (3/5) or higher.

The patient's age and ability to follow commands are important considerations when assessing strength. It is generally accepted that formal manual muscle testing can be accurately performed at age 5 years and above, depending on the child's cognition, ability to follow commands, and participation.[31,58,60] This strength assessment should remain relatively consistent into adulthood.[58] The physical therapist can still obtain strength measurements prior to the age of 5 years to guide interventions and determine motor levels. Strength measurements can be accurately assigned for infants and young children up to a fair (3/5) range, whereas others recommend describing strength as full, weak, or absent in infants. This can be completed with

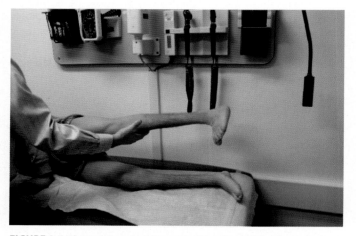

FIGURE 9-7 **Therapist and adolescent with spina bifida. Therapist is performing manual muscle examination.**

observation of active movements and palpation of muscle groups.[57,58,60] If the infant or child is able to perform muscle activation against applied resistance, you can grade that muscle as at least a fair plus (3+/5) grade or "apparently normal."[58] If the child is unable to complete a full active range of motion in a gravity-minimized plane, that is considered poor minus (2–/5) or weak strength. Strength testing of the anterior tibialis has been shown to remain consistent from infancy into childhood as an indicator of identifying motor levels.[58]

SENSATION

A thorough sensory examination can help to determine sensory levels including both sides through all dermatomes. It is imperative to identify any areas that may be impaired with sensation. Sensory levels may differ from motor levels. Sensory testing may occur formally with monofilaments for light touch or pinpoint testing for sharp/dull sensation.

INTEGUMENTARY

While completing a thorough sensory examination, the skin should also be assessed for areas of injury, irritation, or poor skin integrity to identify either current skin injury or areas of potential injury. Skin injury may be due to poor skin integrity or bony prominences over an insensate area of skin. A person may not be sensate and aware of the area where the breakdown is occurring; therefore, the skin should be visualized regularly. Areas of erythema indicating pressure or irritation can be addressed with positioning, adjustment of orthosis, or other protective measures. Caregiver education for daily skin inspection, especially areas that are at risk of injury, is essential. As the child grows, this responsibility should transition to the child to promote independence with self-care. Wounds with prolonged healing times may require referral to a wound care specialist.

TONE

Children with spina bifida may present with flaccid paraplegia, spasticity, or mixed paraplegia and spasticity.[7] Spasticity is present if the individual has abnormal posturing with increased muscular tension, a catch and release with motion, resistance through passive range, or clonus.[8,31,59] The presence of hypertonia increases the risk for joint contracture and may benefit from a stretching and positioning program. Hypotonia may impact the child's positioning, posture, or ability to participate in developmental activities.[57] Any changes in tone could be indicative of a change in neurologic status, such as a tethered cord, and should prompt a referral to the medical team.

MOBILITY

Mobility includes the ability to move within an individual's environment and creates the foundation for learning in young children. Research supports that mobility impacts physical, cognitive, and psychosocial factors of development.[62] A comprehensive mobility assessment should always be completed when working with a child with spina bifida. Benefits of participation in mobility activities include contracture management, benefits of cardiovascular and strength exercise, bone density, motility, participation in household and community activities, participation in ADLs, pressure reduction or redistribution, improvements in pain, and stress reduction.[62]

Typical motor development occurs in a cephalocaudal direction. Postural control is obtained through opportunities to move against gravity.[63] Children with spina bifida will generally follow typical developmental sequencing, but often at a slower rate compared to children without spina bifida, and may require adaptive supports to meet developmental milestones.[62] Developmental skill attainment is correlated with level of lesion; however, developmental skills can vary in children with the same lesion level.[57] Children with spina bifida and lipomyelomeningocele have been shown to perform worse on the Pediatric Evaluation of Disability Inventory (PEDI) compared to age-matched norms.[7,60] The presence of motor paralysis, cognitive delays, neurologic impairments, or bowel and bladder dysfunction also has a negative impact on motor development.[7] Understanding typical motor development can help guide therapists in facilitating skills and mobility.[63]

Standardized developmental assessments used with this population have included the BSID, PEDI, and Pediatric Functional Independence Measure.[23] Any orthoses or assistive devices used during testing should be documented. If the child is not achieving age-appropriate milestones, additional supports may be considered. For example, if a child is not sitting independently, the physical therapist may incorporate additional seating support, such as a positional chair or spinal orthosis. If a child has not yet achieved good trunk control with appropriate righting reactions in sitting, ambulation should not yet be a focus. The ability to bear weight is a good indicator of a child's readiness to begin gait training.[57] If a child has not begun to bear weight during the first year, additional supports to promote weight bearing may be introduced, such as a supine or prone stander.

Gait assessment should include the quality of gait, the speed of gait, level of ambulation, and any type of assistive device or orthosis required. The attainment of gait is associated with improved quality of life.[23] Achieving some level of ambulation during a child's life can help to minimize the negative effects from non–weight bearing, such as bone demineralization, fractures, pressure ulcers, and contractures.[64] As with motor development, children with spina bifida of all levels will likely achieve ambulatory skills but at a slower rate than age-matched peers.[12,14,23,32,35,57] Nearly 90% of children with mid-lumbar level lesions or lower achieve a form of ambulation by the age of 2 and continue to work on ambulatory skills up to the age of 6.[13,57]

Hoffer describes the following levels of ambulation in spina bifida: community ambulator, household ambulator, nonfunctional ambulator, and nonambulator. The Hoffer Functional Ambulation Scale is currently the most consistently used measure for walking ability and was specifically created for use in patients with spina bifida (**Table 9-8**).[23,26,31,59]

Many factors contribute to achieving ambulation for children with spina bifida. Most agree that the level of the lesion is one of the best predictive factors of level of ambulation achieved.[3,6,7,23,31,35,40,42,43,59] The level of lesion is inversely correlated with the level of ambulation. That is, the lower the level of lesion, the more likely it is that a higher level of ambulation will be achieved. The higher the level of lesion, the more support may be

TABLE 9-8 • Hoffer Classification for Ambulation		
Classification	**Level of Ambulation**	**Associated Neurologic Level**
Community ambulator	Ambulates with or without assistive device or orthoses in the community May use wheelchair for longer distances	Sacral Low lumbar
Household ambulator	Ambulates with assistive device and/or orthoses in the home Wheelchair for all community mobility	Low lumbar Mid lumbar
Nonfunctional ambulator	Ambulates with assistive device and/or orthoses in therapy Wheelchair for all community mobility	Mid lumbar High lumbar
Nonambulator	Uses wheelchair for all mobility	High lumbar Thoracic

required to achieve ambulation.[4,6,7,17,23] Approximately 20% to 50% of children with thoracic or high lumbar lesions achieved ambulation by the age of 4 to 5 years, but most did not maintain this past the age of 10.[12,14,32] Children with this level of lesion typically rely on a wheelchair as primary mode of mobility.[6] Approximately 60% of children with mid-lumbar lesions achieve ambulation by the age of 5, although age of onset of walking and type of support are highly variable in this group.[32,57] Over 80% of children with low lumbar lesions and 90% of children with sacral level lesions achieved ambulation by 2 to 4 years of age. Nearly all children with low lumbar or sacral level lesions who achieved ambulation were able maintain this function past the age of 9 years.[12,14,32] The majority (>90%) of individuals with sacral level lesions with dorsiflexion strength (grade 4/5 or 5/5) and the presence of hip abductor strength achieve community level ambulation.[60] Reports have shown independent ambulation in 93% of children with sacral level lesions, 91% with low lumbar (L5 level) lesions, 54% with L4 level lesions, and no patients with thoracic or high lumbar level lesions.[19]

Approximately 60% of children will achieve their predicted level of ambulation based on their motor level, whereas the other 40% do not.[59] Factors negatively impacting ambulatory potential include obesity, impaired cognitive status, balance or coordination deficits, presence of musculoskeletal deformities, presence of spasticity, and presence of other neurologic factors, such as hydrocephalus or upper motor neuron involvement.[31,35,57,59,64] Spasticity appears to have the greatest negative impact on ability to ambulate if present in the hip or knee joints.[8,59] Spasticity at the hip and knee can also contribute to flexion contractures, which may further impact ambulatory status.[59] Increased energy requirements may negatively impact ambulatory potential. The presence of musculoskeletal deformities and compensatory movements to achieve gait increases energy expenditure.[7,14,23,59]

Highest level of ambulation may not be maintained into adulthood.[40,65] Cessation of walking skills in adulthood may be related to increases in size, weight, energy expenditure, weight of orthotics, or neurologic changes.[6,32] Up to 40% of individuals with mid-lumbar level lesions and below showed a decline in ambulation into adulthood with increased reliance on a wheelchair.[14,64] Individuals with lower lumbar or sacral level lesions may continue to ambulate into adulthood.[18] Maintaining community level ambulation is most associated with level of lesion, no history of shunting, and no history of hip or knee flexion contracture surgery.[11] Children who were household ambulators were not likely to maintain this into adulthood.[18,40,45] Prediction of ambulatory status into adulthood is most accurate for those with high lumbar or sacral level lesions, and is variable for those with L3-L5 lesions.[65] A wheelchair is often more efficient, and use is increased into adolescence and adulthood.[6]

AEROBIC CAPACITY AND ENDURANCE

Cost of energy for mobility should be considered when assessing a patient. The physical therapist should consider whether the amount of support is appropriate or if increasing/decreasing support would have a positive impact on energy expenditure. Cardiovascular and endurance training can promote more independence with activities. Encouraging participation in various activities (recreational or sport) has positive benefits on overall health and wellness as well.

■ ORTHOTICS AND ASSISTIVE DEVICES

Orthotics and assistive devices can provide the child with the opportunity to be more upright by providing additional support and joint protection or preventing deformity. They can counterbalance abnormal forces or compensatory movements but also require increased effort to move due to the weight and rigidity of the support. Selection of an appropriate orthosis should take into careful consideration the child's current and anticipated level of function. Orthotic use may be impacted by any musculoskeletal deformities or neurologic involvement, such as spasticity or hypotonia.[57] Orthoses can either correct or accommodate a deformity, but there are limitations with the amount of correction that can be achieved. Often, assistive devices, such as forearm crutches or a reverse rolling walker, will be used with orthotics.

Orthosis selection is highly correlated with the child's motor level, with higher-level lesions requiring more support (**Table 9-9**). For children with no muscle activity of the lower limbs, a standing device may be considered to allow the child to be fully upright and in a weight-bearing position. Readiness to participate in supported standing requires activation of trunk extensors and can be demonstrated with the ability to reach the hand outward while in prone position.[57] The use of a standing frame is most associated with thoracic lesions, and these individuals are often considered nonambulators based on the Hoffer scale.

Reciprocal gait orthoses (RGOs) are used by individuals with thoracic and high lumbar level lesions or by those who benefit from assistance with performing limb advancement. RGOs provide support through the ankle, knee, hip, and trunk and facilitate advancement of the lower extremities to promote a reciprocal gait pattern.[33] RGOs have a cable system that facilitates reciprocal advancement of the lower extremities and are ideal for individuals who have weak hip flexion function.[43,57] An assistive device is required while using an RGO in order to provide additional stability or upright positioning. Posterior (reverse-facing) rolling walkers or forearm crutches are preferred to counterbalance extensor weakness while promoting more upright posture. Although this style of orthotic

TABLE 9-9 • Orthotic Use With Associated Neurologic Levels

Motor Level	Associated Muscle Involvement	Orthotics	Assistive Device
Thoracic	No motor activation below the umbilicus May have weak abdominals or paraspinals	Reciprocating gait orthosis	Posterior walker Wheelchair
High lumbar (L1/L2)	Strong iliopsoas Weak quadriceps	Hip-knee-ankle-foot orthosis	Posterior walker Forearm crutches Wheelchair
Mid lumbar (L3)	Normal iliopsoas Normal quadriceps	Knee-ankle-foot orthosis Ankle-foot orthosis (AFO)	Posterior walker Forearm crutches May use wheelchair
Low lumbar (L4/L5)	Normal iliopsoas Normal quadriceps Strong anterior tibialis Weak to strong hamstrings	AFO	None or forearm crutches May use wheelchair
Sacral	Normal iliopsoas Normal quadriceps Normal anterior tibialis Normal hamstring Weak to strong gluteus medius and maximus Weak gastrocnemius-soleus	AFO Supramalleolar orthosis None	None May use wheelchair for community

does provide opportunity for ambulation, it requires increased energy expenditure. Children who require RGOs will likely achieve household or nonfunctional level ambulation and will likely not maintain this level of ambulation into adulthood.[57]

Hip-knee-ankle-foot orthoses (HKAFOs) are beneficial for individuals with high lumbar (L1-L2) lesions or with the presence of good to normal hip flexion and weak knee extensors.[43] Active hip flexion is required for reciprocal limb advancement or use of momentum to generate a swing-through gait pattern. The hip and knee components of the brace may be locked or unlocked depending on the amount of support required. Locking the hip component will provide more upright support, but will make it more difficult to advance the lower extremities. Another indication for use of HKAFOs is controlling foot placement during limb advancement and weight acceptance. Weakness of the hip abductors contributes to difficulty controlling pelvis in stance and leads to excessive lateral trunk motion or variable foot placement during weight acceptance. HKAFOs will maintain the hip and pelvis alignment and minimize abnormal forces during gait. A child should demonstrate independent sitting position prior to initiating use of HKAFOs.[57] As with the use of RGOs, a posterior walker or forearm crutches are beneficial when using HKAFOs to promote upright alignment and counterbalance extensor weakness. Those who use HKAFOs for ambulation will likely achieve household or nonfunctional level ambulation and otherwise require the use of a wheelchair.[57,65]

Knee-ankle-foot orthoses (KAFOs) can provide stability through the knee joint in the transverse and frontal plane.[57,61] KAFOs can minimize knee hyperextension moments, especially through terminal stance, which is a common gait deviation seen in the presence of weak quadriceps. This style of bracing can also be useful for controlling varus or valgus forces through the knee joint. A knee valgus force may occur with internal hip rotation secondary to proximal hip weakness or femoral anteversion and knee flexion in a crouch gait secondary to gastrocnemius-soleus weakness.[61] KAFOs have a knee joint that can be locked or unlocked based on the amount of support needed but do not provide stability through the hips or pelvis as with HKAFOs. This style of brace can be beneficial for joint protection measures and maintaining long-term joint health.

Ankle-foot orthoses (AFOs) are widely used with children with spina bifida and can help improve alignment and pathologic forces through the ankles and knees. They can also help to improve cost of energy with ambulation and prevent deformities.[20,66] AFOs are most often used in individuals with mid to low lumbar level of involvement who may be able to achieve community ambulation with or without the use of an assistive device.[33,43,57,65] An AFO provides stability through the ankle joint by maintaining a neutral position. This allows for improved foot clearance in the absence of active dorsiflexion. The design of the AFO can also be considered to control forward translation of the tibia to provide additional control of a crouch gait pattern.[20,61] A crouch gait secondary to gastrocnemius-soleus weakness can be fatiguing and lead to knee pain, overuse syndromes, or development of knee flexion contractures. Ground reaction (floor reaction) AFOs or carbon fiber dynamic assist AFOs can be beneficial because they provide additional knee extensor moment through mid-stance.[66] An articulated AFO, or an AFO with a flexible ankle joint, provides the benefit of some additional ankle motion but will not limit anterior translation of the tibia. It should be used selectively for children who do not exhibit a crouch pattern or risk of knee flexion contracture development.

Submalleolar orthoses (SMOs) are often used to provide additional medial/lateral control of the calcaneus. This may be seen with collapsing of the mid-foot arch with calcaneal valgus or a high arch position with calcaneal varus. If additional support is required through the ankle, this cannot be achieved with an SMO alone and an AFO should be considered. SMOs are most often used by individuals with sacral level innervation (Table 9-9).[65]

Many children with spina bifida use some form of wheeled mobility. The timing of introducing wheeled mobility may vary for each individual.[63] For many children, especially if delayed in crawling, early introduction of wheeled mobility can be beneficial by providing an alternative form of independence while promoting cognitive development and environmental exploration. Early introduction of a wheelchair has been shown to benefit cognitive and social development and improve quality of life.[63] Ambulatory children, especially those who use orthoses or assistive devices, may still benefit from a wheelchair for community distances due to the high cost of energy with ambulatory skills. If not previously used, a wheelchair may be introduced in adolescence with increased growth and body size. There is a high incidence of wheelchair use after the onset of adolescence in those who have a mid-lumbar level or higher lesions. Regardless of timing of introduction of a wheelchair, the physical therapist should always emphasize proper wheelchair setup and independence with wheelchair mobility skills within all environments. A power wheelchair or a power assist wheelchair may be beneficial to prevent overuse injuries in adolescence and adulthood and allow improved access to the community environment with energy conservation.

▮ PHYSICAL THERAPY CONSIDERATIONS THROUGHOUT LIFE

The physical therapist has the opportunity to maximize an individual's function, independence, and self-esteem while minimizing family stresses. Interventions focus on achieving independent mobility while minimizing or preventing deformities or secondary complications. The physical therapist also has the unique role of promoting wellness, participation, and quality of life. Multidisciplinary care promotes improved outcomes, with providers collaborating to address the child's complex and multisystem involvement. Identifying baseline function can help identify any changes in neurologic status that could be detrimental to the child's function or health, help to predict functional outcomes, and guide therapeutic interventions.[63] When considering functional prognosis, consider the child's motor level, the presence of upper motor neuron involvement, the ability to achieve age-appropriate milestones, the presence of any deformities or potential

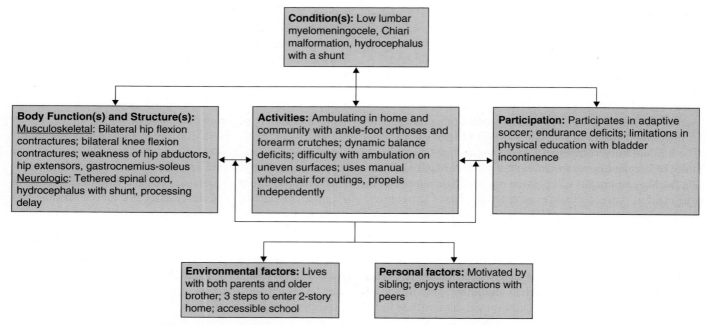

FIGURE 9-8 Example of International Classification of Functioning, Disability, and Health (ICF) model for decision-making.

deformities, the child's skin integrity, the bowel and bladder status and any environmental factors. The International Classification of Functioning, Disability, and Health (ICF) model can also help guide decision-making (**Figure 9-8**). The physical therapist may work closely with the orthopedic surgeon and/or physiatrist to maximize functional independence for the child throughout their life.

NEONATE

The physical therapist may become involved with the neonate shortly after the initial closure of the NTD; often, this may occur in a neonatal intensive care unit (NICU). The primary goal at this age is to identify motor levels, address any congenital deformities, and facilitate participation in developmental skill attainment and interactions.[57] Standardized assessments can help to identify baseline function and monitor for changes in neurologic status.[63] Primary treatment objectives include increasing range of motion, increasing active movement, promoting developmental positioning, and achieving developmental milestones. Range of motion can either be active or passive and considered for areas with restricted motion or at risk for contracture development. Infants with spina bifida have been shown to have decreased spontaneous leg movements compared to age-matched peers within the first 6 months of life.[12] The physical therapist can help facilitate leg movements to promote motor development skill obtainment. Positioning can be used to protect the skin, minimize postural deformities or contractures, and promote participation in developmental interactions.

Caregiver education is essential at this phase. It can be extremely stressful to have a medically complex infant. Parents may be unsure of how to hold, feed, or interact with their infant, which can have a negative impact on social development and bonding. Education is focused around skin care and protection,

any modifications to standard child care based on medical complexity or precautions, development promotion, and discharge planning. A developmental education program within the hospital environment and in anticipation of transitioning to home includes recommendations for range of motion, positioning, handling, and facilitation of age-appropriate activities. A referral to an early intervention or birth-to-3 program is often indicated to promote early involvement with physical and occupational therapy.[63]

INFANCY (UP TO 12 MONTHS)

Infancy is focused on the attainment of age-appropriate skills with the goal of achieving an upright position, whether sitting or standing. Motor development should prioritize alignment and movements against gravity to promote postural control.[63] Mobility can be progressed through prone play, crawling, quadruped, and creeping, which provide the foundation for future motor planning skills. This is also a period of progressing transitional movements such as rolling, pushing to sitting, and pulling to standing.

If a child is not participating in age-appropriate skills due to weakness, poor trunk control, or delayed postural reactions, the physical therapist may consider additional supports. A child presenting with poor trunk control could benefit from additional trunk or seating support. A dynamic trunk orthosis allows for support through the trunk while still allowing participation in developmental skills and activation of core musculature. A more rigid orthosis may be considered if the child needs additional postural support for upright positioning but does not promote core strength development. Other seating devices that may be considered include activity chairs or commercially available seating devices. Stability through the trunk allows for participation and development of fine motor control.

PRESCHOOL AGE

The primary goal for this age group is the attainment of independent mobility. Goals focus on obtaining weight-bearing positions and promoting ambulation.[23] Participation in physical therapy with emphasis on developmental skills and incorporating orthotic support when indicated can help the child achieve their anticipated level of function.[57,63] Treatment interventions may focus on transitional skills, weight-bearing activities, and preambulatory skills. If a child has not yet achieved a weight-bearing position due to weakness, additional supports may be considered. This can include the use of a stander, RGOs, or HKAFOs. AFOs can provide additional ankle support and protection while in a standing device or be used for foot and ankle positioning when sitting in a wheelchair. Range of motion should continue to be prioritized to promote adequate fit into orthotics or devices and prevent contractures. Initiation of wheelchair use is common at this age to promote independent mobility in preparation for transition to school.

SCHOOL AGE

The primary goal for the school-aged child is to achieve functional independence with mobility and ADLs. Independence with mobility includes the ability to transfer, wheelchair propulsion, ambulation, or a combination of skills.[63] This may or may not include orthoses or assistive devices. Children may benefit from additional supports for mobility or learning needs, which could be addressed in an individualized education plan (IEP) or 504 Americans with Disabilities (ADA) plan. Independence with ADLs and self-care is important to emphasize during this age as well.[63] The child should work on skills related to dressing and donning and doffing braces. This can also incorporate learning to assess their skin and perform independent pressure-relief activities. Independence with bowel and bladder management can also significantly increase a child's independence and self-esteem. Allowing children to participate in a CIC program can be empowering and promote continence.

Participation in peer interactions is essential for social and emotional development. Assessment of personal and environmental factors associated with physical activity can help to promote an active and healthy lifestyle.[2]

ADOLESCENCE

Adolescence is a period of rapid growth and gaining independence. There is a focus on developing life skills and prevocational training in anticipation of transitioning into adulthood. The physical therapist can play an integral role during this age by supporting ongoing independence. With the onset of increased body size/rapid growth, the child's previous level of mobility may be impacted by higher energy consumption. There may be increased reliance on wheeled mobility options at this age. Education and training may be required for wheelchair skills as well as performing routine skin checks or pressure relief.[63] Powered mobility options may also be introduced in adolescence or adulthood for school, community, and employment.

Another priority during this age may be learning how to independently manage health care needs. Health literacy has been defined as "the degree to which individuals have the capacity to obtain, process and understand basic health information and services need to make appropriate health decisions."[67] Adolescents with spina bifida have been shown to have poorer health literacy than their peers.[67] The individual's cognitive status and ability to participate in life skills will have an impact on transition to independent living and the adult health care system. Difficulty navigating medical systems can lead to poorer compliance and outcomes.[67] Adolescents may require additional support regarding medical care, community living, employment, and self-management given intellectual or executive functioning challenges.[68] Multidisciplinary care can support preparation for transition and navigating the medical complexities associated with spina bifida. Readiness for transition includes understanding of condition, engagement in medical appointments and discussions, and compliance with treatments.[67]

ADULTHOOD

Improvements in coordinated pediatric care have contributed to up to 85% of children with spina bifida surviving into adulthood.[56] Adults with spina bifida have complex physical, cognitive, and social needs.[69] The care of adults has improved, but there continue to be challenges around having a multidisciplinary and coordinated approach for adults with spina bifida. Transition planning in early adolescence can help make this more successful. Challenges facing the adult with spina bifida include a lack of coordinated care, challenges with insurance coverage, separation from parents, locating independent living options, and obtaining meaningful employment.

Overuse injuries are common in adults with spina bifida. These may result from prolonged use of wheeled mobility or weight bearing through their upper extremities during ambulation or transfers. These are often managed through episodes of outpatient physical therapy by addressing mechanical stressors to that joint. The physical therapist should assess how the individual is participating in mobility and provide any recommendations or modifications to prevent further injury. This also may be a time to consider powered mobility to prevent overuse injuries.

Secondary health conditions become more prevalent in adulthood. Ongoing issues with urinary and fecal incontinence, pain, and obesity can impact outcomes for adults with spina bifida.[69] Common secondary health conditions associated with spina bifida include osteoporosis, osteoarthritis, decreased cardiovascular fitness, obesity or difficulty with weight management, depression, and issues with skin integrity. Nearly 40% of hospitalizations in young adults are related to potentially preventable conditions, such as urinary tract infections or pressure sores.[5] According to *Healthy People With Disabilities 2020*, health outcomes are related to an "individual's ability to take part in meaningful daily activities that add to their growth, development, fulfillment, and community contribution."[70] Adults can benefit from ongoing follow-up care and support services to achieve this.[69] The physical therapist can help promote community participation opportunities when working with individuals with spina bifida.

■ CONCLUSION

Healthy People With disabilities 2020 strives to "maximize health, prevent chronic disease, and improve social and environmental living conditions."[70] It also calls to "promote community participation, choice, health equity and quality of life among individuals with disabilities of all ages."[70] Improved survival rates require ongoing coordinated care from health care professionals throughout the life span.[71] The goal is to maximize physical and mental health for individuals with spina bifida and prevent any secondary health complications.[68] The physical therapist can play an integral role when working with individuals with spina bifida throughout the entire life span. It is important for the physical therapist to collaborate as a part of a multidisciplinary team because this condition has multisystem involvement and children can present with a wide spectrum of abilities.[4,6] Emphasis on preventing complications associated with hydrocephalus, urologic issues, musculoskeletal deformities, and pressure sores has improved life expectancy and contributed to improved quality of life for individuals with spina bifida.[35] The goal for health promotion is to prevent secondary conditions, maintain independence, provide opportunities for participation, and enhance the individual's quality of life.[72] Individuals with deficits in functional mobility and participation in self-care activities have been shown to have decreased quality of life.[8] The physical therapist has the unique role to foster independence and promote participation and activities with peers. In doing so, many individuals with spina bifida can lead an engaged and fulfilling life.

Case 1

Andrew is a 14-month-old boy with spina bifida that was closed after birth, Chiari II malformation, hydrocephalus managed with a ventriculoperitoneal shunt, and neurogenic bowel and bladder. He demonstrates good activation of his quadriceps. His left leg demonstrates partial activation against gravity of his anterior tibialis and absent activation on the right. He has partial activation of hamstrings in gravity-minimized plane. He is able to sit independently with good head and trunk control. He is able to pull to kneeling and standing. His standing posture is significant for hip internal rotation, knee flexion, calcaneal valgus with midfoot collapse, and forefoot abduction.
1. What is a musculoskeletal deformity that Andrew is at risk for developing based on his level of paresis?
2. What orthosis might be considered?
3. What is Andrew's anticipated level of ambulation?

Case 2

Steve is an 8-year-old boy with high lumbar level spina bifida. He has bilateral hip flexion contractures with a right hip dislocation, bilateral knee flexion contractures, and scoliosis. He ambulates with a reverse rolling walker and HKAFOs during therapy sessions. He otherwise uses a manual wheelchair, which he can propel independently. He is working on independent transfers. Recently, Steve has noted increased leaning toward one side while seated in his wheelchair. His right foot is turning in more,

making it difficult to fit into his orthosis. He has had recent episodes of incontinence while in school.
1. What is an important consideration for the physical therapist working with Steve?

Case 3

Kelly is a 20-year-old woman with low lumbar level spina bifida. She ambulates in the community with ground reaction AFOs and forearm crutches. She is a junior in college and lives independently on campus. She reports recent weight gain.
1. What are important activities of daily living for Kelly to participate in to maintain independent living?
2. How might the physical therapist promote an active lifestyle and participation for Kelly to promote wellness?

STUDY QUESTIONS

1. What are potentially preventable secondary conditions associated with spina bifida that the physical therapist should consider?
2. How can the physical therapist promote activity and participation in an individual with spina bifida at each neuromotor level?
3. List ways that orthosis may help support energy expenditure with ambulation?
4. What are considerations when deciding on appropriate timing for use of wheeled mobility?
5. Why might one consider a posterior walker over an anterior walker or forearm crutches over axillary crutches?
6. What factors may have an impact on the highest level of ambulation achieved by a child?
7. List some clinical findings that may indicate a referral to a medical provider

References

1. Koh CJ, DeFilippo RE, Borer JG, Khoshbin S, Bauer SB. Bladder and external urethral sphincter function after prenatal closure of myelomeningocele. *J Urol.* 2006;176:2232-2236.
2. Bloemen MA, Verschuren O, van Mechelen C, et al. Personal and environmental factors to consider when aiming to improve participation in physical activity in children with Spina Bifida: a qualitative study. *BMC Neurol.* 2015;15(11):1-11.
3. Crandall RC, Birkebak RC, Winter RB. The role of hip location and dislocation in the functional status of the myelodysplastic patient. *Orthopedics.* 1989;12(5):675-684.
4. Ellas ER, Hobbs N. Spina bifida: sorting out the complexities of care. *Comtemp Pediatr.* 1998;15(4):156-171.
5. Mahmood D, Dicianno B, Bellin M. Self-Management, preventable conditions and assessment of care among young adults with myelomeningocele. *Child Care Health Dev.* 2011;37(6):861-865.
6. Thompson DNP. Postnatal management and outcome for neural tube defects including spina bifida and encephalocoeles. *Prenat Diagn.* 2009;29:412-419.

7. Tsai PY, Yang TF, Chan RC, Huang PH, Wong TT. Functional investigation in children with spina bifida: measured by the Pediatric Evaluation of Disability Inventory (PEDI). *Child Nervous Syst.* 2002;18:48-53.

8. Danielsson AJ, Bartonek A, Levey E, McHale K, Sponseller P, Saraste H. Associations between orthopeadic findings, ambulation and health-related quality of life in children with myelomeningocele. *J Child Orthop.* 2008;2:45-54.

9. Sandler AD. Children with spina bifida: key clinical issues. *Pediatr Clin N Am.* 2010;57:879-892.

10. Burmister R, Hannay HJ, Copeland K, Fletcher JM, Boudousquie A, Dennis M. Attention problems and executive functions in children with spina bifida and hydrocephalus. *Child Neuropsychol.* 2005;11:265-283.

11. Castillo J, Lupo PJ, Tu DD, Agopian AJ, Castillo H. The National Spina Bifida Patient Registry: a decade's journey. *Birth Defects Res.* 2019;111(14):947-957.

12. Rademacher N, Black DP, Ulrich BD. Early spontaneous leg movements in infants born with and without myelomeningocele. *Pediatr Phys Ther.* 2008;20(2):137-145.

13. Aguilera S, Soothill P, Denbow M, Pople I. Prognosis of spina bifida in the era of prenatal diagnosis and termination of pregnancy. *Fetal Diagn Ther.* 2009;26(2):68-74.

14. Teulier C, Smith BA, Kubo M, et al. Stepping responses of infants with myelomeningocele when supported on a motorized treadmill. *Phys Ther.* 2009;89(1):60-72.

15. Adzick NS, Thom EA, Spong CY, et al. A randomized trial of prenatal versus postnatal repair of myelomeningocele. *N Engl J Med.* 2011;10:1-12.

16. Spina Bifida Association Information Sheets. Spina bifida occulta: a mild form of spina bifida. Accessed November 1, 2018. http://spinabifidaassociation.org/project/spina-bifida-occulta/.

17. Biggio JR, Owen J, Wenstrom KD, Oakes WJ. Can prenatal ultrasound findings predict ambulatory status in fetuses with open spina bifida? *Am J Obstet Gynecol.* 2001;185(5):1016-1020.

18. Davis WA, Zigler CK, Crytzer TM, et al. Factors associated with ambulation in myelomeningocele: a longitudinal study from the National Spina Bifida Patient Registry. *Am J Phys Med Rehabil.* 2020;99(7):586-594.

19. Sacco A, Ushakov F, Thompson D, et al. Fetal surgery for open spina bifida. *Obstet Gynaecol.* 2019;21(4):271-282.

20. Malas BS. What variables influence the ability of an AFO to improve function and when are they indicated? *Clin Orthop Relat Res.* 2011;469(5):1308-1314.

21. Kinderer K, Hinderer O, Walker W, Shurtleff D. Myelodysplasia. In: *Campbell's Physical Therapy for Children.* 5th ed. Elsevier; 2017:542-582.

22. Yamashiro KJ, Galganski LA, Hirose S. Fetal myelomeningocele repair. *Semin Pediatr Surg.* 2019;28(4):150823.

23. Bisaro DL, Bidonde J, Kane KJ, Bergsma S, Musselman KE. Past and current use of walking measures for children with spina bifida: a systematic review. *Arch Phys Med Rehabil.* 2015;96(8):1533-1543.e31.

24. Warf BC, Wright EJ, Kulkarni AV. Factors affecting survival of infants with myelomeningocele in southeastern Uganda. *J Neurosurg Pediatr.* 2011;7:1-7.

25. Omar AT, Espiritu AI, Spears J. Endoscopic third ventriculostomy with or without choroid plexus coagulation for myelomeningocele-associated hydrocephalus: systematic review and meta-analysis. *J Neurosurg Pediatr.* 2022;29(4):435-443.

26. Danzer E, Thomas NH, Thomas A, et al. Long-term neurofunctional outcome, executive functioning, and behavioral adaptive skills following fetal myelomeningocele surgery. *Am J Obstet Gynecol.* 2016;214(2):269e1-269e8.

27. Simpson JL, Greene MF. Fetal surgery for myelomeningocele? *N Engl J Med.* 2011;364(11):1076-1077.

28. Blount JP, Bowman R, Dias MS, Hopson B, Partington MD, Rocque BG. Neurosurgery guidelines for the care of people with spina bifida. *J Pediatr Rehabil Med.* 2020;13(4):467-477.

29. Farmer DL, Thom EA, Brock JW, et al. The management of myelomeningocele study: full cohort 30-month pediatric outcomes. *Am J Obstet Gynecol.* 2018;218(2):256.e1-256.e13.

30. Dewan MC, Wellons JC. Fetal surgery for spina bifida. *J Neurosurg Pediatr.* 2019;24(2):105-114.

31. Bartonek A, Saraste H, Knutson LM. Comparison of different systems to classify the neurological level of lesion in patients with myelomeningocele. *Dev Med Child Neurol.* 1999;41(12):796-805.

32. Williams EN, Broughton NS, Menelaus MB. Age-related walking in children with spina bifida. *Dev Med Child Neurol.* 1999;41(7):446-449.

33. Battibugli S, Gryfakis N, Dias L, et al. Functional gait comparison between children with myelomeningocele: shunt versus no shunt. *Dev Med Child Neurol.* 2007;49(10):764-769.

34. Warf B, Campbell J. Combined endoscopic third ventriculostomy and choroid plexus cauterization as primary treatment of hydrocephalus for infants with myelomeningocele: long-term results of a prospective intent-to-treat study in 115 East African infants. *J Neurosurg Pediatr.* 2008;2:310-316.

35. Llopis ID, Munoz MB, Agullo EM, Martinez AL. Ambulation in patients with myelomeningocele: a study of 1500 patients. *Paraplegia.* 1993;31:28-32.

36. Warf B, Kulkarni A, Ampeire M, Mulondo R. Neurocognitive outcome and ventricular volume in children with myelomeningocele treated for hydrocephalus in Uganda. *J Neurosurg Pediatr.* 2009;4:564-570.

37. Dias MS, Wang M, Rizk EB, et al. Tethered spinal cord among individuals with myelomeningocele: an analysis of the National Spina Bifida Patient Registry. *J Neurosurg Pediatr.* 2021;28(1):21-27.

38. Jasien JM, Mikati MA, Kolarova M, Smith B, Thera S, Lee P. Cognitive and motor function in adults with spina bifida myelomeningocele: a pilot study. *Child Nerv Syst.* 2021;37(4):1143-1150.

39. Conklin MJ, Kishan S, Nanayakkara CB, Rosenfeld SR. Orthopedic guidelines for the care of people with spina bifida. *J Pediatr Rehabil Med.* 2020;13(4):629-635.

40. Lorente Moltó FJ, Martínez Garrido I. Retrospective review of L3 myelomeningocele in three age groups: should posterolateral iliopsoas transfer still be indicated to stabilize the hip? *J Pediatr Orthopaed Part B.* 2005;14(3):177-184.

41. Frawley PA, Broughton NS, Menelaus MB. Anterior release for fixed flexion deformity of the hip in spina bifida. *J Bone Joint Surg Br.* 1996;78-B(2):299-302.

42. Yildirim T, Gursu S, Bayhan İA, Sofu H, Bursali A. Surgical treatment of hip instability in patients with lower lumbar level myelomeningocele: is muscle transfer required? *Clin Orthop Relat Res.* 2015;473(10):3254-3260.

43. Correll J, Gabler C. The effect of soft tissue release of the hips on walking in myelomeningocele. *J Pediatr Orthop Part B.* 2000;9(3):148-153.

44. Alman BA, Bhandari M, Wright JG. Function of dislocated hips in children with lower level spina bifida. *J Bone Joint Surg.* 1996;78-B(2):294-298.

45. Stillwell A, Menelaus MB. Walking ability in mature patients with spina bifida. *J Pediatr Orthop.* 1983;3:184-190.

46. Thompson RM, Foley J, Dias L, Swaroop VT. Hip Status and long-term functional outcomes in spina bifida. *J Pediatr Orthop.* 2019;39(3):E168-E172.

47. Høiness PR, Kirkhus E. Grice arthrodesis in the treatment of valgus feet in children with myelomeningocele: a 12.8-year follow-up study. *J Child Orthop.* 2009;3(4):283-290.

48. Patel J, Talwalker VR, Milbrandt TA. Correlation of spine deformity, lung function, and seat pressure in spina bifida. *Clin Orthop Relat Res.* 2011;469:1302-1307.

49. Berven S, Bradford DS. Neuromuscular scoliosis: causes of deformity and principles for evaluation and management. *Semin Neurol.* 2002;22(2):167-178.

50. Schoenmakers MAGC, Gulmans VAM, Gooskens RHJM, Pruijs JEH, Helders PJM. Spinal fusion in children with spina bifida: influence on ambulation level and functional abilities. *Eur Spine J.* 2005;14:415-422.

51. Bowen RE, Abel MF, Arlet V, et al. Outcome assessment in neuromuscular spinal deformity. *J Pediatr Orthop.* 2012;32(8):792-798.

52. Beierwaltes P, Church P, Gordon T, Ambartsumyan L. Bowel function and care: guidelines for the care of people with spina bifida. *J Pediatr Rehabil Med.* 2020;13(4):491-498.

53. Beierwaltes P, Munoz S, Wilhelmy J. Integument: guidelines for the care of people with spina bifida. *J Pediatr Rehabil Med.* 2020;13(4):543-548.

54. Szalay EA, Cheema A. Children with spina bifida are at risk for low bone density. *Clin Orthop Relat Res.* 2011;469(5):1253-1257.

55. Aliatakis N, Schneider J, Spors B, et al. Age-specific occurrence of pathological fractures in patients with spina bifida. *Eur J Pediatr.* 2020;179(5):773-779.

56. Meneses V, Parenti S, Burns H, Adams R. Latex allergy guidelines for people with spina bifida. *J Pediatr Rehabil Med.* 2020;13(4): 601-609.

57. Bartonek Å. Motor development toward ambulation in preschool children with myelomeningocele—a prospective study. *Pediatr Phys Ther.* 2010;22(1):52-60.

58. McDonald CM, Jaffe KM, Shurtleff DB. Assessment of muscle strength in children with meningomyelocele: accuracy and stability of measurement over time. *Arch Phys Med Rehabil.* 1986;67:855-861.

59. Bartonek Å. Factors influencing ambulation in myelomeningocele: a cross-sectional study. *Dev Med Child Neurol.* 2001;43: 253-260.

60. Schoenmakers MAGC, Gulmans VAM, Gooskens RHJM, Helders PJM. Spina bifida at the sacral level: more than minor gait disturbances. *Clin Rehabil.* 2004;18(2):178-185.

61. Gutierrez EM, Bartonek Å, Haglund-Åkerlind Y, Saraste H. Characteristic gait kinematics in persons with lumbosacral myelomeningocele. *Gait Posture.* 2003;18(3):170-177.

62. Wilson PE, Mukherjee S. Mobility guidelines for the care of people with spina bifida. *J Pediatr Rehabil Med.* 2020;13(4):621-627.

63. Wilson PE, Mukherjee S. Mobility guidelines for the care of people with spina bifida. *J Pediatr Rehabil Med.* 2020;13(4):621-627.

64. Pauly M, Cremer R. Levels of mobility in children and adolescents with spina bifida-clinical parameters predicting mobility and maintenance of these skills. *Eur J Pediatr Surg.* 2013;23(2): 110-114.

65. Seitzberg A, Lind M, Biering-Sørensen F. Ambulation in adults with myelomeningocele. Is it possible to predict the level of ambulation in early life? *Child Nerv Syst.* 2008;24(2):231-237.

66. Wolf SI, Alimusaj M, Rettig O, Döderlein L. Dynamic assist by carbon fiber spring AFOs for patients with myelomeningocele. *Gait Posture.* 2008;28(1):175-177.

67. Lightfoot MA, Cheng JW, Hu X, et al. Assessment of health literacy in adolescents with spina bifida and their caregivers: a multi-institutional study. *J Pediatr Urol.* 2020;16(2):167.e1-167.e6.

68. Fremion E, Kanter D, Turk M. Health promotion and preventive health care service guidelines for the care of people with spina bifida. *J Pediatr Rehabil Med.* 2020;13(4):513-523.

69. Bendt M, Gabrielsson H, Riedel D, et al. Adults with spina bifida: a cross-sectional study of health issues and living conditions. *Brain Behav.* 2020;10(8):e01736.

70. HealthyPeople.gov. Healthy People 2020: health and disability. US Department of Health and Human Services. Published 2014. Accessed November 1, 2023. https://www.healthypeople.gov/2020/topics-objectives/topic/disability-and-health.

71. van Speybroeck A, Beierwaltes P, Hopson B, et al. Care coordination guidelines for the care of people with spina bifida. *J Pediatr Rehabil Med.* 2020;13(4):499-511.

72. Rimmer JH. Health promotion for people with disabilities: the emerging paradigm shift from disability prevention to prevention of secondary conditions. *Phys Ther.* 1999;79(5):495-501.

10

Spinal Cord Injury

Catherine Maher, PT, DPT, and Genevieve Pinto Zipp, PT, EdD

■ INTRODUCTION

Working with a child with a spinal cord injury (SCI), whether traumatic or atraumatic requires that physical therapists embrace the dynamic systems theory as a framework to drive therapeutic practice that supports a child's functional abilities and level of participation. Physical therapists must consider the individual intrinsic and extrinsic factors that influence the child with an SCI developmental journey. Constraints in subsystems that result in impairments that limit function must be continuously addressed and managed. Opportunities for the child to exploit affordances in the environment, practice meaningful functional tasks, explore diverse movement strategies, and engage in extensive practice that manipulates control parameters in order to drive developmental learning are foundational to providing a rich learning environment for children with SCI.[1] This introduction provides background regarding the prevalence and impact of SCI on health care, society, family, and the child and offers insights regarding advances in management and promotion of knowledge translation practices.

■ EPIDEMIOLOGY AND ADVANCES IN RECOVERY

EPIDEMIOLOGY

The management of pediatric SCIs has unique challenges to address the physical, cognitive, and social development of the child who has neuromuscular skeletal damage to the developing spinal column. Pediatric physical therapy must not only focus on the immediate needs of the child and family but also plan for and address the far-reaching implications across the patient's life span. SCI in infants, children, and adolescents is a rare occurrence, representing less than 5% of the total population of individuals injured per year according to The National Spinal Cord Injury Statistical Center (NSCISC). However, SCI impacts children and their families across the patient's life span, impacting psychological, social, and motor development.[2] In addition, health care costs and resources extend beyond the initial injury and include prevention of secondary complications (eg, scoliosis, hip dysplasia, pressure ulcers) and environmental modifications to ensure transition into adulthood. The application of the evidence supporting plasticity in the spinal cord has the potential to improve long-term outcomes and goals of childhood SCIs.

Efforts to coordinate the care and rehabilitation of individuals with SCI in the United States resulted in the development of SCI model systems across the country in the 1970s, with initially 7 institutions, which has now increased to 18 to advance the care and research for adults with SCI. The SCI Model System is run by the US Department of Health and Human Services, National Institute on Disability, Independent Living and Rehabilitation Research (NIDILRR) to track SCI. The National Spinal Cord Injury Statistical Center, in conjunction with the University of Alabama at Birmingham, has compiled over 45 years of data on individuals with SCI regarding age, race, gender, mechanism of injury, and death. The 2022 report on the national aggregate variable of age at the time of spinal injury indicates less than 5% of individual were 18 years old compared to the mean age of 36.1 (SD 17.4). The common causes of SCI in the pediatric population are motor vehicle accidents followed by violence and sports-related injuries (**Table 10-1**). Other causes of SCI in children include birth injuries and child abuse. Damage to the spinal cord and its development are also seen in neurologic dysfunction such as spina bifida, skeletal dysplasia resulting in spinal stenosis, and upper cervical spine instability with Down syndrome, which is discussed in this chapter.[3,4]

The Healthcare Cost and Utilization Project (HCUP) of the Agency for Healthcare Research and Quality (AHRQ) compiles

TABLE 10-1 • Grouped Etiology of Spinal Cord Injury by Age at Injury

Etiology n (%)	Age at Injury						
	<15	16-30	31-45	46-60	61-75	≥ 76	Total
Vehicular	362 (36.9)	7,261 (46.3)	3,332 (44.5)	1,927 (37.7)	755 (27.9)	159 (20.5)	13,796
Violence	226 (23.1)	3,735 (23.8)	1,229 (16.4)	330 (6.5)	63 (2.3)	8 (1.0)	5,591
Sports	236 (24.1)	2,224 (14.2)	544 (7.3)	232 (4.5)	73 (2.7)	7 (0.9)	3,316
Falls	78 (8.0)	1,671 (10.7)	1,717 (22.9)	1,960 (38.4)	1,404 (51.9)	509 (65.7)	7,339
Med/Surg	27 (2.8)	107 (0.7)	122 (1.6)	315 (6.2)	298 (11.0)	62 (8.0)	931
Other	51 (5.2)	659 (4.2)	536 (7.2)	330 (6.5)	104 (3.8)	22 (2.8)	1,702
Unkn	0 (0.0)	16 (0.1)	11 (0.1)	11 (0.2)	6 (0.2)	8 (1.0)	52
Total	980	15,673	7,491	5,105	2,703	775	32,727

Etiology n (%)	Age at Injury						
	<15	16-30	31-45	46-60	61-75	76-98	Total
Vehicular	368 (36.8)	7,760 (46.1)	3,654 (44.3)	2,253 (38.0)	914 (27.3)	170 (18.6)	15,119
Violence	232 (23.2)	4,120 (24.5)	1,363 (16.5)	369 (6.2)	69 (2.1)	10 (1.1)	6,163
Sports	239 (23.9)	2,374 (14.1)	618 (7.5)	272 (4.6)	102 (3.0)	8 (0.9)	3,613
Falls	79 (7.9)	1,774 (10.5)	1,881 (22.8)	2,295 (38.7)	1,799 (53.7)	623 (68.2)	8,451
Med/Surg	27 (2.7)	111 (0.7)	135 (1.6)	358 (6.0)	335 (10.0)	74 (8.1)	1,040
Other	52 (5.2)	690 (4.1)	577 (7.0)	367 (6.2)	123 (3.7)	25 (2.7)	1,834
Unkn	2 (0.2)	16 (0.1)	15 (0.2)	13 (0.2)	6 (0.2)	3 (0.3)	55
Total	999	16,845	8,243	5,927	3,348	913	36,275

Source: *Reproduced with permission from 2022 Annual Report. National Spinal Cord Injury Statistical Center; 2023.*

discharge data on pediatric patients from the community, non-rehabilitation hospital sample in the United States every 3 years. The Kids' Inpatient Database (KID) has been used to estimate the epidemiology of SCI between 1997 and 2012.[5] Data sets for children hospitalized for SCI are coded as spinal fracture with or without SCI or spinal dislocation or SCI without evidence of damage. Rates of injury for children age 0 to 14 and adolescents age 15 to 17 have decreased from 1997 to 2012, with adolescents being hospitalized more frequently. These trends may be related to motor vehicle regulations in children safety laws, use of bicycle helmets, or sports injury awareness. The location of spinal injury in the cervical region among children and adolescents accounted for the highest percentage of admissions, at 60% and 56.9%, respectively, from 1997 to 2012.

The 2016 American College of Surgeons Pediatric Report of the National Trauma Data Bank (NTDB) issued comprehensive data on children in 3 age groups (0-2, 3-12, and 13-20 years old) admitted to 85 hospitals or trauma centers in the United States and Canada that voluntarily submit reports. Patterns associated with race, economic status, and age identify disparities among ethnic and socioeconomic groups in children with SCI. The severity of injury based on the Injury Severity Score was higher among black patients and those with Medicaid or no insurance. Black children had the highest rate of SCI associated with firearms (23.9%) compared to white (1.0%) or Hispanic (8.6%) children, according to the NTDB 2016 report. SCI in children was also reported to be associated with brain injury (38.8%), a Glasgow coma Scale score of 4 or lower (10%), and facial injuries.[4] The coordination of rehabilitation for children and adolescents through multicenter standards has been proposed and instituted at several of the leading pediatric centers across the United States. Pediatric clients require rehabilitation services that focus on patient- and family-centered care because the parents and caregivers are integral to the development of the child, especially when the unique needs from SCI impact not only motor but also psychological and social development as the individual transitions to adulthood.

CHALLENGES FOR THE PEDIATRIC POPULATION

The development of the spinal cord and the bony structures of the spine continues until the child reaches approximately 9 years of age.[6] Pediatric spine mobility, stability, and development allow children to be flexible to resist injury during motor development activities but also to be susceptible to injury due to the spine's hypermobility, a larger head size compared to the body, and underdeveloped cervical muscle strength.[7] Compared to the adult spine, children have ligamentous laxity, shallow facet angles, anterior wedging, and incomplete ossification of the vertebrae, which impact the unique features of pediatric SCI.[8]

Because of the ongoing development of the spine, different regions are more at risk for trauma and injury at various ages (infants/toddlers 0-3 years, preschool/young children 4-9 years, preadolescents 10-13 years, and adolescents 14-17 years).[6]

The cervical spine (C1-C7) appears to be more susceptible to injury in children during the adolescent years.[7] Delineating the regions of the upper (C1-C4) and lower cervical spine (C5-C7), injury in the upper region occurs more frequently in infants/toddlers (70%) and preschool/young children (74%) compared to preadolescents (52%) and adolescents (40%). The mobility in the cervical spine at C1 to C3 in children younger than 9 years places them at risk for upper cervical spinal injury. Atlanto-axial rotatory injuries are frequently the result of dislocations and subluxations.[9] Subaxial injuries include body and burst fractures and ligamentous injuries.[9] Lower cervical spine injuries (C5-C7) have increased in those greater than 9 years old. Injuries of the thoracic spine followed by lumbar spine are less frequent and associated with increasing age into adolescence.

The ligamentous laxity of the pediatric spinal column allows for the stretch and distraction of the cord causing injury without fracture or dislocation and may result in neurologic dysfunction without radiographic abnormality. SCI without radiographic abnormality (SCIWRA) has been related to sensory or motor changes, with a lack of radiographic changes (x-rays or computed tomography [CT]) often seen in injuries associated with sports.[10] Recent use of magnetic resonance imaging (MRI) with SCIWRA indicates that hematomas, edema, endplate fractures, and ligament injury may be present, which need to be monitored for clinical presentation over time.[8] Spinal injuries as a result of vigorous shaking can cause high-velocity hyperextension/hyperflexion injuries in infants and children not only at the cervical spine but also at the thoracic and lumbar spine.[7] Compression fractures in the thoracic and lumbar spine may be asymptomatic but are the result of forceful pushing. Unfortunately, children with axial injuries have a higher rate of mortality compared to those with subaxial injuries. Pediatric patients with additional trauma, especially head and traumatic brain injuries, with SCI have poorer outcomes.

CLASSIFICATION OF LEVELS OF INJURY

Tetraplegia, previously identified as quadriplegia, is the term used to identify individuals with spinal injuries that impact both upper and lower extremity function, whereas paraplegia indicates individuals with spinal injuries that affect the lower extremities but not upper extremities, although the level of trunk involvement is not addressed with these terms. The efforts to coordinate care and research for individuals with SCI lead to the need to have a standardized assessment of motor and sensory levels. Determination of the neurologic level of injury in spinal cord trauma has been established for the adult population (>18 years of age) by the International Standards for Neurological and Functional Classification of Spinal Cord Injury (ISNCSCI) and endorsed by the American Spinal Injury Association (ASIA). The level of SCI is defined as the most caudal segment intact for both sensory and motor function on each side of the body. Sensory testing uses pinprick and light touch on both the left and right side of the body with a 3-point scale. Motor testing uses standard manual muscle testing of key muscle groups using a 5-point scale with intact muscle group determined by a grade of 3/5 (antigravity strength) with the next cephalic level having at least a 4/5 grade.

At the initial onset of SCI, there is spinal shock during which sensory and motor function is absent or unable to be determined. The presence of this sacral sparing may indicate that the injury is incomplete. SCI injuries are classified as being complete or incomplete lesions. A complete lesion indicates no sensory or motor function is preserved in the sacral segment S4-5 as there is no deep anal pressure sensation an no voluntary anal contraction. An incomplete lesion has some preservation of sensory and/or motor function. To determine the corresponding neurological level of injury the most caudal segment of the spinal cord will have intact sensation and at least a grade of 3 or more on muscle testing. Together this determines the ASIA Impairment Scale (AIS) grade of A- E.ASIA A with the corresponding spinal level at which no motor or sensory functions exist more than an incomplete lesion. The available sensory and motor function further classifies incomplete injuries. ASIA B indicates there is a sensory function but no motor function below the neurologic level. ASIA C means incomplete motor function below the neurologic level and more than half the key muscles have a muscle grade of less than 3. ASIA D denotes motor function is preserved below the neurologic level, and more than half of the key muscles have a muscle grade of 3 or more. ASIA E indicates normal sensory and motor function. The use of ASIA scale testing is used on initial assessment and reevaluation to determine neurologic status resolution or change.[7] In children younger than 6 years old, the reliability of assessment of anal sensation and rectal motor function as a component of the ISNCSCI has been shown to have limitations.[11,12] The use of sensory assessment of pinprick has been demonstrated as stress-inducing to children under 10 years old, and therefore, modification is recommended until the child matures. Refer ISNCSCI Description of Asia Levels and Worksheet (see ISNCSCI link) https://asia-spinalinjury.org/wp-content/uploads/2016/02/International_Stds_Diagram_Worksheet.pdf

Within the category of incomplete lesions are several syndromes that have unique features. Anterior cord syndrome is the result of flexion injuries that compromise the anterior and anterolateral aspects within the spinal cord, specifically the anterior and lateral spinothalamic tracts and corticospinal tracts. The clinical presentation includes loss of motor function, pain, and temperature sensation, but light touch sensations remain.

Central cord syndrome is the result of hyperextension injuries within the cervical spine. The centrally located spinal cord tracts influence upper extremity (UE) movement with the peripheral tracts that affect lower extremities. Bowel and bladder function is also less affected and may be spared.

Posterior cord syndrome is rare and affects the posterior tracts responsible for proprioception, pain, and light touch below the level of the lesion, but motor function is retained.[7]

Brown-Séquard syndrome is the result of gunshot or stab wound to one side of the body. The clinical presentation affects both the left and right sides of the spinal column. The lateral column impact results in abnormal reflexes with clonus and positive Babinski sign with weakness and spasticity on the same side. The dorsal column damage results in loss of proprioception, kinesthesia, and vibratory sense ipsilateral to the damage. The contralateral side presents with loss of pain and temperature sensations.

Cauda equina syndrome affects the tail of the spinal cord and results in flaccid lower extremity and bowel and bladder motor function, resulting in incontinence.

PATHOPHYSIOLOGY OF SPINAL CORD DAMAGE

Notwithstanding the mechanism of trauma causing damage to the spinal cord, the body responds by initiating a cascade of cellular and hormonal responses to the injury. While the response is typical, this occurs at the already damaged cord and creates a secondary mechanism of spinal injury. The inflammatory response and clot formation are followed immediately by the release of proteins and neurotoxic agents, leading to edema and increasing interstitial pressure. The accumulation of protein and toxins results in vasospasm and ischemia to the spinal cord tissue, producing further damage. Interventions to reduce primary and secondary damage to the spinal cord through early surgical intervention and administration of new neuroprotective and neuroregenerative agents may reduce the extent of the initial motor and sensory loss.[13] Animal model research with the immature spinal cord has demonstrated spontaneous repair and recovery and less destruction from the secondary response. This possibility for recovery and regeneration along with developing pediatric therapeutic interventions modeled after the neurologic recovery models for adults with SCI may improve outcomes in the pediatric population.[14,15]

■ DYNAMIC SYSTEMS PERSPECTIVE

MOVEMENT SYSTEMS DIAGNOSIS

As discussed in Chapter 4 on movement systems, based on the child's abilities and capabilities to integrate information between and among the various systems, the child's dynamic system, which is influenced by specific task demands and environmental constraints, produces a solution to address the movement problem. The movement solution that emerges may or may not be the most ideal or optimal movement solution. Thus, the solution should be seen as the learner's attempt to self-organize the motor outcome with an acceptable degree of error and minimization of metabolic energy expenditure.[16] As part of the integrated person-centered health care team, the physical therapist (PT) gathers information via the examination process that is synthesized during the evaluation process to formulate what is termed the movement systems diagnosis and prognosis. As discussed in Chapter 4, although the American Physical Therapy Association (APTA) endorses the development of a movement system diagnosis that contributes to the PT's ability to properly and effectively manage movement disorders, the work to ensure a valid and reliable universally acknowledged movement system framework is in its infancy. Thus, the PT must ensure that, as they look to address movement system issues, they gather information during the examination process from

TABLE 10-2 • Potential Secondary Impairments Associated With Spinal Cord Injury
Impairment
Autonomic dysreflexia
Deep vein thrombosis
Hypercalcemia
Pathologic fractures
Heterotopic ossification
Orthostatic hypotension
Thermoregulatory dysfunction
Syringomyelia
Spasticity
Pressure ulcers
Contractures
Respiratory dysfunction
Pain

Source: Adapted from Palisano R, Orlin M, Schreiber J. Campbell's Physical Therapy for Children. 5th ed. Saunders; 2016.

all systems (cognitive, cardiovascular, pulmonary, endocrine, integumentary, nervous, and musculoskeletal) that interact to move the body.

To examine the child with an SCI, we must acknowledge that the emergence of a movement is dependent on the individualized interactions among the developing child (learner), task, and environmental constraints. The age, development, and maturation level of the child at the time of the injury and the time of the examination must be considered as the team designs and executes the examination process. Information discovered during the history, systems review, and test and measures must be synthesized to formulate a movement system diagnosis that reflects the child's abilities and capabilities within the testing setting. The PT must recognize that the child with SCI is also at risk for secondary conditions that may further affect their movement system (**Table 10-2**). Therefore, the PT must screen for the presence or impact of secondary issues on motor development and movement system diagnosis.

Gathering information during the examination that can be used to prepare the child with SCI, like any child, with the abilities and capabilities to meet future task and environmental demands required for meaningful participation is fundamental to addressing foreground questions that direct plans of care.

SYSTEMS REVIEW

Respiratory System

Patients with an acute SCI, particularly those with high cervical spine injuries, are at high risk for respiratory failure.[17] Dysfunction of the muscles of inspiration and expiration caused by damage to the spinal cord may be exacerbated by pulmonary conditions such as asthma or atelectasis. Vigilance for signs of impending respiratory failure is imperative in early management, and ventilatory support is required. Depending on the level of spinal injury, respiratory functions are often compromised, especially in the immature musculoskeletal system of the pediatric client, leading to an increased work of breathing.[18]

Respiratory function after SCI is impacted by respiratory muscle weakness and the resulting immobility during acute care. Pulmonary function testing is used to assess residual respiratory muscle function and vital capacity or the volume that can be exhaled (forced vital capacity and forced expiratory volume). Forced maneuvers in a standardized respiratory assessment are rarely used for children under the age of 5 because they are believed to unable to perform the maneuvers in a valid assessment protocol. In a comparison of age-matched children with SCI and typically developing children, respiratory functional capacity is primarily impacted by the age at which injury occurred, indicating the development of altered mechanics of breathing.[19] Damage to the high cervical region (C1-C4) impacts the innervation of the diaphragm and the muscles of expiration, placing the child at risk for respiratory failure. At the highest level (C1-C2), the child will require mechanical ventilator support full time. Those with injury at C3-C4 may demonstrate partial innervation of the diaphragm and the availability of accessory muscles of breathing (sternocleidomastoid, scalenes, levator scapula, and trapezius muscle) to assist in the work of breathing. Individuals may be weaned from mechanical ventilator support but will need monitoring for the appearance of an increase in the work of breathing (increased respiratory rate and hypercapnia or carbon dioxide). Altered breathing patterns such as glossopharyngeal breathing and accessory muscle training have been used with high cervical injury.[20]

In a retrospective study by Padman et al,[18] a critical pathway is presented that addresses weaning children with SCIs off ventilator support. At the lower cervical level of C5-C7, the diaphragm remains innervated, and the pectoralis muscle group and serratus muscle assist in stabilizing the scapula to assist with ventilation. However, without the abdominal muscle tone and intercostal muscles, there are altered biomechanics of breathing known as the paradoxical breathing pattern. Without abdominal muscle tone, the abdominal contents are not supported and shift forward, changing the orientation of the diaphragm muscle. As the diaphragm contracts during inspiration, the rib cage is displaced inward rather than outward. The neck muscles will contract to increase chest expansion, but this compensatory pattern tends to be inefficient. The child with a lower level of cervical injury will continue to have reduced vital capacity but not need ventilator support. The loss of abdominal muscle tone reduces the effectiveness of a cough (expiration) and results in reduced airway clearance for those with thoracic spine injuries as well. Patients and caregiver are instructed in assisted coughing techniques to improve effectiveness.

Breathing patterns, inhalation with movement requiring trunk extension, and exhalation with movements of trunk flexion are used as part of movement strategies for individuals with SCIs and can be incorporated in the pediatric population. Recent advances in technology to alter synaptic transmission have led to the use of implantable devices such as diaphragmatic pacing and phrenic nerve pacing to generate programmed signals to the diaphragm to override fatigue or stimulate the muscle, thus reducing the need for external ventilator support.[21-24] Pediatric PTs working with children requiring mechanical ventilator support should become familiar with both invasive (tracheostomy) and noninvasive intermittent positive-pressure ventilators and the respiratory care team. Mechanical assisted cough may also be incorporated to reduce saliva aspiration and need for suction management, which requires additional training for the practicing clinician.

Cardiovascular System

Upon initial injury to the spinal cord, the cardiovascular system is challenged by the disruption of the autonomic nervous system sympathetic outflow from upper thoracic to lumbar levels. The autonomic nervous system influences heart rate, blood pressure, peripheral vascular tone, heart muscle contraction, and coronary blood flow. The disruption of sympathetic outflow results in hypotension and tachycardia, especially with higher-level thoracic and cervical spine injuries. The acute management of fluctuations in blood pressure and heart rate typically involves medication and fluid monitoring. Infants, children, and preadolescents have higher baseline heart rates and blood pressures than adults, which must be considered throughout the rehabilitation process.[25] Typically, blood pressure increases and heart rate decreases from infancy to adolescence. These changes occur in children age 0 to 18 with SCIs. However, individuals with higher cervical injuries have lower systolic blood pressures. This lower blood pressure correlates with complete lesion (ASIA A) to incomplete ASIA C.

Orthostatic hypotension (OH) is also a result of autonomic nervous system disruption and presents with a decrease in systolic blood pressure of 20 mm Hg or a decrease in diastolic blood pressure of 10 mm Hg within 3 minutes of transitioning from supine or sitting to standing. Individuals with SCI often experience OH during the early transition of rehabilitation as they assume an upright position. Symptoms include lightheadedness, dizziness, headache, or syncope. Management of OH consists of gradual transition to the upright position often on a tilt table, while gradually increasing the degrees of tilt and close monitoring of blood pressure response. Abdominal binders and lower extremity compression stockings or bandaging are useful to promote venous return for those with OH.

Autonomic dysreflexia (AD) presents as a sudden rise in blood pressure with bradycardia as a result of disruption to sympathetic reflex in patients with cervical and high thoracic level injuries. The coordination of the sympathetic and parasympathetic system allows for a rise in blood pressure followed by vasodilation responses. For individuals with spinal injuries above the T6 level, this coordination of sympathetic and parasympathetic responses does not occur. The rapid rise in blood pressure is triggered by noxious stimuli, not apparent to the person with SCI. The increase in blood pressure of 20 to 40 mm Hg is often perceived as a severe headache, along with a drop in heart rate. In addition, profuse sweating and flushing of the skin above the level of the lesions, stuffy nose, blurry vision, and piloerection or "goose bumps" are common signs.[26] Hickey et al[27] reported on a similar presentation of

AD in patients age 0 to 21 with SCIs, although headaches and piloerection were less frequent in children young than 5 years old. The most frequent triggers for AD were urologic or bowel impaction, as well as fever or systemic infection. The increase in blood pressure is an emergent concern and requires determination of the cause or trigger, such as a catheter tube that is restricted causing urinary backflow, a pressure ulcer that has developed, or even clothing that is too tight. If possible, the child should be positioned upright, and the trigger should be addressed immediately. Implementing and maintaining a bowel and bladder program has been found to reduce the incidence of AD.[26]

Temperature Dysregulation

Children with SCI have difficulty regulating body temperature as a result of disruption of neural pathways from the periphery to the hypothalamus and cannot respond to ambient changes with shivering or sweating. This places individuals at risk for hypothermia during cold weather and hyperthermia during warmer weather or physical exertion. Individuals and caregivers should be instructed to be aware of clothing for the appropriate climate and the need for hydration during times of physical activity or exposure to higher temperatures. Autonomic dysfunction may also indicate an underlying infection with or without a rise in body temperature or fever.

Integumentary System

As with all individuals who are immobilized or hospitalized, the risk of developing pressure ulcers increases not only from limited movement but also from shear and friction, such as repositioning in bed. Pressure ulcers develop over areas of bony prominences as a result of tissue hypoxia. Children with SCI have a similar incidence of pressure ulcer over the greater trochanter, ankles, elbows, and scapular as the adult with SCI. Because of differences in biomechanical tissue properties and body dimension and proportions such as larger head size compared to the body, children are also at risk of developing pressure ulcers at the occiput and ears.[28] Infants and newborns are at higher risk from deformation-induced pressure ulcers from the tubes and wires from medical-related devices.[27] The National Pressure Ulcer Advisory Panel has instituted criteria for the staging of pressure ulcers, and the criteria have been used for the pediatric population. Based on the stage of the ulcer, there are treatment interventions such as dressing selections and topical and enzymatic agents to promote wound healing; however, there is lack of evidence-based clinical guidelines for infants and children. Prevention is the key to avoiding pressure ulcers, and screening should be implemented for infants and children to identify those at risk. The Braden Q Scale and Modified Braden Q Scale assess risk factors for developing pressure ulcers in the pediatric population.[29]

Care must be instituted to provide pressure-relieving redistribution and support surfaces and a program for manual repositioning, not only over bony prominences but also for medical-related device attachments. There are a variety of mattresses and cushions that are either pressure reducing or pressure relieving that should be incorporated into the equipment needs of children with SCI. Pressure relief techniques should be incorporated into patient, family, and caregiver education and training early to unweight bony prominences and to reduce friction and shear during position changes. If the child has incontinence episodes, removal of damp or wet clothing is necessary to reduce moisture maceration of the skin. Older children should be instructed in repositioning and unweighting techniques such as seated pushups and lateral and forward lean in the wheelchair every 15 to 30 minutes.

The pain management protocol during dressing changes and wound interventions needs to be appropriate to the medical and cognitive status of infants and children to reduce undue stress. The use of technology for pressure mapping can indicate a specific area of pressure and shear. As the child continues to grow, the support surface must be monitored to assure it meets their changing needs.

Urogenital System

Bladder

After SCI, the sensory and motor coordination that signals the storage of urine in the bladder and the need to void is disrupted by the disconnection of the central and peripheral signals. The coordination of the signals occurs at the S2-S4 spinal segments and the spinal cord and relays a signal to the pons. With normal bladder function, the internal sphincter muscles close the outlet from the bladder, the detrusor muscle of the urinary bladder relaxes to allow for filling, and the external sphincter muscle contracts to maintain continence. During the spinal shock period following trauma, the bladder muscle does not contract, and sphincter muscles do not respond to stimuli. If the cauda equina or sacral segments are injured, the result is a lower motor neuron or areflexic bladder (and bowel), whereas injury above the sacral segment results in an upper motor neuron or reflexic bladder (and bowel).

Neurogenic bladder is a broad term that describes incoordination of bladder filling and voiding voluntarily as a result of neurologic dysfunction. The immediate medical management of the urologic system involves an indwelling catheter to monitor fluid intake and urine output. When the patient is medically stable, the urologic system is evaluated using imaging of bladder and kidneys, as well as blood tests for renal function. The urodynamic assessment determines filling and emptying capacity, urine flow rates, postvoid residual volume, and voiding pressure. Individuals with SCI are at risk for lower urinary tract infections and bladder and kidney stones and will require ongoing monitoring. The goal for management of bladder dysfunction is to reduce the use of an indwelling catheter and to empty the bladder to low postresidual volumes. Patients and caregivers are instructed in intermittent catheterization techniques at hourly intervals while monitoring fluid intake and output. For males, there is also an external condom catheter that can be used. Surgical options are also available if renal systems are compromised or frequent infections occur. Functional electrical stimulation devices are also being investigated for bladder function. Depending on the age of the child and hand function, self-catheterization techniques can be taught to those developmentally age 5 to 7 years old.[30]

Bowel

Like the bladder, bowel function requires the coordination of the central and autonomic nervous systems in conjunction with gut and colon function to maintain continence. After the period of spinal shock, anal tone and sacral reflexes are assessed. The neurogenic bowel requires manual evacuation by nursing staff initially until a program of bowel management can be established. Bowel management programs are individualized to address timing, position, and techniques for evacuation of bowels, equipment, and medication. A bowel program is initiated for children at approximately 3 years old, and children and adolescents may be capable of starting, managing, or instructing caregivers on their bowel program. Individuals with SCI do not perceive the need for defecation or loss of continence and must be aware that impaction can be a trigger for autonomic dysfunction.

Musculoskeletal System

Scoliosis

Although idiopathic scoliosis is commonly seen in the pre-adolescent and adolescent population, children with SCI can present with neuromuscular scoliosis as a result of damage to the vertebral column and the loss of trunk muscle strength. Development and progression of neuromuscular scoliosis are related to the onset of injury and the timing of skeletal growth. Those who sustained injury before puberty are at risk for spinal deformity. The presence of a spinal curve is determined by the Cobb angle measurement with spinal radiography. As in typically developing children, this angle measurement is reassessed at intervals to monitor any progression of the spinal curve. Age at the time of injury (before skeletal maturation) is the strongest predictor of the worsening or progression of the curve for children with SCI. Options for intervention include the use of a thoracolumbar orthosis to limit curve progression and surgical procedures to fuse the spine. Surgical procedures have inherent risks for all patients, but children with SCI are at risk for integumentary and respiratory complications.[31]

Heterotopic Ossification

Heterotopic ossification (HO), or abnormal formation of bone in soft tissue typically around joints, often develops following SCI. The clinical symptoms are usually a loss of a previous range of motion at the joint and pain. For individuals with loss of sensation, other signs are hyperemia and swelling. Previous literature indicated the frequency of HO in pediatric SCI as between 3% and 18%, and it develops later after the injury, up to 14 months. The diagnosis of HO is confirmed by x-ray, CT scan, or bone scan and elevated serum alkaline phosphatase. Treatment options for pediatric SCI are the same as those for adults with SCI, including reducing aggressive and passive range of motion at the joint and monitoring for bone maturation. Surgical excision is considered when joint limitation restricts functional activities and the heterotopic bone matures.[32]

Osteoporosis

During normal growth and development of children, bone growth, both architecture and mineralization, is enhanced by the mechanical strain applied to the skeletal system with weight bearing and muscle stress. Children with SCI may lose the ability to stand upright and walk and to generate sufficient muscle forces, placing them at risk for osteoporosis. Osteoporosis is caused by disruption of the coupling of bone formation and reabsorption leading to demineralization of bones, especially in the lamellar or long bones. In adults with SCI, these processes appear to begin with 1 to 2 years after injury. Lauer et al[33] reviewed bone mineral density (BMD) in children with SCI and noted lower BMD in the hips, similar to previous findings at the knee, compared to typically developing children. Osteoporosis is diagnosed by assessing bone mineral content in the femur and radius using a dual-energy x-ray absorptiometry scan. Also considered in the diagnosis is the presence of vertebral fractures and multiple long bone fractures. Treatment options for adults include pharmacologic management with bisphosphonates and vitamin D and engagement in weight-bearing activities. Although medication management for children with osteoporosis is an option, emphasis on weight-bearing activities or position and engaging in activities that produce muscle force are important strategies for children with SCI.[33,34]

Hip Disorder

Children under the age of 10 who have SCI are at increased risk for hip dysfunction including hip subluxation and dislocation. These hip disorders are suspected to influence the development of neuromuscular scoliosis. The PT should be aware of this increased risk and monitor muscle tone, positioning when seated, and range of motion of children with SCI. Hip subluxations are nonsurgically managed with hip orthosis to maintain the head of the acetabulum within the focus. Chronic subluxations or dislocations may require surgical repair; however, the evidence is limited but it may be considered for children with the potential for ambulation after SCI.[35]

Spasticity

Spasticity is associated with upper motor neuron lesions and is commonly seen with SCIs at the thoracic level and above. The manifestation of spasticity is a result of disruption of normal efferent and afferent inputs causing reflex hyperexcitability, often flexor spasticity initially and then extensor spasticity. The Modified Ashworth Scale (MAS) is a tool for quantifying spasticity in adult and pediatric clients by grading resistance to passive range of motion at upper and lower extremity joints. The Tardieu Scale and pendulum test are also available measures for spasticity. Spasticity can be triggered by noxious stimuli or muscle reflex. The physical therapy plan of care can address spasticity using a passive range of motion program, stretching, and positioning to reduce triggers. However, spasticity can interfere in movement and stability. Baclofen is the pharmacologic agent for management, initially given orally or intrathecally if unresponsive to oral agents. Implanted pumps, usually placed in the abdominal wall of children, will deliver small amounts of the medication directly to the spinal cord, decreasing nerve reactivity. Other medications such as diazepam (Valium), dantrolene sodium, and clonidine have been used in adults with SCI but are not recommended for children. If spasticity is localized to a muscle or muscle groups, a chemical nerve block using botulinum toxin or phenol is used on a recurrent basis, typically every 3 to 6 months.

■ TESTS AND MEASURES

A wide variety of tests and measures are used by the PT to assist in gathering information that reflects the constraints and demands of the learner, task, and environment. The reliability of data secured from many standardized testing protocols is often questionable based on the child's ability to process information and adhere consistently to formal testing protocols. Therefore, the PT must wisely use tests and measures that result in information that is meaningful and assists in developing and assessing the child's plan of care. To help the PT in recognizing the vast array of tests and measures, the American Academy of Pediatrics organized a document of tests and measures published or revised after 1990 by the domains of the International Classification of Functioning, Disability, and Health (ICF) model. The academy states the following: "Tools on this list are commonly used, but the inclusion of a tool does not equate with an endorsement or statement of reliability and validity. Users must access manuals and research reports for more details" (http://pediatricapta.org). PTs must recognize that the majority of the tests and measures listed have not been specifically tested in the pediatric SCI population; thus, the validity and reliability of the outcomes obtained from these tests are questionable but may offer insight.

INTERNATIONAL CLASSIFICATION OF FUNCTIONING, DISABILITY, AND HEALTH

Body Structure and Function Impairment Tests

In 1982, a multidisciplinary group of experts in the field of SCI from ASIA established standards for neurologic and functional classification of SCI in adults.[36] In 2011, this classification system was revised and retitled "American Spinal Injury Association: International Standards for Neurological Classification of Spinal Cord Injury (ISNCSCI)."[36] Clinicians following the ISNCSCI form conduct a standardized examination of both dermatomes and myotomes, which results in a valid determination of both sensory and motor levels for both right and left sides of the body and classification of the injury as either complete or incomplete. Based on the data from the ISNCSCI form, an ASIA level of impairment is assigned and used universally across the health care team supporting person-centered plans of care. Data support that the ASIA Impairment Scale and worksheet can be used reliably with children with SCI who are at least 6 years of age and can discriminate between light touch and pinprick to the cheek.[37,38] During the period of neurologic recovery, some individuals with SCI have skipped levels on the scale. In the year following the SCI injury, the greatest degree of significant recovery is expected. However, recovery has been shown up to 5 years after initial injury.[36] The ASIA Impairment Scale level provides insight into the child's present status and the possibility for change and thus should be used to continually reassess the child's level.

Activity and Participation Tests

Given our greater understanding regarding the nervous system's plasticity, tests and measures must be capable of evaluating both functional ability and improvement and the neuromuscular capacity of the child with SCI. Neuromuscular capacity is a subdomain of the activity domain of the ICF framework and represents the individual's ability to perform a specific task in a standardized environment.[39]

Global Measures

Establishing baseline data, which can then be used to monitor progress in the child's abilities and functional activity levels, is critical to guiding the plan of care. However, no one test has been found to be useful to measure change in children with SCI. Several pediatric assessments that have been used to describe the child with SCI's level of function include the Functional Independence Measure for Children (WeeFIM), Pediatric Evaluation of Disability Inventory (PEDI), Pediatric Quality of Life (PQL), and Canadian Occupational Performance Measure (COPM). Given the absence of standardized functional outcome measures for the pediatric client with SCI, PTs use outcome measures found to be valid and reliable for adults with SCI. The Modified Barthel Index (MBI), Functional Independence Measure (FIM), Quadriplegic Index of Function (QIF), Walking Index for Spinal Cord Injury II (WISCI-II), and Spinal Cord Independence Measure III (SCIM-III) can aide in identifying potential functional outcomes of the child with SCI.

Specific Measures

In 2015, the SCIM-III self-report (SR) was exposed to formal cognitive testing with 17 youths with SCI using the "think aloud methodology," which records participants' responses specific to how items were understood and interpreted. Items on the scale were adjusted based on participant responses. Concurrently, a modified Delphi technique was employed using expert therapists to critically review the SCIM-III SR for pediatric utilization. After 3 iterative Delphi rounds, 80% agreement was achieved on all items on the scale. SCIM-III SR-Youth (SCIM-III SR-Y) is now the formal pediatric version of the scale.

In 2017, the WISCI-II was found to have high intra- and interrater reliability (among 4 PTs) for 52 children with SCI age 2 to 17 years who were ambulatory (intraclass correlation coefficient [ICC] = 0.997, confidence interval [CI] = 0.995-0.998, and ICC = 0.97, CI = 0.95-0.98, respectively).

In 2016, the Neuromuscular Recovery Scale (NRS) pediatric version was developed and the initial validation completed. Using a Delphi method, the changes made to the NRS were reviewed by 12 pediatric experts. Once 80% agreement was reached by experts, the revised Pediatric NRS was field-tested on a sample of children with SCI (n = 5) and without SCI (n = 7), resulting in the Pediatric NRS, which consists of 13 items scored on a 12-point scale. By design, the Pediatric NRS is a measure of motor capacity, and the scale is not intended as the sole indicator of a child's function. Also, the scale is not designed to assess the developmental sequence of motor development. Rather, the intent of the scale is to capture incremental improvements in neuromuscular capacity associated with therapeutic interventions.[40] The items and scoring of the Pediatric NRS were designed to provide a valid indicator of a child's neuromuscular recovery capacity. The instrument could be used as a baseline assessment before initiating an intervention, to detect progression of recovery after a designated number of therapy sessions, and at discharge. Although motivated by the implementation of activity-based therapies targeting recovery (eg, locomotor training or neuromuscular electrical stimulation in children after SCI), the Pediatric NRS may also be useful in evaluating the effectiveness of other physiologic, pharmacologic, medical, or surgical interventions on neuromuscular capacity without compensation.[41] Future work addressing the responsiveness of the Pediatric NRS is needed to support its use in the clinic and research settings.

Given the constraints surrounding psychometric testing associated with tool validation, item response theory (IRT) is being applied in clinical and research settings. IRT is a set of statistical models that analyzes categorical variables that measure the same concept. Via a computer adaptive testing (CAT) program that houses extensive item banks, each respondent's ability level is tested. Mid-range ability questions are employed first, allowing for fewer items to be administered while gaining precise information regarding an individual's placement along a continuum of abilities. SCI-specific CATs can be used to monitor a child's progression specific to general mobility, activities of daily living, and functional participation levels (**Table 10-3**).[42]

Exploring and documenting how and with what type of assistance the child with SCI accomplishes developmental age-appropriate tasks that require varying degrees of mobility, stability, controlled mobility, and skill is essential to provide a full view of the child's abilities and capabilities as the PT seeks to develop a person-centered plan of care (**Table 10-4**). PTs must stay aware of advances in tests and measures specifically for the child with SCI to ensure that the most effective and efficient tests and measures are employed to help develop and direct a plan of care. As with all things, the 2 most important words we must embrace as PTs are "it depends." Embracing the words "it depends" reminds us of the

TABLE 10-3 • Assistance Level Required for Functional Task Completion

Level	Description
Unable to complete/dependent	The child completes <25% of the task.
Maximal	The child completes 25%-49% of the task.
Moderate	The child completes 50%-74% of the task.
Minimal	The child completes 75% or more of the task.
Supervision	The child completes 100% of the task, but the presence of another person is required for safety concerns.
Independent	The child completes 100% of the task but may require aids or assistive devices.

Source: Adapted from Palisano R, Orlin M, Schreiber J. Campbell's Physical Therapy for Children. 5th ed. Saunders; 2016.

TABLE 10-4 • Motor Skill Category

Motor Skill Category	Child Demonstrates the Ability to:	Task Examples
Mobility (transitional mobility)	• Move from one place to another, changing BOS and/or COM	• Sit to stand • Roll • Transfer
Stability	• Maintain body stability with COM over BOS, which is stable	• Modified plantigrade • Prone on elbows • Tall kneeling • Half-kneeling • Standing
Controlled mobility	• Maintain body stability with COM over BOS, which is stable, *but* some body parts are in motion	• Manipulating with UE or LE while maintaining modified plantigrade • Prone on elbows • Tall kneeling • Half-kneeling • Standing
Skill	• Perform coordinated purposeful movement consistently with UE and LE; BOS is changing, and COM is in motion	• Grasp and manipulate • Locomote

Abbreviations: BOS, base of support; COM, center of mass; LE, lower extremity; UE, upper extremity.
Source: Adapted from Chapter 23 by Zipp and Simpkins.

importance of integrating critical thinking and evidence-based practice for the promotion of person-centered care.

INTERVENTIONS

MEDICAL INTERVENTIONS

Emergent Care
Children suspected of having traumatic SCIs should be managed as outlined in the systematic approach to evaluation and assessment under the Advanced Trauma Life Support (ATLS) guidelines for trauma patients.

Stabilization
Management of patients with possible SCI begins before transitioning to medical care with assessment, immobilization, and resuscitation. The improvements in emergency medical services have reduced the incidence of trauma to the spine as a result of delayed transportation or lack of stabilization. Stabilization requires having appropriate-sized backboards and padding to maintain a neutral position of head and neck of infant's and children's larger head-to-body size and the inherent ligamentous laxity in the pediatric population. In addition, the assessment must address airway stabilization to maintain ventilation, oxygen, and perfusion levels. Individuals with cervical and thoracic injuries often present with shock as evidenced by bradycardia and vascular hypotension.[7] Restoration of adequate ventilation and perfusion is an immediate concern of triage. Depending on the level of injury, the

muscle control for respiration innervation can be compromised, especially at the higher cervical level (C1-C4), or be dampened at the lower cervical level (C5-C7). In addition, trauma to the thoracic region such as rib fractures, atelectasis, or concomitant multitrauma injury, especially traumatic head injury, may be present. Attention must be given to the potential for respiratory failure through airway support and sufficient ventilator support.[13]

Spinal Shock

At the time of injury, the function of the spinal cord below the level of injury/impact becomes depressed, which indicates a period of "spinal shock" with loss of voluntary control, flaccidity, and absence of deep tendon reflexes, as well as changes in the autonomic sympathetic system with depressed blood pressure. The proposed mechanism for the clinical presentation is the loss of descending neural projection, which reduces the excitation of the spinal neurons. Spinal shock may last for a few hours, days, or weeks. The autonomic nervous system responsible for bowel and bladder continence returns and indicates the resolution of spinal shock. Spinal reflexes may return within hours, days, or weeks of the initial injury

Imaging

Spinal radiographs in the anterior-posterior (AP) and lateral views are the first imaging studies, followed by CT scans and MRI recommended for adults with suspected SCI according to the National Emergency X-Radiography Utilization Study (NEXUS) criteria. For children, these imaging studies of AP and lateral radiographs should be performed plus the addition of open mouth for potential odontoid fractures in children greater than 9 years old. CT scans should be limited to identify bony abnormalities at specific levels or in the case of possible atlanto-occipital dislocation. MRI scan is indicated to identify ligamentous injury. Imaging studies are not recommended for children who are greater than 3 years of age, alert, and verbal without any midline cervical tenderness, painful distracting injury, or any unexplained hypotension and who are not intoxicated.[43]

Surgical Management

Surgery is indicated for decompression of the spinal cord and stabilization of the spinal column. Decompression of the spinal cord addresses the secondary mechanism of injury as a result of the inflammatory response to the compression and contusion caused by a fracture or dislocation. Because the occurrence of pediatric SCI is rare, the evidence on criteria for surgical selection and outcomes for children is limited.[43] Pediatric injuries are often treated nonsurgically. Indications for surgery include reduction of deformities, decompression of the spinal cord, and ligamentous instability. Spinal instability as a result of ligamentous laxity or bony disruption, if untreated, can lead to additional neurologic impairment. In a retrospective review of 540 children receiving services at Pediatric Emergency Care Applied Research Network hospitals, the application of halo fixation was more common for axial injuries and internal fixation for subaxial injuries. A rigid collar was frequently used when surgery was not indicated.[9]

REHABILITATION AND HABILITATION

Compensation Versus Restoration

Basic science and clinical research on SCI combined with the public interest in recovery has challenged the rehabilitation community to address basic assumptions about SCI. The notion that an injured spinal cord is permanently damaged with no capability of recovery has been replaced with the potential of nerve regeneration and neuroplasticity of the spinal cord. The recognition of central pattern generators, a set of neural circuitry within the spinal cord that can be accessed by specific task training and result in motor recovery, has redirected therapeutic interventions.[14] Emerging innovation with the use of stem cells and gene translation and functional electrical stimulation has renewed hope that recovery is possible. The current physical therapy intervention strategies for individuals with SCI can be classified as compensatory, restorative, or preventative. Compensatory interventions focus on adapting a strategy to achieve a task in a new manner, such as using momentum to initiate rolling in bed when the lower body is paralyzed or using a lower extremity orthotic to maintain legs in extension during standing. Preventative strategies focus on minimizing or eliminating potential problems such as instructing in weight-shifting activities while sitting in a wheelchair to reduce pressure. Restorative intervention strategies look to design interventions that eliminate substitution and restore optimum recovery of function such a locomotor training paradigm for SCI.[44-46] Pediatric PTs involved with individuals with SCI must consider all these strategies to meet the unique needs of infants, children, and adolescents. One must address the child's current developmental stage and plan for their continued growth and development as they transition into adulthood.

Functional Mobility: Physical Therapy Examination

PTs working in pediatrics assess children's motor skill across the developmental sequence using a variety of tests and measures such as Gross Motor Function Measure (GMFM), Alberta Infant Motor Scale (AIMS), or WeeFIM or FIM (for adolescents) (www.pediatriapta.org). Evaluation of the motor performance of children should consider both their chronologic and developmental age. The age and development of the child at the time of spinal injury as well as the level and completeness of the lesion will impact the child's performance on these tests and measures compared to typically developing children.

Activity-based task analysis of movement is also needed for comprehensive examination. Tasks can be grouped into categories of basic activities of daily living (ADLs) and instrumental ADLs for community engagement. The SCIM-III has looked at tasks of functional ability in 3 categories: self-care, respiratory and sphincter management, and functional mobility. It has been evaluated for reliability and validity to assess physical functioning of children with SCI greater than 6 years old.[35] Functional mobility describes motor tasks such as the ability to move in bed, transition from one position to another, transfer from one surface to another, and locomotion within the environment. Tasks can also be categorized by the motor control needed during the performance, transitional mobility, stability or static postural control, dynamic postural control, and skill.[47,48] During the assessment of functional mobility, the therapist analyzes critical elements of movement, postural stability, and mobility and coordinated effort to achieve the task.[49] Among the functional mobility skills (FMSs) following SCI that are critical to independence in basic ADL bed mobility are rolling, supine to sit, sit to supine, bridging, scooting, and sitting unsupported. Additional FMSs are transfers from one surface to another, standing, stepping, walking, and stair climbing. For children, skills such as bouncing a ball, running, hopping, skipping, and jumping are essential skills for play and engagement. The assessment of these skills needs to consider where the developmental sequence was in the child before the injury. Although there are published guidelines as to the expectation of achieving independence in FMSs based on level and completeness of injury, the notion of neuroplasticity, especially in the immature neuromotor system, should encourage pediatric PTs to consider incorporation of compensatory and restorative strategies within the plan of care. The application of motor learning principles for practice and feedback is useful for engaging and motivating the child during physical therapy. **Table 10-5** provides a systematic way to view functional task-oriented activities for training upright mobility for children with incomplete SCI based on task progression and complexity.

Compensatory Training Strategies: Functional Mobility Skills

Several compensatory movement strategies for adults with SCI can be incorporated for pediatric clients. These movement strategies use the biomechanical advantages of momentum, head-hip relationship, muscle substitution, and breathing to assist or move the weak or paralyzed body parts. Momentum is easily demonstrated by the use of rocking motion of the head, neck, and arms to roll from supine to side lying or prone and back. Use of proprioceptive neuromuscular facilitation UE patterns can guide the incorporation of the head to generate a sufficient momentum force to bring the lower body around the axis of motion.

To move across surfaces such as transfers from bed to wheelchair, the sit-pivot technique can be taught. This technique uses the head-hip relationships to produce lift and rotation of buttocks. The posterior connective tissue linking the head to the lumbosacral spine allows the head and upper trunk to move in the opposite direction to the lower trunk and buttocks. When the UEs is placed forward of the pelvis on the support surface, as the trunk flexes or leans forward, the pelvis is unweighted. Combined with scapular depression and protraction, the buttocks is lifted off the support surface, followed by a descent phase when the buttocks is lowered down to the surface. When trunk flexion is combined with rotation, the hips will unweight and move in the opposite/lateral direction, allowing the individual to transfer to a wheelchair or commode.

Therapeutic Exercise

When planning therapeutic exercise for aerobic conditioning, strengthening, and flexibility for individuals with SCI, the pediatric PT must consider the range of motion. Typically, active and passive range of motion activities look to restore full joint and soft tissue flexibility. However, there are certain advantages to a shortened range, especially at hamstrings and finger extensors, for those with SCI. Those with high tetraplegia (C6 and above) have limited or no isolated finger motion for grasp and release in the hand, which interferes with fine and gross motor hand skills. An alternative strategy is the use of a tenodesis grasp, extension of the wrist with subsequent thumb and finger flexor shortening, producing an alternative passive grasp and lateral prehension, for tasks such as holding a cup. Maintaining a shortened range of motion of the thumb and finger flexors is therefore important for this activity, and aggressive stretching should be limited. A shortened range of motion in the hamstring muscles, coupled with some tightness in the spine musculature, allows individuals to maintain a long sitting posture, a position used in ADL activities such as dressing and bed mobility. Strengthening and aerobic conditioning programs can be designed after an appropriate screening of ability to perform the activity safely and progressed according to the FITT principle (frequency, intensity, type, and time). For infants and children, the activities should engage them in age-appropriate activities that are fun and enjoyable to begin a lifelong appreciation of physical activity as part of a healthy lifestyle despite challenges. Adolescents should also be engaged in physically challenging therapeutic exercise programs with attention to endurance, strength, and power for independence in school and community environments (**Figs. 10-1 to 10-8**).

Upper Extremity Function

The pediatric PT must engage with the occupational therapist to focus on complementary interventions to enhance UE capabilities for functional skills. UE orthotics are used to prevent limb contracture and preserve joint integrity and muscle length and assist in the performance of ADLs for individuals with tetraplegia. During the acute phase of medical care, resting or positional UE orthotics are indicated to maintain a functional hand position. As care begins to focus on strategies to compensate for the loss of UE function, additional supports may be indicated such as mobile arm and suspension supports for individuals with high cervical injuries. A universal cuff can hold a variety of items essential for independent ADLs such as a toothbrush, comb, or utensils. UE tendon transfers are a strategy to restore function and include deltoid or bicep to triceps for elbow extension or the brachioradialis muscle transferred to wrist extension or thumb flexion. Individuals undergoing tendon transfers require periods of immobilization followed by mobilization and retraining. Technology and assisted technology can help achieve UE function through alternatives. A joystick, head controls, or eye movement capture technology can allow independent power wheelchair control for individuals with high cervical injuries. Functional electrical stimulation devices are being designed to replicate functional hand movement. Promoting restoration of UE function for individuals with high-level tetraplegia and incomplete injuries has shifted with the advent of technology; however, the evidence is limited in the rare pediatric SCI population.[50,51]

TABLE 10-5 • Functional Task-Oriented Activities for Training Upright Mobility for Children With Incomplete Spinal Cord Injury (SCI)

Task	Modifications/Progression to Vary Task Complexity	Example of Low Complexity → High Complexity
Kicking with lower extremity: Position of foot (DF or PF) and specified hip and knee position to make contact with **an object**	• Incorporate variability in object size, shape, and distance from individual and stationary or moving object, with or without UE support unilaterally or bilaterally. • Incorporate modifications to speed, vision, and attentional demands, degree of intertrial variability, externally or internally paced, and continuous or noncontinuous performance.	A stationary object → a moving object
Sliding of the lower extremity: Position of foot (DF or PF) and specified hip and knee position for **directional sliding**	• Incorporate variability in direction, required distance traveled of the sliding foot from the stationary foot, with or without UE support unilaterally or bilaterally. • Incorporate modifications to speed, vision, and attentional demands, degree of intertrial variability, externally or internally paced, and continuous or noncontinuous performance.	Unidirectional sliding → bidirectional sliding
Standing and reaching with upper extremity: Pointing to or grasping **an object**	• Incorporate variability in object size, shape, and distance from individual, stationary or moving object, position of feet (tandem, narrow, or wide base of support), specified hip and knee position, unidirectional, bidirectional, unilateral or bilateral reaching, required distance traveled of the reaching arm, with or without UE support unilaterally or bilaterally. • Incorporate modifications to speed, surface firmness, vision, and attentional demands, degree of intertrial variability, externally or internally paced, and continuous or noncontinuous performance.	Stationary object → moving object
Lifting: Lifting **an object**	• Incorporate variability in object size, shape, weight, and distance from individual, stationary or moving object, position of feet (tandem, narrow, or wide base of support), specified hip and knee position, unidirectional, bidirectional, unilateral or bilateral lifting, required distance traveled of the reaching arm, with or without UE support unilaterally or bilaterally. • Incorporate modifications to speed, vision, and attentional demands, degree of intertrial variability, externally or internally paced, and continuous or noncontinuous performance.	Stationary object → moving object
Pushing: Pushing **an object.**	• Incorporate variability in object size, weight, shape, and distance from individual, stationary or moving object, position of feet (tandem, narrow, or wide base of support), specified hip and knee position, unidirectional or bidirectional stepping, unilateral or bilateral lifting, required distance traveled pushing, with or without UE support unilaterally or bilaterally. • Incorporate modifications to speed, vision, and attentional demands, degree of intertrial variability, externally or internally paced, and continuous or noncontinuous performance.	Stationary object → moving object
Pulling: Pulling **an object**	• Incorporate variability in object size, weight, shape, and distance from individual, stationary or moving object, position of feet (tandem, narrow, or wide base of support), specified hip and knee position, unidirectional or bidirectional stepping, unilateral or bilateral lifting, required distance traveled pulling, with or without UE support unilaterally or bilaterally. • Incorporate modifications to speed, vision, and attentional demands, degree of intertrial variability, externally or internally paced, and continuous or noncontinuous performance.	Stationary object → moving object
Marching: Marching with specified ankle, hip, and knee position **in specified directions**	• Incorporate variability in direction, with or without UE support unilaterally or bilaterally, carrying objects unilaterally or bilaterally, weighted LEs. • Incorporate modifications to speed, surface firmness, vision, and attentional demands, degree of intertrial variability, externally or internally paced, and continuous or noncontinuous performance.	Forward → backward or sideways, unidirectional or bidirectional

(Continued)

TABLE 10-5 · Functional Task-Oriented Activities for Training Upright Mobility for Children With Incomplete Spinal Cord Injury (SCI) *(Continued)*		
Task	**Modifications/Progression to Vary Task Complexity**	**Example of Low Complexity → High Complexity**
Bending: Bending with specified position of foot, hip, and knee and **varying UE support**	• Incorporate variability with unilateral or bilateral UE support. • Incorporate modifications to speed, vision, and attentional demands, degree of intertrial variability, externally or internally paced, and continuous or noncontinuous performance.	With UE support → without UE support
Stepping: Stepping (1 step) while **varying UE support**	• Incorporate variability in step height, depth, length, direction of ascent and descent (forward, backward, sideways), UE support unilaterally or bilaterally, carrying objects unilaterally or bilaterally. • Incorporate modifications to speed, surface firmness, vision, and attentional demands, degree of intertrial variability, externally or internally paced, and continuous or noncontinuous performance.	With UE support → without UE support
Kicking in upright position: Kicking **an object**	• Incorporate variability in object weight, height, and shape, required distance traveled, and direction. • Incorporate modifications to speed, surface firmness, vision, and attentional demands, degree of intertrial variability, externally or internally paced, and continuous or noncontinuous performance.	Light object weight → heavier object weight
Sit to stand: Sit to stand **from chairs with differing stability**	• Incorporate variability in chair type, chair height, depth, number, with or without UE support unilaterally or bilaterally, carrying objects unilaterally or bilaterally. • Incorporate modifications to speed, surface firmness, vision, and attentional demands, degree of intertrial variability, externally or internally paced, and continuous or noncontinuous performance.	Standard chair → rolling chair
Side stepping: Side stepping while **varying UE support**	• Incorporate variability with unidirectional or bidirectional stepping, specified ankle, hip, and knee position, UE support unilaterally or bilaterally, carrying objects unilaterally or bilaterally, weighted LEs. • Incorporate modifications to speed, surface firmness, vision, and attentional demands, degree of intertrial variability, externally or internally paced, and continuous or noncontinuous performance.	With UE support → without UE support
Walking: Walking **on different surfaces**	• Incorporate variability including obstacles (over, around, under, through), dual tasking with cognitive or motor tasks, pace (internal and external), with or without UE support unilaterally or bilaterally, carrying objects unilaterally or bilaterally, weighted LEs. • Incorporate modifications to speed, surface firmness, vision, and attentional demands, degree of intertrial variability, externally or internally paced, and continuous or noncontinuous performance.	Level surfaces → unleveled surfaces
Treadmill: Treadmill ambulation **in various directions**	• Incorporate variability including direction of ambulation, treadmill width, length, speed, incline, with or without UE support unilaterally or bilaterally, carrying objects unilaterally or bilaterally. • Incorporate modifications to speed, vision, and attentional demands, degree of intertrial variability, externally or internally paced, and continuous or noncontinuous performance.	Forward → sideways and backward
Ramps: Ambulation on ramps or inclines **in various directions**	• Incorporate variability including direction of step, ramp height, width, depth, length, with or without UE support unilaterally or bilaterally, carrying objects unilaterally or bilaterally. • Incorporate modifications to speed, vision, and attentional demands, degree of intertrial variability, externally or internally paced, and continuous or noncontinuous performance.	Forward → sideways and backward
Stair: Ambulate on stairs **in various directions and in dual task**	• Incorporate variability including pace, internal and external, step height, depth, length, number, direction of ascent and descent (forward, backward, sideways), dual task incorporation, with or without UE support unilaterally or bilaterally, carrying objects unilaterally or bilaterally, weighted LEs. • Incorporate modifications to speed, surface firmness, vision, and attentional demands, degree of intertrial variability, externally or internally paced, and continuous or noncontinuous performance	Ascend, descend, side step, backward → dual tasking (cognitive and motor)

(Continued)

TABLE 10-5 • Functional Task-Oriented Activities for Training Upright Mobility for Children With Incomplete Spinal Cord Injury (SCI) *(Continued)*

Task	Modifications/Progression to Vary Task Complexity	Example of Low Complexity → High Complexity
Curbs: Stepping up on a curb while **varying UE support**	• Incorporate variability including stepping direction (forward, sideways, backward), distance, speed, UE support unilaterally or bilaterally, carrying objects unilaterally or bilaterally. • Incorporate modifications to speed, vision, and attentional demands, degree of intertrial variability, externally or internally paced, and continuous or noncontinuous performance.	With UE support → without UE support
Braiding: Ambulation with a weaving pattern of the LEs while **varying UE support**	• Incorporate variability in direction (forward, backward, or sideways, unidirectional or bidirectional), UE support unilaterally or bilaterally, carrying objects unilaterally or bilaterally, weighted LEs. • Incorporate modifications to speed, vision, and attentional demands, degree of intertrial variability, externally or internally paced, and continuous or noncontinuous performance.	With UE support → without UE support
Obstacle course: Ambulation through an obstacle course **in various directions**	• Incorporate variability in direction (forward, sideways, backward, figure-of-8), distance, speed, with or without UE support unilaterally or bilaterally, obstacle height, length, width, depth, and number, carrying objects unilaterally or bilaterally. • Incorporate modifications to speed, vision, and attentional demands, degree of intertrial variability, externally or internally paced, and continuous or noncontinuous performance.	Forward, sideways → backward, figure-of-8
Hopping: Hopping **in various directions**	• Incorporate variability in intended location (stationary or to a new location), direction of hop, distance (height of the hop), speed, with or without UE support unilaterally or bilaterally, carrying objects unilaterally or bilaterally, bilateral or 1-legged. • Incorporate modifications to speed, vision, and attentional demands, degree of intertrial variability, externally or internally paced, and continuous or noncontinuous performance.	Forward → backward
Skipping: Skipping **in various directions**	• Incorporate variability in direction (forward, backward), distance, speed, with or without UE support unilaterally or bilaterally, carrying objects unilaterally or bilaterally. • Incorporate modifications to speed, vision, and attentional demands, degree of intertrial variability, externally or internally paced, and continuous or noncontinuous performance.	Forward → backward
Jogging: Jogging **in various directions**	• Incorporate variability in direction (forward, backward), distance, speed, with or without UE support unilaterally or bilaterally, carrying objects unilaterally or bilaterally. • Incorporate modifications to speed, vision, and attentional demands, degree of intertrial variability, externally or internally paced, and continuous or noncontinuous performance.	Forward → Backward
Running: Running **in various directions**	• Incorporate variability in direction (forward, sideways, backward), distance, speed, with or without UE support unilaterally or bilaterally, carrying objects unilaterally or bilaterally. • Incorporate modifications to speed, vision, and attentional demands, degree of intertrial variability, externally or internally paced, and continuous or noncontinuous performance.	Forward → sideways, backward

Source: Reproduced with permission from Dennis Fell, Karen y Lunnen, et al. Lifespan neurorehabilitation: A patient-centered approach from examination to interventions and outcomes, 1e. F.A Davis Company; 2018.

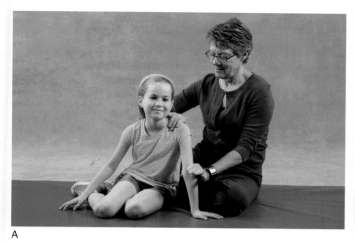
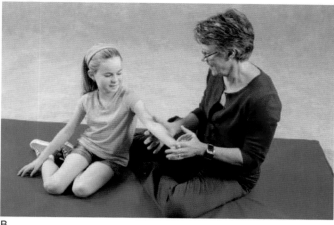

A   B

FIGURE 10-1 PNF using joint approximation through upper extremity. (Reproduced with permission from Dennis W. Fell, Karen Y. Lunnen, Reva P. Rauk, *Lifespan neurorehabilitation: A patient-centered approach from examination to intervention and outcomes*. F. A. Davis Company; 2018.)

Locomotion Training

The abilities to be upright and ambulating are important considerations for children with SCI and their families for physical and psychological development. Upright standing can be achieved for children using a mobile stander and standing frames beginning as young as age 12 months when upright cruising begins to emerge. These devices have a base for foot placement and support for lower extremities and trunk to maintain an upright posture. Trays can be added for UE support or activities. For ambulation, various configurations of orthotics can be used based on the availability of lower extremity and trunk control. An ankle-foot orthosis can be used if there is sufficient strength at the knees and hips, whereas a knee-ankle-foot orthosis controls ankle and knee motion but allows hip movement. Hip-knee-ankle-foot orthoses (HKAFOs) control ankle, knee, and hip motion and are indicated for

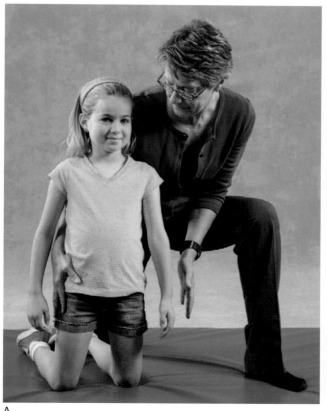
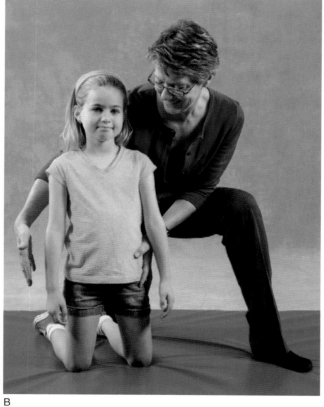

A   B

FIGURE 10-2 Proprioceptive neuromuscular facilitation. (Reproduced with permission from Dennis W. Fell, Karen Y. Lunnen, Reva P. Rauk, *Lifespan neurorehabilitation: A patient-centered approach from examination to intervention and outcomes*. F. A. Davis Company; 2018.)

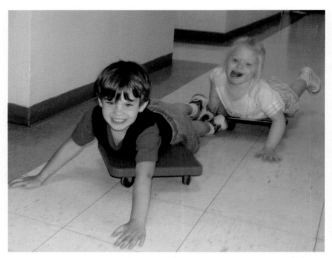

FIGURE 10-3 Children on scooter board that provide proprioceptive and vestibular inputs. (Reproduced with permission from Dennis W. Fell, Karen Y. Lunnen, Reva P. Rauk, *Lifespan neurorehabilitation: A patient-centered approach from examination to intervention and outcomes.* F. A. Davis Company; 2018.)

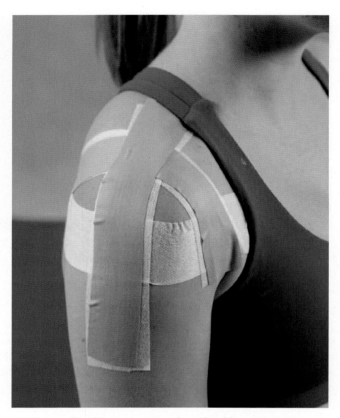

FIGURE 10-5 Shoulder taping to reduce shoulder subluxation. (Reproduced with permission from Dennis W. Fell, Karen Y. Lunnen, Reva P. Rauk, *Lifespan neurorehabilitation: A patient-centered approach from examination to intervention and outcomes.* F. A. Davis Company; 2018.)

thoracic-level lesions. Depending on the neurologic level, children often need bilateral orthotics, which increases the energy expenditure of ambulation. A reciprocal gait orthosis is a bilateral HKAFO with a cable system that coordinates hip flexion on one limb with the hip extension on the opposite limb for more efficiency. Orthotics can be designed with a variety of joints, which will assist, restrict, or stop motion depending on the muscle force the individual is capable of generating. Training with an orthosis begins with temporary devices in the parallel bars to gain skill for static and dynamic balance training, weighting and unweighting lower extremity, forward progression, turning, and backward steps, as well as sit to stand and stand to sit with and without assistive devices (**Figs. 10-9 and 10-10**). Swing-to and swing-through patterns and the use of crutches and canes can be explored for

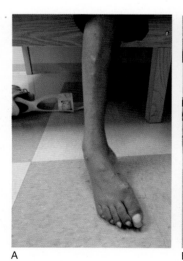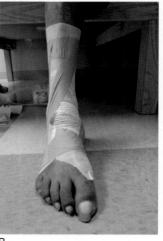

A   B

FIGURE 10-4 Taping of ankle to improve support prior to use of AFO. (Reproduced with permission from Dennis W. Fell, Karen Y. Lunnen, Reva P. Rauk, *Lifespan neurorehabilitation: A patient-centered approach from examination to intervention and outcomes.* F. A. Davis Company; 2018.)

efficiency and energy expenditure. Training should include instruction to the parent and/or child on how to don and doff the orthotics, inspection of skin for irritations, and fit. The final choice of components requires a team approach of the patient and parent with the PT, orthoptist, and physician. Monitoring of an orthotic device is required to adjust for growth. Prognosis for continued use of orthotics for ambulation for children with SCI has been linked to quadriceps strength of at least a 3/5 manual muscle testing grade.[37,52]

Restorative Training Strategies: Locomotor Training

The advances associated with the NeuroRecovery Network (NRN) activity-based locomotor training for adults with incomplete SCI have begun to filter into adapting the training paradigm for children with SCI.[41,53] Locomotor training should not be confused with terms such as body weight–supported treadmill training or overground assisted ambulation, which reference the tools used for training.[54] Activity-based locomotor training incorporates specific manual sensory cues to facilitate a stepping pattern.[15] Limb loading is maximized while fostering trunk and pelvis upright alignment through overhead harness support (**Fig. 10-11**). Recent systematic reviews of literature on pediatric SCI locomotor training summarized the current findings and concerns and recommended how to improve outcomes for children.[55,56] The studies identified a range of training parameters, include time and frequency of training per week,

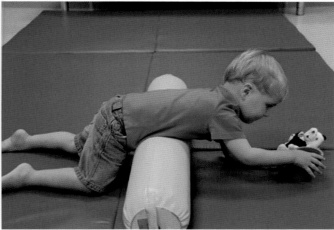

A

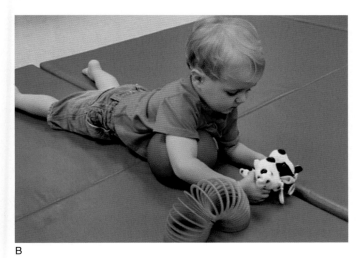

B

FIGURE 10-6 Use of bolster and balls for trunk support while child plays. (Reproduced with permission from Dennis W. Fell, Karen Y. Lunnen, Reva P. Rauk, *Lifespan neurorehabilitation: A patient-centered approach from examination to intervention and outcomes.* F. A. Davis Company; 2018.)

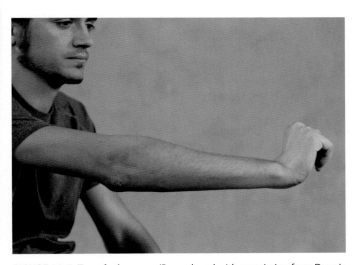

FIGURE 10-7 Tenodesis grasp. (Reproduced with permission from Dennis W. Fell, Karen Y. Lunnen, Reva P. Rauk, *Lifespan neurorehabilitation: A patient-centered approach from examination to intervention and outcomes.* F. A. Davis Company; 2018.)

the total number of weeks, and outcome measures. Measures include the WISCI-II, 10-Minute Walk Test (10MWT), and 6-Minute Walk Test (6MWT). The studies reviewed had small populations, ranging from single subjects to 32 children, consistent with the rarity of pediatric SCI. The majority of subjects were greater than 10 years old, although children as young as 4 years old have participated in locomotor training. No conclusions based on the level of injury, completeness of injury, or optimal timing of initiating training following injury could be recommended because the number of subjects was small and not always reported. Continued study of children with SCI participating in locomotor training to restore recovery of walking will expand the appreciation of the role of activity-based training.[57-59]

Electrical Stimulation and Technology

Technology plays an increasing role in the daily lives of children with SCIs. The use of assistive technologies available on electronic devices, computers, phones, and environmental systems allows interaction with the environment and communities despite physical challenges. Eye gaze, trackball, and head point mouse technology can enable individuals with tetraplegia to engage through computer systems in both the classroom and community.[60] The use of bioengineering tools such as voice recognition software and wireless technology enables both commercial and customized adaptation for individual needs. The pediatric PT should engage closely with the occupational therapist and biomedical engineering professional to seek an assistive technology solution for their pediatric client.

Electrical stimulation (ES) is a modality used in physical therapy for pain management, muscle recruitment, and biofeedback. There are a variety of types of ES, including neuromuscular electrical stimulation (NMES), functional electrical stimulation (FES), and transcutaneous electrical stimulation (TENS). TENS is used for pain management. Neuropathic pain has been associated with SCIs, but the evidence for the use of TENS for pediatric SCI as an intervention strategy is limited. FES combines ES with a task-specific activity, such as cycling or UE movements. Surface electrodes deliver low-voltage stimuli to the muscle group with peripheral innervation for muscle recruitment, task training, or motor relearning. ES systems need to have parameters of pulse width, duration, and frequency to be sufficient to produce a muscle contraction via an intact peripheral nerve. Candidates include those with tetraplegia and incomplete SCIs. Evaluation of potential pediatric candidates needs to consider not only muscle groups but also the cognitive level to understand sensory stimulation and desired output or task. Commercially available FES systems integrate surface electrodes into UE and lower extremity orthoses, which can be used during task-specific training such as grasp and release or standing and walking.[60-63] Although the systems were developed for adults, modifications are being made for pediatric patients based on size and application parameters. FES with stationary lower extremity cycling has been reported to have benefits on BMD, muscle strengthening, cardiovascular fitness, and quality of life parameters for children with SCI.[33,64]

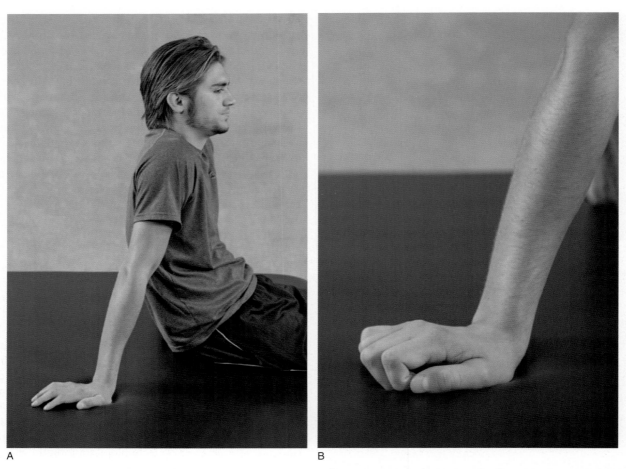

FIGURE 10-8 Preservation of Tenodesis grasp. (Reproduced with permission from Dennis W. Fell, Karen Y. Lunnen, Reva P. Rauk, *Lifespan neurorehabilitation: A patient-centered approach from examination to intervention and outcomes*. F. A. Davis Company; 2018.)

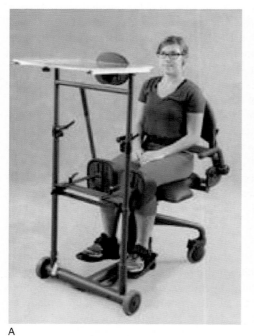
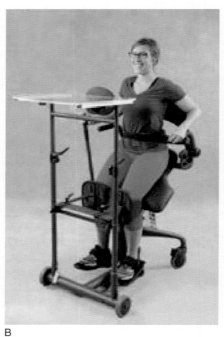
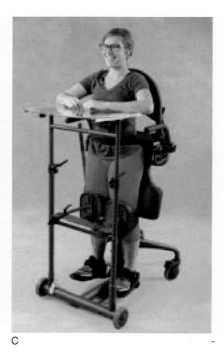

FIGURE 10-9 Sit to stand frame. (Reproduced with permission from Dennis W. Fell, Karen Y. Lunnen, Reva P. Rauk, *Lifespan neurorehabilitation: A patient-centered approach from examination to intervention and outcomes*. F. A. Davis Company; 2018.)

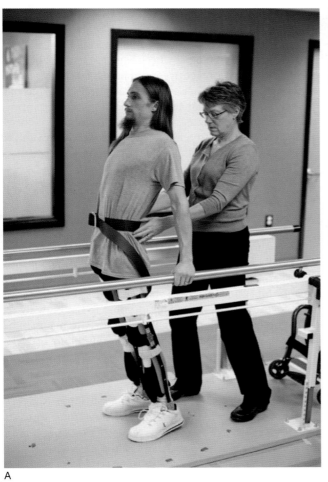 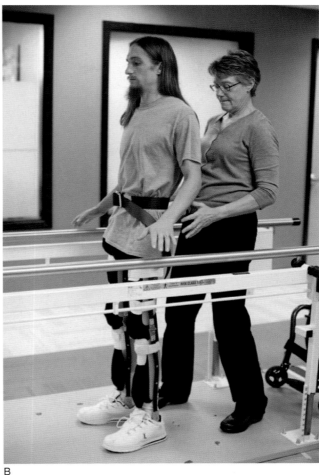

A

B

FIGURE 10-10 Learning to Balance with KAFO in parallel bars. (Reproduced with permission from Dennis W. Fell, Karen Y. Lunnen, Reva P. Rauk, *Lifespan neurorehabilitation: A patient-centered approach from examination to intervention and outcomes.* F. A. Davis Company; 2018.)

The dosage and timing for optimal training outcomes for adults and children with SCI have not been determined.[65] Implantable FES systems, known as neuroprostheses, are being developed to directly stimulate the muscle through electrodes that are connected to external control units.[33] Continued refinement of prototypes has identified units for UE and lower extremity function, phrenic nerve stimulation for diaphragm pacing, and bowel and bladder function.[51] Research and development of neuroprostheses focus on the adult population with SCI because pediatric populations are typically excluded from investigational research and pilot studies. The ability to implant a device in a child who has not yet achieved full body maturation needs to be addressed.

Wheelchairs

Children with complete (ASIA A) and incomplete (ASIA B-D) SCIs will require the use of a wheelchair for mobility because ambulation is limited, especially in the acute recovery phase. The type of wheelchair prescribed should be specific to the unique needs of the child and family and consider the level of injury, functional abilities, financial resources, and environmental conditions.[42] The prescriptive wheelchair must be reassessed periodically because body size, mobility, and functional capabilities of the child may change.[37,66,67]

The basic options for manual and power wheelchairs include frame and wheelbase, tires, seat selection, and leg and armrest options. Add-ons such as tilt in space, lateral supports, headrests, and wheel projection can also be incorporated. The addition of a seat cushion for pressure relief and supports to prevent spinal deformities or reduce spasticity must also be considered. Sports-specific wheelchairs are also available for pediatric clients. For infants and toddlers, a stroller is often used until the child can begin self-propulsion of either the manual or power chair.

Manual wheelchairs are designed with either a rigid frame or a folding frame, which is easier to transport. Seat height and depth should support the child's body and allow for UE propulsion while maintaining the trunk in an optimal position. Manual controls for a tilt-in-space option can be added to a manual wheelchair. Pushrim-activated power assist wheelchairs (PAPAWs) combine manual and power chair options with a motor linked to the pushrim, allowing the user to use less motor output and energy expenditure for propulsion. Although evidence supports the positive response

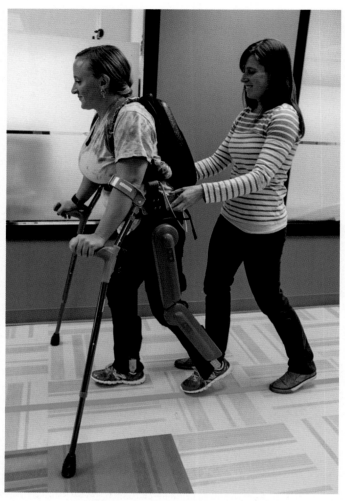

FIGURE 10-11 **Patient and therapist with ReWalk exoskeletal system.** (Reproduced with permission from Dennis W. Fell, Karen Y. Lunnen, Reva P. Rauk, *Lifespan neurorehabilitation: A patient-centered approach from examination to intervention and outcomes.* F. A. Davis Company; 2018.)

of adult SCI patients using PAPAW, there have been limited reports of similar responses from pediatric SCI users. The power wheelchair offers additional options for the wheelbase, seat functions, and drive control. Drive controls include sip and puff, mouth sticks, head switches, and joysticks that can be customized to allow an individual to engage the electronic controls for acceleration, deceleration, turning, reversing, and stopping, as well as positioning the seat or leg rests. Tilt/recline-in-space options with power seats allow the individual to adjust their seat to allow pressure relief and positional changes throughout the day. Power chairs also have the ability to tilt the seat forward while blocking knee and hip movement for upright standing and weight bearing. This option is especially important for children with SCI for peer interaction. Mobility options include manual and power all-terrain chairs to allow children to explore challenges such as sand and rugged environments.[42]

Training for both manual and power wheelchair use requires skills and endurance essential for efficiency and independence. The Wheelchairs Skill Test (WST) for adult manual wheelchair users is currently being revised for a pediatric version.[67]

The Functional Mobility Assessment (FMA) has been adapted to a family-centered pediatric version (FMA-FC) to focus on how wheeled mobility affects children and families.[68] Adults with SCI who use manual wheelchairs are known to be at risk for developing UE repetitive use injuries, but little is known if the risk is similar for those with pediatric-onset SCI, given their potential for long-term use. Investigations are exploring the particular joint mechanics used in children and adolescents for manual propulsion to address preventive measures to reduce injuries and improve biomechanics for long-term preservation of UE function.[69]

Wellness and Fitness

The overwhelming evidence supports the importance of physical activity as a component of wellness, prevention, and health programs for all individuals. In addition, physical activity can potentially help manage or prevent the development of obesity, heart disease, and type 2 diabetes. The US Department of Health and Human Services published Physical Activity Guidelines for Americans in 2008 in response to the growing recognition of the importance of physical activity to maintain health and reduce the burden of health care from many lifestyle diseases such as cardiovascular disease, type 2 diabetes, and obesity (www.health.gov/Paguidelines).

Exercise recommendations for persons with SCI from the American Congress of Rehabilitation Medicine Spinal Cord Injury–Interdisciplinary Special Interest Group Fitness and Wellness Task Force were published in 2015.[70] The recommendations address cardiovascular health, muscle strength and endurance, and flexibility and range of motion, as well as safety considerations specific to persons with SCI such as AD and heart rate responses. These guidelines follow the published evidence-based guidelines for informed physical activity published by SCI Action Canada in 2011.[50] These recommendations do not address any special considerations for children and adolescents with SCI. The APTA Section on Pediatrics provides evidence for the role of PT to design, implement, and evaluate health promotion land fitness programs for youth with disabilities.[71] When designing a program of health promotion and fitness, the pediatric PT should consider examination findings using the ICF Framework for Children and Youth. The task force recommends using the US Department of Health and Human Services Physical Activity Guidelines for Americans from 2008. These guidelines were updated in 2015 with evidence-based recommendations including guidelines for preschool children age 3 through 5 and children and adolescents age 6 through 17.[72]

Children with disabilities face barriers to participation in organized activities, and physical activities that are inclusionary and mainstream for all children should be promoted.[71,73,74] Community and recreational programs may be available in communities but lack the resources and awareness of the needs of children with SCI to promote inclusion.[75,76] There are sports-specific programs for children with SCI, but participation may be limited by families' resources, finances, or geographic access. A pediatric PT can serve as a facilitator to advocate for the importance of physical activities and fitness for children at the local, state, and national levels. The PT can provide opportunities to play and engage in activities such as wheelchair sports or adaptive activities or sports to explore possibilities before transitioning from the health care system.

Educate parents, caregivers, and children on the recommended guidelines for physical activity for preschool children to adolescents. Discuss the health-related benefits of physical activity as part of developing a healthy lifestyle as children with physical disabilities move toward becoming adults. Explore the family's community resources and offer to serve as a consultant to community-based programs that support the inclusion of children with disabilities. Serve as a liaison to school districts on children's capabilities in physical education classes. Recognize the importance of a pediatric PT to promote health and fitness in pediatric patients with SCI.[77]

Case Studies

To integrate the material explored in this chapter, the following case studies have been developed. First, carefully read each case scenario. Develop your individual responses to each case. Once you have written down your responses, we ask that you engage in a peer-to-peer learning experience. Share your responses with a classmate and together come up with one response that both of you agree is the most effective and appropriate response. Then take that peer-to-peer response to each case and engage in a class discussion exploring the similarity and differences among the class responses.

Case 1

Lily

A 14-year-old girl (Lily) was involved in a motor vehicle accident 4 months ago, resulting in C6 American Spinal Injury Association (ASIA) Impairment Scale C tetraplegia with a relatively uncomplicated medical course. The car that Lily was driving in with her 2 friends and her mom, who was the driver, was sideswiped by an out-of-control car. Lily's car was forced into the steel road divider and flew into the air, landing on the wrong side of the highway. Lily's 2 friends who were passengers in the car died at the scene of the accident due to internal injuries. Lily's mom, the driver of the car, was not injured. Lily is now preparing to leave inpatient rehabilitation and to return to a split-level home with her parents, who work full time. In addition, she plans to resume her studies at her local high school, which is a 3-story high school.

Questions for Case 1
1. Describe the neurologic level of injury, motor level, and sensory level.
2. Formulate a physical therapy problem list for each of the following:
   A. Direct impairments
   B. Indirect impairments
   C. Composite impairments (combined effects of both direct and indirect impairments)

3. Determine which standardized tests and measures for examination would be appropriate and why.
4. Identify 2 goals and 2 objectives for each goal to address activity limitations.
5. Consider the potential for household or community locomotion either by ambulation or wheelchair. Determine an appropriate wheelchair.
6. Discuss treatment options/interventions that can be used during this transition period. Provide a rationale to justify your choices.
7. Design a daily exercise program that Lily can engage in and that would be appropriate to the patient and her goals.
8. What type of school-based services do you believe Lily should receive and why?
9. What community resources might be available for Lily?

Case 2

John

John, an 18-year-old male college student, was injured in a varsity football game resulting in a T6 compression fracture. He initially appeared to have a complete motor injury, but after 48 hours, he was classified as AISA C, and now after 5 months of intense rehabilitation services at a nationally recognized center, he is classified as ASIA D. At his weekly team meeting, the team is trying to decide what should be the next step for John. The rehabilitation center is 200 miles away from his college and 400 miles away from his parents' home.

Questions for Case 2
1. Describe the neurologic level of injury, motor level, and sensory level.
2. Formulate a physical therapy problem list for each of the following:
   A. Direct impairments
   B. Indirect impairments
   C. Composite impairments (combined effects of both direct and indirect impairments)
3. Determine which standardized tests and measures for examination would be appropriate at this time to employ and why.
4. Identify 2 goals and 2 objectives for each goal to address activity limitations.
5. Consider the potential for household or community locomotion either by ambulation or wheelchair. Determine an appropriate wheelchair (be specific in recommendations).
6. Formulate a plan of care based on John's current status and previous rehab history. Provide a rationale to justify your choices.
7. Design a daily exercise program that John can engage in and that would be appropriate to the patient and his goals.
8. Describe the parameters for locomotor training that are available for this patient.

Case 3

Jade

Jade, a 2-year-old girl, fell out of a first-floor window landing onto the front porch of the child's home 3 months ago. Her 10-year-old sibling found her lying on the porch and not responding to her name. The sibling ran back into the home and brought her mom out to her sister. The mom quickly picked up the child and carried her into the house and sat her up on the family couch and contacted 911. In the emergency room (ER), the child was initially classified as C5 ASIA B by the attending ER physician. Jade was transported within 42 hours to a pediatric rehabilitation center from an acute care hospital and is now classified as a C7 level ASIA C and ready to begin inpatient rehabilitation services.

Questions for Case 3

1. Describe the neurologic level of injury, motor level, and sensory level.
2. Formulate a physical therapy problem list for each of the following:
   A. Direct impairments
   B. Indirect impairments
   C. Composite impairments (combined effects of both direct and indirect impairments)
3. Determine which standardized tests and measures for examination would be appropriate at this time to employ and why.
4. Identify 2 goals and 2 objectives for each goal to address activity limitations.
5. Consider the potential for household or community locomotion either by ambulation or wheelchair. Determine an appropriate wheelchair (be specific in recommendations).
6. Formulate a plan of care based on Jade's current status and previous rehabilitation history. Provide a rationale to justify your choices.
7. Design a daily exercise program that Jade can engage in and that would be appropriate to the patient and her goals.
8. Describe the parameters for locomotor training that are available for this patient.

References

1. Spittle A, Orton J, Anderson PJ, Boyd R, Doyle LW. Early developmental intervention programmes provided post hospital discharge to prevent motor and cognitive impairment in preterm infants. *Cochrane Database Syst Rev.* 2015;2015(11):CD005495.

2. Wang MY, Hoh DJ, Leary SP, Griffith P, McComb JG. High rates of neurological improvement following severe traumatic pediatric spinal cord injury. *Spine.* 2004;29(13):1493-1497. doi:10.1097/01.BRS.0000129026.03194.0F

3. Powell A, Davidson L. Pediatric spinal cord injury: a review by organ system. *Phys Med Rehabil Clin N Am.* 2015;26(1):109-132. doi:10.1016/j.pmr.2014.09.002

4. Shin JI, Lee NJ, Cho SK. Pediatric cervical spine and spinal cord injury: a national database study. *Spine.* 2016;41(4):283-292. doi:10.1097/BRS.0000000000001176

5. Piatt J, Imperato N. Epidemiology of spinal injury in childhood and adolescence in the United States: 1997-2012. *J Neurosurg Pediatr.* 2018;21(5):441-448. doi:10.3171/2017.10.PEDS17530

6. Mohseni S, Talving P, Branco BC, et al. Effect of age on cervical spine injury in pediatric population: a National Trauma Data Bank review. *J Pediatr Surg.* 2011;46(9):1771-1776. doi:10.1016/j.jpedsurg.2011.03.007

7. Mathison DJ, Kadom N, Krug SE. Spinal cord injury in the pediatric patient. *Clin Pediatr Emerg Med.* 2008;9(2):106-123. doi:10.1016/j.cpem.2008.03.002

8. Osorio M, Reyes M, Massagli T. Pediatric spinal cord injury. *Curr Phys Med Rehabil Rep.* 2014;2(3):158-168. doi:10.1007/s40141-014-0054-1

9. Leonard JR, Jaffe DM, Kuppermann N, Olsen CS, Leonard JC; Pediatric Emergency Care Applied Research Network (PECARN) Cervical Spine Study Group. Cervical spine injury patterns in children. *Pediatrics.* 2014;133(5):e1179-e1188. doi:10.1542/peds.2013-3505

10. Knox J. Epidemiology of spinal cord injury without radiographic abnormality in children: a nationwide perspective. *J Child Orthop.* 2016;10(3):255-260. doi:10.1007/s11832-016-0740-x

11. Mulcahey MJ, Gaughan J, Betz RR, Johansen KJ. The International Standards for Neurological Classification of Spinal Cord Injury: reliability of data when applied to children and youths. *Spinal Cord.* 2007;45(6):452-459. doi:10.1038/sj.sc.3101987

12. Samdani AF, Ames RJ, Kimball JS, et al. Anterior vertebral body tethering for idiopathic scoliosis: two-year results. *Spine.* 2014;39(20):1688-1693. doi:10.1097/BRS.0000000000000472

13. Witiw CD, Fehlings MG. Acute spinal cord injury. *J Spinal Disord Tech.* 2015;28(6):202-210. doi:10.1097/BSD.0000000000000287

14. Field-Fote EC, Yang JF, Basso DM, Gorassini MA. Supraspinal control predicts locomotor function and forecasts responsiveness to training after spinal cord injury. *J Neurotrauma.* 2017;34(9):1813-1825. doi:10.1089/neu.2016.4565

15. Hubli M, Dietz V. The physiological basis of neurorehabilitation—locomotor training after spinal cord injury. *J Neuroeng Rehabil.* 2013;10(1):5. doi:10.1186/1743-0003-10-5

16. Sparrow WA, Newell KM. Metabolic energy expenditure and the regulation of movement economy. *Psychon Bull Rev.* 1998;5(2):173-196. doi:10.3758/BF03212943

17. Tatka J, Elbayer J, Vojdani S, Pallotta N, Malik A. Pediatric spinal cord injury. *J Spine Surg.* 2016;7:2.

18. Padman R, Alexander M, Thorogood C, Porth S. Respiratory management of pediatric patients with spinal cord injuries: retrospective review of the duPont experience. *Neurorehabil Neural Repair.* 2003;17(1):32-36. doi:10.1177/0888439003251751

19. Singh G, Behrman AL, Aslan SC, Trimble S, Ovechkin AV. Respiratory functional and motor control deficits in children with spinal cord injury. *Respir Physiol Neurobiol.* 2018;247:174-180. doi:10.1016/j.resp.2017.10.006

20. Warren VC. Glossopharyngeal and neck accessory muscle breathing in a young adult with C2 complete tetraplegia resulting in ventilator dependency. *Phys Ther.* 2002;82(6):590-600. doi:10.1093/ptj/82.6.590

21. Hormigo KM, Zholudeva LV, Spruance VM, et al. Enhancing neural activity to drive respiratory plasticity following cervical spinal cord injury. *Exp Neurol.* 2017;287(Pt 2):276-287. doi:10.1016/j.expneurol.2016.08.018

22. Hoh DJ, Mercier LM, Hussey SP, Lane MA. Respiration following spinal cord injury: evidence for human neuroplasticity. *Respir Physiol Neurobiol.* 2013;189(2):450-464. doi:10.1016/j.resp.2013.07.002

23. Bach JR. Noninvasive respiratory management of high level spinal cord injury. *J Spinal Cord Med.* 2012;35(2):72-80. doi:10.1179/2045772311Y.0000000051

24. Berlowitz DJ, Wadsworth B, Ross J. Respiratory problems and management in people with spinal cord injury. *Breathe (Sheff)*. 2016;12(4):328-340. doi:10.1183/20734735.012616

25. Hwang M, Zebracki K, Betz RR, Mulcahey MJ, Vogel LC. Normative blood pressure and heart rate in pediatric spinal cord injury. *Top Spinal Cord Inj Rehabil*. 2013;19(2):87-95. doi:10.1310/sci1902-87

26. Eldahan KC, Rabchevsky AG. Autonomic dysreflexia after spinal cord injury: systemic pathophysiology and methods of management. *Auton Neurosci*. 2018;209:59-70. doi:10.1016/j.autneu.2017.05.002

27. Willock J, Maylor M. Pressure ulcers in infants and children. *Nurs Stand*. 2004;18(24):56-60, 62. doi:10.7748/ns2004.02.18.24.56.c3556

28. Hickey K, Anderson C, Vogel L. Pressure ulcers in pediatric spinal cord injury. *Top Spinal Cord Inj Rehabil*. 2000;6(suppl 1):85-90. doi:10.1310/1C86-7L96-1JAR-7Y3N

29. Curley MA, Razmus IS, Roberts KE, Wypij D. Predicting pressure ulcer risk in pediatric patients: the Braden Q Scale. *Nurs Res*. 2003;52(1):22-33. doi:10.1097/00006199-200301000-00004

30. McLaughlin JF, Murray M, Van Zandt K, Carr M. Clean intermittent catheterization. *Dev Med Child Neurol*. 1996;38(5):446-454. doi:10.1111/j.1469-8749.1996.tb15102.x

31. Mulcahey MJ, Gaughan JP, Betz RR, Samdani AF, Barakat N, Hunter LN. Neuromuscular scoliosis in children with spinal cord injury. *Top Spinal Cord Inj Rehabil*. 2013;19(2):96-103. doi:10.1310/sci1902-96

32. Biering-Sørensen F, Burns AS, Curt A, et al. International spinal cord injury musculoskeletal basic data set. *Spinal Cord*. 2012;50(11):797-802. doi:10.1038/sc.2012.102

33. Lauer R, Johnston TE, Smith BT, Mulcahey MJ, Betz RR, Maurer AH. Bone mineral density of the hip and knee in children with spinal cord injury. *J Spinal Cord Med*. 2007;30(Suppl 1):S10-S14. doi: 10.1080/10790268.2007.11753962

34. Grover M, Bachrach LK. Osteoporosis in children with chronic illnesses: diagnosis, monitoring, and treatment. *Curr Osteoporos Rep*. 2017;15(4):271-282. doi:10.1007/s11914-017-0371-2

35. Calhoun Thielen C, Sadowsky C, Vogel LC, et al. Evaluation of the Walking Index for Spinal Cord Injury II (WISCI-II) in children with spinal cord injury (SCI). *Spinal Cord*. 2017;55(5):478-482. doi: 10.1038/sc.2016.142

36. Kirshblum SC, Burns SP, Biering-Sorensen F, et al. International standards for neurological classification of spinal cord injury (revised 2011). *J Spinal Cord Med*. 2011;34(6):535-546. doi:10.1179/204577211X13207446293695

37. Chafetz RS, Gaughan JP, Calhoun C, et al. Relationship between neurological injury and patterns of upright mobility in children with spinal cord injury. *Top Spinal Cord Inj Rehabil*. 2013;19(1):31-41. doi:10.1310/sci1901-31

38. Mulcahey MJ, Calhoun Thielen C, Dent K, et al. Evaluation of the graded redefined assessment of strength, sensibility and prehension (GRASSP) in children with tetraplegia. *Spinal Cord*. 2018;56(8):741-749. doi:10.1038/s41393-018-0084-0

39. Marino RJ. Domains of outcomes in spinal cord injury for clinical trials to improve neurological function. *J Rehabil Res Dev*. 2007;44(1):113-122. doi:10.1682/JRRD.2005.08.0138

40. Behrman AL, Ardolino E, Vanhiel LR, et al. Assessment of functional improvement without compensation reduces variability of outcome measures after human spinal cord injury. *Arch Phys Med Rehabil*. 2012;93(9):1518-1529. doi:10.1016/j.apmr.2011.04.027

41. Ardolino EM, Mulcahey MJ, Trimble S, et al. Development and initial validation of the pediatric neuromuscular recovery scale. *Pediatr Phys Ther*. 2016;28(4):416-426. doi:10.1097/PEP.0000000000000285

42. Calhoun CL, Mulcahey MJ. Pilot study of reliability and validity of the Walking Index for Spinal Cord Injury II (WISCI-II) in children and adolescents with spinal cord injury. *J Pediatr Rehabil Med*. 2012;5(4):275-279.

43. Rozzelle CJ, Aarabi B, Dhall SS, et al. Management of pediatric cervical spine and spinal cord injuries. *Neurosurgery*. 2013;72(3)(suppl 2):205-226. doi:10.1227/NEU.0b013e318277096c

44. Mehrholz J, Kugler J, Pohl M. Locomotor training for walking after spinal cord injury. *Cochrane Database Syst Rev*. 2012;11:CD006676. doi:10.1002/14651858.CD006676.pub3

45. Gollie JM, Guccione AA. Overground locomotor training in spinal cord injury: a performance-based framework. *Top Spinal Cord Inj Rehabil*. 2017;23(3):226-233. doi:10.1310/sci2303-226

46. Donenberg JG, Fetters L, Johnson R. The effects of locomotor training in children with spinal cord injury: a systematic review. *Dev Neurorehabil*. 2019;22(4):272-287. doi:10.1080/17518423.2018.1487474

47. Shumway-Cook A, Woollacott MH. *Motor Control: Translating Research Into Clinical Practice*. 4th ed. Lippincott Williams and Wilkins; 2011.

48. Behrman AL, Velozo C, Suter S, Lorenz D, Basso DM. Test-retest reliability of the Neuromuscular Recovery Scale. *Arch Phys Med Rehabil*. 2015;96(8):1375-1384. doi:10.1016/j.apmr.2015.03.022

49. O'Sullivan S, Schmitz T, Falk T. *Physical Rehabilitation Assessment and Treatment*. 6th ed. F.A. Davis Company; 2013.

50. Martin Ginis KA, Ma JK, Latimer-Cheung AE, Rimmer JH. A systematic review of review articles addressing factors related to physical activity participation among children and adults with physical disabilities. *Health Psychol Rev*. 2016;10(4):478-494. doi:10.1080/17437199.2016.1198240

51. Memberg WD, Polasek KH, Hart RL, et al. Implanted neuroprosthesis for restoring arm and hand function in people with high level tetraplegia. *Arch Phys Med Rehabil*. 2014;95(6):1201-1211.e1. doi:10.1016/j.apmr.2014.01.028

52. Crozier KS, Cheng LL, Graziani V, Zorn G, Herbison G, Ditunno JF Jr. Spinal cord injury: prognosis for ambulation based on quadriceps recovery. *Paraplegia*. 1992;30(11):762-767. doi:10.1038/sc.1992.147

53. Harkema SJ, Schmidt-Read M, Lorenz DJ, Edgerton VR, Behrman AL. Balance and ambulation improvements in individuals with chronic incomplete spinal cord injury using locomotor training-based rehabilitation. *Arch Phys Med Rehabil*. 2012;93(9):1508-1517. doi:10.1016/j.apmr.2011.01.024

54. Prosser LA. Locomotor training within an inpatient rehabilitation program after pediatric incomplete spinal cord injury. *Phys Ther*. 2007;87(9):1224-1232. doi:10.2522/ptj.20060252

55. Gorski K, Harbold K, Haverstick K, Schultz E, Shealy SE, Krisa L. Locomotor training in the pediatric spinal cord injury population: a systematic review of the literature. *Top Spinal Cord Inj Rehabil*. 2016;22(2):135-148. doi:10.1310/sci2202-135

56. Gandhi P, Chan K, Verrier MC, Pakosh M, Musselman KE. Training to improve walking after pediatric spinal cord injury: a systematic review of parameters and walking outcomes. *J Neurotrauma*. 2017;34(9):1713-1725. doi:10.1089/neu.2016.4501

57. Forrest GF, Sisto SA, Barbeau H, et al. Neuromotor and musculoskeletal responses to locomotor training for an individual with chronic motor complete AIS-B spinal cord injury. *J Spinal Cord Med*. 2008;31(5):509-521. doi:10.1080/10790268.2008.11753646

58. Damiano DL, DeJong SL. A systematic review of the effectiveness of treadmill training and body weight support in pediatric

rehabilitation. *J Neurol Phys Ther*. 2009;33(1):27-44. doi:10.1097/NPT.0b013e31819800e2

59. Calhoun CL, Schottler J, Vogel LC. Recommendations for mobility in children with spinal cord injury. *Top Spinal Cord Inj Rehabil*. 2013;19(2):142-151. doi:10.1310/sci1902-142

60. Bryden AM, Ancans J, Mazurkiewicz J, McKnight A, Scholtens M. Technology for spinal cord injury rehabilitation and its application to youth. *J Pediatr Rehabil Med*. 2012;5(4):287-299.

61. Sharif Razavian A, Azizpour H, Sullivan J, Carlsson S. CNN features off-the-shelf: an astounding baseline for recognition. In: *Proceedings of the IEEE Conference on Computer Vision and Pattern Recognition Workshops*. 2014. Accessed November 6, 2023. https://arxiv.org/abs/1403.6382.

62. Miller A, Fisch A, Dodge J, Karimi AH, Bordes A, Weston J. Key-value memory networks for directly reading documents. 2016. Accessed November 6, 2023. https://arxiv.org/abs/1606.03126.

63. Saensook W, Phonthee S, Srisim K, Mato L, Wattanapan P, Amatachaya S. Ambulatory assistive devices and walking performance in patients with incomplete spinal cord injury. *Spinal Cord*. 2014;52(3):216-219. doi:10.1038/sc.2013.120

64. Costello LC, Franklin RB, Reynolds MA, Chellaiah M. The important role of osteoblasts and citrate production in bone formation: "osteoblast citration" as a new concept for an old relationship. *Open Bone J*. 2012;4:4. doi:10.2174/1876525401204010027

65. Haapala SA, Faghri PD, Adams DJ. Leg joint power output during progressive resistance FES-LCE cycling in SCI subjects: developing an index of fatigue. *J Neuroeng Rehabil*. 2008;5(1):14. doi:10.1186/1743-0003-5-14

66. Krey CH. Special seating considerations for the child with a spinal cord injury. *Int J Ther Rehabil*. 2005;12(2):84-86. doi:10.12968/ijtr.2005.12.2.17460

67. Sol ME, Verschuren O, de Groot L, de Groot JF; Fit-For-the-Future! Consortium. Development of a wheelchair mobility skills test for children and adolescents: combining evidence with clinical expertise. *BMC Pediatr*. 2017;17(1):51. doi:10.1186/s12887-017-0809-9

68. Beavers DB, Holm MB, Rogers JC, Plummer T, Schmeler M. Adaptation of the adult Functional Mobility Assessment (FMA) into a FMA-Family Centred (FMA-FC) paediatric version. *Child Care Health Dev*. 2018;44(4):630-635. doi:10.1111/cch.12571

69. Schnorenberg AJ, Slavens BA, Wang M, Vogel LC, Smith PA, Harris GF. Biomechanical model for evaluation of pediatric upper extremity joint dynamics during wheelchair mobility. *J Biomech*. 2014;47(1):269-276. doi:10.1016/j.jbiomech.2013.11.014

70. Evans N, Wingo B, Sasso E, Hicks A, Gorgey AS, Harness E. Exercise recommendations and considerations for persons with spinal cord injury. *Arch Phys Med Rehabil*. 2015;96(9):1749-1750. doi:10.1016/j.apmr.2015.02.005

71. Rowland JL, Fragala-Pinkham M, Miles C, O'Neil ME. The scope of pediatric physical therapy practice in health promotion and fitness for youth with disabilities. *Pediatr Phys Ther*. 2015;27(1):2-15. doi:10.1097/PEP.0000000000000098

72. Piercy KL, Troiano RP, Ballard RM, et al. The physical activity guidelines for Americans. *JAMA*. 2018;320(19):2020-2028. doi:10.1001/jama.2018.14854

73. Murphy NA, Carbone PS; American Academy of Pediatrics Council on Children With Disabilities. Promoting the participation of children with disabilities in sports, recreation, and physical activities. *Pediatrics*. 2008;121(5):1057-1061. doi:10.1542/peds.2008-0566

74. Carey H, Long T. The pediatric physical therapist's role in promoting and measuring participation in children with disabilities. *Pediatr Phys Ther*. 2012;24(2):163-170. doi:10.1097/PEP.0b013e31824c8ea2

75. Ross SM, Bogart KR, Logan SW, Case L, Fine J, Thompson H. Physical activity participation of disabled children: a systematic review of conceptual and methodological approaches in health research. *Front Public Health*. 2016;4:187. doi:10.3389/fpubh.2016.00187

76. Rimmer JH, Vanderbom KA. A call to action: building a translational inclusion team science in physical activity, nutrition, and obesity management for children with disabilities. *Front Public Health*. 2016;4:164. doi:10.3389/fpubh.2016.00164

77. Ginis KA, Hicks AL, Latimer AE, et al. The development of evidence-informed physical activity guidelines for adults with spinal cord injury. *Spinal Cord*. 2011;49(11):1088-1096. doi:10.1038/sc.2011.63

11

Autism Spectrum Disorder

Melissa Moran Tovin, PT, PhD

■ INTRODUCTION

Autism spectrum disorder (ASD) is a developmental disability characterized by social, communication, intellectual, and behavioral challenges.[1-3] The term *spectrum* denotes the broad range of conditions and levels of severity that affect individuals with this diagnosis. Children diagnosed with ASD often struggle with delayed motor development, impaired balance and coordination, and sensorimotor impairments that can impact function, limit physical activity, inhibit participation, and ultimately affect the potential for independence as an adult.

Over the past 2 decades, the incidence of ASD has increased at an alarming rate, both in the United States and around the world. The impact of this dramatic rise has far-reaching effects, extending well beyond the individual diagnosed with the disorder. According to recent studies, the growing number of children diagnosed with ASD has resulted in a significant economic burden from both direct and indirect costs. During childhood, most of these costs include medical care, behavioral intervention, special education, and lost parental productivity. As adults, the financial impact is mostly attributed to residential care, supported living, and individual loss of productivity.[4,5]

Individuals with ASD and their caregivers can benefit greatly from physical therapists' knowledge, expertise, and guidance throughout their life course to improve function and participation, prevent secondary impairments, assist with postsecondary transitions, facilitate improved health and wellness, and improve the potential for independent living. This chapter provides an overview of ASD, including diagnostic testing and clinical presentation, a review of the role of the physical therapist

as a member of the interprofessional team, a description of evidence-based outcomes measures, and physical therapy (PT) evaluation procedures, support strategies, and interventions. Case studies and videos further explore the role of PT through the life course for individuals with ASD.

■ ETIOLOGY

Over the past 2 decades, the number of children diagnosed with ASD has increased dramatically. According to the Centers for Disease Control and Prevention (CDC), the incidence of ASD in the United States jumped from a rate of 1 in 150 in the early 1990s, to a rate of 1 in 36 in the most recent surveillance report from 2020.[6,7] Individuals diagnosed with ASD represent all racial, ethnic, and socioeconomic groups, and males are 4 times more likely to have autism than females.[6] The contribution of diagnostic changes and early identification to the rising incidence is unclear. There are currently ongoing large epidemiologic and longitudinal studies to identify the causes of ASD.[8-11]

There is no single cause for ASD, and not all causes are known. Nevertheless, there is evidence to support that a combination of environmental factors, characteristics, and genetic predispositions contributes to the development of ASD. Several studies have identified many perinatal and neonatal factors as contributing to the development of autism, suggesting that there is a critical period before, during, and immediately after birth.[12] Speculation about the role of environmental exposures has led to studies on the effect of various substances such as perinatal supplements, heavy metals, chemicals (eg, pesticides, flame retardants), and pollutants during critical periods of development.[8,13,14] Recent controversy over the potential role of childhood vaccines (ie, measles-mumps-rubella, hepatitis B) in the development of ASD sparked many studies to examine the relationship between vaccines and ASD. Nevertheless, there is no evidence to date that supports an association between vaccines and ASD.[15]

Evidence supports strong genetic influences on the development of autism.[16] A percentage of children with ASD have genetic alterations in the same chromosomal region as other genetic disorders such as Prader-Willi syndrome, Angelman syndrome, and Rett syndrome. A diagnosis of ASD with another genetic condition accounts for approximately 10% of children diagnosed with ASD.[17,18] Some of these disorders were considered within the same diagnostic spectrum of disorders under the previous version of the *Diagnostic and Statistical Manual of Mental Disorders*.[19] With publication of the fifth edition of the *Diagnostic and Statistical Manual of Mental Disorders* (DSM-5) in 2013, for example, Rett syndrome is no longer considered part of ASD. Children with these genetic disorders share some signs and symptoms with ASD, such as toe walking, loss of language and motor skills, and repetitive behaviors. Some research suggests that ASD screenings (eg, Ages and Stages Questionnaire [ASQ]) alone to determine presence of ASD in this population are misleading and a more sensitive diagnostic tool is indicated (eg, Autism Diagnostic Observation Schedule [ADOS]).[20]

Further examination of the many genetic and environmental factors identified in the literature is beyond the scope of this chapter. Refer to **Table 11-1** for the factors and characteristics strongly supported by the research to date.

■ DIAGNOSTICS

The diagnosis of ASD is based on a set of criteria published by the American Psychiatric Association in the DSM-5.[39] In the DSM-5 (2013), 4 previously distinct diagnoses are merged under the umbrella diagnosis of ASD: autistic disorder, Asperger disorder, childhood disintegrative disorder, and pervasive developmental disorder not otherwise specified (**Table 11-2**).[39] These criteria fall into 2 main domains required for the diagnosis: (1) deficits in social communication and interaction, and (2) restricted, repetitive behaviors, interests, or activities. The child must meet a specified number of criteria in both domains (**Figure 11-1**).

The child's level of impairment in these domains and need for support and the impact on overall function are used to determine the severity of ASD for diagnostic, prognostic, and intervention planning (**Figure 11-2**). Moreover, the DSM-5 facilitates the use of historical information, as well as specifiers, to document the presence of individual clinical characteristics such as intellectual disability, genetic disorders, behavioral disorders, and structural language impairment (**Table 11-3**). In this way, an individualized diagnosis and clinical description can be formulated (**Figure 11-3**).[39] It is important to remember that no 2 children diagnosed with ASD present the same, as each has a unique set of challenges, strengths, and needs. There is evidence that the revised conceptualization of ASD in the DSM-5 provides greater diagnostic sensitivity and specificity in preschool children than the previous edition.[40]

Diagnosis is determined through a range of clinical tests and measures, developmental screenings, and observational reports. Members from several medical and rehabilitation

TABLE 11-1 • Some Factors and Characteristics Associated With the Development of Autism Spectrum Disorder (ASD)

Identical twin with ASD	54%-88% chance both twins will have ASD[21-23]
Nonidentical twins with ASD	25%-31% chance both twins will have ASD[21-23]
Sibling with ASD	5%-25% chance another child sibling will have ASD[22,24-27]
Parental age	Advanced parental age[28,29]
Preterm delivery Low birth weight (LBW) and very low birth weight (VLBW)	Preterm babies are 10 times more likely to develop ASD than full-term babies[30-33] Small for gestational age, LBW, and VLBW are associated with increased risk of ASD[29,34,35]
	Cesarean delivery[33]
Presence of genetic or chromosomal disorder	Approximately 10% of children with ASD have another genetic disorder such as Down syndrome, fragile X syndrome, tuberous sclerosis, Prader-Willi syndrome, Angelman syndrome, or phenylketonuria[17,18,36]
Prenatal exposure to drugs	The prescription drug valproic acid has been linked with a higher risk of ASD[37] Preconception exposure to opiates[38] Small for gestational age[33]

TABLE 11-2 • Disorders Included Under the Diagnosis of Autism Spectrum Disorder (ASD)[39]

Disorder	Symptom Severity
Autistic disorder	Significant language delays Social and communication challenges Unusual behaviors and interests May have intellectual disability
Childhood disintegrative disorder	Loss or regression in language, social function, and motor skills following a period of apparently normal development for at least first 2 years after birth[41,42]
Pervasive developmental disorder, not otherwise specified (PDD-NOS)	Meet some of the criteria for autistic disorder or Asperger syndrome, but not all Usually have fewer and milder symptoms than those with autistic disorder The symptoms might cause only social and communication challenges
Asperger syndrome	Milder symptoms of autistic disorder Have social challenges and unusual behaviors and interests Typically do not have problems with language or intellectual disability

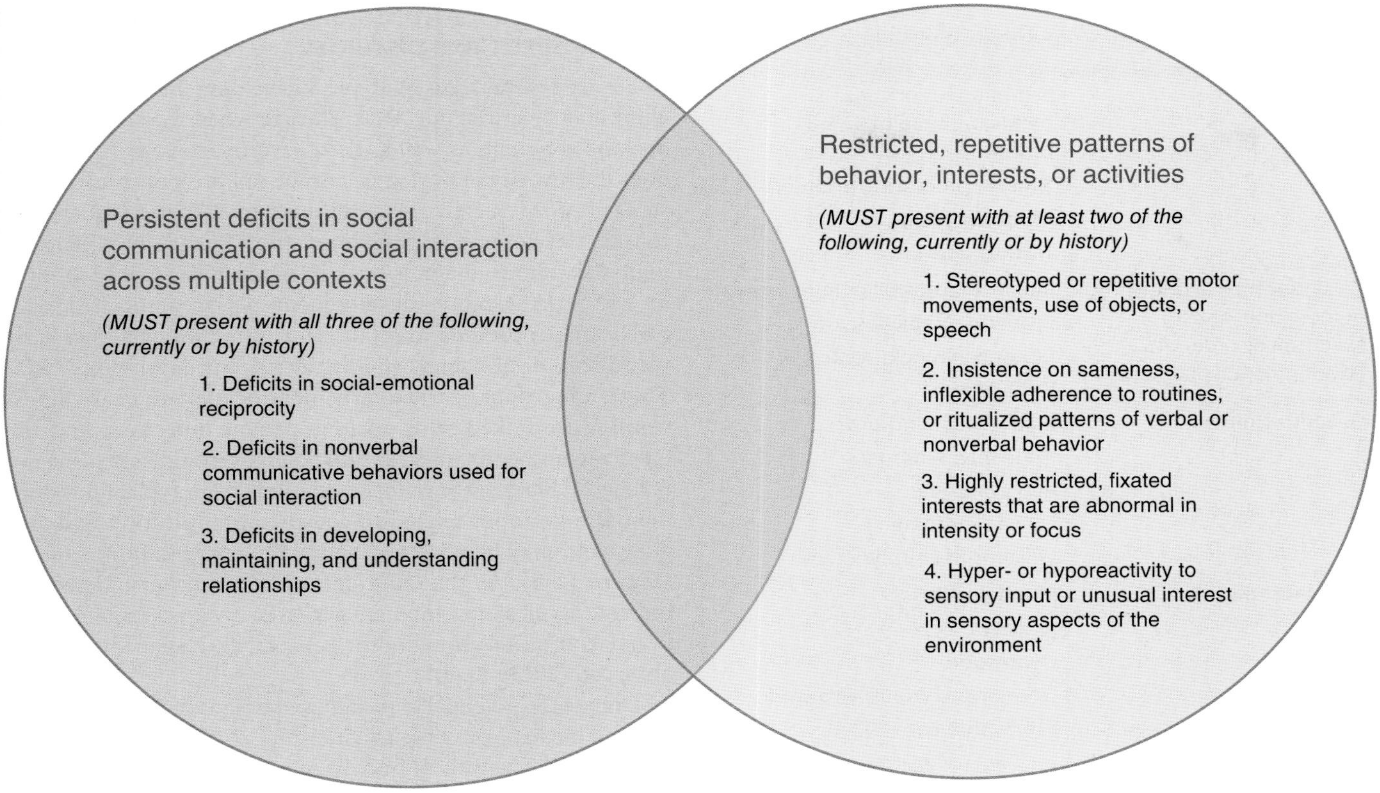

Persistent deficits in social communication and social interaction across multiple contexts

(MUST present with all three of the following, currently or by history)

    1. Deficits in social-emotional reciprocity

    2. Deficits in nonverbal communicative behaviors used for social interaction

    3. Deficits in developing, maintaining, and understanding relationships

Restricted, repetitive patterns of behavior, interests, or activities

(MUST present with at least two of the following, currently or by history)

    1. Stereotyped or repetitive motor movements, use of objects, or speech

    2. Insistence on sameness, inflexible adherence to routines, or ritualized patterns of verbal or nonverbal behavior

    3. Highly restricted, fixated interests that are abnormal in intensity or focus

    4. Hyper- or hyporeactivity to sensory input or unusual interest in sensory aspects of the environment

FIGURE 11-1 *Diagnostic and Statistical Manual of Mental Disorders, Fifth Edition,* **diagnostic criteria for autism spectrum disorder.**[39]

Severity Level

Level 1-High Functioning	Level 2-Moderate	Level 3-Severe
Requires support for social communication	Requires substantial support	Requires very substantial support
Difficulty initiating social interactions	Social impairments are apparent	Severe deficits in verbal and nonverbal social communication
Atypical responses to social advances of others	Marked deficits in verbal and nonverbal social communication skills	Very limited ability to initiate and respond to social interactions and situations
May appear to have decreased interest in social interactions	Social impairments are apparent even with supports in place	All aspects of function are severely limited by restrictive/repetitive behaviors
Attempts to make friends are odd and typically unsuccessful	Limited initiation of social interactions	Rigid behavior, extreme difficulty coping with change
Inflexibility of behavior causes significant interference with functioning in one or more contexts	Reduced/abnormal responses to social advances from others	
Problems of organization and planning hamper independence	Inflexibility, difficulty coping with change, or other restricted/repetitive behaviors frequently interfere with functioning in a variety of contexts	

FIGURE 11-2 **Severity levels of autism spectrum disorder related to social communication and behavior domains.**

TABLE 11-3 • Examples of Specifiers Denoting Presence of Clinical Features and Characteristics[39]

Behavior disorder	Self-injurious or aggressive behavior; head banging or biting
	Sensory processing disorders
	Sleep disorders
	Tic disorders
Co-occurrence of one or more non–autism spectrum disorder (ASD) developmental diagnoses	Intellectual disability/impairment
	Learning disabilities
	Motor planning disorders or dyspraxia
Genetic disorders	Prader-Willi syndrome
	Angelman syndrome
	Rett syndrome
	Down syndrome
	Williams-Beuren syndrome
Psychiatric disorders	Mood disorders
	Anxiety
	Depression
	Obsessive-compulsive disorder
	Schizophrenia
Medical	Attention-deficit/hyperactivity disorder (ADHD)
	Epilepsy
	Gastrointestinal (GI) disorders
	Obesity
	Phenylketonuria (PKU)

disciplines may contribute to the diagnosis, including a psychologist, psychiatrist, developmental pediatrician, neurologist, physical therapist, occupational therapist, speech-language pathologist, and special educator.

EARLY IDENTIFICATION: SIGNS AND SYMPTOMS OF AUTISM SPECTRUM DISORDER

There are several signs of atypical development that indicate a child may be at risk for ASD. The age when the signs of ASD become apparent, as well as their severity, can vary greatly, as does the severity of the signs. For the majority of children, the signs of ASD typically appear by age 2 to 3. With adequate and routine developmental screening and diligent surveillance of high-risk infants, diagnosis can be made as early as 18 months of age. Furthermore, development delays associated with ASD can be observed in infancy for some, which allows early identification of babies who are at risk for developing ASD.[3] This is important because early identification and early intervention are linked with positive patient outcomes, and the CDC recommends intervention begin even if diagnosis is not reached.[43] Early signs reflect deviations from typical developmental milestones related to social communication and language and may be observed between 6 and 24 months of age (**Figure 11-4**). As the child gets older, additional signs that indicate atypical development across many areas (social, emotional, communication, motor, sensory, and behavior) may be observed (**Table 11-4**).

Despite the potential to recognize the signs of ASD at an early age, the median age most children first receive the diagnosis is 52 months.[44] The time of first diagnosis appears to be related to the severity of ASD, as the average age children with a less severe subtype (eg, subtype previously known as Asperger disorder) are diagnosed is 5 years and 7 months, and the average age for children with a more severe subtype (eg, subtype previously known as autistic disorder) is 3 years and 10 months.[44] Moreover, some children with ASD may not show all the signs required for a diagnosis, supporting the need for adequate screening, surveillance, and referral. The CDC has developed an "Act Early" campaign, with evidence-based and free online information and educational resources (eg, milestone tracker app) for parents and providers (https://www.cdc.gov/ncbddd/actearly/index.html). The goal is

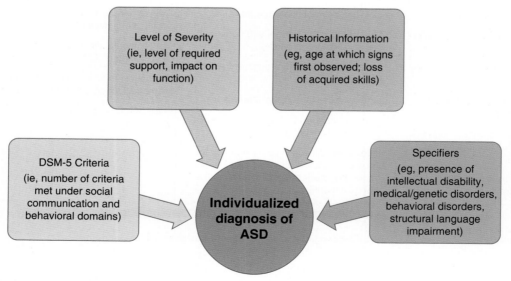

FIGURE 11-3 Building an individualized diagnosis and clinical description of autism spectrum disorder (ASD).

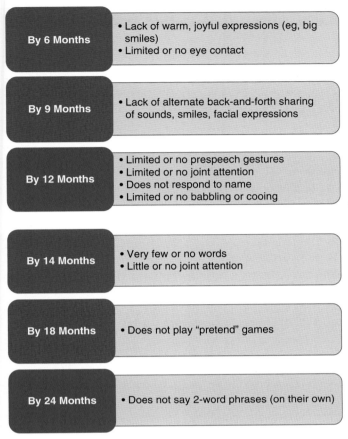

By 6 Months	• Lack of warm, joyful expressions (eg, big smiles) • Limited or no eye contact
By 9 Months	• Lack of alternate back-and-forth sharing of sounds, smiles, facial expressions
By 12 Months	• Limited or no prespeech gestures • Limited or no joint attention • Does not respond to name • Limited or no babbling or cooing
By 14 Months	• Very few or no words • Little or no joint attention
By 18 Months	• Does not play "pretend" games
By 24 Months	• Does not say 2-word phrases (on their own)

FIGURE 11-4 Hallmark signs of autism spectrum disorder.[43,45]

to promote *action* (eg, referral for further testing, access early intervention programs, strategies to promote development) if there are *any* concerns about a child's development, even before the formal diagnosis of ASD is made.

TABLE 11-4 • Additional Signs of Autism Spectrum Disorder[43,45]
Delayed development of speech, language, and social skills
Avoids eye contact and prefers to be alone
Loss of language or social skills already acquired
Trouble relating to others or understanding other people's feelings
Appear unaware when people talk to them or call their name
Repeats or echoes words or phrases (echolalia)
Difficulty adapting to changes in routine
Avoids being held or cuddled, or might cuddle only on their terms
Restricted interests and/or repetitive behaviors
Unusual or intense reactions to sensory input (under- or oversensitive)
Shows little safety or danger awareness
Reversal of pronouns
Deficits and/or delays in motor skills, coordination, praxis, and postural control
Motor stereotypes (eg, flapping, rocking, twirling)

EARLY DIAGNOSIS

Developmental Screening

In an effort to identify children at risk for ASD, the American Academy of Pediatrics (AAP) and CDC's National Center on Birth Defects and Developmental Disabilities (NCBDD) currently recommends that all children undergo broad developmental screening during well-child visits at 9, 18, and 24 (or 30) months of age, and autism-specific screening at 18 and 24 months of age using evidence-based tools. Moreover, the AAP recommends social-emotional screening at regular intervals. Additional screening is indicated if a child is at high risk for developmental delays for the following reasons: preterm birth, low birth weight, having a sibling with ASD, or if behaviors associated with ASDs are present. Many different developmental screening tools are available. The AAP STAR Center (Screening Technical Assistance and Resource Center) provides information and resources on a variety of evidence-based screening tools in an effort to promote healthy development. Selected examples of screening tools for general development and ASD are listed in **Table 11-5**.

Comprehensive Diagnostic Evaluation

Once a child is identified through developmental screening as delayed, the parent or caregiver should be guided to early intervention assessment and/or services (**Figure 11-5**). Those identified as at risk for ASD should be referred to a specialist (eg, developmental pediatrician, child neurologist, child psychologist) for further, more comprehensive diagnostic evaluation. There is evidence that the stability of an early diagnosis of autism and early identification are predictive of later diagnosis.[26,47-49]

Comprehensive diagnostic testing includes the use of evidence-based diagnostic tools to gather information about the child's development from parents or caregivers and the tester's observation of the child's behavior. A list of selected evidence-based diagnostic tools is provided in **Table 11-6**. No one single tool should be the basis for an ASD diagnosis. Rather, it should be used along with other tests and measures (eg, audiology testing, vision testing, genetic testing, neurologic testing, other medical testing) and consideration of the diagnostic criteria put forth in DSM-5[39] to create an individualized clinical picture of the child's development and ASD diagnosis, as previously described in this chapter. It is important to note that in many cases and settings, physical therapists are not typically the clinicians who administers these the diagnostic tools listed. Rather, physical therapists may be more involved in the administration of screening tools that can lead to referral and diagnostic testing (see Figure 11-5).[50]

■ PATIENT MANAGEMENT FOR THE PHYSICAL THERAPIST

INTERNATIONAL CLASSIFICATION OF FUNCTIONING, DISABILITY, AND HEALTH (ICF)

Functioning and disability for individuals with ASD has traditionally been viewed from a behavioral and social communication perspective. The rapid and substantial increase in the incidence of autism and subsequent research has led

TABLE 11-5 • Selected Examples of Developmental and Autism-Specific Screening Tools

Ages and Stages Questionnaires (ASQ)	Screening purpose: General development[46] Age range: 1 month to 5 years 6 months Administration: Parent-completed age-specific questionnaire Time: 10-15 minutes Focus areas: Communication, gross motor, fine motor, problem solving, and personal adaptive skills Notes: Online option
Communication and Symbolic Behavior Scales (CSBS)	Screening purpose: Language development[46] Age range: 6-24 months Administration: Parent-completed screening tool (checklist). Time: 15-20 minutes Focus areas: 7 language predictors (emotion and eye gaze, communication, gestures, sounds, words, understanding, and object use) https://brookespublishing.com/product/csbs-dp/
Parents' Evaluation of Developmental Status (PEDS)	Screening purpose: General development[46] Administration: Parent interview; single response form Time: 5-10 minutes Age: Birth to 8 years Focus areas: Behavior, language development, motor, problem solving, social-emotional development Notes: Identifies developmental and behavioral problems needing further evaluation; useful as a surveillance tool[46] "Elicits and addresses parents' concerns about children's language, motor, self-help, early academic skills, behavior and social-emotional/mental health. PEDS tells you when parents' concerns suggest problems requiring referral and which concerns are best responded to with advice or reassurance." https://pedstest.com/AboutOurTools/LearnAboutPEDS/IntroductionToPEDS.html
Modified Checklist for Autism in Toddlers (MCHAT)	Screening purpose: Identify children at risk for autism in the general population[46] Administration: Parent-completed questionnaire Age: 16-30 months of age Notes: Administered to parents/guardians and interpreted by pediatric providers in the context of developmental surveillance
Screening Tool for Autism in Toddlers and Young Children (STAT)	Purpose: Identify ASD in children when developmental concerns are suspected[46] Administration: Provider facilitates 12 interactive activities Time: 20 minutes Age: 24-36 months Focus areas: Play, communication, and imitation skills

investigators and clinicians to recognize the role of personal, social, and environmental factors on health-related functioning for individuals with ASD. The International Classification of Functioning, Disability, and Health (ICF) provides a framework for a more holistic approach to systemizing function and factors that impact everyday life and functioning for individuals with a disability. Moreover, the Children and Youth version of the ICF (ICF-CY) includes additional categories to capture characteristics and factors that impact function for developing children. The ICF-CY can be effectively applied to children and youth with ASD to develop a more comprehensive description of individual strengths, contextual challenges (eg, environmental factors), and support needs, and how these positively or negatively impact daily function. It can guide intervention planning and facilitate more accurate calculation of health-related service costs.[51] The ICF-CY can also improve communication between clinicians, researchers, patients, families, and community stakeholders that impact, or are impacted by, children and adults with ASD.

The ICF-CY consists of 1685 second-level categories: 531 body functions, 329 body structures, 552 activities and participation, and 273 environmental factors. This can be overwhelming for users, as only a small percentage of second-level categories apply to a given health condition. ICF Core Sets are short lists of ICF second-level categories for specific health conditions in an effort to streamline and facilitate its use in certain populations. ICF Core Sets are available for some other neurodevelopmental disabilities like cerebral palsy (see Chapter 7) and attention-deficit/hyperactivity disorder (ADHD).

Development of an ICF Core Set for ASD was initiated in 2014, and the first version, published in 2019, was created through a rigorous multistep research and consensus-building process.[51] The initial version consists of a comprehensive ICF Core Set for individuals with ASD (111 categories), a brief ICF Core Set for preschool-aged children (73 categories), a brief ICF Core Set for school-aged children and adolescents (81 categories), and a brief ICF Core Set for older adolescents

Pediatric Developmental Screening Flowchart

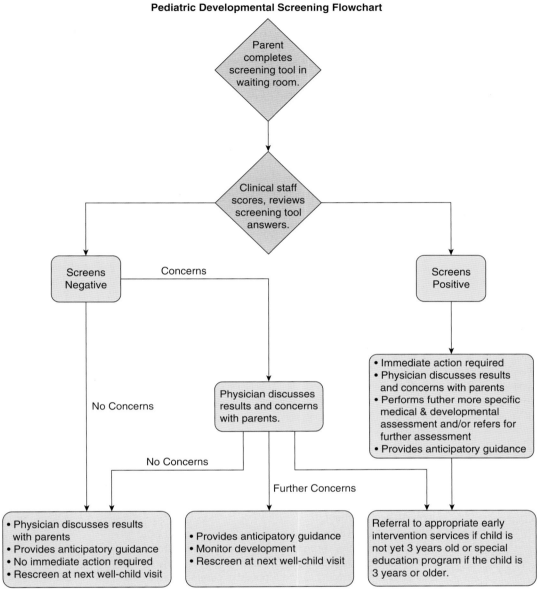

FIGURE 11-5 **Pediatric Developmental Screening Flowchart.** (Centers for Disease Control and Prevention (CDC). Screening and Diagnosis of Autism Spectrum Disorder for Healthcare Providers. https://www.cdc.gov/ncbddd/autism/hcp.html. Published 2022. Updated April 07, 2022. Accessed August 04, 2022.)

and adults (79 categories). A more focused condition-specific set of categories helps highlight the functional abilities of individuals with ASD and other neurodevelopmental conditions, complement diagnostic information with functional data, promote individualized service plans, and ensure appropriate environmental modifications (**Figure 11-6**).[52] For more information on ICF Core Sets, refer to Chapter 3.

EXAMINATION

History

As with all patient populations, a thorough history is an important component of the evaluation. Medical and other pertinent information should be gathered from medical records and referral documentation, as well as from individuals who are involved in the child's day-to-day care (eg, family members,

caregivers, and educators) using intake forms, questionnaires, or interviews. These individuals can provide valuable insight into personal factors (eg, personal interests, motivators, priorities, and goals) and environmental factors (eg, support system, behavioral issues in context, social and adaptive functioning, family roles, home and school environments, and resources). Refer to **Figure 11-7** for examples of information that should be gathered from various resources.[2,53-56]

Systems Review and Impact on ASD

ASD impacts the individual across several systems, resulting in many impairments, activity limitations, and participation restrictions (**Table 11-7**). While some of the impairments and activity limitations listed are not typically and/or specifically addressed through PT intervention (behavioral, educational, communication, and sensory perceptual), they may

TABLE 11-6 • Selected Examples of Diagnostic Tools[50]

Autism Diagnosis Interview–Revised (ADI-R) Source: https://www.wpspublish.com/adi-r-autism-diagnostic-interviewrevised.html	Description: A clinical autism spectrum disorder (ASD) diagnostic instrument Age: Children/adults with mental age >18 months Time: 90-150 minutes Focus areas: Reciprocal social interaction; communication and language; restricted/repetitive behaviors and interests	Administration requirements: A master's degree (MA, MS, MSW, CAGS) in psychology, school counseling, occupational therapy, speech-language pathology, social work, education, special education, or related field; *or* a bachelor's degree (BA, BS) in fields listed above *and* license or certification from an agency/organization that requires training and experience in assessment
Autism Diagnostic Observation Schedule–Second Edition (ADOS-2) Source: https://www.wpspublish.com/store/p/2648/ados-2-autism-diagnostic-observation-schedule-second-edition	Description: Semi-structured, direct assessment designed to elicit the symptoms of autism Age: 12 months to adulthood Time: 45 minutes-1 hour Focus areas: Social reciprocity; nonverbal and verbal communication; stereotypical behaviors and interests Special notes: Considered the "gold standard"; requires initial training and regular reliability checks; provides prognostic information on severity level	Administration requirements: A master's degree (MA, MS, MSW, CAGS) in psychology, school counseling, occupational therapy, speech-language pathology, social work, education, special education, or related field; *or* a bachelor's degree (BA, BS) in fields listed above *and* license or certification from an agency/organization that requires training and experience in assessment
Childhood Autism Rating Scale–Second Edition (CARS-2) Source: https://www.wpspublish.com/store/p/2696/cars-2-childhood-autism-rating-scale-second-edition	Description: Brief 15-item behavioral rating scale developed to compare a child's behavior to same-aged peers without autism; utilizes information from various sources (eg, parent/teacher reports, school/clinic observations) Age: 2 years and up Time: 5-10 minutes Special notes: 2 versions of the scale come with the new edition; the standard version (CARS2-ST) is for young children or children with communication or intellectual impairments; the high-functioning version (CARS2-HF) is for verbally fluent children older than 5 years and/or children without intellectual impairment Focus areas (based on test version): Relating to people; body/object use; emotional response/regulation; adaptation to change/restricted interests; sensory stimulation response and use; nervousness/anxiety; verbal/nonverbal communication; activity level; cognition/intellectual response	Administration requirements: A master's degree (MA, MS, MSW, CAGS) in psychology, school counseling, occupational therapy, speech-language pathology, social work, education, special education, or related field; or a bachelor's degree (BA, BS) in fields listed above *and* license or certification from an agency/organization that requires training and experience in assessment
Gilliam Autism Rating Scale–Third Edition (GARS-3) Source: https://www.pearsonassessments.com/store/usassessments/en/Store/Professional-Assessments/Behavior/Gilliam-Autism-Rating-Scale-%7C-Third-Edition/p/100000802.html?tab=product-details	Description: Designed for use by teachers, parents, and clinicians to help diagnose autism and estimate its severity Age: 3-22 years Time: 5-10 minutes Focus areas: Restrictive and repetitive behaviors, social interaction, social communication, emotional responses, cognitive style, maladaptive speech	Administration requirements: A master's degree (MA, MS, MSW, CAGS) in psychology, school counseling, occupational therapy, speech-language pathology, social work, education, special education, or related field; *or* a bachelor's degree (BA, BS) in fields listed above *and* license or certification from an agency/organization that requires training and experience in assessment

pose significant challenges to successful implementation of PT interventions, goal attainment, and participation across the life span. This section will highlight impairments in cognition and behavior, motor, sensory perceptual, and social communication systems that are relevant to PT evaluation and intervention. Comorbidities will also be presented.

Motor Impairments

Children with ASD often present with motor impairments in balance, gait, and coordination. Delayed motor performance is characteristic in this population at an early age,[57] and weak motor skills have been shown to predict deficits in adaptive behavior skills.[58] Furthermore, early motor delays in children with ASD

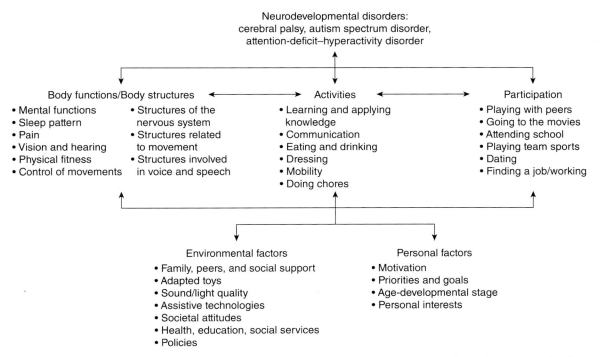

FIGURE 11-6 International Classification of Functioning, Disability, and Health (ICF) Bio-Psychosocial Model applied to neurodevelopmental disorders. (Reproduced with permission from Schiariti V, Mahdi S, Bölte S. International Classification of Functioning, Disability and Health Core Sets for cerebral palsy, autism spectrum disorder, and attention-deficit-hyperactivity disorder. *Dev Med Child Neurol.* 2018;60[9]:933-941.)

under 2 years of age contribute to social impairments,[59] and motor delays in children age 2 to 6 years is associated with problematic behaviors and reduced quality of life.[60] Recent research comparing children with ASD and typically developing peers revealed various motor performance and motor planning deficits across the spectrum of ASD, regardless of severity and IQ.[61] These findings underscore the importance of comprehensive motor evaluation and early intervention to address motor delays.

Medical Records and Reports	Family/Caregiver	Educator

• Diagnosis
• Reason for referral to PT
• Current health status
• Services currently receiving in school and/or through community-based providers (eg, PT, OT, SLP, behavior management, counseling, social skills training)
• Prior PT evaluation or intervention
• Significant medical history
  • Comorbidities (eg, seizure disorder, anxiety disorder, ADHD)
  • GI dysfunction
    • Special diet (food allergies)
  • Prior hospitalizations; surgeries
• Immunizations
• Medications
• Complimentary or alternative medicine/therapy (dietary supplements, herbal remedies, music therapy, Auditory Integration Training, chelation, hyperbaric oxygen therapy)
	• Reason for referral
	• Household members; family roles
	• Primary language spoken in the home
	• Social history
	• Support system
	• Cultural preferences
	• Child's strengths, interests
	• Developmental history
	  • Including perinatal history
	  • Motor milestones
	  • Communication
	  • Social-emotional
	  • Timing and severity of signs and symptoms
	• Sleep disturbances
	• Family history of ASD or related disorders
	• Behavioral issues/concerns
	  • Any current behavioral strategies
	• Other interventions (present or past)
	  • Outcomes
		• Curriculum and school environment (ie, requirements and expectations for functional mobility, motor skills, and play or work skills)
		• Classroom schedule
		• Teacher's concerns (eg, issues during specific activities)
		• The child's educational goals (including social and behavioral)
		• Child's strengths (motivating factors, functional abilities, academic abilities)
		• Ability to follow school routines and rules (eg, follow in line, observe and imitate movements, behavior management)
		• Gross motor skills (eg, type and amount of support needed to perform movements)
		• Senory seeking or avoidance behaviors
		• Safety concerns (for child or others)
		• Willingness and ability to participate in classroom motor activities
		• Attention to task (eg, length of time, postural control, adaptations)

FIGURE 11-7 History components and sources.[2,53-56] ADHD, attention-deficit/hyperactivity disorder; ASD, autism spectrum disorder; GI, gastrointestinal; OT, occupational therapist; PT, physical therapist; SLP, speech-language pathologist.

TABLE 11-7 • Children with ASD Present with a Wide Range of Impairments and Activity Limitations. While not all are Directly Addressed in PT, They can Significantly Impact PT Interventions, Goal Attainment, and Participation Across the Life Span.[52,56,101,210]

Involved Body Functions/Structures	Impairments	Activity Limitations	Participation Restrictions

• Brain structure
• Mental function
• Structures of the nervous system
• Sensory-perceptual function
• Musculoskeletal system function
• Structures of the cardiovascular system
• Structures involved in voice and speech
• Structures involved in vision and hearing
• Structures of the movement system
	Cognitive impairments
	• Executive function impairment
	• Restricted interests
	• Attention
	  ◦ Shifting
	  ◦ Non-social preferences
	• Lack of empathy and insight
	• Delayed/limited intellectual function
	• Impaired working memory
	• Limited/restricted imaginative play
	• Diminished energy, drive, and motivation
	Social communication impairments
	• Delayed/limited speech and language skills
	• Delayed/limited communication
	  ◦ Verbal
	  ◦ Non-verbal
	• Poor integration of eye gaze and language
	Sensory processing impairments
	• Atypical/enhanced auditory and visual perception
	• Impaired proprioception
	• Sensory modulation difficulties (hyper- or hypo- responsiveness to auditory, visual, olfactory, tactile, and vestibular stimuli)
	• Atypical pain responses
	• Impaired sleep function
	Motor impairments
	• Uncoordinated gait
	• Atypical weight bearing during toe-walking
	• Impaired balance
	• Decreased strength
	• Atypical muscle tone
	• Decreased endurance
	• Apraxia/dyspraxia
	• Difficulty completing complex movement sequences
	  ◦ during imitation
	  ◦ on verbal command
	  ◦ during everyday tool use
		• Poor academic achievement
		• Impaired problem-solving ability
		• Impaired adaptive function
		• Limited social reciprocity during social interactions
		• Poor communication of needs, feelings, and interest
		• Poor communication of pain, discomfort, illness, change in health status
		• Sensory seeking or avoidance behaviors
		• Sensorimotor stereotypies
		• Unexplained loss in abilities
		• Fine and gross motor delays
		• Motor incoordination
		• Poor motor imitation
		• Difficulty performing
		• functional/ADL tasks
		• Decreased physical activity levels
			• Participation in educational programming
			• Participation in paid employment
			• Societal integration
			• Peer relationships
			• Participation in extracurricular interests, particularly in group or social contexts
			• Participation in self-care in home and community settings
			• Carry out daily routines independently
			• Maintaining health and wellness

Gait deviations that are characteristic of children with ASD include reduced stride length, increased step width, increased stance time, decreased ankle and knee range of motion during gait, and increased hip flexion, as well as a reduction in ground reaction forces at toe-off.[62]

There is an increased prevalence of toe walking in children with ASD; however, the etiology is unclear. Toe walking has been attributed to sensory processing impairments and persistent tonic labyrinthine reflex.[63]

Sensory Processing Impairments

Sensory processing, also called sensory integration, is the ability of the central nervous system (CNS) to correctly interpret information received through various senses, integrate it with information stored from previous experiences, and make a meaningful, context-appropriate motor or behavioral response (**Figure 11-8**). More simply, the CNS organizes incoming sensory and motor information for immediate or future use or action.[64]

Many, if not most, individuals with ASD show symptoms of impaired sensory processing, causing many of the stereotypic "autistic" behaviors.[65,66] Sensory impairments and related behaviors are distinguishing symptoms of ASD[39,67] and are included in the DSM-5 diagnostic criteria.[39] Since publication of the DSM-5 in 2013, there has been a steady increase in the number of studies related to sensory processing symptoms, assessment, and intervention in individuals with ASD.[66,68-70]

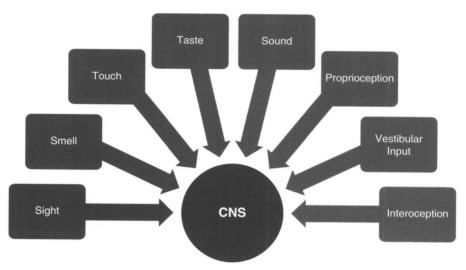

FIGURE 11-8 The central nervous system (CNS) processes and integrates sensory information received through various senses.

Sensory impairments impact individuals with ASD in numerous ways and manifest in a wide range of symptoms, severity, and functional deficits. For some, symptoms are mild and do not interfere with function and participation, while others are severely limited. Young children with ASD have greater sensitivities to tactile, taste, olfactory, and auditory input than young children with other developmental disabilities.[67] Moreover, recent research indicates that individuals with ASD demonstrate atypical interoception, the subjective experience of internal sensation processing,[71] which can have ramifications for pain perception and pain management.[72]

Sensory processing impairments can lead to a variety of sensory modulation difficulties, as well as atypical activity levels, behavioral and emotional problems, and developmental delays. Sensory processing is complex, and it can be difficult for clinicians to determine a child's specific sensory processing impairments, as no 2 children present exactly the same. Moreover, there may be variability in a child's sensory processing and related behaviors from one day to the next and even within a therapy session. Miller et al[73] proposed a diagnostic taxonomy to account for the wide range of clinical presentations in individuals with sensory processing disorder (SPD), consisting of 3 main patterns of impairment. These patterns include sensory modulation disorder, sensory discrimination disorder, and sensory-based motor disorder (**Figure 11-9**). The clinician can use sensory symptoms and behaviors to determine the pattern or patterns of sensory processing impairments and for treatment planning purposes. The patterns and symptoms are presented in **Table 11-8**.

Some literature suggests that SPD and ASD are distinct disorders and that SPD is a comorbidity seen in the majority of children with ASD.[73] Children with ASD often present with modulation disorders in the underresponsive or overresponsive subtypes,[74] with greater tendencies toward sensory overresponsiveness.[69] Although sensory impairments typically peak in childhood,[69,75] they can persist into adulthood. Findings from a recent study that examined the presence of SPD symptoms and autistic traits in adults with and without ASD indicate that symptoms of overresponsivity are experienced by adults with ASD to a high degree and are positively

correlated with autistic traits,[76] whereas there is some evidence that the severity of sensory symptoms is inversely related to the severity of ASD.[77,78] In other words, adults who demonstrate higher functional and cognitive levels (eg, Asperger syndrome) present with less severe sensory processing impairments, symptoms, and behaviors. Given this evidence, PT evaluation should include sensory processing assessment in individuals with ASD across the life course. Moreover, because physical therapists are often among the first health professionals to evaluate children at risk for developmental delay and disorders, they can play a role in enhancing early identification of ASD by recognizing symptoms of SPD.[79]

SPD may impact function and participation in many daily and social activities including typical development and play, self-care, independent living, social engagement, community

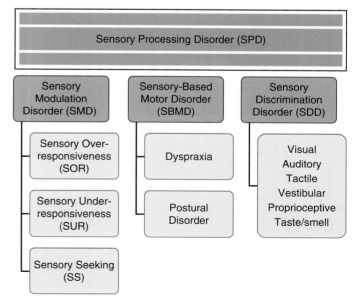

FIGURE 11-9 **Taxonomy of sensory processing disorder.** (Adapted, with permission, from Miller LJ, Anzalone ME, Lane SJ, Cermak SA, Osten ET. Concept evolution in sensory integration: a proposed nosology for diagnosis. *Am J Occup Ther.* 2007;61[2]:135-140.)

TABLE 11-8 • Sensory Processing Patterns and Symptoms[73]

Main Pattern	Description	Subtypes	Signs and Symptoms
Sensory modulation disorder (SMD)	Difficulty responding to sensory input with behavior (emotional and attentional) that is appropriate for the demands of the situation	Sensory overresponsiveness (SOR)	Response to stimuli is faster, more intense, and longer than typical Can involve one system (tactile defensiveness) or multiple systems (sensory defensiveness) Difficulties in new situations or transitions; individual is rigid and controlling Exaggerated fight, flight, fright response Emotional responsiveness: irritability, moodiness, inconsolability
		Sensory underresponsiveness (SUR)	Disregard or do not respond to sensory stimuli Fail to respond to pain Clumsy Poor body scheme Withdrawn, difficult to engage, inattentive, self-absorbed, lethargic
		Sensory seeking (SS)	Crave unusual amount or type of sensory input Engage in actions to add intensity Social inappropriateness (eg, touching others) Unsafe behaviors; constant moving; impulsiveness Can be explosive/aggressive if can't satisfy need SS often interferes with function Often occurs with attention-decicific/hyperactivity disorder
Sensory discrimination disorder (SDD)	Difficulty interpreting qualities of sensory input or discriminating between stimuli Can involve one or more systems (eg, auditory only or combination)	Not applicable	Slow performance Learning or language disability Low self-confidence Frequently occurs with SUR or SOR
Sensory-based motor disorder (SBMD)	Poor postural and volitional movement as a result of sensory problems	Postural disorder	Difficulty stabilizing body during movement or at rest Inappropriate muscle tone (hyper, hypo, poor control) Poor stability, poor righting and equilibrium reactions Poor ocular motor control Avoids movement because of instability and fear (not overreactivity) Can be active but with poor control, unsafe
		Dyspraxia	Poor coordination Poor motor planning Awkward movement Delays Usually in presence of SOR, SUR, and SDD

mobility and access, safety, family/patient/teacher understanding and support, and use of resources. Impact and severity can vary over time, with changes in environment or demands placed on the individual, during times of transition (eg, high school to adulthood, school to employment), and maturation and development of coping strategies. Given the variability of symptoms and severity of SPD, evaluation should consist of a combination of interviews (ie, parent, caregiver, teacher, child/individual), standardized assessment tools, and observation (**Figures 11-10 to 11-11**).[80-89] Additionally, age specific symptoms checklists are available online (e.g., Star Institute: https://sensoryhealth.org/basic/symptoms-checklist).[85] While not diagnostic, checklists can identify the need for additional testing when a parent, caregiver, or teen/adult indicates the presence of more than a few atypical sensory related behaviors.

Social Communication Abilities
As noted previously in this chapter, difficulty with social communication is a hallmark sign of ASD. The level at which a child with ASD can communicate in a social context greatly

Interview	Observation	Questionaires	Evidence-Based Outcome Measures
• Parent/Caregiver • Teacher • Child	• Clinic • Home • Community • School	• Sensory Profile • SPD Checklist (STAR Institute) • Sensory Experience Questionnaire • Sensory Perception Quotient	• Sensory Integration and Praxis Tests (SIPT) • Sensory Performance Analysis (SPA) • Sensory Processing Assessment (SPA) • Sensory Processing Scale Inventory • Sensory Processing Scale Assessment • The Miller Assessment for Preschoolers (MAP)

FIGURE 11-10 Components and tools for sensory processing evaluation.[81,83-89]

impacts their functional ability and participation across domains. For example, some children have difficulty developing language skills (receptive and/or expressive) and/or the ability to communicate with others nonverbally through eye contact, facial expressions, and gestures. They may have difficulty adjusting volume, tone, and rhythm of their speech, or they may misinterpret vocal tones or situational meanings words may carry. Some children with ASD are not able to communicate at all, whereas others have rich vocabularies and are able to participate in conversations. The level of communication ability impacts a child's ability to function in social contexts such as school, community, family gatherings, and as they get older, work settings.

Recently, Di Rezze et al[90] developed a classification system of social communication functioning for children and youth diagnosed with ASD. Development of the system was based on a research study that included perspectives from a variety of stakeholders via focus groups and surveys.[90] The findings contributed to development and validation of the Autism Classification System of Functioning: Social Communication (ACSF:SC).[91-93] Similar to the Gross Motor Function Classification System,[94] the ACSF:SC facilitates assessment of a child's social communication abilities (ie, what they can do) across 5 levels of functioning, in which level V is the most severe. The tool and user guide are freely available on the CanChild website (https://www.canchild.ca/en/resources/254-autism-classification-system-of-functioning-social-communication-acsf-sc).

Pharmacologic Management of Symptoms and Comorbidities

Children with ASD often present with various comorbidities and emotional and behavioral disorders (eg, seizure disorder, anxiety disorder, ADHD, obsessive-compulsive disorder) that can amplify symptoms and functional impairments or threaten the safety of the child and those around the child. Management of these often includes prescription medications that have side effects that may impact other systems. For example, mood stabilizers such as risperidone or gabapentin can cause dystonia, fatigue, and ataxia, ultimately affecting balance, movement, and gait. It is essential to obtain information regarding current medications, monitor the presence and potential impact of such side effects, educate caregivers, and communicate changes to the health care team. Refer to **Table 11-9** for a list of commonly prescribed medications and side effects.

Tests and Measures

A variety of tests and measures are reliable and valid for use with individuals with ASD throughout the life course. Tests and

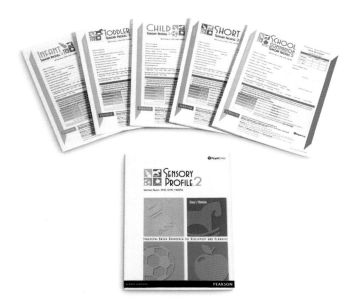

FIGURE 11-11 Sensory Profile-2 consists of a range of products for purchase including test booklets (eg, self-report and observer questionnaires) and supporting materials (eg, manuals and complete) kits for infant, toddler, child, school companion, and adolescent/adult assessment. https://www.pearsonassessments.com/store/usassessments/en/Store/Professional-Assessments/Motor-Sensory/Sensory-Profile-2/p/100000822.html?tab=product-details

TABLE 11-9 • Common Medications to Treat Target Behaviors and Symptoms of ASD and Their Side Effects[56]

Category	Purpose	Medication	Possible Side Effects*
Antipsychotics and mood stabilizers	Aggressive, self-injurious, and manic behaviors	• Risperdal (risperidone) • Zyprexa (olanzapine) • Geodon (ziprasidone) • Abilify (aripiprazole) • Seroquel (quetiapine)	Dystonia, tardive dyskinesia, other movement side effects (muscle spasms or cramping, pacing, restlessness, inability to sit still, weight gain, sedation
		• Neurontin (gabapentin)	Sedation, fatigue, dizziness, ataxia
Stimulants and alpha agonists	hyperactivity, impulsivity, short attention span	• Ritalin, Concerta, Daytrana, Metadate, Methylin (methylphenidate) • Adderall (mixed amphetamine salts) • Dexedrine (dextroamphetamine) • Vyvance (lisdexamfetamine) • Focalin (dexmethylphenidate)	Anxiety, depression, tics, irritability, repeated thoughts, increased blood pressure, changes in heart rate and rhythm, difficulty falling asleep, decreased appetite, growth inhibition,
		• Strattera Atomoxetine	Sleepiness gastrointestinal problems, thoughts of harming self or suicide
		• Tenex, Intuniv (guanfacine)	Dizziness, low blood pressure, sleeplessness, sedation
		• Catapres, Kapvay (clonidine)	Sedation
Selective serotonin reuptake inhibitors (SSRIs)	depression, anxiety, and obsessive-compulsive thoughts and behaviors	• Anafranil (clomipramine hydrochloride) • Prozac (fluoxetine) • Paxil (paroxetine) • Lexapro (escitalopram) • Effexor (venlafaxine) • Cymbalta (duloxetine) • Wellbutrin (bupropion) • Luvox (fluvoxamine) • Zoloft (sertraline) • Celexa (citalopram)	Gastrointestinal problems, sedation, agitation, difficulty falling asleep, weight gain, hyperactivity, changes in heart rhythm, thoughts of harming self or suicide, serotonin syndrome
Melatonin, alpha agonists, or antihistamines	sleep disturbances	• Melatonin	Sedation
		• Elavil (amitriptyline)	Sedation
		• Desyrel (trazodone)	Headache, gastrointestinal problems, allergic skin reactions
		• Zanaflex (tizanidine)	Seizures, orthostasis, arrhythmias
		• Catapres (clonidine)	Orthostasis, sedation, dizziness, dry mouth, weakness, gastrointestinal problems
Anti-seizure medications and steroids	Seizures, aggression, self-injury	• Depakene, Depakote (valproic acid) • Tegretol, Carbatrol (carbamazepine) • Lamictal (lamotrigine) • Trileptal (oxcarbazepine) • Topamax (topiramate)	Rash, sedation, gastrointestinal problems, weight gain or loss, temporary hair loss, bone marrow suppression, hepatitis
		• Keppra (levetiracetam)	Sedation, dizziness, confusion, headache, generalized weakness

Source: Autism and Medication: Safe and Careful Use—An Autism Speaks ATN/AIR-P Tool Kit. Accessed online at https://www.autismspeaks.org/tool-kit/atnair-p-autism-and-medication-safe-and-careful-use) *For more details on side effects, visit Medline Plus. Drugs, Herbs, and Supplements. https://medlineplus.gov/druginformation.html.

measures provide objective and subjective information that can be categorized within the components of the ICF and will inform further testing, treatment planning, and intervention. They can also be used to track progress, determine the need for additional services, and identify resources based on individual and family needs and goals. Outcome measures in pediatrics are addressed in Chapter 3. A number of evidence-based tests and measures are especially useful in obtaining baseline measures, tracking progress, and documenting outcomes in children with ASD. Physical therapists should select the most appropriate tests and measures based on the clinical presentation and other information gathered in the examination and based on

TABLE 11-10 • Select Tests and Measures for Children With Autism Spectrum Disorder

- Motor assessment
  ○ Developmental screening, under 3 years
    • Ages and Stages Questionnaire (ASQ)
    • Modified Checklist of Autism in Children (MCHAT)
  ○ Developmental assessments
    • Bayley Scales of Infant Development–Fourth Edition (Bayley-4)
    • Batelle Developmental Inventory–Second Edition (BDI-2)
    • Vineland Adaptive Behavior Scales–Second edition (VABS-2)
  ○ Hand strength
    • Hand grip dynamometer
  ○ Overall motor performance measures
    • Peabody Developmental Motor Scales-Third Edition (PDMS-3)
    • Bruininks-Oseretsky Test of Motor Proficiency–Second Edition (BOTMP-2)
  ○ Praxis and imitation
    • Modified Florida Apraxia Battery (FAB)
    • Sensory Integration and Praxis Tests (SIPT)
    • The Miller Assessment for Preschoolers (MAP)
  ○ Motor coordination
    • Movement Assessment Battery for Children–Second Edition (MABC-2)
- Functional performance and participation measures
  ○ Pediatric Evaluations of Disability Inventory (PEDI)
  ○ School Functional Assessment (SFA)
  ○ Miller Function and Participation Scales (M-FUN)
- Participation in recreation and leisure activities outside of school
  ○ Children's Assessment of Participation and Enjoyment (CAPE)
  ○ Preferences for Activities of Children (PAC)
- Physical fitness/physical activity
  ○ Body mass index
  ○ Pedometers and accelerometers
  ○ 6-Minute Walk Test[95]
- Quality of life
  • Pediatric Quality of Life Inventory (PedsQL)[96]
  • World Health Organization Quality of Life–Brief (WHOQoL-BREF)[97]
  • Ankylosing Spondylitis Quality of Life Questionnaire (ASQoL)[97]
- Other
  ○ Goal Attainment Scaling[98,99]

each child's unique clinical and functional profile. Diagnostic test results and ICF Core Sets for ASD should inform decision-making. For a list of tests and measures particularly useful in children and adults with ASD to address impairments, activity limitations, and participation restrictions typically seen in this population, see **Table 11-10**.

■ INTERVENTION

Children with ASD present with impairments across multiple systems and functional domains that contribute to activity limitations and participation restrictions at varying levels of severity.[51,52,100,101] There is adequate evidence to support the effectiveness of a broad range of PT interventions for movement-related impairments

and activity restrictions commonly seen in children with ASD and other childhood disorders. Many of these interventions are covered elsewhere in this textbook. Impairments across multiple systems (eg, sensory, motor, metabolic, gastrointestinal) and developmental domains (eg, social-emotional, communication/language, cognitive, behavioral, self-care/adaptive, physical) seen in many children with ASD, however, make administering PT interventions challenging. The remainder of this chapter will focus on impairments and other issues more unique to ASD and present a variety of interventions, support strategies, and resources for physical therapists to consider when working with this population.

IMPAIRED SENSORY PROCESSING

As stated earlier in this chapter, sensory impairment is included in the current diagnostic criteria for ASD. There is mounting evidence to support the presence and impact of sensory processing impairment on daily activities and participation across functional domains. Impaired sensory processing affects sleep,[102] eating,[103-105] attention,[66] language,[106] adaptive behavior, and social participation.[66,106-111] Sensory impairment, particularly overresponsivity, is associated with the presence of anxiety[112] and restrictive and repetitive behaviors in individuals with ASD.[113] Moreover, symptoms and behaviors related to impaired sensory processing contribute to caregiver and family stress,[114,115] which may impact services and supports, as well as opportunities for growth, development, participation, and community engagement.

With physical therapists' focus on participation, it is important to understand the impact of sensory processing on participation across domains (eg, social, self-care, activities of daily living, occupation). Furthermore, there is evidence that sensory overresponsivity interferes with activity participation outside the home, more than inside the home, which is theorized to be caused by (1) sensory symptoms (seeking and avoiding) and behaviors that stem from anxiety surrounding unexpected sensory input,[116] and (2) caregiver stress of participation (eg, peer bullying, tantrum or other problematic behaviors, safety concerns) that outweighs the benefits of the activity (**Figure 11-12A**).[114,115] The potential for children with ASD to have diminished levels of participation outside the home due to sensory issues raises concerns about long-term participation goals and outcomes. Children who have opportunities to engage in community and social activities can use these experiences to build skills for successful participation (**Figure 11-12B**).[116] Participation barriers related to sensory processing and/or caregiver stress should be addressed within the intervention plan. Interventions such as caregiver education and training (eg, support strategies, access to programs, community resources) for supporting participation during childhood may have a significant impact on participation levels into adulthood.[117]

Given the impact of sensory processing on most individuals with ASD, treatment planning should address sensory processing based on individualized assessment, patient and caregiver needs and goals, and evidence for best practice. Interventions

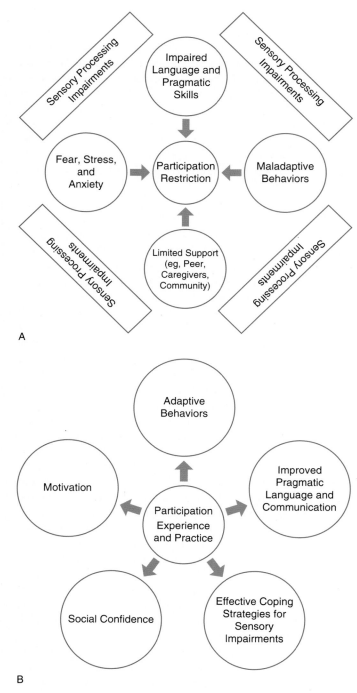

A

B

FIGURE 11-12 A. Impairments caused by sensory processing disorder can restrict participation. B. Opportunities to practice social engagement build skills for successful participation.

for impaired sensory processing are used by therapy professionals, educators, and parents in an effort to manage the behaviors, activity limitations, and participation restrictions that stem from sensory issues. High-level research treatment effectiveness in this area, however, has been slow to emerge due to a variety of limitations in design, method, and sample size. Over the past several years, a number of randomized controlled studies have emerged.[118,119]

Interventions for sensory processing impairments may be incorporated in the PT treatment to support and facilitate attention and focus, modulation and regulation in order to work on motor development, skill acquisition, function, and participation. There are 2 main frameworks for sensory processing intervention: *sensory integration therapy* (SIT) and *sensory-based intervention* (SBI).

SIT, developed by Jean Ayres, is a clinic-based intervention that uses play activities and sensory-enhanced interactions to elicit the child's adaptive responses. The therapy consists of individualized sensorimotor activities based on the unique sensory needs of the child identified during assessment and aimed to facilitate participation. It is traditionally provided in a clinic with specially designed equipment (eg, swings, therapy balls, inner tubes, trampolines, and climbing walls) that can provide vestibular and proprioceptive challenges embedded in playful, goal-directed activities. The goal of SIT is to increase the child's ability to integrate sensory information, thereby demonstrating more organized and adaptive behaviors, including increased joint attention, social skills, motor planning, and perceptual skills.

SBI consists of structured, adult-directed sensory strategies that are integrated into the child's daily routine to improve behavioral regulation. SBIs are often single-sensory strategies or a combination of sensory strategies briefly applied to the child, most often in the school environment. Examples include weighted products (eg, weighted vest, weighted blanket, weighted lap/shoulder pad), pressure products (eg, squeeze machine, pressure body garments), Body Sox, sensory brushes, and vibration products. Often, these strategies are implemented throughout the day to promote sensory modulation in the form of an individualized home and school program, referred to as a *sensory diet*.

Over the past decade, there has been an increasing number of studies looking at the effectiveness of either SBI or SIT for improving a range of behaviors and functions impacted by impaired sensory processing, such as reduction in sensory symptoms, reduction in problematic behaviors, improved language and social engagement, better sleep, and increased joint attention. A systematic review of sensory interventions compared existing research on the effectiveness of SIT and SBI.[120] The findings provide evidence that SIT for children with ASD and sensory processing problems has positive effects on the child's individualized goals. This systematic review did not generate support for effectiveness of SBI, however, because the studies included lacked rigor and consisted of protocols that varied widely. Nevertheless, there is some evidence of effectiveness of SBI in some contexts and with some individuals that should be considered by therapists, and the program should be selected based on patient and caregiver goals, patient response, and therapeutic goals to facilitate skill acquisition and ultimately participation. For example, there is evidence that weighted apparel is not effective for reducing problematic behaviors[121-123] or improving engagement,[124] but parents perceive calmer behavior with its use and that SIT strategies are important for their child.[125] Some study findings also support deep pressure modalities (eg, squeeze machine and deep pressure brushing protocol) for improving mood and reducing sensory-related symptoms.[126] Music-based therapy (eg, playing music, singing, or movement to music) has been shown to reduce sensory and ASD symptom severity, reduce challenging behaviors, and improve social engagement and motor performance.[70]

There is mounting evidence to support the effectiveness of SIT,[119] including studies that implement rigorous randomized controlled trial designs.[118] Physical therapists should continually assess and reassess a child's response to SIT and SBI to support implementation on a case-by-case basis. It is important to note that SIT and SBI may be challenging for some families and caregivers to implement due to time and financial constraints.[117] Furthermore, some interventions that are not sensory based are proven more effective to achieving specific goals. Indeed, better outcomes may be achieved through strategies that focus on optimizing participation by building coping strategies and self-regulation skills.[117] Behavioral intervention, for example, is more effective than SIT for treatment of challenging behaviors (eg, self-injurious).[121] Therefore, it is essential for the physical therapist to consider all options and weigh evidence for best practice, family resources and needs, and patient response when selecting interventions.

Sensory processing assessment and clinical decision-making can be complex and challenging. It may be helpful to use a worksheet or guide to categorize assessment findings according to symptoms and/or systems involved and identify impact on function and participation. An example of a decision guide for therapists working with children who have sensory processing impairments is provided in **Figure 11-13**.[127]

A collaborative, team-based approach is important for successful outcomes of sensory and other intervention for ASD. Pediatric physical therapists should seek parent, caregiver, and teacher input when determining the need for sensory support, feasibility and resources, and the effectiveness of sensory interventions on improving function, participation, and family quality of life. There is often variation in treatment results and also in preferences by the child or individual for sensory intervention.[126] Parents and caregivers can share their experiences living with and managing the sensory symptoms of ASD and are a valuable source of information.[128] Likewise, it is critical to provide education and training for parents, caregivers, siblings, teachers, peers, and others who interact with the child. Providing awareness and information about the child's sensitivities and unique sensory needs can foster improved understanding and tolerance.[65] When appropriate, the child

autism spectrum AUSTRALIA — Name: ________ Date: / / Who is in the team? ________ — aspect practice (autism practice that works)

VISION	SOUND	TOUCH	ORAL SENSORY	SMELL/TASTE	MOVEMENT (VESTIBULAR)	BODY (PROPRIOCEPTION)

Problems with Participation

Are you sure it's sensory? YES/NO — If YES, approach with a sensory lens. If NO, alternative assessment or intervention

Bystander	Seeker	Avoider	Sensor

Is good autism practice in place? (structure, routine, predictability, visual supports etc.)

Proactive Strategies:	Teaching Coping Strategies:	Logistics:
Environmental changes Sensory activities		Where, when, how?? Plan Review Date:

FIGURE 11-13 A Sensory Form to guide treatment. (Reproduced, with permission, from Mills CJ, Michail E, Bye RA. A survey of occupational therapists on a new tool for sensory processing. *Occup Ther Int*. 2020;28:2020:5909347.)

should be included in education and training for building awareness and capacity for coping with sensory impairment in age-appropriate and culturally acceptable ways, and this becomes especially important as the child grows older and during life transitions. There is evidence that many adults with ASD have developed their own strategies to cope with and manage their sensory processing, including both positive and maladaptive strategies.[117]

BEHAVIORAL INTERVENTIONS

A number of behaviors are associated with ASD, including tantrums, self-aggression, aggression toward others, restrictive and repetitive behavior, and elopement. These behaviors vary in type and severity and may be dictated by the level of severity of ASD,[129] as well as a variety of factors such as underlying sensory impairments (eg, sensory over- or underresponsive), language or communication impairments, feelings of anxiety and frustration, and psychiatric disorders (eg, obsessive-compulsive disorder, mood disorder).[113,130] Some behaviors (eg, aggression, elopement, impulsivity) may threaten the safety of the child and/or those around them. Regardless, any behavior can be disruptive and interfere with function and participation in the community, school, home, and during therapy sessions. Although direct behavioral intervention is not the priority for physical therapists, strategies to manage behaviors are essential for success and positive patient outcomes. Examples of evidence-based strategies that may be implemented by a physical therapist include positive reinforcement, augmentative and alternative communication, visual aids, social stories, and applied behavior analysis (ABA). Some strategies require some level of training (eg, ABA), but with consultation and collaboration with other professionals (eg, behavior analysis, psychologist, special education teacher, speech-language pathologist), these strategies can be applied during PT to facilitate a positive therapist-child relationship and a more productive session. Additionally, therapists who work with a child who is exhibiting behaviors that are difficult to manage should consult other members of the team. It is important to identify the strategies that work for a child and apply them consistently across disciplines for maximum effectiveness.

Positive Reinforcement

A positive reward or reinforcement is an action or object that follows a desired behavior (eg, social participation, attention to a therapeutic task, following instructions, task completion). Used correctly, rewards or reinforcements can increase the likelihood of that behavior occurring again and can motivate the child to improve behavior and participation. Conversely, negative reinforcement occurs when an object is removed or there is a consequence following an unwanted behavior, with the goal of minimizing unwanted behaviors and facilitating desired behaviors. While negative reinforcers are sometimes successful, evidence suggests the use of positive reinforcement. There are different types of reinforcers, such as tangible, social, and activity based (**Table 11-11**).

Initially, the reinforcement should be provided immediately and consistently after the target (eg, desired) behavior

TABLE 11-11 • Examples of Types of Positive Reinforcements

Tangible	Social	Activity Based

• Food or drink
  ○ Pretzels
  ○ Candies
  ○ Popcorn
  ○ Juice
• Toys
• Money
• Stickers
• Hand stamp
• Bubbles
• Treasure box
	• Verbal praise
	• Hugs
	• High fives
	• Thumbs up
	• Tickle time
	• Special job
	  ○ Line leader
	  ○ Teacher's helper
		• Play with preferred toys, child's choice activity or game, screen time
		  ○ Can include preferred sensory-based activities (water play, swing, ball pit, vibrating toy, sensory room)
		  ○ May be increments of time (time to engage in the task) or an earned finite activity (read a book, trip to the zoo, movie, sports event)

is exhibited. Some children may require verbal prompts to remind them of the target behavior and reward using a *first-then* strategy (eg, "*First* bicycle, *then* coloring"). As the child is able to manage their behavior, reinforcements can be weaned to intermittent or delayed. It is also important to accompany the reinforcement with specific and positive feedback, rather than nonspecific feedback or feedback focused on the unwanted behavior (**Figure 11-14**). Consistency is critical to using reinforcements successfully, and it is therefore important that family, caregivers, and other professionals on the team use the same approach to managing behaviors. If the behavior continues or is severe or injurious to the child or others, it is important to consult a behavior specialist for guidance.

Augmentative and Alternative Communication

According to the American Speech-Language-Hearing Association, augmentative and alternative communication (AAC) simply refers to ways to communicate without talking.[131] There are 2 main types of AAC, aided and unaided, and an individual may use a combination of AAC to communicate effectively. Unaided AAC includes gestures, body language, facial expressions, and sign language. Aided AAC includes the use of a tool or device and can be basic or high-tech. An example of a basic aided AAC system is pointing to letters, words, or pictures on a board, whereas touching letters or pictures on a computer screen that speaks for you is an example of a high-tech aided system.[131]

Previous research findings indicate that over 25% of children with ASD are minimally verbal,[132] and the potential benefits of AAC to improve and facilitate functional communication for children and adults with ASD are well-documented.[70,133] Of the various types of AAC, evidence indicates that both low-tech and high-tech aided AAC systems, such as picture exchange–based AAC and speech-generating devices, are the most effective for individuals with ASD.[134] Moreover, the use of AAC may reduce unwanted behaviors by providing a means of communication.[70,134] The physical therapist should determine if the child is using AAC at home, in school, or with another service provider and if the AAC is effective

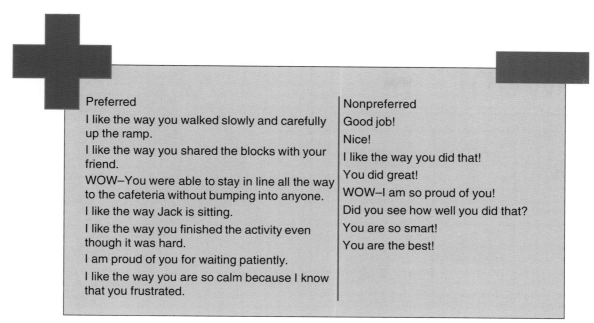

Preferred	Nonpreferred
I like the way you walked slowly and carefully up the ramp.	Good job!
I like the way you shared the blocks with your friend.	Nice!
WOW–You were able to stay in line all the way to the cafeteria without bumping into anyone.	I like the way you did that!
I like the way Jack is sitting.	You did great!
I like the way you finished the activity even though it was hard.	WOW–I am so proud of you!
I am proud of you for waiting patiently.	Did you see how well you did that?
I like the way you are so calm because I know that you frustrated.	You are so smart!
	You are the best!

FIGURE 11-14 Examples of preferred and nonpreferred feedback.

for improving communication and managing behavior. If so, AAC systems can be easily integrated into the PT sessions. One example commonly used with very young children with ASD is the Picture Exchange Communication System (PECS) (**Figure 11-15**). PECS can be effectively used during a session to manage behavior and facilitate engagement and performance. PECS can be displayed and effectively used in various ways depending on resources and context, such as magnetic boards, Velcro strips, tablet applications, and card rings.[135] Nevertheless, the therapist must participate in some level of training to use PECS to the full potential (ie, for more than object requesting). Additional and more detailed information about AAC is presented in Chapter 20.

Visual Aids

Some behaviors, such as tantrum behaviors, may be caused by intolerance of uncertainty and anxiety.[136] Children with ASD commonly desire rigid or predictable schedules and respond well to external structure. Providing a detailed visual schedule (consisting of words, pictures, or both) or checklist of activities at the start of each session can help alleviate anxiety by letting the child know what is next and providing a sense of accomplishment when tasks are completed. Visual schedules can be used to improve cooperation and motivation and can also be used outside of therapy to facilitate self-management in older children, adolescents, and adults (**Figure 11-16**).[137]

Social Stories

Social stories, as a form of social narrative intervention, were first developed in 1991 by Carol Gray, former teacher for students with ASD, as a "social learning tool that supports the safe and meaningful exchange of information between parents, professionals, and people with autism of all ages."[138] The aim of a Social Story is to explain confusing or difficult social concepts, interactions, or situations in a meaningful way for the individual, and it can be used for children through adults. Each story is individualized and uniquely based on the needs of the person who will use it. Stories are brief and written collaboratively by the therapist, individual, and caregiver, but from the perspective of the individual who will use it. See **Table 11-12** for the basic format and structure of Social Stories according to Gray's Social Stories 10.4 Criteria. Social stories have been used predominately with children who have ASD and can have a positive impact not only on social interaction but also on managing behaviors in specific situations or social conexts.[139] There are several books and resources to assist parents and professionals in creating individualized and effective social stories. Refer to supplemental material for a video example of a social story to ease the transition from classroom to PT.

Although additional research on the effectiveness of social stories is needed, there is evidence to suggest that social stories can be an effective tool to improve attention, social engagement, communication, and adaptive skills, as well as facilitate self-regulation behaviors and increase independence in children with ASD.[70,140]

Applied Behavior Analysis

ABA is a form of therapy based on the science of learning and behavior and has been used with children with ASD for more than 5 decades.[141] The aim of ABA is to increase desired behaviors to facilitate learning and reduce behaviors that negatively impact learning. ABA programs can increase language, communication, attention, focus, memory, academics, and social skills, and decrease problem behaviors in children with ASD.[142] ABA is flexible and adapted to meet the needs of the child, in any context, to improve skills in the areas mentioned above, as well as self-care, play skills, and motor skills. ABA applies strategies of positive reinforcement in a framework

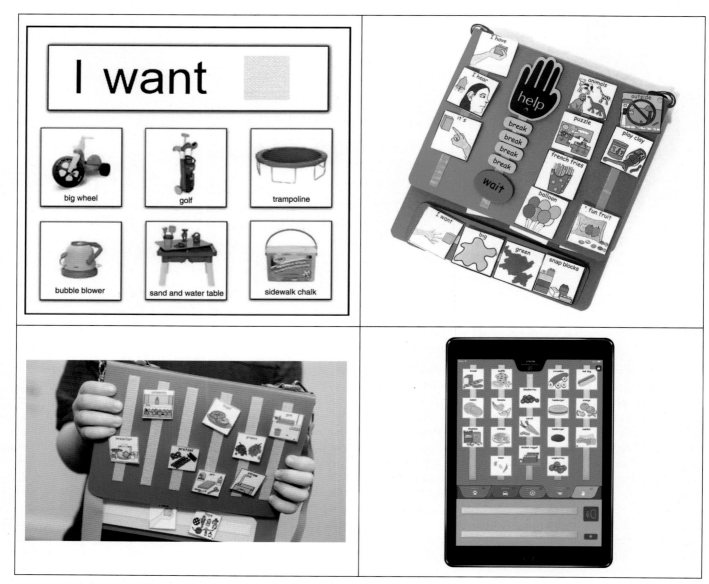

FIGURE 11-15 **Examples of ways to use the Picture Exchange Communication System (PEC).**

of antecedent-behavior-consequence to impact behavior and learning. During ABA sessions, target skills are broken down into smaller steps, progressing from simple to more complex. ABA programs should be developed and led by a board-certified behavior analyst (BCBA), who will supervise behavior therapists or technicians who implement the program. The ABA team works with parents, caregivers, and other members of the team (eg, physical therapist, occupational therapist, teacher) to achieve individualized goals. Data are collected during each ABA therapy session and used to determine progress toward goals and to modify or develop new goals.

ABA is evidence-based and proven to be effective when performed correctly and supervised by a trained BCBA. These services may or may not be covered by insurance,[142] and the intensity of the programs for effectiveness (20-40 hours per week)[141] makes it cost prohibitive for some families. ABA strategies can prove beneficial during PT sessions, particularly when

the child is receiving ABA services. The physical therapist should consult with the BCBA to determine effective learning strategies for the child and to reinforce ABA goals within the PT session. Autism Speaks provides an ABA family toolkit for free at their website (https://www.autismspeaks.org/sites/default/files/2018-08/Applied%20Behavior%20Analysis%20Guide.pdf).

Complementary and Alternative Medicine

Several complementary and alternative medicine (CAM) treatments are commonly explored by families and used in the treatment of autism, and previous studies indicate that up to 74% of families with a child who has ASD has used some type of CAM.[55] A detailed exploration of the various treatments is beyond the scope of this chapter; however, it is important for physical therapists to have a basic knowledge of the various treatments in order to effectively provide

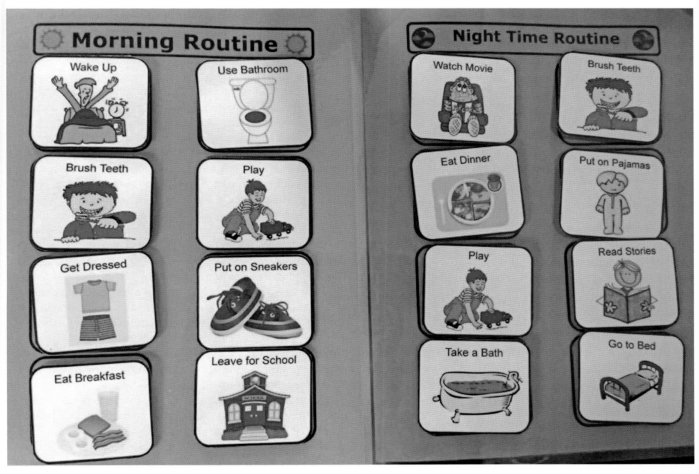

FIGURE 11-16 Examples of visual schedules.

information and guidance to families. Some treatments may be administered by physical therapists (eg, SIT, SBI, hippotherapy, aquatherapy, yoga), while some are administered by other medical and health professionals (eg, special diets, acupuncture, chelation). These treatments have differing levels of supporting evidence, associated costs, provider credentials, and safety considerations. Families are often eager and sometimes desperate to explore potential treatments for their child with ASD. Physical therapists should provide factual, unbiased information and provide credible resources and referrals for families to make informed decisions. Refer to **Table 11-13** for a list of commonly used CAM treatments for children with ASD.

TABLE 11-12 • Basic Structure and Format of Social Stories	
One Title	Meaningfully represents the topic
Two Sentence Types	*Descriptive:* accurately describes relevant aspects of context, including external and internal factors
	Coaching: gently guide with descriptions of effective responses of team players (e.g., parent, teacher, professional) and child, adolescent or adult audience
Three Parts	*Introduction:* describes topic
	Body: provides detail
	Conclusion: reinforces and summarizes information

Adapted from Gray C, Faherty C, Timmins S, Lanou A. 2023. Social Stories 10.4 Criteria.

■ TRANSITION TO ADULTHOOD

DIMINISHED ACCESS TO HEALTH AND HUMAN SERVICES

Each year, approximately 70,700 to 111,000 youth with ASD turn 18 each year.[144] Between 18 and 22 years of age, individuals enrolled in public education will age out of school-based autism services and resources.[145,146] These emerging adults face many challenges that threaten their present and future quality of life. This transition is at time fraught with anxiety and fear due to limited educational or employment opportunities,[147,148] diminished access to health and human services, an increased risk for obesity and related health conditions, and a switch to the adult health service model in which professionals may not have the knowledge and skills to serve their unique needs. The paucity of services available to these individuals limits their participation

TABLE 11-13 • Examples of Complementary and Alternative Medicine Treatments Used by Families for Children With Autism Spectrum Disorder[55,128]

Hippotherapy; equine-assisted therapy

Dolphin-assisted therapy

Aquatherapy

Sensory integration therapy (SIT)

Sensory-based intervention (SBI)

Dietary intervention
• Dietary supplements (omega-3, probiotics)
• Gluten- and casein-free diet
• Feingold diet

Chelation

Hyperbaric oxygen therapy

Acupuncture

Auditory integration therapy

Music therapy

Yoga[143]

Traditional Chinese medicine

and potential contributions to society. As a result, an increasing number of children with ASD will become adults and "age out" of childhood services. This has led to a growing concern nationwide for successful transition to adulthood, improved quality of life, and cost containment. Research on the economic impact of ASD reveals a lifetime cost of up to $3.6 million per individual, with the greatest costs incurred in adulthood related to residential care, supported living, productivity loss, and medical expenses.[4,149-153] These young adults are transitioning from a pediatric family-centered model of health care to an underfunded and fragmented system of adult health care. As they age out of school-based services, they face a paucity of services and affordable programming. This is an adjustment not only for the patients and families but also for health professions who may not have the knowledge or skills to communicate with and support these patients' unique needs. Additionally, these young adults lack the skill sets to navigate the complex health care environment and communicate effectively with their medical providers. Research demonstrates high levels of service disengagement, social isolation, and poor outcomes across multiple domains among adults with ASD.[154,155] Inadequate community-based interventions and scarce interprofessional supports further restrict community participation.[155,156]

OBESITY, HEALTH, AND WELLNESS CONCERNS

Along with inadequate services and supports, there are growing concerns over the declining health status of adults with ASD. Health disparities for this population include diminished access to services; greater risk for obesity, heart disease, early parkinsonism, chronic gastrointestinal problems, mental disorders, seizures, and persistent sleep disturbances; and shorter life expectancy (up to 36 years shorter) than cohorts without ASD.[145,157,158] Health disparities are greater for individuals who are disadvantaged related to their race, ethnicity, culture, socioeconomic status, environment, geography, sex, or gender.[159,160]

While poor health status is a contributing factor to increasing costs in adulthood, it also impacts the quality of life for the individuals and their family members.

As already discussed, children and adults with ASD often struggle with SPD, dyspraxia, overweight and obesity, social communication impairments, anxiety, and impaired cognition and executive functioning. The complex nature of the disorder and the challenge of impairments across multiple systems often result in difficulty participating in recreational physical activity alone or with peers.[161-163] Moreover, obesity has a higher prevalence within the ASD population, particularly teens and young adults, for whom opportunities for physical activity engagement are greatly diminished. The risk for obesity is compounded by sedentary behaviors, dietary restrictions, medications that cause weight gain, metabolic abnormalities, and lack of knowledge or awareness.[95,145,161,164,165] There is also indication that the risk of overweight and obesity trends upward with increased ASD severity level among adolescents.[166] Increased risk for obesity can have significant ramifications as children with ASD transition into adulthood, such as the development of diabetes or other obesity-related health issues.

The importance of physical activity to overall wellness for individuals with ASD is well-documented to improve motor function, exercise capacity, social and communication skills, attention, motivation, self-esteem, and desire to participate in community peer activities.[70,95,161,167] Barriers to participation in community-based physical activity programs include behavior, impaired executive functioning, safety concerns, financial limitations, time, fear of bullying, lack of staff training and support, and lack of information.[164,168] Diminished funding, lack of programming, and barriers to participation further increase stress and anxiety, ultimately impacting overall health, well-being, and quality of life. Moreover, the social communication challenges that adults with autism experience frequently lead to loneliness, anxiety, depression, and unemployment or underemployment. High rates (up to 70%) of depression and anxiety have been documented in young adults with autism.[169,170] As such, there is a need for community-based wellness and prevention programs and initiatives that specifically address and support the unique needs of this growing population.

COMMUNITY ENGAGEMENT: CHALLENGES AND OPPORTUNITIES

As youth with ASD age out of school and mature into adulthood, communities face the increasingly urgent challenge of integrating them into programs and services designed to support health and wellness.[171] While young adults with autism have difficulty accessing and being successful in community programs, they also have higher rates of comorbidities that make accessing community programs even more important than it is for the general population.[130,170,172,173] Overall quality of life appears to be reduced in this population.[174,175] It is not surprising, then, that young adults with autism have high rates of social isolation. Research indicates that up to 47% do not connect with friends and 48% are not invited to participate in social activities and that approximately 33% do not participate in community activities, classes, or lessons.[148,176] Physical therapists can assist in identifying and creating opportunities for community engagement by identifying community partners, consulting with businesses and staff, and building capacity through staff education and training. There is recent evidence that peer-guided PT activity programs have positive physical and social outcomes.[177,178] Moreover, not only is remote delivery of physical activity intervention feasible and acceptable among young adults with ASD, but some prefer this mode of delivery to in-person programming.[179] Other studies support a variety of program strategies and considerations that facilitate physical activity and social participation in this population, such as activity trackers and wearable technologies, SMART (specific, measurable, achievable, realistic, and timely) goal setting, gamification, social media, personalization, and more.[180-187]

INTERPROFESSIONAL TRAINING AND COLLABORATION FOR TRANSITION PLANNING

Health care professionals, such as physical and occupational therapists, speech-language pathologists, athletic trainers, and physicians, can play a significant role in reducing costs and improving potential for independent living, paid employment, quality of life, and community participation. Moreover, evidence highlights the importance of interprofessional collaboration and early transition planning.[188,189] With improved outcomes, young adults with ASD have a variety of transition options, including college, vocational school, degree program for independent living, directly entering the workforce, or supported employment.[190]

Physical therapists can support many aspects of transition for individuals with ASD and their families through individual and family education, training, identification of resources, and advocacy. Additionally, physical therapists may be instrumental in developing much-needed community-based physical activity programs, vocational training, and consultation/training for staff development at community centers, postsecondary institutions, and the workplace. There is evidence to suggest that adults with ASD need more supportive social contexts to improve their quality of life, and it is important to consider social, psychological, and sensory processing needs when designing programs for adults with ASD.[175] The role of PT in transitions of adults with developmental disabilities, including ASD, is discussed in greater detail in Chapter 22.

■ FAMILY AND CAREGIVER CHALLENGES

Family members and caregivers experience high levels of stress and significant challenges on a daily basis.[191] There are many aspects of caring for a child, adolescent, or adult with ASD that are emotionally challenging, physically demanding, time consuming, and financially draining. Previous research identifies stigma and financial burden as significant challenges experienced by parents.[192] In addition, parents have reported that their child's behaviors disrupt daily routine and social order and that they observe negative public perception of the disorder.[193]

One of the biggest challenges reported by families is the financial burden associated with caring for a child with ASD. There are 6 types of ASD costs described in the literature: medical and health care services, therapy services, special education, loss of income for adults with ASD, loss of income for family or caregivers, and the costs associated with respite care and out-of-pocket expenses.[150] Out-of-pocket health care costs are significantly higher for children with ASD than those without ASD.[194] Families are often financially responsible for high deductibles, high copays, capitated services, or noncovered medication (eg, psychotropic drugs, stimulants), psychiatric treatment, and therapy services (eg, PT, occupational therapy, speech therapy, behavior therapy/ABA). According to a recent report by Autism Speaks, autism costs an estimated $60,000 a year through childhood, most of which is attributed to the cost of special services and lost wages associated with the burden of care on one or both parents.[145,191] This cost is greater in the presence of intellectual disability. Although there has been some recent legislation and some programs that can alleviate the financial and caregiver burden (eg, Achieving a Better Life Experience Act, insurance legislation to cover ASD-related treatment and therapy, and Medicaid Waiver, Supplemental Security Income, and Work Incentives Planning and Assistance program), not all families or caregivers are aware of the existence of the programs or that their child may be eligible.

In addition to time and financial burden, raising a child with ASD can be an overwhelming experience. Parents experience a shift to a child-centered life, with very little personal time.[195] Family members feel isolated[164,196] or withdraw socially due to sensory behaviors.[197] This is not without impact on the health of the family. There is evidence of increased rate of separation and divorce among parents with children diagnosed with ASD compared to parents of typically developing children.[198,199] This increased rate persists from childhood through adulthood because, unlike some childhood disorders, the burden of care often continues through the life span.

Evidence is building that having a child with ASD significantly impacts the quality of life for parents and family members. In fact, parents of children with ASD experience increased levels of stress and are at greater risk for developing anxiety and depression than parents of children without ASD, including children with other disabilities.[200-202] Parental stress is greater when the child exhibits higher levels of social disability and lower levels of adaptive functioning.[203,204]

Physical therapists, in collaboration with other members of the health care team, can assist caregivers in effectively managing stress and challenges by providing training and education guidance, support, and resources to the caregivers, as well as training and consultation to other support personal and community program staff (eg, teachers, coaches, in-home support staff, respite workers, supervisors, and employers).[196] Parent/caregiver coaching and training can reduce stress and anxiety.[205] Support should be focused not only on the child (eg, behavioral management training) but on also reducing parental stress. Respite care and social support can reduce psychological stress and depression.[206] Many communities have local centers for autism and related disabilities that provide free resources, programs, and referral services for individuals with autism and their families. (https://www.centerforautism.com/locations/; http://florida-card.org/). In the absence of a local center, families and professionals can contact their local or state chapter of the Autism Society. Support groups for caregivers, parents, and siblings provide opportunities for emotional support, as well as information and resource sharing.[196] Many family members report limited knowledge and access to social programs, and preparing and orienting them to local resources could facilitate more satisfying social participation.[207] Refer to Appendix 11-1 for a list of resources.

■ CONCLUSION

ASD is a complex developmental disorder with a broad spectrum of clinical presentations. It is typically diagnosed in childhood and persists through adulthood. Severity of the disorder varies greatly, and no 2 children with ASD present exactly the same. The disorder affects several systems, impacting function and participation across various domains, and can greatly impact an individual's capacity for independent living and quality of life. Sensorimotor impairments are common and affect physical function as well as social engagement.

The rapid growth in the number of children diagnosed with ASD presents numerous opportunities for physical therapists to play a vital role in research, education, clinical practice, and advocacy for ASD.[208] There is a mounting body of evidence for best practice regarding evaluation, treatment, and support strategies to improve PT outcomes for this population.[70,209] The physical therapist works collaboratively with the family, caregivers, and other members of the team to address and support the unique needs of these children and to attain their greatest potential for independence, health, and wellness.

Case 1

Connor

Background Information and Past Medical History

Connor is a 5-year-old boy diagnosed with autism spectrum disorder (ASD). His parents report an uncomplicated birth but describe sensitivity to auditory stimulus, lack of eye contact, and delays in motor milestone achievement noted as early as 6 months old. Other than a metatarsal fracture as a result of a fall from an elevated surface on a playground, Connor has no other significant medical history. He currently takes no prescribed medications and has no dietary restrictions or allergies, although a gluten-free diet was trialed around the age of 3 years old. Connor was able to sit independently at 10 months, stand and cruise along furniture at 14 months, and began ambulating independently at 18 months. He has frequent episodes of balance impairments and falls when traversing change of surfaces and crowded areas. Connor is nonverbal currently but does vocalize noises when excited and when attempting to express wants and needs. The speech therapist has recently introduced him to a Picture Exchange Communication System (PECS). He attends a local, public prekindergarten program that adheres to an Individualized Education Plan (IEP) to improve his learning and development, independent functioning, and social skills. He receives accommodations such as a compression vest for sensory regulation, cube chair for seated activities, and modified utensils for feeding. His parents are concerned about his transition to kindergarten next year due to the larger environment and higher ratio of teacher and aides to students in the classroom.

Observation and Systems Review

Connor has a body mass index of 32.2 and also appears to be taller than most of his peers. Connor requires multimodal cueing for task initiation and maintenance of attention. He generally plays away from peers and will not engage in age-appropriate play. Review of systems does not reveal any other observable concerns or impairments.

Sensory Processing and Behavior Management

Connor's parents have expressed difficulty with managing his behaviors and understanding ways to fulfill his sensory needs and self-regulation. Some of his behaviors include elopement, mouthing inedibles, and dropping to the ground during transitions or nonpreferred tasks. Rarely do his behaviors escalate to tantrums and "breakdowns"; however, his parents recall 3 episodes in the past 6 months where he needed more than 30 minutes in public settings to cease crying and screaming after being presented with an unfavored choice. He enjoys listening to sing-a-long tasks, the iPad, and playing in sand.

Neuromuscular and Gross Motor Assessment

Upon assessment, the following impairments are present:
- Tone
  - Widespread hypotonia in all 4 extremities and trunk
- Range of motion
  - Grossly normal range of motion except for hyperextension in bilateral knees and elbows
- Strength
  - Functional testing shows muscular weakness most notably in proximal groups of upper and lower extremities, as well as core and trunk.
  - Connor has difficulty carrying a 3-pound object across the room.
- Posture
  - Connor demonstrates rounded shoulders and protruding abdomen.
  - He stands in a wide base of support and sits with flexed trunk and posterior pelvic tilt in all types of chairs.
- Sensation
  - No sensation deficits are noted to light or sharp touch.
  - Proprioception and kinesthetic awareness are impaired during static and dynamic tasks.
- Balance
  - Connor demonstrates excessive postural sway and compensatory recovery strategies. He demonstrates delayed righting reactions in response to perturbations or dynamic surface activities.
  - He has difficulty completing tandem or single leg stance activities, including the balance beam or stepping over objects.
  - Multiple episodes of loss of base of support and/or balance are noted during sitting and standing activities of durations greater than 2 minutes.
- Gait and endurance
  - Connor is able to ambulate community distances independently; however, he demonstrates intermittent poor foot clearance during swing phase with episodes of loss of

balance. He relies on adult hand-held assist for safety and negotiation of crowded spaces and obstacles.

- He requires minimal assistance for safe ascent and descent of stairs, demonstrating fair eccentric control with a step-to pattern and cueing necessary to safely use handrail for support.
- Connor's endurance is fair due to body habitus. He requires rest periods in community or active settings after 6 minutes of exertion.

Questions for Case 1

1. One of Connor's parents is most concerned about his over-weight appearance. Given his difficulty attending to tasks and activities for long periods of time, what are 2 examples of exercises that can be used to induce cardiovascular changes?
   a. Can you think of one exercise that his parents can per-form at home that would help achieve their goal of weight management?
   b. What are some dietary factors that could be contributing to his increased weight?
2. Connor has difficulty transitioning to nonpreferred tasks. He will attempt to elope during physical therapy sessions. His prekindergarten teacher has considered requesting a func-tional behavioral assessment (FBA) but wonders if you have any ideas.
   a. What is one tool you could use during therapy sessions that may reduce his behaviors during task transition?
   b. Do you think this would be effective at home and in the classroom as well? If not, what is a different tool that you could suggest his parents and teacher use?
3. Ascending and descending stairs is a challenge for Con-nor for many reasons. Can you conceptualize an exer-cise or activity for each of the body systems that needs improvement?
   a. Lower body strength
   b. Single leg balance
   c. Motor planning and synchronized movements

Case 2

Brandon

Background Information and Past Medical History

Brandon is a 9-year-old boy diagnosed with autism spec-trum disorder (ASD). Parents report typical motor milestones through the age of 2 but a delay in language development, aversion to many food items, and stereotypic movements for the majority of the day. He has been attending outpatient phys-ical, occupational, and speech therapy services consistently for 6 years. His verbal communication has improved significantly so that he can convey his wants and needs; however, he fre-quently scripts and speaks out of context. He is integrated into a general education classroom for specials, math, and science but remains in an exceptional student education classroom for language arts and composition. Brandon's parents report that although he is very active and plays well with peers, they notice him toe walking 75% of the time. They would like for him to participate in a community-based sports league, but

they are concerned his toe walking will get worse and that the coach may not know how to instruct him properly. He also has a younger sister at home.

Observation and Systems Review

Brandon appears to be of age-appropriate weight and height. He demonstrates fidgeting, rapid hand movements, and tap-ping during 35% of observation. Review of systems does not reveal any other observable concerns or impairments.

Sensory Processing and Behavior Management

Brandon is a pleasant and inquisitive child. He requires inter-mittent verbal or gestural cueing to maintain attention to long-duration tasks, but overall, he does very well with follow-ing commands. His parents report that he has been prescribed risperidone since he was 5 years old. There is concern for his development of age-appropriate vocational skills and execu-tive function, as well as social communication in appropriate settings with peers and adults. Although he does not elope, he does lack situational and environmental awareness, especially in parking lots. Brandon responds well to being presented with choices and rewards in a "first-and-then" method.

Neuromuscular and Gross Motor Assessment

Upon assessment, the following impairments are present:

- Tone
  - Hypertonic palpation noted in gastrocnemius and soleus complex and hamstrings group of bilateral lower extremities
- Range of motion
  - Range of motion is normal in all major joints except for bilateral ankles as measured:
    - Right ankle dorsiflexion: 5 degrees
    - Left ankle dorsiflexion: 8 degrees
  - Straight leg raise is measured in supine with contralateral leg flexed and relaxed:
    - Right straight leg raise: 65 degrees
    - Left straight leg raise: 70 degrees
- Strength
  - Functional testing and movement analysis shows no obvi-ous impairments to strength
- Posture
  - Brandon demonstrates loss of normal lumbar lordosis alignment in standing.
  - He maintains a normal base of support and will keep flat foot contact when stationary.
- Sensation
  - Brandon demonstrates sensitivity to change in surface and flooring.
  - Proprioception and kinesthetic awareness are impaired during dynamic movements and activities.
- Balance
  - Brandon can maintain single leg stance for approximately 10 seconds on each foot before postural sway initiates.
  - He can only maintain tandem stance for approximately 6 seconds before loss of balance.
  - He demonstrates delayed righting reactions at ankle, knee, and hip and compensates with upper extremity movement and postural sway.

- Gait and endurance
  - Brandon is able to ambulate community distances independently but demonstrates impaired quality of gait. He engages in excessive arm swing and decreased heel strike in stance phase for the vast majority of the time.
  - He ascends and descends stairs with step-over pattern and no handrail necessary. Heel strike is decreased during both sequences, and there is occasional circumduction to clear the step.
  - Brandon demonstrates good cardiovascular endurance and enjoys sport-related activities.

Questions for Case 2

1. Brandon's parents are most concerned with his toe walking and expect growth spurts to become more problematic as he ages. Other parents have talked to them about ankle-foot orthotics (AFO), but they are unsure what is the best option for him.
   a. What are 2 components of a home exercise program (HEP) that you can educate his parents on?
   b. What are 2 examples of sensory integration activities that you can use as intervention to reduce toe walking during your sessions?
2. After a couple of sessions, you notice that Brandon has some weakness in his proximal stabilizers of the pelvis and hips. You wonder if this is contributing to some of his gait dysfunction and ability to navigate stairs with compensatory motions.
   a. What are 3 interventions you can focus on that will address this new finding?
3. Brandon does a pretty good job of staying on task and following commands. However, his scripting and stereotypical movements are interrupting your sessions at times. His parents report that his teachers have also noted an increase in these movements lately, although his toe walking has begun to improve.
   a. What sensory integration strategy can you recommend to his teacher to help improve his focus during class activities?
   b. Why might a shift in sensory-seeking behaviors be seen if toe walking is improving?

Case 3

Diana

Background Information and Past Medical History

Diana is a 15-year-old girl diagnosed with autism spectrum disorder (ASD). She was diagnosed in prekindergarten after her teacher noticed she lacked awareness to classmates nearby, moved in a clumsy manner on the playground, and transitioned between tasks poorly. Since then, she has received a variety of therapy services in the school and outpatient settings. She is able to verbalize a majority of her wants and needs but struggles with communicating with unfamiliar peers and adults and maintaining appropriate context and volume. Although she has done well with integrating into some school groups, her parents remain vigilant to bullying and other age-appropriate social scenarios. Diana demonstrates dyspraxia with many activities. Her parents are concerned with advancing her skills to best prepare

her for community integration, vocational roles, and early adulthood. Diana enjoys art and creative activities but does not embrace physical exercise as much.

Observation and Systems Review

Diana is overweight, with a body mass index of 28.4. Her parents report that they noticed a 10-pound weight gain in the past 6 months, which they relate to puberty and adjustments to her dosage of olanzapine. Review of systems does not reveal any other observable concerns or impairments.

Sensory Processing and Behavior Management

Diana is attentive and quiet. She makes minimal eye contact and shies away from sustained conversation or human contact. Intermittently she will cover her ears in response to auditory stimulus and sing songs at inappropriate times. Parents report labile emotions, but she typically responds well to a positive reinforcement plan via preferred activities as reinforcers. Tangible reinforcers have been less effective due to her preference for only select food items and textures.

Neuromuscular and Gross Motor Assessment

Upon assessment, the following impairments are present:
- Tone
  - Hypotonic presentation in all extremities and trunk
- Range of motion
  - Range of motion is within normal limits in all major joints.
- Strength
  - Functional testing and movement analysis show weakness in core and proximal groups during squats, sit-ups, step-ups, lifts, and carries of objects greater than 8 pounds.
- Posture
  - Diana presents with a forward head, rolled shoulders, wide base of support, and externally rotated hips in static sitting and standing positions.
  - Mild right convexity is palpable along the lower thoracic spine.
- Sensation
  - Diana demonstrates sensitivity to and withdrawal from textures such as sand and grass.
  - Proprioception and kinesthetic awareness are impaired during all dynamic movements and activities.
- Balance
  - Diana demonstrates fair righting reactions and balance recovery strategies during single leg and tandem stance activities.
  - Postural sway is present upon initiation of any dynamic movement.
- Gait and endurance
  - Diana is able to ambulate in the community without physical assistance. She can become overwhelmed in crowded, loud environments and requires adult supervision to negotiate those areas safely.
  - She has fair cardiovascular endurance and responds with auditory self-stimulation when she begins to sweat.

Questions for Case 3

1. Diana appears to be demonstrating multiple subtypes of sensory processing disorder that are impacting her ability to participate in activities.

a. What are 2 tools of sensory integration therapy (SIT) that would be effective in addition to your plan of care?

b. What is a tool that may negatively affect Diana's adaptive responses?

2. As Diana continues to age, her parents want to focus on maximizing her potential to participate in the community. There are some vocational programs that cater to her specific accommodations, but they worry if she can physically perform the tasks without hurting herself.

a. Much like an adult work hardening program, what are 3 essential body mechanics and safety techniques that Diana and her parents need to be educated on?

3. Improving Diana's cardiovascular endurance is a priority for body systems management and prevention of obesity. However, she reverts to behaviors and auditory stimulation when on a treadmill or bicycle for longer than 4 minutes.

a. How can you use positive reinforcement to achieve longer durations of exercise?

STUDY QUESTIONS

1. Compare and contrast the various diagnostic and screening tools used for children with ASD.

2. Discuss the early signs of ASD, and the recommendations for early identification and intervention. What is the role of the physical therapist?

3. Describe the system-specific impairments commonly seen in children with ASD and their impact on behavior, movement, and participation. Complete the following table as a guide:

System	1.	2.	3.	4.
Commonly seen impairments	a.	a.	a.	a.
	b.	b.	b.	b.
	c.	c.	c.	c.
	d.	d.	d.	d.
	e.	e.	e.	e.
	f.	f.	f.	f.
	g.	g.	g.	g.

4. Using the ICF as a framework, categorize the various tests and measures that can be used for children with ASD. What evidence-based measures can be used to assess body structure and function, activity and activity limitations, participation and participation restrictions, and personal and environmental contextual factors? How can these inform the plan of care and guide treatment?

5. Describe how sensory and behavioral needs may be addressed during PT intervention? Provide specific examples of assessment and treatment strategies and how they may be incorporated to facilitate achievement of PT goals.

References

1. Centers for Disease Control and Prevention (CDC). What is autism spectrum disorder? Autism Spectrum Disorder (ASD) website. Updated March 31, 2022. Accessed August 4, 2022. https://www.cdc.gov/ncbddd/autism/facts.html.

2. Centers for Disease Control and Prevention (CDC). Autism spectrum disorder (ASD). Updated May 2, 2022. Accessed August 5, 2022. https://www.cdc.gov/ncbddd/autism/index.html.

3. Autism Speaks. What is autism? Updated 2022. Accessed August 4, 2022. https://www.autismspeaks.org/what-autism.

4. Buescher A, Cidav Z, Knapp M, Mandell DS. Costs of autism spectrum disorders in the United Kingdom and the United States. *JAMA Pediatr.* 2014;168(8):721-728.

5. Shimabukuro TT, Grosse SD, Rice C. Medical expenditures for children with an autism spectrum disorder in a privately insured population. *J Autism Dev Disord.* 2008;38(3):546-552.

6. Maenner MJ, Warren Z, Williams AR, et al. Prevalence and Characteristics of Autism Spectrum Disorder Among Children Aged 8 Years — Autism and Developmental Disabilities Monitoring Network, 11 Sites, United States, 2020. MMWR Surveill Summ 2023;72(No. SS-2):1-14. http://dx.doi.org/10.15585/mmwr.ss7202a1.

7. Centers for Disease Control and Prevention (CDC). Data & Statistics on Autism Spectrum Disorder. Centers for Disease Control and Prevention. Autism Web site. https://www.cdc.gov/ncbddd/autism/data.html. Updated April 4, 2023. Accessed December 4, 2023.

8. Hertz-Picciotto I, Croen LA, Hansen R, Jones CR, van de Water J, Pessah IN. The CHARGE study: an epidemiologic investigation of genetic and environmental factors contributing to autism. *Environ Health Perspect.* 2006;114(7):1119-1125.

9. ASD Research Project aims to collect 50,000 DNA samples. *ASHA Leader.* 2016;21(7):10.

10. DiGuiseppi C, Levy SE, Sabourin KR, et al. Injuries in children with autism spectrum disorder: Study to Explore Early Development (SEED). *J Autism Dev Disord.* 2018;48(2):461-472.

11. SPARK Foundation. SPARK: Simons Powering Autism Research. Published 2022. Updated 2022. Accessed August 5, 2022. https://sparkforautism.org/portal/page/about-spark/.

12. Gardener H, Spiegelman D, Buka SL. Perinatal and neonatal risk factors for autism: a comprehensive meta-analysis. *Pediatrics.* 2011;128(2):344-355.

13. Hertz-Picciotto I, Schmidt RJ, Walker CK, et al. A prospective study of environmental exposures and early biomarkers in autism spectrum disorder: design, protocols, and preliminary data from the MARBLES study. *Environ Health Perspect.* 2018;126(11):117004-117015.

14. Campbell KA, Hickman R, Fallin MD, Bakulski KM. Prenatal exposure to metals and autism spectrum disorder: current status and future directions. *Curr Opin Toxicol.* 2021;26:39-48.

15. Centers for Disease Control and Prevention (CDC). Research on autism spectrum disorder. Updated April 2, 2022. Accessed August 5, 2022. https://www.cdc.gov/ncbddd/autism/research.html#ref.

16. Frazier T, Thompson L, Youngstrom E, et al. A twin study of heritable and shared environmental contributions to autism. *J Autism Dev Disord.* 2011;41(9):2013-2025.

17. Woodbury-Smith M, Scherer SW. Progress in the genetics of autism spectrum disorder. *Dev Med Child Neurol.* 2018;60(5):445-451.

18. Devlin B, Scherer SW. Genetic architecture in autism spectrum disorder. *Curr Opin Genet Dev.* 2012;22(3):229-237.

19. American Psychiatric Association. *Diagnostic and Statistical Manual of Mental Disorders, Fourth Edition, Text Revision.* American Psychiatric Association; 2000.

20. Dykens EM, Roof E, Hunt-Hawkins H, et al. Diagnoses and characteristics of autism spectrum disorders in children with Prader-Willi syndrome. *J Neurodev Disord*. 2017;9:18.

21. Rosenberg RE, Law JK, Yenokyan G, McGready J, Kaufmann WE, Law PA. Characteristics and concordance of autism spectrum disorders among 277 twin pairs. *Arch Pediatr Adolesc Med*. 2009;163(10):907-914.

22. Sandin S, Lichtenstein P, Kuja-Halkola R, Larsson H, Hultman CM, Reichenberg A. The familial risk of autism. *JAMA*. 2014; 311(17):1770-1777.

23. Hallmayer J, Cleveland S, Torres A, et al. Genetic heritability and shared environmental factors among twin pairs with autism. *Arch Gen Psychiatry*. 2011;68(11):7.

24. Kumar A, Juneja M, Mishra D. Prevalence of autism spectrum disorders in siblings of Indian children with autism spectrum disorders. *J Child Neurol*. 2016;31(7):873-878.

25. Ozonoff S, Young GS, Carter A, et al. Recurrence risk for autism spectrum disorders: a Baby Siblings Research Consortium study. *Pediatrics*. 2011;128(3):8.

26. Ozonoff S, Young GS, Landa RJ, et al. Diagnostic stability in young children at risk for autism spectrum disorder: a baby siblings research consortium study. *J Child Psychol Psychiatry*. 2015;56(9):988-998.

27. Hansen SN, Schendel DE, Francis RW, et al. Recurrence risk of autism in siblings and cousins: a multinational, population-based study. *J Am Acad Child Adolesc Psychiatry*. 2019;58(9): 866-875.

28. Durkin MS, Maenner MJ, Newschaffer CJ, et al. Advanced parental age and the risk of autism spectrum disorder. *Am J Epidemiol*. 2008;168(11):1268-1276.

29. Itzchak EB, Lahat E, Zachor DA. Advanced parental ages and low birth weight in autism spectrum disorders-Rates and effect on functioning. *Res Dev Disabil*. 2011;32(5):1776-1781.

30. Bokobza C, Van Steenwinckel J, Mani S, Mezger V, Fleiss B, Gressens P. Neuroinflammation in preterm babies and autism spectrum disorders. *Pediatr Res*. 2019;85(2):155-165.

31. Joseph RM, Korzeniewski SJ, Allred EN, et al. Extremely low gestational age and very low birthweight for gestational age are risk factors for autism spectrum disorder in a large cohort study of 10-year-old children born at 23-27 weeks' gestation. *Am J Obstet Gynecol*. 2017;216(3):304.e301-304.e316.

32. Limperopoulos C, Bassan H, Sullivan NR, et al. Positive screening for autism in ex-preterm infants: prevalence and risk factors. *Pediatrics*. 2008;121(4):758-765.

33. Schieve LA, Tian LH, Baio J, et al. Population attributable fractions for three perinatal risk factors for autism spectrum disorders, 2002 and 2008 autism and developmental disabilities monitoring network. *Ann Epidemiol*. 2014;24(4):260-266.

34. Lampi KM, Lehtonen L, Tran PL, et al. Risk of autism spectrum disorders in low birth weight and small for gestational age infants. *J Pediatr*. 2012;161(5):830-836.

35. Schieve L, Clayton H, Durkin M, Wingate M, Drews-Botsch C. Comparison of perinatal risk factors associated with autism spectrum disorder (ASD), intellectual disability (ID), and co-occurring ASD and ID. *J Autism Dev Disord*. 2015;45(8): 2361-2372.

36. Cohen D, Pichard N, Tordjman S, et al. Specific genetic disorders and autism: clinical contribution towards their identification. *J Autism Dev Disord*. 2005;35(1):103-116.

37. Christensen J, Grønborg TK, Sørensen MJ, et al. Prenatal valproate exposure and risk of autism spectrum disorders and childhood autism. *JAMA*. 2013;309(16):1696-1703.

38. Rubenstein E, Young JC, Croen LA, et al. Brief report: maternal opioid prescription from preconception through pregnancy and the odds of autism spectrum disorder and autism features in children. *J Autism Dev Disord*. 2019;49(1):376-382.

39. American Psychiatric Association. *Diagnostic and Statistical Manual of Mental Disorders*. 5th ed. American Psychiatric Association; 2013.

40. Wiggins LD, Rice CE, Barger B, et al. DSM-5 criteria for autism spectrum disorder maximizes diagnostic sensitivity and specificity in preschool children. *Soc Psychiatry Psychiatr Epidemiol*. 2019;54(6):693-701.

41. Charan SH. Childhood disintegrative disorder. *J Pediatr Neurosci*. 2012;7(1):55-57.

42. Rosman NP. Childhood disintegrative disorder: part of the autism spectrum? *Dev Med Child Neurol*. 2019;61(5):503-503.

43. Centers for Disease Control and Prevention (CDC). Learn the signs. Act early. Published 2019. Updated February 18, 2021. Accessed August 4, 2022. https://www.cdc.gov/ncbddd/actearly/concerned.html.

44. Baio J, Wiggins L, Christensen D, et al. Prevalence of autism spectrum disorder among children aged 8 years: autism and developmental disabilities monitoring network, 11 sites, United States, 2014. *MMWR Surveill Summ*. 2018;67(6):1-23.

45. Autism Speaks. What are the signs of autism? Published 2019. Accessed August 2019. https://www.autismspeaks.org/learn-signs-autism.

46. American Academy of Pediatrics (AAP). Screening Technical Assistance and Resource Center (STAR). Published 2017. Updated 2017. Accessed September 19, 2019. https://screening-time.org/star-center/#/screening-tools#top.

47. Lord C, Risi S, DiLavore PS, Shulman C, Thurm A, Pickles A. Autism from 2 to 9 years of age. *Arch Gen Psychiatry*. 2006;63(6): 694-701.

48. Kantzer A-K, Fernell E, Westerlund J, Hagberg B, Gillberg C, Miniscalco C. Young children who screen positive for autism: stability, change and "comorbidity" over two years. *Res Dev Disabil*. 2018;72:297-307.

49. Bieleninik Ł, Posserud M-B, Geretsegger M, Thompson G, Elefant C, Gold C. Tracing the temporal stability of autism spectrum diagnosis and severity as measured by the Autism Diagnostic Observation Schedule: a systematic review and meta-analysis. *PLoS One*. 2017;12(9):e0183160-e0183160.

50. Centers for Disease Control and Prevention (CDC). Screening and diagnosis of autism spectrum disorder for healthcare providers. Published 2022. Updated April 7, 2022. Accessed August 4, 2022. https://www.cdc.gov/ncbddd/autism/hcp.html.

51. Bölte S, Mahdi S, de Vries PJ, et al. The Gestalt of functioning in autism spectrum disorder: results of the international conference to develop final consensus International Classification of Functioning, Disability and Health core sets. *Autism* 2019; 23(2):449-467.

52. Schiariti V, Mahdi S, Bölte S. International Classification of Functioning, Disability and Health Core Sets for cerebral palsy, autism spectrum disorder, and attention-deficit-hyperactivity disorder. *Dev Med Child Neurol*. 2018;60(9):933-941.

53. Academy of Pediatric Physical Therapy (APPT). Physical Therapy Evaluation of Children with Autism Spectrum Disorder: Practice Recommendations for the School-Based Physical Therapist. chrome-extension://efaidnbmnnnibpcajpcglclefindmkaj/https://pediatricapta.org/includes/fact-sheets/pdfs/FactSheet_EvaluationofChildrenwithASD-PracticeRecommendationsfor-School-BasedPTs_2014.pdf.

54. Centers for Disease Control and Prevention (CDC). Treatment and intervention services for autism spectrum disorder. Published 2020. Updated March 9, 2022. Accessed August 4, 2022. https://www.cdc.gov/ncbddd/autism/treatment.html.

55. Brondino N, Fusar-Poli L, Rocchetti M, Provenzani U, Barale F, Politi P. Complementary and alternative therapies for autism spectrum disorder. *Evid Based Complement Alternat Med.* 2015; 2015:258589.

56. Bhat A, Bubela D. *Autism Spectrum Disorder in Children: Clinical Summary.* American Physical Therapy Association; 2017.

57. Lane A, Harpster K, Heathcock J. Motor characteristics of young children referred for possible autism spectrum disorder. *Pediatr Phys Ther.* 2012;24(1):21-29.

58. MacDonald M, Lord C, Ulrich D. The relationship of motor skills and adaptive behavior skills in young children with autism spectrum disorders. *Res Autism Spectr Disord.* 2013; 7(11):1383-1390.

59. Bhat AN, Landa RJ, Galloway JC. Current perspectives on motor functioning in infants, children, and adults with autism spectrum disorders. *Phys Ther.* 2011;91(7):1116-1129.

60. Hedgecock JB, Dannemiller LA, Shui AM, Rapport MJ, Katz T. Associations of gross motor delay, behavior, and quality of life in young children with autism spectrum disorder. *Phys Ther.* 2018; 98(4):251-259.

61. Kaur M, Srinivasan S, Bhat A. Comparing motor performance, praxis, coordination, and interpersonal synchrony between children with and without autism spectrum disorder (ASD). *Res Dev Disabil.* 2018;72:79-95.

62. Kindregan D, Gallagher L, Gormley J. Gait deviations in children with autism spectrum disorders: a review. *Autism Res Treat.* 2015;2015:1-8.

63. Accardo PJ, Barrow W. Toe walking in autism: further observations. *J Child Neurol.* 2015;30(5):606-609.

64. STAR Institute. About SPD. Published 2020. Accessed January 11, 2020. https://www.spdstar.org/basic/about-spd.

65. Hazen EP, Stornelli JL, O'Rourke JA, Koesterer K, McDougle CJ. Sensory symptoms in autism spectrum disorders. *Harv Rev Psychiatry.* 2014;22(2):112-124.

66. Dellapiazza F, Vernhet C, Blanc N, Miot S, Schmidt R, Baghdadli A. Links between sensory processing, adaptive behaviours, and attention in children with autism spectrum disorder: a systematic review. *Psychiatry Res.* 2018;270:78-88.

67. Wiggins LD, Robins DL, Bakeman R, Adamson LB. Brief report: sensory abnormalities as distinguishing symptoms of autism spectrum disorders in young children. *J Autism Dev Disord.* 2009;39(7):1087-1091.

68. DuBois D, Lymer E, Gibson BE, Desarkar P, Nalder E. Assessing sensory processing dysfunction in adults and adolescents with autism spectrum disorder: a scoping review. *Brain Sci.* 2017;7(8):108.

69. Ben-Sasson A, Gal E, Fluss R, Katz-Zetler N, Cermak SA. Update of a meta-analysis of sensory symptoms in ASD: a new decade of research. *J Autism Dev Disord.* 2019;49(12):4974-4996.

70. Steinbrenner JR, Hume K, Odom SL, et al. *Evidence-Based Practices for Children, Youth, and Young Adults with Autism.* The University of North Carolina at Chapel Hill, Frank Porter Graham Child Development Institute, National Clearinghouse on Autism Evidence and Practice; 2020.

71. DuBois D, Ameis SH, Lai M-C, Casanova MF, Desarkar P. Interoception in autism spectrum disorder: a review. *Int J Dev Neurosci.* 2016;52:104-111.

72. Mieres AC, Smallwood V, Nicholson SK. Retrospective case report: evaluation of pain in a child with pervasive developmental disorder. *Pediatr Phys Ther.* 2011;23(2):194-200.

73. Miller LJ, Anzalone ME, Lane SJ, Cermak SA, Osten ET. Concept evolution in sensory integration: a proposed nosology for diagnosis. *Am J Occup Ther.* 2007;61(2):135-140.

74. STAR Institute. Co-morbidity: SPD and other disorders. Published 2019. Accessed August 2019. https://www.spdstar.org/basic/co-morbidity#spdandautism.

75. Little LM, Dean E, Tomchek S, Dunn W. Sensory processing patterns in autism, attention deficit hyperactivity disorder, and typical development. *Phys Occup Ther Pediatr.* 2018;38(3): 243-254.

76. Tavassoli TM, Schoen SA, Nielsen DM, Baron-Cohen S. Sensory over-responsivity in adults with autism spectrum conditions *Autism.* 2013;18(4):5.

77. Ben-Sasson A, Hen L, Fluss R, Cermak SA, Engel-Yeger B, Gal E. A meta-analysis of sensory modulation symptoms in individuals with autism spectrum disorders. *J Autism Dev Disord.* 2009;39(1):1-11.

78. Sanz-Cervera P, Pastor-Cerezuela G, Fernández-Andrés M-I, Tárraga-Mínguez R. Sensory processing in children with autism spectrum disorder: relationship with non-verbal IQ, autism severity and attention deficit/hyperactivity disorder symptomatology. *Res Dev Disabil.* 2015;45-46:188-201.

79. Ben-Sasson A, Atun-Einy O, Yahav-Jonas G, Lev-On S, Gev T. Training physical therapists in early ASD screening. *J Autism Dev Disord.* 2018;48(11):3926-3938.

80. Tavassoli T, Brandes-Aitken A, Chu R, et al. Sensory over-responsivity: parent report, direct assessment measures, and neural architecture. *Mol Autism.* 2019;10(1):4.

81. Schoen SA, Miller LJ, Sullivan J. The development and psychometric properties of the Sensory Processing Scale Inventory: a report measure of sensory modulation. *J Intellect Dev Disabil.* 2017;42(1):12-21.

82. Kirby AV, Dickie VA, Baranek GT. Sensory experiences of children with autism spectrum disorder: in their own words. *Autism.* 2015;19(3):316-326.

83. Dunn W. Sensory Profile 2. Pearson. Published 2014. Accessed November 5, 2023. https://www.pearsonclinical.com/therapy/products/100000566/sensory-profile.html.

84. Ayres J. Sensory Integration Praxis Test (SIPT). WPS: Educational and Psychological Assessments. Published 1989. Accessed August 2019. https://www.wpspublish.com/store/p/2971/sipt-sensory-integration-and-praxis-tests.

85. STAR Institute. Symptoms Checklist. Published 2020. Accessed November 5, 2023. https://www.spdstar.org/basic/symptoms-checklist.

86. Baranek GT, David FJ, Poe MD, Stone WL, Watson LR. Sensory Experiences Questionnaire: discriminating sensory features in young children with autism, developmental delays, and typical development. *J Child Psychol Psychiatry.* 2006;47(6): 591-601.

87. Little LM, Freuler AC, Houser MB, et al. Psychometric validation of the Sensory Experiences Questionnaire. *Am J Occup Ther.* 2011;65(2):207-210.

88. Schoen SA, Miller LJ, Sullivan JC. Measurement in sensory modulation: the Sensory Processing Scale Assessment. *Am J Occup Ther.* 2014;68:522-530.

89. Tavassoli T, Hoekstra RA, Baron-Cohen S. The Sensory Perception Quotient (SPQ): development and validation of a new sensory questionnaire for adults with and without autism. *Mol Autism.* 2014;5(1):1-16.

90. Di Rezze B, Rosenbaum P, Zwaigenbaum L, et al. Developing a classification system of social communication functioning of preschool children with autism spectrum disorder. *Dev Med Child Neurol.* 2016;58(9):942-948.

91. Di Rezze B, Rosenbaum P, Zwaigenbaum L, et al. Autism Classification System of Functioning: Social Communication (ACSF:SC). CanChild. Published 2021. Accessed November 5, 2023. https://www.canchild.ca/en/resources/254-autism-classification-system-of-functioning-social-communication-acsf-sc.

92. Di Rezze B, Gentles SJ, Hidecker MJC, et al. Adaptation, content validity and reliability of the Autism Classification System of Functioning for Social Communication: From Toddlerhood to Adolescent-Aged Children with Autism. *J Autism Dev Disord.* 2022;52(12):5150-5161.

93. Tajik-Parvinchi D, Rosenbaum P, Hidecker MJC, et al. Construct validity of the Autism Classification System of Functioning: Social Communication (ACSF:SC) across childhood and adolescence. *J Autism Dev Disord.* 2023;53(8):3246-3256.

94. Palisano R, Rosenbaum P, Bartlett D, Livingston M. Gross Motor Function Classification System–Expanded & Revised. CanChild. Published 1997. Accessed November 5, 2023. https://canchild.ca/en/resources/42-gross-motor-function-classification-system-expanded-revised-gmfcs-e-r.

95. Srinivasan SM, Pescatello LS, Bhat AN. Current perspectives on physical activity and exercise recommendations for children and adolescents with autism spectrum disorders. *Phys Ther.* 2014;94(6):875-889.

96. Ikeda E, Hinckson E, Krägeloh C. Assessment of quality of life in children and youth with autism spectrum disorder: a critical review. *Qual Life Res.* 2014;23:1069-1085.

97. McConachle H, Mason D, Parr J, Garland D, Wilson C, Rodgers J. Enhancing the validity of a quality of life measure for autistic people. *J Autism Dev Disord.* 2017;48:15.

98. McDougall JK, King G. Goal *Attainment Scaling: Description, Utility, and Applications in Pediatric Therapy Services.* 2007. Accessed November 5, 2023. https://mississaugahalton.rehabcareontario.ca/Uploads/ContentDocuments/gasmanual_.pdf.

99. Ruble L, McGrew J, Toland M. Goal Attainment Scaling as an outcome measure in randomized controlled trials of psychosocial interventions in autism. *J Autism Dev Disord.* 2012; 42(9):10.

100. Randolph-Gips M, Srinivasan P. Modeling autism: a systems biology approach. *J Clin Bioinforma.* 2012;2(1):17.

101. de Schipper E, Mahdi S, de Vries P, et al. Functioning and disability in autism spectrum disorder: a worldwide survey of experts. *Autism Res.* 2016;9(9):959-969.

102. Mazurek MO, Dovgan K, Neumeyer AM, Malow BA. Course and predictors of sleep and co-occurring problems in children with autism spectrum disorder. *J Autism Dev Disord.* 2019;49(5): 2101-2115.

103. Cermak SA, Curtin C, Bandini LG. Food selectivity and sensory sensitivity in children with autism spectrum disorders. *J Am Diet Assoc.* 2010;110(2):238-246.

104. Leader G, Tuohy E, Chen JL, Mannion A, Gilroy SP. Feeding problems, gastrointestinal symptoms, challenging behavior and sensory issues in children and adolescents with autism spectrum disorder. *J Autism Dev Disord.* 2020;50(4):1401-1410.

105. Zobel-Lachiusa J, Andrianopoulos MV, Mailloux Z, Cermak SA. Sensory differences and mealtime behavior in children with autism. *Am J Occup Ther.* 2015;69(5):6905185050.

106. Tomchek SD, Little LM, Dunn W. Sensory pattern contributions to developmental performance in children with autism spectrum disorder. *Am J Occup Ther.* 2015;69(5): 6905185041-690518504010.

107. Miguel H, Sampaio A, Martínez-Regueiro R, et al. Touch processing and social behavior in ASD. *J Autism Dev Disord.* 2017;47(8):2425-2433.

108. Kojovic N, Ben Hadid L, Franchini M, Schaer M. Sensory processing issues and their association with social difficulties in children with autism spectrum disorders. *J Clin Med.* 2019;8(10):1508.

109. Williams KL, Kirby AV, Watson LR, Sideris J, Bulluck J, Baranek GT. Sensory features as predictors of adaptive behaviors: a comparative longitudinal study of children with autism spectrum disorder and other developmental disabilities. *Res Dev Disabil.* 2018;81:103-112.

110. Glod M, Riby DM, Honey E, Rodgers J. Psychological correlates of sensory processing patterns in individuals with autism spectrum disorder: a systematic review. *Rev J Autism Dev Disord.* 2015;2:199-221.

111. Ismael N, Lawson LM, Hartwell J. Relationship between sensory processing and participation in daily occupations for children with autism spectrum disorder: a systematic review of studies that used Dunn's sensory processing framework. *Am J Occup Ther.* 2018;72(3):1-9.

112. Green SA, Ben-Sasson A, Soto TW, Carter AS. Anxiety and sensory over-responsivity in toddlers with autism spectrum disorders: bidirectional effects across time. *J Autism Dev Disord.* 2012;42(6):1112-1119.

113. Schulz SE, Stevenson RA. Sensory hypersensitivity predicts repetitive behaviours in autistic and typically-developing children. *Autism.* 2019;23(4):1028-1041.

114. Kirby AV, White TJ, Baranek GT. Caregiver strain and sensory features in children with autism spectrum disorder and other developmental disabilities. *Am J Intellect Dev Disabil.* 2015; 120(1):32-45.

115. Bagby MS, Dickie VA, Baranek GT. How sensory experiences of children with and without autism affect family occupations. *Am J Occup Ther.* 2012;66(1):78-86.

116. Little L, Ausderau K, Sideris J, Baranek G. Activity participation and sensory features among children with autism spectrum disorders. *J Autism Dev Disord.* 2015;45(9):2981-2990.

117. Ashburner JK, Rodger SA, Ziviani JM, Hinder EA. Optimizing participation of children with autism spectrum disorder experiencing sensory challenges: a clinical reasoning framework: Optimiser la participation des enfants atteints d'un trouble du spectre autistique ayant des troubles. *Can J Occup Ther.* 2014;81(1):29-38.

118. Randell E, McNamara R, Delport S, et al. Sensory integration therapy versus usual care for sensory processing difficulties in autism spectrum disorder in children: study protocol for a pragmatic randomised controlled trial. *Trials.* 2019; 20(1):113.

119. Weitlauf AS, Sathe N, McPheeters ML, Warren ZE. Interventions targeting sensory challenges in autism spectrum disorder: a systematic review. *Pediatrics.* 2017;139(6):1-22.

120. Case-Smith J, Weaver LL, Fristad MA. A systematic review of sensory processing interventions for children with autism spectrum disorders. *Autism.* 2015;19(2):133-148.

121. Devlin S, Healy O, Leader G, Hughes B. Comparison of behavioral intervention and sensory-integration therapy in the treatment of challenging behavior. *J Autism Dev Disord.* 2011;41(10):1303-1320.

122. Leew SV, Stein NG, Gibbard WB. Weighted vests' effect on social attention for toddlers with autism spectrum disorders. *Can J Occup Ther.* 2010;77(2):113-124.

123. Davis TN, Dacus S, Strickland E, et al. The effects of a weighted vest on aggressive and self-injurious behavior in a child with autism. *Dev Neurorehabil.* 2013;16(3):210-215.

124. Zimmerman KN, Ledford JR, Severini KE. Brief report: the effects of a weighted blanket on engagement for a student with ASD. *Focus Autism Other Dev Disabl.* 2019;34(1):15-19.

125. Peña M, Ng Y, Ripat J, & Anagnostou E. Brief Report: Parent Perspectives on Sensory-Based Interventions for Children with Autism Spectrum Disorder. Journal of autism and developmental disorders. *J Autism Dev Disord* 20.21;51(6):2109-2114. https://doi.org/10.1007/s10803-020-04644-8.

126. Bestbier L, Williams TI. The immediate effects of deep pressure on young people with autism and severe intellectual difficulties: demonstrating individual differences. *Occup Ther Int.* 2017;24(1):1-7.

127. Mills CJ, Michail E, Bye RA. A survey of occupational therapists on a new tool for sensory processing. *Occup Ther Int.* 2020;28:2020:5909347.

128. Hopf KP, Madren E, Santianni KA. Use and perceived effectiveness of complementary and alternative medicine to treat and manage the symptoms of autism in children: a survey of parents in a community population. *J Altern Complement Med.* 2016;22(1):25-32.

129. De Giacomo A, Craig F, Terenzio V, Coppola A, Campa MG, Passeri G. Aggressive behaviors and verbal communication skills in autism spectrum disorders. *Glob Pediatr Health.* 2016;3:2333794X16644360.

130. Hofvander B, Delorme R, Chaste P, et al. Psychiatric and psychosocial problems in adults with normal-intelligence autism spectrum disorders. *BMC Psychiatry.* 2009;9:35.

131. American Speech-Language-Hearing Association (ASHA). Augmentative and alternative communication (AAC). Accessed September 29, 2019. https://www.asha.org/public/speech/disorders/AAC/#about.

132. Rose V, Trembath D, Keen D, Paynter J. The proportion of minimally verbal children with autism spectrum disorder in a community-based early intervention programme. *J Intellect Disabil Res.* 2016;60(5):464-477.

133. Logan K, Iacono T, Trembath D. A systematic review of research into aided AAC to increase social-communication functions in children with autism spectrum disorder. *Augment Altern Commun.* 2017;33:1(1):51-64.

134. Ganz JB. AAC interventions for individuals with autism spectrum disorders: state of the science and future research directions. *Augment Altern Commun.* 2015;31(3):203-214.

135. Agius MM, Vance M. A comparison of PECS and iPad to teach requesting to pre-schoolers with autistic spectrum disorders. *Augment Altern Commun.* 2016;32(1):58-68.

136. Boulter C, Freeston M, South M, Rodgers J. Intolerance of uncertainty as a framework for understanding anxiety in children and adolescents with autism spectrum disorders. *J Autism Dev Disord.* 2014;44(6):1391-1402.

137. Tovin MM. Children and teens with autism spectrum disorder: considerations and basic guidelines for health and fitness professionals. *Strength Condition J.* 2013;35(4):31-37.

138. Gray C, Faherty C, Timmins S, Lanou A. 2023. Social Stories 10.4 Criteria.

139. Samuels R, Stansfield J. The effectiveness of Social Stories™ to develop social interactions with adults with characteristics of autism spectrum disorder. *Br J Learn Disabil.* 2012;40(4): 272-285.

140. Thompson RM, Johnston S. Use of social stories to improve self-regulation in children with autism spectrum disorders. *Phys Occup Ther Pediatr.* 2013;33(3):271-284.

141. Linstead E, Dixon DR, French R, et al. Intensity and learning outcomes in the treatment of children with autism spectrum disorder. *Behav Modif.* 2017;41(2):229-252.

142. Autism Speaks. Applied Behavior Analysis (ABA). Published 2019. Accessed September 30, 2019. https://www.autismspeaks.org/applied-behavior-analysis.

143. Kaur M, Bhat A. Creative yoga intervention improves motor and imitation skills of children with autism spectrum disorder. *Phys Ther.* 2019;99(11):1520-1534.

144. Shattuck PT, Garfield T, Roux AM, et al. Services for adults with autism spectrum disorder: a systems perspective. *Curr Psychiatry Rep.* 2020;22(3):13.

145. Autism Speaks. *Autism and Health: A Special Report by Autism Speaks. Advances in Understanding and Treating the Health Conditions that Frequently Accompany Autism.* Autism Speaks; 2017.

146. Roux AM, Shattuck PT, Cooper BP, Anderson KA, Wagner M, Narendorf SC. Postsecondary employment experiences among young adults with an autism spectrum disorder. *J Am Acad Child Adolesc Psychiatry.* 2013;52(9):931-939.

147. Taylor J, Seltzer M. Employment and post-secondary educational activities for young adults with autism spectrum disorders during the transition to adulthood. *J Autism Dev Disord.* 2011;41(5):566-574.

148. Orentliher M, Schefkind S, Gibson R. *Transitions Across the Lifespan: An Occupational Therapy Approach.* AOTA Press; 2015.

149. Ganz M. The lifetime distribution of the incremental societal costs of autism. *Arch Pediatr Adolesc Med.* 2007;161(4): 343-349.

150. Rogge N, Janssen J. The economic costs of autism spectrum disorder: a literature review. *J Autism Dev Disord.* 2019;49(7): 2873-2900.

151. Cidav Z, Lawer L, Marcus S, Mandell D. Age-related variation in health service use and associated expenditures among children with autism. *J Autism Dev Disord.* 2013;43(4):924-931.

152. Wang L, Leslie DL. Health care expenditures for children with autism spectrum disorders in Medicaid. *J Am Acad Child Adolesc Psychiatry.* 2010;49(11):1165-1171.

153. Cakir J, Frye RE, Walker SJ. The lifetime social cost of autism: 1990–2029. *Res Autism Spectr Disord.* 2020;72:101502.

154. Friedman NDB, Warfield ME, Parish SL. Transition to adulthood for individuals with autism spectrum disorder: current issues and future perspectives. *Neuropsychiatry.* 2013;3(2):181-192.

155. Shattuck PT, Wagner M, Narendorf S, Sterzing P, Hensley M. Post-high school service use among young adults with an autism spectrum disorder. *Arch Pediatr Adolesc Med.* 2011;165(2): 141-146.

156. Anderson KA, Shattuck PT, Cooper BP, Roux AM, Wagner M. Prevalence and correlates of postsecondary residential status among young adults with an autism spectrum disorder. *Autism.* 2014;18(5):562-570.

157. Croen LA, Zerbo O, Qian Y, et al. The health status of adults on the autism spectrum. *Autism.* 2015;19(7):814-823.

158. Li YJ, Xie XN, Lei X, Li YM, Lei X. Global prevalence of obesity, overweight and underweight in children, adolescents and adults with autism spectrum disorder, attention-deficit hyperactivity disorder: a systematic review and meta-analysis. *Obes Rev.* 2020;21(12):e13123.

159. Bishop-Fitzpatrick L, Kind A. A scoping review of health disparities in autism spectrum disorder. *J Autism Dev Disord.* 2017;47(11):3380-3391.

160. Iadarola S, Pérez-Ramos J, Smith T, Dozier A. Understanding stress in parents of children with autism spectrum disorder: a focus on under-represented families. *Int J Dev Disabil.* 2019;65(1):20-30.

161. Rimmer JH, Yamaki K, Lowry BMD, Wang E, Vogel LC. Obesity and obesity-related secondary conditions in adolescents with intellectual/developmental disabilities. *J Intellect Disabil Res.* 2010;54(9):787-794.

162. Curtin C, Anderson SE, Must A, Bandini L. The prevalence of obesity in children with autism: a secondary data analysis using nationally representative data from the National Survey of Children's Health. *BMC Pediatr.* 2010;10:11.

163. Macdonald M, Esposito P, Ulrich D. The physical activity patterns of children with autism. *BMC Res Notes.* 2011;4:422.

164. Tovin MM, Braunius C. *Physical Activity, Obesity Risk, and Physical Therapy for Autism Spectrum Disorder: Parent Perspectives.* APTA Combined Sections Meeting; 2015.

165. Pan CY, Tsai CL, Chen FC, Chow BC, Chen CC, Chu CH. Physical and sedentary activity patterns in youths with autism spectrum disorder. *Int J Environ Res Public Health.* 2021;18(4):1739.

166. McCoy SM, Morgan K. Obesity, physical activity, and sedentary behaviors in adolescents with autism spectrum disorder compared with typically developing peers. *Autism.* 2020;24(2):387-399.

167. Ruggeri A, Dancel A, Johnson R, Sargent B. The effect of motor and physical activity intervention on motor outcomes of children with autism spectrum disorder: a systematic review. *Autism.* 2020;24(3):544-568.

168. Stanish H, Curtin C, Must A, Phillips S, Maslin M, Bandini L. Enjoyment, barriers, and beliefs about physical activity in adolescents with and without autism spectrum disorder. *Adapt Phys Activ Q.* 2015;32(4):302-317.

169. Eaves LC, Ho HH. Young adult outcome of autism spectrum disorders. *J Autism Dev Disord.* 2008;38(4):739-747.

170. White SW, Oswald D, Ollendick T, Scahill L. Anxiety in children and adolescents with autism spectrum disorders. *Clin Psychol Rev.* 2009;29(3):216-229.

171. Orsmond G, Shattuck P, Cooper B, Sterzing P, Anderson K. Social participation among young adults with an autism spectrum disorder. *J Autism Dev Disord.* 2013;43(11):2710-2719.

172. Cage E, Monaco J, Newell V. Experiences of autism acceptance and mental health in autistic adults. *J Autism Dev Disord.* 2018;48(2):473-484.

173. van Steensel F, Bögels S, Perrin S. Anxiety disorders in children and adolescents with autistic spectrum disorders: a meta-analysis. *Clin Child Fam Psychol Rev.* 2011;14(3):302-317.

174. Ayres M, Parr JR, Rodgers J, Mason D, Avery L, Flynn D. A systematic review of quality of life of adults on the autism spectrum. *Autism.* 2018;22(7):774-783.

175. Ling-Yi Lin, Pai-Chuan Huang. Quality of life and its related factors for adults with autism spectrum disorder. *Disabil Rehabil.* 2019;41(8):896-903.

176. Roux A, Shattuck P, Rast J, Rava J, Anderson K. *National Autism Indicators Report: Transition Into Adulthood.* Drexel University; 2015.

177. Temple VA, Stanish HI. The feasibility of using a peer-guided model to enhance participation in community-based physical activity for youth with intellectual disability. *J Intellect Disabil.* 2011;15(3):209-217.

178. Nunez-Gaunaurd A, Agahan D, Asta A, Leon S, Sequeira D, Tovin M. Effectiveness of a peer guided physical activity via telehealth program (PACT) in adults with autism: a pilot randomized controlled trial. *Medicine & Science in Sports & Exercise:* 2022;54(9S):298-299. doi:10.1249/01.mss.0000878760.95064.d3.

179. Tovin MM & Nunez-Gaunaurd A. Implementation of peer-assisted physical activity via telehealth for autistic adults:

a feasibility study. *Phys Ther.* 2024; pzae005, https://doi.org/10.1093/ptj/pzae005

180. Bolaños-Boudreau M. Person-centered physical training programs for individuals with intellectual disabilities: stimulating motivation and participation as essential components of program development. Ann Arbor, University of North Florida; 2020. Accessed November 5, 2023. https://digitalcommons.unf.edu/cgi/viewcontent.cgi?article=1993&context=etd.

181. Hamm J, Yun J. The motivational process for physical activity in young adults with autism spectrum disorder. *Disabil Health.* 2018;11(4):644-649.

182. de Nocker YL, Toolan CK. Using telehealth to provide interventions for children with ASD: a systematic review. *Rev J Autism Dev Disord.* 2023;10(1):82-112.

183. Healy S, Marchand G. The feasibility of project CHASE: a Facebook-delivered, parent-mediated physical activity intervention for children with autism. *Int J Disabil Dev Educ.* 2020;67(2):225-242.

184. Sehlin H, Hedman Ahlström B, Andersson G, Wentz E. Experiences of an internet-based support and coaching model for adolescents and young adults with ADHD and autism spectrum disorder: a qualitative study. *BMC Psychiatry.* 2018;18(1):15.

185. Srinivasan SM, Su WC, Cleffi C, Bhat AN. From social distancing to social connections: insights from the delivery of a clinician-caregiver co-mediated telehealth-based intervention in young children with autism spectrum disorder. *Front Psychiatry.* 2021;12:700247.

186. Pérez-Cruzado D, Cuesta-Vargas AI. Smartphone reminder for physical activity in people with intellectual disabilities. *Int J Technol Assess Health Care.* 2017;33(1):442-443.

187. Garcia JM, Leahy N, Brazendale K, Quelly S, Lawrence S. Implementation of a school-based Fitbit program for youth with autism spectrum disorder: a feasibility study. *Disabil Health J.* 2021;14(2):100990.

188. Crabtree LA, Demchick BB. Young adults on the autism spectrum: perceived effects of participation in a university-based challenge course program in the community. *Occup Ther Mental Health.* 2015;31(3):253-265.

189. Perryman T, Ricks L, Cash-Baskett L. Meaningful transitions: enhancing clinician roles in transition planning for adolescents with autism spectrum disorders. *Lang Speech Hear Serv Sch.* 2020;51(4):899-913.

190. vanSchalkwyk G, Volkmar FR. Autism spectrum disorders: challenges and opportunities for transition to adulthood. *Child Adolesc Psychiatr Clin N Am.* 2017;26(2):329-339.

191. Grace NR, Golden CT, Mala KK, Kanniammal C, Arulappan J. Exploration of challenges faced by caregivers of children with autism spectrum disorder. *Int J Nursing Educ.* 2018;10(3): 125-130.

192. Gona JK, Newton CR, Rimba KK, et al. Challenges and coping strategies of parents of children with autism on the Kenyan coast. *Rural Remote Health.* 2016;16(2):1-12.

193. Desai MU, Divan G, Wertz FJ, Patel V. The discovery of autism: Indian parents' experiences of caring for their child with an autism spectrum disorder. *Transcult Psychiatry.* 2012;49(3/4):613-637.

194. Lavelle TA, Weinstein MC, Newhouse JP, Munir K, Kuhlthau KA, Prosser LA. Economic burden of childhood autism spectrum disorders. *Pediatrics.* 2014;133(3):e520-e529.

195. Hsu YC, Tsai SL, Hsieh MH, Jenks MS, Tsai CH, Hsu MT. On my own: a qualitative phenomenological study of mothers of young children with autism spectrum disorder in Taiwan. *J Appl Res Intellect Disabil.* 2017;30(1):147-156.

196. Tovin MM. *A Place for Me: The Lived Experience of Special Olympics for Young Adults With ASD*. APTA Combined Sections Meeting Nova Southeastern University; 2017.

197. Schaaf RC, Toth-Cohen S, Johnson SL, Outten G, Benevides TW. The everyday routines of families of children with autism: examining the impact of sensory processing difficulties on the family. *Autism*. 2011;15(3):373-389.

198. Karst JS, Van Hecke AV. Parent and family impact of autism spectrum disorders: a review and proposed model for intervention evaluation. *Clin Child Fam Psychol Rev*. 2012;15(3):247-277.

199. Kousgaard SJ, Boldsen SK, Mohr-Jensen C, Lauritsen MB. The effect of having a child with ADHD or ASD on family separation. *Soc Psychiatry Psychiatr Epidemiol*. 2018;53(12):1391-1399.

200. Schieve LA, Blumberg SJ, Rice C, Visser SN, Boyle C. The relationship between autism and parenting stress. *Pediatrics*. 2007;119:S114-S121.

201. Hayes S, Watson S. The impact of parenting stress: a meta-analysis of studies comparing the experience of parenting stress in parents of children with and without autism spectrum disorder. *J Autism Dev Disord*. 2013;43(3):629-642.

202. Estes A, Olson E, Sullivan K, et al. Parenting-related stress and psychological distress in mothers of toddlers with autism spectrum disorders. *Brain Dev*. 2013;35(2):133-138.

203. Postorino V, Gillespie S, Lecavalier L, et al. Clinical correlates of parenting stress in children with autism spectrum disorder and serious behavioral problems. *J Child Family Studies*. 2019;28(8): 2069-2077.

204. Thullen M, Bonsall A. Co-parenting quality, parenting stress, and feeding challenges in families with a child diagnosed with autism spectrum disorder. *J Autism Dev Disord*. 2017;47(3):878-886.

205. Estes A, Vismara L, Mercado C, et al. The impact of parent-delivered intervention on parents of very young children with autism. *J Autism Dev Disord*. 2014;44(2):353-365.

206. Falk N, Norris K, Quinn M. The factors predicting stress, anxiety and depression in the parents of children with autism. *J Autism Dev Disord*. 2014;44(12):3185-3203.

207. Turcotte P-L, Côté C, Coulombe K, Richard M, Larivière N, Couture M. Social participation during transition to adult life among young adults with high-functioning autism spectrum disorders: experiences from an exploratory multiple case study. *Occup Ther Mental Health*. 2015;31(3):234-252.

208. Mieres AC, Kirby RS, Armstrong KH, Murphy TK, Grossman L. Autism spectrum disorder: an emerging opportunity for physical therapy. *Pediatr Phys Ther*. 2012;24(1):31-37.

209. Wong C, Odom S, Hume K, et al. Evidence-based practices for children, youth, and young adults with autism spectrum disorder: a comprehensive review. *J Autism Dev Disord*. 2015;45(7):1951-1966.

210. Hayden-Evan, M, Evans K, Milbourn B, et al. Validating the International Classification of Functioning, Disability and Health Core Sets for Autism in a Sample of Australian School-Aged Children on the Spectrum. *J Autism Dev Disord*. 2024. https://doi.org/10.1007/s10803-024-06295-5.

12

Developmental Coordination Disorder

Jennifer Parent-Nichols, DPT, EdD

LEARNING OBJECTIVES

Upon completion of this chapter, the reader will be able to:

- Use the clinical practice guideline from the Academy of Pediatric Physical Therapy of the American Physical Therapy Association to inform the examination, evaluation, and treatment of individuals with a diagnosis of developmental coordination disorder (DCD).
- Describe the standardized and nonstandardized tests and measures used to identify impairments in body functions and structures, functional limitations, and participation restrictions for an individual with a diagnosis of DCD.
- Integrate information regarding pathophysiology, diagnostic criteria, and potential differential and associated diagnoses to develop a prognosis for individuals with a diagnosis of DCD.
- Implement findings of tests and measures to generate appropriate child/adolescent and family-centered goals for an individual with a diagnosis of DCD.
- Develop an evidenced-based plan of care to maximize outcomes for an individual with the diagnosis of DCD.
- Construct management strategies to promote learning for individuals with the diagnosis of DCD.
- Identify appropriate referrals for individuals with a diagnosis of DCD, including engagement in community activities.

Case Study

Ryan is an 8-year-old who is in second grade at his neighborhood elementary school. His classroom teacher has asked Ryan's school team to discuss concerns with academic progress and awareness of his body in space. The school nurse and counselor; the school-based physical, speech, and occupational therapists; and the classroom teacher are all present for this meeting. Because of concerns about the quality of Ryan's movement, the physical education (PE) teacher also has been invited to this meeting. The classroom teacher notes that Ryan has difficulty organizing himself and that his desk frequently has items "spilling out." He reports that Ryan requires consistent cues to initiate tasks and support to complete activities, especially tasks that require writing. His PE teacher has noticed that Ryan tends to "move to the back of the room" and "frequently moves into his peers' space." He frequently requires redirection and seems to want to "do his own thing."

INTRODUCTION

The development of motor skills allows children to maximize their access to the world. Such skills are necessary to engage in self-care, play, and educational and social activities. Individuals with developmental coordination disorder (DCD) demonstrate challenges with the performance of the motor tasks required for successful self-management, academic engagement, and participation in social and recreational activities. The diagnosis of DCD may also be referred to as developmental dyspraxia,[1] or specific developmental disorder of motor function.[2] Symptoms of this neurodevelopmental condition emerge over the developmental period.

Individuals with DCD experience the symptoms associated with this diagnosis to varying degrees. As the diagnostic term indicates, coordination difficulties are a hallmark of DCD. Typically, activities that require organization, prioritization, and generalization of motor output present challenges. Individuals with DCD may require a longer time to learn motor skills and require consistent practice to maintain those skills. While coping strategies may be developed to accommodate movement difficulties, challenges with motor output may continue over the life span as new skills are required to meet the increasing demands of life.

COORDINATION AND THE SENSORY-MOTOR LOOP

Execution of coordinated movement requires accurate input from the sensory system and output from the motor system. This sensory input and motor output must work together efficiently if the mover is to be successful. First, sensory information from the environment is received and interpreted. The individual uses these data to select from a series of established motor plans. Motor output is then executed. The sequence, speed, force, and direction of these motor plans must all be modulated for the movement to be effective. Finally, the executed plan must be adapted to meet the needs of the environment. Each of these steps contributes to coordinated movement.

Individuals with DCD may experience delays in the acquisition, refinement, and generalization of fine and gross motor skills. Adapting those skills to meet changing environmental demands may also be challenging. Delays in reception and interpretation of information from the body or from the environment may negatively affect motor performance. Specific deficits in motor planning and coordination, postural control, and gait activities have been linked to deficits in the organization of sensory information.[3] For example, children with DCD may have delayed execution of balance reactions when bumped on the playground, resulting in a fall. Decreased or delayed proprioceptive input may result in unintendingly moving into peers' personal space.

Difficulties managing sophisticated movements may result in challenges with peer interaction. Children and adolescents with DCD may not be sought out to join playground or community-based activities with their peers. They may begin to avoid activities that require motor output, limiting opportunities to participate in physical activity and to socialize with peers. These negative experiences contribute to lower levels of physical and health-related fitness and increased risk for low self-esteem.

Physical therapists (PTs) are well suited to address the impairments, functional limitations, and participation restrictions commonly experienced by children and adults with a diagnosis of DCD. PTs can provide information to promote self-advocacy, create opportunities for skill practice and generalization, and help to develop strategies to meet the evolving needs of individuals with this diagnosis.

■ PATHOPHYSIOLOGY

The pathophysiology of DCD is not well understood. Several explanations for this neurodevelopmental diagnosis continue to be investigated. Male sex and prematurity (birth prior to 37 weeks' gestation) may be contributors to this diagnosis with gestational age at birth inversely associated with frequency of the diagnosis.[4] White matter abnormalities, which are common in prematurity, may be a possible explanation for the symptoms related to DCD.[5] On a larger scale, alterations in networks, the way the brain communicates with itself, are seen when comparing children with DCD with their typically developing peers.[6] Diagnostic imaging shows specific differences in activation patterns across the cerebrum and cerebellum during motor tasks.[7,8] Impairments in balance, coordination, dexterity, and spatial processing common to this diagnosis may be related to these brain differences.[9]

■ DIAGNOSIS

Ideally, diagnosis of DCD should include input from a team of individuals familiar with the individual. Information may be solicited from parents, teachers, health care providers, and

the child. Comprehensive examination of medical, neuromotor, behavioral, and sensory function should occur to rule out other potential diagnoses. An individual receiving the diagnosis of DCD must demonstrate behaviors meeting the diagnostic criteria set in the fifth edition of the *Diagnostic and Statistical Manual of Mental Disorders* (DSM-V).[10] These criteria include the following:

1. Acquisition and performance of motor skills are below those expected at their chronological age. Skill performance may be described as slow, inaccurate, or clumsy. Deficits or delays in these skills remain even after adequate exposure and opportunity to develop these skills.
2. The challenges with acquisition and performance of motor skills impact the ability to execute age-appropriate participation in life skills including academic, prevocational, vocational, and recreational activities.
3. The onset of symptoms occurred during the developmental period.
4. Motor challenges cannot be attributed to intellectual disability, visual impairment, or an alternative neurologic condition.

■ REFERRAL TO PHYSICAL THERAPY

The early school years bring about demands for increased organizational and motor skills. As such, teachers and support staff may be the first to recognize challenges for the child in this environment. Teachers may report concerns to a child-centered team at the school where these concerns can be discussed and next steps determined. Alternatively, primary care physicians or parents may recognize early challenges in motor skill acquisition or refinement or in completion of activities of daily living. Identification of these concerns may result in referral to the school or to an outpatient facility for evaluation. Emerging evidence supports that early intervention benefits children with a diagnosis of DCD.[11]

■ PATIENT MANAGEMENT FOR THE PHYSICAL THERAPIST

INTERNATIONAL CLASSIFICATION OF FUNCTIONING, DISABILITY, AND HEALTH

The International Classification of Functioning, Disability, and Health (ICF) categorizes patient function in the context of a health condition. ICF classification emphasizes health and ability and provides consistent language with which professionals may communicate. The ICF model recognizes the dynamic interaction of the health condition(s), the environment including personal supports, and the individual themselves. The identified categories of body functions and structures, activities, and participation aid the PT with organization of the examination, evaluation, and plan of care. Individuals with DCD frequently demonstrate differences in all categories of the ICF.

The *Guide to Physical Therapist Practice 3.0* is consistent with language of the ICF. This guide serves as a primary reference for best practice for the PT.[12] Components of proper patient management of children and adults with the diagnosis of DCD include examination, evaluation, diagnosis, prognosis, intervention, and outcome assessment. The ICF model can help to inform decision-making around appropriate tests and measures, development and assessment of goals, and appropriate interventions.

In 2020, the Academy of Pediatric Physical Therapy of the American Physical Therapy Association (APTA) published a clinical practice guideline (CPG) informing clinicians and families about the management of DCD. The CPG provides recommendations based on current evidence for examination, referral, intervention, and discharge.[13]

EXAMINATION

Accurate examination of the patient with DCD requires measurements of potential deficits across many domains of function. Gaining information from as many sources as possible is important to develop a full picture of the child or adult. Initial data may be collected through purposeful interviewing of parents, teachers, and the child. Interviews should include a detailed history of the child's development, acquisition of motor milestones, co-occurring diagnoses, and current concerns. Details about previous bouts of intervention and past strategies that have been either successful or unsuccessful in teaching and learning can inform interactions between the therapist and child. Specific goals of the family and child should always be discussed.

Checklists and screenings may also provide important information. Parent and teacher checklists appropriate for the pediatric population include the Movement Assessment Battery for Children-2 (MABC-2) Checklist, the Children Activity Scale for Teachers (ChAS-T) and Parents (ChAS-P), and the Motor Observation Questionnaire for Teachers (MOQ-T). Other checklists may be used directly with the children. Examples of these child-centered checklists are the Children's Self-Perceptions of Adequacy in and Predilection for Physical Activity (CSAPPA) scale, the Children's Assessment of Participation and Enjoyment (CAPE), and Preferences for Activities of Children (PAC). These tools may also provide information regarding participation in leisure activity outside of school.

The PT should remain aware of any yellow or red flags that become evident through the history and systems review process and at any time during the examination. Yellow and red flags should signal a referral to the child's primary care physician.

Case Study

At the request of the PT on the child-centered school team, Ryan's classroom teacher, his PE teacher, and his parents all completed the Movement Assessment Battery for Children-2 Checklist. While his classroom teacher's scores on this checklist indicated slightly higher function, all 3 checklists indicated concerns with coordination and motor performance. All the completed checklists indicated concerns with Ryan's ability to modify his movements in response to changes in his environment.

Screening

A screening tool for DCD has been developed for children age 5 to 15 years. The Developmental Coordination Disorder Questionnaire Screening 2007 (DCDQ'07) provides caregivers with an opportunity to rate the motor performance of their child as compared to the child's peers. The DCDQ'07 includes 15 items related to control during movement, fine motor and handwriting, and general coordination. Because the DCDQ'07 is a screening tool, it is not intended to be used in isolation to identify and diagnose DCD, but rather to identify children who are suspect for the diagnosis of DCD. This tool is available at no cost at the following website: www.dcdq.ca.[14] Information regarding the properties and purchase of these checklists and screenings is provided in **Table 12-1**.

TABLE 12-1 • Properties of Checklists and Screening Tools Common to Developmental Coordination Disorder			
Tool	**Age Range**	**Administration**	**Website or Reference**
Movement Assessment Battery for Children-2 Checklist	5-12 years	Parents and teachers	https://www.pearsonclinical.com/therapy/products/100000433/movement-assessment-battery-for-children-second-edition-movement-abc-2.html
Children Activity Scale for Teachers and Parents (ChAS-P/T)	4-8 years	Parents and teachers	Rosenblum[15]
Motor Observation Questionnaire for Teachers (MOQ-T)	5-11 years	Teachers	Giofre et al[16]
Children's Self-Perceptions of Adequacy in and Predilection for Physical Activity (CSAPPA) Scale	9-16 years	Children	Hay[17]
Children's Assessment of Participation and Enjoyment (CAPE) Preferences for Activities of Children (PAC)	6-21 years	Children	https://www.pearsonassessments.com/store/usassessments/en/Store/Professional-Assessments/Behavior/Adaptive/Children%27s-Assessment-of-Participation-and-Enjoyment-and-Preferences-for-Activities-of-Children/p/100000481.html
Developmental Coordination Disorder Questionnaire Screening 2007 (DCDQ'07)	5-15 years	Parents	http://www.dcdq.ca/

Case Study

Ryan's parents also completed the DCDQ'07. On this instrument, his parents indicated differences in Ryan's movement control, fine motor skills, and coordination. Ryan's score on the DCDQ'07 was 35 out of 75, revealing an indication or suspicion for DCD.

Tests and Measures

Once interviews, checklists, and screening have been completed, a decision regarding whether to conduct a full physical therapy examination must be made. Data from these tools are assessed to determine if gross motor deficits contribute to the reported challenges with function. If further physical therapy examination is warranted, observation of the child's function in their natural environment can provide important information regarding function. The therapist should observe the child engaging in activities in their natural environments (ie, the environments where those activities are expected to occur). If observation is not possible, the PT should inquire about specific challenges the child experiences. Information gathered from these observations and interviews can be used to determine the most appropriate objective measures to follow.

Systems Review

A comprehensive systems review should be a part of the physical therapy examination. For individuals with a diagnosis of DCD, it is common for these screenings to indicate the need for further investigation into multiple systems. Concerns with integumentary system function are not common with a diagnosis of DCD. However, bruising and abrasions from bumping and falling should be noted. Cardiovascular and pulmonary systems review may indicate limitations in exercise tolerance. Common indications in the musculoskeletal system include postural deviations and impairments in ranges of motion, strength, power, and muscular endurance. Neuromuscular system review may be positive for lower than expected muscle tone for children of the same age. Coordination deficits may also be observed. Review of cognition may reveal differences in learning.

Case Study: Systems Review for Ryan

Integumentary system: Bruising medial left knee, 2 inches × 3 inches. Abrasion left medial elbow, 2 inches × 2 inches. Healing with scabbing noted.

Cardiovascular and pulmonary systems: Observed to require frequent rest periods, in excess when compared to peer performance, during recess play.

Musculoskeletal system: Greater than expected passive range of motion in upper and lower extremities, except bilateral hamstrings. Forward head, upper thoracic kyphosis, anterior pelvic tilt, bilateral genu recurvatum, bilateral foot pronation.

Neuromuscular system: Symmetrical but lower than expected tone in trunk and extremities. Coordination (toe tapping, heel to shin, and finger to nose): Able to demonstrate accuracy with coordination activities only when slows movement significantly. When moving at a faster rate of speed, requires corrections to contact target. Noted a delayed (~2 seconds) response to tactile stimulation during attempts at facilitation. Cognition/learning preference: Benefits from whole/part/whole learning. Visual demonstration and multiple repetitions help with direction following.

Primary and Secondary Impairments in Body Structure and Function

DCD presents with common primary and secondary impairments in body function and structure. Primary impairments are problems arising directly from the identified health concern. Differences in sensory processing, sensory integration, motor control, and motor learning represent primary impairments in DCD. Challenges with reception, organization, and interpretation of sensory information from visual, tactile, and vestibular input are common.[18,19] The PT must keep these impairments in mind when conducting an examination for individuals with this diagnosis.

In the face of improper sensory function, efficient control of motor output becomes challenging. Execution of rhythmic, coordinated movement requires increased effort for the individual with DCD. Motor control deficits can result in decreased propulsive power, explosive strength, and general tolerance of exercise.[20] For this reason, children with DCD may be described as having awkward or clumsy movement. These challenges may be increasingly apparent as requirements for speed increase. Higher-level coordination skills like skipping and jumping rope are especially challenging.

Delayed or reduced responses to postural challenges further contribute to movement difficulties.[3] Deficits in postural control can be seen with anticipated and unanticipated balance challenges. Latent balance corrections require larger responses, resulting in a greater risk of falls.[21] Limitations in the ability to adapt motor plans to meet changing environmental demands can result in tripping and loss of balance. Individuals with DCD frequently adopt compensatory strategies to allow for safe participation in activities that require balance control.

Deficits in skills requiring executive function, including working memory and attention to task, can directly influence motor output. Efficient learning, planning, and motor skill execution require executive function.[22] Visual-spatial tasks, such as handwriting and negotiation through complex or cluttered environments, require greater cognitive effort for the individual with DCD. Distraction and divided attention during these tasks, as could occur in the classroom, further complicate successful execution. Primary impairments in executive functioning can persist over the life span of the individual with DCD, and compensatory strategies may be necessary.

Secondary impairments are problems arising from a diagnosis that become apparent as time passes. Secondary impairments in body structure and function that are associated with a diagnosis of DCD include limitations in endurance, strength, and flexibility.[23] Movement challenges associated with DCD contribute to feelings of decreased competence when participating in motor activities.[24] Individuals with DCD are more likely not to choose to engage in these activities. Inactivity associated with DCD can result in decreased exercise tolerance and limitations in muscle strength and flexibility. Children with DCD experience

TABLE 12-2 • Task Analysis Form

Student:											
Analysis of Task: Going to the playground											
Cleans up current project.											
Moves to personal belonging area.											
Removes and dons necessary items for recess.											
Gets into line.											
Stands in line to wait.											
Walks in line to door to playground.											
Opens and walks through door to playground.											
Manages curb from door to playground.											

1–Dependent for task
2–Moderate assistance (50% teacher/50% student)
3–Minimum assistance (25% caregiver/75% student)
4–Supervision, may include verbal reminders
5–Independent with task

decreased levels of overall physical and health-related fitness as compared to peers who are typically developing.[25]

Decreased confidence in motor skill execution may also influence the secondary impairments of social isolation. Fear of failure can contribute to withdrawal from peer interaction. Social challenges may be a factor in higher than expected rates of anxiety, depression, and low self-esteem for children with DCD. These secondary impairments in DCD may influence engagement in activities related to physical therapy.[26] Developing short-term goals and identifying opportunities for participation should be considered. Monitoring mood or behavioral changes outside of what is expected during adolescence is important. Significant mood or behavioral changes may warrant referral to a mental health care provider.

Understanding common primary and secondary impairments related to DCD promotes appropriate decision-making with regard to examination. The ICF model provides a framework from which to manage physical therapy examination for this global diagnosis. Relevant tests of body structure and function may include measures of sensory processing, balance, posture, visual-motor performance, strength, range of motion, and aerobic capacity.[13] Coordination is of special consideration in this diagnosis. Specific tests of coordination such as the Clinical Observation of Motor and Postural Skills (COMPS) and the Florida Apraxia Screening Test–Revised (FAST-R) may provide important information relating to deficits in body structure and function.

Activity Limitations
Information regarding activity limitations can be gathered using any of the screenings and checklists reviewed earlier in this chapter. Examination of performance at the ICF level of activity may include measures of mobility and play skills. Global assessments covering more than one domain of performance may provide helpful insight into limitations in academic, self-care, and social-behavioral skills common

in DCD. Activities requiring sustained attention to task and sequencing of tasks are frequently challenging for individuals with DCD. Specifically, self-care tasks such as dressing, meal preparation, and packing for school or work may present unique challenges.[27] Performing task analyses for these activities may help with determining strengths and challenges. **Table 12-2** shows an example of a task analysis form.

Examination of the potential limitations in the activity domain of the ICF may also be completed using standardized measures. The Movement Assessment Battery for Children-2 (MABC-2) is a multidomain, standardized, norm-referenced test that has demonstrated sensitivity to the diagnosis of DCD and is recommended by the CPG.[13] Activities on the MABC-2 relate to the areas of manual dexterity, balance, and ball skills for 3 age ranges: 3 to 6, 7 to 10, and 11 to 16 years. Children whose performance falls below the 15th percentile may benefit from intervention. Children whose performance falls between the 6th and 15th percentiles are identified as being at risk for DCD. Children whose motor performance is at or below the 5th percentile and meet additional criteria are identified as having DCD.[28] More information may be found at the following website: https://www.pearsonassessments.com/store/usassessments/en/Store/Professional-Assessments/Motor-Sensory/Movement-Assessment-Battery-for-Children-%7C-Second-Edition/p/100000433.html.

Participation Restriction
Development of skill is highly related to participation in life activities, particularly in leisure activities.[29] Examination of the individual's participation in the life activities level of the ICF model may include the use of the CPG-recommended Children's Assessment of Participation and Enjoyment (CAPE) and Preferences for Activities of Children (PAC) (CAPE/PAC), Canadian Occupational Performance Measure (COPM),[13] or

TABLE 12-3 • Tests and Measures for the Examination of Developmental Coordination Disorder

ICF categories	Test or Measure
Impairments in body structure and function	
Sensory processing	Sensory Integration and Praxis Test (SIPT) Sensory Profile
Balance/posture	Timed Up and Down Stairs (TUDS) Pediatric Balance Scale (PBS)
Visual motor performance	Developmental Test of Visual Motor Integration (VMI)
Strength	Manual Muscle Testing (MMT)
Range of motion	Active and passive goniometry measurements
Aerobic capacity	6-Minute Walk Test (6MWT)
Coordination	Clinical Observation of Motor and Postural Skills (COMPS) Florida Apraxia Screening Test-Revised (FAST-R)
Activity restrictions	
Gait	Observational Gait Scale (OGS)
Global activity assessment	Movement Assessment Battery for Children-2 (MABC-2)[a] Bruininks-Oseretsky Test of Motor Proficiency-2 (BOT-2)[a]
Participation restrictions	
Life activities	Children's Assessment of Participation and Enjoyment (CAPE) and Preferences for Activities of Children (PAC)[a] (CAPE/PAC) Canadian Occupational Performance Measure (COPM)[a] Participation and Environment Measure–Children and Youth (PEM-CY)
Quality of life	Pediatric Quality of Life Inventory (PEDS QL)
Health status assessment	Child Health Questionnaire (CHQ)

[a]*Recommended by clinical practice guideline of the Academy of Pediatric Physical Therapy of the American Physical Therapy Association.*[13]

the Participation and Environment Measure–Children and Youth (PEM-CY). Each of these tools is a self-reported, client-centered measure that reveals the individual's perception of their level of participation. The PEM-CY is unique in that the measure also accounts for environmental factors related to participation.

Quality of life assessments such as the Pediatric Quality of Life Inventory (PEDS QL) and health status assessments such as the Child Health Questionnaire (CHQ) may illuminate specific challenges in participation for children with DCD. Adults working with individuals with DCD must be acutely aware of and responsive to the potential impact on the quality of life from this diagnosis. Participation restrictions persist and evolve across the life span for individuals with DCD. As a child ages, challenges associated with DCD may have a greater, lesser, or just different impact on their ability to participate and enjoy that participation. Participation restrictions are linked to an increased risk of mental health concerns, especially in late adolescence and especially for girls.[30] Proactive programs designed to address social communication skills and self-esteem should be considered[30] and should consider the individual, the family, and the community.[31] Refer to **Table 12-3** for a more comprehensive list of potential measures in the examination of DCD.

Comprehensive evaluation of each of the ICF levels (body structure and function and activity and participation restriction) is necessary to develop an appropriate physical therapy diagnosis, goals, and a plan of care. PTs working with children and adolescents with a diagnosis of DCD should be mindful of the need to assess evolving challenges as aging occurs. Successful management includes planning for meeting the increasingly complex demands of academic, vocational, and social situations.

Case Study

An educationally based physical therapy evaluation was agreed upon by Ryan's family and his school team. The following information was obtained during this evaluation:

Ryan reports that he does not really have friends and that he wants to be good at running.

Strength: Unable to control midrange motion in squat. Moves to floor sitting position rather than returning to standing. Uses support surfaces to pull to stand from floor sitting.

Range of motion: Lacking 15 degrees of knee extension bilaterally during straight leg raise. Patient has greater than expected ranges of passive motion at all other joints.

Posture: Bilateral foot pronation, valgus position of the lower extremities, anterior pelvic tilt, bilateral genu recurvatum, rounded shoulders, and forward head.

Balance: Single leg stance: left: 2 seconds, right: 3 seconds. Requires multiple steps to stop movement and change direction. Chooses to crash to ground to stop forward movement.

During expected and unexpected perturbations in sitting and standing, demonstrates later and larger postural corrections.

Gait: Wide base of support, inconsistent foot placement. Limited trunk rotation and arm swing during fast gait and running activities. Reciprocal upper and lower extremity movement <25% of the time during gait activities, more notable as speed increased.

Propulsion: Able to jump forward one time for >12 inches. Asymmetry of push noted with increased reliance on right side. Able to clear both feet from surface. Lands in very low squat and uses hands on ground to assist with balance. When attempting multiple, consecutive jumps, patient assumes a gallop with right leg leading.

Stairs: Heavy reliance on railing when ascending stairs. Uses step-to pattern with right leg leading. Demonstrates variable toe clearance and foot placement on tread. Turns to face railing when descending. Step-to pattern with left leg lead. Timed Up and Down Stairs (TUDS): 13.32 seconds for 12 stairs (>2 standard deviations from norm).

Motor control: During novel movement activities, relies heavily on vision to assist with movement. Uses a wide base of support during postural transitions and seeks boundaries when holding static positions, such as moving up against a bookcase or peer during floor sitting activities.

Sensory: Slow to respond to sensory stimulation, taking up to 2 seconds before reporting feeling light touch stimulation of lower and upper extremities. Less than 50% accurate with proprioception activities and unable to accurately reproduce upper and lower extremity positions.

Coordination: Able to touch target during finger to nose activities with 50% accuracy. Slows movement when approaching target. Heel to shin activities are slowed and movement occurs only 75% of range. During jumping jack activities, patient moves legs, corrects position, and then moves arms. Able to attempt 2 jumping jacks before moving quickly with little accuracy for remainder of attempts.

Endurance: 6-Minute Walk Test: 375 m.

MABC-2: 8th percentile.

PROGNOSIS

The prognosis for individuals with DCD is varied and dependent on a range of factors. The severity of the challenges experienced by the individual and how early intervention occurs to address those challenges influence functional outcomes. While some individuals may experience resolution of symptoms as they mature, many continue to experience evolving challenges across their life span. Developing positive strategies to identify and address these challenges fosters independent function. Understanding strategies that have worked for the child in the past can inform choices for strategies that may be successful in the future.

Co-occurring diagnoses complicate the ability to develop an accurate prognosis for patients. Learning disabilities, attention-deficit disorder, and attention-deficit disorder with hyperactivity have significant overlap with the diagnosis of DCD. However, these diagnoses represent distinctly separate conditions and therefore require specific evaluation and treatment.[32]

Case Study

Plan: Discussed with family that child may require periodic episodes of care as he grows.

Frequency: High-frequency practice at 3-4 times per week for 10 weeks. Encourage community-based activity such as swimming or martial arts. Develop engaging home exercise program with frequent practice.

Assessment: Ryan presents with decreased strength, endurance, and motor control. These challenges negatively affect his ability to participate safely and successfully in his school day. Ryan has no coexisting diagnoses, is motivated to "be a better runner," and has a supportive family and school team. Ryan is a good candidate for physical therapy to address these findings. Use of metronome during activities requiring timing, repetition, and/or coordination supports performance for Ryan.

GOAL SETTING

Because symptoms and the impact of those symptoms may vary in individuals with DCD, goal setting must be individualized. Involving the individual in the process of goal setting helps to establish relevance. The Perceived Efficacy and Goal Setting (PEGS) system may prove useful in the development of child-centered goals and is recommended by the CPG.[13] This system has a set of cards that allows children age 5 to 6 years to report their perceived competence in self-care, school, and leisure activities. Goals are then set based on the child's interest. Caregiver and educator questionnaires provide additional data and opportunities for collaboration. This tool is available for purchase at the following website: https://canchild.ca/en/shop/5-pegs-2nd-edition-complete-kit.[33]

Use of the COPM can help to establish priorities and assist with accurate measurement of the outcomes of intervention. The COPM is intended for use by occupational therapists but is also appropriate to use in a multidisciplinary team setting. The COPM identifies self-perception of skills in the areas of self-care, leisure, and productivity across the life span. Goals for the bout of intervention can be developed in relation to the individual's perception of strengths and challenges. The COPM can be purchased at the following website: http://www.thecopm.ca/buy/.

An alternative method to assess functional goal attainment can be through use of the Goal Attainment Scale (GAS). GAS allows for the measurement of criterion-referenced, individualized, functional goal achievement. The 5-point rating scale of the GAS ranges from −2 (outcome much less than expected) to +2 (outcome much greater than expected). GAS goals should be written so that the interval between scores −2 and −1 are the same as scores between +1 and +2. A score of 0 represents achievement of the intended goal. Therapist training in GAS goal writing is recommended to improve accuracy and reliability.[34]

PEGS, COPM, and GAS are all recommendations from the APTA Academy of Pediatric Physical Therapy's CPG.[13]

Case Study

Goals for Ryan include the following:

Goal 1	
+2	Ryan can jump forward 15 inches for more than 8 consecutive jumps, demonstrating bilateral foot clearance in each jump.
+1	Ryan can jump forward 15 inches for 8 consecutive jumps, demonstrating bilateral foot clearance in each jump.
0	Ryan can jump forward 15 inches for 5 consecutive jumps, demonstrating bilateral foot clearance in each jump.
−1	Ryan can jump forward 15 inches for 3 consecutive jumps, demonstrating bilateral foot clearance in each jump.
−2	Ryan can jump forward 15 inches for 1 jump, demonstrating bilateral foot clearance.

Goal 2	
+2	Ryan can ascend and descend 20 stairs using a reciprocal gait pattern without the use of a rail during a change of class with high traffic.
+1	Ryan can ascend and descend 15 stairs using a reciprocal gait pattern without the use of a rail during a change of class with high traffic.
0	Ryan can ascend and descend 10 stairs using a reciprocal gait pattern without the use of a rail during a change of class with high traffic.
−1	Ryan can ascend and descend 5 stairs using a reciprocal gait pattern without the use of a rail during a change of class with high traffic.
−2	Ryan can ascend and descend 5 stairs using a reciprocal gait pattern with the use of a rail during a change of class with high traffic.

Goal 3	
+2	Ryan can independently get up and down from the floor while holding an item with both hands, using a 1/2 kneel to stand pattern within 3 seconds, without touching another object or person.
+1	Ryan can independently get up and down from the floor, using a 1/2 kneel to stand pattern without touching another object or person during the transition within 3 seconds.
0	Ryan can independently get up and down from the floor, using a 1/2 kneel to stand pattern without touching another object or person during the transition within 5 seconds.
−1	Ryan can independently get up and down from the floor, using a 1/2 kneel to stand pattern without touching another object or person during the transition within 7 seconds.
−2	Ryan can independently get up and down from the floor, using one hand on chair to push up moving through a 1/2 kneel to stand pattern without touching another object or person during the transition within 7 seconds.

Goal 4	
+2	Ryan can maintain pace with peers while walking in line from drop off to the classroom (350 ft), stopping and starting as necessary without stepping out of line or bumping into peers.
+1	Ryan can maintain pace with peers while walking in line to the cafeteria (250 ft), stopping and starting as necessary without stepping out of line or bumping into peers.
0	Ryan can maintain pace with peers while walking in line to the playground (150 ft), stopping and starting as necessary without stepping out of line or bumping into peers.
−1	Ryan can maintain pace with peers while walking in line to the playground (150 ft), stepping out of line or bumping into peers no more than 2 times.
−2	Ryan can maintain pace with peers while walking in line to the playground (150 ft), stepping out of line or bumping into peers more than 2 times.

Goal 5	
+2	Ryan can run 100 ft, demonstrating reciprocal arm swing and flight phase of gait on the school playground (wood chips) on 2 separate occasions during 1 recess period without a loss of balance or fall.
+1	Ryan can run for 75 ft, demonstrating reciprocal arm swing and flight phase of gait on the school playground (wood chips) on 2 separate occasions during 1 recess period without a loss of balance or fall.
0	Ryan can run for 50 ft, demonstrating reciprocal arm swing and flight phase of gait on the school playground (wood chips) on 2 separate occasions during 1 recess period without a loss of balance or fall.
−1	Ryan can run for 25 ft, demonstrating reciprocal arm swing and flight phase of gait on the school playground (wood chips) on 2 separate occasions during 1 recess period without a loss of balance or fall.
−2	Ryan can walk quickly for 50 ft, demonstrating reciprocal arm swing on the school playground (wood chips) on 2 separate occasions during 1 recess period without a loss of balance or fall.

INTERVENTION

General Teaching and Learning Strategies

Individuals with DCD require specific teaching strategies to meet their unique learning needs. There are 2 general methods to approach the treatment of DCD. A bottom-up approach uses the process of the motor task as the focus for teaching. Components of the task are broken down. Task analysis (see example in Table 12-2) can help to identify challenges and organize interventions. Bottom-up approaches treat the underlying deficit. Sensory integration or perceptual motor therapies are an example of such an approach.

In a top-down approach, the functional task is the focus. The top-down approach uses cognition to drive motor output.[32,35,36] Specific attention to successful task completion is the hallmark of a top-down approach. Successful programs incorporate a multifaceted approach to treatment that includes attention to both the execution of the components of a task and the whole task.

Improved outcomes in the treatment of DCD have been related to large training doses and skill practice at high frequencies.[13,37] Intervention programs with frequent practice (4-5 times per week) and those that lasted longer than 9 weeks significantly increased motor performance.[37] These findings are in line with the challenges in learning and generalization that individuals with DCD experience. While there is significant evidence that motor intervention yields strong immediate effects, longer term effects are not sustained. Consistent practice is necessary to maintain newly developed skills.[37]

Typically, individuals with DCD are not able to acquire skills simply by watching others perform that skill. Strategies that include direct teaching and task-specific training have been shown to be of benefit in promoting motor skills.[36] Suggestions for successful teaching include the following:

- Practice of skills in a part-to-whole sequence. This sequence involves practice of the component parts of a skill with advancement of practice toward the ultimate skill.
- Practice the concrete skill. If the goal is for the individual to learn to catch and throw, design the intervention to use an object to catch and throw. If the goal is to learn to independently swing on a swing, the intervention should include that specific skill.
- Encourage attention to the important aspects of the motor skill. Attending to one aspect of the skill at a time may be helpful to decrease frustration and increase success.
- Talk through requisite components of the skill with the individual. Ask probing questions, such as the following: "What do you think you will need to do to be successful at this skill?" "What parts do you think might be challenging for you?" "What strategies might you use to address those challenges?" This approach leverages the verbal skills of this population and increases movement toward independent function.
- Provide opportunities for generalization. Try the skill in a variety of places and under a variety of conditions.
- Celebrate success, no matter how small.

Treatment

Successful treatment includes direct teaching of the expected skill. Early practice may need to occur within a closed environment with limited distraction. Later practice should occur in the environment in which this skill is expected because generalization can be challenging. As the individual demonstrates improved proficiency with each task, variability in the task should become the priority. Changing the speed, postural position, or weight-bearing surface; varying the distance or size of the target; or altering the materials and/or environment may all contribute to task variability. Studies have suggested that greater success is seen when the task has a competitive component and includes the need to develop a strategy for successful completion. These strategies may optimize motor learning and skill acquisition.[38] Task-specific intervention has been shown to have an immediate impact on those specific activities. However, additional investigation needs to take place to determine if this approach has a positive effect on participation in physical activity and well-being.[39]

Purposeful incorporation of tasks requiring a cognitive component during intervention has also been shown to improve results. Cognitive orientation to daily occupational performance has been shown to improve task knowledge of children with DCD.[40-42] This evidence-based program addresses skill acquisition in child-chosen tasks, the development of cognitive strategies associated with those tasks, and generalization of those tasks across environments.[43]

Use of task visualization and imagery may enhance improvements in motor function.[44] Individuals with DCD have difficulty with the ability to predict necessary movement, leading to challenges with accurate motor planning. Use of guided imagery or developing a clear mental representation of the motor task may help individuals with DCD to develop improved motor control.[45] Practice includes imagining successful completion of all the components of a motor task from beginning to end.

Attention to the developmental level of the individual should be given when incorporating visualization and imagery. The ability to participate successfully in imagery increases throughout childhood but does not reach adult levels until mid to late adolescence.[46] Use of visual imagery has been successful in pediatric rehabilitation in typically developing children as young as 5 years of age. It has also been used successfully in populations with disabilities.[46]

Practice and experience should be designed to alter the sensory-motor loop to drive reorganization. This reorganization can be encouraged through sensory-rich play. Strategies may include use of mirrors, heavy work, body weight training, and other sensory-based activities. Engaging in sensory-rich activities may enhance the ability to effectively receive, interpret, and respond to incoming information. Sensory integration activities may also promote greater awareness of body in space and opportunities for self-monitoring.[47] When these activities are selected and applied to patients based on their unique needs, motor outcomes may be improved (**Table 12-4**).[33,48]

TABLE 12-4 • Examples of Vestibular/Proprioceptive Activities

Potential Vestibular/ Proprioceptive Activities	Ideas for the Classroom
Weight bearing: Creeping and bear walking activities	Wrap resistance bands around the legs of the classroom chair to provide sensory input
Wheelbarrow or crab walking activities: progress to movement over a variety of surfaces	Carry "weighted" items to other classrooms/office Push open and hold doors
Bouncing: on a ball, half ball, trampoline	Wall or chair push ups
Working on suspended equipment: stretchy swings, platform swings, bouncing swings, body weight suspension	Use an inflatable or gel-filled wedge or cushion in the child's desk chair
Use of scooter boards: sitting, supine, push/pull	Use of a weighted lap pad or vest
Balance activities: on balls, tilt boards, foam	Stretching or yoga poses
Climbing: up and down playground equipment	Use of a rocking chair
Rolling: log or egg rolling	Head, neck, and shoulder rolls

Case Study

During his examination, it was found that Ryan's response to sensory stimulation was delayed. For this reason, preparatory sensory-based activities occurred at the start of each physical therapy session. These activities included use of the vibration plate, jumping on a trampoline, swinging on suspended equipment, use of stretchy tunnels, and pushing/pulling/carrying heavier items when helping to set up during the therapy session. All these activities were of high interest to Ryan and compliance was easily gained.

Therapeutic Interventions

Direct instruction and direct practice of the specific skill will be utilized as teaching strategies. Initial skill practice will occur in the closed environment of the therapy room. Generalization of skill will be supported by progressive introduction into the open environment of the school building and playground.

Activities

At a minimum, one activity during session will be of patient's choice. Sessions will include some activities that are familiar to Ryan.

Obstacle course to include: planning for movement execution, transitions between postures, and balance activities. Ryan will help to set up.

Functional strengthening activities to include: squatting to standing, lift and carry, up and down from ground, wheelbarrow/bear/tiptoe and heel walking. Attention will be given to midrange control and endurance.

Practice of functional skills to include: stairs, jumping, climbing, running, throw/catch/kick.

Practice of higher-level coordination skills to include: hop, skip, rope jumping, bike riding, and mountain climbers/jumping jacks.

All activities to include repetition of movement patterns.

Equipment: scooter boards, wedges, foam surfaces, ladders (floor and upright), suspended equipment, bolsters, floor targets, balls, metronome, stopwatch, free weights, weighted vest.

CONSULTATION

Because the challenges experienced by individuals with DCD can influence function across many settings, consultation is an important part of any plan of care. Establishing consistent expectations for function and intervention in all environments fosters generalization of skills. Sharing of successful strategies enhances efficient movement toward established goals. Consultation with and education of teachers, support staff, families, coaches, and the children with a diagnosis of DCD may promote understanding and create additional opportunities for skill practice throughout the day.[39]

Providing individuals with DCD with environmental modifications may enhance successful participation. In the classroom, providing opportunities for movement breaks, preferential seating, placing the individual's cubby or locker at the edge of the room, providing support for floor sitting activities, providing a seat for dressing/undressing, and allowing additional time to "get ready" may help.

For physical education class and recess, provide direct teaching of expected skills. Preteaching of more challenging motor skills may be necessary to maximize participation. Providing auditory cues for attention to specific, important portions of the skill to be executed may help. An example of this strategy might be saying "hands up" when expected to catch a ball. Visual cues may also be used to aid in awareness. Providing brightly colored dots for stationary tasks or for movement tasks requiring accuracy may assist with training to use external cues for performance. Use of a peer model may also promote increased participation. Self-assessment may also promote awareness of performance. Asking "How did that go?" and following up with "What do you think you might do to make that even better?" may facilitate greater independence in function. Asking these questions should occur with attention to sensitivity and encouraging continued participation. Using materials that slow down skills like catching, throwing, and kicking may increase successful participation. Beanbags, foam balls, and larger balls and racquets can be helpful. Engagement and effort should be the focus of physical education class.

Participation in community settings is important to establish active lifelong leisure activities. Research has shown that children with DCD become older children and adults who participate less frequently in physical activity and demonstrate lower tolerance for exercise. Slight adaptations may enhance success and enjoyment in community participation. Establishing appropriate activities that allow successful participation and access to peers will improve compliance. Open communication can help to establish interests. Adults can help to identify supports in the community to promote inclusion in a positive, reinforcing manner. Individual sports, such as walking, swimming, and karate,[12] may be best for children and adults in this population. Evidence supporting the efficacy of these interventions is sufficient to support their recommendation. Evidence for other interventions, such as the active gaming systems, core stability training, table tennis, and aquatic therapy, is not as strong. Therefore, their use cannot be recommended at this time.[47]

Understanding how the individual's impairments are linked to observable challenges with activities can empower adults to provide appropriate supports. Providing education to community partners, such as coaches, teachers, and activity instructors, can be helpful in promoting success. This education may take the form a well-designed pamphlet or as part of a lunch-and-learn series. Team sports where the coach is well informed regarding the diagnosis of DCD and is able to accommodate potential needs can also facilitate a positive experience. Appropriate support of children and adolescents over the course of development is necessary to maximize outcomes.

Case Study

The school PT discussed Ryan's plan of care and expectations with this school-based team, including his parents. The team discussed necessary supports and potential barriers to implementing the proposed plan of care. Together, the team was able to identify possible solutions to maximize outcomes. Ryan's teachers were provided a list of activities for Ryan and the rest of his class to engage in for movement breaks. These activities were offered multiple times during the school day. Ryan's teacher has commented that they seem to make a "big difference" in attention for all the children in the class.

■ CONCLUSION

DCD is a neurodevelopmental condition that describes individuals who have difficulty completing tasks that are common to everyday function. Challenges with planning and sequencing of these tasks are common. Impairments in strength, motor planning, coordination, and executive function contribute to these challenges. While there are evidenced strategies that assist children with functional limitations associated with DCD, difficulties may persist as life demands evolve. Children with DCD become adults with DCD. For this reason, intervention should be carried out with an eye toward life transitions. Planning for transitions to new schools, driving, and developing skills related to vocation and avocations should be at the center of the plan of care. Modifications to plans, schedules, tools, and worksites may be necessary to maximize success.

Individuals with DCDs should be involved in all aspects of decision-making across the life span. Goals and activities should be designed to maximize independent function and promote quality of life. By using modified teaching approaches to meet the needs of children with DCD, effective strategies can be established to minimize the impact of this diagnosis in later childhood, adolescence, and adulthood. Education and consultation are necessary components of care. When the community surrounding the child understands and is empowered, outcomes can be maximized.

STUDY QUESTIONS

1. What are strategies that might be used to educate teachers, parents, health care providers, and children about developmental coordination disorder (DCD) to promote appropriate recognition and referral?

2. What specific activities of daily living would likely be challenging for children with DCD? What are strategies for addressing those challenges?

3. Is a group therapy setting appropriate for children with DCD? Under what circumstances and for what reasons?

4. How might challenges with generalization be approached within the school as the child ages?

5. What are potential suggestions for preparing for transitions to:
   a. Middle school
   b. High school
   c. College/workplace

6. For a child with DCD who is challenged with participating in a physical education unit on jump rope, what are specific strategies/interventions that would be appropriate to try? What consultation/education would be necessary?

7. What information is important for parents to know? How might they be encouraged to carry over expectations to the home environment?

8. What might a home exercise program look like for a child with DCD at the following ages?
   a. At age 6
   b. At age 10
   c. At age 16

9. When do social-emotional challenges rise to the level of requiring a referral to a mental health care professional?

10. What are potential challenges for the adult with DCD? How might they be addressed through physical therapy?

References

1. Miyahara M, Register C. Perceptions of three terms to describe physical awkwardness in children. *Res Dev Disabil.* 2000;21(5): 367-376.
2. World Health Organization. Specific developmental disorder of motor function F82. In: *International Classification of Diseases.* World Health Organization; 1992:250-252.
3. Wilson PH, Ruddock S, Smits-Engelsman B, Polatajko H, Blank R. Understanding performance deficits in developmental coordination disorder: a meta-analysis of recent research. *Dev Med Child Neurol.* 2013;55:217-228.
4. Van Hoorn JF, Schoemaker MM, Stuive I, et al. Risk factors in early life for developmental coordination disorder: a scoping review. *Dev Med Child Neurol.* 2021;63(5):511-519.
5. Zhu JL, Olsen J, Olesen AW. Risk for developmental coordination disorder correlates with gestational age at birth. *Paediatr Perinatal Epidemiol.* 2012;26(6):572-577.
6. Wilson PH, Smits-Engelsman B, Caeyenberghs K, et al. Cognitive and neuroimaging findings in developmental coordination

disorder: new insights from a systematic review of recent research. *Dev Med Child Neurol.* 2017;59(11):1117-1129.

7. Caçola P, Getchell N, Srinivasan D, Alexandrakis G, Liu H. Cortical activity in fine-motor tasks in children with developmental coordination disorder: a preliminary fNIRS study. *Int J Dev Neurosci.* 2018;65:83-90.

8. Hyde C, Fuelscher I, Williams J, et al. Corticospinal excitability during motor imagery is reduced in young adults with developmental coordination disorder. *Res Dev Disabil.* 2018;72:214-224.

9. Hannant P, Cassidy S, de Weyer Van R, Mooncey S. Sensory and motor differences in autism spectrum conditions and developmental coordination disorder in children: a cross-syndrome study. *Hum Move Sci.* 2018;58:108-118.

10. American Psychiatric Association. *Diagnostic and Statistical Manual of Mental Disorders.* 5th ed. American Psychiatric Association; 2013.

11. Zwicker JG, Lee EJ. Early intervention for children with/at risk of developmental coordination disorder: a scoping review. *Dev Med Child Neurol.* 2021;63(6):659-667.

12. American Physical Therapy Association. *Guide to Physical Therapy Practice 3.0.* American Physical Therapy Association; 2019:3.

13. Dannemiller L, Mueller M, Leitner A, Iverson E, Kaplan SL. Physical therapy management of children with developmental coordination disorder: an evidence-based clinical practice guideline from the Academy of Pediatric Physical Therapy of the American Physical Therapy Association. *Pediatr Phys Ther.* 2020;32(4):278-313.

14. Wilson BN, Crawford SG, Green D, Roberts G, Aylott A, Kaplan BJ. Psychometric properties of the revised developmental coordination disorder questionnaire. *Phys Occup Ther Pediatr.* 2009;29(2):184-204.

15. Rosenblum S. The development and standardization of the Children Activity Scales (ChAS-P/T) for the early identification of children with developmental coordination disorders. *Child Care Health Dev.* 2006;32(6):619-632.

16. Giofre D, Cornoldi C, Schoemaker MM. Identifying developmental coordination disorder: MOQ-T validity as a fast screening instrument based on teachers' ratings and its relationship with praxis and visuospatial working memory deficits. *Res Dev Disabil.* 2014;35(12):3518-3525.

17. Hay JA. Adequacy in and predilection for physical activity. *Clin J Sport Med.* 1992;2(3):192-201.

18. Tseng YT, Tsai CL, Chen FC, Konczak J. Position sense dysfunction affects proximal and distal arm joints in children with developmental coordination disorder. *J Mot Behav.* 2019;51(1):49-58.

19. Goyen TA, Lui K, Hummel J. Sensorimotor skills associated with motor dysfunction in children born extremely preterm. *Early Hum Dev.* 2011;87(7):489-494.

20. Farhat F, Hsairi I, Baiti H, et al. Assessment of physical fitness and exercise tolerance in children with developmental coordination disorder. *Res Dev Disabil.* 2015;45-46:210-219.

21. Wilson PH, Smits-Engelsman B, Caeyenberghs K, et al. Cognitive and neuroimaging findings in developmental coordination disorder: new insights from a systematic review of recent research. *Dev Med Child Neurol.* 2017;59(11):1117-1129.

22. Bernardi M, Leonard HC, Hill EL, Botting N, Henry LA. Executive functions in children with developmental coordination disorder: a 2-year follow-up study. *Dev Med Child Neurol.* 2018;60(3):306-313.

23. Farhat F, Masmoudi K, Cairney J, Hsairi I, Triki C, Moalla W. Assessment of cardiorespiratory and neuromotor fitness in children with developmental coordination disorder. *Res Dev Disabil.* 2014;35(12):3554-3561.

24. Yu J, Sit CH, Capio CM, Burnett A, Ha AS, Huang WY. Fundamental movement skills proficiency in children with developmental coordination disorder: does physical self-concept matter? *Disabil Rehabil.* 2016;38(1):45-51.

25. Farhat F, Hsairi I, Baiti H, et al. Assessment of physical fitness and exercise tolerance in children with developmental coordination disorder. *Res Dev Disabil.* 2015;45:210-219.

26. Crane L, Sumner E, Hill EL. Emotional and behavioural problems in children with developmental coordination disorder: exploring parent and teacher reports. *Res Dev Disabil.* 2017;70:67-74.

27. Harrowell I, Hollén L, Lingam R, Emond A. The impact of developmental coordination disorder on educational achievement in secondary school. *Res Dev Disabil.* 2018;72:13-22.

28. Blank R, Smits-Engelsman BO, Polatajko H, Wilson P. European Academy for Childhood Disability (EACD): recommendations on the definition, diagnosis and intervention of developmental coordination disorder (long version). *Dev Med Child Neurol.* 2012;54(1):54-93.

29. Green D, Lingam R, Mattocks C, Riddoch C, Ness A, Emond A. The risk of reduced physical activity in children with probable developmental coordination disorder: a prospective longitudinal study. *Res Dev Disabil.* 2011;32(4):1332-1342.

30. Gagnon-Roy M, Jasmin E, Camden C. Social participation of teenagers and young adults with developmental co-ordination disorder and strategies that could help them: results from a scoping review. *Child Care Health Dev.* 2016;42(6):840-851.

31. Tamplain P, Miller HL. What can we do to promote mental health among individuals with developmental coordination disorder? *Curr Dev Disorders Rep.* 2021;8(1):24-31.

32. Goulardins JB, Rigoli D, Licari M, et al. Attention deficit hyperactivity disorder and developmental coordination disorder: two separate disorders or do they share a common etiology. *Behav Brain Res.* 2015;292:484-492.

33. Missiuna C, Pollock N, Law M, Walter S, Cavey N. Examination of the Perceived Efficacy and Goal Setting System (PEGS) with children with disabilities, their parents, and teachers. *Am J Occup Ther.* 2006;60(2):204-214.

34. Turner-Stokes L. Goal attainment scaling (GAS) in rehabilitation: a practical guide. *Clin Rehabil.* 2009;23(4):362-370.

35. Smits-Engelsman B, Vinçon S, Blank R, Quadrado VH, Polatajko H, Wilson PH. Evaluating the evidence for motor-based interventions in developmental coordination disorder: a systematic review and meta-analysis. *Res Devel Disabil.* 2018;74:72-102.

36. Smits-Englesman BO, Blank R, Van Der Kaay AC, et al. Efficacy of interventions to improve motor performance in children with developmental coordination disorder: a combined systematic review and meta-analysis. *Dev Med Child Neurol.* 2013;55(3):229-237.

37. Jane JY, Burnett AF, Sit CH. Motor skill interventions in children with developmental coordination disorder: a systematic review and meta-analysis. *Arch Phys Med Rehabil.* 2018;99(10):2076-2099.

38. Lucas BR, Elliott EJ, Coggan S, et al. Interventions to improve gross motor performance in children with neurodevelopmental disorders: a meta-analysis. *BMC Pediatr.* 2016;16(1):193.

39. Offor N, Ossom Williamson P, Caçola P. Effectiveness of interventions for children with developmental coordination disorder in physical therapy contexts: a systematic literature review and meta-analysis. *J Mot Learn Dev.* 2016;4(2):169-196.

40. Mandich A, Polatajko HJ. *Enabling Occupation in Children: The Cognitive Orientation to Daily Occupational Performance*

(CO-OP) Approach. Canadian Association of Occupational Therapists; 2004.

41. Sangster CA, Beninger C, Polatajko HJ, Mandich A. Cognitive strategy generation in children with developmental coordination disorder. *Can J Occup Ther.* 2005;72(2):67-77.

42. Rodger S, Brandenburg J. Cognitive Orientation to (daily) Occupational Performance (CO-OP) with children with Asperger's syndrome who have motor-based occupational performance goals. *Aust Occup Ther J.* 2009;56(1):41-50.

43. Missiuna C, Mandich AD, Polatajko HJ, Malloy-Miller T. Cognitive Orientation to Daily Occupational Performance (CO-OP) part I: theoretical foundations. *Phys Occup Ther Pediatr.* 2001; 20(2-3):69-81.

44. Adams IL, Smits-Engelsman B, Lust JM, Wilson PH, Steenbergen B. Feasibility of motor imagery training for children with developmental coordination disorder: a pilot study. *Front Psychol.* 2017;8:1271.

45. Williams J, Omizzolo C, Galea MP, Vance A. Motor imagery skills of children with attention deficit hyperactivity disorder and developmental coordination disorder. *Hum Move Sci.* 2013;32(1):121-135.

46. Spruijt S, van der Kamp J, Steenbergen B. Current insights in the development of children's motor imagery ability. *Front Psychol.* 2015;6:787.

47. Preston N, Magallón S, Hill LJ, Andrews E, Ahern SM, Mon-Williams M. A systematic review of high quality randomized controlled trials investigating motor skill programmes for children with developmental coordination disorder. *Clin Rehabil.* 2017;31(7):857-870.

48. El Shemy SA, Mohamed NE. Effect of sensory integration on motor performance and balance in children with developmental coordination disorder: a randomized controlled trial. *Int J Ther Rehabil Res.* 2017;6(1):1-9.

49. Hunt J, Zwicker JG, Godecke E, Raynor A. Awareness and knowledge of developmental coordination disorder: a survey of caregivers, teachers, allied health professionals and medical professionals in Australia. *Child Care Health Dev.* 2021;47(2):174-183.

13

Vestibular Disorders

Jennifer Parent-Nichols, DPT, EdD

■ INTRODUCTION

For the human balance system to function at its most efficiently, it relies on contributions from proprioceptive, visual, and vestibular components. The vestibular system is composed of central and peripheral components that provide information necessary for spatial orientation.

CENTRAL COMPONENTS

Information regarding the estimation of head orientation is sent from the peripheral nervous system to the central vestibular system, where it is processed and output is provided to the ocular muscles and spinal cord. Three primary vestibular responses result from this output. The vestibulo-ocular reflex (VOR) stabilizes visual images on the fovea. This reflex allows vision to remain clear when the head is in motion. Should the VOR be impaired, complaints of double vision or dizziness may occur (**Figure 13-1**). The vestibulospinal reflex (VSR) helps to maintain postural stability, especially during head movement. When the VSR is affected injury, an individual may be observed to lean toward the side of involvement. This posture results from unilateral input regarding head position from the uninjured side. The vestibulocollic reflex (VCR) works to maintain head position on the neck by stabilizing the neck muscles. The VOR works closely with the VCR. Should the VOR not work adequately to stabilize visual images, the VCR may become overactive in an attempt to limit head movement.

PERIPHERAL COMPONENTS

The peripheral vestibular system (**Figure 13-2**) is made up of a membranous labyrinth housed in each of the 2 temporal bones. Each labyrinth contains 3 semicircular canals. These organs detect the angular acceleration of the head in space and are filled with endolymph that moves freely in response to head rotation and tilting. These 3 canals are oriented in a (1) horizontal, (2) anterior, and (3) posterior orientation and are labeled according to that orientation. The left and right anterior and posterior canals have a more vertical orientation, so there is greater redundancy in the information received from head movement in these planes. When symptoms of vestibular dysfunction do occur, they are more likely to result from horizontal canal involvement because there is less redundancy in information.

To detect linear acceleration of the head in space and head tilt, each labyrinth also contains 2 otolith organs: the utricle and the saccule. The utricle has open communication with the semicircular canals and provides information regarding orientation to gravity and movement in the horizontal plane. This information contributes to postural control. The role of the saccule is less understood, but it may detect vertical movement of the head in space, such as when riding in an elevator.

The vestibular portion of the eighth cranial nerve (CN8) is also considered part of the peripheral vestibular system. The left and right side of the vestibulocochlear nerve have an established resting firing rate. In normal function, when one side of this

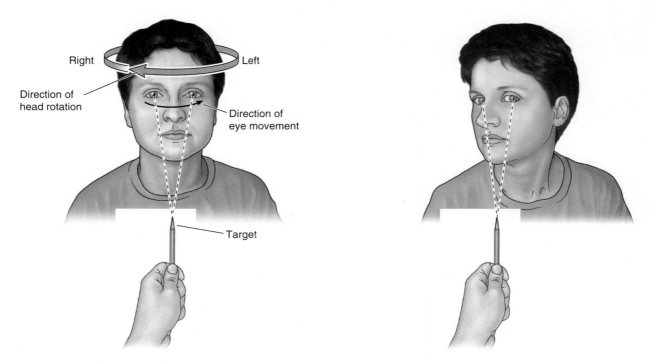

FIGURE 13-1 **The vestibulo-ocular reflex.** (Reproduced with permission from Martin J. *Neuroanatomy Text and Atlas*. 4th ed. McGraw Hill; 2012.)

nerve is excited, the contralateral side is equally inhibited. This equivalent excitation and inhibition occur because of endolymph flow in the semicircular canals. An enlarged area at the end of each semicircular canal, the ampulla, contains a gelatinous barrier that holds sensory hair cells. Angular head acceleration causes the endolymph in the semicircular canals to move in a direction opposite of head movement. This flow causes the hair cells in the ampulla to bend, like the bending of seaweed caused by ocean waves. The hairs are deflected toward the largest hair

filament on the side to which rotation is occurring, the ipsilateral side. This deflection causes an increased firing rate of CN8. Contralateral to the head motion, hairs are deflected away from the largest filament, decreasing the firing rate. In summary, when the vestibular system is functioning properly, the firing rate of CN8 increases on the side to which the head is turned and decreases on the side to which the head is turned away. The resulting difference in firing rates from the right and left side lets the brain know the head is in motion.

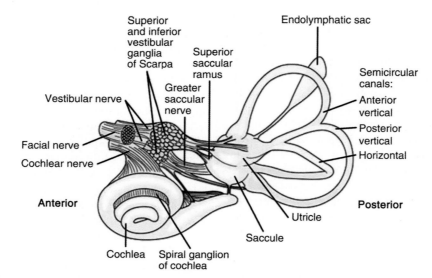

FIGURE 13-2 **Vestibular labyrinths. This schematic illustrates the relationship of the cochlea and the components of the vestibular labyrinth: the vestibule with its saccule and the utricle and the 3 semicircular canals.** (Reproduced with permission from Kandel ER, Schwartz JH, Jessell TM, Siegelbaum SA, Hudspeth AJ. *Principles of Neural Science.* 4th ed. McGraw Hill; 2000.)

VESTIBULAR DYSFUNCTION IN THE PEDIATRIC POPULATION

Dizziness in the pediatric population occurs with approximately a 5% to 10% prevalence, making the diagnosis not infrequent.[1-3] For many of these children, the source of these challenges is related to vestibular dysfunction. In children, disorders of the vestibular system may result in vertigo, challenges with balance, and delays in motor development. Challenges with schoolwork, physical activity, and social interactions are common.[4] Younger children may have difficulty describing the symptoms associated with vestibular dysfunction. Instead, observation of their behaviors may provide important information. Resisting up and down or rotational movements, holding tight to parents, eye closing during movement, and "shutting down" or falling asleep during movement activities may indicate the child is experiencing dizziness. Feelings of falling when not and sensation of the room moving around them may be described by older children.

Pathologies of the vestibular system, or vestibulopathies, may be of central or peripheral origin. Those vestibulopathies arising from central origin may require a longer time to rehabilitate.[5] Specific pediatric diagnoses may present more frequently with central vestibular dysfunction, including cerebral palsy, myelomeningocele, vestibular migraine, attention-deficit/hyperactivity disorder, developmental coordination disorder, concussion, childhood cancer, congenital muscular torticollis, and autism.[6] Sources of central vestibulopathies can be found in **Table 13-1**.

Vestibulopathies originating in the peripheral vestibular system may be unilateral or bilateral. Peripheral pathology of the vestibular system typically results in a change in the resting firing rate of CN8 on one side (unilateral) or both sides (bilateral). In the case of unilateral vestibular dysfunction, the resting firing rate of the affected side of CN8 is decreased when compared to the healthy, contralateral side. This lower rate of firing is referred to as unilateral vestibular hypofunction (UVH). This difference in firing rate results in an information mismatch and the potential for the perception that the head is moving when, in fact, it is not. Individuals with UVH will report that they experience *vertigo*, a sensation of turning, even when they are standing still.

Remember that the rate of firing increases on the ipsilateral side to which the head is turned (**Figure 13-3**). Because of the mismatch in firing rate in UVH, the individual perceives that

TABLE 13-1 • Sources of Central Vestibulopathy[7-9]

Acquired brain injury, including concussion
Cerebellar degeneration
Cerebral vascular accident (CVA; stroke)
Demyelinating disease
Migraine, including vestibular migraine
Seizure disorder
Tumors

they are always turning toward the side of healthy vestibular function even when at rest. In the case of bilateral vestibular hypofunction, it is possible that the individual will not report vertigo if firing from both sides is equally decreased. Sources of peripheral vestibulopathy can be found in **Table 13-2**.

It is important to note that benign paroxysmal positional vertigo (BPPV) is a mechanical issue and does not result from damage to the peripheral nervous system. Peripheral dysfunction of the vestibular system responds quite well to intervention, with the treatment of BPPV having the greatest success.[11,12]

Central and peripheral vestibular dysfunction typically differ in evolution, symptom experience, and test and measure outcomes. It is important to distinguish the etiology of signs and symptoms commonly experienced with these diagnoses so that proper intervention can be developed. **Table 13-3** delineates general signs and symptoms of central versus peripheral dysfunction. **Table 13-4** provides examples of pediatric diagnoses that may lend themselves to central and peripheral vestibular dysfunction.

THE INTERNATIONAL CLASSIFICATION OF FUNCTIONING, DISABILITY, AND HEALTH MODEL

With vestibular dysfunction, common impairments in body structure and function can be seen in balance, oscillopsia, dizziness, vertigo, motion sensitivity, and limited range of motion and strength of the cervical spine. Depending on the type and severity of symptoms experienced by individuals diagnosed with vestibulopathy, activity restrictions may include limitations in activities of daily living, vocational or avocational activities, and driving. Fear avoidance may cause individuals with vestibular dysfunction not to participate in community activities when their movement or the movement of others may increase their symptoms.[17,18]

VESTIBULOPATHIES AND PHYSICAL THERAPY

The skill set of physical therapists (PTs) fits well with the examination, evaluation, and management of individuals with vestibulopathy.[19] A moderate level of evidence supports the use of specific exercise techniques to target identified impairments or functional limitations. The same level of evidence supports supervised vestibular rehabilitation by clinicians. General recommendations include patient education aimed at understanding programmatic goals and increasing patient independence in managing their specific symptoms. As in other diagnoses, an effective home exercise program is critical to patient success.[20]

> **Note**
>
> Before engaging in evaluation and/or treatment of the vestibular system, it is of great importance that clinicians assess the stability of the cervical ligaments and patency of the vertebrobasilar artery. Clearing of these structures must occur before moving patients into positions that may create risk for them should integrity be compromised.[21]

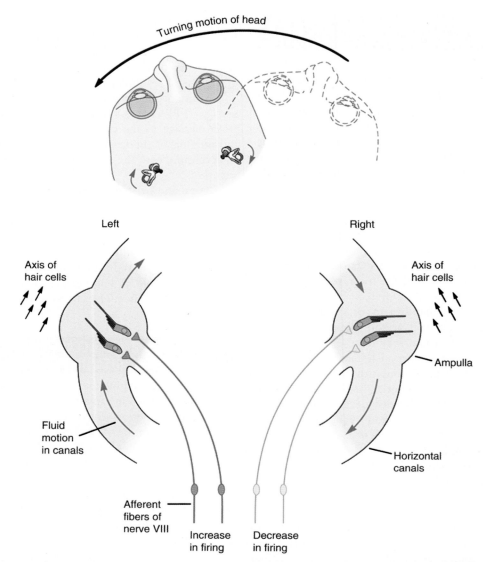

FIGURE 13-3 Complimentary function between the pairs of semicircular canals (SCCs). This schematic illustrates the push-pull relationship of the complimentary SCC pairings. With a slight head turn to the left, the left hair cells are excited, moving toward the kinocilium while the hair cells in the right canal are inhibited (moving away from the kinocilium) in association with the movement of the endolymph. (Reproduced with permission from Kandel ER, Schwartz JH, Jessell TM, Siegelbaum SA, Hudspeth AJ. Principles of Neural Science. 5th ed. McGraw Hill; 2013.)

TABLE 13-2 • Sources of Peripheral Vestibulopathy[4,7,8]
Vestibular schwannoma (acoustic neuroma)
Ototoxicity (damage occurs to the vestibulocochlear nerve resulting from exposure to drugs or chemicals; typically, bilateral presentation)
Ménière disease
Perilymphatic fistula
Vestibular neuritis/labyrinthitis
Benign paroxysmal vertigo of childhood (BPCV) (Recurrent episodes of acute dizziness typically are seen in children <6 years old. BPCV does not usually result in nystagmus.)
Chronic otitis media[10]
Benign paroxysmal positional vertigo (BPPV)

■ WHAT APPEAR TO BE VESTIBULAR SYMPTOMS ARE NOT ALWAYS VESTIBULAR IN ORIGIN

It is always important to conduct a thorough differential diagnosis (**Table 13-5**). This indication is particularly true when assessing potential vestibular dysfunction. Ligamentous instability, vascular disorders, and cervicogenic dysfunction must first be ruled out. These diagnoses present similarly but require significantly different interventions from those aimed at the treatment of vestibulopathy.

Symptoms like vestibulopathy may also be experienced with cervicogenic dysfunction (CGD). Impairments in the cervical spine may create a sensory mismatch among the proprioceptive, visual, and vestibular systems. These symptoms can result from either acquired or traumatic cervical spine dysfunction.

TABLE 13-3 • General Signs and Symptoms of Central Versus Peripheral Vestibular Dysfunction[11,12]

Central	Peripheral
More insidious onset of symptoms	Sudden onset
Vague symptoms	True vertigo
Consistent reports of subjective vertigo (feeling of spinning within own head)	Head movement–provoked symptoms lasting <2 minutes
Direction-changing nystagmus	Direction-fixed nystagmus
Post–head shake nystagmus, primarily vertical or torsional	Post–head shake, increased nystagmus in the horizontal direction, increased speed when looking in direction of nystagmus (Alexander's law)
Increased likelihood of abnormal pursuit and saccade testing	Normal pursuit and saccade testing, abnormal vestibulo-ocular reflex testing

Symptoms indicating CGD may include cervical spine pathology with headache and/or neck pain, complaints of dizziness without true experience of vertigo (spinning), decreased active cervical range of motion, decreased cervical muscle strength, and abnormal postural control.[21,22] Tests and measures to examine CGD and related interventions are listed in **Table 13-6**.

An adequate examination of potential vestibulopathy requires a thorough subjective history. Past medical history questions should include clarification of complaints. Understanding symptom onset, duration, activation, and activities that exacerbate or dampen symptoms is important to developing an accurate working diagnosis. The Motion Sensitivity Quotient (MSQ) is a free survey that can enhance data collection about symptoms of dizziness. This measure evaluates 16 different head and body positions in which the patient indicates the intensity and duration of symptoms of dizziness. Scores for these attributes are summed, and a motion sensitivity quotient is calculated.[25]

The Pediatric Vestibular Symptom Questionnaire (PVSQ) has been developed to quantify subjective self-reported symptoms of vestibular dysfunction. Initial investigation into the psychometric properties of this questionnaire has found that it discriminates between healthy children and those with vestibulopathies and could be used to identify and quantify vestibular symptoms.[26]

TABLE 13-4 • Other Pediatric Diagnoses Associated With Vestibular Dysfunction

Diagnosis	Source
Cerebral palsy	Ghai et al[13]
Cochlear implant	Licamelli et al[14]
Congenital cytomegalovirus	Bernard et al[15]
Late prematurity	Eshaghi et al[16]
Traumatic brain injury	Ghai et al[13]

TABLE 13-5 • Tests and Measures to Assess Common Ligamentous and Vascular Disorders

Tests of Ligament Stability/Upper Cervical Spine Stability

• Transverse ligament stress test: Assess for hypermobility of C1-C2 articulation
• Sharp-Purser test: Assess the integrity of the transverse ligament
• Alar ligament test: Assess the integrity of alar ligaments

Test of Vertebrobasilar Artery Blood Flow

• Vertebral artery test: Assess blood flow from the right and left vertebrobasilar artery. Positive symptoms include the 5 Ds: dizziness, diplopia, dysarthria, dysphagia, and drop attacks.

Note: Negative findings for this test do not definitively rule out insufficiency.

■ OCULOMOTOR EXAM

Vestibular assessment should include an examination of the ocular system. Smooth pursuit, or the ability to track a moving object in all directions, should be evaluated. Saccadic movements, or the ability to accurately move the visual gaze from one target to another, should also be included. Near point of convergence, or when the ability to see an object clearly as it approaches the eyes is lost, is another measurement of interest. All 3 of these oculomotor tests can be conducted using the tip of a pen or any small object of visual interest to the child.

Evaluation of the function of the VSR would include measures of postural control. The Modified Clinical Test of Sensory Interaction on Balance (mCTSIB), the Fukuda Stepping Test, the Dynamic Gait Index (DGI), and the Pediatric Balance Scale (PBS) may be helpful tools to measure VSR function.

The function of the VOR may reveal important deficits in vestibular function. The VOR is responsible for maintaining a clear image on the fovea when the head is in motion. This clarity is achieved when the eyes move in an equal and opposite direction to the head. This movement must occur both vertically and horizontally. For the VOR to work properly, it needs to achieve this equal and opposite movement with at least 90% accuracy. Less accuracy results in oscillopsia, or image blurring.

TABLE 13-6 • Cervicogenic Dysfunction: Tests and Measures and Related Interventions[21]

Tests and Measures	Related Interventions
Cervical spine stability and vascular insufficiency tests	Referral to doctor
Postural control tests (sensory organization test)	Postural control training
Smooth pursuit torsion test	Range of motion and proprioception training
Cervical spine passive/active ranges of motion and strength Cervical spine joint mobility	Manual therapy[23,24] Cervical spine strengthening
Cervical joint position error testing	Cervical spine proprioception training

Testing of the VOR may include head thrust, dynamic visual acuity testing (DVA), and head shaking tests.

Tests aimed at provoking the vestibular system through movement may result in nystagmus. Nystagmus is an involuntary oscillation of the eyes in a back and forth, up and down, or torsional direction. Nystagmus has a slow and quick phase. Nystagmus is an involuntary oscillation of the eyes in a back and forth, up and down, or torsional direction. Nystagmus has a slow and quick phase and is labeled for the direction of the quick phase. Sometimes therapists will find that Frenzel lenses will improve their ability to detect nystagmus. Frenzel lenses block the patient's ability to visually fixate on a stationary object, because fixation may dampen or stop nystagmus. If Frenzel lenses are not available, having the patient look in the direction of the quick phase may increase the nystagmus momentarily to aid in detection. It is possible, however, that individuals with vestibulopathies may experience nystagmus without moving at all, especially in the acute stages. Additionally, patients with vestibulopathies may not demonstrate nystagmus. Use of a mirror during therapeutic assessment or interventions can be a useful tool for the therapist to identify activities and/or positions that may provoke nystagmus while the child is playing.

Nystagmus can tell therapists a great deal. Qualities of eye nystagmus, including direction, intensity, duration, activities or movements that either increase or decrease nystagmus, and whether fixating gaze on a singular object can extinguish nystagmus, assist with appropriate physical therapy diagnosis and plan of care. For example, when nystagmus is seen in a downbeating-only direction, central impairment is indicated. Horizontal nystagmus can indicate either central or peripheral issues. Up and down beating combined is typically seen with peripheral issues, most commonly BPPV.

> **Note**
>
> It is not uncommon for children without vestibulopathy to experience nystagmus when at the end range of eye motions.

■ BENIGN PAROXYSMAL POSITIONAL VERTIGO

BPPV is a relatively common cause of dizziness in the pediatric population. In BPPV, it is suspected that otoconia (located in the otoliths organs; **Figure 13-4**) have become dislodged and worked their way into the semicircular canals, blocking the free flow of endolymph. This blockage causes inappropriate signaling from the peripheral vestibular system. Blockages in specific canals bring about symptoms when those canals are engaged during head movements. BPPV may be suspected in cases where the patient reports experiencing vertigo when moving into or out of specific positions. Therefore, testing for BPPV includes attempts to reproduce symptoms by placing the patient in provocatory positions. Such positions are typically held for up to a minute because symptoms may not emerge immediately. When patients with BPPV are placed in these positions, symptoms of vertigo and nausea are elevated, and nystagmus is frequently, but not always, seen. See **Table 13-7** for information regarding assessment of nystagmus direction and associated canal involvement. The Dix-Hallpike maneuver (Figure 13-4) is used to assess the anterior and posterior canals because the test position engages those canals. Modifications

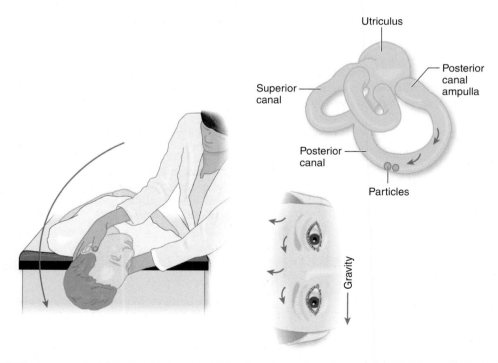

FIGURE 13-4 Dix-Hallpike maneuver. With benign paroxysmal positional vertigo of the right posterior semicircular canal, when the patient's head is turned over the right shoulder and the patient is brought into the supine position, upbeat torsional nystagmus occurs with the rotatory component in the direction of the ground. (Reproduced with permission from Ropper A, Samuels M, Klein J. *Adams and Victor's Principles of Neurology.* 10th ed. McGraw Hill; 2014.)

TABLE 13-7 • Nystagmus Assessment and Associated Canals[28]

Direction	Canal
Vertical (upbeat)/torsional	Posterior canal
Vertical (downbeat)/torsional	Anterior canal
Horizontal/torsional	Horizontal canal

Note: The posterior canal is the most commonly involved in benign paroxysmal positional vertigo (91%).

such as placing a folded pillow under the thoracic spine may be used if cervical extension off the bed is uncomfortable for the patient. Further, a side-lying position (Figure 13-4) can be used if supine is not possible.

To engage the horizontal canals, the roll test may be used.[27] The provocation of symptoms indicates a positive test result for both the Dix-Hallpike and roll tests.

Canalithiasis occurs when otoconia are free flowing within the semicircular canal, causing nystagmus that appears after a latency of approximately 10 seconds and typically resolves within 60 seconds. Canalithiasis is responsive to the Epley maneuver. Cupulolithiasis occurs when otoconia adhere to the cupula and cause an immediate response of nystagmus that persists for between 10 and 60 seconds. Cupulolithiasis is responsive to the Semont maneuver.[29]

BPPV is quite responsive to treatment. In fact, the appropriate treatment may result in immediate positive effects for the patient. Interventions are planned according to the canal determined to be involved. For posterior canal involvement, either the Epley repositioning maneuver or the Semont liberatory maneuver may be used. Horizontal canal involvement may be treated with the barbeque maneuver, the Appiani maneuver, or the Gufoni/Casani maneuver.

Postmaneuver restrictions where patients were asked to remain in upright sitting for a period are no longer recommended as they are not supported by research.[30] The creation of a home exercise program that includes self-maneuvers is important because recurrence is common.[31] It is important to note that children who experience BPPV may experience relative resistance to therapy and may be at a higher risk for recurrence. This relative risk is increased for children with a concurrent diagnosis of vestibular migraine.[32]

Case 1

Benign Paroxysmal Positional Vertigo

Charlene is a 12-year-old who arrives at an outpatient physical therapy clinic for evaluation and treatment. She reports that she "feels like she is falling" when rolling over her right shoulder in bed and when sitting up. She reports she feels better after less than 1 minute if she rests and stares at something not moving in the room. She reports throwing up following one episode. Her mother reports no history of this happening before and no past medical history that would explain her symptoms. Her goals are to manage her school day without feeling terrible and returning to her running program because cross-country training begins in 4 weeks.

Objective Measures

Vertebrobasilar artery tests are negative.

Cervical instability tests are negative.

Strength and sensation are determined to be within normal limits.

Active ranges of motion in upper and lower extremities are within normal limits.

Cervical range of motion: Left rotation is within normal limits, right cervical rotation to 25 degrees before patient reports initial feelings of dizziness.

Vital signs are as follows: Sitting: heart rate (HR) 78 bpm, resting respiration (RR) 16 breaths/min, blood pressure (BP) 95/75 mm Hg. Sitting following therapy: HR 80 bpm, RR 13 breaths/min, BP 93/75 mm Hg.

Oculomotor tests show smooth pursuits, near-point convergence, and saccades all within normal limits.

Sitting and standing postures are remarkable for bilateral shoulder elevation, rounded shoulders, and cervical flexion. Little head rotation is noted during the history taking and systems exam.

Dix-Hallpike to the right provokes up-beating and torsional nystagmus, indicating posterior canal involvement. Onset is 7 seconds in position and extinguishes at 15 seconds. Patient reports that these "are her symptoms." Dix-Hallpike for the left and roll test are both negative.

Assessment and Intervention

From these tests and measures, the PT determines that the patient likely has BPPV involving the right posterior canal. The PT determines the best course of action is to perform the Epley maneuver. The PT asks the patient to move into a long sitting position on the table. The PT turns the patient's head 45 degrees toward her right side. Holding onto the therapist, the patient is lowered to a supine position with her head in the 45-degree turn and her neck in a semi-extended position over the head of the bed. The patient is held here until symptoms abate. This usually occurs within 1 minute. For this patient, all symptoms were abolished by 35 seconds. The patient's head was then rotated 90 degrees toward her left (unaffected side), and the patient was rolled onto her left side with her chin tucked so that she ended up looking toward the ground. In this position, her symptoms were slightly elevated again, and she was held here until these symptoms were abolished. Once the symptoms had cleared, the patient was helped to return to a seated position while maintaining a chin tuck position.

Outcomes

After the patient was given a short rest period, she reported that her symptoms improved. A Dix-Hallpike retest was done and was negative for provocation. The patient was seen for 2 more treatments and was successfully discharged with a home exercise program that included the Epley maneuver. The maneuver was videotaped on the child's phone to allow for reference for accuracy in performance.

■ TREATMENT OF NON–BENIGN PAROXYSMAL POSITIONAL VERTIGO VESTIBULAR DYSFUNCTION: HYPOFUNCTION AND CENTRAL VESTIBULAR DYSFUNCTION

In 2022, the Academy of Neurologic Physical Therapy of the American Physical Therapy Association (APTA) updated their clinical practice guideline (CPG) for the treatment of vestibular hypofunction. CPGs are evidence-based statements regarding optimizing outcomes for patient management. While, as suggested by the CPG, clinical trials including the pediatric population are necessary, the information included in the CPG is helpful in the examination, evaluation, and management of the pediatric patient.[33]

The goal of treatment of non-BPPV vestibular hypofunction and central vestibular dysfunction is not to restore function, but rather to assist the central nervous system in compensating for the loss of function. Treatment can be creative and must be completely patient-centered. It involves graded experience to challenge the central nervous system to patient tolerance. Based on patient presentation, therapists must decide to use adaptation/habituation or substitution as a compensatory strategy. Gradual exposure to the movement that exacerbates symptoms to a level tolerable to the patient would be an example of adaptation/habituation. Substitution requires the forced use of intact sensory modalities other than vestibular. Substitution is employed when visual or proprioceptive input is specifically trained to increase their contribution to balance to make up for the vestibular loss. For example, a patient with limited vestibular function would be trained to rely on their vision and/or proprioception to provide information regarding balance. This type of intervention is sometimes referred to as *up-training* or *up-regulating*.

In the case of VOR dysfunction, adaptation/habituation exercises would include changes in movement speed, movement direction, the complexity and size of the target on which individual is attempting to fixate visually. Elements of interventions that may be modified include increasing/decreasing the busyness of the environment, altering the patient's base of support, dividing the patient's attention, and adding/eliminating had and body movement into the exercises. All exercises would increase in complexity based on patient tolerance.[20,34] Recommended treatment frequency and duration is one time per week for 2 to 3 weeks for acute UVH and one time per week for 4 to 6 weeks for chronic UVH. In the case of bilateral vestibular hypofunction, recommended frequency is one time per week for a duration of 5 to 7 weeks.[20,33,35] Home exercise programs should include gaze stabilization exercises and static and dynamic balance exercises.

■ SUMMARY

Vestibular dysfunction can result in impairments in body functions and structures, functional limitations, and participation restrictions. Understanding the anatomy of the vestibular system and the contributors to the balance system are necessary to choose appropriate tests and measures to correctly identify sources of dizziness, imbalance, and motion intolerance and determine whether physical therapy intervention is indicated. Use of an individualized, evidence-based plan of care can maximize outcomes for individuals with a diagnosis of vestibular dysfunction and use of the APTA CPG for vestibular dysfunction can assist PTs' decision-making.

Case 2

Central Vestibular Dysfunction

Alex is an 18-month-old female with a diagnosis of spastic quadriplegic cerebral palsy and periventricular leukomalacia. Alex resists rolling to her left and right and transitional movements between postures. She can demonstrate independent head control and upper trunk control in supported sitting. Her family reports that her "eye shaking" during movement and that they are not always sure what she is looking at. They report that this shaking happens more after moving but sometimes happens spontaneously. The family's goals include maximizing Alex's participation in movement, including doing some stepping in their home when supported. They are willing to help her in whatever way they can.

Objective Measures

Previous imaging shows intact cervical spine ligaments.

Musculoskeletal: Modified Ashworth Scale: 3 for elbow, wrist, and knee extension bilaterally, hip abductors, hamstrings, and plantar flexors bilaterally.

Minor deficits in passive range of bilateral elbow and knee extension and dorsiflexion.

Noted ability to move all extremities against gravity.

Able to bear weight on lower extremities when supported.

Oculomotor: Able to track the general movement of colorful object 12 to 15 inches from eyes in a full arc during sitting activities.

Noted direction-changing nystagmus at end range. Also noted bouts of spontaneous nystagmus that included a rotatory component. Nystagmus was not dampened when offered a preferred, stable object on which to fixate.

Nystagmus of variable duration.

Motor control:

Rolling supine to prone: Able to demonstrate lateral head righting and assist with upper and lower extremity movement during rolling supine to prone to the left and right. Patient demonstrating initial resistance to rolling, but with slow facilitation at trunk and encouragement, patient is able to complete the activity to the left and to the right. Requires moderate assist at the trunk for initiating and completion of the first third of roll, then minimal assist to complete rolling. Requires assistance for completion of upper extremity placement to allow for elbow under the shoulder when moving into a prone position. Noted vertical and rotatory nystagmus following rolling, slowing within 20 seconds and extinguished in 35 seconds.

Side lying to sitting: Patient engages in very slow movement during this activity. Patient able to right head during this activity and assist with pushing with upper extremities. Requires moderate assistance at hip to initiate and complete transition and is resistant to movement. Nystagmus was noted during this activity in vertical and rotatory directions. Extinguished within 15 seconds with visual fixation on a favorite toy.

Sitting balance: Patient requires moderate assistance to maintain upright balance in sitting at edge of stepstool with feet on the floor.

Plan of Care

Practice with facilitated movement between positions to improve tolerance to increasing speed and increasing upright positioning. The use of a therapy ball may help to allow for the graduated introduction of positional changes. Use of visually stimulating toys to promote visual tracking/stabilization activities in all positions may be useful. Seated balance can be addressed in a variety of environments and conditions by changing hip and knee angles, varying seating surfaces, and incorporating reaching tasks. All activities will be to patient tol-erance. Referrals to vision therapy will be made.

Note: Close attention should be paid to facial expressions, vocalizations, and body positions that may indicate discomfort or resistance. Adaptations to the approach, intensity, and frequency of any given intervention should be made based on the "whole patient" response. Sensitivity to intervention may vary both within and between sessions. It is also important to check with the patient and family upon the next visit to determine if any latent response to intervention was experienced.

Outcomes

Patient was seen for a course of therapy 2 times per week for 6 months. The family was extremely compliant with the home exercise program, and patient participated in a community aquatic program throughout. Patient required minimal assistance to complete rolling from prone to supine and supine to prone to clear upper extremities. Static sitting balance improved to allow for sitting at the edge of stepstool with feet on floor for up to 10 seconds independently. Training with a gait trainer was initiated, and patient was able to take up to 2 steps before facilitation was required. Nystagmus decreased in both duration and frequency following treatment.

Case 3

Peripheral Vestibular Dysfunction

Marcus is a 9-year-old swimmer who reports "feeling weird" over the past 4 weeks. He comes to outpatient physical therapy because his symptoms of motion sensitivity and blurry vision are interfering with his training and beginning to interfere with his daily life. The subjective portion of his examination is as follows:

Patient reports feeling "spinny" and "bumps into doors and counters." He also reports that these symptoms worsen when he turns his head, like when breathing during the freestyle stroke. Walking in between classes, riding the bus to school, and the chaos of the pool during competition exacerbate his symptoms. He reports that it feels like objects are "blurry" or "move." Closing his eyes makes his symptoms better. These symptoms were not present prior to the last 4 weeks. He does report having a bad cold and attributed his initial symptoms to this illness; however, his cold has resolved, and his symptoms continue. His past medical history is not significant for issues that may be contributing to his present symptoms.

Objective Measures

Vertebrobasilar artery testing: negative.
Cervical instability testing: negative.

Musculoskeletal: Ranges of motion and strength are within expected limits for age. Slight tightness is noted through hamstrings but reports he has grown quite a bit in the last few months. Palpable, tender muscular nodules in bilateral upper trapezius and levator scapulae. Increased tension in suboccipital region.

Cervical joint position error testing: Target at 90 cm, 10 degrees from target after turning to the right.

Oculomotor:

Smooth pursuit: Within normal limits.

Saccadic movement: Reports dizziness with this activity but can accurately reach target.

Postural stability testing: Modified Clinical Test of Sensory Integration on Balance

Condition 1: 30 seconds
Condition 2: 30 seconds
Condition 3: 28 seconds
Condition 4: 24 seconds
Condition 5: 8 seconds
Condition 6: 4 seconds

Fukuda Stepping Test (50 steps): Turning 40 degrees to the right.

VOR:

Head thrust: Noted corrective saccade to the right.

DVA (30 degrees cervical flexion, 2 Hz): 3-line difference on Snellen chart.

Head-shaking nystagmus (20 seconds at 2 Hz): No nystagmus noted.

Tests and measures indicate vestibular hypofunction on the right and limitations in cervical joint proprioception that contribute to balance challenges.

Plan of Care

Plan of care included VOR training × 1 moving to × 2 on a variety of surfaces using printed superhero pictures, reading from one target to another from word cards held by the therapist, walking with head turning to read messages at eye level in a hallway, and progressive balance training on increasingly compliant surfaces to include dense foam squares and beams, tilt boards, and mini-trampoline. Manual therapy techniques to address trigger points in the cervical spine were initiated, and self-stretches were encouraged in a home exercise program. Cervical proprioception training was performed by fixing a laser headlamp on the patient's head and encouraging the use of the laser to complete a variety of mazes hung on the wall. A home exercise program was developed for the patient that included targeted interventions that the patient was able to safely and independently control such as identifying pictures in a book while turning his head side to side and up and down and balance activities while standing at his bedroom desk.

Outcomes

Patient was seen over a course of therapy one time per week for 4 weeks. Patient returned to swimming training and school activities with minimal provocation of dizziness and was independent with a home exercise program. Follow-up occurred 6 weeks after discharge. Patient reported feeling back to 100%.

■ GOAL WRITING

Goal writing for patients with vestibular dysfunction should focus on a return to participation in vocational and avocational activities. Examples of goal writing are as follows:

- Patient will report a dizziness rating of 0/10 when moving to standing from laying on their bed.
- Patient will improve score on the Pediatric Balance Scale from ____ to ____ to allow functional community ambulation.

- Patient will be independent with home exercises for improving balance and stability with gait.
- Patient will turn to look over their right or left shoulder while walking in the school hallways without exacerbation of symptoms.
- Patient will walk 100 ft down a busy hallway without report of increased symptoms.

STUDY QUESTIONS

1. Abbey is a 14-year-old patient who arrives for physical therapist (PT) examination and evaluation with a diagnosis of vestibular dysfunction. The PT finds the following on examination: severe ataxia, abnormal smooth pursuits, and acute vertigo that does not go away when the patient is able to fixate visually on an object. She also experiences direction-changing nystagmus. Abbey's likely diagnosis is which of the following?
   a. Central vestibular dysfunction
   b. Chronic otitis media
   c. Ménière disease
   d. Peripheral vestibular dysfunction

2. A 6-year-old female patient comes into a physical therapy clinic for evaluation after complaints of increasing dizziness. The PT conducts testing to determine potential causes of this dizziness. The first test conducted involves the patient long sitting on the plinth. The patient is instructed to turn her head to the right and relax while the PT quickly lowers the patient onto her back with her neck in some extension. The therapist then evaluates the nystagmus and symptoms the patient experiences. What test is this?
   a. The barbeque maneuver
   b. The Vestibular/Ocular Motor Screening
   c. The Epley maneuver
   d. The Dix-Hallpike maneuver

3. A 6-year-old female patient comes into a physical therapy clinic for evaluation after complaints of increasing dizziness. The PT conducts testing to determine potential causes of this dizziness. The first test conducted involves the patient long sitting on the plinth. The patient is instructed to turn their head to the right and relax while the PT quickly lowers the patient onto their back with their neck in some extension. The therapist then evaluates the nystagmus and symptoms the patient experiences. This test is sensitive to which diagnosis?

   a. Benign paroxysmal positional vertigo
   b. Vestibulocochlear tumor
   c. Vestibular hypofunction
   d. Central vestibular dysfunction

4. An 11-year-old male patient comes to a PT clinic with complaints of dizziness. The results of the head thrust testing are as follows: noted inability to keep his eyes steady on the target when head is turned to the left. A corrective saccade is noted back to the visual target. This result indicates which of the following?
   a. Benign paroxysmal positional vertigo on the left
   b. Benign paroxysmal positional vertigo on the right
   c. Vestibular hypofunction on the left
   d. Vestibular hypofunction on the right

5. A 12-year-old patient arrives for PT evaluation with complaints of feeling woozy. She reports being a passenger in a motor vehicle accident last week. She did not require medical attention. Dix-Hallpike is negative. Roll test does not provoke nystagmus. The patient can stabilize her eyes on a target with head thrust test. What is the most likely diagnosis for this patient?
   a. Benign paroxysmal positional vertigo
   b. Central vestibular dysfunction
   c. Cervicogenic dysfunction
   d. Vestibular hypofunction

6. A middle school football player has the position of wide receiver. He can run down the field and keep his eyes on the pass at the same time. For this reason, he can catch the ball and score the winning touchdown. The reflex that allows for images to remain stable on the fovea when the head is moving is referred to as which reflex?
   a. Opticokinetic reflex
   b. Vestibulocollic reflex
   c. Vestibulo-ocular reflex
   d. Vestibulospinal reflex

(Continued)

STUDY QUESTIONS (*CONTINUED*)

7. A 4-year-old child experiences episodes of vertigo that are not connected to her movement or position. The child does not report ringing in her ears with the onset of vertigo but will sometimes experience vomiting. No nystagmus is noted during these episodes, and hearing is normal. The child is most likely experiencing which of the following?

a. Benign paroxysmal vertigo of childhood

b. Ototoxicity related to medications

c. Unilateral otitis media

d. Vestibular migraine

8. Which of the following statements is accurate regarding pediatric patients born with or developing bilateral vestibular hypofunction soon after birth?

a. They do not experience any differences in development because the issue is bilateral.

b. They experience a spinning sensation that lasts for hours at a time.

c. They experience significant delays in developing balance and other motor abilities.

d. They have a greater likelihood of experiencing migraines as adolescents.

9. A PT is evaluating a 15-year-old boy after he sustained a blow to the head following a lacrosse game. The patient reports dizziness and visual changes. During the transverse ligament stress test, the patient reports a feeling of a lump in his throat. What is the PT's most appropriate course of action?

a. Begin manual therapy for the cervical spine.

b. Conduct the head impulse test.

c. Execute the Dix-Hallpike maneuver.

d. Refer patient for imaging immediately.

10. True or false? Pediatric athletes who experience prolonged symptoms following a concussion are likely to have vestibular symptoms on physical therapy evaluation.

a. True

b. False

References

1. Brodsky JR, Lipson S, Bhattacharyya N. Prevalence of pediatric dizziness and imbalance in the United States. *Otolaryngol Head Neck Surg.* 2020;162:241-247.

2. Duarte JA, Leão EM, Fragano DS, et al. Vestibular syndromes in childhood and adolescence. *Int Arch Otorhinolaryngol.* 2020;24:e477-e481.

3. Gioacchini FM, Alicandri-Ciufelli M, Kaleci S, Magliulo G, Re M. Prevalence and diagnosis of vestibular disorders in children: a review. *Int J Pediatr Otorhinolaryngol.* 2014;78(5):718-724.

4. Rine RM, Christy JB. *Part I: Pediatric Vestibular Disorders.* Vestibular Disorders Association; 2016.

5. Brown KE, Whitney SL, Marchetti GF, Wrisley DM, Furman JM. Physical therapy for central vestibular dysfunction. *Arch Phys Med Rehabil.* 2006;87(1):76-81.

6. Christy JB. Considerations for testing and treating children with central vestibular impairments. *Semin Hear.* 2018;39(3): 321-333.

7. Thompson TL, Amedee R. Vertigo: a review of common peripheral and central vestibular disorders. *Ochsner J.* 2009;9(1): 20-26.

8. Cha Y-H. Acute vestibulopathy. *Neurohospitalist.* 2011;1(1): 32-40.

9. Strupp M, Mandalà M, López-Escámez JA. Peripheral vestibular disorders: an update. *Curr Opin Neurol.* 2019;32(1):165-173.

10. Mostafa BE, Shafik AG, Makhzangy AM, Taha H, Mageed HM. Evaluation of vestibular function in patients with chronic suppurtive otitis media. *ORL J Otorhonolaryngol Relat Spec.* 2013; 75:357-360.

11. Muncie HL, Sirmans SM, James E. Dizziness: approach to evaluation and management. *Am Fam Phys.* 2017;95(3):154-162.

12. Shepard N. Signs and symptoms of central vestibular disorders. *Access Audiol.* 2009;8:1.

13. Ghai S, Hakim M, Dannenbaum E, Lamontagne A. Prevalence of vestibular dysfunction in children with neurological disabilities: a systematic review. *Front Neurol.* 2019;10:1294.

14. Licamelli G, Zhou G, Kenna MA. Disturbance of vestibular function attributable to cochlear implantation in children. *Laryngoscope.* 2009;119:740-745.

15. Bernard S, Wiener-Vacher S, Van den Abbeele T, Teissier N. Vestibular disorders in children with congenital cytomegalovirus infection. *Pediatrics.* 2015;136:1-10.

16. Eshaghi Z, Jafari Z, Shaibanizadeh A, Jalaie S, Ghaseminejad A. The effect of preterm birth on vestibular evoked myogenic potentials in children. *Med J Repub Iran.* 2014;28:75.

17. Dunlap PM, Sparto PJ, Marchetti GF, et al. Fear avoidance beliefs are associated with perceived disability in persons with vestibular disorders. *Phys Ther.* 2021;101(9):pzab147.

18. Mueller M, Schuster E, Strobl R, Grill E. Identification of aspects of functioning, disability and health relevant to patients experiencing vertigo: a qualitative study using the international classification of functioning, disability and health. *Health Qual Life Outcomes.* 2012;10:75.

19. Shiozaki T, Ito T, Wada Y, Yamanaka T, Kitahara T. Effects of vestibular rehabilitation on physical activity and subjective dizziness in patients with chronic peripheral vestibular disorders: a six-month randomized trial. *Front Neurol.* 2021;12:656157

20. Hall CD, Herdman SJ, Whitney SL, et al. Vestibular rehabilitation for peripheral vestibular hypofunction: an evidence-based clinical practice guideline: from the American Physical Therapy Association Neurology Section. *J Neurol Phys Ther.* 2016;40(2):124

21. Berliner JM. *Cervicogenic Dizziness*. American Physical Therapy Association Section of Neurology; 2013:25.

22. Schneider KJ, Meeuwisse WH, Nettel-Aguirre A, et al. Cervicovestibular rehabilitation in sport-related concussion: a randomised controlled trial. *Br J Sports Med*. 2014;48(17):1294-1298.

23. De Vestel C, Vereeck L, Reid SA, Van Rompaey V, Lemmens J, De Hertogh W. Systematic review and meta-analysis of the therapeutic management of patients with cervicogenic dizziness. *J Man Manip Ther*. 2022;30(5):273-283.

24. Reid SA, Callister R, Snodgrass SJ, Katekar MG, Rivett DA. Manual therapy for cervicogenic dizziness: long-term outcomes of a randomised trial. *Man Ther*. 2015;20(1):148-156.

25. Akin FW, Davenport MJ. Validity and reliability of the Motion Sensitivity Test. *J Rehabil Res Dev*. 2003;40(5):415-422.

26. Pavlou M, Whitney S, Alkathiry AA, et al. The pediatric vestibular symptom questionnaire: a validation study. *J Pediatr*. 2016;168:171-177.

27. Von Brevern M, Bertholon P, Brandt T, et al. Benign paroxysmal positional vertigo: diagnostic criteria. *J Vestib Res*. 2015;25(3, 4):105-117.

28. Korres S, Balatsouras DG, Kaberos A, Economou C, Kandiloros D, Ferekidis E. Occurrence of semicircular canal involvement in benign paroxysmal positional vertigo. *Otol Neurotol*. 2002;23:926-932.

29. Hain TC, Squires TM, Stone HA. Clinical implications of a mathematical model of benign paroxysmal positional vertigo. *Ann N Y Acad Sci*. 2005;1039(1):384-394.

30. Roberts RA, Gans RE, DeBoodt JL, Lister JJ. Treatment of benign paroxysmal positional vertigo: necessity of postmaneuver patient restrictions. *J Am Acad Audiol*. 2005;16(06):357-366.

31. Pérez P, Franco V, Cuesta P, Aldama P, Alvarez MJ, Méndez JC. Recurrence of benign paroxysmal positional vertigo. *Otol Neurotol*. 2012;33(3):437-443.

32. Brodsky JR, Lipson S, Wilber J, Zhou G. Benign paroxysmal positional vertigo (BPPV) in children and adolescents: clinical features and response to therapy in 110 pediatric patients. *Otol Neurotol*. 2018;39(3):344-350.

33. Hall D, Herdman S, Whitney S, et al. Vestibular rehabilitation for peripheral vestibular hypofunction: an updated clinical practice guideline from the Academy of Neurologic Physical Therapy of the American Physical Therapy Association. *J Neurol Phys Ther*. 2022;46(2):118-177.

34. Whitney SL, Sparto PJ. Principles of vestibular physical therapy rehabilitation. *Neurorehabilitation*. 2011;29(2):157-166.

35. MacDowell S, Farrell L, D'Silva L. Clinical practice guideline: vestibular rehabilitation for peripheral vestibular hypofunction. Academy of Neurologic Physical Therapy. Accessed October 8, 2018. http://www.neuropt.org/docs/default-source/vsig-english-pt-fact-sheets/cpg-vestibular-rehab-for-peripheral-vestibular-hypofunction.pdf?sfvrsn=23625743_2.

Genetic Disorders

Kay Tasso, PT, PhD, Eric Shamus, PT, DPT, PhD, and Sarah Fabrizi, OTR/L, PhD

LEARNING OBJECTIVES

Upon completion of this chapter, the reader will be able to:

- Analyze the history and objective assessment to identify functional short-term and long-term goals for pediatric patients with genetic disorders.
- Evaluate a child's developmental skills to discern the appropriate interventions needed.

- Create interventions to assist children with developing and progressing functional, age-appropriate skills.
- Evaluate children with genetic disorders to teach family/caregivers appropriate care and home activities.

INTRODUCTION

The incidence of infants and children diagnosed with genetic disorders has increased since completion of the Human Genome Project in 2001.[1] These disorders are a leading cause of infant mortality and affect approximately 3% of births in the United States.[2] Many genetic disorders result in infants and toddlers exhibiting gross motor skill delay, prompting pediatricians to refer to physical therapy. As experts in movement, physical therapists (PTs) may be the first to recognize atypical developmental signs that warrant a recommendation to the referring physician for a consultation with neurology, orthopedics, and genetics.[3] Once an infant or child has been diagnosed with a genetic disorder, the therapist often assists the family with digesting the medical information provided by the physicians and material the parents or caregivers discern from the Internet.[4] PTs must collaborate with occupational therapists, speech-language pathologists, physicians, and genetic specialists for ongoing understanding to benefit the patients and their families.[5]

A fetus receives 23 chromosomes from each parent for a total of 46 chromosomes, each of which contains genes. Chromosome pairs numbered 1 through 22 are referred to as autosomes with the remaining pair of sex-linked chromosomes consisting of XX for females and XY for males. Genetic disorders can occur for a variety of reasons either on the autosome or sex-linked chromosomes and may be either dominant or recessive. An autosomal dominant defect means that an affected chromosome or gene from only one parent causes the disorder. When the autosomal defect is recessive, both parents must carry the defect but typically do not have the disorder. Sex-linked genetic defects can be dominant or recessive as well. In an X-linked dominant disorder, females or males can have the disorder. Because males only have one X chromosome, if that one contains a recessive defect, the male will have the disorder. **Figure 14-1** illustrates the inheritance patterns for X-linked genes.

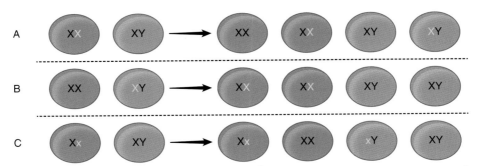

FIGURE 14-1 X-linked inheritance. (A) Trait manifested in mother as a dominant gene; all children have a 50% chance of inheriting the trait. (B) Dominant trait carried by father on the X chromosome will be manifested in all daughters. (C) When a recessive trait is carried by mother, 50% of the daughters will be carriers and 50% of the sons will have the disorder. X = normal X chromosome; x = trait carrying; left side of diagram: pink oval = mother's genes; blue oval = father's genes. Right side of diagram = genetic possibilities for offspring (pink = girls; blue = boys). (Reproduced with permission from Deborah S. Nichols Larsen.)

The mechanisms for genetic disorders include the following:

- **Autosomal dominant** such as achondroplasia, DiGeorge syndrome, neurofibromatosis, and tuberous sclerosis
- **Autosomal recessive** such as cystic fibrosis, sickle cell anemia, and Tay-Sachs disease
- **Sex-linked**
  - X-linked recessive such as Duchenne muscular dystrophy and hemophilia[6]
  - X-linked dominant such as in fragile X syndrome and Rett syndrome
- **Additions** such as an extra chromosome like trisomy 21 in Down syndrome or Klinefelter syndrome caused by an extra X or Y chromosome
- **Deletions,** whether partial or complete, such as cri-du-chat and Turner syndrome
- **Translocation** (a piece of one gene attaches in the wrong place)
- **Nondisjunction** (the chromosomes do not separate)
- **Inversion** (a piece of the gene is upside down)
- **Mosaic** (contains some normal and some abnormal cells)
- **Variants** (previously referred to as mutations)
- **Multifactorial** disorders, such as teratogenic exposure, and mitochondrial disorders inherited from the mother[7]

Some genetic disorders can result from more than one method of transmission. For example, Down syndrome most often occurs due to an additional chromosome 21 but can also result from a nondisjunction, translocation, or mosaicism. Similarly, CHARGE (coloboma of the eye, heart defects, atresia of the nasal choanae, restricted growth and/or development, genital and/or urinary abnormalities, and ear abnormalities and deafness) syndrome can result from a variant, which is not inherited, or an autosomal dominant gene. Osteogenesis imperfecta can occur due to autosomal dominant, autosomal recessive, or X-linked recessive defects.

Because parents are aware they contribute their genetic makeup to their progeny, therapists should recognize that parents may feel guilty and responsible for causing their child's special needs. As a result, PTs can assist in supporting the family by reassuring them that their child's condition is not their fault.

Although most genetic disorders cannot be cured, research has led to tremendous progress in treating spinal muscular atrophy with gene therapy and disease-modifying medications.[8]

■ DESCRIPTION

Genetic disorders frequently present with their own unique combination of characteristic facial and physical features. Stereotypical facial features such as micrognathia, cleft lip or cleft palate, and small ears may be one of the first signs that leads a therapist to suspect a genetic disorder. Feeding difficulty as an infant, developmental delay, hypotonia, joint laxity, or other orthopedic anomalies frequently occur in babies and young children with genetic disorders. Associated conditions may include intellectual disability, vision or hearing deficits, and cardiac, pulmonary, or gastrointestinal involvement.

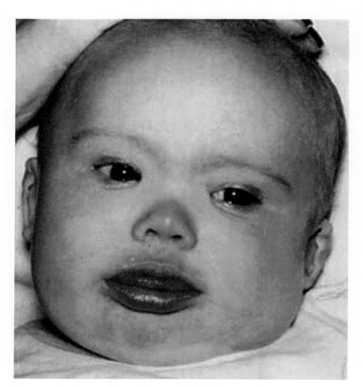

FIGURE 14-2 Down syndrome, showing upward-slanting eyes, a flat profile, and protuberant tongue. (Reproduced with permission from Chandrasoma P, Clive R. *Taylor, Concise Pathology,* 3e. New York: McGraw Hill; 1998.)

Down syndrome is one of the most common genetic disorders PTs treat; the infant is typically referred after the genetic diagnosis has been confirmed. Characteristics of Down syndrome may include developmental delay, hypotonia, joint laxity, a Simian crease, upward-slanting eyes, and a protruding tongue (**Figure 14-2**). These children often have an intellectual disability and short stature. They may also have congenital heart defects, congenital cataracts, or hypothyroidism. PTs should use caution as children with Down syndrome have a risk of atlantoaxial instability, although they are not routinely screened for this anomaly and have an increased risk of leukemia as children and Alzheimer disease as adults.[9-11]

Rett syndrome is another genetic disorder commonly treated by PTs. Due to the genetic transmission as X-linked dominant, only females manifest this disorder. Initially, babies and toddlers develop typically but then their gross and fine motor skills and speech and language begin to regress. As a result, the child is often referred to physical therapy for developmental delay prior to receiving a diagnosis. The young child often exhibits stereotypical hand movements such as wringing or tapping. Children with Rett syndrome may also have cardiac, pulmonary, or gastrointestinal involvement and often develop scoliosis, seizures, and intellectual disability.[12,13]

Table 14-1 contains a list of some of the more common genetic disorders encountered in pediatric physical therapy and the genetic origin of each disorder. Other less common

TABLE 14-1 • Common Genetic Disorders, Characteristics, and Genetic Origin		
Name of Genetic Disorder	**Characteristics**	**Genetic Origin**
Achondroplasia[7,14]	Macrocephaly Characteristic facial features Short stature Short extremities Hypotonia Joint laxity Chronic ear infections Gross motor delay Obstructive sleep apnea	Autosomal dominant
Angelman syndrome[9]	Intellectual disability Characteristic facial features Ataxic gait Epilepsy Stereotypical laugh	Partial deletion of chromosome 15 from mother or variant
CHARGE syndrome[15,16]	**C**oloboma **H**eart defects **A**tresia Choanal atresia **R**estricted growth and development **G**enital abnormality **E**ar anomalies CNS defects Cranial nerve involvement Feeding difficulties Gross motor delay Fine motor delay Speech delay Endocrine involvement Pulmonary involvement	Autosomal dominant or variant
Cri-du-chat[7,17,18]	Microcephaly Intellectual disability Stereotypical cry Stereotypical facial features Micrognathia Feeding difficulties Hypotonia Balance, coordination, motor-planning impairments Orthopedic abnormalities Behavioral issues Gross motor delay Fine motor delay Speech/language impairments	5p deletion
Cystic fibrosis[9,19,20]	Frequent pulmonary infections Gastrointestinal involvement Pancreas involvement Liver involvement Developmental delay	Autosomal recessive

(Continued)

TABLE 14-1 • Common Genetic Disorders, Characteristics, and Genetic Origin (*Continued*)		
Name of Genetic Disorder	**Characteristics**	**Genetic Origin**
DiGeorge syndrome[9]	Cardiovascular involvement Facial and palate anomalies Thymus involvement Parathyroid involvement Mental illness	Autosomal dominant
Down syndrome[9-11]	Intellectual disability Stereotypical facial features Hypotonia Joint laxity Short stature Congenital heart defects Atlantoaxial instability Increased risk of leukemia Vision issues such as esotropia or myopia Congenital cataracts Decreased hearing Seizures Pes planus Diastasis recti Hypothyroidism Increased risk of Alzheimer disease	Trisomy 21 by nondisjunction, translocation, mosaicism
Duchenne muscular dystrophy[9]	Only affects males Progressive muscle weakness Contractures Loss of mobility Cardiac involvement Cognitive involvement in some	X-linked recessive
Ehlers-Danlos syndrome[9]	(Different types) Hypotonia Scoliosis Hypermobile joints	Autosomal dominant or autosomal recessive or X-linked recessive
Fragile X syndrome[9,20]	Intellectual disability Stereotypical facial features Hypotonia Developmental delay	X-linked dominant
Hemophilia[6]	Primarily males Excessive bleeding into muscles, joints, cranium, or genitourinary system from injury, surgery, or trauma Painful	X-linked recessive
GATAD2B-associated neurodevelopmental disorder (GAND)[21]	Intellectual disability Macrocephaly Hypotonia Feeding difficulty Global developmental delay Speech involvement Atypical facial features Joint laxity Eye involvement Gastroesophageal reflux	Variant

(*Continued*)

TABLE 14-1 • Common Genetic Disorders, Characteristics, and Genetic Origin (*Continued*)

Name of Genetic Disorder	Characteristics	Genetic Origin
Klinefelter syndrome[9]	Small testes and penis Infertile Decreased body hair Increased risk for breast cancer	Extra X or Y chromosome
Low γ-glutamyl-transferase cholestasis, acute liver failure, and neurodegeneration syndrome (CALFAN)[22]	Ataxia Intellectual disability Speech involvement Peripheral neuropathy Liver failure Scoliosis Hip dysplasia Orthopedic anomalies	Autosomal recessive
Myotonic dystrophy[9]	Inability to release muscle activation after use Weakness Facial muscle atrophy Eye involvement Cardiovascular involvement	Autosomal dominant
Neurofibromatosis[9]	Neurofibromas (may become malignant) Café-au-lait spots Eye involvement Hearing involvement	Autosomal dominant
Osteogenesis imperfecta[23-25]	Many different types with varying involvement Fragile bones resulting in frequent, spontaneous fractures Macrocephaly Hypotonia Eye involvement Joint laxity Hearing loss Growth retardation Scoliosis	Autosomal dominant, autosomal recessive, or X-linked recessive
Pierre-Robin sequence[26,27]	Cleft palate Micrognathia Glossoptosis Airway obstruction Feeding difficulties	Autosomal dominant or multifactorial
Potocki-Lupski syndrome[28,29]	Intellectual disability Hypotonia Feeding difficulties Failure to thrive Gross motor delay Speech delay Neuropsychiatric involvement Cardiovascular involvement Failure to thrive Micrognathia	Autosomal dominant

(Continued)

TABLE 14-1 • Common Genetic Disorders, Characteristics, and Genetic Origin (*Continued*)

Name of Genetic Disorder	Characteristics	Genetic Origin
Prader-Willi syndrome[7,9,30,31]	Intellectual disability Inability to regulate eating resulting in obesity Short height Small gonads Hypothalamic-pituitary involvement Stereotypical facial features Small hands and feet Behavior issues Hypotonia Gross motor delay Scoliosis Hip dysplasia	Partial deletion of chromosome 15 from father or Autosomal dominant or variant
Rett syndrome[12,13]	Primarily females Develop typically as infant and young toddler Intellectual disability Regression in gross motor skills Regression in fine motor skills Stereotypical hand wringing Regression in speech Pulmonary involvement Limited mobility Feeding difficulty Gastrointestinal involvement Cardiac involvement Seizures Scoliosis Behavior issues Decreased bone mineral density	X-linked dominant
Sickle cell anemia[25]	Abnormal red blood cell shape resulting in painful vaso-occlusive crises Severe anemia Increased risk of infection Painful	Autosomal recessive
Spinal muscular atrophy[32,33]	4 types Hypotonia Muscle weakness Muscle atrophy Feeding difficulty Pulmonary involvement Contractures Scoliosis Hip dysplasia	Autosomal recessive or X-linked

(Continued)

TABLE 14-1 • Common Genetic Disorders, Characteristics, and Genetic Origin (*Continued*)

Name of Genetic Disorder	Characteristics	Genetic Origin
Tay-Sachs disease[34,35]	Progressive damage to central nervous system Hearing loss Vision loss No gag reflex Progressive muscle weakness Ataxia Hypotonia Seizures Intellectual disability Regression of motor skills Exaggerated startle reflex Mental illness	Autosomal recessive[34]
Tuberous sclerosis[9]	Eye involvement Seizures Intellectual disability Cardiovascular involvement Renal involvement Hypopigmentation areas on skin	Autosomal dominant
Turner syndrome[9,36]	Short in height Webbed neck Abnormal shaped kidney Cardiac defects Renal involvement Liver involvement Hearing disorder Ovarian involvement Short stature	Incomplete X chromosome

genetic disorders are also listed and will be discussed in patient scenarios.

■ DIAGNOSIS

Obstetricians may recommend prenatal genetic testing when the family has a history of genetic disorders or due to advanced maternal age as both factors contribute to an increased risk in the fetus. Prenatal screening may include chorionic villus sampling, amniocentesis, or a sonogram (diagnostic ultrasound). Chorionic villus sampling typically occurs between 10 and 13 weeks' gestation. This method is less accurate than an amniocentesis and has a greater risk of complications but can be used earlier during the pregnancy should termination be a consideration.[10] An amniocentesis is considered the gold standard to test for chromosomal abnormalities between 14 and 16 weeks' gestation since it has almost 100% accuracy.[10] Fetal percutaneous umbilical blood sampling is another option but is associated with an increased risk of complications.[10] Sonograms assist in prenatal testing and can detect Down syndrome through nuchal translucency (measurement of the neck), osteogenesis imperfecta[23] at 15 to 18 weeks' gestation,[37] and other anomalies between 11 and 14 weeks' gestation (**Figure 14-3**).[10] Other special tests

include pre- or postnatal fluorescence in situ hybridization (FISH),[10] karyotype analysis,[10] maternal α-fetoprotein or other biomarkers,[10] chromosomal microarray,[28] or genome sequencing analysis.[21]

Postnatally, a pediatrician may refer an infant or child to a geneticist in the presence of atypical facial or physical features or due to unexplained global developmental delay.[38] The geneticist completes a physical examination, child and family medical history, and laboratory testing. The physical examination includes measurements of head circumference, distance between the eyes, and arm and leg length. Diagnostics may include radiographs, computed tomography (CT), magnetic resonance imaging (MRI), and diagnostic procedures such as an electrocardiogram to rule out congenital heart defects. Genetic testing consists of DNA sequencing to determine the order of the strands to assess for additions, deletions, translocation, variations, or other deviations discussed earlier.[39] In some cases such as a family with a medical history of sickle cell disease, a single gene test or a genetic panel will suffice.[40] The first round of genetic testing examines the presence of the most common genetic defects. Additional genetic panels test for less common disorders. Testing may include exome sequencing, which examines the whole exome, or genome sequencing, which examines

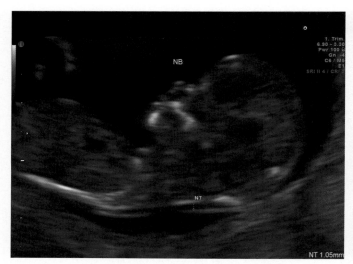

FIGURE 14-3 Fetal nuchal translucency measurement at 12 weeks' gestation. The nuchal translucency refers to the echolucent space underneath the skin at the back of the neck. In this case, the nuchal translucency measurement was normal. In this figure, also note that the nasal bone is imaged. It is seen as a line underneath and parallel to the skin that is of equal or greater echogenicity than the skin. (Reproduced, with permission, from Gupta S, Roman AS. Imaging in obstetrics. In: DeCherney AH, Nathan L, Laufer N, Roman AS, eds. *CURRENT Diagnosis & Treatment: Obstetrics & Gynecology.* 11th ed. McGraw-Hill; 2013.)

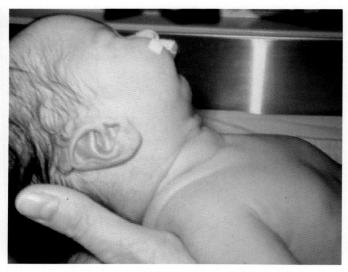

FIGURE 14-4 Pierre Robin syndrome. Hypoplastic mandible associated with a ventricular septal defect. (Reproduced, with permission, from Fuster V, Walsh RA, Harrington RA. *Hurst's The Heart.* 13th ed. New York, NY: McGraw-Hill; 2011.)

the entire DNA sequence, for children suspected of having an undiagnosed genetic disorder.[40] Other types of testing involve looking at the chromosomes or gene expression tests.[40] The more extensive the search of the genome, the more expensive the testing and the less likely that health insurance will cover the cost. When the more common genetic panels fail to determine a diagnosis, families may consider participating in research studies such as the Undiagnosed Diseases Network, where the costs will be covered. Establishing a differential diagnosis contributes significantly to developing an appropriate plan of care that targets the current and projected impairments and assists the family with planning how to maximize the child's potential.

Physicians use the following categories when describing dysmorphic features[41]:

- Malformation: Intrinsic developmental anomaly, a defect of an organ or body part resulting from an abnormal developmental process (eg, spina bifida, cleft lip).
- Disruption: An event disrupting intrinsically normal development (eg, amniotic bands)
- Deformation: External force altering the shape or form of development (eg, clubfoot or face shape due to abnormal intrauterine positioning secondary to oligohydramnios)
- Dysplasia: A defect involving abnormal organization of cells into tissues (eg, hemangioma, achondroplasia)
- Sequence: A defect with secondary structural changes (eg, Pierre Robin sequence with primary defect of mandibular development that produces a small jaw and cleft palate; **Figure 14-4**)
- Syndrome: A pattern of multiple malformations due to a single cause (eg, trisomy 13 syndrome)

■ PHYSICAL THERAPY EXAMINATION

Many of the major categories for examination of the pediatric patient are the same as those for the adult patient. In general, PTs must examine range of motion, muscle tone, muscle performance/strength, sensation, posture, and function. Young children require increased emphasis on assessment of their developmental motor skills. **Figure 14-5** is an example of a typical evaluation for an infant or young child.

HISTORY

When possible, obtaining the child's diagnosis prior to the appointment provides the therapist time to research the specific genetic disorder to ascertain the anticipated physical therapy implications prior to the child's arrival. In general, the therapist obtains the history from the parent, caregiver, or legal guardian from the intake form (see Figure 14-5) or medical record. When a medical record is not available, one should be conscientious yet sensitive in questioning a parent about this history because of the emotional stress that may be associated with these questions.

OBJECTIVE DATA

Tests and measures: Chapter 3 of this book contains the tests and measures available for the pediatric population. Only spinal muscular atrophy has assessment tools specifically designed for that diagnosis including the Children's Hospital of Philadelphia Infant Test of Neuromuscular Disorders (CHOP-INTEND) and Hammersmith-2. For infants and young children with cystic fibrosis (CF), the Prechtl General Movement Assessment (GMA) and Bayley Scales of Infant and Toddler Development–Third Edition (Bayley-III) detected decreased or absent fidgety movement and developmental motor, language, and cognitive delay, respectively.[19] The GMA statistically is not yet predictive for

Pediatric History

Child's:

Last name:	First name:	Middle initial:	DOB:	Age:

Gestational age: _____   Gender: ____ female ____ male

ID#:   Tel#:   Address:

City: State: Zip:

If client is minor: name of parent or responsible party:

Telephone and address if different than minor's: Primary language: _____

                                                        Second language: _____

Social : Parents are: ____married ____separated ____divorced ___single

Child lives with: _____

Does the child have siblings? _____no _____yes If yes, number and ages _____
Was this child one of a multiple birth? _____no _____yes If yes, please indicate: ____twins ____triplets ____quads ____quints

Is primary caregiver responsible for the care of others in the home? ____no ____yes Explain:

Dwelling: Do you have to negotiate stairs into or inside your home? ____no ____yes

Do you have transportation available? _____yes _____no

Reason for PT: Please indicate if you know the child's medical diagnosis:

Did the physician indicate there were problems? ____yes ____no

Did the caregiver perceive there were any problems? ____yes ____no

Please indicate if birth mother had any of the following problems during the pregnancy:

_____pre-eclampsia   _____excessive weight gain : _____pounds gained

_____diabetes   _____dehydration

_____thyroid problems   _____premature labor

_____edema

How many pregnancies did the birth mother have? _____   How many live births? _____

Did the birth mother:
Smoke during the pregnancy?

Drink alcohol during the pregnancy?

Take drugs during the pregnancy that were over the counter?

Take drugs that were prescribed?

Take dietary supplements?   Please indicate: _____

Please indicate the type of diet the birth mother was on during the pregnancy:

FIGURE 14-5 Pediatric history form. (Reproduced with permission from Shamus E, Stern D, McGehee WF, Gainer K. *Communicating Clinical Decision-Making Through Documentation: Coding, Payment, and Patient Categorization.* New York: McGraw Hill; 2021.)

Does the child have: vision impairment _____no _____yes If yes, describe: _____

hearing impairment _____no _____yes If yes, describe: _____

Family history: Are there any other family members with similar problem? _____yes _____no

If yes, please describe:

Please check as appropriate for each category:

Birth history	Where did the birth take place? _____hospital _____home _____birthing center _____other: Please explain:

Type of delivery: _____vaginal _____C-section   Did the baby present breech? _____yes _____no

Were forceps used? _____yes _____no   Was vacuum extraction used? _____yes _____no

What was the baby's birth weight? _____	What was the baby's APGAR score?	How long was the baby in the hospital? Was the baby in the NICU?
What was the baby's birth length? _____	Did the baby need ventilator support? _____yes _____no	How long was the mother in the hospital?

Please indicate any diagnostic tests the baby/child has had:

Please check as applicable	No	Yes	Describe
Respiratory Problems			
Seizures			
Muscle spasms			
Head injury			
Falls			
High fevers			
Hearing problems			
Shunt placement			
Failure to thrive			
Loss of consciousness			
Dehydration			
Abnormal bleeding &/or bruising			
Abnormal growth			
Loss of weight			
Diabetes			
Thyroid dysfunction			
Urinary or bowel problems			
Gastrointestinal			
HIV			

FIGURE 14-5 (*Continued*)

Wheezing, coughing during or after activity			
Agitation			
Excessive sleeping			
Allergies			
Other			
Development of child: ___normal ___delayed			

Recent weight changes: ____weight gain ____weight loss   Describe:

Recent memory or cognitive changes: ____yes ____no   If yes, please describe:

Medications: Prescription:

        Over the counter:

General nutrition: Is the child breastfed: now _____yes _____no   Was the child breastfed? _____yes _____no   How long?_____

Is the child bottle fed? _____yes _____no   Combination breast/bottle: _____yes _____no

If on formula, what type? _____

Diet/dietary supplements: Please indicate if child is on solid food: _____yes _____no
Other:

Please indicate any other information that may be important or you wish to discuss:

The above information is accurate and true to the best of my knowledge, and I give my consent for the evaluation to be performed.

Signature of responsible party if client is a minor: _____Date: _____
Printed Name: Relationship to the child:

FIGURE 14-5 (*Continued*)

infants with CF but may be beneficial in early identification of motor delay.

State of alertness: The behavioral or emotional state of the infant/child should be noted since it will affect muscle tone and motor performance. Typical descriptors include deep sleep, light sleep, drowsy, quiet alert, active alert, or crying.[57]

Asymmetries related to movement: Observe if the infant or child prefers to weight bear on one side more than the other, reach with one arm more than the other, shift weight better to one side than the other, or transition (change position) only in one direction.

Postural alignment: Assess the infant or young child for head and trunk control and postural alignment, especially in sitting and standing.

Muscle tone: Babies with genetic disorders often present with hypotonia. Note the severity and location of any abnormal muscle tone.

Range of motion: As the child ages, some genetic disorders such as Duchenne muscular dystrophy and spinal muscular atrophy have patterns of loss of flexibility that may result in plantar flexor contractures.

Muscle performance/strength: Many genetic disorders often involve muscle weakness. Although standard muscle testing

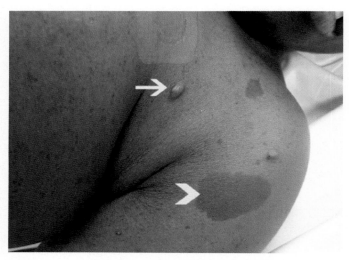

FIGURE 14-6 Neurofibromatosis café-au-lait spots. This patient had type 1 neurofibromatosis. Note the cutaneous neurofibromas (arrow) and café-au-lait spots (arrowhead). (Reproduced with permission from Chapter 6. Genetic Disorders. In: Kemp WL, Burns DK, Brown TG, eds. *Pathology: The Big Picture.* McGraw Hill; 2008.)

should not be performed in infants and young children under the age of 7 years old, inferences regarding strength may be made based on the child's ability to move against gravity.

Sensation and perception: Does the infant or child exhibit tactile defensiveness gravitational insecurity, or other sensory or perceptual challenges?

REVIEW OF SYSTEMS

Integumentary: Children with hemophilia may have redness or increased warmth of a joint. Neurofibromatosis can result in café-au-lait spots or visible masses on or below the skin (**Figure 14-6**).

Cardiovascular and pulmonary status: Some genetic disorders such as Down, CHARGE, or DiGeorge syndrome cause congenital heart defects and CF affects the pulmonary system.

Neurologic: Most genetic disorders primarily affect the neurologic system, which will be discussed further in this chapter.

Musculoskeletal: Many genetic disorders such as Ehlers-Danlos syndrome, Rett syndrome, and spinal muscular atrophy result in scoliosis. Others such as achondroplasia, cri-du-chat, and osteogenesis imperfecta result in orthopedic anomalies.

Genitourinary: Most genetic disorders do not affect this system.

Gastrointestinal: Infants and children with hypotonia due to a genetic disorder often have constipation and may have gastroesophageal reflux.

Endocrine: Most genetic disorders do not affect this system.

REFLEXES AND REACTIONS

Emphasis on assessment of reflexes and reactions has declined. PTs should consider whether primitive reflexes such as the asymmetric tonic neck reflex persist and interfere with function.

GROSS MOTOR DEVELOPMENT

Motor skills for infants and toddlers should be assessed in supine, prone, sitting, and standing including the ability to roll, commando crawl, creep on hands and knees, and transfer in and out of positions. For toddlers and young children, the therapist should assess gait, stair climbing, the primary method of mobility, balance in all positions, running, jumping, hopping on one leg, skipping, kicking a ball, catching a ball, and the length of time the child can stand on one leg.

If no occupational or speech therapy evaluations are scheduled, the therapist should screen for fine motor, oral motor, vocalizations, difficulty feeding, and eating age-appropriate food, such as baby food or table food, and if there are any foods the child refuses to eat. Excessive drooling or frequent emesis should also be noted. Difficulty in these areas warrants a referral to the appropriate therapist.

■ ASSESSMENT

SUMMARY STATEMENT

One strategy for beginning the assessment portion of an evaluation is to begin with a one-sentence summary of the therapist's findings. For example, "18-month-old female recently diagnosed with Rett syndrome." The International Classification of Disease, Disability, and Function (ICF) Model may be used to categorize the information based on body structure and function, impairments, activity limitations, and participation restrictions.

EVALUATION CODES:

The evaluation current procedural terminology (CPT) codes must be documented. Determining the correct CPT code depends on the number of personal factors and/or comorbidities involved with the child, the number of elements included in the examination of the body systems, stability of the child's clinical presentation, and the amount of time spent during the evaluation. Specifically, CPT codes from least complex to most complex include 97161, 97162, and 97163.[56]

REHABILITATION POTENTIAL/PROGNOSIS

Rehabilitation potential refers to the progress the child will make with intervention and a rationale for the rating. For example, "good rehab potential as evidenced by ability to achieve quadruped with facilitation today." The statement may also include a reference to the child's level of motivation, such as: "good rehab potential as evidenced by child's strong desire to interact with environment while observed reaching for objects and babbling to therapist." Prognosis, as described in the *Guide to Physical Therapist Practice*,[42] refers to a more long-term determination of progress.

GOALS/FUNCTIONAL OUTCOMES

In the pediatric practice setting, goals should be documented in the same fashion as physical therapy goals for adults. Goals should be measurable, include what is to be achieved, the time frame for achieving it, under what conditions or criteria, and functional.

PLAN/PLAN OF CARE

As with the initial examination and evaluation of an adult, the plan should include the frequency and duration the child will be treated; any recommendations for additional consultations, such as referral to occupational therapy (OT), speech-language pathology, or an orthotist; what interventions will be used; and how the findings and plan will be communicated to the referring physician.

■ IMPAIRMENTS

The impairments caused by genetic disorders vary depending on the specific defect. Some common impairments include hypotonia, joint laxity, wide-based gait, ataxia, sensory defensiveness, and decreased strength, balance, coordination, range of motion, or endurance.

■ FUNCTIONAL IMPLICATIONS

Infants with genetic disorders may have difficulty with breastfeeding or drinking from a bottle, may have poor head and trunk control, and may refuse to bear weight on their feet. Developmental delays in gross motor function may result in learning to roll, sit, commando crawl, creep on hands and knees, or walk independently much later than expected. Activity limitations may also include progressive loss or delay in mobility, especially independent ambulation; an ataxic or wide-based gait; frequent falls; and delayed acquisition of advanced gross motor skills such as jumping, catching a ball, single leg stance, or riding a bike.

Some children have movement patterns typical of a specific genetic disorder. For example, children with Rett syndrome exhibit an almost constant wringing of the hands when awake. Children with Down syndrome often transfer from prone to sitting or sitting to prone using extreme hip abduction ("a split").

A few research studies document the typical pattern of development for some genetic disorders.[43,44] For example, Palisano et al[43] created motor growth curves that illustrate the age at which children with Down syndrome achieve functional skills such as sitting independently by 12 to 18 months old and walking by 30 to 36 months old. For Rett syndrome, the age at which stages of the disorder typically progress assists the PT with developing and modifying the plan of care.[44] Likewise, the type of muscular dystrophy or spinal muscular atrophy and respective research provide important information in treatment planning. During the active period of sickle cell disease or hemophilia, health care providers focus on pain control, diminishing symptoms, maintaining or slowing the degradation of quality of life, and returning to maximal participation.

Identifying and recognizing clinical patterns in pediatrics contribute to assisting the pediatrician with establishing the child's medical diagnosis especially for an undiagnosed genetic disorder. The following are 2 examples to illustrate this point.

A 15-month-old male evaluated in the home through a local early intervention program presented with a history of a full-term birth weighing 6 lb, 2 oz. The child had already tested negative for muscular dystrophy. Both parents and paternal grandparents lived in the home; the mother thought the child was delayed due to an overprotective grandmother. The child appeared to have micrognathia with an atypical shape of his maxilla. He could not commando crawl, creep on hands and knees, cruise at furniture, or ambulate. He exhibited significant separation anxiety and had emesis when overly anxious. He could ring sit independently when placed on the floor but would not reach outside of the base of support and could not transfer himself into or out of sitting. While sitting, he had spinal flexion, a hypomobile spine on palpation, and a panicked appearance. He rolled as his primary method of mobility, stood with support, and ambulated 2 to 3 ft with his hands held overhead. The PT recommended consultations with orthopedics, neurology, and genetics to the pediatrician. Neither orthopedics nor neurology reported any unusual findings. The mother initially declined a genetics consultation but, 8 months later, agreed to it, and the child was diagnosed with Potocki-Lupski syndrome, duplication of gene 17. The key physical findings that led the therapist to recommend a genetics evaluation included atypical facial features, a hypomobile spine, and an atypical pattern of gross motor skill development.

The second example involves an 8-month-old female evaluated in the home in conjunction with the local early intervention program. She lived with both parents and sister who was a few years older. She had atypical facial features, was hypotonic, and had muscle weakness, joint laxity, and global developmental delay. Her hypotonia was so severe that when held, it felt like she would "slip through" your hands. Her muscle weakness was so severe that when placed in prone, her cervical extensors would fatigue quickly, resulting in her losing eccentric control and, thus, hitting her head on the surface. She was unable to roll, sit independently when placed, or bear weight on her lower extremities when supported in standing. She had significant feeding difficulties including allergies to most food. The family and pediatrician pursued a genetic consultation that required multiple rounds of genetic testing. Ultimately, the family enrolled in a research study by the Undiagnosed Diseases Network, which completed extensive genetic sequencing that would otherwise have been cost prohibitive. At 4.5 years old, she was diagnosed with a rare genetic disorder referred to as GATAD2B-associated neurodevelopmental disorder (GAND). The key indicators that led the therapist to recommend a genetic consult included atypical facial features and a severe degree of hypotonia, weakness, difficulty feeding, and food allergies.

When a therapist suspects a possible genetic disorder in a child diagnosed generically with "developmental delay," the treatment plan will address the body structure and function, impairments, activity restrictions, participation restrictions, and functional limitations present. In other words, the therapist treats the presenting signs and symptoms until the genetic disorder is identified. Once the specific genetic diagnosis is determined, the therapist conducts research to learn the common growth and development associated with that disorder. After discerning the physical therapy implications of the defect, the therapist implements a treatment plan to prevent the anticipated complications or secondary impairments typically associated with that genetic disorder such as plantar flexor contractures.

■ INTERVENTIONS

Physical therapy interventions for infants and children with genetic disorders strive to maximize function and participation, educate the child and family, recommend any needed adaptive equipment, and coordinate services.

Babies from birth to 3 years old may qualify for early intervention services provided in the natural environment, which typically includes at home, daycare, or parks. Based on this model, PTs use the toys and equipment the family or caregiver has available. Consequently, therapists use their body and household furniture as equipment, toys, books, balls, and the child's family as motivation. PTs and families may find this model offers too few therapy services from all disciplines. While many infants, young children, families, and caregivers prefer this model, others may find that the child participates better or requires more equipment typically available in the outpatient arena. Consequently, families may choose therapy services outside of the early intervention model, selecting instead to attend an outpatient clinic that contains benches, therapy balls, developmentally appropriate toys, and other therapeutic equipment such as a treadmill, functional electrical stimulation, or serial casting. The family may also choose to supplement or substitute therapy with hippotherapy, aquatics, motorized ride-on child cars, community fitness programs, or adaptive sports.

Therapists collaborate with families to integrate the desired motor skills into their child's normal routines, often during parent and child play activities.[45] Valvano[45] investigated activity-focused motor interventions for infants and young children with neurologic conditions. According to this model, the therapist, as a member of the intervention team, develops activity-related goals in collaboration with the child's family.

Key Concepts

The therapist plans activity-focused interventions by (1) using guidelines based on principles from motor learning and motor development; (2) adapting these guidelines, when necessary, to address the young child's individual strengths and needs; and (3) integrating impairment-focused interventions with activity-focused interventions, optimally within the context of everyday routines and activities.[45]

■ ADAPTIVE EQUIPMENT

Depending on the child's mobility, the progressive nature of the specific genetic disorder, and the family's needs, the PT may recommend adaptive equipment. This can include positioning devices for supported sitting or feeding or mobility devices such as walkers, gait trainers, standers, or wheelchairs. Occupational and speech therapists may recommend additional equipment to help with feeding and communication. Each therapist educates team members to reinforce and follow through with the recommendations so that each discipline is supporting the other, the caregiver, and the child with integrating the recommendations. For example, the PT may recommend and assist with acquiring a seat for positioning during feeding. The OT may recommend use of specific cause-effect toys that the PT incorporates during therapy. The speech therapist may recommend use of sign language that the PT and OT incorporate during their therapy. The PT must be cognizant of the expense incurred when recommending equipment and ensure the family's willingness to consistently use the equipment prior to proceeding with its purchase. When possible, a trial with loaner equipment helps determine the child's tolerance to and family's follow through with use of the equipment. Unfortunately, vendors seldom stock equipment for trial use. Consequently, therapists often find the piece of equipment, such as a stander, that was recommended, agreed to, and purchased gathering dust in the corner of the home because the child resists its use, so the family abandons the device.

■ AQUATICS

Physical therapy using therapeutic activities in a swimming pool, or aquatics, allows children with genetic disorders to exercise or move in a safer, gravity-eliminated environment. As a result, the child may move through a greater range of motion, with greater ease and less pain, and with less risk of joint damage or a fracture while also improving strength endurance. See **Figure 14-7**A&B. Aquatics have been recommended as a physical therapy intervention for children with Down syndrome, spinal muscular atrophy,[32] Prader-Willi syndrome,[30] and osteogenesis imperfecta.[24]

■ BODY WEIGHT–SUPPORTED LOCOMOTOR TRAINING

Body weight–supported locomotor training (BWSLT) consists of straps suspended from overhead that support the child to allow for partial or full weight bearing during ambulation either with or without manual assistance of the lower extremities. See **Figure 14-8**. Many families do not have the option of using the equipment needed for BWSLT in the home, but instead, the adult can support the young child's weight while the child ambulates on a treadmill. Families without treadmills at home may use the same technique at their local gym. Otherwise, this treatment technique occurs most frequently in the outpatient setting. The ultimate purpose of BWSLT is to transition the child toward independent ambulation on a level surface in the natural environment. In one study, research on

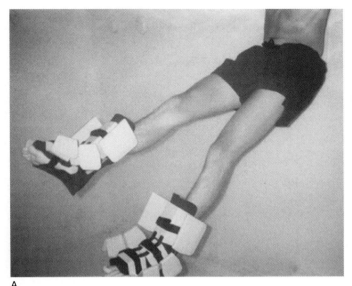

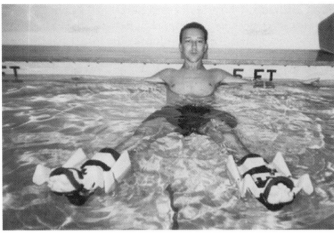

A   B

FIGURE 14-7 Aquatic exercises. (Reproduced, with permission, from Canavan PK. *Rehabilitation in Sports Medicine:* A Comprehensive Guide. New York, NY: Appleton & Lange; 1998.)

young children with Down syndrome who received therapy incorporating a treadmill ambulated independently 101 days sooner than their peers with Down syndrome who did not use a treadmill.[46] Young children with Down syndrome exercising

at a higher intensity produced a significantly longer stride length, learned to walk earlier, and elicited more advanced gait patterns.[47]

CONSTRAINT-INDUCED MOVEMENT THERAPY

Therapists primarily select constraint-induced movement therapy (CIMT) for children who have hemiplegia. CIMT involves use of a sling, mitten, or cast on the strong arm to force use of the weaker arm. Although most research on CIMT is based on children with hemiplegia due to cerebral palsy, it may be efficacious for children with hemiplegia resulting from a genetic disorder such as sickle cell disease.

MODIFIED ADELI SUIT THERAPY

The Adeli suit was originally developed for the fitness of Russian astronauts. The suit includes a special vest, shorts, knee pads, and footwear linked together with adjustable ties. Modified Adeli suit therapy (MAST) uses a client-centered, goal-oriented approach with an emphasis on play while wearing the suit. Research on MAST primarily involves children with cerebral palsy and small sample sizes. The presence of only 4 randomized controlled trials limits evidence-based support for the applicability and effectiveness of this strategy.[47]

ORTHOTICS

Children with genetic disorders may benefit from orthotics to compensate for hypotonia, in the case of Down syndrome or spinal muscular atrophy, or for joint protection, such as in osteogenesis imperfecta.[24] Therapists should read Chapter 19 of this textbook for an in-depth discussion of lower extremity orthoses for children.

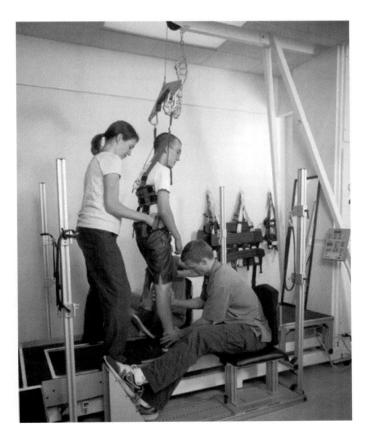

FIGURE 14-8 Body-weight-support treadmill training (BWSTT) with an adolescent. (Reproduced, with permission, from Pelletier ES, Jobst EE. *Physical Therapy Case Files*: Pediatrics. New York: McGraw Hill; 2015.)

■ SENSORY INTEGRATION THERAPY

Sensory integration (SI) therapy incorporates child-directed sensory stimulation (proprioceptive, vestibular, and tactile) activities to elicit adaptive responses to assist the child with learning to organize sensory information in a constructive, pleasurable manner. Although therapy sessions exclusively designed for SI purposes are typically provided by OTs, PTs should incorporate the principles of addressing sensory hyper- or hypofunction into the child's plan of care to optimize function. An example of SI therapy includes the use of swings, other suspended equipment, or therapy balls for vestibular stimulation in all planes of movement with the child in a variety of positions. In sitting or prone, children can use scooter boards to propel themselves for strengthening and vestibular activities. Sensory bins filled with a variety of objects in rice, beans, or water foster tactile stimulation and stereognosis. Likewise, playing in a ball pit provides tactile and proprioceptive input.

Difficulty with processing sensory information, or sensory processing disorder, may occur in some children with genetic disorders such as Down syndrome[48] or fragile X syndrome. Children with sensory processing disorders tend to become easily overwhelmed with the amount of sensory input that most people can filter out and ignore. Symptoms of sensory processing disorders include hyperactive behavior, tactile defensiveness when touched or wearing certain clothing (including socks or shoes), refusing to walk barefooted on the grass, reduced eye contact, and "picky eaters."

■ WHOLE-BODY VIBRATION

Originally designed for astronauts, whole-body vibration (WBV) increases muscle power and strength in adults.[49] In children with Down syndrome, research indicates that WBV improves strength, balance,[11,49] and bone density.[50] See **Figure 14-9.** The methods; duration of the episode of care; and type, design, and parameters of machines varied in each study; therefore, therapists should pay attention to the recommended protocols that primarily include 1 minute on/1 minute off.[49-51] Best practice for the recommended parameters has not been established.[49] WBV is primarily recommended for preadolescent to adolescent children with Down syndrome or children with Rett syndrome who have low bone mineral density.[12] WBV is safe for use in children with Duchenne muscular dystrophy, but no lasting changes were noted in the small study.[52] Low-quality evidence[53] exists for use of WBV for children with osteogenesis imperfecta. In a systemic review and meta-analysis conducted in 2019, no randomized controlled trials existed. WBV was found to positively affect bone mineral density but failed to result in clinical outcomes.[53]

Case 1

Down Syndrome

A PT receives a referral for a 7-month-old male diagnosed with Down syndrome who is enrolled in an early intervention

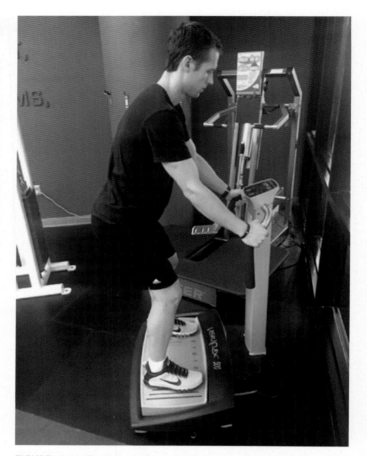

FIGURE 14-9 Vibration platform. (Reproduced, with permission, from Shamus E, Shamus J. *Sports Injury Prevention & Rehabilitation*, 2e. New York: McGraw Hill; 2017.)

program. The parents report that the baby was diagnosed in utero and was born full term. He is hypotonic and not yet rolling. He can achieve prone on elbows but not prone on extended arms. In supine, the baby exhibits decreased activity when reaching against gravity or kicking his legs. There is a mild head lag when pulled into sitting and mild trunk flexion when supported in sitting. When held in supported standing, the baby does not take weight on the legs.

Interventions

- Encourage tummy time for play: Practice assisting him from prone on elbows to prone on extended arms; place toys slightly out to the sides to encourage him to reach and to begin moving in prone.
- Encourage increased kicking: While supervised in supine, loosely tie a balloon to his leg to improve his antigravity leg strength and endurance.
- Facilitate rolling: In supine, gently traction one arm or leg across his trunk to activate the abdominals to encourage rolling while reaching for a toy or family member. In side lying, use a toy to encourage reaching to transfer into prone or supine; this activity can also be completed on a medium- or large-size ball with the therapist's hands on the baby's trunk to control the speed of rolling.

- Encourage weight bearing through the legs: Place him in prone on a small therapy ball and support his trunk with your trunk, hold his knees straight, and bring his feet toward the floor to accept weight. While you are sitting down, have the baby facing you for a hug while you hold his knees straight and place his feet on the floor to accept some weight.
- When he begins to accept weight on his legs, if the family is interested, explore the possibility of body weight–supported locomotor training either at home or in an outpatient clinic to facilitate ambulating independently.

Case 2

Down Syndrome

At birth, a female baby presented with signs of Down syndrome including the typical facial features and hypotonia. The diagnosis was confirmed several weeks later. The baby was enrolled in the local early intervention (EI) program at 3 months old. The EI team included a PT and OT and a speech-language pathologist. The PT served as the primary service provider of the EI team and worked with the baby's family to develop a home program to facilitate her development. At 5 months of age, the baby had heart surgery to correct a congenital atrioventricular septal defect, from which she recovered well. She developed her gross motor skills in a time frame typical for children with Down syndrome. She started rolling at 6 months, sitting independently at 12 months old, creeping on hands and knees at 16 months old, and walking independently at 28 months.[54]

Now at 38 months old, she is starting preschool. She walks up to 250 ft and is beginning to run, but she quickly fatigues. She climbs up and down stairs in a step-to-step pattern with both hands held for support. At preschool, her family wants her to sit with her friends in circle time on the floor, sit at the table during snack time, and keep up with her friends on the playground. Her preschool also has a variety of tricycles available to use on the playground, although she never attempted to use one before. She is shy with new people but eventually warms up and is very social. The family's goals are to improve her play with her peers and participation in family outings.

Interventions

- Use social games (singing, dance, yoga) with her and/or other children to improve her coordination, proprioception, and imitation.
- Assist her on the playground equipment such as using a slide; walking up the slide with her hands held; climbing up and down a ladder; using a toddler swing and then progressing to the child's sling swing; and climbing up and down steps, through tunnels, up the child-sized rock wall, and over and under equipment.
- Help her complete activities and stay on task while participating in physical education with her classmates.
- Create obstacle courses such as walking over a step or on a balance beam or curb, jumping on a mini trampoline,

standing on one foot, and standing up on her toes while reaching to retrieve an object; this activity can include picking up various puzzle pieces, toys, or bean bags with assistance as needed.
- Assist her with using a toddler's riding toy or tricycle; this equipment may need modifications like straps that keep her feet on the pedals.
- Incorporate floor and tabletop motor activities (puzzles, coloring books, reading books) to reinforce sitting endurance.
- Walk on the curb or a 2 in × 4 ft "beam" on the floor to facilitate narrowing her base of support and work on balance and coordination.
- Teach her and her family how to "jump" by holding her hands and encouraging her to bend her knees; use a child's trampoline; practice jumping into ball pit or pool.
- Practice ball skills such as kicking a ball that is stable and then progressing to kicking a rolling ball; practice throwing different size balls; practice catching a ball gently thrown to her from a short distance and progressively move farther away from her; play basketball by placing a ball in a child-size hoop or elevated wastebasket; use a plastic bat to hit a ball off a child's tee-ball stand.
- Instruct the family to practice stair climbing either in the home or out in the community.
- Teach her family to hold her hand to help her learn to "run" with them to increase her speed and endurance.
- Encourage her family to walk with her for progressively longer time periods while out in the community for outings to build her endurance.

Case 3

Rett Syndrome

A 2-year-old female referred to outpatient physical therapy with a diagnosis of developmental delay has an appointment with genetics in a few weeks. The child recently had an electroencephalogram that suggested generalized seizure disorder and an MRI that showed cerebral atrophy. Her mother reports an uncomplicated pregnancy and delivery. She states the child was developing well until she started to regress at 13 months old. The child no longer babbles, pays attention to her family, or holds objects in her hands. The parents' primary goal is for her to walk by herself.

Upon examination, the PT notes the child is hypotonic, "walks" on her knees as her primary method of mobility, and sits independently but does not pull to stand or take weight on her legs when supported in standing. She is nonverbal with very few vocalizations and infrequent eye contact.

Interventions

- Educate the family regarding their rights to and the benefits of enrolling in a local early intervention program, and refer the child if the family is interested.
- Discuss the benefits of a gait trainer with the family; write a letter of medical necessity for the equipment if the family

agrees, and coordinate with a local provider of durable medical equipment to order the device.

- Develop a home program with the family including instructing them on how to help the child stand after diaper changes and when giving her hugs.
- Encourage the use of musical toys that are easily activated to motivate her to use her hands.
- Assist the child with playing in quadruped to inhibit wringing her hands and facilitate upper extremity weight bearing.
- Practice transfers from sitting to standing first from a child's chair by standing in front of her, elevating and gently using traction on both of her arms; progress to transferring from the floor through half kneel to standing by kneeling behind her and helping her push up on the lead leg with one hand on that quadriceps and the other hand on her glutes on the opposite side.
- Assist her with standing by kneeling behind her using your trunk to extend her hips and hands on the anterior lower portion of her quadriceps to facilitate weight bearing; passively weight shift with her in this position and/or actively encourage her to reach for her mother.
- Consider ankle-foot orthoses to maintain her foot and ankle in good alignment in standing, if needed.
- Assist with weight bearing in standing with a universal exercise unit (known as the "monkey cage" or the "spider cage") that is available in some outpatient clinics. This device uses a system of pulleys that isolate muscles, allowing for strengthening of specific muscle groups based on exercises performed. The spider cage is made up of a system of bungee cords that allow for more independent movements including weight bearing and weight shifting. Games should be incorporated with the exercise unit that allow the child to use her upper extremities to play while weight bearing through her lower extremities.
- Explore the possibility of body weight–supported locomotor training on a treadmill either at home or in an outpatient clinic to facilitate ambulating if the family is interested.
- Incorporate music and dance into interventions to enhance motor skills.[55]

Case 4

Prader-Willi Syndrome

A 3-month-old male is referred to physical therapy due to hypotonia. The mother reports no difficulty with the pregnancy or delivery. The infant is diagnosed with failure to thrive and difficulty feeding, resulting in placement of a gastrostomy tube (G-tube) to assist with weight gain and growth. Upon examination, the infant has poor head control and is unable to achieve prone on elbows. The infant is referred to a geneticist and is ultimately diagnosed with Prader-Willi syndrome.

Interventions

- Teach the family how to help the baby sit on their lap with one hand supporting his abdominals and the other hand supporting his back with both hands close to the head while allowing enough movement for him to practice head control; this same strategy may be used with him on a therapy ball.
- Encourage the family to carry the baby up at their shoulder with support at the upper back or to carry him against their trunk with him facing forward with one arm supporting his hips and knees in flexion and their other arm around his trunk to allow him to practice holding his head up while looking around.
- Place him in prone with an adult or child in front of him calling his name; the G-tube is usually not uncomfortable in this position unless it was recently placed, in which case, a pillow can be placed above and below the G-tube to prevent bearing weight on the device.
- Place him prone on elbows with a U-shaped nursing pillow or towel roll horizontally under his axilla with support at his shoulders and toys to entertain him for motivation to lift his head. Educate the family on the importance of supervising the child in this position and prohibiting sleeping in this position due to risk of apnea.
- Facilitate lower extremity weight bearing by holding him in supported standing after each diaper change or when hugging him with his feet on the adult's legs or on a supporting surface.
- Since he presents with hypotonia and developmental delay, the treatment strategies previously discussed for the 7-month-old child with Down syndrome may be appropriate for this baby as well, especially as he progresses.

Case 5

CHARGE Syndrome

A 9-year-old boy was born at 32 weeks' gestational age. After genetic testing, he received a primary diagnosis of CHARGE syndrome. He has multiple congenital anomalies including a ventricular septal defect and gastroesophageal reflux disease. He has disturbances in sensory processing involving all senses, in addition to hearing and vision impairment and difficulties with communication, balance, and mobility. The child currently lives with his father who wants him to receive every opportunity in therapy to participate at home and in school as much as possible. The child is in special education and has an Individualized Education Program. He is followed by a special education teacher and OT and has had services recommended by a PT for proprioception and mobility. He was not able to complete standardized testing, and during observation, he appeared to have poor safety and judgment when ambulating, including attempting to leave the area with evidence of frustration and agitation during challenging tasks.

Interventions

- Educate the teachers regarding the importance of structure and routine; encourage them to assist the child with independent mobility in the classroom and around the school as much as possible.
- Assess the appropriateness of his classroom chair to ensure the required amount of support is provided; modify seating and make recommendations accordingly to minimize fatigue.
- Assist him with standing on a Bosu ball with one or both feet or on a rocker board with contact guard or close stand-by supervision while playing a game or singing to improve his dynamic balance.
- Practice standing on one leg for as long as possible; place a sticker on his foot or shoe during this task or encourage him to step on bubbles blown by the therapist.
- Practice ball skills to increase his coordination including kicking a ball rolled to him, playing soccer, and teaching him how to drop-kick a ball (like punting a football), dribble a ball, throw a tennis ball into a trash can, catch different-sized balls thrown from progressively greater distances, and play volleyball with a balloon or beach ball.
- Walk throughout the school and/or playground for progressively longer time periods to increase his endurance; include stair climbing if available.
- Use an obstacle course that incorporates jumping over a line taped on the floor, walking on a balance beam, and pulling himself in prone on a scooter board and other similar activities that incorporate other targeted impairments or functional limitations.
- Monitor flexibility and strength and address as needed.
- Incorporate following directions with an emphasis on safety during all activities.

Case 6

Potocki-Lupski Syndrome

As introduced earlier in this chapter, a 15-month-old male could ring sit independently when placed on the floor but would not reach outside of the base of support and could not transfer himself into or out of sitting. While sitting, he had spinal flexion, a hypomobile spine on palpation, and a panicked appearance. He rolled as his primary method of mobility, but could not commando crawl, creep on his hands and knees, or cruise at furniture. He stood with support and ambulated 2 to 3 ft with his hands held overhead.

Interventions

- Place toys progressively out of his reach in sitting to encourage him to reach outside of his base of support with manual assistance provided to reduce his anxiety.
- Provide manual assistance at his trunk to facilitate spinal mobility into trunk flexion, extension, and rotation while in ring sitting or sitting on the therapist's leg.

- Place him on hands and knees assisting him with support surrounding his trunk, including weight shifting anteriorly and posteriorly as well as laterally to increase tolerance to movement.
- Assist him with pulling up into standing at furniture with assistance at his hips and help him slowly lower himself into sitting.
- Sit him on the therapist's lap while on a therapy ball with gentle anterior, posterior, and lateral rocking to increase his tolerance to movement while feeling safe and secure. Progressively move him further away from the therapist's body, and eventually help him sit on the ball with only contact guard assistance for safety.
- Ambulate with his hands held overhead for progressively increased distances. He may respond best when ambulating toward a family member or preferred toy.

Case 7

GATAD2B-Associated Neurodevelopmental Disorder

At 7 years old, a child continues to exhibit generalized hypotonia. She has decreased strength in the lower extremities especially in right quadriceps and gluteals as evidenced by transferring from the floor to standing through half kneeling consistently leading with left leg and using her hands on floor to push up into standing. She exhibits gravitational insecurity by refusing to ride a trike or bike with pedals and dislikes the child's swing in the park. She sits straddled on a child's electric riding toy (like a horse) if her brother rides behind her but falls off backward if he does not and is fearful of riding alone. She runs slowly in an awkward manner and is not yet able to jump in place.

Interventions

- Transfer from half kneel to standing leading with the right lower extremity while holding a toy to prevent her from using her arms and with manual assistance to complete the task.
- Ascend a large step with manual assistance at her trunk or by holding her hands leading with the right lower extremity to increase muscle strength.
- Help her learn to jump using a small trampoline with a handlebar that family possesses.
- Practice riding electric toy horse that she operates with close stand-by assistance at her trunk to prevent falls.
- Sit her on a therapy ball with firm manual assistance to instill security and slowly increase the speed to improve her tolerance to vestibular stimulation.
- Stand on one leg "like a ballerina" with hands held with progressively less assistance and for progressively longer periods of time.
- Run holding her hand while chasing and kicking a ball.

CHAPTER SUMMARY

- A PT partnership with families and other health care professionals is necessary to coordinate the enhancement of coping skills, educational planning, health care, and respite services.[4]

- PTs may be the first provider to recognize a possible genetic disorder and to recommend genetic testing to the primary care provider.

- Genetic disorders can be classified as single-gene, dominant, or recessive. There are autosomal dominant disorders, autosomal recessive disorders, X-linked dominant disorders, and X-linked recessive disorders.

- Many genetic disorders affect stages of development and result in global developmental delay, such as Down syndrome, while others result in purely motor symptoms such as muscular dystrophy.

- Obstetricians may recommend prenatal genetic testing when there is a family history of a known genetic disorder or due to advanced maternal age, both of which are associated with an increased risk for a genetic defect.

- A genetic disorder is usually diagnosed through a combination of a physical examination, personal medical history, family medical history, and laboratory testing.

- Genetic disorders may be characterized by cognitive impairment, orthopedic anomalies, stereotypical facial features, and physical features.

- Common impairments of a genetic disorder include hypotonia, ligamentous laxity, decreased strength, decreased balance, decreased coordination, pes planus when standing, wide base of support during gait, ataxia, and sensory defensiveness.

- The main purposes of interventions for infants and children with genetic disorders are to improve participation and function, prevent secondary impairments, educate the child and family, and coordinate services.

STUDY QUESTIONS

1. Which of the following is characteristic of children with Rett syndrome?
   a. Micrognathia
   b. Wringing of hands
   c. Fractures
   d. Nystagmus

2. Constraint-induced movement therapy would be *most* appropriate for children with which of the following deficits?
   a. Bilateral lower extremity spasticity
   b. Poor head and trunk control
   c. Upper extremity hemiplegia
   d. Inability to stand with support

3. A physical therapist is preparing to evaluate a 3-year-old diagnosed with Down syndrome. The therapist should anticipate which of the following findings?
   a. Decreased strength and flexibility
   b. Excessive range of motion and joint pain
   c. Gross motor delay and contractures
   d. Hypotonia and ligamentous laxity

4. Osteogenesis imperfecta most often results in which of the following?
   a. Spontaneous fractures and death as an infant
   b. Normal height and use of a wheelchair for mobility
   c. Spontaneous fractures and scoliosis
   d. Normal height and life span

5. Pierre Robin sequence is characterized by which of the following?
   a. Ear infections
   b. Hearing impairment
   c. Musculoskeletal anomalies
   d. All of the above

6. Family education for a 3-month-old infant with Prader-Willi syndrome should include which of the following instructions?
   a. Avoid placing the baby in prone because it is too difficult at this age.
   b. Teach the parents how to carry the baby to facilitate improved head control.
   c. Restrict the daily caloric intake to prevent the tendency for obesity.
   d. Use the infant seat often for positioning for the baby.

7. The typical genetic makeup of a fetus contains which of the following?
   a. 1 Y chromosome
   b. 23 genes
   c. 24 autosomes
   d. 46 chromosomes

(Continued)

STUDY QUESTIONS (*CONTINUED*)

8. Which of the following is the *most* appropriate action for a physical therapist who suspects a young child has an undiagnosed genetic disorder?

a. Stop physical therapy until the child is properly diagnosed.

b. Inform the parent that the child has an undiagnosed genetic disorder.

c. Contact the pediatrician to recommend a genetic consult.

d. Instruct the parent to contact a geneticist for a consultation.

9. Which of the following techniques for assessing genetic disorders in utero is considered the *most* accurate?

a. Amniocentesis

b. Chorionic villus sampling

c. Radiograph

d. Sonogram

10. A physical therapist is scheduled to evaluate a young child who has a genetic disorder with which the therapist is unfamiliar. Which of the following is the MOST appropriate strategy for the therapist?

a. Ask the parents to educate you about the disorder.

b. Contact the geneticist to inquire about the disorder.

c. Read research articles about the disorder prior to the appointment.

d. Refer the family to a therapist with more knowledge of the disorder.

References

1. Johnson M, Gallagher K. *One in a Billion*. New York: Simon & Schuster; 2016.

2. Centers for Disease Control and Prevention. *Data and Statistics on Birth Defects*. Accessed November 25, 2023. https://www.cdc.gov/ncbddd/birthdefects/data.html.

3. Smith M, Danoff J, Jain M, Long T. Genetic disorders: implications for allied health professionals: two case studies. *Int J Allied Health Sci Pract*. 2007;5:4.

4. American Academy of Pediatrics Committee on Children With Disabilities. General principles in the care of children and adolescents with genetic disorders and other chronic health conditions. *Pediatrics*. 1997;99(4):643-644.

5. Sanger WG, Dave B, Stuberg W. Overview of genetics and role of the pediatric physical therapist in the diagnostic process. *Pediatr Phys Ther*. 2001;13(4):164-18.

6. Orphanet. *Hemophilia*. Accessed November 25, 2023. https://www.orpha.net/consor/cgi-bin/Disease_Search.php?lng=EN&data_id=646&Disease_Disease_Search_diseaseGroup=Hemophilia&Disease_Disease_Search_diseaseType=Pat&Disease(s)/group%20of%20diseases=Hemophilia&title=Hemophilia&search=-Disease_Search_Simple.

7. Effgen SK. Child development. In: Effgen SK, Fiss AL, eds. *Meeting the Physical Therapy Needs of Children*. 3rd ed. McGraw Hill; 2021.

8. Al-Zaidy SA, Mendell JR. From clinical trials to clinical practice: practical considerations for gene replacement therapy in SMA Type 1. *Pediatr Neurol*. 2019;100:3-11.

9. Kemp WL, Burns DK, Brown TG, eds. Genetic disorders. In: *Pathology: The Big Picture*. McGraw Hill; 2008.

10. Medscape. *Down Syndrome Workup*. Accessed November 23, 2023. https://emedicine.medscape.com/article/943216-workup#c6.

11. Saquetto MB, Pereira FF, Queiroz RS, da Silva CM, Conceicao CS, Gomes-Neto M. Effects of whole-body vibration on muscle strength, bone mineral content and density, and balance and body composition of children and adolescents with Down syndrome: a systematic review. *Osteoporos Int*. 2018;29(3):527-533.

12. Afzal SA, Wender AR, Jones MD, Fung EB, Pico EL. The effect of low magnitude mechanical stimulation (LMMS) on bone density in patients with Rett syndrome: a pilot and feasibility study. *J Pediatr Rehabil Med*. 2014;7(2):167-178.

13. Orphanet. *Rett Syndrome*. Accessed November 23, 2023. https://www.orpha.net/consor/cgi-bin/Disease_Search.php?lng=EN&data_id=3164&Disease_Disease_Search_diseaseGroup=rett-syndrome&Disease_Disease_Search_diseaseType=Pat&Disease(s)/group%20of%20diseases=Atypical-Rett-syndrome&title=Atypical%20Rett%20syndrome&search=Disease_Search_Simple.

14. Orphanet. *Achondroplasia*. Accessed November 3, 2023. https://www.orpha.net/consor/cgi-bin/Disease_Search.php?lng=EN&data_id=148&Disease_Disease_Search_diseaseGroup=Achondroplasia&Disease_Disease_Search_diseaseType=Pat&Disease(s)/group%20of%20diseases=Achondroplasia&title=Achondroplasia&search=Disease_Search_Simple.

15. Genetic and Rare Diseases Information Center. *CHARGE Syndrome*. Accessed November 5, 2023. https://rarediseases.info.nih.gov/diseases/29/charge-syndrome.

16. Orphanet. *CHARGE Syndrome*. November 5, 2023. https://www.orpha.net/consor/cgi-bin/Disease_Search.php?lng=EN&data_id=110&Disease_Disease_Search_diseaseGroup=charge-syndrome&Disease_Disease_Search_diseaseType=Pat&Disease(s)/group%20of%20diseases=CHARGE-syndrome&title=CHARGE%20syndrome&search=Disease_Search_Simple.

17. National Human Genome Research Institute. *A Brief Guide to Genomics*. Accessed November 25, 2023. https://www.genome.gov/about-genomics/fact-sheets/A-Brief-Guide-to-Genomics.

18. National Organization for Rare Diseases. *Cri-du-chat*. Accessed November 2, 2023. https://rarediseases.org/rare-diseases/cri-du-chat-syndrome/.

19. Tekerlek H, Yardımcı-Lokmanoglu BN, Inal-Ince D, Özçelik U, Mutlu A. Developmental functioning outcomes in infants with cystic fibrosis: a 24- to 36-month follow-up study. *Phys Ther*. 2022;102(6):pzac037.

20. Centers for Disease Control and Prevention. *Genomics 101*. Accessed November 25, 2023. https://www.cdc.gov/genomics/about/basics.htm#:~:text=Genetics%20research%20studies%20how%

20individual,promoting%20health%20and%20preventing%20disease.

21. Yigit S, Albayrak HM, Yücel PP, Usgu S, Yakut Y. The outcomes of an individualized physical therapy program in CAL-FAN syndrome: a case report. *Pediatr Phys Ther.* 2022;34(3):432-437.

22. Shieh C, Jones N, Vanle B, et al. *GATAD2B*-associated neurodevelopmental disorder (GAND): clinical and molecular insights into a NuRD-related disorder. *Genet Med.* 2020;22(5):878-888.

23. Orphanet. *Osteogenesis Imperfecta.* Accessed October 3, 2023. https://www.orpha.net/consor/cgi-bin/Disease_Search.php?lng=EN&data_id=654&Disease_Disease_Search_diseaseGroup=osteogenesis-imperfecta&Disease_Disease_Search_diseaseType=Pat&Disease(s)/group%20of%20diseases=Osteogenesis-imperfecta&title=Osteogenesis%20imperfecta&search=Disease_Search_Simple.

24. Medscape. *Osteogenesis Imperfecta (OI).* Accessed November 23, 2023. https://emedicine.medscape.com/article/1256726-overview.

25. Quinonez SC, Barsh G. Genetic disease. In: Hammer GD, McPhee SJ, eds. *Pathophysiology of Disease: An Introduction to Clinical Medicine.* 8th ed. McGraw Hill; 2019.

26. Orphanet. *Isolated Pierre Robin Syndrome.* Accessed November 30, 2023. https://www.orpha.net/consor/cgi-bin/Disease_Search.php?lng=EN&data_id=562&Disease_Disease_Search_diseaseGroup=Isolated-Pierre-Robin-Syndrome&Disease_Disease_Search_diseaseType=Pat&Disease(s)/group%20of%20diseases=Isolated-Pierre-Robin-syndrome&title=Isolated%20Pierre%20Robin%20syndrome&search=Disease_Search_Simple.

27. Medscape. *Pierre Robin Sequence.* Accessed November 30, 2023. https://emedicine.medscape.com/article/995706-overview.

28. Potocki L, Neira-Fresneda J, Yuan B. Potocki-Lupski syndrome. 2017 Aug 24. In: Adam MP, Mirzaa GM, Pagon RA, et al, eds. *GeneReviews®.* University of Washington, Seattle; 1993-2022. Accessed November 30, 2023. https://www.ncbi.nlm.nih.gov/books/NBK447920/.

29. Orphanet. *Potocki-Lupski Syndrome.* Accessed November 30, 2023. https://www.orpha.net/consor/cgi-bin/Disease_Search.php?lng=EN&data_id=1160&Disease_Disease_Search_diseaseGroup=Potocki-Lupski-Syndrome&Disease_Disease_Search_diseaseType=Pat&Disease(s)/group%20of%20diseases=17p11-2-microduplication-syndrome&title=17p11.2%20microduplication%20syndrome&search=Disease_Search_Simple.

30. Orphanet. *Prader-Willi Syndrome.* Accessed November 30, 2023. https://www.orpha.net/consor/cgi-bin/Disease_Search.php?lng=EN&data_id=139&Disease_Disease_Search_diseaseGroup=Prader-Willi-syndrome&Disease_Disease_Search_diseaseType=Pat&Disease(s)/group%20of%20diseases=Prader-Willi-syndrome&title=Prader-Willi%20syndrome&search=Disease_Search_Simple.

31. Callanen A, Richman S. *Prader-Willi Syndrome: Physical Therapy.* CINAHL Rehabilitation Guide; January 3, 2020.

32. Matlick D, Richman S. *Spinal Muscular Atrophy: Physical and Occupational Therapy.* CINAHL Rehabilitation Guide; September 17, 2021.

33. MedlinePlus. *X-linked Infantile Spinal Muscular Atrophy.* Accessed November 30, 2023. https://medlineplus.gov/genetics/condition/x-linked-infantile-spinal-muscular-atrophy/.

34. MedlinePlus, National Library of Medicine. *Tay-Sachs Disease.* Accessed October 30, 2023. https://medlineplus.gov/genetics/condition/tay-sachs-disease/.

35. Orphanet. *Tay-Sachs Disease.* Accessed October 30, 2023. https://www.orpha.net/consor/cgi-bin/Disease_Search.php?lng=EN&data_id=888&Disease_Disease_Search_diseaseGroup=Tay-Sachs-disease&Disease_Disease_Search_diseaseType=Pat&Disease(s)/group%20of%20diseases=Tay-Sachs-disease&title=Tay-Sachs%20disease&search=Disease_Search_Simple.

36. Orphanet. *Turner Syndrome.* Accessed October 30, 2023. https://www.orpha.net/consor/cgi-bin/Disease_Search.php?lng=EN&data_id=44&Disease_Disease_Search_diseaseGroup=Turner-syndrome&Disease_Disease_Search_diseaseType=Pat&Disease(s)/group%20of%20diseases=Turner-syndrome&title=Turner%20syndrome&search=Disease_Search_Simple.

37. Medscape. *Osteogenesis Imperfecta (OI) Workup.* Accessed October 30, 2023. https://emedicine.medscape.com/article/1256726-workup#c6.

38. Mithyantha R, Kneen R, McCann E, Gladstone M. Current evidence-based recommendations on investigating children with global developmental delay. *Arch Dis Child.* 2017;102(11):1071-1076.

39. National Human Genome Research Institute. *A Brief Guide to Genomics.* Accessed November 29, 2023. https://www.genome.gov/about-genomics/fact-sheets/A-Brief-Guide-to-Genomics.

40. Centers for Disease Control and Prevention. *Genomics and Precision Health*: Genetic Testing. Accessed October 29, 2023. https://www.cdc.gov/genomics/gtesting/genetic_testing.htm.

41. Hunter AGW. Medical genetics: 2. The diagnostic approach to the child with dysmorphic signs. *CMAJ.* 2002;167(4):367-372.

42. American Physical Therapy Association. *APTA Guide to Physical Therapist Practice, 3.0.* American Physical Therapy Association. Accessed October 29, 2023. http://guidetoptpractice.apta.org/.

43. Palisano RJ, Walter SD, Russell DJ, et al. Gross motor function of children with Down Syndrome: creation of motor growth curves. *Arch Phys Med Rehabil.* 2001;82:(4):494-500.

44. Medscape. *Rett Syndrome.* Accessed October 1, 2023. https://emedicine.medscape.com/article/916377-overview.

45. Valvano J. Activity-focused motor interventions for children with neurological conditions. *Phys Occup Ther Pediatr.* 2004;24(1-2):79-107.

46. Ulrich DA, Ulrich BD, Angulo-Kinzler RM, Yun J. Treadmill training of infants with Down syndrome: evidence-based developmental outcomes. *Pediatrics.* 2001;108(5):E84.

47. Wu J, Looper J, Ulrich BD, Ulrich DA, Angulo-Barroso RM. Exploring effects of different treadmill interventions on walking onset and gait patterns in infants with Down syndrome. *Dev Med Child Neurol.* 2007;49(11):839-845.

48. Uyanik M, Bumin G, Kayihan H. Comparison of different therapy approaches in children with Down syndrome. *Pediatr Int.* 2003;45(1):68-73.

49. Swolin-Eide D, Magnusson P. Does whole-body vibration treatment make children's bones stronger? *Curr Osteoporos Rep.* 2020;18(5):471-479.

50. Ibrahim MM, Abdullah GA. Effect of whole body vibration versus treadmill training on bone mineral density in children with Down Syndrome. *Indian J Physiotherapy Occupat Ther.* 2015;9(2):97-101.

51. Matute-Llorente Á, González-Agüero A, Gómez-Cabello A, Tous-Fajardo J, Vicente-Rodríguez G, Casajús JA. Effect of whole-body vibration training on bone mass in adolescents with and without Down syndrome: a randomized controlled trial. *Osteoporosis Int.* 2016;27(1):181-191.

52. Söderpalm A-C, Kroksmark A-K, Magnusson P, Karlsson J, Tulinius M, Swolin-Eide D. Whole body vibration therapy in patients with

Duchenne muscular dystrophy: a prospective observational study. *J Musculoskelet Neuronal Interact.* 2013;13(1):13-18.

53. Leite HR, Camargos ACR, Mendonc VA, Lacerda ACR, Soares BA, Oliveira VC. Current evidence does not support whole body vibration in clinical practice in children and adolescents with disabilities: a systematic review of randomized controlled trial. *Braz J Phys Ther.* 2019;23(3):196-211.

54. Kim HI, Kim SW, Kim J, Jeon HR, Jung DW. Motor and cognitive development profiles in children with Down syndrome. *Ann Rehabil Med.* 2017;41(1):97-103.

55. Wigram T, Lawrence M. Music therapy as a tool for assessing hand use and communicativeness in children with Rett syndrome. *Brain Dev.* 2005;27(suppl 1):S95-S96.

56. American Physical Therapy Association. *Evaluation Codes.* Accessed November 20, 2023. https://www.apta.org/contentassets/d3065561ef7643ad9a88f282c6083faa/apta-evalcodes-pocketguide.pdf

57. Brazelton TB. *Neonatal Behavioral Assessment Scale.* Spastics International Publications: Clinics in Developmental Medicine. 3rd ed. Monograph no. 137. Cambridge: Cambridge University Press; 1973. Accessed November 20, 2023. Brazelton-1995-BNBAS-3rd-Edition-Whole-Book.pdf (nidcap.org)

Additional Resources

- Martin K, Natarus M, Martin J, Henderson S. Minimal detectable change for TUG and TUDS test for children with Down syndrome. *Pediatr Phys Ther.* 2017;29(1):77-82.
- Martins E, Oliveira R, Letras S, et al. Efficacy of suit therapy on functioning in children and adolescents with cerebral palsy: a systematic review and meta-analysis. *Dev Med Child Neurol.* 2016;58(4):348-360.
- National Human Genome Research Institute. *Genetic Disorders.* Accessed November 30, 2023. https://www.genome.gov/For-Patients-and-Families/Genetic-Disorders.
- Schoen SA, Lane SJ, Mailloux Z, et al. A systematic review of Ayres Sensory Integration intervention for children with autism. *Autism Res.* 2019;12(1);6-19.
- Steinbrenner JR, Hume K, Odom SL, et al. *Evidence-based Practices for Children, Youth, and Young Adults with Autism.* University of North Carolina at Chapel Hill, Frank Porter Graham Child Development Institute, National Clearinghouse on Autism Evidence and Practice Review Team. 2020. Accessed November 30, 2023. https://ncaep.fpg.unc.edu/sites/ncaep.fpg.unc.edu/files/imce/documents/EBP%20Report%202020.pdf

15

Juvenile Idiopathic Arthritis

Eric Shamus, PT, DPT, PhD, and Jennifer Shamus, DPT, PhD

LEARNING OBJECTIVES

Upon completion of this chapter, the reader will be able to:

- Evaluate signs and symptoms including joint soreness, stiffness, and inflammation related to juvenile idiopathic arthritis.
- Design interventions to protect the joints and maximize function.
- Evaluate activities of daily living to determine if adaptive equipment is indicated.

- Analyze the biomechanics of movement to assist in developing a comprehensive physical therapy plan of care.
- Educate families on juvenile idiopathic arthritis and provide resources on how medical intervention can improve long-term prognosis.

INTRODUCTION

Juvenile arthritis is the most common childhood disease with a prevalence of 1 per 1000 children.[1-3] Juvenile idiopathic arthritis (JIA) (formerly known as juvenile rheumatoid arthritis or pediatric rheumatoid arthritis) refers to a group of autoimmune and inflammatory disorders acquired in children before the age of 16 years with chronic inflammation of one or more joints for more than 6 weeks.[4] The common signs and symptoms include fatigue, rash, morning stiffness, joint redness, swelling, pain, and tenderness unilaterally or bilaterally.[5-13] JIA is characterized by acute and chronic episodes and can affect one or multiple areas of the body. If not detected in the early stages, permanent damage can occur. There is no known etiology[10] and no known cure.[11] Primary treatment includes different medications to reduce inflammation, pain, and prevent joint degradation. The condition can go into remission. Secondary treatment is directed at joint protection and maximizing function.

DIAGNOSIS

JIA is an exclusion diagnosis is made through a combination of methods. Taking a thorough subjective history is very important and can assist the physician in the differential diagnosis. A traditional physical exam that examines joint range of motion is important. Blood work is commonly ordered to investigate markers such as antinuclear antibodies (ANA), rheumatoid factor (RF), and many others. Imaging is often ordered to confirm the diagnosis and identify if any joint damage has occurred. Plain radiography can be used to look at joint space and congruence when evaluating the presence of degradation of the joint in relation to JIA (**Figure 15-1**).[14] Magnetic resonance imaging can detect synovial hypertrophy and articular

cartilage abnormalities.[14] Biochemical changes can be detectable with magnetic resonance spectroscopy even before structural changes within the joint are detectable.[14]

CLASSIFICATION

The 1995 International League of Associations for Rheumatology (ILAR) classification describes the 7 different types of JIA.[4] The categories are defined by the number of joints involved, the presence or absence of extra-articular manifestations, and the presence or absence of clinical laboratory

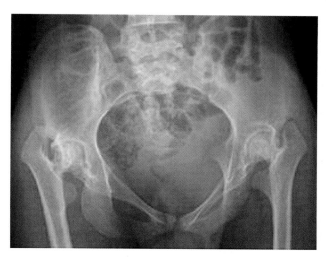

FIGURE 15-1 Juvenile idiopathic arthritis. Anteroposterior view of the pelvis in an 18-year-old male shows concentric narrowing of the hip joints with shortening and erosion of the femoral necks bilaterally. (Reproduced, with permission, from Tehranzadeh J. *Basic Musculoskeletal Imaging*. New York: McGraw Hill; 2014.)

TABLE 15-1 • Subgroups of Juvenile Idiopathic Arthritis (JIA)

JIA Subgroup	Oligoarticular	Polyarticular Negative	Polyarticular Positive	Systemic Onset	Juvenile Psoriatic	Enthesitis-Related (ERA)
Percentage of all JIA	40%	20%	15%	10%–20%	≤10%	≤10%
Age at onset and gender	<8 years g >b	8–12 years g = b	Teen years g >b	Any age	Any age	8–12 years b >g
No. of joints involved	<5	Many	Many	Varies	Varies	Varies
Pattern	Asymmetric	Varies	Symmetric	Asymmetric	Asymmetric	Lower extremity joints
Hips involved	Rarely	No	No	Occasionally	Sometimes	Yes
Back pain	No	No	No	Myalgic	Sometimes	Yes
Clinical features	Painless iridocyclitis Requires regular slitlamp examination	Poor weight gain	Aggressive course Nodules Poor weight gain	Fever Evanescent rash Serositis Lymphadenopathy Hepatosplenomegaly MAS Complications can be fatal	DIP joints Nail pitting Psoriatic rash or positive family history Dactylitis Can look like polyarticular JIA or ERA	Enthesitis Heel pain Sausage digits Abnormal Schober test Sacroiliitis Oral ulcers
Distinguishing lab abnormalities	Antinuclear antibody positive	Rheumatoid factor positive	Rheumatoid factor negative	Increased ESR, WBC, CRP, ferritin, platelets Anemia Abnormal LFTs	None	HLA–B27 positive

Abbreviations: g, girls; b, boys; CRP, C-reactive protein; ESR, erythrocyte sedimentation rate; HLA, human leukocyte antigen; WBC, white blood cell count; LFTs, liver function tests; DIP, distal interphalangeal; MAS, macrophage activation syndrome.

Source: Reproduced with permission from Imboden J, Hellmann DB, Stone JH. Current Rheumatology Diagnosis & Treatment. 2nd ed. New York: McGraw Hill LLC; 2007. and Reproduced with permission from Eric Shamus. The Color Atlas of Physical Therapy. New York: McGraw Hill LLC; 2015.

measures. The 7 classifications are oligoarthritis (persistent or extended), polyarthritis RF positive, polyarthritis RF negative, systemic arthritis, psoriatic arthritis (PsA), enthesitis-related arthritis, and undifferentiated arthritis. Each of the categories is described in the following text and **Table 15-1**.

Oligoarticular JIA (oligoarthritis) is defined as affecting 4 or fewer joints in the first 6 months of diagnosis.[12] This is the most common type of juvenile arthritis, accounting for 50% to 80% of cases involving the large joints (eg, knees, ankles, elbows).[13] The subcategories of persistent or extended oligoarthritis are applied after the first 6 months depending on the number of joints involved at that time. It is persistent if 4 or fewer joints are involved or extended if more than 4 joints become involved.[9] Symptoms tend to be unilateral, and the knee is the most affected joint. It can also impact the ankles, hands, and elbows. Often, the first sign is a limp. Cases can include involvement of the temporomandibular joints (TMJs) and the cervical spine. Oligoarticular JIA can also cause inflammation of the eye that can cause blindness if not detected. The age of onset is typically around 2 to 4 years old, and it occurs more frequently in females.[10]

Polyarticular JIA (polyarthritis) is defined as 5 or more inflamed joints in the first 6 months of the disease and often occurs bilaterally.[12] It accounts for approximately 25% to 35% of JIA cases and is broken down into RF positive or RF negative.

The RF-positive type is more destructive and similar to the adult form. It primarily affects females from 2 to 4 years old or 6 to 12 years old.[10] The RF-negative type primarily occurs in children younger than 6 years old and is more common in females than males. This type of arthritis can affect both the large and small joints of the body including the knees, wrists, TMJ, and cervical spine. Children with polyarthritis can also have involvement of the eye, lymph nodes, spleen, and liver.[10]

Systemic JIA accounts for 5% to 15% of JIA cases, can occur anytime in childhood, and affects boys and girls equally.[13] It is characterized by a high spiking fever (>102-103°F) once or twice a day that can last up to 2 weeks with a macular rash. Systemic JIA affects the entire body and not just the joints. It commonly impacts the skin and the organs.[9] Children with Systemic JIA can have hepatosplenomegaly, leukocytosis, and lymphadenopathy.[12]

Psoriatic arthritis (PsA) generally occurs in 2- to 4-year-olds and 9- to 11-year-olds. It is more common in females than males and impacts both joints and skin. Children will usually have at least 2 of the following 3 symptoms: dactylitis, nail pitting or onycholysis, and psoriasis in a first-degree relative, see **Figure 15-2**. There is usually a scaling red rash on the elbows, knees, eyelids, umbilicus, and behind the ears. Psoriatic arthritis may affect one or more joints.

Enthesitis-related JIA (spondyloarthritis) involves joint swelling and tenderness at the junction between the tendon or

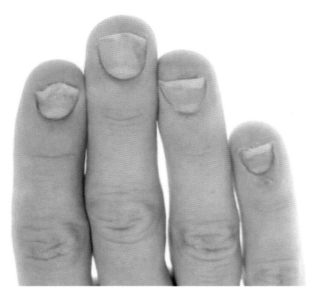

FIGURE 15-2 Typical appearance of nails in a patient with psoriatic arthropathy. (Reproduced, with permission, from Brukner P, Clarsen B, Cook J, et al. *Brukner & Khan's Clinical Sports Medicine: Injuries,* Volume 1, 5e. New York: McGraw Hill; 2017.)

TABLE 15-2 • Impairments in Juvenile Idiopathic Arthritis
• Pain
• Morning stiffness
• Fatigue
• Decreased range of motion or joint contractures in extremities, axial skeleton, and temporomandibular joint
• Decreased strength or muscle atrophy
• Decreased function
○ Transfers
○ Stairs
○ Activities of daily living
• Decreased balance and proprioception[16]
• Impaired coordination
• Vision issues (an appointment with an ophthalmologist is recommended early on for assessment of uveitis)
• Decreased physical fitness[17]
• Decreased physical activity[18]

ligament and the bone. It is frequently seen in the feet, knees, and hips but can impact the fingers, elbows, digestive tract (Crohn disease), spine (ankylosing spondylitis), and pelvis. This type of JIA occurs more often in male children over 6 years old[1] or adolescents (8-15 years old).[10] Cardiovascular or cerebrovascular involvement may occur.[13]

Undifferentiated arthritis is the category used when the symptoms do not fit perfectly into any other category. It can include symptoms that span more than 2 of the previously discussed types. Inflammation in one or more joints must be present.

It is suggested that some of the categories are homogenous while others are heterogeneous.[5] RF-negative polyarthritis and PsA have been shown to be heterogeneous. RF-negative polyarthritis and PsA include a subset of patients characterized by early onset and ANA positivity, a more homogeneous entity observed only in childhood.[5-8] Therefore, the number of joints and the presence of psoriasis may not represent reliable classification for JIA.[5]

In 2019, the Pediatric Rheumatology International Trials Organization (PRINTO) proposed revisions of the current JIA ILAR classification criteria with an evidence-based approach to distinguish those forms of chronic arthritis that are typically seen in children from those that represent the childhood counterpart of diseases observed in adults.[5]

With the revisions, it is recommended that:

- JIA does not represent a single disease; it is a group of different disorders.[5]
- The presence of arthritis is no longer required because patients without arthritis have been included in the definition of systemic JIA.[5]
- Presence of arthritis for 6 or more weeks is now mentioned in pertinent criteria.[5]
- Onset of the disease has been changed to before 18 years of age to distinguish between children and adults in many countries.[5]

FUNCTIONAL IMPLICATIONS

When pain and/or inflammation are present, children with JIA often have difficulty with activities of daily living. Transfers such as getting out of bed or rising from a chair may be difficult. The first few steps in the morning can be very stiff, and walking can be impacted. Climbing or descending stairs can be challenging if the joints of the lower extremity are affected. Fastening buttons or writing can be difficult if the hands are stiff and inflamed. Children often need modification in their school environment depending on the extent of the impairments. Without proper treatment, there is a risk of long-term joint damage that can cause ongoing impaired quality of life.[15] **Table 15-2** provides a list of common impairments seen in JIA.

TESTS AND MEASURES

There are many objective questionnaires and scales that can be used with children with JIA to identify areas of impairment and assess improvement. See **Table 15-3**.

Rashed et al[19] examined the association of handgrip strength with disease activity, disability, and quality of life in children and adolescents with JIA. The research found significant weakness in hand grip strength in the children with JIA when compared to age- and sex-matched controls. Grip strength also had a significant inverse correlation with the Juvenile Arthritis Disease Activity Score, Juvenile Arthritis Functional Assessment Scale, and Pediatric Quality of Life Inventory. Handgrip strength was detected as an independent predictor of disease activity, disability, and quality of life in JIA patients in multivariate linear regression.

PRIMARY MEDICAL INTERVENTION

The primary treatment for JIA is pharmaceutical intervention. If the medications are effective, the pain and swelling will be resolved and further joint damage abated. Initially, a corticosteroid or nonsteroidal anti-inflammatory (NSAID) may be prescribed for the initial relief of inflammation. Following that,

TABLE 15-3 • Objective Questionnaires And Scales That Can Be Used With Children With Juvenile Idiopathic Arthritis

- Childhood Arthritis Health Questionnaire
- Juvenile Arthritis Quality of Life Questionnaire
- Pediatric Quality of Life Questionnaire
- Juvenile Arthritis Functional Assessment Scale
- Juvenile Arthritis Functional Assessment Reports for Parents (JAFAR) (**Figure 15-3A&B**)
- Childhood Health Assessment Questionnaire
- Juvenile Arthritis Functional Assessment Index
- Pediatric Pain Questionnaire
- Visual analog scale (VAS)
- Peabody Developmental Motor Scales–2
- Bruininks-Oseretsky Test of Motor Proficiency
- School Function Assessment
- Canadian Occupational Performance Measure[10]
- Juvenile Arthritis Functional Status Index[10]
- Pediatric Escola Paulista de Medicina Range of Motion Scale[10]
- Pediatric Quality of Life Inventory[17]
- Health-Related Quality of Life[17]
- Childhood Health Questionnaire[17]
- Harvard Step Test[17]
- 6-Minute Walk Test[17]
- Disability Index[17]
- Juvenile Arthritis Disease Activity Score (JADAS)[20]
- Activities Scale for Kids[21]
- Pediatric Outcomes Data Collection Instruments[21]
- Quality of My Life Questionnaire[21]
- Joint Count–Limitation of Motion[21]
- Joint Count–Pain on Motion[21]
- Joint Count–Tenderness[21]
- Functional Reach Test[22]
- Flamingo Balance Test[23]
- Numeric Rating Scale[23]
- Articular Severity Score
- Global Range of Motion Score
- Hand Grip Strength (HGS)[20]

it is common to try a disease-modifying antirheumatic drug (DMARD) such as methotrexate. Methotrexate can be a liquid or injectable form and is normally administered on a weekly basis. If that is insufficient in eliminating the inflammation, a biologic such as adalimumab (Humira) is recommended. The goal of biologics is to suppress the inflammatory pathways without affecting natural defenses. It is not uncommon to combine drug therapies in an attempt to eliminate symptoms and inflammation.

For the physical therapist, it is important to know the side effects of these medications. With the NSAIDs, DMARDs, and biologics, the ability of the immune system to fight infection is reduced. Exposure to people who are ill should be avoided when possible. The NSAIDs and corticosteroids can cause increased bruising. Prolonged usage is rare because it can lead to osteoporosis. Other common side effects of medications can be headache, fever, chills, loss of appetite, fatigue, and nausea. On the day of treatment and the following day, the child may not have the same energy level. Treatment may need to be modified on the day of the physical therapy visit. In addition, if the

medication is administered via injection, there may be injection site pain to take into consideration.

■ PHYSICAL THERAPY INTERVENTION

The need for physical therapy is based on the physician's assessment of loss of range of motion, strength, and function. If the JIA is detected and treated early, physical therapy may not be indicated. When it is ordered, the physical therapist must conduct a thorough history. It is important to know how many and which joints are involved, if articular cartilage damage has occurred, if swelling is present in the joint, the medication regimen, what activities of daily living are limited, and if the child has pain. It is important to note if the disease process is in a period of exacerbation or remission.

The appropriate intervention is dependent on understanding these answers. If swelling is present, the treatment approach must be gentler. If the JIA is in remission, the treatment has few limitations. During an acute flare-up of JIA, the goal is pain control through rest, active range of motion, and modalities like cryotherapy. In the presence of little to no inflammation, intervention can be more comprehensive and based on the physical exam. The physical exam includes the traditional components. Range of motion, strength, gait, balance, and palpable tenderness should all be assessed.

A comprehensive treatment approach is recommended if tolerated. This includes active/active-assisted range of motion, gentle stretching, strengthening, functional activities, and physical fitness. Passive range of motion is normally avoided because it can cause unnecessary stress to the joint. When active and active-assisted range of motion is combined with manual therapy, increased range of motion can be achieved without increasing inflammation. Patient and family education is essential to long-term success with this condition. Joint protection strategies will help prevent further damage to the joints. For example, if the TMJ is involved, learning the proper resting position of the tongue and cutting food into smaller pieces will promote improved joint health and reduce pain. If the wrists and hands are involved, using a pen with a larger grip and avoiding painful end-range positions such as during a push up are important. Proper posture and learning the resting position of each joint can relieve unnecessary stress on the joints. Including age-appropriate activities as part of therapy and a home program can increase the likelihood of adherence to the plan of care.

Splinting is a controversial topic for the child with JIA. In cases where the joint is unstable or an acute injury has been sustained to a ligament, a brief course of splinting may be appropriate to allow for proper healing and to protect the area. Prolonged immobilization can be detrimental to a joint that has active inflammation. It can lead to significant loss of range of motion that is not easily regained. On the other hand, if contractures are present or the goal is to prevent them, resting night splints can be used effectively.

The Ottawa panel evidence-based clinical practice guidelines for structured physical activity in the management of JIA made the following recommendations based on high-quality randomized controlled trials.[24] Pilates was effective for improving quality of life, pain, functional ability, and range of motion

Juvenile Arthritis Functional Assessment Report for Parents (JAFAR)

For children 7 and older with JRA

Patient's
Name (print) _____   **Date of Office Visit**:_____
          First   MI   Last
Patient Date of Birth: _____   **Date this Form Completed:** _____

Part 1   Ability Scale

On this questionnaire, we are interested in learning how your child's illness affects her/his ability to function in daily life. Please feel free to add any comments on the back of this page.
Please check the one response which best describes your child's usual abilities **OVER THE PAST WEEK.**

please answer all questions
In the past week, was Patient able to:

		All the time	Sometimes	Almost never
1	Take shirt off hanger	___	___	___
2	Button shirt	___	___	___
3	Pull on sweater over head	___	___	___
4	Turn on water faucet	___	___	___
5	Sit on floor, then stand up	___	___	___
6	Dry back with towel	___	___	___
7	Wash face with wash cloth	___	___	___
8	Tie shoelaces	___	___	___
9	Pull on socks	___	___	___
10	Brush teeth	___	___	___
11	Stand up from chair without using arms	___	___	___
12	Get into bed	___	___	___
13	Cut food with knife and fork	___	___	___
14	Lift empty glass to mouth	___	___	___
15	Reopen previously opened food jar	___	___	___
16	Walk 50 feet without help	___	___	___
17	Walk up 5 steps	___	___	___
18	Stand on tiptoes	___	___	___
19	Reach above head	___	___	___
20	Get out of bed	___	___	___
21	Pick up something from floor from standing position	___	___	___
22	Push open door after turning knob	___	___	___
23	Turn head and look over shoulder	___	___	___

A

FIGURE 15-3A & B Juvenile Arthritis Functional Assessment Report for Parents. (A. Modified with permission from Howe S, Levinson J, Shear E, et al; Development of a disability measurement tool for juvenile rheumatoid arthritis. The juvenile arthritis functional assessment report for children and their parents. *Arthritis & Rheumatology.* 2005;34(7):873-880. **B.** Reproduced with permission from Eric Shamus. *The Color Atlas of Physical Therapy.* New York, NY: McGraw-Hill, 2015.)

2   **Aids or Devices**

Please check any AIDS or DEVICES that your child uses for any of these activities

		Have Used	**Have not used**
1	Cane	_____	_____
2	Walker	_____	_____
3	Crutches	_____	_____
4	Wheelchair	_____	_____
5	Built-up pencil	_____	_____
6	Button hook	_____	_____
7	Zipper Horn	_____	_____
8	Shoe horn	_____	_____
9	Special eating utensils	_____	_____
10	Special chair	_____	_____
11	A special kind of toilet seat	_____	_____
12	Bathtub seat	_____	_____
13	Jar opener	_____	_____
14	Bathtub bar	_____	_____
15	Reacher	_____	_____

Does your child use any other kind of special tool, appliance, aid or device that helps him or her do things more easily?

IF YES: Could you describe it?   _____

_____

3   **Help from Others**

Please check any categories for which your child needs HELP FROM ANOTHER PERSON.

		No Help	**Some Help**
1	Get dressed in the morning	_____	_____
2	Get washed in the morning	_____	_____
3	Get in and out of bed	_____	_____
4	Eat dinner	_____	_____
5	Move around the house	_____	_____
6	Get in and out of chairs	_____	_____
7	Reach and get things for you	_____	_____

4   **Pain Scale**

We are also interested in learning whether or not your child has been affected by pain because of his/her illness.
How much pain do you think your child has had because of his/her illness IN THE PAST WEEK?
Place a mark on the line below to indicate the severity of the pain.

0	100
No Pain	Very Bad Pain

Comments:_____

_____

_____Jafar1.doc

Return to: Researcher **Suzanne L. Bowyer, Riley Hospital For Children, Rm 5863, 1 Children's Square, Indianapolis, Indiana 46202**

B

FIGURE 15-3A & B **(Continued)**

(grade A). The use of a home exercise program improved the quality of life and functional ability (grade A). Aquatic aerobic fitness helped decrease the number of active joints (grade A). Cardio-karate aerobic exercise for improving range of motion and decreasing the number of active joints was slightly less effective (grade C+).[24] The letter A means that the data came from a meta-analysis or many randomized clinical trials. The letter B means that the data came from one randomized or non-randomized studies. The letter C indicates that the data came from an opinion or case study.

Klepper et al[25] performed a systematic review investigating the effects of structured exercise training in children and adolescents with JIA. The focus was on the safety and efficacy of exercise training to improve physical fitness, pain, functional capability, and quality of life. The research produced moderate-quality evidence supporting STOTT Pilates and underwater knee-resistance exercise. The research determined that 30 to 50 minutes of exercise therapy, 2 to 3 times per week, for 12 to 24 weeks helped decrease pain and improve range of motion, knee strength, functional capability, and quality of life in children and adolescents with JIA. In the systematic review, no adverse effects of exercise training were reported.[25]

Bayraktar et al[26] investigated the effects of a controlled trial 8-week water-running program on exercise capacity in children with JIA. The 8-week trial found improved anaerobic capacity but found that 8 weeks was not long enough to significantly improve aerobic exercise capacity.[26]

Houghton et al[27] investigated the feasibility and safety of a 6-month exercise program to increase bone and muscle strength in children with JIA. The researchers saw fatigue lessen, but there were no other sustained improvements in muscle, bone, or clinical outcomes. However, adherence to the exercise program was low (47%). Children with JIA safely participated in a home-based exercise program designed to enhance muscle and bone strength, but the design of the program did not promote adherence.[27]

Heale et al[28] performed a pilot study on wearable activity tracker intervention for promoting physical activity in adolescents aged 12 to 18 years with JIA. The participants' activity level was logged on their smartphone application for 72% of the intervention period. The standard deviation of the change in mean metabolic equivalents (METs) per day was 12.15, and the standard deviation for mean moderate-to-vigorous physical activity was 3.14 blocks per day over the study period. Heale et al[28] concluded that a wrist-worn activity tracker is feasible to use in adolescent patients. See **Table 15-4** for a list of interventions for JIA.

■ FUNCTIONAL GOAL EXAMPLES

1. The child will be able to perform single leg balance for 10 seconds to promote donning pants.
2. The child will show increased endurance as measured on the 6-minute walk test to promote ambulation at school.
3. The child will be able to fasten a button in less than 20 seconds for dressing.

TABLE 15-4 • Interventions for Juvenile Idiopathic Arthritis

- Massage
- Aquatic therapy[22]
- Splinting of short duration
- Range of motion (active or active-assisted)
- Gentle stretching
- Grade 1 and 2 mobilizations for pain control and fluid movement
- Grade 3 mobilization for joint ROM
- Gait training
- Strengthening (limit high-impact activities)
- Aerobic activity (when arthritis controlled): 30-50 minutes, 2 times per week, for at least 12 weeks[17]
- Pilates[17,22]
- Dance[21]
- Tai chi[21]
- Balance and proprioceptive activities: single limb stance, balance board, mini-trampoline (**Figure 15-4**)[23]
- Cycling
- Patient/family education including joint protection and energy conservation
- Recommendations for adaptive equipment and accommodations as needed
- Home exercise program[12]
- Ice as necessary

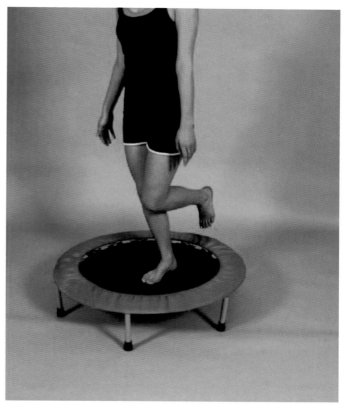

FIGURE 15-4 Mini trampoline standing on one leg. (Reproduced with permission, from Mark Dutton. *Dutton's Orthopaedic Examination, Evaluation, and Intervention*, 4e. New York: McGraw Hill; 2017.)

Case 1

A 3-year-old girl is hospitalized due to bilateral severe knee pain, unwillingness to weight bear, and daily fevers. Following a medical exam including imaging and bloodwork, she is diagnosed with juvenile idiopathic arthritis (JIA). Upon examination, the therapist notes erythema, edema, and tenderness to palpation of both knees. The child has decreased active knee extension and is unable to stand without support.

Intervention

Because this child is in the acute phase of JIA, her physical therapy intervention should include parent education regarding the use of rest, gentle active range of motion, and joint protection strategies. Utilization of proper positioning will be included to prevent knee flexion contractures. At the time of discharge, outpatient physical therapy will be recommended for range of motion, strengthening, gait training and to educate the child and family on the appropriate monitoring and progression of activities to ensure return to the prior level of function, age-appropriate motor skills, and physical fitness.

Case 2

An 11-year-old boy is referred to outpatient physical therapy for decreased ankle and knee passive and active range of motion associated with chronic polyarthritis resulting in pain and fatigue. He currently uses a manual wheelchair at home, at school, and in the community, and he wants to get back to playing soccer with his friends. His medications have recently been changed due to poor response.

Intervention

Physical therapy interventions will include low load stretching for decreased knee flexion, self-stretching for decreased ankle dorsiflexion, aquatic therapy for gravity-eliminated mobility and aerobic activity, and gait training. Ball skills will be added to the treatment plan as the patient progresses. Patient and family education will include reviewing joint protection, a home program for stretching and ambulation, and a discussion regarding how to reduce dependence on the wheelchair and increase stamina at home, at school, and in the community.

■ PATIENT RESOURCES

- Ten Tips for Parents of Children Living with JIA. Arthritis in Children. American College of Rheumatology. https://rheumatology.org/patient-blog/ten-tips-for-parents-of-children-living-with-jia
- Juvenile Arthritis. Arthritis Foundation. https://www.arthritis.org/about-arthritis/types/juvenile-arthritis/
- Juvenile Idiopathic Arthritis. https://kidshealth.org/en/parents/jra.html

CHAPTER SUMMARY

- JIA refers to a group of autoimmune and inflammatory disorders acquired in children before the age of 16 years with chronic inflammation of one or more joints for more than 6 weeks.[4]
- The categories of JIA are oligoarthritis (persistent or extended), polyarthritis RF positive, polyarthritis RF negative, systemic arthritis, psoriatic arthritis, enthesitis-related arthritis, and undifferentiated arthritis.
- Children with JIA often have difficulty with activities of daily living and may need modifications in their school environment.
- The primary treatment is pharmaceutical intervention such as NSAIDs and DMARDs to decrease pain and swelling and prevent further joint damage.
- Secondary treatment is physical therapy. Understanding the disease process assists the physical therapist in selecting appropriate treatment interventions. Education, joint protection, and activity modification are all important components of the plan of care in the acute phases. As inflammation improves, range of motion, strengthening, gait training, balance training, functional activities, and use of a home program are indicated.

STUDY QUESTIONS

1. What are the most common signs and symptoms of juvenile idiopathic arthritis?
   a. Ligament laxity
   b. Morning stiffness, swelling, and pain
   c. Irritable bowel syndrome and headaches
   d. Diminished taste
2. Which form of juvenile idiopathic arthritis (JIA) involves 4 or fewer joints, typically the knees, ankles, and elbows?
   a. Systemic JA
   b. Enthesitis-related JA
   c. Polyarthritis
   d. Oligoarticular arthritis
3. What is the overall goal for treatment of Juvenile arthritis?
   a. Joint protection and reduction of symptoms
   b. Pushing through pain and building muscle
   c. Increasing aerobic capacity
   d. Increasing range of motion in joints

(Continued)

4. To be included in the classification criteria of juvenile arthritis, which of the following is the least amount of time required?
   a. Presence of arthritis of ≥6 weeks
   b. Presence of arthritis of ≥2 weeks
   c. Presence of arthritis of ≥12 weeks
   d. Presence of arthritis is not required

5. Which of the following special tests is most associated with disease activity, disability, and quality of life in children and adolescents with juvenile idiopathic arthritis (JIA)?
   a. 6-Minute walk test
   b. Hand grip strength
   c. Timed Get Up and Go
   d. Sit and reach test

6. Which type of of medication is most commonly prescribed after an anti-inflammatory medication?
   a. Nonsteroidal anti-inflammatory drug (NSAID)
   b. β-Blocker
   c. Disease-modifying antirheumatic drug (DMARD)
   d. Analgesic

7. During an acute flare-up of JIA, what is the main intervention goal?
   a. Strengthening
   b. Stretching
   c. Endurance exercise
   d. Pain control

8. Long-term joint instability is best addressed through which of the following?
   a. Splinting
   b. Weight loss
   c. Closed-chain exercises
   d. Medications

9. Which of the following techniques would be indicated for a child with JIA that has loss of knee joint range of motion?
   a. Passive stretching to the point of pain
   b. Gentle knee joint mobilization
   c. Plyometrics
   d. High weight, low repetitions resistance training

10. Which of the following senses should be evaluated early on with certain types of JIA?
    a. Hearing
    b. Vision
    c. Taste
    d. Smell

References

1. Mielants H, Veys EM, Maertens M, et al. Prevalence of inflammatory rheumatic diseases in an adolescent urban student population, age 12 to 18, in Belgium. *Clin Exp Rheumatol.* 1993;11(5): 563-567.

2. Danner S, Sordet C, Terzic J, et al. Epidemiology of juvenile idiopathic arthritis in Alsace, France. *J Rheumatol.* 2006;33(7): 1377-1381.

3. Hanova P, Pavelka K, Dostal C, Holcatova I, Pikhart H. Epidemiology of rheumatoid arthritis, juvenile idiopathic arthritis, and gout in two regions of the Czech Republic in a descriptive population-based survey in 2002-2003. *Clin Exp Rheumatol.* 2006;24(5):499-507.

4. Petty RE, Southwood TR, Manners, et al. International League of Associations for Rheumatology classification of juvenile idiopathic arthritis: 2nd revision, Edmonton, 2001. *J Rheumatol.* 2004;31(2):390-392.

5. Martini A, Ravelli A, Avcin T, Beresford MW, Burgos-Vargas R. Toward new classification criteria for Juvenile Idiopathic Arthritis: first steps, Pediatric Rheumatology International Trials Organization International Consensus. *J Rheumatol.* 2019;46(2):190-197.

6. Martini A. Are the number of joints involved or the presence of psoriasis still useful tools to identify homogeneous disease entities in juvenile idiopathic arthritis? *J Rheumatol.* 2003; 30(9):1900-1903.

7. Martini A. It is time to rethink juvenile idiopathic arthritis classification and nomenclature. *Ann Rheum Dis.* 2012;71(9): 1437-1439.

8. Raveli A, Felici E, Magni-Manzoni S, et al. Patients with antinuclear antibody-positive juvenile idiopathic arthritis constitute a homogeneous subgroup irrespective of the course of joint disease. *Arthritis Rheum.* 2005;52:826-832.

9. Rheumatology Image Bank. Systemic juvenile idiopathic arthritis: rash. Accessed November 23, 2023. https://images.rheumatology.org/bp/#/assets.

10. van der Net J, Helders PJM, Takken T. Juvenile idiopathic arthritis. In: Palisano RJ, Orlin MN, Schreiber J, eds. *Campbell's Physical Therapy for Children.* 6th ed. Elsevier; 2023.

11. Joint Health. Spotlight on idiopathic juvenile arthritis. Accessed November 24, 2023. https://jointhealth.org/aboutarthritis-diseasespotlight.cfm?id=5&locale=en-CA.

12. Soep JB. Chapter 29. Rheumatic diseases. In: Hay W, Levin MJ, Sondheimer JM, Detering RR, eds. *CURRENT Diagnosis & Treatment: Pediatrics.* 24th ed. McGraw-Hill; 2018.

13. Giancan G, Consolaro A, Lanni S, Davi S, Schiappapietra B, Ravelli A. Juvenile idiopathic arthritis: diagnosis and treatment. *Rheumatol Ther.* 2016;3(2):187-207.

14. Graham TB, Blebea JS, Gylys-Morin V, Passo MH. Magnetic resonance imaging in juvenile rheumatoid arthritis. *Semin Arthritis Rheum.* 1997;27(3):161-168.

15. Seid M, Opipari L, Huang B, Brunner HI, Lovell DJ. Disease control and health-related quality of life in juvenile idiopathic arthritis. *Arthritis Rheum.* 2009;61(3):393-399.

16. Houghton KM, Guzman J. Evaluation of static and dynamic postural balance in children with juvenile idiopathic arthritis. *Pediatr Phys Ther.* 2013;25(2):150-157.

17. Klepper S, Mano Khong TT, Klotz R, Gregorek AO, Chan YC, Sawade S. Effects of structured exercise training in children and adolescents with juvenile idiopathic arthritis. *Pediatr Phys Ther*. 2019;31(1):3-21.

18. Bos GJ, Lelieveld OT, Armbrust W, Sauer PJ, Geertzen JH, Dijkstra PU. Physical activity in children with juvenile idiopathic arthritis compared to controls. *Pediatr Rheumatol Online J*. 2016;14(1):42.

19. Rashed AM, Abdel-Wahab N, Moussa EMM, Hammam N. Association of hand grip strength with disease activity, disability, and quality of life in children and adolescents with juvenile idiopathic arthritis. *Adv Rheumatol*. 2018;58(1):11.

20. Bohr AH, Nielsen S, Muller K, Karup Pedersen F, Anderson LB. Reduced physical activity in children and adolescents with juvenile idiopathic arthritis despite satisfactory control of inflammation. *Pediatr Rheumatol Online J*. 2015;13:57-66.

21. Ginter CL, Vogel LF. Juvenile idiopathic arthritis and other rheumatic disorders. In: Spearing EM, Pelletier ES, Drnach, eds. *Tecklin's Pediatric Physical Therapy*. 6th ed. Lippincott Williams and Wilkins; 2021.

22. Kuntze G, Nesbitt C, Whittaker JL, et al. Exercise therapy in juvenile idiopathic arthritis: a systematic review and meta-analysis. *Arch Phys Med Rehabil*. 2018;99(1):178-193.

23. Baydogan SN, Tarakci E, Kasapcopur O. Effect of strengthening versus balance-proprioceptive exercises on lower extremity function in patients with juvenile idiopathic arthritis: a randomized, single-blind clinical trial. *Am J Phys Med Rehabil*. 2015;94(6):417-424, quiz 425-428.

24. Cavallo S, Brosseau L, Toupin-April K, et al. Ottawa panel evidence-based clinical practice guidelines for structured physical activity in the management of juvenile idiopathic arthritis. *Arch Phys Med Rehabil*. 2017;98(5):1018-1041.

25. Klepper S, Mano Khong TT, Klotz R, Gregorek AO, Chan YC, Sawade S. Effects of structured exercise training in children and adolescents with juvenile idiopathic arthritis. *Pediatr Phys Ther*. 2019;31(1):3-21.

26. Bayraktar D, Savci S, Altug-Gucenmez O, et al. The effects of 8-week water-running program on exercise capacity in children with juvenile idiopathic arthritis: a controlled trial. *Rheumatol Int*. 2019;39(1):59-65.

27. Houghton KM, Macdonald HM, McKay HA, Guzman J, Duffy C, Tucker L; LEAP Study Investigators. Feasibility and safety of a 6-month exercise program to increase bone and muscle strength in children with juvenile idiopathic arthritis. *Pediatr Rheumatol Online J*. 2018;16(1):67.

28. Heale LD, Dover S, Goh YI, Maksymiuk VA, Wells GD, Feldman BM. A wearable activity tracker intervention for promoting physical activity in adolescents with juvenile idiopathic arthritis: a pilot study. *Pediatr Rheumatol Online J*. 2018;16(1):66.

29. Catania H, Fortini V, Cimaz R. Physical exercise and physical activity for children and adolescents with juvenile idiopathic arthritis: a literature review. *Pediatr Phys Ther*. 2017;29(3):256-260.

ADDITIONAL RESOURCES

• Cimaz R, Maioli G, Calabrese G. Current and emerging biologics for the treatment of juvenile idiopathic arthritis. *Expert Opin Biol Ther*. 2020;20(7):725-740.

• Demirkaya E, Ozen S, Bilginer Y, et al. The distribution of juvenile idiopathic arthritis in the eastern Mediterranean: results from the registry of the Turkish Paediatric Rheumatology Association. *Clin Exp Rheumatol*. 2011;29(1):111-116.

• Doğru Apti M, Kasapçopur Ö, Mengi M, Özturk G, Metin G. Regular aerobic training combined with range of motion exercises in juvenile idiopathic arthritis. *Biomed Res Int*. 2014;2014:748972.

• Flodén A, Broström EW, von Heideken J, Rostlund S, Nilsson R. A qualitative study examining the validity and comprehensibility of physical activity items: developed and tested in children with juvenile idiopathic arthritis. *Pediatr Rheumatol Online J*. 2019;17(1):16.

• Giannini MJ, Protas EJ. Aerobic capacity in juvenile rheumatoid arthritis patients and healthy children. *Arthritis Care Res*. 1991;4(3):131-135.

• Henderson CJ, Lovell DJ, Specker BL, Campaigne BN. Physical activity in children with juvenile rheumatoid arthritis: quantification and evaluation. *Arthritis Care Res*. 1995;8(2):114-119.

• Iversen MD, Weidenhielm-Broström E, Wang R, Esbjörnsson AC, Hagelberg S, Åstrand P. Self-rated walking disability and dynamic ankle joint stiffness in children and adolescents with juvenile idiopathic arthritis receiving intraarticular corticosteroid joint injections of the foot. *Gait Posture*. 2019;67:257-261.

• Kalden JR. Expanding role of biologic agents in rheumatoid arthritis. *J Rheumatol Suppl*. 2002;66:27-37.

• Lelieveld OT, van Brussel M, Takken T, van Weert E, van Leeuwen MA, Armbrust W. Aerobic and anaerobic exercise capacity in adolescents with juvenile idiopathic arthritis. *Arthritis Rheum*. 2007;57(6):898-904.

• Manners PJ, Bower C. Worldwide prevalence of juvenile arthritis why does it vary so much? *J Rheumatol*. 2002;29(7):1520-1530.

• Petty RE, Laxer RM, Lindsley CB, Wedderburn L, Fuhlbrigge RC, Melins ED. *Textbook of Pediatric Rheumatology*. 8th ed. Saunders; 2021.

• Ravelli A, Martini A. Juvenile idiopathic arthritis. *Lancet*. 2007;369(9563):767-778.

• Ringold S, Angeles-Han ST, Beukelman T, et al. 2019 American College of Rheumatology/Arthritis Foundation Guideline for the treatment of juvenile idiopathic arthritis: therapeutic approaches for non-systemic polyarthritis, sacroiliitis, and enthesitis. *Arthritis Rheumatol*. 2019;71(6): 717-734.

• Schneider R, Passo MH. Juvenile rheumatoid arthritis. *Rheum Dis Clin North Am*. 2002;28(3):503-530.

• Takken T, van der Net J, Kuis W, Helders PJ. Aquatic fitness training for children with juvenile idiopathic arthritis. *Rheumatol*. 2003;42(11):1408-1414.

• Tarkianinen M, Tynjala P, Vahasalo P, Kroger L, Aalto K, Lahdenne P. Health-related quality of life during early aggressive treatment in patients with polyarticular juvenile idiopathic arthritis: results from randomized control trial. *Pediatr Rheumatol Online J*. 2019;17(1):80.

• van Brussel M, Lelieveld OT, van der Net J, Engelbert RH, Takken T. Aerobic and anaerobic exercise capacity in children with juvenile idiopathic arthritis. *Arthritis Rheum*. 2007;57(6):891-897.

• van Brussel M, van Doren L, Timmons BW, et al. Anaerobic-to-aerobic power ratio in children with juvenile idiopathic arthritis. *Arthritis Rheum*. 2009;61(6):787-793.

• Weiss, JE, Ilowite NT. Juvenile idiopathic arthritis. *Pediatr Clin North Am*. 2005;52(2):413-442.

16

Cardiopulmonary Dysfunction in Pediatrics

Eric Shamus, PT, DPT, PhD, and Jamie Dyson, PT, DPT

LEARNING OBJECTIVES

Upon completion of this chapter, the reader will be able to:

- Identify signs and symptoms of respiratory distress.
- Understand normal development changes in blood pressure and heart rate.
- Discuss radiologic consideration in cardiovascular problems.
- Describe functional limitations in children with asthma.
- Understand steps of airway clearance.
- Discuss progression of rehabilitation for children with cardiovascular dysfunction.
- Explain the effects of COVID-19 in children.
- Discuss manual therapy techniques to improve lung function.

Case Study

A 7-year-old boy complains of a 3-month history of a nonproductive cough that is worse at night and with exercise. He does not have fevers or other symptoms to suggest infection. He is normotensive, and his lungs are clear to auscultation bilaterally, except for an occasional expiratory wheeze on forced expiration. A chest radiograph is read as normal.

■ INTRODUCTION

Children with cardiopulmonary dysfunction can have a combination of impairments and decreased function including decreased proximal upper-limb strength, limited endurance capacity, limited active range of motion, inability to ambulate independently, dependent for transfers, and developmental delay. They may also have activity and exercise limitations, excess loss of salts/electrolytes from sweating, and shortness of breath.

As a physical therapist with direct access, it is important to recognize signs of cardiopulmonary dysfunction (**Table 16-1**).

■ PHYSICAL THERAPY ASSESSMENTS

If the child has a history of cardiopulmonary issues, the physical therapist should assess the child's vital signs including heart rate, blood pressure, temperature, and oxygen saturation levels (pulse oximetry); capillary refill time; height; and weight. Assessments of functional limitations of decreased

TABLE 16-1 • Signs of Cardiopulmonary Dysfunction

Heart and respiratory rate increased
Skin color changes related to hypoxia
Mucus in the lungs
Dehydration
Chest tightness, limited rib cage mobility
Fatigue
Malnutrition
Constipation
Clubbing of fingertips
Wheezing
Sinusitis
Chronic cough
Shoulder raised to allow increased airflow to lungs
Shortness of breath
Tensed muscles from dyspnea
Anxiety
Postural abnormality
Depression
Salty sweat
Cyanosis
Syncope
Carbon dioxide retention

TABLE 16-2 • Resting Heart Rate Values in Children
Newborns 0-1 month old: 70-190 bpm
Infants 1-11 months old: 80-160 bpm
Children 1-2 years old: 80-130 bpm
Children 3-4 years old: 80-120 bpm
Children 5-6 years old: 75-115 bpm
Children 7-9 years old: 70-110 bpm
Children ≥10 years and adults (including seniors): 60-100 bpm

Source: MedlinePlus. https://medlineplus.gov/ency/article/003399. htm#:~:text=Children%201%20to%202%20years,to%20110%20beats%20per%20minute.

activity level and exercise tolerance are key assessments. Disabling dyspnea can cause malnutrition and fatigue and limit functional ability when performing simple tasks. Lung function or pulmonary function tests include spirometry, body plethysmography, and peak expiratory flow. It is important to determine and document if the infant or child has any unrepaired heart defects or cardiopulmonary pathology, precautions, or contraindications. Indications should include if the child requires oxygen or ventilator support, and the child's aerobic capacity and endurance should be noted, including any shortness of breath observed.

HEART RATE VALUES IN CHILDREN

Resting heart rate values in children are listed in **Table 16-2**.

BLOOD PRESSURE VALUES IN CHILDREN

Information regarding blood pressure values and practices in children are provided in **Tables 16-3, 16-4**, and **16-5**.

PULSE OXIMETRY

Pulse oximetry measures the ratio of hemoglobin to oxyhemoglobin. Normal values are greater than 90%. A finger pulse

TABLE 16-3 • Definitions of Blood Pressure (BP) Categories and Stages	
For Children Aged 1 to <13 Years	**For Children Aged ≥13 Years**
Normal BP: <90th percentile	Normal BP: <120/<80 mm Hg
Elevated BP: ≥90th percentile to <95th percentile or 120/80 mm Hg to <95th percentile (whichever is lower)	Elevated BP: 120/<80 to 129/<80 mm Hg
Stage 1 hypertension (HTN): ≥95th percentile to <95th percentile + 12 mm Hg, or 130/80 to 139/89 mm Hg (whichever is lower)	Stage 1 HTN: 130/80 to 139/89 mm Hg
Stage 2 HTN: ≥95th percentile + 12 mm Hg, or ≥140/90 mm Hg (whichever is lower)	Stage 2 HTN: ≥140/90 mm Hg

Source: Flynn JT, Kaelber DC, Baker-Smith CM, et al. AAP clinical practice guideline for screening and management of high blood pressure in children and adolescents. Pediatrics. 2017;140(3):e20171904.

TABLE 16-4 • Screening Blood Pressure (BP) Values Requiring Further Evaluation

Age, years	BP, mm Hg			
	Boys		**Girls**	
	Systolic	Diastolic	Systolic	Diastolic
1	98	52	98	54
2	100	55	101	58
3	101	58	102	60
4	102	60	103	62
5	103	63	104	64
6	105	66	105	67
7	106	68	106	68
8	107	69	107	69
9	107	70	108	71
10	108	72	109	72
11	110	74	111	74
12	113	75	114	75
≥13	120	80	120	80

oximeter can be used, or an infrared sensor is placed on a child's finger, toe, or earlobe (**Figure 16-1**).

EXERCISES TESTING

"Cardiopulmonary exercise testing (CPET) quantitates and qualitates the integrated physiological response of a person to incremental exercise and provides additional information compared to static lung function tests alone."[1]

CPET provides information on respiratory abilities to perform exercise and functional activities. There are specific studies of exercise testing for children.[1-3] Takken et al[1] provide clinical recommendations for CPET in children with respiratory diseases. Radtke et al[2] examined maximal exercise capacity in children with cystic fibrosis. Silverman and Anderson[3] examined standardization of exercise tests in asthmatic children.

From childhood to adolescence, specific developmental aspects occur regarding ventilation during exercise. With growth, an increase in minute ventilation ($\dot{V}E$) and efficiency of $\dot{V}E$ occurs.[3] The change in efficiency is from an increase in tidal volume, coinciding with a decreasing in breathing frequency.[4]

Static lung function tests are useful for diagnosis and management but are not able to predict exercise capacity of a patient.[5]

CPET is an essential tool to assess cardiorespiratory fitness (CRF) in children.[6-8] Testing can be performed on a bicycle (ergometer) or a treadmill. When testing the children, a small facemask or mouthpiece is needed, along with child-sized blood pressure cuffs, oxygen saturation devices for small fingers, and airflow meters.[9,10]

TABLE 16-5 • Best Blood Pressure (BP) Measurement Practices
1. The child should be seated in a quiet room for 3-5 min before measurement, with the back supported and feet uncrossed on the floor.
2. BP should be measured in the right arm for consistency, for comparison with standard tables, and to avoid a falsely low reading from the left arm in the case of coarctation of the aorta. The arm should be at heart level, supported, and uncovered above the cuff. The patient and observer should not speak while the measurement is being taken.
3. The correct cuff size should be used. The bladder length should be 80%-100% of the circumference of the arm, and the width should be at least 40%.
4. For an auscultatory BP, the bell of the stethoscope should be placed over the brachial artery in the antecubital fossa, and the lower end of the cuff should be 2-3 cm above the antecubital fossa. The cuff should be inflated to 20-30 mmHg above the point at which the radial pulse disappears. Overinflation should be avoided. The cuff should be deflated at a rate of 2-3 mmHg per second. The first (phase I Korotkoff) and last (phase V Korotkoff) audible sounds should be taken as systolic BP and diastolic BP. If the Korotkoff sounds are heard to 0 mmHg, the point at which the sound is muffled (phase IV Korotkoff) should be taken as the diastolic BP, or the measurement should be repeated with less pressure applied over the brachial artery. The measurement should be read to the nearest 2 mmHg.
5. To measure BP in the legs, the patient should be in the prone position, if possible. An appropriately sized cuff should be placed midthigh and the stethoscope placed over the popliteal artery. The systolic BP in the legs is usually 10%-20% higher than the brachial artery pressure.

Source: Adapted from Pickering TG, Hall JE, Appel LJ, et al. Recommendations for blood pressure measurement in humans and experimental animals: part 1: blood pressure measurement in humans: a statement for professionals from the Subcommittee of Professional and Public Education of the American Heart Association Council on High Blood Pressure Research. Circulation. 2005;111(5):697-716.

For reproducible peak oxygen consumption ($\dot{V}O_{2peak}$), the preferred duration for a CPET is between 6 and 10 minutes in children and between 8 and 12 minutes in adolescents.[11,12] When testing clinical populations with low $\dot{V}O_{2peak}$ values, an exercise protocol in which the work rate increases with small increments (so-called ramp protocol) is preferred.[12]

There are limited CPETs with pediatric reference values that are independent of body size and pubertal stage. Blanchard et al[13] provide Z-score equations for several maximal and submaximal CRF parameters derived from a prospectively recruited sample of healthy children.

Cardiopulmonary assessments can be broken down into body structure function tests (**Table 16-6**), activity tests and scales (**Table 16-7**), and participation tests and scales (**Table 16-8**) categorized by the International Classification of Functioning, Disability, and Health (ICF) model.[14]

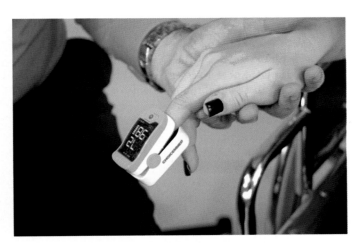

FIGURE 16-1 Pulse oximeter. (Reproduced, with permission, from *Dutton M, Dutton's Orthopaedic Examination, Evaluation, and Intervention.* New York: McGraw Hill; 2022.)

■ IMAGING

Radiography, computed tomography (CT), or a ventilation-perfusion lung scan can provide information on diagnosis and progression of cardiopulmonary disorders. CT and magnetic resonance imaging (MRI) offer a noninvasive way to image cardiovascular anatomy, which can be used in conjunction with echocardiography for diagnosis and treatment planning. CT and MRI can depict the morphology and relationship to surrounding structures better than echocardiography, especially in complex congenital defects.[15]

Echocardiography provides several different image types and measurements such as M-mode, gray scale, color Doppler, strain, and 3-dimensional (3D) images.[16,17] Tissue Doppler, myocardial strain assessment, and 3D echocardiography have expanded the use of echocardiography as a diagnostic tool. 3D images add to the presurgical assessment, particularly in cases of complex intracardiac anomalies, septal defects, and valvular anatomy.[18,19]

■ PULMONARY FUNCTION TESTING

Pulmonary function testing is an important tool in the evaluation of children who have or are suspected of having lung disease (**Table 16-9**). The test provides objective and reproducible measurements, which then can be used to follow the response to therapy. The measurements of air flow and lung volumes are the mechanical pulmonary function tests used most. Measurements of the efficiency of gas exchange also are considered a test of pulmonary function and can be assessed by methods such as arterial blood gas and oximetry. By 6 years of age, these tests can be performed reliably by most, but not all, children with the help of an experienced technician. They are used to verify the presence or assess the severity of abnormalities in a child's pulmonary function. They can help to answer the following questions:

1. Is airflow obstructed?
2. Is lung volume restricted?

TABLE 16-6 • Body Structure Function Tests

Anthropometrics:
- Body composition (body mass index)
- Height/weight
- Leg length

Cardiopulmonary:
- Blood pressure
- Heart rate
- Oxygen saturation, respiratory pattern and rate
- Skin color
- Skin turgor

Coordination:
- Clinical Observation of Motor and Postural Skills (COMPS)
- Florida Apraxia Screening Test
- Gross Motor Performance Measure (GMPM)
- Selective Control Assessment of the Lower Extremity
- Test of Ideational Praxis

Endurance/energy expenditure:
- Early Activity Scale for Endurance (EASE)
- Energy Expenditure Index
- 6-Minute Walk Test
- 30-Second Walk Test

Fitness measures:
- Fitness Gram
- Presidential Physical Fitness Test

Multiple measures:
- Quick Neurological Screening Test–III (QNST-III)

Pain:
- Children's Hospital of Eastern Ontario Pain Scale (CHEOPS)
- CRIES Scale (Cries, Require Oxygen, Increased Vital Signs, Expression, Sleep)
- Faces Pain Scale
- FLACC (Faces, Legs, Activity, Crying, Consolability Behavioral Pain Scale)
- Individualized Numeric Pain Scale (INRS)
- Numeric Scale

Pain (Cont.):
- Oucher Scale
- Visual analog scale

Posture/balance:
- Early Clinical Assessment of Balance (ECAB)
- Movement Assessment of Infants (MAI)
- Pediatric Balance Scale (PBS)
- Pediatric Clinical Test of Sensory Interaction for Balance (PCTSIB)
- Pediatric Reach Test (Pediatric Functional Reach Test)
- Timed Up and Down Stairs Test

Posture/structural integrity:
- Adam forward bend test
- Anterior/posterior drawer test
- Apley's test
- Arch index
- Beighton Scale of Hypermobility
- Craig's test
- Galeazzi sign
- Heel bisector angle
- Lachman's test
- Navicular drop test
- McMurray's test
- Ryder's test
- Talar tilt
- Transmalleolar axis

Range of motion (ROM):
- Ely's test
- Hamstring length test
- Modified Ober test
- Popliteal angle
- Prone hip extension test
- Spinal Alignment and Range of Motion Measure (SAROMM)
- Straight leg test
- Thomas test

3. Is there a change from previous testing?
4. What is the magnitude of the abnormality?

   See Figure 16-2, Interpretation of pulmonary function tests.

LABORATORY TESTS

Laboratory tests should include a complete blood count (CBC), sweat chloride test, sputum culture, and genetic tests, as appropriate (**Table 16-10**).

- **CBC.** CBC measures the size, number, and maturity of the red blood cells, white blood cells, and platelets.[20]
- **Electrolytes.** This test measures the minerals sodium, potassium, calcium, and magnesium. Diuretics may cause electrolyte problems. Potassium levels are needed for healthy heart function.[20]
- **B-type natriuretic peptide (BNP).** The heart's ventricles make the BNP hormone. When the heart must pump harder than usual, BNP levels in the blood are higher. BNP testing can tell if your child has a problem with the heart or lungs.[20]

- **Total protein and albumin.** Total protein and albumin indicate how well the liver is functioning.[20]
- **Genetic blood tests.** These tests may be used to find chromosome problems linked to congenital heart defects.[20]
- **Prothrombin time, partial thromboplastin time, and international normalized ratio.** These assess clotting and how well blood-thinning medicines (anticoagulants) are working. These medicines are taken for various heart problems.[20]
- **Blood gas.** Oxygen, carbon dioxide, and acidity (pH) of the blood are measured. This is a painless, noninvasive test. It measures the amount of oxygen in the blood through a small infrared sensor placed on a child's finger, toe, or earlobe.[20]

MEDICATIONS

Medications in pediatric patients with cardiopulmonary dysfunction can range from β-blockers to vasodilators (**Table 16-11**).

TABLE 16-7 • Activity Tests

Gait/walking:
- Dynamic Gait Index
- Functional Mobility Assessment
- Observational Gait Scale (OGS)
- Standardized Walking Obstacle Course
- Timed Obstacle Ambulation Test
- Timed Up and Down Stairs test
- Timed Up and Go (TUG)

Gross motor:
- Alberta Infant Motor Scales (AIMS)
- Bruininks-Oseretsky Test of Motor Proficiency–3 (BOTP-3)
- Gross Motor Function Measure (GMFM)
- Gross Motor Performance Measure
- High-Level Mobility Assessment Tool (HIMAT)
- Motor Function Measure 2
- Peabody Developmental Motor Scales Third Edition (PDMS-3)
- Test of Gross Motor Development–3 (TGMD-3)
- Test of Infant Motor Performance (TIMP)

Fine motor:
- Bruininks-Oseretsky Test of Motor Proficiency Third Edition (BOTP-3)
- Jebsen Taylor Test of Hand Function
- Nine-Hole Peg Test
- Peabody Developmental Motor Scales Third Edition (PDMS-3)
- Assisting Hand Assessment
- Shriner's Upper Extremity Assessment
- Melbourne Unilateral Upper Limb Function (MUUL)

Play:
- Preschool Play Scale
- Test of Playfulness (ToP)

Developmental screening tools:
- Ages and Stages Questionnaires (ASQ-3)
- Assessment, Evaluation, and Programming System for Infants and Children (AEPS-3) Third Edition
- Bayley Infant Neurodevelopmental Screener (BINS)
- Carolina Curriculum for Infants and Toddlers with Special Needs (CCITSN) Third Edition
- Carolina Curriculum for Preschoolers With Special Needs
- FirstSTEp: Screening Test for Evaluating Preschoolers
- Motor Skills Acquisition in the First Year and Checklist

TABLE 16-8 • Participation Tests

Multidomain:
- Activities Scale for Kids (ASK)
- Battelle Developmental Inventory, Second Edition
- Bayley Scales of Infant Development–III
- Brigance Inventory of Early Development, Revised Edition
- Canadian Occupational Performance Measure (COPM)
- Functional Independence Measure for Children (WeeFIM)
- Harris Infant Motor Test (HINT)
- Hawaii Early Learning Profile (HELP-Strands)
- Merrill-Palmer Scale, Revised
- Miller Assessment of Preschoolers
- Miller Function and Participation Scales
- Movement Assessment Battery for Children (Movement ABC-2)
- Pediatric Evaluation of Disability Inventory (PEDI)
- Pediatric Evaluation of Disability Inventory (PEDICAT)
- POSNA Pediatric Musculoskeletal Functional Health Questionnaire
- School Function Assessment (SFA)
- Toddler and Infant Motor Evaluation (TIME)
- Transdisciplinary Play-Based Assessment, Second Edition (TPBA2)
- Vineland Adaptive Behavior Sales, Third Edition

Quality of life:
- Child Health Index of Life with Disabilities
- Kidscreen
- Pediatric Quality of Life Inventory (PedsQL)
- Pediatric Outcomes Data Collection Instrument (PODCI)
- Quality of Well-Being Scale (QWB)

Health status:
- Child Health and Illness Profile–Adolescent Edition (CHIP-E)
- Child Health Questionnaire (CHQ)
- Child Health Assessment Questionnaire (CHAQ)
- Health Utilities Index–Mark

■ PHYSICAL THERAPY DIFFERENTIAL DIAGNOSIS

Heart disease in children can be congenital (**Table 16-12**) or acquired (**Table 16-13**). Problems can range from a condition that has no symptoms and is never diagnosed to a problem that is severe and potentially life threatening that is apparent at birth.[21]

■ PEDIATRIC HEART TRANSPLANT

In a heart transplant, there is removal of all (orthotopic transplant) or part (heterotopic transplant) of the heart due to end-stage heart failure and replacement with a healthy heart from a clinically dead donor. After the heart transplant, the patient will be deconditioned, have decreased strength and endurance, and be immunosuppressed.[22]

TABLE 16-9 • Terms Used in Pulmonary Function Testing

Terms	Definition
Tidal volume (TV)	The volume of air breathed in and out without conscious effort
Inspiratory reserve volume (IRV)	The additional volume of air that can be inhaled with maximum effort after a normal inspiration
Expiratory reserve volume (ERV)	The additional volume of air that can be forcibly exhaled after normal exhalation
Vital capacity (VC)	The total volume of air that can be exhaled after a maximum inhalation: VC = TV + IRV + ERV
Residual volume (RV)	The volume of air remaining in the lungs after maximum exhalation. The lungs are never completely emptied.
Total lung capacity (TLC)	VC + residual volume
Minute ventilation	The amount of gas inhaled or exhaled in one minute (tidal volume x respiration rate)

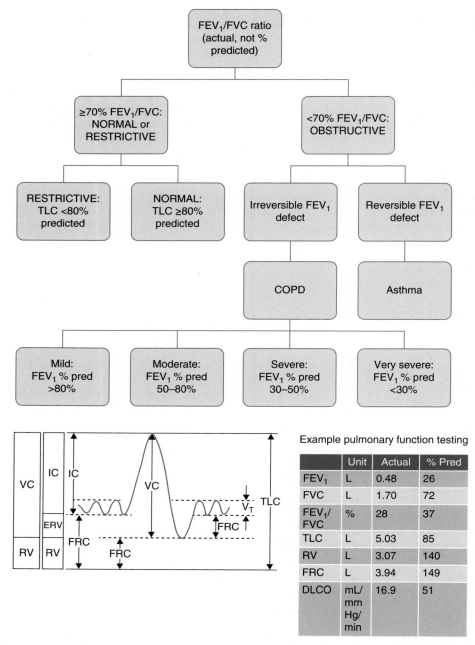

FIGURE 16-2 Interpretation of pulmonary function tests. (Reproduced with permission from Raj Mitra. *Principles of Rehabilitation Medicine*. New York: McGraw Hill Education; 2019; Bottom left panel: Reproduced with permission from Weinberger SE. *Principles of Pulmonary Medicine*, 4th ed. Philadelphia, PA: Saunders 2004.)

The heart is considered denervated following transplantation (due to severing of thoracic and vagus nerves). As a result, the pulse rate can no longer be used as the primary method of assessing intensity of exercise. Circulating catecholamines regulate the heart's response to exercise. A warm-up period prior to exercise and a cool-down period following exercise are crucial to any active exercise program.[23]

When gauging the intensity of the exercise, the Borg or Modified Borg Scale (ie, rating of perceived exertion) should be used to determine the intensity of the session. The distance ambulated only tells you how far the patient was able to walk but not how difficult it was. Heart rate cannot be used to determine intensity since the heart is denervated. Oxygen saturation cannot be used to gauge the intensity of exercise, only the efficiency or effectiveness of the pulmonary system. Electrocardiography (ECG) is also performed routinely after transplant for monitoring.

TABLE 16-10 • Laboratory Tests and Values

Test	Referenced Normal Value
Complete blood count	
Red blood cells	Male: 4.35-5.65 trillion cells/L
	Female: 3.92-5.13 trillion cells/L
Hemoglobin	Male: 13.2-16.6 g/dL
	Female: 11.6-15 g/dL
Hematocrit	Male: 38.3%-48.6%
	Female: 35.5%-44.9%
White blood cells	3.4-9.6 billion cells/L
Platelet count	Male: 135-317 billion/L (135,000-317,000/μL)
	Female: 157-371 billion/L (157,000-371,000/μL)
Basic metabolic panel	
Calcium	9-11 mg/dL
Chloride	95-105 mEq/L
Sodium	135-145 mEq/L
Potassium	3.5-5.0 mEq/L
Creatinine	0.5-1.2 mg/dL
Blood urea nitrogen	10-20
Albumin	3.2-4.8 g/L
Glucose	70-110 mg/dL
Magnesium	1.5-2.5 mEq/L
Anticoagulant and clotting factors	
Prothrombin time	9.0-11.7 seconds
Partial thromboplastin time (heparin monitoring)	55.0-75.0 seconds
International normalized ratio	≤1.1 normal
	(2.0-3.0 is general effective therapeutic range when taking warfarin for atrial fibrillation or blood clot in the leg or lung)
Arterial blood gas values	
pH (blood acid-base balance)	Normal value 7.40
	Normal adult range 7.35-7.45
	Patient will have **acidemia** with pH <7.35 and **alkalemia** with pH >7.45.
$PaCO_2$ (mm Hg) (alveolar hyperventilation value)	Normal value 40
	Normal adult range 35-45 (**eucapnia**)
	Elevated $PaCO_2$ is referred to as **hypercapnia.**
	Low $PaCO_2$ is referred to as **hypocapnia.**
PaO_2 (mm Hg) (alveolar hypoventilation value)	Normal value 97
	Normal range >80
	Low PaO_2 is referred to as **hypoxemia.**
	Hypoxia means a patient has low level of oxygen in tissue yet adequate perfusion of tissue.
HCO_3 (mEq/L) (bicarbonate)	Normal value 24
	Normal adult range 22-28
SaO_2 (percent oxygen saturation of hemoglobin)	95%-98%

TABLE 16-11 • Common Medication in Cardiopulmonary Dysfunction

Immunosuppressants
- Cyclosporin
- Tacrolimus
- Alemtuzumab (Campath)
- Azathioprine (Imuran)
- Mycophenolate mofetil (Cellcept)
- Basiliximab (Simulect)
- Rapamycin
- Sirolimus
- Everolimus

Corticosteroids (eg, methylprednisolone)

Vasodilators (eg, nitroglycerin)

Inotropic agents (eg, digoxin, dopamine)

Pulmonary vasodilators (eg, nitric oxide, sildenafil)

Immunoglobulins (eg, intravenous immunoglobulin)

Calcium channel blockers (eg, amlodipine)

Prophylactic antibiotics
- Ganciclovir
- Valganciclovir
- Nystatin (antifungal)

Diuretics

Angiotensin-converting enzyme inhibitors

TABLE 16-12 • Congenital Heart Conditions in Children

Anomalous coronary arteries/fistulas

Anomalous pulmonary venous return

Aortic stenosis/bicuspid aortic valve

Atrial septal defect

Atrioventricular septal defect

Coarctation of the aorta/interrupted aortic arch

D-Transposition of the great arteries

Ebstein anomaly

Hypoplastic left heart syndrome

L-Transposition of the great arteries

Patent ductus arteriosus

Pulmonary atresia

Pulmonary stenosis

Tetralogy of Fallot

Tricuspid atresia

Truncus arteriosus

Vascular ring/sling

Ventricular septal defect

TABLE 16-13 • Acquired Heart Conditions in Children

Dilated cardiomyopathy

Endocarditis

Hypertrophic cardiomyopathy

Kawasaki disease

Myocarditis

Pericarditis

Rheumatic fever

Hypertension

Following is the Modified Ross classification for pediatric heart failure[24]:

- **Class I:** No symptoms, asymptomatic
- **Class II:** Mild increased respiratory rate (tachypnea) and/or sweating (diaphoresis) during feeding (infant) or shortness of breath (dyspnea) with exertion in older children
- **Class III:** Significantly increased respiratory rate (tachypnea) and/or sweating (diaphoresis) during feeding (infant) or shortness of breath with exertion (older child)
- **Class IV:** Signs and symptoms of heart failure at rest (eg, tachypnea, retractions, grunting, or diaphoresis at rest)

Case Presentation

A 12-month-old girl is referred from an early intervention program for home physical therapy following a heart transplant 5 months ago for a hypoplastic left heart syndrome. She can prop sit but is not rolling, creeping on hands and knees, or transferring in or out of sitting.

▪ MITRAL VALVE PROLAPSE

Mitral valve prolapse is an abnormally thickened mitral valve that becomes displaced into the left atrium during systolic contraction. Complications include mitral valve regurgitation, endocarditis, congestive heart failure, and cardiac arrest. Mitral valve prolapse is usually not diagnosed until adulthood. Mild to moderate mitral valve prolapse generally does not cause symptoms. Severe mitral valve prolapse causes progressive shortness of breath, chest pain, and signs of congestive heart failure. Children with mitral valve prolapse may have symptoms of dizziness, shortness of breath, palpitations, chest pain, and fainting episodes.[25]

Impairments that can be seen are shortness of breath, dyspnea on exertion, limited activity tolerance, and decreased functional capacity. Specific tests and measures can include the 6-Minute Walk Test for mild or non-symptomatic cases, Borg Rating of Perceived Exertion, monitoring of vital signs to include lung auscultations, Short Form-36, and the New York Heart Association Functional Classification Scale.[26] An echocardiogram or ECG will help determine what is causing the sound in the heart. See **Figure 16-3**: A cardiac echocardiogram demonstrating a mitral prolapse without regurgitation in an 8 year old.

Specific interventions include risk factor modification, 3 phases of cardiac rehabilitation, aerobic training, and education on the signs and symptoms. Appropriate warm up and cool down are essential.[27]

Case Presentation

A 13-year-old boy presents with anxiety and dizziness. He states he feels his heart racing. On exam, there is an audible non-ejection click and faint late systolic murmur. On the musculoskeletal exam, there is mild scoliosis.

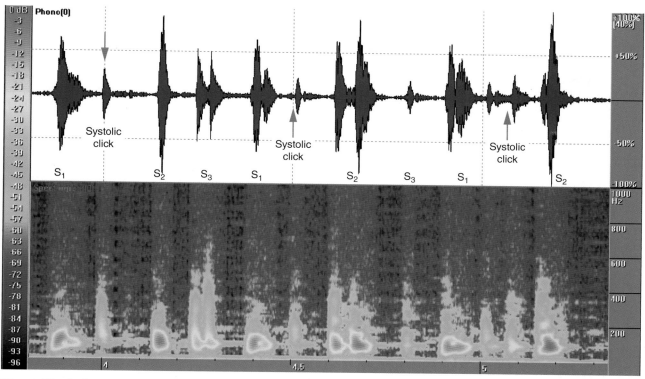

FIGURE 16-3 Mitral valve prolapse cardiac echocardiography (echo). Mitral valve prolapse in an asymptomatic 8-year-old child. The cardiac echo demonstrated a mitral prolapse without regurgitation. Both the phonogram and spectrogram show a systolic mitral click and a diastolic S3 prominent during inspiration. (Reproduced, with permission, from Pahlm O, Wagner GS. *Multimodal Cardiovascular Imaging: Principles and Clinical Applications.* New York: McGraw Hill; 2022.)

PEDIATRIC LUNG TRANSPLANT

A pediatric lung transplant is the removal of diseased or defective lung (single-lung transplant) or lungs (double-lung transplant) or a portion thereof. A healthy partial lung from a living donor or complete donor lung(s) from a deceased person is implanted. Lung transplants are considered when patient death is imminent within 1 to 2 years and all other medical options have been tried.[28,29] The most common causes in children under 1 year of age are congenital heart disease, peripheral vascular disease, and cystic fibrosis. Other causes are surfactant dysfunction, idiopathic pulmonary disorders, bronchiolitis obliterans, chronic lung disease of infancy, pulmonary fibrosis, and pulmonary vein anomalies (**Figure 16-4** shows indications for pediatric lung transplant). The timing of a lung transplant for children over 12 years of age depends on their Lung Allocation Score.[28-30]

Functional implications include deconditioning, developmental delay, being dependent for activities of daily living, and being immunosuppressed. Children will also have decreased upper extremity range of motion, decreased strength, and decreased endurance. Specific tests include the 6-Minute Walk Test, goniometric measurements, pulmonary function tests, spirometry and oximetry, strength assessment, and forced expiratory volume in 1 second (FEV_1).[28-31]

Specific interventions include active range of motion only for upper extremities for the first 6 weeks postoperatively, aerobic activity including walking or the stationary bike, breathing techniques like blowing bubbles and pinwheel, and developmental activities.[30-32]

Case Presentation

A 15-year-old boy is referred to an outpatient physical therapy clinic 4 months after receiving a double-lung transplant secondary to cystic fibrosis. He was receiving physical therapy 3 times a week in the hospital. His goal is to progress to outdoor cycling, and he is working on improving strength and overall endurance.

ASTHMA

Asthma is a form of bronchial disorder associated with airway obstruction that is marked by recurrent attacks of paroxysmal dyspnea, with wheezing due to spasmodic contraction of the bronchi.[33-35]

Asthma is a chronic respiratory disease manifested as difficulty breathing due to the narrowing of bronchial passageways.[3] Asthma inflames and narrows the airways, leading to recurrent periods of wheezing, chest tightness, shortness of breath, and cough. Coughing often occurs at night or early in the morning but may go unnoticed during the day or be considered an allergic response to an inhaled (airborne or environmental) trigger. Allergy testing is usually done in children aged 5 years or older. Environment and adjustments of indoor air quality and environmental pollutants can be modified. Items such as feather pillows and certain smells in fragrance or laundry detergents can be eliminated.[36]

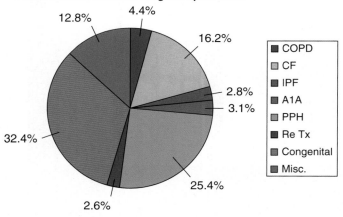

Pediatric indications for lung transplantation

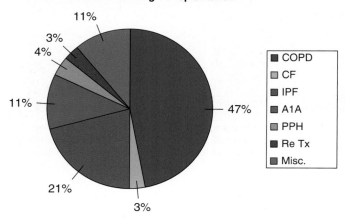

Adult indications for lung transplantation

FIGURE 16-4 Pediatric and adult lung transplant recipients. Indications for transplantation. (Reproduced with permission from Shamus, Eric. *The Color Atlas of Physical Therapy.* New York: McGraw Hill LLC; 2015.)

Asthma affects people of all ages but most often starts during childhood. More than 22 million people are known to have asthma in the United States; nearly 6 million are children. Asthma is the most common chronic lung disease in childhood. Physical impairments seen are decreased lung function, decreased activity or exercise tolerance, and sleep loss. Quality of life and health-related quality of life scales may be diminished with uncontrolled asthma for the patient and family.[37,38]

The goals of pharmacotherapy are to reduce airway constriction or bronchospasm and prevent recurrent inflammation that may lead to irreversible lung damage if not properly controlled. Rescue medication for acute symptoms (bronchoconstriction) include an inhaled short-acting β-agonist, anticholinergics, and systemic corticosteroids (oral or intravenous) (**Figure 16-5**). Controller medications for chronic symptoms (inflammation) include inhaled corticosteroids, long-acting β-agonist, leukotriene modifiers, long-acting bronchodilators (mediator inhibitors), and recombinant antibodies. The combination of an antihistamine and a leukotriene receptor antagonist has been shown to have additive effects. Antihistamines have also been shown to delay or prevent the development of asthma in a subgroup of atopic

children.[39] See **Figure 16-6** for a flow diagram for the treatment of exercise-induced asthma.

Interventions by the physical therapist include patient education and lifestyle changes, chest physical therapy with manual therapy to loosen congestion in the lungs, exercise (eg, aerobic, strength, flexibility, posture, breathing), airway clearance, pursed-lip breathing, teaching coughing techniques, and inspiratory muscle training (IMT).[40]

Children with asthma do not appear to be disproportionately affected by coronavirus disease 2019 (COVID-19).[41] Asthma, particularly when uncontrolled, may be included among the underlying conditions imposing a risk for severe COVID-19.[42]

Case Presentation

A 7-year-old girl complains of a nonproductive cough that is worse at night and with exercise. X-rays for the lungs are clear. She does not have a fever or any other symptoms. She is doing accessory breathing and does not have good diaphragm movement. The lungs are clear to auscultation bilaterally, except for expiratory wheezing on forced expiration.

■ CYSTIC FIBROSIS

Cystic fibrosis is a genetic disease mutation of chromosome 7 that causes lung mucus buildup that blocks the airways. The exocrine glands are affected. Mucus blocks pancreatic digestive enzymes from the small intestines. The intestines cannot absorb fats, proteins, or vitamins, which can cause malnutrition. Overall, this affects the lungs, pancreas, liver, intestines, and sinuses. Bacteria can grow in the built-up mucus. Cystic fibrosis is usually diagnosed in newborns. Children of Caucasian descent are most affected.[43]

The child will usually have disabling dyspnea when performing simple tasks. There is a decrease in exercise tolerance and often malnutrition that causes fatigue. Assessment includes lung function or pulmonary function tests, spirometry, body plethysmography, and peak expiratory flow.[2,4,5]

Specific interventions include airway clearance with chest physical therapy using percussion and postural positioning for drainage of airway clearance and removal of mucus from the 5 different lobes of the lungs. IMT can elicit meaningful improvements in physiologic and patient-centered clinical outcomes. Shei et al[44] investigated the role of IMT in patients with cystic fibrosis. The current evidence indicates improved exercise tolerance and improved health-related quality of life.[44-46]

Case Presentation

A 13-year-old girl presents with cystic fibrosis diagnosed by a sweat chloride test at 1 month old. She is complaining of increased sputum production and decreased activity/exercise tolerance with difficulty walking the necessary distances around school without having shortness of breath. When she is not having an exacerbation, she reports increased coughing with moderately intense activity or exercise and that she participates in a walking program 3 times a week for 20 minutes. She performs airway clearance using vest treatment (high-frequency chest wall

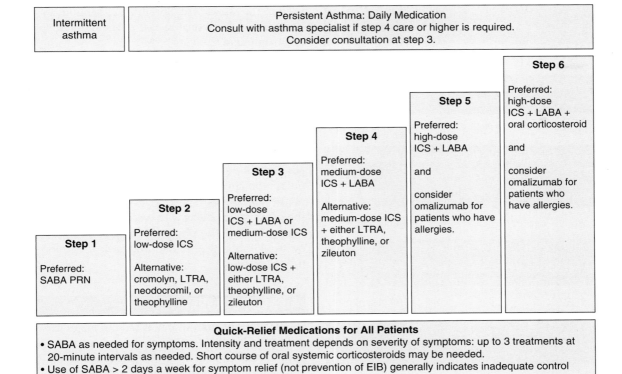

FIGURE 16-5 Stepwise approach for managing asthma in adults and youths 12 years of age or older.
Alphabetical order is used when more than one treatment option is listed within either preferred or alternative therapy.
Notes:
- The stepwise approach is meant to assist, not replace, the clinical decision-making required to meet individual patient needs.
- If alternative treatment is used and response is inadequate, discontinue it, and use the preferred treatment before stepping up.
- Zileuton is a less desirable alternative due to limited studies as adjunctive therapy and the need to monitor liver function. Theophylline requires monitoring of serum concentration levels.
- In step 6, before oral corticosteroids are introduced, a trial of high-dose ICS + LABA + either LTRA, theophylline, or zileuton may be considered, although this approach has not been studied in clinical trials.
- Clinicians who administer immunotherapy or omalizumab should be prepared and equipped to identify and treat anaphylaxis that may occur.
ICS, inhaled corticosteroid; LABA, long-acting inhaled beta2-agonist; LTRA, leukotriene receptor antagonist; SABA, inhaled short-acting beta2-agonist. (From the Guidelines for the Diagnosis and Management of Asthma of the National Asthma Education and Prevention Program (NAEPP) Expert Panel Report 3, 2007.)

oscillation) 2 times per day for 30 minutes at variable frequency. She has nebulizer treatments with dornase alfa (Pulmozyme) and bronchodilators 2 times a day. She has had progressively increasing frequency of hospitalizations over the past 2 years for cystic fibrosis exacerbation and pneumonia. Her past medical history includes positive cultures for *Pseudomonas* and *Burkholderia cepacia*, as well as gastrostomy tube placement. Pulmonary function testing shows an FEV_1 of 85%. Physical exam reveals moderate clubbing of her nail beds and flattened thoracic spine with elevated and forward rounded shoulders. She can complete a 6-Minute Walk Test for a distance of 1700 ft, with oxygen saturation of 89% (97% at rest), increased heart rate from 99 at rest to 118 bpm, and report of dyspnea on the Modified Borg Scale of 3 and perceived rating of exertion on the Modified Borg Scale of 2.

PECTUS EXCAVATUM

Pectus excavatum is a common thoracic deformity where the sternum is depressed, resulting in a sunken appearance (**Figure 16-7**). This structural deformity can cause a right sternal rotation, resulting in the heart shifting to the left. Lung capacity can decrease with the changed rib cage shape. Mitral calve prolapse may be present and associated with congenital heart disease or murmur due to the disrupted blood flow. Patients who have severe symptomatic pectus excavatum are offered minimally invasive repair of pectus excavatum.[47]

The structural deformity can shorten the anterior thoracic muscles and overlengthen the posterior thoracic muscles, causing pain in the back and ribs. Pulmonary function tests can be

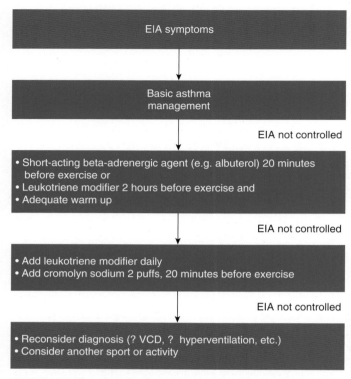

```
┌─────────────────────────────────┐
│         EIA symptoms            │
└─────────────────────────────────┘
                │
                ▼
┌─────────────────────────────────┐
│       Basic asthma              │
│       management                │
└─────────────────────────────────┘
                │        EIA not controlled
                ▼
┌─────────────────────────────────┐
│ • Short-acting beta-adrenergic  │
│   agent (e.g. albuterol) 20     │
│   minutes before exercise or    │
│ • Leukotriene modifier 2 hours  │
│   before exercise and           │
│ • Adequate warm up              │
└─────────────────────────────────┘
                │        EIA not controlled
                ▼
┌─────────────────────────────────┐
│ • Add leukotriene modifier daily│
│ • Add cromolyn sodium 2 puffs,  │
│   20 minutes before exercise    │
└─────────────────────────────────┘
                │        EIA not controlled
                ▼
┌─────────────────────────────────┐
│ • Reconsider diagnosis (? VCD,  │
│   ?  hyperventilation, etc.)    │
│ • Consider another sport or     │
│   activity                      │
└─────────────────────────────────┘
```

FIGURE 16-6 Flow chart for the treatment of exercise-induced asthma (EIA). (Reproduced with permission from Patel DR, Graydanus DE, Baker RJ: *Pediatric Practice Sports Medicine.* New York: McGraw Hill LLC; 2009.)

used in the assessment. Specific interventions include manual therapy and myofascial release to the thoracic spine, rib cage, and diaphragm.[48]

Case Presentation

A 17-month-old child is receiving physical therapy for developmental delay. The physical therapist notes the child has hypotonia and pectus excavatum. The mother states she had a viral illness during her first trimester but a normal vaginal delivery. She reports that the orthopedist states no current surgical intervention is necessary for the pectus excavatum unless the child's respiratory system becomes compromised as the child ages. The physical therapist plans on treating the gross motor delay with weekly therapeutic activities and strengthening. The physical therapist also plans on working on trunk mobility and diaphragmatic breathing for the pectus excavatum.

■ PNEUMOTHORAX

Spontaneous pneumothorax is seen in males between the ages of 10 and 30 years. There is a sudden sharp chest pain and dyspnea. Diagnosis is made by x-ray (**Figure 16-8**). Reoccurrence of pneumothorax is seen in about 30% of patients.

Signs and symptoms of pneumothorax include the following:

- Sudden shortness of breath
- Focal area of absent breath sounds
- Chest pain; worsens with deep breath or cough
- Cyanosis
- Fatigue

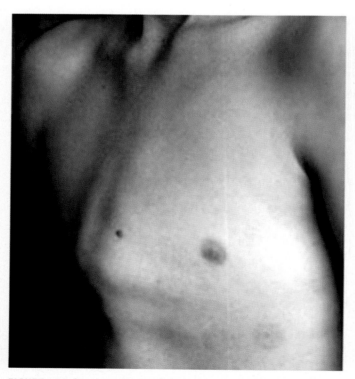
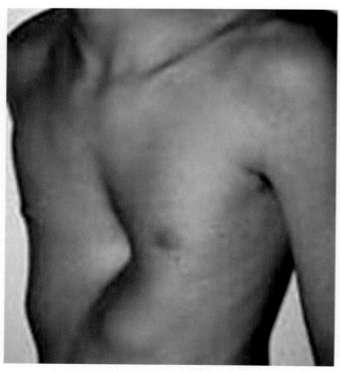

FIGURE 16-7 Pectus carinatum (left) and pectus excavatum (right). (Reproduced, with permission, from Patel DR, Greydanus DE, Baker RJ. *Pediatric Practice: Sports Medicine.* New York: McGraw Hill; 2009.)

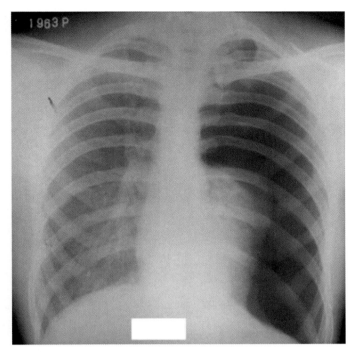

FIGURE 16-8 Left side pneumothorax. (Reproduced, with permission, from Patel DR, Greydanus DE, Baker RJ. *Pediatric Practice: Sports Medicine.* New York: McGraw Hill; 2009.)

- Increased heart rate
- Decreased oxygenation throughout the body
- Nasal flaring
- Hypotension (low blood pressure)
- Chest tightness
- Raising shoulders allows increased lung airflow

Once scarring has occurred, patients can participate in pulmonary rehabilitation to improve exercise capacity. This will include rib cage and thoracic mobility and exercises to improve aerobic condition, strength, flexibility, posture, and diaphragmatic breathing.

COVID-19

The COVID-19 pandemic and public health emergency caused concerns for children of all ages. In neonates (≤28 days old), the following guidance was provided from the Centers for Disease Control and Prevention (CDC).[49]

COVID-19 CARE FOR NEWBORNS (UPDATED MAY 20, 2020)

This guidance is intended to inform healthcare providers about the diagnosis, evaluation, infection prevention and control practices, and disposition of neonates (≤28 days old) with confirmed or suspected COVID-19 or known COVID-19 exposure, including birth to a mother with confirmed or suspected COVID-19.[49]

Routes of transmission

Transmission of SARS-CoV-2, the virus that causes COVID-19, to neonates is thought to occur primarily through respiratory droplets during the postnatal period when neonates are exposed to mothers, other caregivers, visitors, or healthcare personnel with COVID-19. Limited reports have raised concern of possible intrapartum or peripartum transmission, but the extent and clinical significance of vertical transmission by these routes is unclear.

Clinical presentation and disease severity

Data suggest that infants (<12 months of age) may be at higher risk for severe illness from COVID-19 compared with older children; however, information on clinical presentation and disease severity among neonates is limited and based on case reports and small case series.

Reported signs among neonates with SARS-CoV-2 infection include fever, lethargy, rhinorrhea, cough, tachypnea, increased work of breathing, vomiting, diarrhea, and feeding intolerance or decreased intake. The extent to which SARS-CoV-2 infection contributed to the reported signs of infection and complications is unclear, as many of these findings can also be seen commonly in term and preterm infants for other reasons (e.g., transient tachypnea of the newborn or neonatal respiratory distress syndrome). Most term infants (≥37 weeks gestational age) in these case reports had asymptomatic or mild disease and recovered without complication. However, severe disease requiring mechanical ventilation has been reported in COVID-19 positive neonates.

Testing recommendations

Testing is recommended for all neonates born to women with confirmed or suspected COVID-19, regardless of whether there are signs of infection in the neonate. For neonates presenting with signs of infection suggestive of COVID-19 as described above, providers should also consider alternative diagnoses to COVID-19.

Recommended testing

- Diagnosis should be confirmed by testing for SARS-CoV-2 RNA by reverse transcription polymerase chain reaction (RT-PCR). Detection of SARS-CoV-2 viral RNA can be collected using nasopharynx, oropharynx, or nasal swab samples.
- Serologic testing is not recommended at this time to diagnose acute infection in neonates.

When to test

- Both symptomatic and asymptomatic neonates born to mothers with confirmed or suspected COVID-19, regardless of mother's symptoms, should have testing performed at approximately 24 hours of age. If initial test results are negative, or not available, testing should be repeated at 48 hours of age.
- For asymptomatic neonates expected to be discharged <48 hours of age, a single test can be performed prior to discharge, between 24 and 48 hours of age.

Limitations and interpretation of testing

- The optimal timing of testing after birth is unknown. Early testing may lead to false positives (e.g., if the neonate's nares, nasopharynx and/or oropharynx is contaminated by SARS-CoV-2 RNA in maternal fluids) or false negatives (e.g., RNA may not yet be detectable immediately after exposure following delivery).

Infection prevention and control

Given the paucity of information regarding signs of COVID-19 in neonates, all neonates born to mothers with confirmed or suspected COVID-19 should be considered as having suspected SARS-CoV-2 infection when testing results are not available.

Infants with suspected SARS-CoV-2 infection should be isolated from other healthy neonates and cared for according to the Interim Infection Prevention and Control Recommendations for Patients with Suspected or Confirmed Coronavirus Disease 2019 (COVID-19) in Healthcare Settings.

For healthcare personnel, recommendations for appropriate PPE are outlined in the Interim Infection Prevention and Control Recommendations for Patients with Suspected or Confirmed Coronavirus Disease 2019 (COVID-19) in Healthcare Settings.

Mother/neonatal contact

Although it is well recognized that the ideal setting for care of a healthy term newborn while in the hospital is within the mother's room, temporary separation of the newborn from a mother with confirmed or suspected COVID-19 should be strongly considered to reduce the risk of transmission to the neonate. Efforts are under way to address the knowledge gap of transmission between mother and neonate during pregnancy, delivery and in the postpartum period, and recommendations will be updated as new information informing the risk-benefit of maternal-infant separation is available.

Temporary separation in the clinical setting can be achieved in many ways, including a separate room, maintaining a physical distance of ≥6 feet between the mother and neonate, and placing the neonate in a temperature-controlled isolette if the neonate remains in the mother's room. For mothers whose test results are negative, separation precautions may be discontinued.

Although temporary separation of a neonate from a mother with confirmed or suspected COVID-19 should be strongly considered in healthcare settings, it may not always be feasible. For these situations, the risks, and benefits of temporary separation of the mother from her baby should be discussed with the mother by the healthcare team, and decisions about temporary separation should be made in accordance with the mother's wishes. Considerations include:

- Clinical conditions of the mother and neonate
  - Separation may be necessary for infants at higher risk for severe illness (e.g., preterm infants and infants with medical conditions)
- Availability of testing, staffing, space, and PPE in the healthcare facility
- Results of neonatal testing
  - If the neonate tests positive for SARS-CoV-2, separation is not necessary

If separation is not undertaken, measures that can be taken to minimize the risk of transmission from mother to neonate include:

- Mother uses cloth face covering and practices hand hygiene during all contact with the neonate. Cloth face coverings should not be placed on neonates or any children younger than 2 years of age.
- Engineering controls like physical barriers are used (e.g., placing the neonate in a temperature-controlled isolette), and the neonate is kept ≥6 feet away from the mother as much as possible.

Breastfeeding guidance is available at: Interim Guidance on Breastfeeding and Breast Milk Feeds in the Context of COVID-19. Additional information for parents and other caregivers about the importance of well childcare and information regarding feeding can be found on CDC's Pregnancy, Breastfeeding, and Caring for Young Children website. Resources are also available on stress and coping secondary to COVID-19.

COVID-19 CARE IN CHILDREN

The CDC provides current information on COVID-19 in children.[50]

Pediatric cases of COVID-19, caused by severe acute respiratory syndrome coronavirus 2 (SARS-CoV-2), have been reported. However, there are relatively fewer cases of COVID-19 among children compared to cases among adult patients. Recent studies report that children are less likely to get infected after contact with a SARS-CoV-2–positive individual. It has been suggested that children and adolescents have similar viral loads and may therefore be as likely to transmit SARS-CoV-2 as adults. In addition, the viral load may be similar in asymptomatic and symptomatic individuals. However, reassuringly, transmission in schools from children either to other children or to adults has been rare.

Children have a lower prevalence of the comorbidities that have been associated with severe COVID-19 in adults, such as obesity, diabetes, hypertension, and chronic kidney, lung, and heart disease. Even though no definite risk factors have been identified in children, those with chronic lung disease (including asthma), cardiovascular disease, and immunosuppression more often require hospital compared with previously healthy children. Even children with serious medical conditions, who are on immunosuppressive or cancer treatment, are much less affected by COVID-19 than adults.[51]

Symptoms in Pediatric Patients

Illness among pediatric cases appears to be mild, with most cases presenting with symptoms of upper respiratory infection such as:

- Fever
- Cough
- Nasal congestion
- Rhinorrhea
- Sore throat

Outcomes in Pediatric Patients

Relatively few children with COVID-19 are hospitalized, and fewer children than adults experience fever, cough, or shortness of breath. Severe outcomes have been reported in children, including COVID-19–associated deaths. Hospitalization was most common among pediatric patients aged less than 1 year and those with underlying conditions.

Although most cases reported among children to date have not been severe, clinicians should maintain a high index of suspicion for SARS-CoV-2 infection in children and monitor for progression of illness, particularly among infants and children with underlying conditions.

Incubation Period

While data on the incubation period for COVID-19 in the pediatric population are limited, it is thought to extend to 14 days, similar to adult patients with COVID-19. In studies from China, the reported incubation period among pediatric patients ranged from 2 to 10 days.

Clinical Presentation

Pediatric patients with COVID-19 may experience the following signs or symptoms over the course of the disease:

- Fever
- Cough
- Nasal congestion or rhinorrhea
- Sore throat
- Shortness of breath
- Diarrhea
- Nausea or vomiting
- Fatigue
- Headache
- Myalgia
- Poor feeding or poor appetite

The predominant signs and symptoms of COVID-19 reported to date among all patients are similar to other viral respiratory infections, including fever, cough, and shortness of breath. Although these signs and symptoms may occur at any time during the overall disease course, children with COVID-19 may not initially present with fever and cough as often as adult patients. In a report of 9 hospitalized infants in China with confirmed COVID-19, only half presented with fever. Gastrointestinal symptoms, including abdominal pain, diarrhea, nausea, and vomiting, were reported in a minority of adult patients. In one pediatric case of COVID-19, diarrhea was the only symptom reported.

There have been multiple reports to date of children with asymptomatic SARS-CoV-2 infection. In one study, up to 13% of pediatric cases with SARS-CoV-2 infection were asymptomatic.[16] The prevalence of asymptomatic SARS-CoV-2 infection and duration of presymptomatic infection in children are not well understood, as asymptomatic individuals are not routinely tested.

Signs and symptoms of COVID-19 in children may be like those for common viral respiratory infections or other childhood illnesses. It is important for pediatric providers to have an appropriate suspicion of COVID-19 but also to continue to consider and test for other diagnoses, such as influenza (see CDC's Flu Information for Healthcare Professionals [https://www.cdc.gov/flu/professionals/index.htm] for more information).

Clinical Course and Complications in Children

The largest study of pediatric patients (>2000) with COVID-19 from China reported that illness severity ranged from asymptomatic to critical:

- Asymptomatic (no clinical signs or symptoms with normal chest imaging): 4%
- Mild (mild symptoms, including fever, fatigue, myalgia, cough): 51%
- Moderate (pneumonia with symptoms or subclinical disease with abnormal chest imaging): 39%
- Severe (dyspnea, central cyanosis, hypoxia): 5%
- Critical (acute respiratory distress syndrome [ARDS], respiratory failure, shock, or multiorgan dysfunction): 0.6%

Based on these early studies, children of all ages are at risk for COVID-19; however, complications of COVID-19 appear to be less common among children compared with adults based on limited reports from China and the United States. In children, SARS-CoV-2 may have more affinity for the upper respiratory tract (including nasopharyngeal carriage) than the lower respiratory tract.

As of April 2, 2020, infants younger than 1 year old accounted for 15% of pediatric COVID-19 cases in the United States. However, this age group remains underrepresented among COVID-19 cases in patients of all ages (0.3%) compared to their percentage in the US population (1.2%). Relative to adult patients with COVID-19, there were fewer children with COVID-19 requiring hospitalization (6%-20%) and intensive care unit admission (0.6%-2%). Although severe complications (eg, acute respiratory distress syndrome, septic shock) have been reported in children of all ages, they appear to be infrequent. Based on limited data on children with either suspected or confirmed infection with SARS-CoV-2, infants (<12 months of age) may be at higher risk of severe or critical disease compared with older children, with hospitalization being most common among children younger than 1 year old and those with underlying conditions, such as chronic lung disease (including asthma), cardiovascular disease, and immunosuppression. Other reports describe a mild disease course, including in infants.

Long COVID-19 in Children

In children and adolescents, acute COVID-19 is less severe than in adults. Concern among many parents has therefore focused more on the potential long-term effects of SARS-CoV-2 infection. Unfortunately, fewer data are available on long COVID-19 in young people compared with adults. The widely quoted frequency in children is based on a study with a 13% response rate.[52]

The prevalence of long COVID symptoms varies between studies from 4% to 66%. There is also a large variation in the reported frequency of persistent symptoms.

The most common reported symptoms are the following[53]:

- Headache (3%-80%)
- Fatigue (3%-87%)
- Sleep disturbance (2%-63%)
- Concentration difficulties (2%-81%)
- Abdominal pain (1%-76%), myalgia or arthralgia (1%-61%)
- Congested or runny nose (1%-12%)
- Cough (1%-30%)
- Chest tightness or pain (1%-31%)
- Loss of appetite or weight (2%-50%)
- Disturbed smell or anosmia (3%-26%)
- Rash (2%-52%)

Multisystem Inflammatory Syndrome in Children

The CDC is collaborating with domestic and international partners to learn more about multisystem inflammatory syndrome in children (MIS-C) associated with COVID-19.

Patients with MIS-C have presented with a persistent fever and a variety of signs and symptoms including multiorgan (eg, cardiac, gastrointestinal, renal, hematologic, dermatologic, neurologic) involvement and elevated inflammatory markers.

Testing, Laboratory Findings, and Radiographic Findings

Chest x-rays of children with COVID-19 have shown patchy infiltrates consistent with viral pneumonia, and chest CT scans have shown nodular ground-glass opacities; however, these findings are not specific to COVID-19 and may overlap with other diagnoses, and some children may have no radiographic abnormalities. Chest radiograph or CT alone is not recommended for the diagnosis of COVID-19. The American College of Radiology also does not recommend CT for screening or as a first-line test for diagnosis of COVID-19.

Treatment and Prevention

Currently, there are no specific drugs approved by the US Food and Drug Administration (FDA) for treatment or prevention of COVID-19. Treatment remains largely supportive and includes prevention and management of complications. Health care facilities, including pediatric health care facilities, should ensure that infection prevention and control policies, including universal source control, are in place to minimize chance of exposure to SARS-CoV-2 among providers, patients, and families. CDC has published specific guidance, including infection prevention and control considerations, for inpatient obstetric health care settings and the evaluation and management of neonates at risk for COVID-19.

There is limited evidence at this time about which underlying medical conditions in children might increase the risk of severe illness from COVID-19. Current evidence suggests that children who are medically complex, who have serious genetic, neurologic, or metabolic disorders, or who have congenital heart disease might be at increased risk for severe illness from COVID-19. Like adults, children with obesity, diabetes, asthma or chronic lung disease, or immunosuppression might also be at increased risk for severe illness from COVID-19.

Severe complications associated with COVID-19 in pediatric patients have not been well-described. One newly described severe complication, MIS-C, is being investigated by CDC and partners. The treatment of severe and critical cases of pediatric patients with COVID-19 in the hospital may include management of pneumonia, respiratory failure, exacerbation of underlying conditions, sepsis or septic shock, or secondary bacterial infection. Situations in which a patient requires prolonged hospitalization may also result in secondary nosocomial infections.

■ PHYSICAL THERAPY INTERVENTIONS

Physical therapy interventions for cardiopulmonary dysfunction focus on improving respiratory function. This can include airway clearance, pursed-lip breathing, coughing techniques, and chest physical therapy to loosen up mucus (percussion and postural positioning). Manual therapy can be used to improve rib cage, diaphragm, and thoracic spine mobility. Exercises for strengthening and conditioning include aerobic, strength, flexibility, posture, and breathing exercises and IMT. Pulmonary rehabilitation uses a combination of all these techniques along with cardiac monitoring.

AIRWAY CLEARANCE

Manual or mechanical procedures can facilitate mobilization of secretions from the airways. These techniques include postural drainage, percussion, vibration, cough techniques, manual hyperinflation, and airway suctioning. The indications for airway clearance techniques include impaired mucociliary transport, excessive pulmonary secretions, and an ineffective or absent cough. The clinician can facilitate the mobilization of secretions by using one or more airway clearance techniques. Considerations of the pathophysiology and symptoms, the stability of the medical status of the child, and the child's adherence to the technique(s) are all important factors in choosing an optimal airway clearance plan of care.

The goals of airway clearance techniques are as follows:

- Optimize airway patency
- Increase ventilation and perfusion matching
- Promote alveolar expansion and ventilation
- Increase gas exchange

Duration and frequency of the techniques are based on pulmonary reevaluation at each session.

COUGH

An effective cough consists of the following 4 stages:

1. Inspiration greater than tidal volume; 60% of the patient's predicted vital capacity
2. Closure of the glottis
3. Abdominal and intercostal muscle contraction, producing positive intrathoracic pressure

4. Opening of the glottis and the forceful expulsion of the inspired air

Examination of cough effectiveness is vital in determining the amount and type of intervention the patient will need for adequate removal of secretions. An effective cough should maximize the function of each of the 4 stages. The patient should exhibit a deep inspiration combined with trunk extension, a momentary hold, and then a series of sharp expirations while the trunk moves into flexion. Any absence or deficiency in this sequence of events is likely to result in an ineffective cough. This can lead to retained secretions and, if left untreated, can progress to atelectasis, hypoxemia, pneumonia, and potentially respiratory failure. For acutely ill patients with reduced cough effectiveness and the ability to follow instructions, the first line of intervention is positioning and teaching proper coughing technique.

POSTURAL DRAINAGE AND PERCUSSION

Percussion and postural positioning are used for postural drainage of airway clearance and removal of mucus from the 5 different lobes of the lungs. The goal of each position is to have the lung lobe positioned in the downward position to drain (**Figure 16-9**). Once in the position, gravity and a vibration or clapping technique are used to loosen up the mucus. The goal is to loosen the mucus and move it toward larger airways to be coughed out. The techniques are performed for 3 to 5 minutes followed by forced exhalation and coughing to get the mucus out. A treatment session can be performed for 20 to 40 minutes depending on the tolerance of the patient.[54]

SUCTIONING

Airway suctioning is performed routinely for intubated patients to facilitate the removal of secretions and to stimulate the cough reflex. It is indicated for patients with artificial airways who have excess pulmonary secretions and the inability to clear the secretions from the airway. Reserve airway suctioning for those secretions that the patient is unable to clear from the airway independently or with assists; rehabilitation of cough effectiveness can be initiated before extubation. Patients with artificial airways can be instructed in huffing and cough assist techniques to enable them to progress to an effective cough, except for glottal closure. Endotracheal and tracheal tubes prevent glottal closure from contributing to the intubated patient's attempts to clear secretions. The suction catheter can reach only to the level of the mainstem bronchi. When lung secretions are retained in the small airways, postural drainage with percussion and/or vibration should be used to mobilize the secretions centrally, before suctioning.

Recommended Procedure—Tracheal Suctioning[55]:

1. Check baseline vital signs (eg, heart rate, blood pressure, SpO_2) and arterial blood gases.
2. Check equipment to make sure it is operational (vacuum pressure <120 mmHg).
3. Note ventilator settings, increase FiO_2 if baseline SpO_2 <92% to 95%.

4. Check with medical staff regarding need for a PEEP adapter if PEEP ≥10 cmH_2O pressure, if not using an inline catheter.
5. Explain procedure to patient.
6. Don mask, eye protection, gloves.
7. Attach suction catheter to suction tubing.
8. Discontinue patient from oxygen source.
9. Increase ventilation by giving 3-5 breaths with a manual resuscitator bag if the patient is breathing spontaneously.
10. Insert suction catheter into the airway until resistance is felt. Apply suction after withdrawing the catheter a few centimeters. Suction should be continuous, and catheter rotated while withdrawing. Assess vital signs during the procedure.
11. Ventilate with 3-5 breaths from a manual resuscitator bag if indicated. Reattach the patient to the oxygen source, recheck vital signs, if SpO_2 has dropped wait until it returns to baseline. Increase FiO_2 if indicated.
12. Repeat steps 9-11 as indicated for 2-4 suction catheter passes. Change suction catheter if the patient requires more than 3-4 passes of the suction catheter.
13. Suction the mouth.
14. Return FiO_2 to baseline setting and reassess vital signs.
15. Dispose of suction supplies.

MANUAL THERAPY

Manual therapy techniques can be performed to loosen the rib cage, diaphragm, and thoracic spine. Patients with scoliosis can have decreased respiratory function secondary to compression and decreased mobility. Manual therapy techniques like myofascial release, soft tissue mobilization, joint oscillations, and positional release can improve soft tissue and joint mobility.[56-58]

Rib cage mobility can restrict thoracic mobility and rib cage expansion with inspiration and rib cage compression with expiration. During inspiration, the sternum and those ribs attached to it elevate and move further out from the mediastinum as the lungs fill with air. Anteriorly, there is elevation of the ribs in a pump handle direction. Ribs 2 through 5 have an axis of movement through the costovertebral and costotransverse articulations. During inhalation, the anteroposterior diameter of the thorax is increased. The motion is analogous to flexion/extension.[59,60]

In the lateral line of the body, the ribs elevate in a bucket handle direction. During inspiration, as the lungs fill with air, ribs at the lateral-most location move away from the midline. This is seen in ribs 6 to 10. Inhalation increases the transverse diameter of the thorax. The movement is on an axis through the costotransverse and costochondral articulations. The motion is analogous to abduction/adduction.

Evaluation of rib dysfunction is done on the anterior chest wall, the posterior chest wall, and the lateral chest wall. Assessment of rib dysfunctions is done both statically and dynamically. In an inhalation dysfunction, the ribs will move upward into an inhalation position, but during exhalation, they will not drop downward. In an exhalation dysfunction, the ribs will move inferiorly with exhalation, but they will not move upward with inhalation.[57-60]

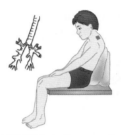

UPPER LOBES Apical segments

Bed or drainage table flat.

Patient leans back on pillow at 30° angle against therapist.

Therapist claps with markedly cupped hand over area between clavicle and top of scapula on each side.

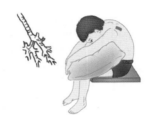

UPPER LOBES Posterior segments

Bed or drainage table flat.

Patient leans over folded pillow at 30° angle.

Therapist stands behind and claps over upper back on both sides.

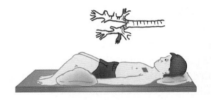

UPPER LOBES Anterior segments

Bed or drainage table flat.

Patient lies on back with pillow under knees.

Therapist claps between clavicle and nipple on each side.

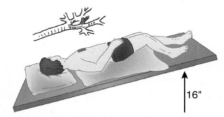

16"

RIGHT MIDDLE LOBE

Foot of table or bed elevated 16 inches.

Patient lies head down on left side and rotates 1/4 turn backward. Pillow may be placed behind from shoulder to hip. Knees should be flexed.

Therapist claps over right nipple area. In females with breast development or tenderness use cupped hand with heel of hand under armpit and fingers extending forward beneath the breast.

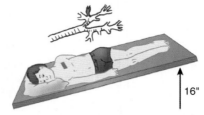

16"

LEFT UPPER LOBE Singular segments

Foot of table or bed elevated 16 inches.

Patient lies head down on right side and rotates 1/4 turn backward. Pillow may be placed behind from shoulder to hip. Knees should be flexed.

Therapist claps with moderately cupped hand over left nipple area. In females with breast development or tenderness use cupped hand with heel of hand under armpit and fingers extending forward beneath the breast.

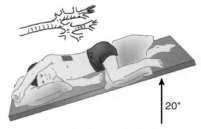

20"

LOWER LOBES Anterior basal segments

Foot of table or bed elevated 20 inches.

Patient lies on side, head down, pillow under knees.

Therapist claps with slightly cupped hand over lower ribs. (Position shown is for drainage of left anterior basal segment. To drain the right anterior basal segment, patient should be on the left side in same posture.)

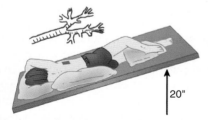

20"

LOWER LOBES Lateral basal segments

Foot of table or bed elevated 20 inches.

Patient lies on abdomen, head down, then rotates 1/4 turn upward. Upper leg is flexed over pillow for support.

Therapist claps over uppermost portion of lower ribs. (Position shown is for drainage of right lateral basal segment. To drain the left lateral basal segment, patient should lie on the right side in the same posture.)

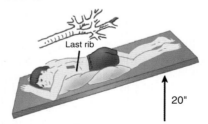

Last rib

20"

LOWER LOBES Posterior basal segments

Foot of table or bed elevated 20 inches.

Patient lies on abdomen, head down, with pillow under hips.

Therapist claps over lower ribs close to spine on each side.

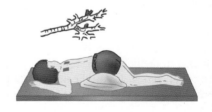

LOWER LOBES Superior segments

Bed of table flat.

Patient lies on abdomen with two pillows under hips.

Therapist claps over middle of back at tip of scapula on either side of spine.

FIGURE 16-9 Gravity assisted drainage positions. (Reproduced with permission from Burke-Doe A, Dutton M. *National Physical Therapy Examination and Board Review.* New York: McGraw Hill LLC; 2019.)

Manual therapy techniques can be performed to increase rib cage mobility. Manual therapy techniques can address autonomics, lymph drainage, and rib cage mobility. Examples are (1) rib raising, (2) thoracic pump, (3) doming of the thoracic diaphragm, and (4) muscle energy for rib 1.[61,62]

Mobilization with movement is a technique that increases mobility of the joints, fascia, muscle, and soft tissue restrictions while performing functional movement. The technique in **Figure 16-10** is used to perform thoracic and rib cage mobility. It is also used to incorporate thoracic rotation.[56] The physical

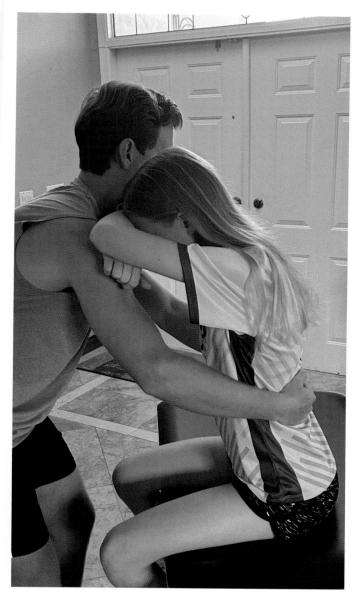

FIGURE 16-10 Seated rib cage manipulation.

therapist can facilitate individual rib mobility or a grouping of ribs.[56]

Patient position: Seated

Physical therapist position: Stand in front of the seated patient

1. The patient crosses their arms in front of the and sits in a flexed trunk posture.
2. The physical therapist places the patient's forearms onto their upper chest. The physical therapist places both of their hands around the patient at the posterior rib angles to facilitate upward rotation.
3. While the physical therapist lifts into trunk extension, the physical therapist places a sweeping force (accessory glide) at the rib angles to facilitate upward rotation of the rib cage.

4. As the physical lifts further into trunk extension, the therapist adds an anterior gliding of the thoracic spine.
5. This is repeated until a greater amount of trunk extension is obtained.

The myofascial manipulation technique in **Figures 16-11A** is used to perform thoracic and rib cage mobility.[56]

Type of manipulation: Myofascial manipulation

Patient position: Supine or prone

Therapist position: Standing on the side of the table

1. The patient lies side lying.
2. The therapist palpates the latissimus dorsi muscles, pectoralis major, and anterior ribs that have limited extensibility.
3. The therapist uses a tissue tension technique to mobilize the fascia.
4. The therapist palpates into the soft tissue and uses the caudad hand to grasp the upper arm and flex the shoulder with upward traction.
5. The therapist uses the cephalad hand on the latissimus dorsi or pectoralis major to engage the restrictive barrier with a light force in the direction of tension, sometimes for up to 3 to 5 minutes.
6. A light pressure on the barrier is held until the tissue barrier softens and relaxes and the myofascial unit elongates.

Notes: Depending on the specific muscle identified, the fiber direction will change.

The myofascial manipulation technique in **Figure 16-11B** is used to perform thoracic and rib cage mobility.

Type of manipulation: Myofascial manipulation

Patient position: Supine or prone

Therapist position: Standing on the side of the table

1. The patient lies side lying or supine.
2. The therapist palpates the latissimus dorsi muscles, pectoralis major, and anterior ribs that have limited extensibility.
3. The therapist uses a tissue tension technique to mobilize the fascia.
4. The therapist uses both hands in opposite directions.
5. A light pressure on the barrier is held until the tissue barrier softens and relaxes and the myofascial unit elongates.

Notes: Depending on the specific muscle identified, the fiber direction will change.

The self-mobilization technique in **Figure 16-12** is used to perform upper thoracic, shoulder, and rib cage mobility.

Type of manipulation: Self-mobilization

Restricted motion: Limited upper thoracic extension and shoulder flexion

Patient position: Hands and knees

1. The patient is on their knees and places their forearms on a foam roller.
2. The patient can hold the stretch statically or can rock back and forth with their knees to increase the thoracic and shoulder stretch.

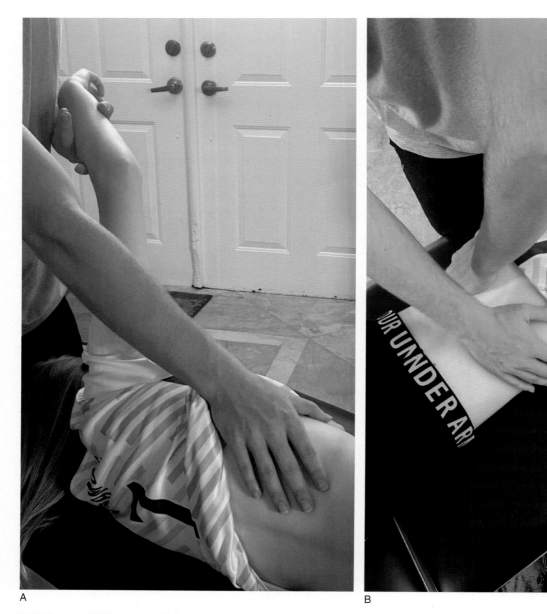

A   B

FIGURE 16-11 (A) Thoracic myofascial manipulation side lying. **(B)** Thoracic myofascial manipulation prone.

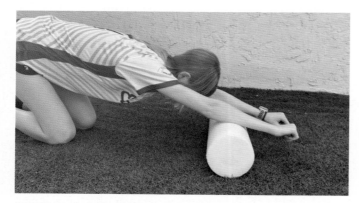

FIGURE 16-12 Self-mobilization of the thoracic spine quadruped over foam roller.

The self-mobilization with movement technique in **Figure 16-13** is used to perform shoulder and clavicle mobility.

Type of manipulation: Self-mobilization

Restricted motion: Limited shoulder abduction, lateral rib cage mobility

Patient position: Side lying

1. The patient lays side lying with the shoulder abducted.
2. The patient places the foam roller under their forearm.
3. The patient uses a tissue tension technique to relax the tissue tension.
4. The patient engages the restrictive barrier with a light force in the shoulder adduction, as the patient relaxes tissue tension is taken up with further shoulder abduction.

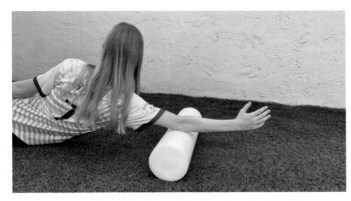

FIGURE 16-13 Self-mobilization of the thoracic spine side lying over foam roller.

5. This is repeated until no further tissue elongation into abduction after the engagement of the restricted barrier.

   Notes: An option is a light pressure on the barrier is held until the tissue barrier softens and relaxes and the myofascial unit elongates.

The diaphragm separates the thoracic cavity from the abdominal cavity. The diaphragm is involved in breathing, blood circulation, and lymphatic flow. The diaphragm assists to create negative and positive pressures. During inhalation, the diaphragm contracts and flattens while the lungs and chest get bigger. The diaphragm contracts to create a vacuum to pull air into the lungs. During exhalation, the diaphragm relaxes and stretches up into a dome shape to exhale all the air out. A dysfunction of the diaphragm is the limited mobility of the diaphragm to move into a dome shape. This creates an inability to push all the air out of the lungs. This causes hyperinflation of the lungs. This will decrease lung function capacity. Diaphragmatic breathing will help facilitate normal action of the diaphragm. The diaphragm can have decreased mobility that can be treated with myofascial release called doming the diaphragm.[59-62]

The myofascial release technique in **Figures 16-14** is used to perform doming of the diaphragm.

Type of manipulation: Self–soft tissue mobilization.

Doming the Thoracic Diaphragm[63,64]

1. With the patient lying in supine, palpate the rib cage bilaterally when the patient inhales and exhales.
2. Stand to either side of patient. Thumbs should be placed inferolateral to the xiphoid process and rest along the anterolateral costal margin below rib 7, which corresponds to muscular attachments of the respiratory diaphragm. The remaining fingers should rest along the inferolateral border of ribs 8 to 10.
3. Have the patient inhale and exhale all the way out. As the patient exhales, follow the diaphragm by pressing thumbs posterior toward the table.
4. Hold this point on the diaphragm as the patient takes the next deep inhalation. During the next exhalation, a cephalad motion of the diaphragm is performed to take up any tissue slack toward doming the diaphragm.

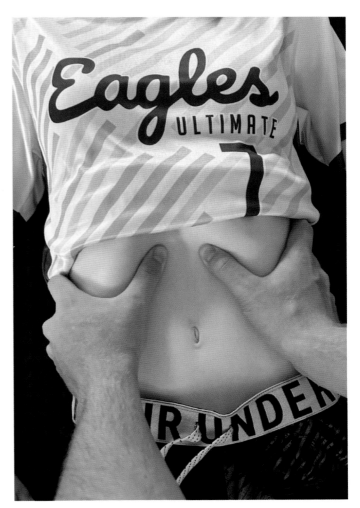

FIGURE 16-14 Doming the diaphragm.

5. Hold the tissue tension until there is relaxation and stretching of the diaphragm. Often one side will be more limited than the other. Focus the pressure on the side of limitation until the diaphragm domes symmetrically or further when exhaling.
6. Reassess by monitoring the diaphragm for improvement in excursion.

WEARABLE

Individuals with cystic fibrosis can wear a device called a Vest[65] for high-frequency chest wall oscillation (vest or oscillator). This inflatable vest wraps around the chest and vibrates at a high frequency. The vibrations loosen and thin the mucus. After 5 minutes of vibration, the person turns off the machine and huff coughs (see later in this chapter for huff coughing). Sessions generally last 20 to 30 minutes.[65]

EXERCISE

Exercise can include aerobic conditioning, strengthening, flexibility, posture, and breathing techniques. Active cycle of breathing techniques (ACBTs) are used to get air behind the mucus so that it can be cleared.[66] ACBTs include the following[66]:

- **Breathing control:** Relaxed upper chest and shoulders.
- **Chest expansion:** Deep breathing causes chest expansion. Sometimes it is done while holding the breath for 3 seconds, and sometimes, it is done with chest clapping or vibrating.
- **Forced expiration:** Huffs for different lengths of time combined with breathing control.

The pursed lip breathing technique[67] is a technique where you position your lips like you were going to whistle and breathe out, or exhale, all the air in your lungs through your mouth slowly and gently through pursed lips. Breathe in (inhale) slowly through your nose for 2 counts, keeping your mouth closed. Do not take a deep breath; take a normal breath while inhaling and counting 1, 2. Pucker or "purse" your lips as if you were going to whistle or gently flicker the flame of a candle. Breathe out (exhale) slowly and gently through your pursed lips while counting to 4. It may help to count to yourself: exhale, 1, 2, 3, 4.[67]

In individuals with low peak expiratory flow, pursed-lip breathing reduces dynamic hyperinflation and improves exercise tolerance, breathing pattern, and arterial oxygenation at submaximal intensity exercise.[68]

Diaphragmatic breathing (belly breathing) is used to focus inspiration and expiration using your diaphragm.[69] When doing diaphragmatic breathing, your chest, clavicle, and upper shoulder should not expand. Place one hand on your belly just below your ribs and the other hand on your chest. Then take a deep breath in through your nose, and let your belly push your hand out. Breathe out through pursed lips as if you were whistling. Feel the hand on your belly go in and use it to push all the air out. Do this breathing 3 to 10 times. Take your time with each breath.[69]

Roll breathing helps you to develop full use of your lungs and to focus on the rhythm of your breathing.[70] It is best to lie on your back with your knees bent.

1. Put your left hand on your belly and your right hand on your chest. Notice how your hands move as you breathe in and out.
2. Practice filling your lower lungs by breathing so that your "belly" (left) hand goes up when you inhale and your "chest" (right) hand remains still. Always breathe in through your nose and breathe out through your mouth. Do this 8 to 10 times.
3. When you have filled and emptied your lower lungs 8 to 10 times, add the second step to your breathing: inhale first into your lower lungs as before, and then continue inhaling into your upper chest. Breathe slowly and regularly. As you do so, your right hand will rise and your left hand will fall a little as your belly falls.
4. As you exhale slowly through your mouth, make a quiet, whooshing sound as first your left hand and then your right hand fall. As you exhale, feel the tension leaving your body as you become more and more relaxed.
5. Practice breathing in and out in this way for 3 to 5 minutes. Notice that the movement of your belly and chest rises and falls like the motion of rolling waves.[70]

COUGHING TECHNIQUE

Coughing is a basic airway clearance technique. It can be used to get rid of mucus in the lungs. Huffing (huff coughing) helps remove mucus from the lungs. It involves taking a breath in, holding it, and actively exhaling. Breathing in and holding your breath enables air to get behind the mucus and separates it from the lung wall so it can be coughed out. Huffing is not as forceful as a cough. Huffing is like exhaling onto a mirror or window to steam it up.

The huff coughing technique is as follows:

- Think about breathing fog onto a mirror or glasses.
- Taking a deep breath through your nose.
- Breathe out forcefully in 3 equal breaths while pulling your abdomen inward to force the air from your lungs.
- Making a "huff" sound in the back of your throat.
- Repeat this 2-3 times followed by a forceful cough.

AUTOGENIC DRAINAGE

Autogenic drainage (self-drainage) helps move the mucus from the smaller to large airways. This technique requires training, hard work, and practice. It can take from 20 to 45 minutes. It is generally only used for ages 8 and up.[71] Autogenic drainage is a 3-phase breathing technique. Inhale at different lung volume levels and then adjust the exhalation to maximize airflow and move mucus. The goal is to reach high airflows in different areas of the lung. This can help loosen mucus from the bronchial walls and move the mucus from the small to large airways.[71]

The 3 phases of autogenic drainage are as follows:

1. Loosening secretions: Low lung volume level
2. Collecting secretions: Mid lung volume level
3. Evacuating secretions: High lung volume level

The autogenic drainage techniques is performed as follows:

- Begin breathing at a low lung volume level.
- Breathe in slowly through your nose using the diaphragm and/or lower chest.
- Hold your breath for 1 to 3 seconds, keeping the glottis (voice box) open. This helps the lungs fill evenly and allows air to get behind the mucus. Exhale as quickly and forcefully as possible while keeping an open glottis. Exhalation should be as fast as possible, but not tightening the airway.
- Continue breathing at a low lung volume level. Raise your breath from low to mid to high lung volume when you hear and feel crackles (mucus). High-frequency crackles indicate secretions in the smaller airways. Low-frequency crackles indicate secretions in the upper airways. Breathe at each level for 3 minutes.[72]

VENTILATORY MUSCLE TRAINING

Ventilatory muscle training (VMT) is one component of respiratory rehabilitation.[73,74] VMT is performed to enhance respiratory muscle function that can potentially reduce the severity of breathlessness and improve exercise tolerance.[73]

Inspiratory Muscle Training

With training, IMT can result in decreases in exercise-induced increases in heart rate, oxygen uptake (VO_2/kg), and rating of perceived exertion. The Threshold-IMT (HealthScan, New Jersey) device comprises a plastic tube incorporating a spring-loaded valve occluding the inspiratory orifice at one end and a mouthpiece at the other end. When the subject breathes through the mouthpiece, they must generate sufficient vacuum pressure to open the spring-loaded valve and initiate airflow; exhalation is unloaded. The amount of resistance can be adjusted by varying the compression of the spring-loaded valve. Training can be performed at 30% of maximal inspiratory muscle strength for 15 minutes twice daily.

Expiratory Muscle Training

Suzuki et al[74] reported that expiratory muscle training (EMT) increased expiratory muscle strength and decreased sensation of respiratory effort during exercise, and Akiyoshi et al[75] indicated that EMT increased both expiratory and inspiratory muscle strength. A Souffle (Kayaku, Tokyo, Japan) device comprises a central container with a dead space of 400 or 800 mL, a mouthpiece, and a metal positive end-expiratory pressure (PEEP) plate elastic-loaded valve occluding the expiratory orifice. When subjects exhale through the mouthpiece, they must generate positive pressure equivalent to 5, 10, or 15 cm H_2O to open the PEEP plate elastic-loaded valve. Training can be performed at 30% of maximal expiratory muscle strength for 15 minutes twice daily.[74,75]

PULMONARY REHABILITATION

A pulmonary rehabilitation program is a multidisciplinary approach individualized to optimize function. Pulmonary rehabilitation services include evaluation, physical reconditioning, and psychological support.[2] A team including a doctor, nurse, respiratory therapist, physical therapist, psychologist, exercise physiologist, and registered dietitian/nutritionist usually make up the interprofessional team.

Pulmonary rehabilitation can be used for improvement and restoration of function or as a preventive measure. Children with chronic obstructive lung disease, interstitial lung disease (sarcoidosis or hypersensitivity pneumonitis), pulmonary hypertension, asthma, and other chronic lung diseases can have decreased lung function.[1] Decreased lung function and reserves can cause dyspnea or shortness of breath. Goals of pulmonary rehabilitation are to improve shortness of breath, build aerobic capacity for exercise and activity, and reduce anxiety and depression.

Pulmonary rehabilitation includes the monitoring of heart rate, blood pressure, blood oxygen saturation, and exercise exertion, and often ECG monitoring. Endurance training, breathing training, muscle strengthening and flexibility, and nutrition are also included.[76]

■ SUMMARY

Children with cardiopulmonary dysfunction can have a combination of impairments and decreased function, including decreased proximal upper limb strength, limited endurance capacity, limited active range of motion, inability to ambulate independently, dependency for transfers, and developmental delay. Physical therapists play an integral role in the management, training, and conditioning of children so that they are able to function at their highest level.

STUDY QUESTIONS

1. Name 4 signs and symptoms of respiratory distress.
2. What would normal blood pressure and heart rate be in a 6-year-old child and a 12-year-old child?
3. What radiologic device would be beneficial for a child with a heart transplant?
4. List 4 functional limitations in children with asthma.
5. List the steps of airway clearance for a child with cystic fibrosis.
6. How do you determine the level of intensity of exercise for a child with a heart transplant?
7. Are children more susceptible to COVID-19?
8. How do you dome the diaphragm to improve exhalation?

References

1. Takken T, Sonbahar Ulu H, Hulzebos EHJ. Clinical recommendations for cardiopulmonary exercise testing in children with respiratory diseases. *Expert Rev Respir Med.* 2020;14(7):691-701.
2. Radtke T, Hebestreit H, Gallati S, et al. CFTR genotype and maximal exercise capacity in cystic fibrosis: a cross-sectional study. *Ann Am Thorac Soc.* 2018;15(2):209-216.
3. Silverman MA, Anderson SD. Standardization of exercise tests in asthmatic children. *Arch Dis Child.* 1972;47(256):882-889.
4. Saynor ZL, Barker AR, Oades PJ, Williams CA. Reproducibility of maximal cardiopulmonary exercise testing for young cystic fibrosis patients. *J Cyst Fibros.* 2013;12(6):644-650.
5. Klijn PHC, van der Net J, Kimpen JL, Helders PJM, van der Ent CK. Longitudinal determinants of peak aerobic performance in children with cystic fibrosis. *Chest.* 2003;124(6):2215-2219.
6. Ohuchi H, Negishi J, Noritake K, et al. Prognostic value of exercise variables in 335 patients after the Fontan operation: a 23-year single-center experience of cardiopulmonary exercise testing. *Congenit Heart Dis.* 2015;10(2):105-116.
7. Myers J. Applications of cardiopulmonary exercise testing in the management of cardiovascular and pulmonary disease. *Int J Sports Med.* 2005;26(Suppl 1):S49-S55.
8. Guazzi M, Bandera F, Ozemek C, Systrom D, Arena R. Cardiopulmonary exercise testing: what is its value? *J Am Coll Cardiol.* 2017;70(13):1618-1636.
9. Cooper DM, Weiler-Ravell D, Whipp BJ, Wasserman K. Aerobic parameters of exercise as a function of body size during growth in children. *J Appl Physiol Respir Environ Exerc Physiol.* 1984;56(3):628-634.
10. Blais S, Berbari J, Counil FP, Dallaire F. A systematic review of reference values in pediatric cardiopulmonary exercise testing. *Pediatr Cardiol.* 2015;36(8):1553-1564.
11. Hebestreit H. Exercise testing in children: what works, what doesn't, and where to go? *Paediatr Respir Rev.* 2004;5(Suppl A): S11-S14.
12. Takken T, Bongers BC, van Brussel M, Haapala EA, Hulzebos EHJ. Cardiopulmonary exercise testing in pediatrics. *Ann Am Thorac Soc.* 2017;14(Suppl 1):S123-S128.

13. Blanchard J, Blais S, Chetaille P, et al. New reference values for cardiopulmonary exercise testing in children. *Med Sci Sports Exerc.* 2018;50(6):1125-1133. Published correction appears in *Med Sci Sports Exerc.* 2019;51(7):1571.

14. Academy of Pediatric Physical Therapy. *List of Pediatric Assessment Tools Categorized by ICF model.* American Physical Therapy Association. Accessed November 24, 2023. https://pediatricapta.org/includes/fact-sheets/pdfs/13%20Assessment&screening%20tools.pdf.

15. Opfer E, Shah S. Advances in pediatric cardiovascular imaging. *Mo Med.* 2018;115(4):354-360.

16. Lai WW, Geva T, Shirali GS, et al. Guidelines and standards for performance of a pediatric echocardiogram: a report from the Task Force of the Pediatric Council of the American Society of Echocardiography. *J Am Soc Echocardiogr.* 2006;19(12):1413-1430.

17. Nagueh SF, Quinones MA. Important advances in technology: echocardiography. *Methodist Debakey Cardiovasc J.* 2014;10(3):146-151.

18. Mertens L, Ganame J, Eyskens B. What is new in pediatric cardiac imaging? *Eur J Pediatr.* 2008;167(1):1-8.

19. Shirali GS. Three-dimensional echocardiography in congenital heart defects. *Ann Pediatr Cardiol.* 2008;1(1):8-17.

20. Stanford Children's Health. Blood tests and your child's heart. Accessed November 24, 2023. https://www.stanfordchildrens.org/en/topic/default?id=blood-tests-and-your-childs-heart-90-P01769.

21. The Society for Cardiovascular Angiography and Interventions. Common heart conditions in children. Accessed November 24, 2023. http://www.secondscount.org/pediatric-center/conditions-children#.XybnAiqSnIU.

22. Masarone D, Valente F, Rubino M, et al. Pediatric heart failure: a practical guide to diagnosis and management. *Pediatr Neonatol.* 2017;58(4):303-312.

23. Bock M. Pediatric heart transplant. Medscape, June 30, 2022. Accessed November 24, 2023. http://emedicine.medscape.com/article/1011927-overview.

24. Ross RD. The Ross classification for heart failure in children after 25 years: a review and an age-stratified revision. *Pediatr Cardiol.* 2012;33(8):1295-1300.

25. Delling FN, Vasan RS. Epidemiology and pathophysiology of mitral valve prolapse: new insights into disease progression, genetics, and molecular basis. *Circulation.* 2014;129(21):2158-2170.

26. Janiec I, Werner B, Sieminska J, Ravens-Sieberer U. Quality of life of children with mitral valve prolapse. *Qual Life Res.* 2011;20(4):537-541.

27. American Academy of Pediatrics Committee on Sports Medicine and Fitness. Mitral valve prolapse and athletic participation in children and adolescents. *Pediatrics.* 1995;95(5):789-790.

28. Wu B, Hu C, Chen W, et al. China lung transplantation developing: past, present, and future. *Ann Transl Med.* 2020;8(3):41.

29. Hirche TO, Knoop C, Hebestreit H, et al. Practical guidelines: lung transplantation in patients with cystic fibrosis. *Pulm Med.* 2014;2014:621342. Published correction appears in *Pulm Med.* 2015;2015:698460.

30. Benden C. Pediatric lung transplantation. *J Thorac Dis.* 2017;9(8):2675-2683.

31. Wickerson L, Rozenberg D, Janaudis-Ferreira T, et al. Physical rehabilitation for lung transplant candidates and recipients: an evidence-informed clinical approach. *World J Transplant.* 2016;6(3):517-531.

32. Yeung JC, Keshavjee S. Overview of clinical lung transplantation. *Cold Spring Harb Perspect Med.* 2014;4(1):a015628.

33. National Heart, Lung, and Blood Institute, National Institute of Health. What Is Asthma? Accessed November 24, 2023. https://www.nhlbi.nih.gov/health/asthma.

34. AccessMedicine. Asthma. Quick Answers to Medical Diagnosis and Therapy. McGraw-Hill. Accessed November 24, 2023. https://accessmedicine.mhmedical.com/content.aspx?bookid=3109&sectionid=261295149.

35. National Asthma Education and Prevention Program. *Guidelines for the Diagnosis and Management of Asthma.* Expert Panel Report 3: National Institutes of Health Pub. No. 08-4051. Bethesda, MD; 2007. Accessed November 24, 2023. https://www.nhlbi.nih.gov/health-topics/guidelines-for-diagnosis-management-of-asthma.

36. Rangachari P, May KR, Stepleman LM, et al. Measurement of key constructs in a holistic framework for assessing self-management effectiveness of pediatric asthma. *Int J Environ Res Public Health.* 2019;16(17):3060.

37. Yavuz ST, Koc O, Gungor A, et al. 4th Pediatric Allergy and Asthma Meeting (PAAM). *Clin Transl Allergy.* 2016;6(Suppl 1):1-60.

38. Papadopoulos NG, Čustović A, Cabana MD, et al. Pediatric asthma: an unmet need for more effective, focused treatments. *Pediatr Allergy Immunol.* 2019;30(1):7-16.

39. Wilson AM. The role of antihistamines in asthma management. *Treat Respir Med.* 2006;5(3):149-158.

40. Caruso FR, Trimer R, da Luz Goulart C, et al. Thoracoabdominal mobility evaluation of asthmatic patients in physiotherapy practice: intra-rater reliability. *Physiother Res Int.* 2020;25(3):e1837.

41. Papadopoulos NG, Custovic A, Deschildre A, et al. Impact of COVID-19 on pediatric asthma: practice adjustments and disease burden. *J Allergy Clin Immunol Pract.* 2020;8(8):2592-2599.

42. CDC COVID-19 Response Team. Coronavirus disease 2019 in children—United States, February 12-April 2, 2020. *Morb Mortal Wkly Rep.* 2020;69(14):422-426.

43. Athanazio RA, Silva Filho LVRF, Vergara AA, et al. Brazilian guidelines for the diagnosis and treatment of cystic fibrosis. *J Bras Pneumol.* 2017;43(3):219-245.

44. Shei RJ, Dekerlegand RL, Mackintosh KA, Lowman JD, McNarry MA. Inspiration for the future: the role of inspiratory muscle training in cystic fibrosis. *Sports Med Open.* 2019;5(1):36.

45. Shei RJ, Mackintosh KA, Peabody Lever JE, McNarry MA, Krick S. Exercise physiology across the lifespan in cystic fibrosis. *Front Physiol.* 2019;10:1382.

46. Button BM, Wilson C, Dentice R, et al. Physiotherapy for cystic fibrosis in Australia and New Zealand: a clinical practice guideline. *Respirology.* 2016;21(4):656-667.

47. Nuss D, Obermeyer RJ, Kelly RE Jr. Pectus excavatum from a pediatric surgeon's perspective. *Ann Cardiothorac Surg.* 2016;5(5):493-500.

48. Brochhausen C, Turial S, Müller FK, et al. Pectus excavatum: history, hypotheses and treatment options. *Interact Cardiovasc Thorac Surg.* 2012;14(6):801-806.

49. Centers for Disease Control and Prevention (CDC). COVID-19 care for newborns. US Department of Health and Human Services. Accessed November 24, 2023. https://public4.pagefreezer.com/browse/CDC%20Covid%20Pages/11-05-2022T12:30/https://www.cdc.gov/coronavirus/2019-ncov/hcp/caring-for-newborns.html.

50. Centers for Disease Control and Prevention (CDC). COVID-19 care for children. US Department of Health and Human Services. Accessed October 1, 2022. https://www.cdc.gov/coronavirus/2019-ncov/hcp/pediatric-hcp.html.

51. Zimmermann P, Curtis N. Why is COVID-19 less severe in children? A review of the proposed mechanisms underlying the

age-related difference in severity of SARS-CoV-2 infections. *Arch Dis Child*. 2020;106(5):429-439.

52. Asadi-Pooya AA, Nemati H, Shahisavandi M, et al. Long COVID in children and adolescents. *World J Pediatric*. 2021;17(5):495-499.

53. Zimmermann P, Pittet LF, Curtis N. How common is long COVID in children and adolescents? *Pediatr Infect Dis*. 2021;40(12):e482.

54. Cystic Fibrosis Foundation. Chest physical therapy. Accessed October 1, 2022. https://www.cff.org/managing-cf/chest-physical-therapy.

55. DeTurk WE, Cahalin LP. *Cardiovascular and Pulmonary Physical Therapy: An Evidence-Based Approach, 3e*. Copyright © 2018 by McGraw-Hill Education.

56. Shamus E, van Duijn AJ. *Manual Therapy of the Extremities*. Jones and Bartlett Learning; 2016.

57. Bordoni B, Marelli F, Morabito B, Sacconi B. Manual evaluation of the diaphragm muscle. *Int J Chron Obstruct Pulmon Dis*. 2016;11:1949-956.

58. González-Álvarez FJ, Valenza MC, Torres-Sánchez I, Cabrera-Martos I, Rodríguez-Torres J, Castellote-Caballero Y. Effects of diaphragm stretching on posterior chain muscle kinematics and rib cage and abdominal excursion: a randomized controlled trial. *Braz J Phys Ther*. 2016;20(5):405-411.

59. Nair A, Alaparthi GK, Krishnan S, et al. Comparison of diaphragmatic stretch technique and manual diaphragm release technique on diaphragmatic excursion in chronic obstructive pulmonary disease: a randomized crossover trial. *Pulm Med*. 2019;2019:6364376.

60. Yao S, Hassani J, Gagne M, George G, Gilliar W. Osteopathic manipulative treatment as a useful adjunctive tool for pneumonia. *J Vis Exp*. 2014;87:50687.

61. Noll DR, Degenhardt BF, Fossum C, Hensel K. Clinical and research protocol for osteopathic manipulative treatment of elderly patients with pneumonia. *J Am Osteopath Assoc*. 2008;108(9):508-516.

62. Hruby RJ, Hoffman KN. Avian influenza: an osteopathic component to treatment. *Osteopath Med Prim Care*. 2007;1:10.

63. DiGiovanna E, Amen CJ, Burns DK. *An Osteopathic Approach to Diagnosis and Treatment*, Fourth Edition. Lippincott Williams & Wilkins; 2020.

64. Chila A, Carreiro JE, eds. *Foundations of Osteopathic Medicine, Third Edition*. Lippincott Williams & Wilkins; 2011:797-803.

65. Airway Clearance. Cystic Fibrosis Foundation. High-frequency chest wall oscillation (the Vest). Accessed November 24, 2023. https://www.cff.org/managing-cf/high-frequency-chest-wall-oscillation-vest.

66. Cystic Fibrosis Foundation. Active cycle of breathing techniques. Accessed November 24, 2023. https://www.cff.org/managing-cf/active-cycle-breathing-technique-acbt.

67. Cleveland Clinic. Pursed lip breathing. Accessed November 24, 2023. https://my.clevelandclinic.org/health/articles/9443-pursed-lip-breathing.

68. Cabral LF, D'Elia Tda C, Marins Dde S, Zin WA, Guimarães FS. Pursed lip breathing improves exercise tolerance in COPD: a randomized crossover study. *Eur J Phys Rehabil Med*. 2015;51(1):79-88.

69. Healthwise Staff. Stress management: breathing exercise for relaxation. Healthwise. Michigan Medicine. University of Michigan, June 25, 2023. Accessed November 24, 2023. https://www.uofmhealth.org/health-library/uz2255.

70. Healthwise Staff. Stress management: breathing exercises. Peace Health. June 25, 2003. Accessed November 24, 2023. https://www.peacehealth.org/medical-topics/id/ug1812.

71. Autogenic Drainage (AD). Cystic Fibrosis Foundation. Accessed October 1, 2023. https://www.cff.org/managing-cf/autogenic-drainage-ad

72. Intermountain Healthcare. Breathing exercises: autogenic drainage. Intermountain Healthcare, 2018. Accessed November 24, 2023. https://intermountainhealthcare.org/ckr-ext/Dcmnt?ncid=529596859#:~:text=Autogenic%20drainage%20(AD)%20is%20a,mucus%20may%20benefit%20from%20AD.

73. Sasaki M, Kurosawa H, Kohzuki M. Effects of inspiratory and expiratory muscle training in normal subjects. *J Jpn Phys Ther Assoc*. 2005;8(1):29-37.

74. Suzuki S, Sato M, Okubo T. Expiratory muscle training and sensation of respiratory effort during exercise in normal subjects. *Thorax*. 1995;50(4):366-370.

75. Akiyoshi F, Takahashi H, Sugawara K, Satake M, Shioya T. The effect of expiratory muscle training on respiratory muscle strength. *Rigaku Ryohogaku*. 2001;28:47-52.

76. Medline Plus. Pulmonary rehabilitation. Accessed November 24, 2023. https://medlineplus.gov/pulmonaryrehabilitation.html.

Pediatric Orthopedic and Sports Injuries

Eric Shamus, PT, DPT, PhD, Caroline Ubben, PT, DPT, and Steven Walczak, PT, DPT

LEARNING OBJECTIVES

Upon completion of this chapter, the reader will be able to:

- Understand skeletal developmental issues and effect on rehabilitation.
- Discuss how open growth plates change the rehabilitation process.

- Discuss progression of rehabilitation for general orthopedic injuries.
- Create and structure physical therapy interventions for children with orthopedic injuries.
- Evaluate and provide treatment to individuals with sports injuries.

INTRODUCTION

Orthopedic injuries in the pediatric population require several considerations that differ from an adult with a mature musculoskeletal system. As the child grows, there are physiologic differences in bone development, cognitive development, neurological development, and biomechanical alignment. An estimated 30 million American youths participate in organized sports. This number is in part driven by public health initiatives that promote sports participation for physical and psychological benefits.[1-3] Sports participation has been linked to improved self-esteem and school outcomes, as well as decreased alcohol and drug use among youths.[4,5] However, sports are one of the leading causes of injury in adolescents.[6,7]

Once played recreationally, youth sports have become increasingly competitive. Training camps for sports performance are targeting an even younger population. The prevalence of year-round sports participation is also increasingly popular. There is no longer an off season to build strength and coordination. The popularity of youth sports has created many challenges for the physical therapist. It is important to have a greater understanding of developmental changes and how overuse often plays a direct role in injuries that occur.

Child abuse can be a cause of orthopedic injuries. Common injuries are skull, facial, sternum, rib, and spinous fractures. There can be multiple fractures in different healing stages. Burns and bruising as different stages of healing should also be considered.

PHYSIOLOGIC CONSIDERATIONS IN SKELETAL DEVELOPMENT AND DYSFUNCTIONS

Skeletal development can be seen in the skeletal maturity and remodeling of the bones, muscles, tendons, and ligaments. In child development, there is chronologic age but also biologic or physiologic age. Skeletal maturation is different within each child and occurs differently between males and females. Females have an earlier onset of puberty than males. Females usually start puberty around age 11, a year or 2 earlier than males. Puberty can last between 2 and 5 years. Peak bone mass is usually seen in the early 20s in females and later 20s for males. During this development, there are changes in the shape and strength of the bones.

BONE DEVELOPMENT AND INJURIES

Major regions of the bone include the epiphysis (end of the bone), physis (growth plate), metaphysis (region between the growth plate and the shaft of the bone), and the diaphysis (shaft of the long bone). Ossification of the bones is a gradual process that can be seen on x-ray as growth plates close. Within these changes of ossification and growth of the skeletal structure, bone angles change along with the density of the bones. Physiologic differences are seen as the periosteum is thicker and stronger with the bones being more porous. The pediatric bone has less density and is composed of a higher percentage of cartilage.

Growth plates (physis) are made up of cartilage and are near the ends of long bones. Growth plates are weaker than the surrounding muscles and ligaments. Growth plates add to the size of the bones (length and width) and usually close around the end of puberty (13-15 years old for females and 15-17 years old for males), depending on the location of the bone. It is not uncommon to see a later growth spurt for males. Once a growth plate closes (closed growth plate), the bone will no longer grow. With injuries around the growth, there is concern about premature growth plate closure. Prior to the growth plates closing, growth hormone therapy may be considered for those that have a hormonal deficiency.

GROWTH PLATE INJURIES

Growth plate injuries can occur over time from repetitive stress or from a single-force trauma.

> ### Key Concept
> The incidence of growth plate injuries is highest during adolescence. About a quarter of all fractures in children are seen at the growth plates. These injuries are commonly seen in sports such as gymnastics, football, basketball, biking, skateboarding, and soccer. Serious problems can occur with growth plate injuries if they are not addressed quickly. Most growth plate fractures can heal and not interrupt bone growth development.

Physeal (Growth Plate) Fractures

About 15% of childhood fractures involve the growth plate. Peak growth plate fractures occur between 10 and 12 years of age and are usually in the upper extremity. There are 5 different types of growth plate fractures. Upon assessment of tenderness and pain at the distal ends of long bones, growth plate injuries should be considered. The most common sign is tenderness at a single point over the growth plate. There may be a visual deformity and an inability to move or place weight through the bone. Swelling, warmth, and tenderness along with nighttime pain, are common associated symptoms. See **Figure 17-1** for growth plate fractures according to the Salter-Harris classification. Salter Harris type 3 fractures are the most common. The treatment for growth plate injuries begins with immobilization in casts and/or splints. It is important to consider limiting any stress on the growth plate until it heals. This would include therapeutic ultrasound that creates vibrations. If the bone is out of alignment, surgery is a consideration to restore alignment. Untreated, the bone may grow out of alignment, causing a visible deformity and a length change.

A slipped capital femoral epiphysis (SCFE) can occur in preteens and teens while they are still growing.[8] It is more common in boys than girls. This injury occurs during a rapid growth spurt or can occur after a fall. It can happen gradually over a few weeks or months with no history of trauma. The specific cause is not known. Some hypotheses are excessive body weight, family history, or a metabolic disorder. Assessment includes pain with extremes of hip range of motion (ROM), limited hip internal rotation, and muscle guarding/increased tone/spasm. X-rays will show the head of the femur

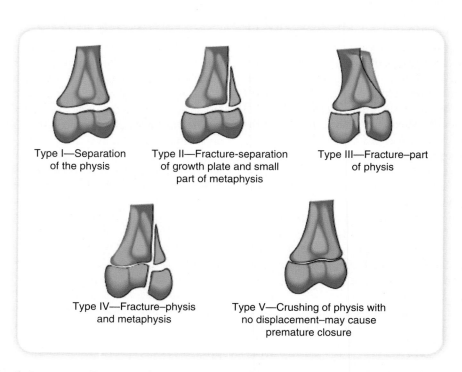

Type I—Separation of the physis

Type II—Fracture-separation of growth plate and small part of metaphysis

Type III—Fracture–part of physis

Type IV—Fracture–physis and metaphysis

Type V—Crushing of physis with no displacement–may cause premature closure

FIGURE 17-1 Growth plate fractures according to the Salter-Harris classification. (A) Type I. (B) Type II. (C) Type III. (D) Type IV. (E) Type V.
(Reproduced with permission from Barbara J. Hoogenboom, Voight ML, Prentice WE. Considerations for the Pediatric Patient: Musculoskeletal Interventions: Techniques for Therapeutic Exercise, 3ed. New York: McGraw Hill; 2013.)

slipping off the neck of the femur. Factors to consider during the rehabilitation process:

- Excessive loading
  - Obesity: If weight bearing is initially painful, an aquatic program may be beneficial in the early stages. Mat-based exercises for core and lower extremity strengthening are also a good place to start. Patient education on finding an activity that they enjoy doing 3 to 5 times per week is very important. Use your time in the clinic once the child progresses to explore various sports and physical activities in session to find an interest for increased carryover. As always, the goal is that the patient can independently continue working on their goals after discharge.
    - It is also beneficial to encourage family fitness plans. This may include family walks, backyard games, and so on. The goal is to work on improving the overall activity level of the child.
  - Jumping mechanics: Once the child has good core and lower extremity strength and pain-free, the program can be advanced. Most children enjoy standing and jumping off everyday items. Their sport may also require jumping. Physical therapy can work on decreasing the forces placed through the hips via drop jump training. Have the child stand on a small box and have them step down from the box with cues to have "quiet" landings, by flexing the hips and knees and maintaining proper positioning of knees over toes. Once landing is mastered, add a vertical or horizontal jump after landing. You can progress to higher surfaces as they improve their skills.[9]
- Contracture: Hip musculature shortening
  - It is important to know if the deformity of the femur will limit the hip range of motion or if there is capsular tightness or muscle shortening that is part of the limitation. If there is a bony deformity, avoid forced end range of motion. If there is capsular or muscle tightness, joint mobilization and positioning are beneficial. The therapist can encourage the child to spend time on the floor. Prone lying with a progression to prone on elbows assists with hip flexor lengthening. Side sitting and criss-cross sitting can assist with hip rotator tightness. Playing or coloring during these positions helps the time go by. Myofascial release and prolonged stretching can be used as well.
- Hip musculature and core weakness
  - Hip musculature: Be sure to target all the muscles of the hip including the flexors, extensors, adductors, abductors, hip internal rotators, and hip external rotators. Depending on the acuteness of the injury, exercises may start on a mat and progress to standing. Functional movements such as sit-to-stand transfers and squatting are important to train, as well as, stair climbing. Core musculature: Bridging: Start on a mat, and have them extend their hips into a glute bridge. Progress to marching or using 1 leg. They can progress to having their legs on a gymnastic ball. Upper extremity movements can be incorporated as well. Side planks can be fun. They can progress by performing rhythmic stabilization or catching an object with the unsupported arm to make it harder. Quadruped opposite

arm and leg raises are also good for rotational stability. For some children, the exercise may have to start with just 1 limb prior to combining the arm and the leg.

Case 1

A 13-year-old boy with autism presents to your clinic after falling off his bike with a subsequent traumatic olecranon fracture at the growth plate of his left arm. He has had emergency surgery with hardware placement to maintain stability of his ulna. He presents to your clinic after 6 weeks of casting with significant limitations of his left arm. He is unable to fully bend or extend his elbow due to pain and reports pain with wrist motion in all directions. He is lacking 50 degrees of elbow flexion and 60 degrees of elbow extension. He presents with hypersensitivity at his scar and is tactically defensive to passive ROM of his left arm. The therapist is unable to test his strength. He wants to get back to eating meals with both his hands, playing video games, and riding his bike.

Take a moment to review the case in relation to the material discussed in this section. Consider the following:
- What are the most important pieces of information?
  - Lack of range of motion, hypersensitive scar, tactically defensive
  - Patient goals: eating, video games, riding his bike
- What impairments should be prioritized?
  - Tactile defensiveness
  - Scar desensitization
  - Range of motion
  - Weakness
  - Functional activities
- What should the plan of care progression look like?
  - Address the tactile defensiveness with particle immersion in a ball pit if available, so passive and active-assisted range of motion will be tolerated
  - Ball rolling and other activities to promote active range of motion are beneficial
  - Wrist mazes are a fun way to regain range of motion of the wrist

Growth Plates Overuse Injuries

There are many common overuse injuries that include the growth plate in children. They lead to stress reactions. Sever's disease, Osgood-Schlatter disease (jumper's knee),[10] Little League shoulder, and Little League elbow are examples of these. The periosteum is the dense fibrous membrane covering the surface of the bones. There is an outer fibrous layer and an inner cellular layer. The outer layer is mostly collagen and has many nerve fibers. Periosteal issues may be seen if growth in bones and muscle length does not occur at the same time. Tendon and ligament attachment points can be impacted by overuse or excessive force production. Interventions commonly include ice, anti-inflammatory medication, load management, orthoses, and physical therapy.

Calcaneal apophysitis (Sever's disease) is an example of inflammation at the heel growth plate. This is commonly seen in 8- to 14-year-olds. The calcaneus is not fully calcified, and too much stress on the growth plate from the Achilles tendon results in remodeling of the bony structure. This can be seen on

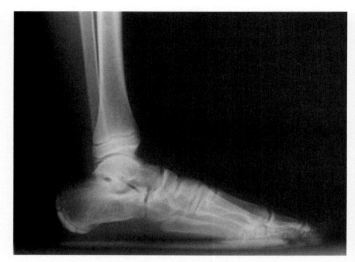

FIGURE 17-2 X-ray in case of Sever disease typically shows the normal appearing posterior calcaneal apophysis. (Reproduced, with permission, from Dilip R. Patel, Donald E. Greydanus, Robert J. Baker, *Pediatric Practice: Sports Medicine.* New York: McGraw Hill; 2009.)

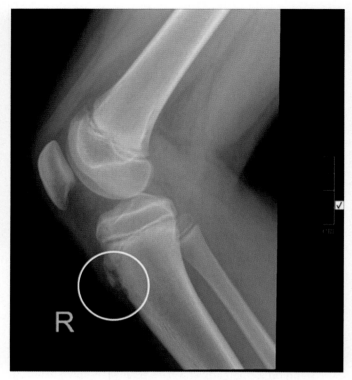

FIGURE 17-3 Radiographic appearance of Osgood-Schlatter disease. (Reproduced, with permission, from Peter Brukner, Ben Clarsen, Jill Cook, Ann Cools, Kay Crossley, Mark Hutchinson, Paul McCrory, Roald Bahr, Karim Khan, *Brukner & Khan's Clinical Sports Medicine: Injuries,* Volume 1, 5e. New York: McGraw Hill; 2017.)

an x-ray (**Figure 17-2**). Appropriate shoe wear, lower extremity muscle detonification, activity modification, joint mobilization, and appropriate rest are important interventions for Sever's disease. Treatment should include heel lifts for the shoes, lower extremity neural tension glides, and non-weight bearing exercises like bike riding or swimming.

Osgood-Schlatter disease is a common knee problem in growing adolescents.[10] It can be the result of an imbalance following a growth spurt or from repetitive loading. Many children will complain of pain during running, jumping, and open-chain knee extension. The apophysitis pain occurs where the patellar tendon attaches to the tibia. The repetitive pull of the patellar tendon on the tibial tuberosity can result in remodeling of the bone and can lead to excess bone growth; see **Figure 17-3** for an x-ray demonstrating the appearance of Osgood-Schlatter disease.

Treatment interventions include the following:[10]

- Phase 1: Ice, over the counter non-steroidal anti-inflammatory drugs (NSAIDs), immobilization and activity modification to limit running and jumping until the area is non-painful to palpation. The quadricep may be inhibited, and quadricep setting is a good exercise to introduce early on. Address hip weakness with 4-way Straight Leg Raises (SLRs) exercises with a resistance band for hip internal and external rotation. Check hamstring strength and determine if there is a muscle strength imbalance between the quadriceps and the hamstrings. It is also important to avoid static stretching, as this places additional pull on the area of inflammation.
- Phase 2: Progressive pain free closed chain strengthening with mini-squats, leg press, wall sits, and forward and lateral step-ups. Additional exercises can include resisted band walking, side stepping, and single leg balance progression. Open chain knee extension exercises should be avoided.
- Phase 3: Dynamic stretching to include high knees, butt kicks, hip ins and outs, karaoke's, forward, lateral, and

backward jogging. Graded exposure to return to sport activities to progress to high-impact activities or running by following this progression:

- Jump on trampoline
- Jump on soft mat
- Bilateral jump on ground
- Unilateral jump on ground
- Run on treadmill

Case 2

A 12-year-old girl reports progressively increasing knee pain at her tibial tubercle. She previously only had pain with activity but now has pain all the time. The pain began shortly after starting an after-school "Girl's on the Run" running program with her classmates, running 5 days a week after school on the sidewalk. She notes that she has grown 4 inches in the past 8 months and gained 20 pounds. She presents to your clinic with the goal of getting rid of the pain and participating in her after-school program.

Take a moment to review the case in relation to the material discussed in this section. Consider the following:

- What are the most important pieces of information?
- What impairments should be prioritized?
- What should the plan of care progression look like?
- What does intermittent pain progressing to constant pain mean?
- Discuss running surface, shoe wear, height growth, weight gain, and progressive training.

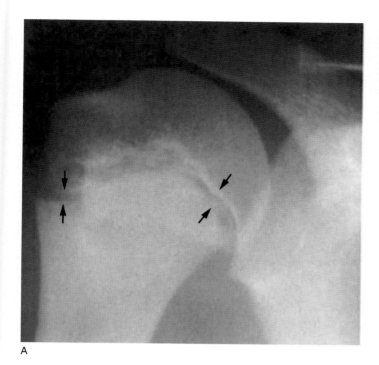
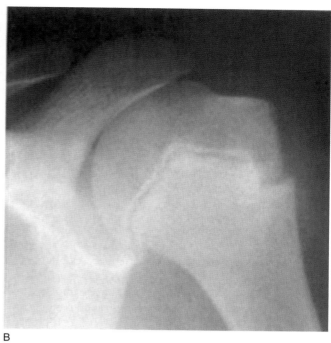

A   B

FIGURE 17-4 X-ray of stress injury of proximal humeral physis shows widening of the physis (A) compared to the normal side (B). (Used with permission from DeLee JC, Drez D Jr, Miller MD, eds. *DeLee and Drez's Orthopedic Sports Medicine.* Saunders Elsevier Imprint; 2003: Figure 21M2-7, p 1136.)

Thrower's shoulder/epiphysiolysis (Little League shoulder) is an overuse of the throwing shoulder in 11- to 16-year-olds. Widening of the proximal physis is seen, resulting in a Salter-Harris type I fracture (**Figure 17-4**). The epiphyseal plates are still developing, and the external rotation creates too much torque on the bone. It commonly occurs with early specialization in the pitcher's position and year-round practice of one sport (ie, baseball). Monitoring pitch count and overall volume of throwing can help prevent injuries. Pitch counts, rest days, and types of pitches thrown need to be considered. Curve balls should not be thrown prior to 15 years of age. Common factors are repeated overhead throwing without proper rest, improper pitching mechanics, and upper girdle weakness. Counting the number of pitches thrown will help determine the number of days of rest. US baseball has pitch limit recommendations per day and days of rest needed per number of pitches thrown:

Under 20 pitches thrown	0 days of rest
21 to 40 pitches	1 day of rest
41 to 60 pitches	2 days of rest
61+ pitches	3 days of rest

Depending on the player's age, there are also pitch limits per day:

10 or under	75 pitches
11 to 12	85 pitches
13 to 16	95 pitches
17 to 18	105 pitches

Exercises should focus on eccentric external rotation of the shoulder and may include proprioceptive neuromuscular facilitation (PNF) diagonal patterns with tubing, scaption plane exercises to shoulder height, prone horizontal abduction, and prone rowing. Core strengthening with a focus on trunk and leg drive.

Elbow medial epicondyle apophysitis (Little League elbow) is seen with overthrowing at a young age with open growth plates. This can occur from improper mechanics or trying to throw pitches that create too much torque, such as curve balls. Proper pitching coaches are critical at this point to teach the children the types of pitches that are appropriate for their age. These children usually have a lack of strength, improper mechanics, repeated throwing without rest time between throwings, and/or too great of a volume of pitches. (See earlier information on pitch counts and rest days.) Both parent and child education and buy-in are essential for success. It is important to help families understand the long-term effects on growth and performance and explain that this shorter-term investment will bring long-term results. Common issues seen are pain, fatigue, or changes in pitching control. Upper extremity neural tension glides should be included in treatment. Stretching of the wrist flexors should occur with the elbow straight and bent. Tubing or weighted stick exercises are used to strengthen wrist flexion and extension, radial and ulnar deviation, and pronation and supination.

BIOMECHANICAL ALIGNMENT INJURIES AND DYSFUNCTION

As the child develops, there are biomechanical changes in the alignment that occur. Some of the common lower extremity issues seen are flexible flat feet, toe walking, and patellofemoral syndrome. Babies are born with flexible flat feet. Pes planus (flat feet) will fluctuate throughout early childhood for typically developing children. Toddlers younger than 16 months have flat feet. Arch formation in the feet fully develops around age 6 to 8. Barefoot walking is great for kids to develop the musculature in the feet. Obesity and ligamentous laxity may lead to concern for deformity. Severe cases are identified when the foot is either rigid or so severe that a child is unable to attain subtalar neutral in a weight-bearing position. Treatment should include activity modification, proper shoe wear, orthotics, and exercises.

Clubfoot (tales equinovarus, TEV) is a birth defect that causes twisting of the foot inward toward the other leg. The components of clubfoot include: pes cavus and adductus in the midfoot; and varus and equinus in the rearfoot. Clubfoot can be diagnosed by ultrasound between 13- and 24-weeks gestation. This may occur unilaterally or bilaterally. Clubfoot can be caused by a shortened achilles tendon and is twice as common in boys as in girls. Once treated with surgery, club foot is now addressed with serial casting and bracing, known as the Ponseti method. Exercises like swimming and bicycle riding are better early on than impact activities like running and jumping.

The knee (tibiofemoral) angle in the lower extremity changes throughout development. The tibiofemoral angle changes from a genu varus (usually not present past 2 years of age) to genu valgum (peak at about 6 years of age of about 8 degrees, with >10-12 degrees being of concern; after age 10, it averages about 4 to 5 degrees). If genu valgum persists after age 8, further investigation and treatment intervention should be considered. Long-term dysfunction in biomechanics can persist with a myriad of musculoskeletal dysfunctions. This should be considered when performing gait evaluations in these age ranges. Hip rotation and knee strength are important to limit lower-extremity internal rotation and excessive pronation.

Congenital conditions like cerebral palsy and muscular dystrophy can cause changes in the formation of the feet and arches. An issue that is often treated at a younger age is heel cord tightness. Walking on your toes does not automatically mean the heel cord is tight, which can be idiopathic. Toe walking can be a result of a short achilles tendon, autism, cerebral palsy, or muscular dystrophy. Orthotics can play an important role in rehabilitation for pain modulation and correction of biomechanical alterations up the lower extremity movement chain.[11,12] Intrinsic toe strengthening can support the arch. Toe crunches and marble pick-ups are good beginning exercises to facilitate intrinsic muscle contraction. Progression to weight shifting in standing to forefoot, resistance tubing, and standing toe exercises coming up to a ballet point are useful. Strengthening of the intrinsic muscles is key (**Figure 17-5**).

During walking, in toeing (pigeon-toed) can be seen. In the majority of children, this resolves around 8 years of age. The 3 parts of intoeing include metatarsus adductus, tibial torsion, and femoral anteversion (seen with W-sitting). Metatarsus adductus will frequently spontaneously resolve in infants and young children with a basic stretching home exercise program. Early treatment when bones are more cartilaginous (younger age) allows for greater influence of musculoskeletal structure. Intoeing causes can result from developmental and genetic problems.

Impairments include the following:

- Posterior chain weakness
  - Animal walks are a fun way to promote strengthening for children without them realizing they are doing work at all. Below are some examples of animal walks that will promote hip, knee, and ankle strengthening for children, subsequently influencing the lower extremity alignment associated with intoeing.
    - Penguin walks: Walking with feet facing out, promoting out-toeing position with ambulation.
    - Crab holds: Maintaining a high bridge/tabletop with arms extended and legs bent at knees for hip extension and core strengthening. The child pretends to be a bridge where cars roll under or practices "crab" position to warm up for crab walks.
    - Crab walks: Using the high bridge/tabletop positions, race a distance while maintaining the bottom off the ground for dynamic hip extension and core strengthening.

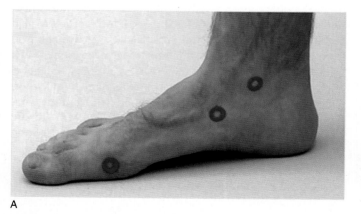
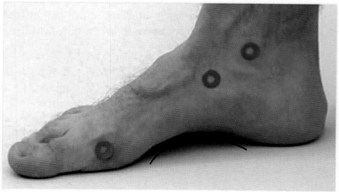

A   B

FIGURE 17-5 **Short foot concept, which is used to enhance and strengthen the foot intrinsic muscles. The patient is instructed to shorten the foot from front to back while keeping the toes straight. The metatarsal heads should stay in contact with the ground. The physical therapist can palpate the foot intrinsic muscles and will notice a raised longitudinal arch with a flexible foot type. The shortened foot should be maintained at all times while in the exercise sandals.** (Reproduced, with permission, from Barbara J. Hoogenboom, Michael L. Voight, William E. Prentice, *Musculoskeletal Interventions: Techniques for Therapeutic Exercise*, 4e. New York: McGraw Hill; 2021.)

– Flamingo walks: Standing on one foot for hip abduction strengthening with progression to single leg hopping like a flamingo to hop on dots on the ground.
– Frog jumps: Keeping hands and feet on the ground in a deep squat position, while jumping on and off the ground like a frog to promote out-toeing with squat jumping.

- Core weakness
  - W-sitting is a common movement pattern used by children to provide increased stability in sitting. By using sticker charts to promote self-awareness for a variety of sitting patterns, the child gets a sticker every time they point out to their parents that they are sitting in a different way than W-sitting.
  - Animal walks can also be used to promote core strengthening for children without them realizing they are doing work.
    – Octopus: Maintaining a crunch or V-up position while moving arms and legs to pretend to be an octopus and seeing how long they can keep their "tentacles" off the ground.
    – Whale: Pretending to be a whale in the water by performing "superman" exercise in prone by lifting arms and legs off the ground while rocking for back extensor strengthening.
  - Physioball: Playing on the dynamic surface of the physioball can increase core activation while rolling on top of the ball.
    – The patient maintains a prone position on top of the ball and walks their hands out away from the ball to collect puzzle pieces one at a time for multiple repetitions of core strengthening with ball walkouts.
- Ankle/foot impairments
  - Metatarsus adductus can be addressed with daily stretching of the foot into forefoot alignment. For, forefoot stretching, maintain hindfoot positioning while stretching the forefoot into abduction to promote neutral position of the forefoot while maintaining neutral position of hindfoot.

Case 3

A 5-year-old girl presents to therapy with concerns of intoeing and frequent tripping at the playground. Parents report that she has always walked with her feet turned in, but since her last birthday, she has been falling more around the house and on trips to the park. At the clinic, she is playing in a W-sit position but can sit crisscross when asked. She presents with no increased femoral anteversion upon Craig's test of her hips, but when you take her shoes off, you notice her forefoot is turning in relative to her hindfoot. She cannot stand on one foot for 3 seconds on either foot. She has difficulty jumping with both feet off the ground at the same time and is unable to hop on one foot.

Take a moment to review the case in relation to the material discussed in this section. Consider the following:
- What are the most salient pieces of information?

- What impairments should be prioritized?
- What should the plan of care progression look like?

At the knee, Patellofemoral syndrome is commonly seen with changes or lack of changes in the femoral angle. This is seen with quadriceps weakness, an increased Q-angle, overuse, tight lateral structures (eg, iliotibial band and biceps femoris), and dysfunctional patellar tracking.[13] The Q-angle is a line drawn from the anterior superior iliac spine (ASIS) on the pelvis to the center of the patella. The second line is drawn from the center of the patella to the tibial tuberosity. At birth, the Q-angle is about 10 to 15 degrees. The Q-angle decreases between ages 2 and 8 to about 5 to 7 degrees. After puberty, the Q-angle should be less than 18 degrees in girls and 22 degrees in boys. Patellofemoral syndrome is more common in females because of their anatomic differences in the pelvis (wider hips). Rehabilitation progress should include an initial rest period, followed by correction of patellar tracking. Specific interventions will be needed to address any impairments found during the examination. This may include the correction of muscular strength and flexibility imbalances. Bracing, taping, proper shoe wear, and NSAIDs can also be helpful.[13,14] The increased Q-angle will create a lateral pull on the knee extensor mechanism. Tight lateral structures like the iliotibial band or tensor fascia latae will also increase the lateral pull. The use of myofascial release on the iliotibial band, along with the use of a foam roller, can be beneficial. The lateral release surgical procedure has been used to increase lateral laxity, but often the scar tissue reforms, and there are not many long-term benefits. Strengthening of the vastus medialis oblique (VMO) can help counterbalance the lateral pull. Knee extension exercises with lateral tibial rotation can facilitate VMO activity. Surface biofeedback can be used to facilitate contraction of the VMO. Patellofemoral taping is used to mechanically pull the patella medially (**Figure 17-6**), or a knee sleeve with a lateral buttress (eg, DonJoy Lateral J brace) can be used for longer-term application. Medial tibial rotation should be assessed for mobility, and intervention with manual therapy can be used to increase internal tibial rotation.

At the hip, development dysplasia of the hip can be a shallow or underdevelopment of the acetabulum. Hip dysplasia is a group of bony abnormalities at the hip joint. The femoral head can be manually dislocated from the acetabulum. The hip may be unstable, malformed, dislocated, dislocateable, or subluxated. The clinical diagnosis is based on a positive Ortolani sign or Barlow maneuver and can be seen on an x-ray or MRI. Congenital hip dysplasia can be from utero posture of hip flexion and abduction, can be linked to the Relaxin hormone, and can be a trait that runs in the family. Acquired hip dysplasia can be a result of a breech birth, swaddling with the use of a cradle board, associated with myelomeningocele, and more common in infants with congenital muscular torticollis, metatarsus adductus, or occur as a result of arthrogryposis.

The demographics of hip dysplasia are a female-to-male ratio of 5:1, approximately 1 in 1000 infants, more common in first-born children, and three times more common in left hip than the right hip. Signs and symptoms include decreased hip abduction while in flexion, asymmetry of skin folds in the

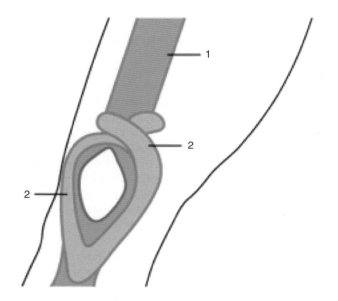

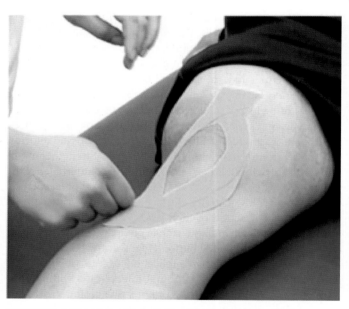

FIGURE 17-6 Kinesio taping technique for patellofemoral pain.
(Reproduced, with permission, from William E. Prentice, *Principles of Athletic Training: A Guide to Evidence-Based Clinical Practice*, 17e, New York: McGraw Hill; 2021.)

superior thigh, medial thigh, or gluteals, and an abnormal gait (Trendelenburg Waddle gait). Infants are usually treated with a brace (Pavlik harness) that holds the convex femur against the socket to help form the deeper round shape. After 6 months of age, a full body cast maybe used or surgery. When the dysplasia is not controlled, an Osteotomy maybe performed to reposition the joint.

■ PEDIATRIC FRACTURES

Fractures in pediatrics have distinct patterns secondary to ossification development. Children are more prone to incomplete fractures as the periosteum is thicker and stronger in children. Bones in children are less dense and more porous, with capillary channels throughout the bone. Younger children with fractures heal faster because of a more active periosteum. Fractures in young children heal in sometimes 3 weeks. With children and teenagers, there is still bone remodeling for 3 to 6 months post fracture. Once diagnosed with an x-ray to see alignment, the fracture can be followed for healing using ultrasonography to reduce radiation.

BOWING FRACTURE (PLASTIC DEFORMATION)

Immature bone usually will bow instead of fully breaking. In the forearm (ulna and radius) and lower leg (fibula), plastic deformation of the bone can be seen. The force on the bone can cause microscopic damage to the bone where the bone becomes bent beyond its plastic limit, but not enough to cause a fracture. As the child grows, the bend in the bone should correct itself, but there may be functional and visual impairments.

BUCKLE FRACTURE

A buckle fracture is a compression of the bone commonly seen in the radius. It occurs between the metaphysis and diaphysis of the bone. A buckle fracture is usually stable and heals on its own with immobilization for about 4 weeks.

GREENSTICK FRACTURE

Greenstick fractures are the most common fracture in children and occurs when the bone is bent and a fracture occurs on the convex side of the bone. The greenstick fracture does not completely go through the bone, and can cause plastic deformation on the concave side. One cortex remains unfractured. It is important to get alignment of the bone and often the concave side of the bow needs to be fractured to achieve union. Greenstick fractures are much more common in children than adults. Common sites in the lower extremity are the foot, ankle, tibial shaft, and femur. In the upper extremity, common fracture sites are the hand, distal radius, elbow, humerus, and clavicle.

STRESS FRACTURE

Stress fractures can be commonly seen in the feet. These can be the result of overuse. Dysfunction and intervention include the following:

- Immobilization atrophy (weakness) of hip, knee, and ankle musculature: Up the chain weakness due to non–weight bearing and decreased activity. Immobilization is necessary to allow the bone to heal.
- Patients may continue to have precautions or non–weight-bearing restrictions of their involved leg but need to continue to strengthen above the injury, potentially without weight bearing on the injured foot. Aquatic therapy can be used to decrease weight bearing.
  - Hip: Playing a board game while kneeling on a higher surface to play a game allows for transitional play in and out of short and tall kneeling for hip extension strengthening without weight bearing on injured foot. Putting all the pieces or cards to a game on the ground but

playing up at a higher surface allows short to tall kneel transitions to maintain hip strengthening.

- Knee: The pulleys can be used to facilitate knee extension and flexion strengthening without weight bearing on injured lower extremity by allowing open-chain knee movement with resistance. Place the patient in a chair with an ankle strap around the shin, with the pulley in front for knee flexion strengthening or with the pulley behind the patient for knee extension strengthening. Playing "Don't Smash the Egg," where there is a plastic egg between the weights of the pulley, allows for an external cue for control with knee extension/flexion to make it more fun.

- Foot intrinsic motor control
  - Arch formation
    - Teach motor pattern or pronation and supination of the foot with a small ball/towel roll/Elastic band/whoopie cushion under arch, where making noises to pronate and supinate foot gives feedback into this isolated movement of the foot.
    - Progression: Take this motor pattern of maintaining the arch in subtalar neutral and then carry it over into functional activities
- Squat: Place items into a bucket while maintaining an arch in the foot during sit to stand transition or squatting.
- Single-leg stance: Perform standing balance on one foot while resisting foot falling into pronation.
  - Foot intrinsic strength: Isolated toe/foot movements
    - Game: Sit at the edge of the mat with a suction cup item stuck onto a whiteboard. Using one foot, pull the suction cup item off the whiteboard with toes while using the other foot to maintain the position of the whiteboard. Then switch roles of the feet. This can then be made more difficult by transitioning to standing on one foot while pulling the suction cup off the board and then hopping on one foot to fill up a bucket.
- Proprioceptive impairments (balance)
  - Dynamic game: Standing on a tilt board and looking at a target drawn on the wall, the patient can squat down to pick up a ball and toss it at a target.

COMPLETE FRACTURES

Some common causes of complete pediatric fractures are birth injuries, Rickets, Osteomyelitis, Copper deficiency, child abuse, and trauma from a fall or impact injury. Birth injuries can occur with a complication of forceps delivery. Common birth fractures can occur at the clavicle, humerus, and femur. Rickets is a vitamin D deficiency or metabolic deficiency and may show with bowing of the lower extremities. Osteomyelitis is an infection of the bone, usually with lesions in the metaphysis seen in the long bones. Fractures associated with child abuse can be seen in the long bones of the femur and humerus.

Colles Fracture

With a fall on an outstretched hand (FOOSH), a Colles fracture can occur when the distal radius fractures at about 1 inch from

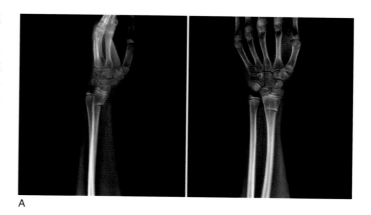

A

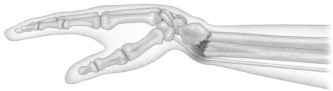

B

FIGURE 17-7 **The x-ray in A shows the deformity typical of a displaced Colles fracture. The illustration in B shows how this deformity can kink the volar neurovascular structures. Similar fracture or dislocation deformities elsewhere in the musculoskeletal system can create neurovascular compromise as well.** (A, Used with permission from Joel Bubble Ben/Shutterstock. B, Reproduced with permission from Edward P. *Practical Orthopedics.* New York: McGraw Hill; 2017.)

the thumb side of the wrist. See **Figure 17-7** for a Colles fracture and the classic dinner-fork deformity.

- Range of motion (ROM) limitations
  - Flexion/extension
    - The patient will be kneeling at the edge of a mat with a wedge or incline on the mat. The patient can roll a ball up and down an incline for active-assisted ROM into wrist sagittal plane motion with the goal of trying to get the ball up to a certain line on the wedge.
    - Standing next to a whiteboard and using dry erase markers, the patient can work on active motion of their arm by trying to make as big a vertical line as possible on the board. The patient's forearm will be stabilized for isolated wrist motion while drawing lines.
  - Radial/ulnar deviation
    - Standing next to a whiteboard and using dry erase markers, the patient can work on active motion of their arm by trying to make as big a horizontal line as possible on the board. The patient's forearm will be stabilized for isolated wrist motion while drawing lines.
    - Window wiping/whiteboard wiping: Patient uses wrist to make circles with sheet on wall in clockwise and counterclockwise motion by wiping off the lines made with expo markers.
  - Shoulder and elbow ROM
    - Include as prevention measures for movement and pain pathologies throughout the upper extremity chain. These exercises will include ROM at the

glenohumeral joint, the scapulothoracic joint, and the rotator cuff, as well as flexion and extension at the elbow.[15]

- Grip strength
  - Rubber band strengthening between fingers, making different shapes/using different-colored bands.
  - Paper football: Flicking various items with different fingers for distance.
  - Play-Doh: General hand ROM by playing with putty and using toys to roll/shape/squeeze Play-Doh. Parents can make their own dough by using flour, water, and salt.
  - Putty: Squeezing putty into various shapes plus active ROM (AROM) of affected upper extremity.
  - Carrying items in the affected hand (eg, a grocery bag, purse, or backpack).
- Upper extremity weight-bearing limitations
  - Graded exposure is an important concept with limitations after an upper extremity injury, and a patient should gradually increase tolerance to arm/wrist/hand weight bearing.
  - The patient is prone on elbows while rolling a weighted ball back and forth with the therapist. As this becomes easy, the patient can progress to prone on extended arms while passing the weighted ball.

Clavicle Fracture

The clavicle is one of the most fractured bones in children. Clavicle fracture is the most common perinatal fracture seen with trauma from birth. Clavicle fractures are commonly treated conservatively, and thus activity limitations, including graded return to activity/sport, backpack-carrying modifications, and overall posture, need to be addressed in education with the patient and their family. The Allman classification is used to describe the location of the fracture. Most clavicle fractures are treated nonoperatively. Scapular positioning and poor posture may influence pain following an injury. Rehabilitation precautions include using a sling to limit movement, most especially overhead movements such as flexion and abduction, but also depression. These precautions can assist with proper reunion of the bone fragments in conservative treatment.[16,17] Pulleys and early pendulum exercises (Codman circumduction exercises) are recommended for early mobility. See **Figure 17-8** for the Codman circumduction exercise.

JUVENILE OSTEPCHONDROSIS

Juvenile osteochondrosis is a dysfunction in normal bone growth and development in children. There is a temporary or permanent disruption in the blood supply to the bones (avascular necrosis). It can occur following cancer treatment. Up to half of the children treated for acute lymphoblastic leukemia (ALL) have some component of necrosis. Children who receive a bone marrow transplant are also at risk. Avascular necrosis can happen in any bone but is more commonly seen in the spine, hip, and knee. In the foot, there can be avascular necrosis (osteonecrosis) to bones in the forefoot in adolescents, called Freiberg's disease. It occurs due to an interruption of blood supply. It most commonly occurs in the second toe but can occur in the 3rd and 4th toes.

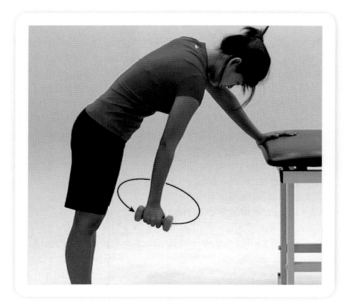

FIGURE 17-8 Codman's circumduction exercise. The patient holds a dumbbell in the hand and moves it in a circular pattern, reversing direction periodically. This technique is useful as a general stretch in the early stages of rehabilitation when motion above 90 degrees is restricted. (Reproduced, with permission, from Hoogenboom BJ, Voight ML, Prentice WE. *Musculoskeletal Interventions: Techniques for Therapeutic Exercise*, 3e. New York: McGraw Hill; 2014.)

In the hip, avascular necrosis (AVN) of the femoral head, or Legg-Calvé-Perthes disease, can be seen with disruption of blood flow to the head of the femur. This condition is more common between the ages of 4 and 8 years old. It is seen in boys 4 times more often than in girls. Usually, soreness or complaints of growing pains in the hip and groin region are seen. Pain management may be challenging in children. Rest and unweighting are used conservatively, along with surgical considerations depending on the necrosis of the bone. Bracing can play an important role in maintaining abduction and external rotation, allowing resumption of blood flow to the femoral head. The A-frame and Scottish Rite abduction orthosis are 2 common brace types for dealing with Legg-Calvé-Perthes disease.[18] Nighttime traction and bracing are other interventions. Educating parents and the child on coping techniques and appropriate compensations for injured hips is essential to maintain function. See **Figure 17-9** for an x-ray of a patient with Legg-Calvé-Perthes disease.

JUVENILE SCOLIOSIS

In the spine, scoliosis is a major concern. Public schools usually perform scoliosis screenings at about 10 to 13 years. Early onset of scoliosis can be seen at age 3 years. Juvenile scoliosis begins between the ages of 3 and 10 years. Adolescent scoliosis begins around age 10 and continues until the bones stop growing. Upon screening for scoliosis, if an abnormal angle is seen, an x-ray will be performed, a Cobb angle measurement will be taken, and the scoliosis will be identified by the convex side.[19] If the angle is less than 15 degrees, physical therapy alone may be sufficient for conservative management.

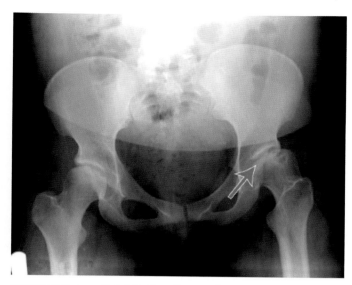

FIGURE 17-9 Legg-Calvé-Perthes disease. Chronic and significant deformity of the left femoral head is apparent (arrow). Subcortical cysts are also present. The joint space is normal. (Reproduced with permission from Shah BR, Lucchesi M. *Atlas of Pediatric Emergency Medicine.* New York: McGraw Hill; 2006.)

If the angle is between 20 and 40 degrees, a back brace is also added to the interventions. There is greater concern and surgical consideration if the angle is greater than 40 degrees. See **Table 17-1** for juvenile scoliosis curve progression.

Long-term issues in pediatric scoliosis can be seen in the respiratory system, along with back pain from nerve compression and stretch. Impairments include the following:

- Muscle imbalance
  - Tightness (active stretch): Have the child side lying over a peanut or exercise ball while you are supporting/balancing them. Have them reach for items placed on the ground

TABLE 17-1 • Juvenile Scoliosis and Curve Progression

- Thoracic curves are at a higher risk for progression compared with thoracolumbar or lumbar curves
- Females have 10 times higher risk for curve progression
- The risk for curve progression is highest during first 2 y of peak height velocity, that is 11–13 y in girls and 13–15 y in boys
- The risk for curve progression is highest during Sexual Maturity Rating 2
- Curve of 30 degrees or more at the onset of puberty progresses rapidly and presents a 100% prognosis of surgery
- Curves between 21 degrees and 30 degrees at the onset of puberty have a 75% prognosis for surgery
- Curve progression velocity of 1 degree per month during pubertal growth represents 100% prognosis for surgery
- Surgery is indicated for curves of 40 degrees or more during peak height velocity
- Curve progression is difficult to predict before onset of puberty
- Fusion of all elbow epiphyses marks the end of pubertal growth, typically at bone age of 13 y in girls and 15 y in boys

Source: Reproduced with permission from Patel DR, Greydanus DE, Baker RJ. Pediatric Practice: Sports Medicine. New York: McGraw Hill; 2009.

below their head and set them on a mat at eye level. You can use blocks or board game pieces, such as Connect 4. Have their curve side down on the ball. This intervention can assist with stretching the concave side of the body.[20,21]

- Weakness (contraction): Perform scapular retractions on the side contralateral to curve; you can perform karate or boxing activities with pulley resistance. Give an external cue to "elbow" a pretend punching bag (eg, bolster, foam pad). This intervention will assist with strengthening the convex side of the body.[22]
- Movement patterns
  - Perform forward punches with pulley resistance. Similar to the last activity, frame it as "karate training" and have the child punch a target. Progress to adding a contralateral step to the punch. The final progression would be to punch with a step and rotation to opposite direction of rotation bias of scoliosis deformity (eg, punch with right arm and left rotation with a right scoliosis/right rotation deformity).
- Breath control: Have the child blow bubbles through a straw with belly breathing, and progress from sitting to standing to walking. You can add extra fun by adding some soap and food coloring to the water, ensuring the child does not drink any.

Case 4

A 10-year-old boy with Noonan syndrome presents to your clinic with his mother. She reports that he was recently diagnosed with 20-degree right-sided scoliosis by their pediatrician. They are concerned that their child will not tolerate bracing because he has some sensory challenges, so they are seeking physical therapy to correct his spine and avoid surgery. On presentation, he has a right-sided rib hump with forward bending, flexible posture, and overall decreased activity tolerance.

Take a moment to review the case in relation to the material discussed in this section. Consider the following:

- What are the most salient pieces of information?
- What impairments should be prioritized?
- What should the plan of care progression look like?

■ MUSCLE AND TENDON INJURIES

Muscle/tendon injuries can be seen during growth spurts and with increased activity levels. Overuse syndromes need education regarding a period of inactivity to decrease inflammation of the injured area, followed by graded return to activity without overloading the tissues. Year-round sports participation in one sport like baseball should be avoided. Cross-training and off-season time are needed.

Soft tissue contusions can occur even in non-contact sports. Interventions for soft tissue contusions include pain-free AROM of the injured tissue, which will promote blood flow to that tissue to speed healing of the contusion. Pulsed ultrasound is a consideration, but there is much controversy regarding the use of ultrasound near growth plates. Lyon and Liu[23] found that high-intensity ultrasound on the physis plate of the rabbit knee joint altered the normal growth plate. Taping techniques can be used for lymphatic drainage. Taping can help control the spread, appearance, and tenderness of the contusion.

Rotator cuff (RTC) injury/tendonitis can be seen in overhead throwing activities. The muscles of the rotator cuff provide the majority of the stability of the shoulder and can frequently be overworked when they are asked to help stabilize and move the shoulder. Progression of therapy should begin with correction of scapulohumeral rhythm.[24–26] Strengthening the RTC muscles along with other muscles that provide scapular stability will help to decrease inflammation in the RTC and should begin after normal scapulohumeral rhythm has been achieved.[26]

The Thrower's 10 Program can be used to increase strength, power, and endurance of the shoulder complex. Exercises include the following:

1A. Diagonal pattern D2 extension

1B. Diagonal pattern D2 flexion

2A. External rotation at 0 degrees of abduction

2B. Internal rotation at 0 degrees of abduction

2C. External rotation at 90 degrees of abduction

2D. Internal rotation at 90 degrees of abduction

3. Shoulder abduction to 90 degrees

4. Scaption, external rotation

5. Side-lying external rotation

6A. Prone horizontal abduction (neutral)

6B. Prone horizontal abduction (full external rotation, 100 degrees of abduction)

6C. Prone rowing

6D. Prone rowing into external rotation

7. Press-ups

8. Push-ups

9A. Elbow flexion

9B. Elbow extension (abduction)

10A. Wrist extension

10B. Wrist flexion

10C. Supination

10D. Pronation

Other common muscle-tendon injuries include the following:

- Low back pain/strain can be common with overuse, sleeping or sitting in poor posture, working out or lifting too much, and school backpacks that do not fit properly or are too heavy. In the acute phase, addressing muscle guarding, pain management, joint mobility, and core stabilization is key.[27]
  - Muscle guarding: Passive ROM (PROM) via therapy ball. Have the child lay on their back and place their feet on the therapy ball. Transition between hip/knee flexion and extension and low trunk rotations. Have the child perform flashcards or various other mentally challenging activities to add distraction to the activity.
  - Modalities: Cryotherapy during acute phase, followed by heat therapy during later phases.[27] If there are radicular symptoms and no centralization with McKenzie

flexion or extension movements, lumbar traction may be helpful.
  - Manual therapy: Joint manipulation and soft tissue mobilization are both useful in managing low back pain.[28]
  - Core stability: Lying supine, the child will complete a straight leg raise on one side while raising the opposite arm. The key is to keep the child's pelvis in neutral, as well as their back flat on the floor.[29]
  - Core motor control/strength: Supermans off a therapy ball onto a crash mat. Have the child lie prone on a therapy ball, reach arms out in front, and extend the hips/spine. Give them a countdown from 3, having them extend each time, and then roll them forward quickly as they extend and "superman" onto the crash pad.
  - Hip strength: Have the child perform a single leg glute bridge, trying to add kicks with the free leg to hit drums/tambourine in rhythm with a song of their choice.
- Hamstring strain
  - Muscle guarding: Massage followed by high-repetition prone hamstring curls/AROM butt kicks. You can use instruments to hit or kick to music beats to keep the child engaged. Massage and light stretching should be used before beginning protected active exercises progressing from open kinetic chain (OKC) to closed kinetic chain (CKC).[30] Neural tension test should be performed to determine neural involvement contribution (**Figure 17-10**).
  - Weakness: While standing, have the child pick up items with their toes and perform a hamstring curl to transfer items to their hands. They can be small items. You can progress with ankle weights as they build strength. Resistance can also be provided using tubing.
  - Eccentric control: Child performs Nordic hamstring curls while kneeling on foam, and the therapist secures lower legs. Have the child lean forward, extending their knees as slowly as they can with their best effort, until their arms help accept weight and push back up.
- Achilles tendinitis/tendinosis
  - Pain/ROM
    - Graded exposure: Education to decrease strain on the Achilles tendon includes monitoring tolerance time to activity with walking to class/participating in sport and slowly increasing tolerance, encouraging pain-free AROM of ankle, avoiding activities that require excessive push-off (jumping), wearing heels or shoes with wedges to decrease the strain on the tendon, and informing about the potential for increased pain on an incline or uphill running. A slight lift inside the heel of the shoe could assist with releasing the tightness of the Achilles tendon during walking.[31]
    - ROM: AROM should be pain-free and should include all motions at the ankle and foot, including inversion, eversion, plantar flexion, dorsiflexion, and toe flexion and extension. Special attention should be paid to stretching the Achilles tendon.[31] Neural tension glides are important to be performed as the neural tension and lumbar dysfunctions at the L5-S1 and sacral levels can mimic achilles tendonitis.

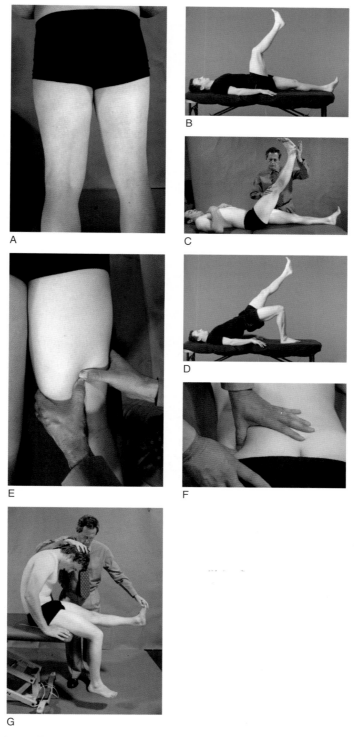

FIGURE 17-10 **Examination of the patient with posterior thigh pain. (A) Observation. Look for wasting, bruising, or swelling of the posterior thigh. Observation of gait is also important. Observation of the lumbar spine may show the presence of excessive lordosis or relative asymmetry. A lateral view may demonstrate excessive lumbar lordosis or anterior pelvic tilt. (B) Active movement—active knee extension. The hip is actively flexed to 90 degrees with the knee initially at 90 degrees also. The knee is then slowly extended until pain is felt and then to the end of range. (C) Passive movement— hamstring muscle stretch. The leg is raised to the point where pain is first felt and then to the end of range, pain permitting. Movement should be compared with the uninjured side. (D) Combined contraction—single leg bridge. A widely used "quick" clinical assessment of resisted hamstring contraction is the single leg bridge. This can be done with the knee fully extended or flexed to 90 degrees (or any angle in between these 2 positions). (E) Palpation. Palpate carefully bearing the underlying anatomy in mind to determine the location of an acute muscle strain (eg, medial vs lateral hamstring, proximal vs distal). (F) Palpation—gluteal muscles. Palpate the gluteal muscles for trigger points that are taut bands, which are usually exquisitely tender locally and may refer pain into the hamstring muscle. (G) Special tests—slump test. The slump test is an essential part of the examination of the patient with posterior thigh pain. It helps the clinician differentiate between hamstring muscle injuries and referred pain to the hamstring region from the lumbar spine.** (Reproduced with permission from *Brukner P, Clarsen B, Cook J, et al. Brukner & Khan's Clinical Sports Medicine: Injuries*, Volume 1, 5e. Australia: McGraw Hill;2017.)

– Heel raises: The patient is standing with hands on a wall and multiple flash cards/pictures overhead. The patient is given a pattern or cards to reach up and touch for Achilles strengthening with heel raises. Progression of this can be assessed during gait.[31]

• Poor motor control (hip/foot): Promote Achilles activation with forward tibial translation.

– The patient is standing with feet together and forward lunging onto a half-ball (Bosu) device. The game is to step on a sticker each time the patient gets into lunge position. The patient then pushes off from a lunged position back into single-leg standing with a goal of trying to keep single leg balance as long as possible after pushing off from the balance device.

• Poor force development

– Obstacle courses with a focus on jumping can help work on strength deficits with the Achilles tendon. Using dots, hurdles, agility ladders, and boxes allows for various forms of double-leg, single-leg and depth jumping in a fun way. Jump rope and eccentric exercises should be performed; one pain-free activity is accomplished. The tendons are made of type 1 collagen and become stronger under tension. Eccentric loading of the achilles tendon can create the highest tension on the tissue. Slow eccentric calf lowering of 3 sets of 15 repetitions, twice a day for 12 weeks, has been shown to assist in the healing process.

Case 5

Elizabeth, a 16-year-old girl, presents to therapy with right hamstring pain. She is a cheerleader and weightlifter who has pain in her right hamstring when running, deadlifting, power

cleaning, and stunting in cheer. Elizabeth presents with no hip and knee ROM limitations or manual muscle test weaknesses with formal testing, except pain at her ischial tuberosity with hip extension. Her pain gets worse after a day of walking around school, and she has not participated in her after-school activities for the past month to decrease irritation of her posterior thigh.

Take a moment to review the case in relation to the material discussed in this section. Consider the following:

• What are the most salient pieces of information?
• What impairments should be prioritized?
• What should the plan of care progression look like?

Ligament injuries can result from rapid growth or minor or major trauma. As a child grows, balance and coordination often take time to catch up. Younger children tend to fracture the bones before spraining a ligament. The ligaments are stronger than the bones. As the child develops and bone density and strength increases ligament injuries become more common. Sprains in children usually affect the ankles, knees, and wrists. Common symptoms include pain, swelling, warmth, bruising, weakness, and instability.

• Annular ligament subluxation/nursemaid's elbow (**Figure 17-11**): Prevention is key with this injury. Families need to understand the anatomy of the elbow and how easily dislocated the radius can be due to only a small ligament holding the bone to the joint. Practice and demonstration with parents on alternative methods to pick their child up besides pulling up on both arms will help prevent this injury and prevent a recurrence if this has already happened. The child may be apprehensive about movement after this happens. Allowing successful reaching and

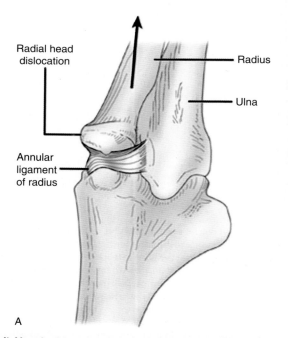
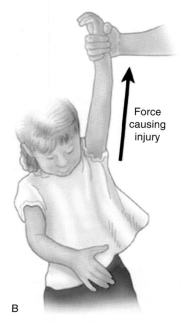

A   B

FIGURE 17-11   Radial head subluxation (nursemaid's elbow). (A) Drawing demonstrating direction of pull. (B) Example of some tractioning the arm that can cause a dislocation of the radial head. (Reproduced with permission From Simon RR, Sherman SC. *Simon's Emergency Orthopedics*, 8th ed. New York: McGraw Hill; 2019.)

playing with that arm following an injury will help return that child to their previous level of play. When the hand or forearm is pulled, the radius can shift out of position and dislocate. Nursemaid elbow makes up 20% of upper arm injuries in young children. Children will complain of pain in the elbow and want to limit pronation or supination of the hand. By flexing the elbow and rotating the arm, the radius can relocate into position. Nursemaid's elbow usually occurs prior to 5 years of age.

- Subluxation of the patella or shoulder is common. The strength surrounding the joints is still developing. Patella subluxation is commonly seen with poor quadriceps activation along with an increased likelihood of recurrent subluxation. Quadriceps motor control training may be needed following a traumatic subluxation of the patella, along with posterior chain training to prevent reinjury. Subluxation and dislocation of the shoulder are most commonly anterior due to limited structural support anteriorly.[32]

- Shoulder dislocation

  - Poor motor control: It is important to establish a proper scapulohumeral rhythm with a slow progression of external rotation of the shoulder first at the side, then in flexion, then in scaption, and then gradually toward combination of external rotation and 90 degrees of shoulder abduction. Exercise focus should be on closed chain (weight bearing) exercises.
    - Closed chain: Push-up. Push-ups are a great way to combine shoulder stability with mobility. By placing a ball on the top of their backs while the patient performs push-ups, the goal is to prevent the ball from rolling down their back to promote proper speed and control while performing push-ups. Progression for push-ups should begin in a gravity-minimized position vertically against the wall and progress to horizontal floor push-ups.
    - Open chain: Throwing. When returning patients to throwing, it is important to promote a mid-range throwing pattern to prevent an aggravating position (excessive external rotation at 90 degrees of horizontal abduction). Start with short-distance targets so the patient can focus on form with throwing and then increase the distance for integration of power into throwing. Using light-up balls can give them visual feedback if they are throwing with enough power to activate the balls.

  - Capsule laxity: Closed chain exercises
    - Planking can be a tedious way to build capsular stability but is a great challenge for patients, especially if good form is required from the patient. Once it is established that the patient can maintain good shoulder and core activation during a plank, they can now do other activities in a plank position. This exercise is most effective later in the progression.
    - Game: Have patients in a plank on their elbows and have them pass a weighted medicine ball back and forth between themselves and the physical therapist, who is also planking. Have patients alternate arms for single upper extremity closed chain

strengthening along with end-range open chain capsular strengthening.

- RTC weakness: Open chain exercises
  - "Minute to Win It" can turn elastic band exercises into a fun competition when isolating strengthening of the rotator cuff. The patient performs scapular rows, internal rotation, or external rotation with an elastic band and competes with themselves or the physical therapist for how many repetitions with good form they can do in 1 minute.

For knee anterior cruciate ligament (ACL) injuries, the most common mechanisms of injury can be either contact or noncontact. Common contact modes of injury (MOIs) include sports injuries and motor vehicle accidents. Noncontact MOIs include sudden deceleration before direction change, hyperextension, and laxity of the hamstrings (**Figure 17-12**).[33] ACL injuries are

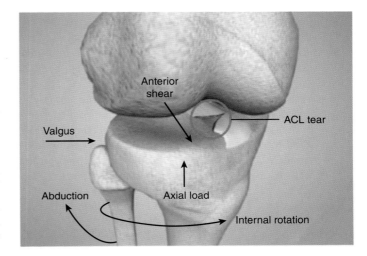

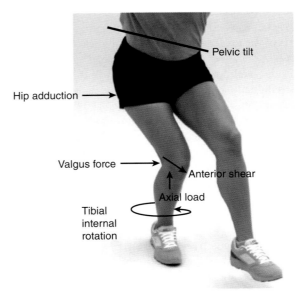

FIGURE 17-12 The primary mechanism of noncontact injury to the anterior cruciate ligament (ACL) involves an axial load with the knee close to extension, a valgus force, anterior shear, internal rotation of the tibia, and adduction of the hip. (Reproduced with permission from Prentice WE, *Principles of Athletic Training: A Guide to Evidence-Based Clinical Practice*, 16e. New York: McGraw Hill; 2017.)

more common in females because of their increased knee valgus and smaller notch area.

- ROM limitations
  - Knee flexion: With both exercises, the competition is how far the patient can flex their knee, but a balloon as a target at their glutes as a cue to try and kick with their feet can be used if they are lacking knee flexion ROM.
    - Open chain exercise: Have the patient lie on their stomach and try to kick their buttocks to promote pain-free AROM into maximal knee flexion.
    - Closed chain exercise: Have the patient in the quadruped position on the mat with a foam pad under the affected knee for increased comfort. Have the patient rock back and forth on all fours to promote pain-free AROM into knee flexion to tolerance.
  - Knee extension
    - Have the patient lie on their back with their feet supported 90/90 on the physioball. Draw a picture on the mat with chalk, and have the patient roll over the picture with the ball to promote facilitation into knee extension.
  - Quad activation
    - Terminal knee extension: The patient sits on a mat with a whoopie cushion under their knee and performs terminal knee extensions with auditory feedback for better quadriceps activation. This same exercise can be transitioned into standing with a whoopie cushion on the wall for a more functional position of the knee. This intervention can begin 4 months after the operation.[34]
    - Quad sets: Begin OKC quad sets, and then begin progression of CKC quadriceps strength exercises, moving into full-strength OKC exercises. These exercises can be assisted by Russian electrical stimulation.[34]
- Motor control impairments
  - Hip extension and abduction strengthening are important parts of the exercise plan to decrease shearing and valgus forces at the knee.
    - Bridge and squat progression can both promote this strengthening, but knee alignment is an important consideration with these exercises. By placing a laser on the knee, there can be a visual target/dot either on the ceiling (for bridges) or on the wall in front of the patient (for squats) to provide external cues on good knee position while also strengthening the posterior chain.
    - Bracing for stability during hip abduction and knee flexion for the first 2 months can be useful.[34]
  - Hamstring control with functional activities
    - Backward or retro walking and running activate the hamstring muscles. The hamstring muscles create a posterior pull on the tibia, protecting the ACL.
  - Quadriceps control with functional activities
    - Step-downs to targets: Have the patient stand on top of a step with different-colored dots or pictures of their favorite show/team/book printed out and spread on the floor. The patient can then be told various colors/pictures for them to tap down with their foot while performing step-downs with cues not to smash

any dots/pictures. This can be progressed by giving the patient a color pattern or picture order to tap and then having them close their eyes and remember where specific colors are.

Ankle sprains are seen on the lateral side of the ankle. The 3 common lateral ligament sprains seen involve the anterior talofibular ligament, posterior talofibular ligament, and calcaneofibular ligament. Inversion ankle sprains are associated with ligamentous laxity after the ankle is forced inward. The talus can be in a dysfunctional position and can be treated with manual therapy. An ankle sprain increases the likelihood of reinjury, as too often an early return to activity limits the ability for the ligament to develop stiffness. Early immobilization is important for healing. Foot intrinsic and dorsiflexion strengthening will help to create muscular stability and allow the healing of ligamentous tissue for increased stability with future activity. When performing plantarflexion, caution should be used for motions greater than 15 degrees as the talus moves anteriorly with dorsiflexion and places too much stress on the anterior talofibular ligament. Other protection of the lateral ankle ligaments includes bracing, limiting ROM at the ankle, and strengthening plantar flexion and dorsiflexion only in protected isometrics, beginning in open chain exercises (OKC) and progressing to closed chain exercises (CKC).[35] On the medial side of the ankle, the medial deltoid ligament is very thick, and avulsion is more of a concern with an eversion ankle movement. The Ottawa ankle rules should be considered when evaluating ankle pain.

- Pain: Spend time educating the parent on how to perform PROM in a pain-free range. Dose with time periods such as the length of songs or during commercial breaks of television shows.
- ROM deficit: Ankle "writing" (eg, name, alphabet). Have the child sit on a bench with a mirror in front. Place shaving cream or a gel on a board below the feet, and then have the patient transfer the substance and spread it onto the mirror via ankle movement. The therapist can ensure ankle strengthening by stabilizing the leg to isolate the ankle instead of hip motion. These exercises should be used later in the progression, after the ligaments have fully healed.[35]
- Motor control: Perform a dissociated stand by having one foot planted on the ground and the other foot elevated anteriorly on a bench. This activity can be progressed with challenging surfaces under the rear foot. While here, the child can play catch or hit a balloon back and forth with the therapist. Balance board and rubber band exercises are important to challenge the child dynamically. (See **Figure 17-13** for strengthening exercises.)

Case 6

A 14-year-old girl comes to your clinic with generalized right ankle pain. She notes that it began 3 weeks ago while playing in a soccer game, where she tried to get around a defender and tripped as she fell onto the outside of her foot. She has diffuse swelling and pain when weight bearing and laterally when moving her ankle into both inversion and eversion actively. She wants to be able to run and return to soccer as soon as possible.

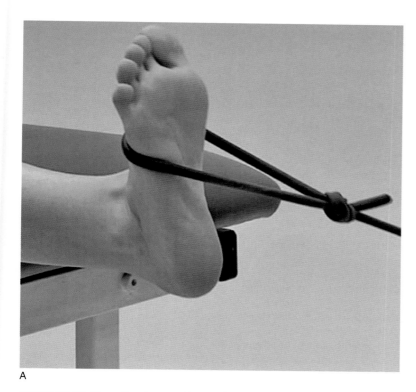
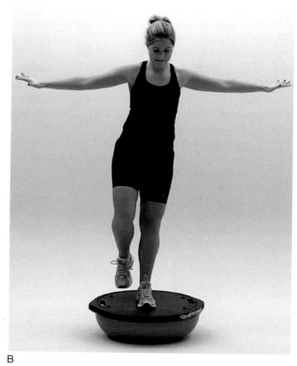

A   B

FIGURE 17-13 **Strengthening exercises are important in prevention of ankle sprains and may be done using (A) surgical tubing resistance or (B) a Bosu Balance Trainer.** (Reproduced with permission from Prentice WE, *Essentials of Athletic Injury Management*, 10e. New York: McGraw Hill; 2016.)

Take a moment to review the case in relation to the material discussed in this section. Consider the following:
- What are the most salient pieces of information?
- What impairments should be prioritized?
- What should the plan of care progression look like?

NERVE ISSUES

Erb palsy (Erb-Duchenne palsy) or Klumpke palsy is caused by an injury to the nerves, usually at the C5-C6 level. Weakness in one arm, loss of feeling, and partial or full paralysis are seen. About 1 in every 1000 babies have this issue because of a difficult delivery. Because children are smaller, they will regain reinnervation faster (shorter peripheral nerve distance). Physical therapy includes ROM to prevent contractures and activity-based exercises to regain strength and coordination. If after 6 months, there is no change, surgical considerations are then considered. Children have much better results after nerve repair than adults.

CONCUSSIONS

Concussion injuries have become a large concern in youth sports. Even in soccer, where heading the ball is a main component of the game, it is being limited or removed from youth age groups. Athletes aged 15 to 19 years have the highest overall incidence of concussions, followed by those aged 10 to 14 years.[36] Many athletes are getting baseline testing on cognition and balance. Immediate Post-Concussion Assessment and Cognitive Testing (ImPACT)[37] and SWAY testing are used for pre- and post-head

injury evaluations. ImPACT testing is Food and Drug Administration cleared for concussion assessment for ages 5 to 59 years of age. There is a format for ages 5 to 11, and then 12 to 59 years of age. The test takes about 25 minutes to perform. The best scenario is to have a baseline test in case a child sustains a head injury. The post-injury exam will help determine if the individual sustained a concussion and whether the individual can return to play. This testing is commonly used on high school, college, and professional teams. If the child scores significantly lower on the exam, active rest is usually the first step in recovery. Absence from school, in addition to missing practice, is often required.[38]

Most concussions can resolve in a few weeks, but some take longer depending on whether the child does not get the proper recovery. Graded progression of activity needs to be monitored closely.[39] Concussions occurring during non-helmet sports resulted in longer recovery times and an increased risk of loss of consciousness on the field.[40] Girls have a longer recovery time than boys.[41] The National Football League (NFL) has a very good concussion protocol. They have a Head, Neck, and Spine Committee that reviews the protocol.[42] Their return to participation is broken down into steps.

Step 1: Rest and recover until signs and symptoms, including cognitive and balance tests, return to baseline

Step 2: Light aerobic exercise and the beginning of dynamic stretching and balance training

Step 3: Continued aerobic exercise and the introduction of strength training

Step 4: Sports-specific activities

Step 5: Return to full activity/clearance[42]

TABLE 17-2 • Pediatric Therapist Competency-Based Goals[43]

University of South Florida

Pediatric Orthopedics – PGY 3

Competency Based Goals and Objectives

Competency 1. Patient Care: Provide family-centered patient care that is developmentally and age appropriate, compassionate, and effective for the treatment of health problems and the promotion of health.

1. Hone skills in identifying key history and exam needed to evaluate children presenting with conditions involving the musculoskeletal systems.
2. Understand the scope and use of diagnostic studies typically used by pediatric orthopedists.
3. Discuss and identify how the pediatric orthopedist and their care team involves the patient and family in decision-making about complex diagnoses and highly sophisticated medical care issues.
4. Screen for developmental dysplasia of the hip in the newborn nursery and at appropriate health maintenance visits:
    a. Use competent physical examination techniques.
    b. Use radiographs and ultrasonography appropriately.
    c. Educate parents about the rationale for screening and referral.
    d. Refer when indicated.
    e. Introduce parents to the management options that the orthopedist may offer.
5. Screen for scoliosis on routine examinations (by exam and scoliometer) and refer as needed.
6. Screen for occult dysraphism.
7. Counsel families regarding risks and prevention of orthopedic injuries sustained from play near motor vehicles, lawn mowers, snow blowers, farm equipment, bicycles, snowmobiles, motorbikes, and all-terrain vehicles.
8. Advise family about optimal weight and style of backpacks in order to prevent back injury.
9. Order and interpret (with the assistance of the radiologist) common diagnostic imaging procedures when evaluating and managing patients with orthopedic conditions: plain radiographs, body magnetic resonance imaging, computed tomography scan, and radionuclide bone scans.
10. Recognize and manage the following conditions, with appropriate referral for physical therapy services for rehabilitation when indicated:
    a. Calcaneal apophysitis
    b. Clavicular fracture
    c. Annular ligament subluxation/nursemaid's elbow
    d. Elbow medial epicondyle apophysitis/Little League elbow
    e. Erb palsy for Klumpke palsy
    f. Femoral anteversion and retroversion
    g. Pes planus (flat feet)
    h. Internal and external tibial torsion
    i. Low back strain
    j. Metatarsus adductus
    k. Muscle strains
    l. Nondisplaced finger and toe fractures
    m. Tibial tuberosity apophysitis (Osgood-Schlatter disease)
    n. Overuse syndromes
    o. Patellofemoral syndrome
    p. Inversion/eversion ankle sprains
    q. Thrower's shoulder/epiphysiolysis
    r. Soft tissue contusion
    s. Subluxation of the patella or shoulder
    t. Rotator cuff injury/tendonitis
11. Recognize and provide initial management of the following conditions:
    a. Avascular necrosis of the femoral head/Legg-Calvé-Perthes disease
    b. Signs of child abuse
    c. Cervical spine injury
    d. Compartment syndrome
    e. Talipes equinovarus
    f. Developmental dysplasia of the hip
    g. Fractures and dislocations not listed above, including stress fractures
    h. Knee ligament and meniscal tears or disruptions
    i. Limb length discrepancies
    j. Osteochondritis dissecans
    k. Osteomyelitis

(Continued)

TABLE 17-2 • Pediatric Therapist Competency-Based Goals[43] (*Continued*)

    l. Scoliosis with >20-degree curve
  m. Septic joint
  n. Slipped capital femoral epiphysis
  o. Spondylolysis or spondylolisthesis
  p. Subluxation of the knee or shoulder
  q. Benign and malignant bone tumors
12. Develop the expected level of proficiency in the following procedures:
    a. Immobilization techniques for common fractures and sprains
    b. Reduction of nursemaid's elbow
    c. Cervical spine immobilization
    d. Reeducation of phalangeal dislocation

Competency 2. Medical Knowledge: Understand the scope of established and evolving biomedical, clinical, epidemiologic, and social-behavioral knowledge needed by a pediatrician; demonstrate the ability to acquire, critically interpret, and apply this knowledge needed by a pediatrician; demonstrate the ability to acquire, critically Interpret, and apply this knowledge in patient care.

1. Demonstrate knowledge of normal variations in foot, knee, and leg development.
2. Know normal variations in gait and posture.
3. Demonstrate if the following presenting signs and symptoms are caused by an orthopedic condition, and if so, treat appropriately:
    a. Limp
    b. Musculoskeletal pain
    c. Refusal to walk or gain disturbance
    d. Refusal to use a limb
    e. Swollen or painful joint
    f. Bowed legs or knock-knees
    g. Intoeing or out-toeing
4. Identify the role and general scope of practice of pediatric orthopedists; recognize situations where children benefit from the skills of specialists training in care of children; and work effectively with these professionals in the care of children with orthopedic conditions.
5. Develop an efficient approach to finding information resources related to the musculoskeletal system (eg, information on the web, in the literature, in textbooks, or PDAs) to obtain rapid information that is relevant to a presenting patient problem.
6. At the beginning and end of a rotation or clinical experience, clarify your learning needs related to this subspecialty.

Competency 3. Communication Skills: Demonstrate interpersonal and communication skills that result in information exchange and partnering with patients, their families, and professional associates.

1. Talk to family members about sensitive issues that relate to a patient's illness (eg, coping with the child's altered needs in their home setting).
2. Write an effective and timely consultation note that summarizes the findings and recommendations of the pediatric orthopedist and clarifies the continued role and responsibility of the consultant.
3. Describe the role of all members of a multidisciplinary team and show respect for the contributions of each.
4. Maintain comprehensive, timely, and legible medical records.

Competency 4. Practice-Based Learning and Improvement: Demonstrate knowledge, skills, and attitudes needed for continuous self-assessment, using scientific methods and evidence to investigate, evaluate, and improve one's patient care practice.

1. Identify standardized guidelines for diagnosis and treatment of complex problems of the musculoskeletal system and learn the rationale for adaptations that optimize treatment.
2. Identify personal learning needs, systematically organize relevant information resources for future references, and plan for continuing data acquisition if appropriate.
3. Seek and incorporate feedback and self-assessment into a plan for professional growth and practice improvement (eg, use evaluations provided by patients, peers, superiors, and subordinates to improve patient care).

Competency 5. Professionalism: Demonstrate a commitment to carrying out professional responsibilities, adherence to ethical principles, and sensitivity to diversity.

1. Be honest and use integrity in your professional duties.
2. Reflect on your own biases toward particular illnesses or patient groups and take steps to assure that these biases do not interfere with the care you deliver.
3. Appreciate the psychosocial impact of diseases commonly seen by the subspecialist (eg, on the child, family, parents' work, school).
4. Respect your patients'/parents' privacy, autonomy, and need to maintain a positive self-concept, irrespective of age, gender, or health belief system, and regardless of acuity of diseases.
5. Be sensitive to the ethical and legal dilemmas faced by providers working with patients with orthopedic problems. Strive to understand how the orthopedist and care team deal with these dilemmas and use such experiences to enhance your own understanding.

(Continued)

TABLE 17-2 • Pediatric Therapist Competency-Based Goals[43] (*Continued*)

Competency 6. System-Based Practice: Understand how to practice quality health care and advocate for patients within the context of the health care system.

1. Describe school-based scoliosis screening programs and the benefits and inherent limitations of such strategies.
2. Clarify how documentation and billing charges differ for consultations versus referrals versus ongoing management of children treated on the pediatric orthopedic service.
3. Explore the difference between fee-for-service referrals and managed care referrals and the office systems needed to support both.
4. Describe patient and system factors that contribute to escalating costs of care in the subspecialty setting, and consider the impact of these costs on families and on the health care system.
5. Recognize and advocate for families who need assistance to deal with systems complexities, such as lack of insurance, multiple medication refills, multiple appointments with long transport times, or inconvenient hours of service.
6. Support community prevention efforts related to pediatric orthopedics by working with a local professional organization or organizing a project to do with colleagues.
7. Consider potential sources of medical error in this subspecialty setting (eg, drug interactions, complex care plans, provider fatigue).

Reproduced with permission from Pediatric Orthopeadics Competency Based Goals and Objectives. University of South Florida. 2022.

■ CONCLUSION

Children are not small adults. It is important to understand the physiologic differences in how and when development changes that occur. Some basic concepts of how the musculoskeletal system (bones, joints, and muscles) develop are important to determine how pediatric orthopedic injuries occur and the rehabilitation progression. With participation in sports at an earlier age, traumatic and overuse injuries can occur. Orthopedic injuries in children can impact their growth and development and have a long-term effect if not treated properly. Finding activities that the children enjoy performing will create a fun environment for the child and physical therapist (**Table 17-2**).

STUDY QUESTIONS

1. At what age should the physical therapist intervene for children who have persistent, larger angles of genu valgum?
   a. 4 years old
   b. 6 years old
   c. 8 years old
   d. 2 years old

2. Which of the following structures is most likely to cause a lateral deviation of the patella?
   a. Strong vastus medialis oblique (VMO)
   b. Tight iliotibial band
   c. Decreased Q-angle
   d. Tear of the lateral patellar retinaculum

3. Patient is a 31-year-old man. He was out walking on a dirt path when he turned his ankle inward and fell. Patient was able to walk home. He saw the physician the next day, who took x-rays that were negative. The physician placed him in a walking boot for 2 weeks to try and get some stability. Patient presents with swelling, pain, and decreased mobility. He is still having difficulty with ambulation. At what functional stability level would this anterior talofibular ligament sprain be, and what special test(s) would be best used to determine the stability level?
   a. Stable grade 1 sprain, anterior drawer test
   b. Unstable grade 3 sprain, Ottawa ankle test and anterior drawer test

   c. Stable grade 2 sprain, talar tilt test
   d. Unstable grade 2 sprain, anterior drawer test and talar tilt test

4. What is the underlying cause for hip and groin impairments with Legg-Calvé-Perthes disease and what is the likely pathogenesis for this?
   a. Hip avascular necrosis (AVN) with possible pathogenesis of injury, synovitis, infection, or vascular abnormalities (either inherited or developed)
   b. Fracture of the proximal femur with possible pathogenesis of injury or impaired bone remodeling
   c. Femoral nerve impingement with possible pathogenesis of injury, structural deformity, or prolonged pressure from activity or abnormal growth
   d. Hip dysplasia with possible pathogenesis of congenital deformity or chronic femoral subluxation

5. For how many degrees of scoliosis is only physical therapy indicated?
   a. <15 degrees
   b. <40 degrees
   c. >20 degrees
   d. <35 degrees

6. By what age is intoeing (pigeon-toed) typically resolved?
   a. 5 years old
   b. 3 years old
   c. 12 years old
   d. 8 years old

(*Continued*)

7. What is the typical mechanism of injury with an annular ligament subluxation?
   a. Fall on an outstretched arm
   b. Overuse from throwing
   c. Pulling on the arm
   d. Fall on the elbow

8. Which of the following people most commonly experience an anterior cruciate ligament (ACL) injury?
   a. Young, active females with large Q-angles
   b. Young, active males with a small Q-angles
   c. Young, sedentary males with tight hamstrings
   d. Young, active females with tight hamstrings

9. A young baseball pitcher is complaining of pain and fatigue in his medial elbow. He states that he has difficulty controlling his pitches, and as an intervention, you give him stretches of the wrist flexors and weighted stick strengthening exercises for the wrist flexors and extensors. What condition does this pitcher most likely have?
   a. Ulnar collateral ligament tear
   b. Lateral epicondylitis
   c. Medial epicondylitis apophyitis
   d. Annular ligament subluxation

10. Which of the following would not be considered an appropriate initial intervention for Osgood-Schlatter disease?
   a. Stretching the quadriceps
   b. Plyometric training
   c. Cryotherapy
   d. Isometric strength training

References

1. Adirim TA, Cheng TL. Overview of injuries in the young athlete. *Sports Med.* 2003;33:75-81.
2. Piercy KL, Dorn JM, Fulton JE, et al. Opportunities for public health to increase physical activity among youths. *Am J Public Health.* 2015;105:421-426.
3. Foss KDB, Myer GD, Hewett TE. Epidemiology of basketball, soccer, and volleyball injuries in middle-school female athletes. *Phys Sportsmed.* 2014;42:146-153.
4. Merkel DL. Youth sport: positive and negative impact on young athletes. *Open Access J Sports Med.* 2013;4:151-160.
5. Eime RM, Young JA, Harvey JT, et al. A systematic review of the psychological and social benefits of participation in sport for children and adolescents: informing development of a conceptual model of health through sport. *Int J Behav Nutr Phys Act.* 2013;10:98.
6. Emery CA. Risk factors for injury in child and adolescent sport: a systematic review of the literature. *Clin J Sport Med.* 2003;13:256-268.
7. Rechel JA, Collins CL, Comstock RD. Epidemiology of injuries requiring surgery among high school athletes in the United States, 2005 to 2010. *J Trauma.* 2011;71:982-989.
8. American Academy of Orthopaedic Surgeons. *Slipped Capital Femoral Epiphysis.* OrthoInfo. Updated: August 2020. Accessed January 30, 2024. https://orthoinfo.aaos.org/en/diseases–conditions/slipped-capital-femoral-epiphysis-scfe.
9. Peck DM, Voss LM, Voss TT. Slipped capital femoral epiphysis: diagnosis and management. *Am Fam Physician.* 2017; 95(12): 779-784.
10. Antich TJ, Brewster CE. Osgood-Schlatter disease: review of literature and physical therapy management. *J Orthop Sports Phys Ther.* 1985;7(1):5-10.
11. Raj MA, Tafti D, Kiel J. Pes planus (flat feet). In: *StatPearls.* StatPearls Publishing; 2020.
12. American Academy of Orthopaedic Surgeons. *Flexible Flatfoot in Children.* OrthoInfo. Updated: April 2022. Accessed January 30, 2024.
13. Dixit S, DiFiori JP, Burton M, Mines B. Management of patellofemoral pain syndrome. *Am Fam Physician.* 2007;75(2):194-202.
14. Leschitz J, Shamus E, Pauley EN. Chondromalacia patellae. In: Shamus E, ed. *The Color Atlas of Physical Therapy.* McGraw-Hill; 2015.
15. Balsky S, Goldford RJ. Rehabilitation protocol for undisplaced Colles' fractures following cast removal. *J Can Chiropr Assoc.* 2000;44(1):29-33.
16. Donnelly TD, Macfarlane RJ, Nagy MT, Ralte P, Waseem M. Fractures of the clavicle: an overview. *Open Orthop J.* 2013;7:329-333.
17. Lenza M, Taniguchi LF, Ferretti M. Figure-of-eight bandage versus arm sling for treating middle-third clavicle fractures in adults: study protocol for a randomized controlled trial. *Trials.* 2016;17(1):229.
18. American Academy of Orthopaedic Surgeons. *Perthes Disease.* OrthoInfo. Updated: February 2023. Accessed January 30, 2024. https://orthoinfo.aaos.org/en/diseases–conditions/perthes-disease.
19. Imran A, Huang C, Tang H, et al. Analysis of scoliosis from spinal X-ray images. April 2020. arXiv:2004.06887v1. Accessed January 30, 2024. https://arxiv.org/abs/2004.06887.
20. Šarčević Z. Scoliosis: muscle imbalance and treatment. *Br J Sports Med.* 2010;44:16.
21. Berdishevsky H, Lebel VA, Bettany-Saltikov J, et al. Physiotherapy scoliosis-specific exercises: a comprehensive review of seven major schools. *Scoliosis* 2016;20:11.
22. Schroth Method. *Schroth Exercises For Scoliosis.* Updated 2021. Accessed January 30, 2024. http://www.schrothmethod.com/scoliosis-exercises.
23. Lyon R, Liu XC. *Effects of Low and High-intensity Ultrasound on the Physis Plate of the Rabbit Knee Joint.* Poster 0349. 48th Annual Meeting of the Orthopaedic Research society. Accessed January 30, 2024. https://www.ors.org/transactions/48/0349.pdf.
24. HEP2GO. *Selected Exercise: Scapular Retraction.* Updated: December 2013. Accessed January 30, 2024. https://www.hep2go.com/exercise_editor.php?exId=15487&userRef=gciaake.
25. HEP2GO. *Selected Exercise: Theraband Protraction With Pronation.* Updated: September 2017. Accessed January 30, 2024. https://www.hep2go.com/exercise_editor.php?exId=51471&userRef=gciaake.
26. Cricchio M, Frazer C. Scapulothoracic and scapulohumeral exercises: a narrative review of electromyographic studies. *J Hand Ther.* 2011;24(4):322-334.

27. Pediatric Orthopaedic Society of North America. *Back Pain in Children*. OrthoKids. Accessed January 30, 2024. https://orthokids.org/conditions/back-pain-in-children/.

28. Hidalgo B, Detrembleur C, Hall T, Mahaudens P, Nielens H. The efficacy of manual therapy and exercise for different stages of non-specific low back pain: an update of systematic reviews. *J Man Manip Ther*. 2014;22(2):59-74.

29. Kordi R, Rostami M. Low back pain in children and adolescents: an algorithmic clinical approach. *Iran J Pediatr*. 2011;21(3):259-270.

30. Gunn LJ, Stewart JC, Morgan B, et al. Instrument-assisted soft tissue mobilization and proprioceptive neuromuscular facilitation techniques improve hamstring flexibility better than static stretching alone: a randomized clinical trial. *J Man Manip Ther*. 2019;27(1):15-23.

31. Mumbleau A. *Physical Therapy Guide to Achilles Tendinopathy*. ChoosePT. American Physical Therapy Association. Updated July 9, 2018. Accessed January 30, 2024. https://www.choosept.com/symptomsconditionsdetail/physical-therapy-guide-to-achilles-tendon-injuries-tendinopathy#HowCanPhysicalTherapistHelp.

32. Sheehan SE, Gaviola G, Gordon R, Sacks A, Shi LL, Smith SE. Traumatic shoulder injuries: a force mechanism analysis-glenohumeral dislocation and instability. *AJR Am J Roentgenol*. 2013; 201(2): 378-393.

33. Boden BP, Dean GS, Feagin JA, et al. Mechanisms of anterior cruciate ligament injury. *Orthopedics*. 2000;23(6):573-578.

34. Makhni EC, Crump EK, Steinhaus ME, et al. Quality and variability of online available physical therapy protocols from Academic Orthopaedic Surgery Programs for Anterior Cruciate Ligament reconstruction. *Arthroscopy*. 2016;32(8):1612-1621.

35. Wells B, Allen C, Deyle G, et al. Management of acute grade II lateral ankle sprains with an emphasis on ligament protection: a descriptive case series. *Int J Sports Phys Ther*. 2019;14(3):445-458.

36. Zhang AL, Sing DC, Rugg CM, et al. The rise of concussions in the adolescent population. *Orthop J Sports Med*. 2016;4: 2325967116662458.

37. Impact Applications. *ImPACT Test*, Version 4. Accessed January 30, 2024. Available at https://impacttest.com/.

38. Collins MW, Kontos AP, Reynolds E, et al. A comprehensive, targeted approach to the clinical care of athletes following sport-related concussion. *Knee Surg Sports Traumatol Arthrosc*. 2014;22:235-246.

39. Koh JO, Cassidy JD, Watkinson EJ. Incidence of concussion in contact sports: a systematic review of the evidence. *Brain Inj*. 2003;17:901-917.

40. Miller JH, Gill C, Kuhn EN, et al. Predictors of delayed recovery following pediatric sports-related concussion: a case-control study. *J Neurosurg Pediatr*. 2016;17:491-496.

41. Giza CC, Hovda DA. The neurometabolic cascade of concussion. *J Athl Train*. 2001;36:228-235.

42. NFL. *Concussion Protocol and Return-to-Participation Protocol: Overview*. NFL Concussion Guidelines. Accessed January 30, 2024. https://www.playsmartplaysafe.com/newsroom/videos/nfl-head-neck-spine-committees-concussion-protocol-overview/.

43. University of South Florida. *Pediatric Orthopaedics Competency Based Goals and Objectives*. Accessed January 30, 2024. https://health.usf.edu/~/media/Files/Medicine/Orthopaedic/Residency/PGY%203%20Pediatric.ashx.

18

Pediatric Wellness and Fitness

Eric Shamus, PT, DPT, PhD, Marla Laufer, MD, Rob Sillevis, PT, DPT, PhD, and Grant Shamus, CPT

LEARNING OBJECTIVES

Upon completion of this chapter, the reader will be able to:

- Identify health promotion strategies.
- Understand the definitions for health promotion and related topics.

- Discuss considerations for health promotion interventions.
- Identify information for children with disabilities.
- Identify information for children who are obese.
- Understand the roles in community settings.

PHYSICAL ACTIVITY

Fitness, wellness, health promotion, and prevention are all key components in the rehabilitation for children. President Bush in 2002, launched a President's HealthierUS Initiative.[1] *Steps to a HealthierUS* was established by the US Department of Health and Human Services to target public education and community-based grants to reduce the burden of diabetes, overweight, obesity, asthma, and to address 3 related risk factors: physical inactivity, poor nutrition, and tobacco use. The president's initiative was designed to improve personal health and fitness. The 4 points of the initiative were to:

- Be physically active every day.
- Eat a nutritious diet.
- Get preventive screenings.
- Make healthy choices.

The president's initiative is based on improving personal fitness and becoming healthier to achieve a better and longer life.[1] See **Figure 18-1** for an example of outdoor city space that encourage fitness activities.[2]

The Surgeon General in 2005 published *The Surgeon General's Call to Action to Improve the Health and Wellness of Persons With Disabilities*.[3] The surgeon general described the challenges to health and well-being faced by persons of all ages with disabilities. The 4 goals for the vision for the future are[3]:

- **Goal 1:** People nationwide understand that persons with disabilities can lead long, healthy, productive lives.
- **Goal 2:** Health care providers have the knowledge and tools to screen, diagnose, and treat the whole person with a disability with dignity.
- **Goal 3:** Persons with disabilities can promote their own good health by developing and maintaining healthy lifestyles.
- **Goal 4:** Accessible health care and support services promote independence for persons with disabilities.

The US Department of Health and Human Services recommends that young people aged 6 to 17 years participate in at least 60 minutes of physical activity daily.[4] See **Table 18-1** for physical activity guidelines for Americans. This is the part of the recommendation the President's Council on Sports, Fitness, and Nutrition has made. The President's Council reports that active children are more likely to become active and healthier adults. Physical activity has an impact on academic performance and social skills. It has been demonstrated that increased physical activity will lead to:

- Improved test scores, grades, and time management skills
- Boosted concentration, memory, and classroom behavior
- Increased self-confidence and self-esteem
- Strengthened social and cooperative skills, such as teamwork and problem solving
- Reduced anxiety and stress

Small bouts of increased physical activity throughout the day can be beneficial. Recess and classroom activity breaks show positive association with indicators of cognitive skills, attitudes, and academic behavior and achievement.[4] When children are active, their blood flow increases, improving memory and concentration, which are essential in the classroom.[5] In addition, hormones are released that can improve their mood and reduce anxiety and stress.[5] Despite the initiatives and recommendations to have at least 60 minutes of physical activity, only 1 in 3 children achieves this minimum amount of physical activity they need each day.[6] Physical activity is particularly important among children with physical disabilities, as 22.5% of children with disabilities are obese compared to 16% of children without disabilities. There is evidence that children of high school age are not very active.

In 2011, 29% of high school students surveyed had participated in at least 60 minutes per day of physical activity on all 7 days before the survey.[7] As society has become technologically

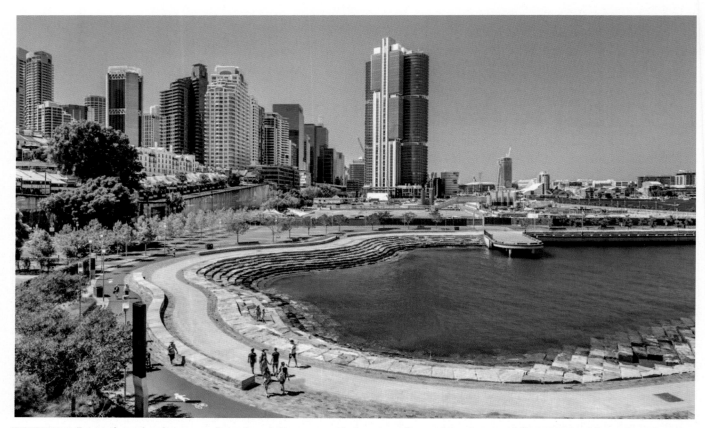

FIGURE 18-1 **Footpaths and cycleways, as shown here in Barangaroo, Sydney, as well as parks and open public spaces provide outdoor places for sport, active recreation, and relaxation, as well as preserving areas of the natural environment, among advancing urban development.** (Used with permission from Leonid Andronov/Shutterstock.)

TABLE 18-1 • Physical Activity Guidelines for Americans[4]	
Age	**Recommendations**
3-5 years	• Preschool-aged children (ages 3 through 5 years) should be physically active throughout the day to enhance growth and development. • Adult caregivers of preschool-aged children should encourage active play that includes a variety of activity types.

6-17 years	• It is important to provide young people opportunities and encouragement to participate in physical activities that are appropriate for their age, that are enjoyable, and that offer variety.
	• Children and adolescents ages 6 through 17 years should do 60 minutes (min)/1 hour or more of moderate-to-vigorous physical activity daily:
	  ◦ Aerobic: Most of the 60 min or more per day should be either moderate- or vigorous-intensity aerobic physical activity and should include vigorous-intensity physical activity on at least 3 days a week.
	  ◦ Muscle strengthening: As part of their 60 min or more of daily physical activity, children and adolescents should include muscle-strengthening physical activity on at least 3 days a week.
	  ◦ Bone strengthening: As part of their 60 min or more of daily physical activity, children and adolescents should include bone-strengthening physical activity on at least 3 days a week.

Note: Moderate-intensity physical activity: Aerobic activity that increases a person's heart rate and breathing to some extent. On a scale relative to a person's capacity, moderate-intensity activity is usually a 5 or 6 on a 0 to 10 scale. Brisk walking, dancing, swimming, or bicycling on a level terrain are examples. Vigorous-intensity physical activity: Aerobic activity that greatly increases a person's heart rate and breathing. On a scale relative to a person's capacity, vigorous-intensity activity is usually a 7 or 8 on a 0 to 10 scale. Jogging, singles tennis, swimming continuous laps, and bicycling uphill are examples. Muscle-strengthening activity: Physical activity, including exercise that increases skeletal muscle strength, power, endurance, and mass. It includes strength training, resistance training, and muscular strength and endurance exercises. Bone-strengthening activity: Physical activity that produces an impact or tension force on bones, which promotes bone growth and strength. Running, jumping rope, and lifting weights are examples.

Source: Adapted from US Department of Health and Human Services. Physical Activity Guidelines for Americans. 2nd ed. US Department of Health and Human Services; 2018. Available at https://health.gov/sites/default/files/2019-09/Physical_Activity_Guidelines_2nd_edition.pdf.[4]

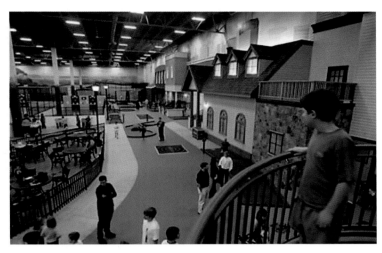

FIGURE 18-2 **This Minnesota school was organized on the layout of a village square with the classroom in a hockey rink and used sit-stand desks and mobile whiteboards and information technology (IT_ equipment). Children were allowed to move throughout the neighborhood during lessons and reached higher daily physical activity levels than children in traditional classrooms—levels equivalent to those among children on their summer holidays.** (Reproduced with permission from Lanningham-Foster L, Foster RC, McCrady SK, et al. Changing the school environment to increase physical activity in children. *Obesity (Silver Spring).* 2008;16[8]:1849-1853.)

driven, children spend more time using technology. They spend an average of more than 7.5 hours a day in front of a screen, inside watching TV, playing video games, or surfing the Internet.[8] As a result, participation in physical activity declines as young people age.[6] See **Figure 18-2** for an innovative school for child activity.[9]

■ OBESITY

Childhood obesity has become a significant health issue. Today, more and more children are being diagnosed with diabetes, hypertension, dyslipidemia, and other comorbid conditions associated with obesity.[10] "The persistence or worsening of childhood cardio-metabolic risk factors and metabolic syndrome into adulthood is assumed to substantially increase the risk for future diseases."[11]

The Obesity Action Coalition[12] is a more than 58,000 member–strong 501(c)(3) national nonprofit organization dedicated to giving a voice to individuals affected by the disease of obesity and helping individuals along their journey toward better health through education, advocacy, and support. The Obesity Action Coalition describes obesity as follows: "Obesity is a complex, multifactorial, and chronic disease that requires a comprehensive medical approach to care. It is the second leading preventable cause of death in the United States and is associated with a large number of comorbid conditions. Care should therefore not be seen as simply having the goal of reducing body weight, but should additionally be focused on improving overall health and quality of life."[12] A child is defined as "affected by obesity" if their body mass index–for-age (or BMI-for-age) percentile is equal to or greater than 95%. A child is defined as "overweight" if their BMI-for-age percentile is greater than 85% and less than 95%.[13] (See **Table 18-2** for the prevalence of obesity at a global level.[13])

CAUSES OF OBESITY

There are many factors that could contribute to the development of obesity. Social determinants of health and physiologic factors could make weight management challenging for a child, especially when a child is troubled by stress.[14]

> ### Key Concept
>
> If the child has a mismatch between energy in and energy out over time, there will be an imbalance. If the calories in are more than the calories burned, this will equal a weight gain.
>
> **Calories in > Calories Burned = Weight Gain**

There could be a hormonal reason why children always feel hungry and therefore consume more. We are surrounded by advertisements that promote the consumption of foods and beverages that are high in calories and fat. Some neighborhoods have little or no access to fresh, healthy foods. Long daily commutes to and from school make it harder to get physical activity. If there is time, not all communities have safe spaces to run, bike, or walk, which will contribute to inactivity and greater participation in in-house activities.

Studies have shown that there is a relationship between how much people sleep and how much people weigh.[15-17] As there has been a societal shift toward children going to bed later and spending the evening hours behind TV, phone, and/or computer screens, the total time available for sleep has decreased. There is a negative linear relationship between sleeping hours and weight.[15-17]

The presence of certain genes will make it more likely that one develops obesity.[18] Despite the fact that one might have these genes, one should still try and lose weight, as it has been shown that even a weight loss of 5% will lead to better health.[18] As more

TABLE 18-2 • Prevalence of Underweight Among Children and Adolescents Aged 2-19 years, by Age and Sex: United States, 1963-1965 Through 2017-2018

Survey period	Sample size (*n*)	Total	2-5 years	6-11 years	12-19 years	Boys	Girls
			Percent (standard error)				
1963-1965	7,047	—	—	5.8 (0.6)	—	—	—
1966-1970*	6,768	—	—	—	4.6 (0.3)	—	—
1971-1974	7,041	5.1 (0.3)	5.8 (0.5)	5.3 (0.5)	4.7 (0.5)	5.0 (0.3)	5.3 (0.5)
1976-1980	7,351	4.5 (0.3)	5.3 (0.4)	4.2 (0.4)	4.4 (0.4)	5.0 (0.4)	4.1 (0.3)
1988-1994	10,777	4.0 (0.3)	4.3 (0.4)	3.9 (0.6)	3.9 (0.6)	4.2 (0.5)	3.8 (0.5)
1999-2000	4,039	4.2 (0.4)	5.1 (1.3)	4.3 (0.9)	3.7 (0.6)	4.9 (0.9)	3.5 (0.7)
2001-2002	4,261	3.4 (0.3)	2.8 (0.8)	3.4 (0.3)	3.7 (0.6)	3.7 (0.5)	3.1 (0.4)
2003-2004	3,961	3.2 (0.3)	3.7 (1.0)	3.0 (0.7)	3.2 (0.7)	3.6 (0.4)	2.9 (0.5)
2005-2006	4,207	3.2 (0.4)	1.9 (0.4)	2.3 (0.7)	4.5 (0.7)	3.7 (0.7)	2.7 (0.4)
2007-2008	3,249	3.7 (0.4)	3.8 (0.9)	3.0 (0.7)	4.2 (0.6)	3.8 (0.8)	3.6 (0.4)
2009-2010	3,408	3.3 (0.4)	3.1 (0.5)	4.2 (0.7)	2.8 (0.6)	3.3 (0.5)	3.4 (0.5)
2011-2012	3,355	3.5 (0.5)	3.2 (0.7)	3.6 (0.8)	3.6 (0.7)	4.2 (1.1)	2.8 (0.5)
2013-2014	3,523	3.8 (0.4)	3.4 (0.8)	4.8 (1.1)	3.2 (0.8)	3.6 (0.6)	4.0 (0.5)
2015-2016	3,340	3.0 (0.6)	2.3 (0.9)	2.5 (0.6)	3.7 (1.0)	3.6 (1.0)	2.5 (0.6)
2017-2018	2,824	4.1 (0.5)	3.4 (0.9)	3.6 (0.7)	4.7 (0.8)	5.0 (0.7)	3.1 (0.6)

Data not available. National Health Examination Surveys (NHES) 1963–1965 did not include boys and girls aged 2–5 and 12–19. NHES 1966–1970 did not include boys and girls aged 2–5 and 6–11.
*Data are for adolescents aged 12–17, not 12–19.
Notes: Underweight is body mass index (BMI) less than the 5th percentile from the sex-specific BMI-for-age 2000 CDC Growth Charts. Pregnant females are excluded from analysis beginning with 1971–1974. Pregnancy status was not available for 1963–1965 and 1966–1970.
Sources: National Center for Health Statistics, National Health Examination Surveys, 1963–1965 and 1966–1970; and National Health and Nutrition Examination Surveys, 1971–1974, 1976–1980, 1988–1994, and 1999–2018.

and more children are increasingly being diagnosed with childhood diseases (including mental illness and allergies), there has been a proportional increase in medication usage. Many of these medications (including antipsychotic, antidepressant, seizure, and steroid medications) have side effects that can lead to weight gain. Even preventative medication such as birth control has weight gain listed as a side effect. Parents should always discuss the risks and benefits of medications with their child's physician, especially if weight gain is a concern.

PHYSICAL ACTIVITY MODIFICATIONS

Physical activity is key to promoting health and wellness. There is expanding evidence that increasing physical activity can not only benefit weight modification but also increase cardiorespiratory fitness as well. It is best to start simple and keep it manageable. Taking a walk around the block after dinner, walking to and from a neighborhood school, parking further away from the store, or engaging with children with exercise can be examples of some more attainable strategies. Before an exercise program is implemented, make sure that there are no reasons why a child should not participate in physical activities. These are easy ways to make physical activity part of someone's day. When making an exercise and physical activity plan for the child, remember to:

• Make it simple.
• Make it realistic.
• Make it happen.
• Make it fun.

Although the US Department of Health and Human Services recommends children and adolescents undertake moderate to vigorous physical activity for an average of 60 minutes per day to improve mental, physical, and cognitive health, there is increasing evidence that most adolescents fall short of this daily average. Burden et al[19] suggest that perhaps only 20 minutes of vigorous physical activity is sufficient to obtain cardiorespiratory fitness.

■ NUTRITION

The *2015-2020 Dietary Guidelines for Americans* focuses on making small shifts in daily eating habits that will improve the child's health over the long run (**Table 18-3**).[20] The *2015-2020 Dietary Guidelines* also emphasize the importance of "eating patterns," which refers to the combination of *all* foods and beverages a person consumes regularly over time, rather than focusing on individual nutrients or foods in isolation.[20] Healthy eating patterns, along with regular physical activity, have been shown in a large body of current science to help people reach and maintain good health while reducing risks of chronic disease throughout their lives. Additionally, healthy eating patterns can be adapted to an individual's budget, taste preferences, traditions, and culture.

Action for Healthy Kids[21] is a nonprofit organization dedicated to fighting childhood obesity, undernourishment, and physical inactivity. Action for Healthy Kids has identified the following key concepts for nutrition:

TABLE 18-3 • Daily Nutritional Goals for Age-Sex Groups Based on Dietary Reference Intakes and *Dietary Guidelines* Recommendations[20]

	Source of goal[a]	Child 1-3	Female 4-8	Male 4-8	Female 9-13	Male 9-13	Female 14-18	Male 14-18
Calorie level(s) assessed		1,000	1,200	1,400, 1,600	1,600	1,800	1,800	2,200, 2,800, 3,200
Macronutrients								
Protein, g	RDA	13	19	19	34	34	46	52
Protein, % kcal	AMDR	5-20	10-30	10-30	10-30	10-30	10-30	10-30
Carbohydrate, g	RDA	130	130	130	130	130	130	130
Carbohydrate, % kcal	AMDR	45-65	45-65	45-65	45-65	45-65	45-65	45-65
Dietary fiber, g	14g/1,000 kcal	14	16.8	19.6	22.4	25.2	25.2	30.8
Added sugars, % kcal	DGA	<10%	<10%	<10%	<10%	<10%	<10%	<10%
Total fat, % kcal	AMDR	30-40	25-35	25-35	25-35	25-35	25-35	25-35
Saturated fat, % kcal	DGA	<10%	<10%	<10%	<10%	<10%	<10%	<10%
Linoleic acid, g	AI	7	10	10	10	12	11	16
Linolenic acid, g	AI	0.7	0.9	0.9	1	1.2	1.1	1.6
Minerals								
Calcium, mg	RDA	700	1,000	1,000	1,300	1,300	1,300	1,300
Iron, mg	RDA	7	10	10	8	8	15	11
Magnesium, mg	RDA	80	130	130	240	240	360	410
Phosphorus, mg	RDA	460	500	500	1,250	1,250	1,250	1,250
Potassium, mg	AI	3,000	3,800	3,800	4,500	4,500	4,700	4,700
Sodium, mg	UL	1,500	1,900	1,900	2,200	2,200	2,300	2,300
Zinc, mg	RDA	3	5	5	8	8	9	11
Copper, mcg	RDA	340	440	440	700	700	890	890
Manganese, mg	AI	1.2	1.5	1.5	1.6	1.9	1.6	2.2
Selenium, mcg	RDA	20	30	30	40	40	55	55
Vitamins								
Vitamin A, mg RAE	RDA	300	400	400	600	600	700	900
Vitamin E, mg AT	RDA	6	7	7	11	11	15	15
Vitamin D, IU	RDA	600	600	600	600	600	600	600
Vitamin C, mg	RDA	15	25	25	45	45	65	75
Thiamin, mg	RDA	0.5	0.6	0.6	0.9	0.9	1	1.2
Riboflavin, mg	RDA	0.5	0.6	0.6	0.9	0.9	1	1.3
Niacin, mg	RDA	6	8	8	12	12	14	16
Vitamin B$_6$, mg	RDA	0.5	0.6	0.6	1	1	1.2	1.3
Vitamin B$_{12}$, mcg	RDA	0.9	1.2	1.2	1.8	1.8	2.4	2.4
Choline, mg	AI	200	250	250	375	375	400	550
Vitamin K, mcg	AI	30	55	55	60	60	75	75
Folate, meg DFE	RDA	150	200	200	300	300	400	400

[a]RDA = Recommended Dietary Allowance, AI = Adequate Intake, UL = Tolerable Upper Intake Level, AMDR = Acceptable Macronutrient Distribution Range, DGA = 2015-2020 Dietary Guidelines recommended limit; 14 g fiber per 1,000 kcal = basis for AI for fiber.
[b]Calcium RDA for males ages 71+ years is 1,200 mg.
[c]Vitamin D RDA for males and females ages 71+ years is 800 IU.
Notes
Source: Institute of Medicine. Dietary Reference Intakes: The essential guide to nutrient requirements. Washington (DC): The National Academies Press; 2006.
Institute of Medicine. Dietary Reference Intakes for Calcium and Vitamin D. Washington (DC): The National Academies Press; 2010.

- Make half of your plate fruits and vegetables.
- Consume 5 servings of fruits and vegetables each day.
- Eating whole fruits is best, but drink 100% juice when choosing fruit juice.
- Make at least half of your grains whole grains.
- Switch to fat-free or low-fat (1%) dairy.
- Consume 3 servings of dairy each day.
- Limit soda and other sugar sweetened beverages.
- Water is the best option!

Some issues that might affect children's eating abilities may include the following:

- Slower oral-motor development
  - Larger tongues, smaller teeth
- Hypothyroidism
- Celiac disease
- Allergies
  - Gluten, egg, dairy, peanut, sesame, shellfish, tree nut, etc.
  - There are fun bracelets children can wear to help identify allergies for other individuals. For example, someone might offer the child a cookie with nuts in it!

Other children's eating resources include the following:

- Kids Eat Right: www.kidseatright.org
- Fruit and Veggies More Matters: www.fruitsandveggiesmore-matters.org
- US Department of Agriculture's ChooseMyPlate: www.choosemyplate.gov

■ STRENGTH (RESISTANCE) TRAINING

For many years, the American Academy of Pediatrics Council on Sports Medicine and Fitness,[22] American College of Sports Medicine,[23] American Orthopaedic Society for Sports Medicine,[24] and the National Strength and Conditioning Association[25] have agreed that a supervised strength (resistance) training program that follows the recommended guidelines and precautions is safe and effective for children. It seems that even children with disabilities benefit from strength training. The Centers for Disease Control and Prevention[6] and the American Academy of Pediatrics[22] recommend school-aged children participate in at least 60 minutes of moderate to vigorous physical activity each day. Strength training can focus on improving muscle strength, increasing power or muscle bulk, and enhancing endurance.

> ### Key Concept
>
> When beginning an exercise and strength program, the focus should be on technique and form without resistance. Emphasizing correct form will decrease the risk for injury. After good form has been achieved, early conditioning should be focused using body weight as resistance instead on adding additional weight.

The ability to control one's own weight is important for daily activities. The focus of training should be on agility, balance, and coordination. Strength training can be used with infants and young children to improve quality of movement and performance in both upper and lower extremities. Examples of strength training for this population include weight bearing on hands and elbows during play, wheelbarrow, prone on swing crawling with arms, crab walk, bear walk, jumping, and standing in a stander for supervised increased periods of time.[26] Another strategy that therapists use with children is heavy work, which consists of having the child push and carry heavy items to increase repetition of movements to build strength.[27]

Strength training can occur once balance and coordination have been mastered and the child can understand instructions, which is usually around the age of 7 to 8.[28] Free weight training should occur after puberty with submaximal exercises being recommended. The American Academy of Pediatrics does not endorse using continuous maximal lifts for youth strength training.[22] Due to high injury risk of single maximal lifts, it is not recommended that children perform these until skeletal maturity is attained. Healthy children with the proper adult supervision can perform single-repetition testing safely with child-sized weight training machines.[29]

For each training session, it is recommended to use about 6 to 8 exercises that will focus and train the major muscle groups (including the chest, shoulders, back, arms, legs, abdomen, and lower back). It is important to balance agonist and antagonist muscle groups with exercise to prevent asymmetry due to 1-sided exercise focus. Balanced exercise effort between the flexing (agonist) and extending (antagonist) muscles and between upper and lower body is important. The goal is to perform 2 to 3 exercises per muscle group in each session. Youth strength training programs should start with 1 to 2 sets per exercise, with 6 to 15 repetitions in each set with muscle fatigue at the end of the set. For children and adolescents, the initial load should be selected so that 10 to 15 repetitions can be completed with some fatigue but no muscle failure. In general, resistance can be increased by 5% to 10% when the child can easily perform 15 repetitions. If the participant fails to complete at least 10 repetitions per set or is unable to maintain proper form, then the weight is probably too heavy and should thus be reduced. It is recommended that there should be a rest time of 1 to 3 minutes in between sets and there should be 2 to 3 days in between training the same muscle groups again. As fatigue occurs during the training, the change increases as a result of improper form. Unless good form can be maintained, the number of sets and/or the resistance during the set should not be increased. Increased strength will lead to improved motor skills, endurance, strength, and flexibility.[28,29] There is evidence that this youth strength training will lead to improved squats, and the vertical and long jump.[28] One must keep in mind that strength training is not the best way to improve overall endurance.[29] Endurance training would be more appropriate to achieve this.

There is a need for a well-designed strength training program following the recommended loads, sets, and repetitions appropriate for the young athlete's age and body type. Strength training can be performed with body weight, machine-based, free weight,

TABLE 18-4 • General Guidelines for a Strength-Training a Program

1. Establish a strength-training program that is both challenging and exciting for children to participate.
2. Qualified strength and conditioning professions such as those certified by the *National Strength and Conditioning Association* should be used for developing strength-training programs for children. Coaches must have the scientific and clinical background in adolescent development to create and develop adequate strength-training programs.
3. Make sure all children have a preparticipation screening prior to any strength-training program by qualified physicians or allied health professionals to examine for preexisting conditions or injuries. A standard health history questionnaire followed by a physical examination that includes flexibility, strength testing for weakness, muscle imbalances, and reflexes will help detect potential risks for strength training.
4. If the preparticipation screening detects physical limitations or strength deficits, a comprehensive program to correct these deficiencies should be addressed as a priority when beginning a strength-training program.
5. Strength-training programs for adolescents should emphasize submaximal efforts, using their body weight or bars with no added weights and concentration on muscular strength and endurance instead of power exercises. The strength-training program should first focus on mastery of technique and motor skills with lightweight before progressing to heavier resistance training and more complex multijoint exercises.
6. Avoid 1 RM lifts.
7. Perform all exercises through a full range of motion and with proper form.
8. Instruct children on the proper methods to breath during exercise and make sure they do not hold their breath.
9. Have an adequate supervision in the strength training facility that includes the use of spotters, if necessary.
10. Make sure the facility is safe, well ventilated, and illuminated properly.
11. Strength training should be performed only two to three times a week with an adequate rest and recovery between sessions. Each session should comprise a general warm-up period, flexibility, resistance training and workout program, specific tasks, and a cool down period.

Reproduced with permission from Patel DR, Greydanus DE, Baker RJ. eds. Pediatric Practice: Sports Medicine. New York: McGraw Hill; 2009.

plyometric, and complex and functional training. Sports such as gymnastics and baseball, which involve repetitive impact and torque, provide a greater risk of epiphyseal injury. Children can improve strength by 30% to 50% after just 8 to 12 weeks of a well-designed strength-training program. Faigenbaum et al[30] found that twice-weekly strength training in boys and girls between the ages of 7 and 12 years produced significant strength gains in the chest press (vs age-matched controls). To achieve muscle hypertrophy, there needs to be circulating testosterone.[31] This is typically missing in children of younger ages. It is believed that children gain strength through neural adaptations, not muscle hypertrophy.[32] Strength training in children likely improves the number and coordination of activated motor neurons, as well as the firing rate and pattern.[33] See **Tables 18-4** and **18-5** for a conceptual model for the implementation of resistance training (RT).

Prepubertal children and postpubertal adolescents respond to strength training differently; namely, adolescents are capable of greater absolute gains owing to higher levels of circulating androgens.[34] It has been demonstrated that physical training has produced an increased cross-sectional area of the erector spinae, multifidus, and psoas musculature, as documented on axial magnetic resonance imaging (MRI) studies, in comparison with age-matched nonathletic controls.[35] An increased muscle cross-sectional area is directly correlated with increased overall muscle strength. This suggests that long-term physical training alone can lead to significant muscular hypertrophy and strength gains in young athletes.[36]

Children with chronic medical conditions face many challenges when considering exercise participation. Compared with their healthy counterparts, they are often discouraged from physical activity or sports participation because of real or perceived limitations imposed by their condition. Examples of activities that can be used are the Nintendo Wii for active video games.[37]

Key Concept

Prescribed exercise should be based on the condition of the child, the effects the disease might have on muscle performance, and the potential for exercise-induced acute or chronic worsening of the condition. Being creative and designing a program that captures the child's attention will aid in compliance and follow-through.

TABLE 18-5 • Special Considerations in Adolescents Athletes

Adolescent growth spurt
Size and weight
Height
Muscle mass and strength
Development of motor skills
Training effects
Change in body composition
Differential growth and strength of bones and connective tissue
Change in musculotendinous flexibility
Presence of growth cartilage
The growth plate—physis
Articular surface
Apophysis
Bone maturation, peak bone mass accumulation
Psychosocial developmental issues

Reproduced with permission from Patel DR, Greydanus DE, Baker RJ. eds. Pediatric Practice: Sports Medicine. New York: McGraw Hill; 2009.

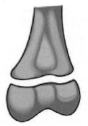
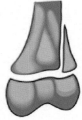
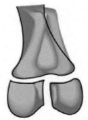

Type I—Separation of the physis

Type II—Fracture–separation of growth plate and small part of metaphysis

Type III—Fracture–part of physis

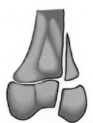
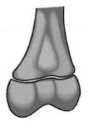

Type IV—Fracture–physis and metaphysis

Type V—Crushing of physis with no displacement–may cause premature closure

FIGURE 18-3 **Salter-Harris classification of physeal (growth plate) fractures.** (Reproduced with permission from William P. *Principles of Athletic Training: A Guide to Evidence-Based Clinical Practice.* New York: McGraw Hill LLC; 2017.)

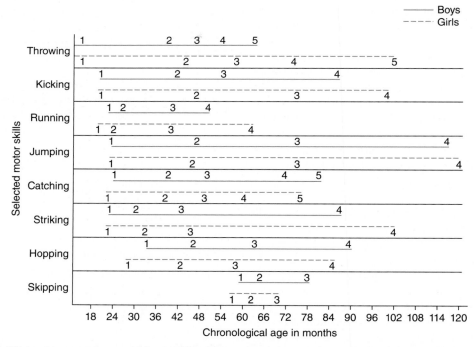

FIGURE 18-4 **Age and skill development. Age at which 60% of the boys and girls were able to perform at a specific developmental level for selected fundamental motor skills. Numbers refer to the developmental stages of that motor skill.** (Reproduced with permission from Patel DP, Greydanus DE, Baker RJ. *Pediatric Practice: Sports Medicine,* New York: McGraw Hill; 2009.)

It was shown that after 6 weeks of an exercise program, there was improved exercise capacity, muscular strength, and overall quality of life.[38] What is more telling is the fact that the effects of exercise on muscle performance and quality of life were still evident after 12 months.[38] Other benefits of strength training include increased strength, lower rates of sports-related injury, increased bone strength index, decreased risk of fracture, and improved self-esteem and interest in fitness.[39]

> *Resistance training (RT) in youth is believed to capitalize on the synergistic effects of physiological adaptations demanded by RT along with the natural proliferation and adaptations due to maturation in the young athlete. During pre-pubescence, youth experience is heightened by neural proliferation and central nervous system (CNS) maturation.[32,40] Increased load and stress on the body provides an added stimulus to the already natural proliferation taking place, resulting in a synergistic increase in neural proliferation compared to youth who do not partake in RT. Studies also show youth and adolescents that undertake initial RT of different forms show increased gains in strength compared to adults undergoing initial RT.[32,40] This disparity between youth and adults also supports the suggestion that increased neural adaptation during normal physiological maturation is synergistic with the physical demands of RT.[39]*

Reproduced with permission from Myers AM, Beam NW, Fakhoury JD. Resistance training for children and adolescents. *Transl Pediatr.* 2017;6(3):137-43.

There might be situations in which strength training is contraindicated, such as in the presence of cardiomyopathy[22] and stage 2 hypertension.[41] For that reason, a medical screening and clearance should be considered before the child partakes in strenuous exercise and strength training. Skeletally immature children have growth plates, areas of rapidly growing cartilage, which eventually promote lengthening of bone. To prevent excessive loading of the child's growth plates, there must be some caution with strength training. Separation of the growth plate (Salter-Harris type 1 fracture) (**Figure 18-3**) can occur. Although most mild degree (type 1) growth plate injuries usually heal well and do not cause long-term growth abnormalities, repetitive injuries can cause deformities over time. Growth plate injuries are more common with free weight strength training. The spine is one of the more common areas for injury with free weights.

In summary, exercise and strength training are beneficial for children and should be considered for every child. Exercise and age-appropriate strength training can reduce injuries.[42] Skeletal maturity should be a guiding factor when determining the use of overload principles. Balance, coordination, and flexibility should be considered prior to the progression into sporting activities.

■ SKILL DEVELOPMENT

As children develop, neurodevelopment maturation occurs. There are key principles of child development to progress from having fun at an activity to sports participation. See **Table 18-6** for key principles of child development.

Infants and toddlers are often started on early activities of swimming. It is important to teach prevention of drowning skills for children ages 1 to 4. The American Academy of Pediatrics recommends that swim lessons for skill development begin after age 4.[43] Acquisition of motor skills occurs rapidly after physical growth slows down after the toddler period. Preschoolers can learn to ride a bicycle without training wheels and catch a ball. See **Figure 18-4** for children's ages when specific skill levels are developed.

Preschool children need to participate in activities of running, jumping, crawling, and climbing to develop balance and control. Playground jungle gyms are great for these activities. There is a development sequence for throwing a ball (**Figure 18-5**). There are also advances in motor development for jumping (**Figures 18-6** and **18-7**).

Participation in activities that develop motor skills, cognitive development, social and emotional development, and visual and motor development is important as the child develops. It is common in Little League soccer when someone kicks the ball for all of the players to run for the ball and bunch up because there is not yet the cognitive development (abstract thought) to learn about the game and about spacing and ball movement. The child's level of development should provide guidance to the participation in the sports activities.

TABLE 18-6 • Key Principles of Child Development

1. Growth and maturation are an ongoing and continuous process.
2. Neurologic, somatic, cognitive, and social development of the child and adolescent progress at the same time as interdependent factors and, therefore, must be considered together as one looks at development and sport participation.
3. Although different developmental milestones are recognized at specific ages, appearance of these milestones often varies considerably in between children.
4. The *sequential* nature of development remains the same in typically developing children (ie, a child must first have neurologic maturity in order to stand and walk; no amount of training will make a child walk before a certain level of neurologic maturity is reached).
5. It is generally well recognized that there will always be children who will be at either end of the developmental spectrum.

Source: Reproduced with permission from Patel DP, Greydanus DE, Baker RJ. Pediatric Practice: Sports Medicine, New York: McGraw Hill; 2009.

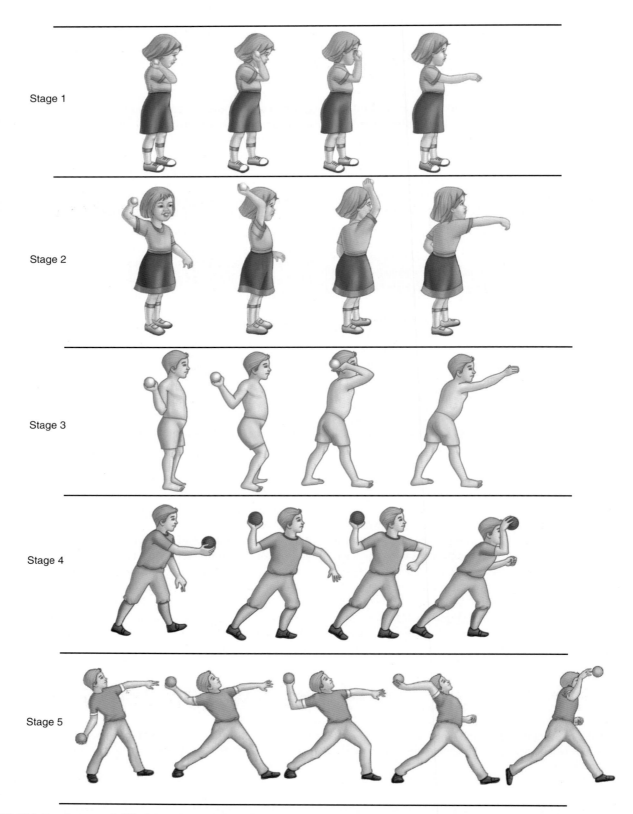

FIGURE 18-5 Developmental skill of throwing. Developmental sequence of throwing behavior. (Reproduced with permission from Patel DP, Greydanus DE, Baker RJ. *Pediatric Practice: Sports Medicine,* New York: McGraw Hill; 2009.)

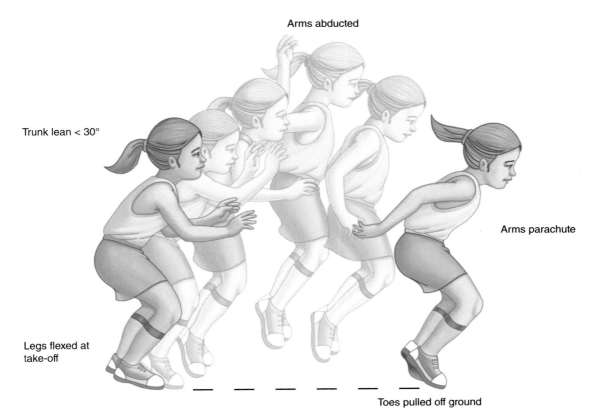

Arms abducted

Trunk lean < 30°

Arms parachute

Legs flexed at
take-off

Toes pulled off ground

FIGURE 18-6 Pattern of long jump in the beginner. (Reproduced with permission from Patel DP, Greydanus DE, Baker RJ. *Pediatric Practice: Sports Medicine,* New York: McGraw Hill; 2009.)

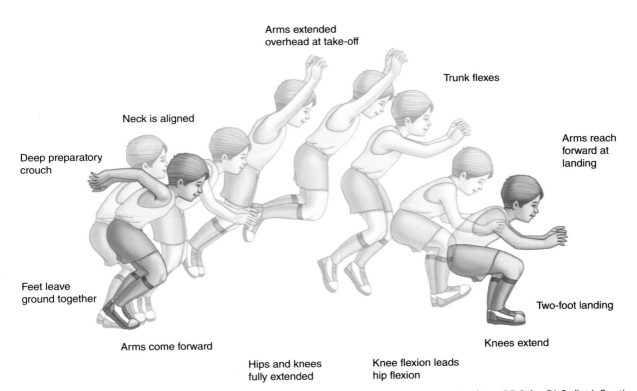

Arms extended
overhead at take-off

Trunk flexes

Neck is aligned

Arms reach
forward at
landing

Deep preparatory
crouch

Feet leave
ground together

Two-foot landing

Arms come forward

Hips and knees
fully extended

Knee flexion leads
hip flexion

Knees extend

FIGURE 18-7 Pattern of long jump in an advanced jumper. (Reproduced with permission from Patel DP, Greydanus DE, Baker RJ. *Pediatric Practice: Sports Medicine,* New York: McGraw Hill; 2009.)

STUDY QUESTIONS

1. Increased physical activity will lead to:
   a. Improved test scores, grades, and time management skills
   b. Increased anxiety and stress
   c. Decreased self-confidence and self-esteem
   d. Deficits in concentration, memory, and classroom behavior

2. What is the recommended minimum amount of physical activity each day for children?
   a. At least 30 minutes a day
   b. At least 60 minutes a day
   c. At least 45 minutes a day
   d. At least 100 minutes a day

3. Over time, how can a child gain weight?
   a. If calories in are more than calories burned
   b. If calories in are equivalent to calories burned
   c. If calories in are less than calories burned
   d. If calories in are equivalent to hydration in milliliters

4. When beginning a strength training exercise program, what should the focus be initially?
   a. Building aerobic endurance
   b. Increasing mobility in the specific joints targeted
   c. Increasing the weight to gain muscle strength
   d. Correct technique and form without resistance

5. What should youth strength training program parameters initially start at?
   a. 3-4 sets, 4-6 reps with muscle failure at the end of the set
   b. 1-2 sets, 6-15 reps with muscle fatigue at the end of the set
   c. 4-6 sets, 4-6 reps with muscle fatigue at the end of the set
   d. 3-4 sets, 15-20 reps with muscle failure at the end of the set

6. What type of fracture can excessive resistance training lead to in children at the growth plate?
   a. Spiral fracture
   b. Buckle fracture
   c. Greenstick fracture
   d. Salter-Harris type 1 fracture

7. Which of the following is not a benefit of strength training?
   a. Increased strength
   b. Higher rates of sports-related injury
   c. Increased bone strength index (BSI)
   d. Decreased risk of fracture

8. At what percentile of their body mass index (BMI) for age is a child considered to be "affected by obesity"?
   a. Greater than 95%
   b. Greater than 85% and less than 95%
   c. Greater than 75% and less than 85%
   d. Greater than 65% and less than 75%

9. Which condition is associated with inflammation at the heel growth plate causing excess bone growth?
   a. Osgood-Schlatter disease
   b. Calcaneal apophysitis
   c. Plantar fasciitis
   d. Salter-Harris fracture

10. How do you define the general relationship between how much people sleep and how much they weigh?
    a. Decreased amount of sleep leads to decreased weight
    b. Increased amount of sleep leads to increased weight
    c. Decreased amount of sleep leads to no change in weight
    d. Decreased amount of sleep leads to increased weight

CHAPTER SUMMARY

1. Fitness, wellness, health promotion, and prevention are all key components in the rehabilitation for children.
2. The US Department of Health and Human Services recommends that young people aged 6 to 17 years participate in at least 60 minutes of physical activity daily.[4]
3. Despite the initiatives and recommendations to have at least 60 minutes of physical activity, only 1 in 3 children achieves this minimum amount of physical activity they need each day.[6]
4. Physical activity is particularly important among children with physical disabilities, as 22.5% of children with disabilities are obese compared to 16% of children without disabilities.
5. When making an exercise and physical activity plan for the child remember to:
   - Make it simple.
   - Make it realistic.
   - Make it happen.
   - Make it fun.

(Continued)

CHAPTER SUMMARY (*CONTINUED*)

6. Healthy eating patterns, along with regular physical activity, have been shown in a large body of current science to help people reach and maintain good health while reducing risks of chronic disease throughout their lives.

7. For many years, the American Academy of Pediatrics Council on Sports Medicine and Fitness,[22] American College of Sports Medicine,[23] American Orthopaedic Society for Sports Medicine,[24] and the National Strength and Conditioning Association[25] have agreed that a supervised strength (resistance) training program that follows the recommended guidelines and precautions is safe and effective for children.

8. For each training session, it is recommended to use about 6 to 8 exercises that will focus and train the major muscle groups (including the chest, shoulders, back, arms, legs, abdomen, and lower back). At first, the program should focus on technique and form without resistance.

9. There might be situations in which strength training is contraindicated, such as in the presence of cardiomyopathy[22] and stage 2 hypertension.[41] For that reason, a medical screening and clearance should be considered before the child partakes in strenuous exercise and strength training.

10. Skeletal maturity should be a guiding factor when determining the use of overload principles.

References

1. The White House. *Steps to a HealthierUS.* Accessed November 26, 2023. https://georgewbush-whitehouse.archives.gov/news/releases/2002/06/20020620-6.html.
2. Brukner P, Khan K. Chapter 27, Physical activity and the built environment, *Brukner & Khan's Clinical Sports Medicine: The Medicine of Exercise, Volume 2, 5e*; 2019. Available at: https://accessphysiotherapy.mhmedical.com/content.aspx?bookid=2667&sectionid=224524923 Accessed: November 26, 2023 Copyright © 2023 McGraw-Hill Education. All rights reserved.
3. Office of the Surgeon General (US); Office on Disability (US). *The Surgeon General's Call to Action to Improve the Health and Wellness of Persons With Disabilities.* Office of the Surgeon General; 2005. Accessed November 20, 2023. https://www.ncbi.nlm.nih.gov/books/NBK44667/.
4. US Department of Health and Human Services. *Physical Activity Guidelines.* 2nd ed. Accessed November 20, 2023. https://health.gov/sites/default/files/2019-09/Physical_Activity_Guidelines_2nd_edition.pdf.
5. Singh A, Uijtdewilligen L, Twisk JR, van Mechelen W, Chinapaw MM. Physical activity and performance at school: a systematic review of the literature including a methodological quality assessment. *Arch Pediatr Adolesc Med.* 2012;166(1):49-55.
6. Centers for Disease Control and Prevention. Youth Risk Behavior Surveillance—United States, 2011. *Morbid Mortal Wkly Rep.* 2012;61:SS-4.
7. Laura K, McManus T, Harris WA, et al. Youth risk behavior surveillance-United States, 2015. *Morbid Mortal Wkly Rep.* 2016;65(6):1-174.
8. Rideout VJ, Foehr UG, Roberts DF. Generation M2: media in the lives of 8- to 18-year-olds. Rep. Menlo Park: Henry J. Kaiser Family Foundation, 2010. Accessed November 20, 2023. https://www.kff.org/other/poll-finding/report-generation-m2-media-in-the-lives/.
9. Lanningham-Foster L, Foster RC, McCrady SK, et al. Changing the school environment to increase physical activity in children. *Obesity.* 2008;16(8):1849-1853.
10. Obesity Action Coalition. *What Is Childhood Obesity?* Accessed November 20, 2023. https://www.obesityaction.org/get-educated/understanding-childhood-obesity/what-is-childhood-obesity/.
11. Reisinger C, Nkeh-Chungag BN, Fredriksen PM, et al. The prevalence of pediatric metabolic syndrome: a critical look on the discrepancies between definitions and its clinical importance. *Int J Obes.* 2021;45:12-24.
12. Obesity Action Coalition. *OAC Position Statements.* Accessed November 20, 2023. https://www.obesityaction.org/our-purpose/about-us/position-statements/.
13. GBD 2015 Obesity Collaborators, Afshin A, Forouzanfar MH, et al. Health effects of overweight and obesity in 195 countries over 25 year. *N Engl J Med.* 2017;377(1):13-27.
14. Yusuf ZI, Dongarwar D, Yusuf RA, et al. Social determinants of overweight and obesity among children in the United States. *Int J MCH AIDS.* 2020;9(1):22-33.
15. Perreault L, Bessesen D. *Obesity In Adults: Etiology And Risk Factors.* Accessed November 20, 2023. https://www.uptodate.com/contents/obesity-in-adults-etiology-and-risk-factors.
16. Taveras EM, Gillman MW, Pena MM, Redline S, Rifas-Shiman SL. Chronic sleep curtailment and adiposity. *Pediatrics.* 2014;133(6):1013-1022.
17. Hart CN, Carskadon MA, Considine RV, et al. Changes in children's sleep duration on food intake, weight, and leptin. *Pediatrics.* 2013;132(6):e1473-e1480.
18. Sicat J. *Obesity And Genetics: Nature And Nurture.* July 23, 2018. Accessed November 20, 2023. https://obesitymedicine.org/obesity-and-genetics/.
19. Burden SJ, Weedon BD, Turner A, et al. Intensity and duration of physical activity and cardiorespiratory fitness. *Pediatrics.* 2022;150(1):e2021056003.
20. US Department of Health and Human Services, US Department of Agriculture. *2015–2020 Dietary Guidelines for Americans.* 8th ed. Appendix 7. December 2015. Accessed November 20, 2023. https://health.gov/dietaryguidelines/2015/guidelines/appendix-7/.
21. Action for Healthy Kids. *Nutrition Education.* Accessed November 20, 2023. http://www.actionforhealthykids.org/tools-for-schools/find-challenges/classroom-challenges/1212-nutrition-education.
22. American Academy of Pediatrics Council on Sports Medicine and Fitness, McCambridge TM, Stricker PR. Strength training by children and adolescents. *Pediatrics.* 2008;121(4):835-840.
23. Faigenbaum AD, Micheli LJ, American College of Sports Medicine. *Current Comment: Youth Strength Training.* American College of Sports Medicine; 2017. Accessed November 20, 2023. https://www.acsm.org/docs/default-source/files-for-resource-library/smb-youth-strength-training.pdf
24. Cahill BR. *American Orthopaedic Society for Sports Medicine: Proceedings of the Conference on Strength Training and the Prepubescent.* American Orthopaedic Society for Sports Medicine; 1998.

25. Faigenbaum AD, Kraemer WJ, Cahill, et al. Youth resistance training: updated position statement paper from the National Strength and Conditioning Association. *J Strength Cond Res.* 2009;23(5 Suppl):S60-S79.

26. Gillingham G. *AUTISM: Handle with Care! Understanding and Managing Behavior of Children and Adults with Autism.* Future Horizons; 1995.

27. Bumin G, Huri M, Salar S, Kayihan. Occupational therapy in Autism. In: Fitzgerald M. *Autism Spectrum Disorder-Recent Advances.* IntechOpen. April 25, 2015. Accessed November 10, 2023. https://www.intechopen.com/books/autism-spectrum-disorder-recent-advances/occupational-therapy-in-autism.

28. Dahab KS, McCambridge TM. Strength training in children and adolescents: raising the bar for young athletes? *Sports Health.* 2009;1(3):223-226.

29. Faigenbaum AD, Milliken LA, Westcott WL. Maximal strength testing in healthy children. *J Strength Cond Res.* 2003;17:162-166.

30. Faigenbaum AD, Milliken LA, Loud RL, Burak BT, Doherty CL, Westcott WL. Comparison of 1 and 2 days per week of strength training in children. *Res Q Exerc Sport.* 2002:73:416-424.

31. Kraemer WJ, Ratamess NA. Hormonal responses and adaptations to resistance exercise and training. *Sports Med.* 2005;35(4):339-361.

32. Negra Y, Chaabene H, Hammami M, Hachana Y, Granacher U. Effects of high-velocity resistance training on athletic performance in prepuberal male soccer athletes. *J Strength Cond Res.* 2016;30(12):3290-3297.

33. Ozmun JC, Mikesky AE, Surburg PR. Neuromuscular adaptations following prepubescent strength training. *Med Sci Sports Exerc.* 1994;26:510-514.

34. Faude O, Rössler R, Petushek EJ, Roth R, Zahner L, Donath L. Neuromuscular adaptations to multimodal injury prevention programs in youth sports: a systematic review with meta-analysis of randomized controlled trials. *Front Physiol.* 2017;8:791.

35. Peltonen JE, Taimela S, Erkintalo M, Salminen JJ, Oksanen A, Kujala UM. Back extensor and psoas muscle cross sectional area, prior physical training, and trunk muscle strength a longitudinal study in adolescent girls. *Eur J Appl Physiol Occup Physiol.* 1998;77:66-71.

36. Ramsay JA, Blimkie CJ, Smith K, Garner S, MacDougall JD, Sale DG. Strength training effects in prepubescent boys. *Med Sci Sports Exerc.* 1990;22(5):605-614.

37. Del Corral T, Cebria I Iranzo MÀ, López-de-Uralde-Villanueva I, Martínez-Alejos R, Blanco I, Vilaró J. Effectiveness of a home-based active video game programme in young cystic fibrosis patients. *Respiration.* 2018;95(2):87-97.

38. Warburton DER, Nicol CW, Bredin S. Health benefits of physical activity: the evidence. *CMAJ.* 2006;174(6):801-809.

39. Myers AM, Beam NW, Fakhoury JD. Resistance training for children and adolescents. *Transl Pediatr.* 2017;6(3):137-143.

40. Lloyd RS, Radnor JM, De Ste Croix MB, Cronin JB, Oliver JL. Changes in sprint and jump performance after traditional plyometric, and combined resistance training in male youth pre- and post-peak height velocity. *J Strength Cond Res.* 2016;30(5):1239-1247.

41. Rice SG, American Academy of Pediatrics Council on Sports Medicine and Fitness. Medical conditions affecting sports participation. *Pediatrics.* 2008;121(4):841-848.

42. Legerlotz K, Marzilger R, Bohm S, Arampatzis A. Physiological adaptations following resistance training in youth athletes: a narrative review. *Pediatr Exerc Sci.* 2016;28(4):501-520.

43. American Academy of Pediatrics Committee on Injury and Poison Prevention and Sports Medicine and Fitness. Swimming programs for infants and children. *Pediatrics.* 2000;105:868-870.

19

Lower Extremity Orthoses for Children

Kathy Martin, PT, DHSc

LEARNING OBJECTIVES

Upon completion of this chapter, the reader will be able to:

- Identify the indications and contraindications for common lower extremity orthoses.
- Design an evaluation specifically for determining lower extremity orthotic needs of a child.
- Compare and contrast how intervention philosophies based on biomechanics and motor learning may

influence orthotic decisions, including when to introduce and dosage.
- Summarize the key concepts for patient/caregiver education when fitting a lower extremity orthosis.
- Appraise the evidence for lower extremity orthotic efficacy for children.

INTRODUCTION

The use of lower extremity orthoses to address standing and gait deficits in children with movement system dysfunction has been a part of the standard of rehabilitation care for decades. However, newer materials (eg, plastics) and application of contemporary understanding of motor learning theories have led to a paradigm shift in the past 10 to 15 years. This chapter will cover the traditional understanding of orthotic intervention as well as newer concepts that are emerging. Various orthotic styles and their indications, precautions, and contraindications will be discussed along with a review of the current evidence for the efficacy of each style of orthosis. Gaps and controversies in our current evidence will also be explored.

Important factors for determining which style of orthosis to be used will be discussed. This will include common examination techniques as well as important biopsychosocial factors to consider in order to provide family-centered care. Outcome measures to monitor the effects of orthotic intervention across all domains of the International Classification of Functioning, Disability, and Health (ICF)[1] will be identified along with their advantages and disadvantages.

The logistics of how to obtain an orthosis and work with an orthotist to obtain the best individual solution for each child will be discussed along with guidelines for how to evaluate the fit, how to educate the patient and caregiver about proper use, and when to refer the family back to an orthotist. Finally, this chapter will explore how an orthotic intervention fits into the bigger picture of the child's physical therapy plan of care.

Several case studies will be included to help the reader apply the concepts in this chapter.

TERMINOLOGY

The word *orthosis* is a noun, and its plural form is *orthoses*. The term *orthotic* is an adjective and frequently used incorrectly. Using the term orthotic to refer to the actual device is slang and technically incorrect. To refer to the specific brace or device, the correct term is orthosis. The adjective form is correctly used when it is describing a noun, such as orthotic device or orthotic intervention. Although this may seem to be a minor point, all physical therapists should strive to use technically correct language. Unfortunately, much of the peer-reviewed literature contributes to the confusion by using the term *orthotic* incorrectly.

Orthoses may be rigid or dynamic. These terms may also be used to describe the patient's impairments of body structure. For example, a rigid, or fixed, deformity is one that cannot be passively or manually corrected. A dynamic, or flexible, deformity can be manually corrected. Identifying the type of body structure impairment a patient has is an important part of the examination and orthotic prescription process. A rigid orthosis is one that does not allow movement and will fully constrain the joints or body segments that it covers. The term *static* may also be used instead of rigid, but the meaning is the same. However, a dynamic orthosis will allow some movement. This may be only one movement and in only one plane, or it may allow some movement in all planes. The term *dynamic orthosis* may be used to describe a wide variety of orthotic devices and, as a result, is often too general to help identify the specific style of orthosis. The only point that can be known for sure when the term *dynamic orthosis* is used is that some movement will be allowed.

Orthoses may be either custom-made or off-the-shelf. Custom-made orthoses are ones that are made to fit one specific patient and are typically fabricated from cast molds of the patient's lower extremities. Occasionally custom-made orthoses can be made from measurements, but a cast mold is more common. Off-the-shelf orthoses are not specific to any particular patient and are usually selected based on the patient's shoe size. There are advantages and disadvantages to both types: custom orthoses usually provide a better fit and thus may provide better control, but they are also much more expensive. Custom orthoses are generally indicated for individuals with rigid deformities or more complex movement dysfunction. Off-the-shelf orthoses may provide adequate results for patients with emerging motor control and those who do not have any joint deformity. Although not ideal, the cost of custom orthoses may be the deciding factor in that some families may only be able to afford an off-the-shelf style and this choice may be better than no orthosis at all.

GOALS OF ORTHOTIC INTERVENTION

The goals of orthotic intervention vary depending on the severity of the child's body structure impairments and activity limitations, but ultimately, orthoses are used to minimize deficits across all domains of the ICF. For cerebral palsy (CP), an international and multidisciplinary conference was convened in 2008 by the International Society of Prosthetics and Orthotics with the goal of reviewing the evidence for orthotic intervention for children with CP and developing consensus recommendations based on that evidence.[2] One outcome of this consensus conference was the identification of specific goals for orthotic intervention for CP based on the Gross Motor Function Classification System (GMFCS). These goals are listed in **Table 19-1**.

Goals of orthotic intervention such as the ones identified for CP have not been specifically identified for other conditions. However, the current standard of care for children with movement disorders implies that orthoses are used to improve or maintain ambulation for children who have that capacity and to improve alignment and prevent deformity for children with more severe impairments and activity limitations. Regardless of whether specific goals have been published in the peer-reviewed

TABLE 19-1 • Cerebral Palsy Goals Based on Gross Motor Function Classification System (GMFCS)

GMFCS Levels I, II, and III
• Improve or maintain efficient gait
• Prevent deformity[2]
GMFCS Levels IV and V
• Prevent spine and hip deformities
• Improve sitting posture
• Enable upright standing and weight bearing[2]

literature or not, every physical therapist should have clear goals identified before initiating orthotic intervention for any child.

NAMING CONVENTION FOR ORTHOSES

The general rule is that lower extremity orthoses are named by the joints that they enclose or constrain. For example, an ankle-foot orthosis (AFO) encloses the foot and ankle, but not the knee. This is perhaps an oversimplification of the way orthoses are named, and not all orthotic names provide an adequate picture of what the device looks like; however, this convention can be a helpful starting point. **Table 19-2** provides the name, indications, and contraindications for the most common lower extremity orthoses in use today, but it is not an exhaustive list of all of the possible orthotic devices available.

INDICATIONS AND CONTRAINDICATIONS

One of the major challenges for pediatric physical therapists and orthotists alike is predicting which type of device will be the most effective for a child. Although Table 19-2 provides general indications, contraindications, and precautions, the efficacy of a device will depend on the quality of the child's motor control, their strength, and other biopsychosocial factors. These factors are often difficult to measure, and thus, there is no simple formula or chart that will accurately predict which orthosis will work the best. The information in Table 19-2 should be considered a general starting point, but there will always be additional considerations.

For devices that go above the knee (hip-knee-ankle-foot orthoses [HKAFOs] and knee-ankle-foot orthoses [KAFOs]), a key consideration will be how to manage knee range of motion. Most orthoses in these 2 categories will have a hinge at the knee joint that allows flexion and extension, but there is also usually a mechanism to control how much flexion is allowed and to lock the knee in full extension to provide stability in stance. The ankle part of the device is often solid, limiting all ankle motion, to limit the degrees of freedom a child has to control. Without this limitation of those degrees of freedom, the child would likely be unable to stand or ambulate. One final consideration is that larger orthoses that constrain more joints like the 2 in this category are more expensive, more challenging to make, and heavier. Their use will be primarily to allow for static standing, household ambulation, or perhaps exercise.

A key decision-making factor when deciding between a KAFO and an AFO will be the severity of genu recurvatum in stance. By design, any AFO that limits plantar flexion (PF) can help prevent genu recurvatum because the device controls the position of the tibia in the stance phase of gait. However, if the genu recurvatum is severe, an AFO will likely not be sufficient, and the better choice will be the KAFO.

With the great variety of AFOs on the market, deciding between various styles can be a challenge. The child's ability to control knee extension in stance is one thing to consider when trying to decide between a solid AFO and a hinged AFO. If the child has a tendency to drop into a crouch or the knee buckles in stance phase, the solid AFO would be a better choice because the hinged AFO will not control DF or help to maintain a

TABLE 19-2 • Orthotic Types

Orthosis	Photo	Indications	Contraindications/ Precautions	Additional Comments
Hip-knee-ankle-foot orthosis (HKAFO)		Poor voluntary motor control of entire lower extremity in stance (eg, upper lumbar myelomeningocele); household ambulation or exercise	Inability to maintain upright trunk, even with upper extremity support (crutches, walker); high energy requirement—not practical for community ambulation	Usually, solid ankle but knee may be free or lockable; will need assistive device such as walker or crutches
Knee-ankle-foot orthosis (KAFO)		Poor voluntary control of the knee, ankle, and foot; control of severe genu recurvatum or knee buckling in stance (eg, L3/L4 myelomeningocele, polio, muscular dystrophy); household ambulation or exercise	Inability to control hip and pelvis in stance; not practical for community ambulation secondary to high energy requirement	Usually, solid ankle but knee may be free or lockable; may need assistive device such as walker or crutches
Solid ankle-foot-orthosis (AFO)		Poor ankle and foot control; maintain neutral ankle position in all planes; prevent equinus gait/toe walking or drop foot; control mild to moderate genu recurvatum in stance	May not be enough to control severe genu recurvatum in stance; limits transitional movements requiring dorsiflexion (DF), such as sit or squat from or to stand and descending stairs	May or may not need assistive device—dependent on postural control
Posterior leaf spring AFO		Similar to solid AFO but with enough voluntary control to maintain knee extension in stance	Similar to solid AFO; may exacerbate crouch gait by allowing increased DF in stance	Posterior strut is flexible enough to bend under child's body weight, allowing some DF in mid and terminal stance
Hinged AFO		Similar to solid AFO but with enough voluntary control to maintain knee extension in stance	Similar to solid AFO; may exacerbate crouch gait by allowing increased DF in stance	May or may not need assistive device—dependent on postural control; hinge adds bulk, weight, and cost

(Continued)

TABLE 19-2 • Orthotic Types (*Continued*)

Orthosis	Photo	Indications	Contraindications/ Precautions	Additional Comments
Ground reaction AFO (GRAFO)		Crouch gait secondary to hypotonia (eg, myelomeningocele); usually solid ankle but occasionally may see hinged to allow limited plantar flexion (PF) and DF	Hip and knee flexion contractures >15 degrees[3]	May also be called anterior shell AFO or floor reaction AFO; may or may not need assistive device
Kiddie Gait AFO	Source: Allard INT/Camp Scandinavia.	Similar to solid AFO, but it does allow some DF and PF	Does not control calcaneus or midfoot so will not control pronation or supination; squatting and descending stairs difficult with minimal DF allowed	Extremely lightweight; some energy return properties and may assist with push-off; consider pairing with SMO for pronation control
Ankle-foot orthosis footwear combination (AFOFC)		Poor ankle and knee control (eg, spastic cerebral palsy); typically, solid AFO with wedge on sole of shoe to accommodate PF contractures	Inability to stand, even with assistive device	See Owen[4] for more comprehensive information on this option
Supramalleolar orthosis (SMO)	Source: Cascade Dafo, Inc.	Poor control of pronation and supination; will allow free PF and DF	Will not control drop foot, toe walking, or genu recurvatum in stance	A wide variety of styles available with variability in degree of control
AFO-SMO combo		Benefits of both a solid AFO and an SMO; can be used together or SMO alone depending on task and child's status	Same as noted for solid AFOs and SMOs	Increased cost but twice the options
Foot orthoses (FOs)		Poor control of pronation; allows free DF and PF	Severe pronation will likely need SMO; will not control toe walking	Typically, not reimbursed by insurance; many off-the-shelf choices

vertical tibia in stance. However, if the child does have voluntary control of the knee, the hinged AFO will make floor transitions and stairs easier because of the free dorsiflexion (DF).

The carbon fiber Kiddie Gait AFO by Allard USA[5] does have some limited flexibility to it because of the materials used to make it. Because the carbon fiber does give a little under the child's body weight, a limited amount of both PF and DF is allowed. Although it is primarily anecdotal information, the Kiddie Gait is suggested to have some energy-returning properties to help with push-off. However, full DF is blocked, so transitions that require ankle DF, such as squatting, getting up from the floor, and descending stairs, will still be challenging with the Kiddie Gait AFO. The one major drawback to the Kiddie Gait is that the hindfoot is open, and thus, it does not provide any calcaneal control or pronation control. This can be remedied by adding a supramalleolar orthosis (SMO) on top of the footplate.

Ground reaction AFOs (GRAFOs) may be the most misunderstood devices. They were developed for low-tone crouch gait, such as seen with myelomeningocele. The GRAFO has often been described as the orthosis of choice for "crouch gait" and has frequently been used with crouch gait secondary to spasticity, such as with spastic diplegic CP. In the presence of hip and knee flexion contractures greater than 15 degrees, this orthosis is not the best choice.[3] Because the GRAFO ankle is solid and maintains the child's ankle in a neutral position, hip and knee flexion contractures will place the child's center of gravity behind their feet. The result is that the child will either fall backward or have to go up on their toes to stay upright. In my opinion, kids with crouch gait secondary to spasticity are probably the most challenging to brace, but the more recent concept of the AFO footwear combination by Elaine Owen[4] may be the better option for children with crouch gait and hip and knee flexion contractures. Owen's approach is beyond the scope of this chapter but has been described in more detail in other texts.

The challenge of deciding between an AFO and an SMO has been made easier by the emergence of AFO-SMO combinations. These devices offer the best of both options and may be ideal for children whose skills are expected to change before they outgrow an orthosis. For example, a child who is working on walking but still uses creeping on the floor as their primary means of mobility would be a good candidate for this device. The SMO could be used alone when the child is moving around the environment independently on the floor, but the AFO shell could be added for assisted standing and walking. These devices may also be helpful for a child with poor muscular endurance for walking. The SMO may be enough for part of the day, but the AFO shell may need to be added once the child begins to fatigue. The physical therapist also has the choice to either increase or decrease the support during a therapeutic activity, depending on the child's need for assistance.

Similar to AFOs, SMOs come in a variety of styles with differences in rigidity of the plastic, trimlines, and length of the footplate. The commonality though is that DF and PF are not limited. The SureStep SMO[6] was specifically designed for children with hypotonia and is made from thin and flexible plastic. The footplate of the SureStep ends proximal to the metatarsal heads, leaving the toes free to flex and extend.[6] This improves the child's ability to run, jump, and use ankle balance strategies. More traditional SMOs often have a full-length footplate and are more rigid.

As noted in Table 19-2, most third-party payors will not pay for custom foot orthoses (FOs). There are many off-the-shelf versions of FOs available, and these are often used because of the lack of payment for custom FOs. There is no evidence to date to indicate whether custom FOs are better than off-the-shelf versions. In addition to using FOs to help control overpronation, usually secondary to hypotonia, FOs may be a good option for the noninvolved side in spastic hemiplegic CP. If the child with spastic hemiplegia needs an orthosis on the involved side, even the thinnest of plastic will create some degree of leg length discrepancy if an orthosis is only used on one side. Putting an FO in the shoe on the noninvolved side can help minimize the leg length discrepancy and subsequent gait deviations that are induced by that difference between sides.

One additional term that is frequently used is dynamic ankle-foot orthosis (DAFO). The concept was originated by Nancy Hylton, PT and licensed orthotist. She was using a full-contact footplate and wraparound 2-part plaster casts in her clinical practice. Don Buethorn, CPO and founder of the Cascade DAFO company, was able to take her concept and create plastic dynamic orthoses.[7] The Cascade DAFO company uses the term DAFO in the name of nearly all of its products, so additional descriptors are needed in order to clearly understand the orthotic device and what it is intended to do. Even though the term DAFO originally described one specific type of device, its meaning is now very ambiguous and can imply any style of orthosis, including various styles of AFOs, SMOs, and FOs. At best, the term DAFO implies that the orthosis is not rigid and will allow some movement.

OTHER FACTORS FOR ORTHOTIC SELECTION

Another consideration for all orthoses, regardless of type, is the length of the footplate. Most orthoses have a full-length footplate, meaning it extends distally to the end of the toes. A full-length footplate will assist with achieving knee extension in stance because it eliminates the toe "break" or toe extension during terminal stance. This effectively moves the line of ground reaction force more forward, producing a stronger extension moment at the knee. Choosing to end the footplate behind the metatarsal heads would restore the toe extension at terminal stance. The length of the footplate should be customized to allow the child the most functional gait pattern.

SHOE CHOICE

One last consideration for choosing an orthotic device is what type of shoe will be worn with the orthosis. A good orthosis in a bad shoe will lead to a poor result. The shoe is the foundation for the orthosis, and if the shoe is worn down, too tight, or even too large, the orthosis will likely not provide the expected outcome. A shoe that is worn down may put the lower extremity in poor alignment, despite the orthosis. A shoe that is too tight may cause pressure points and skin breakdown, whereas a shoe that is too large will add unnecessary weight and length. The added length will change the line of ground reaction force as noted earlier in the discussion of length of the orthotic footplate. For all these reasons, helping the family to choose the right shoe for the orthosis is just as important as choosing the right orthosis.

Shoe fit over an orthosis is a common complaint and frustration for families. Traditionally the orthosis requires 1 to 1½ larger size to accommodate the bulk of the orthosis, depending on its style and thickness. Finding a shoe with a wide enough toe box is usually the issue. Several manufacturers now make shoes designed specifically to go over orthoses. This has minimized the hassle for many families and also allowed the child to have a shoe that is stylish and similar to what their peers wear. One orthotic company, SureStep, has put together a website summarizing the options for parents.[8] A similar resource appears on a digital health community called "The Mighty."[9] Neither of these 2 sources are likely all-inclusive, but a quick Internet search for "shoes that fit over orthoses" will turn up multiple options. The primary point is that shoe manufacturers have realized that this market exists, and they are now creating new designs to meet the needs of these families.

■ NIGHT SPLINTS

One final category of orthoses for patients with CP to consider is night splints. These typically resemble solid AFOs but are intended to be worn during sleep to provide a low-load, prolonged stretch of the calf muscles, and they are not designed for ambulation. They often have straps that can be adjusted with Velcro to vary the intensity of the stretch (**Figure 19-1**). Simple knee immobilizers are often used to provide a low-load stretch to the hamstrings. The theoretical concept for night splints is to prevent or manage contracture that may develop over time as a result of spasticity.[10] As you will read later in this chapter, that

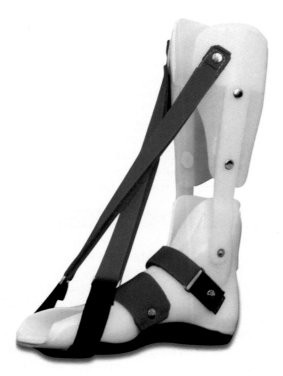

FIGURE 19-1 Nightsplint.

theoretical framework is being questioned by some researchers. A 2016 systematic review by Craig et al[11] concluded that the evidence for the use of orthoses or night splints to prevent contractures was "both insufficient and conflicting." Poor compliance with night splints has been identified as an issue as well, and the effectiveness of the prolonged stretch may be overshadowed by the "hassle factor" if the splints interfere with the child's ability to sleep. Using a stoplight grading system, Craig et al[11] gave the use of orthoses and night splints to prevent contracture a yellow light, meaning that this intervention should be used cautiously and outcomes must be tracked in order assess the effectiveness of the intervention.

■ EVIDENCE FOR ORTHOTIC EFFICACY

CEREBRAL PALSY

Quite a few studies have been published regarding orthotic efficacy in CP, but the methodology is so varied across the studies that generalizations are challenging to make. To efficiently use this literature base, systematic reviews and the documents from the 2008 International Society of Prosthetics and Orthotics conference are the best places to start.[2,12]

The majority of studies use 3-dimensional (3D) gait analysis and indicate that AFOs with a PF stop (ie, solid, hinged, or GRAFO) will effectively improve the ankle position at initial contact to minimize or eliminate toe walking.[2,11,13,14] These studies also show improved gait velocity and stride length.[2,11,13,14] Most researchers have theorized that the velocity and stride length improvements are a result of the better ankle position at initial contact. Interestingly, Morris et al[2] noted that these results are equivocal in studies that focus exclusively on children with spastic diplegic CP. Rogozinski et al[3] found that GRAFOs were able to improve knee extension in mid-stance and velocity and stride length for children who had hip and knee flexion contractures less than 10 degrees, and in their discussion, they propose that hip or knee flexion contractures greater than 15 degrees should be considered a contraindication for GRAFOs.[3]

Studies that have measured energy efficiency have shown less consistent results. The systematic review by Figueiredo et al[13] concluded that AFOs *usually* improve the energy expenditure of gait. Of the studies reviewed by these authors, AFOs decreased energy expenditure in 4 studies, 1 study showed no change, and 1 study showed increased energy expenditure. Figueiredo et al[13] commented that hinged AFOs or posterior leaf spring AFOs improved energy expenditure the most. The reason for this is not clearly identified by the data as the studies were too heterogeneous to directly compare, but these 2 devices allow DF in mid and terminal stance and thus allow some tibial advancement over the foot. Two other studies imply that AFOs improve energy expenditure for children with more severe motor impairments.[15,16] Brehm et al[15] found improved energy expenditure for children with spastic quadriplegic CP, but it was unchanged for children with spastic diplegic and spastic hemiplegic CP. Kerkum et al[16] found that energy expenditure was improved if knee extension in stance was improved, and these authors commented that the best benefit was seen in children with the highest baseline energy cost.

A few studies have used electromyography (EMG) as an outcome measure and shown decreased muscle activation and improved standing endurance with solid AFOs.[15,17,18] Leonard et al[19] found increased standing but not decreased EMG activity in AFOs that optimized shank to vertical (tibia) alignment. An exploratory study by Lindskov et al[20] on the effect of AFOs on muscle activity was conducted with 17 children with unilateral CP. Lindskov et al[20] used EMG to explore the effect of a contoured versus flat AFO footplate on the medial gastrocnemius and anterior tibialis. Although total muscle activity was not significantly different, both types of footplates decreased medial gastrocnemius activity in early stance phase and tibialis anterior activity in swing phase.[20] The contoured footplate led to the greatest decrease in muscle activity. Lindskov et al[20] noted that the AFOs may help decrease the "spastic activation" of the medial gastrocnemius; however, early stance phase requires eccentric gastrocnemius function to help decelerate forward momentum. What remains unanswered is whether this reduction in medial gastrocnemius activity is helpful or hinders gait function. EMG may not be the best tool to answer this question as it is only able to capture activity and not force production.

Based on an observational comparison study, Morris[12] noted significant variation in orthotic prescription and clinician uncertainty about which orthosis would give the best results. Morris[12] went on to comment that children with less severe impairments may benefit more from less restrictive designs, such as SMOs, hinged AFOs, and posterior leaf spring AFOs. However, Morris[12] did not clarify or define what was meant by "less severe impairments." This author and others have found that restricting the ankle joint movement with an orthosis will reduce power generation and absorption at the ankle during gait.[2,12,21] Limpaninlachat et al[22] offer some additional support to the concept that less restrictive designs may be better for some children. In the study by Limpaninlachat et al,[22] hinged AFOs led to better scores on the Functional Reach Test compared to solid AFOs, and children who were able to walk without an assistive device also had greater stride length and velocity with hinged AFOs versus solid AFOs.

Certain orthotic designs have been proposed to decrease muscle tone for individuals with spasticity.[23] These designs include a metatarsal bar, toe extension, positioning in subtalar neutral, and molding the areas surround the Achilles tendon insertion in a way to induce weight bearing. To date, studies have been unable to confirm that these features do influence spasticity.[24,25] Kobayashi et al[24] noted that the quality of the evidence was too low to draw any conclusions. Kobayashi et al[24] also commented that there is currently no definitive method to quantify spasticity and cited this as a barrier to truly evaluating the proposed benefits of these designs. Overall, tone-reducing features do not seem to offer any additional benefit in regard to functional outcomes compared to standard AFOs without these features.[24,25]

The concept that positioning the ankle in subtalar neutral in an orthosis will improve function was evaluated by Westberry et al.[26] Westberry et al[26] retrospectively evaluated standing radiographs of 160 feet (102 children with CP) both barefoot and wearing orthoses. The results indicated some statistically significant changes in the pitch of the calcaneus (sagittal plane), hindfoot varus, and forefoot planus. However, Westberry et al[26] did not find any statistically significant changes in the midfoot and concluded that the statistically significant changes they did find were probably not large enough to be clinically important. The overall conclusion of Westberry et al[26] was that the functional benefits of the orthoses were likely the result of external support and stability and not a result of changes in bony alignment. An earlier and less rigorous study by Ricks and Eilert[27] came to the same conclusion about inhibitory casts; that is, the benefit was not the result of improved bony alignment. A recent study by Jarvis et al[28] with healthy individuals further challenges the concept that subtalar neutral is the key to proper function, but it still seems to be a pervasive basis for orthotic design.

Paradigm Shift?

The theoretical framework that orthoses influence muscle tone and improve alignment has poor support in the literature. The other prevailing concept is that the external support from the orthoses is the reason for gait improvements that have been documented. Admittedly, this rigid support comes at the cost of reduced ankle power generation, but this may be an acceptable compromise for children with severe gait dysfunction.[2] Recent evidence though is beginning to spark questions about whether or not providing rigid external stability is the right approach. Multiple studies have recently shown that a key issue for young children with CP is not spasticity but rather a failure of muscle growth.[29-31] Willerslev-Olsen et al[30] published a study and concluded that passive muscle stiffness was the cause of contracture development, not spasticity. Willerslev-Olsen et al[30] also noted that distinguishing between spasticity and passive muscle stiffness was clinically difficult and that passive muscle stiffness was already present by age 3 years. Herskind et al[29] followed up with a study using magnetic resonance imaging (MRI) and ultrasound that confirmed that, in children with CP, the medial gastrocnemius muscle growth decreases (compared to typically developing children) at the age of 15 months while overall growth remains typical. One of the key findings by Herskind et al[29] was that the sarcomeres of the medial gastrocnemius were actually lengthened. This finding is a game changer because if contractures were the result of spasticity, leading to excessive contraction and shortening of the overall muscle, then sarcomeres should also be shortened. However, if overall bone growth remains similar to typically developing children but muscle growth is limited, then the lengthened sarcomeres make sense. The bone is elongating but the muscle is not keeping pace, resulting in sarcomeres being stretched or pulled apart. Herskind et al[29] stated that their results regarding poor muscle growth in CP supported the hypothesis that contractures were related to a failure of muscle growth and not spasticity.

Herskind et al[29] proposed that the reduced muscle growth was from a lack of neuromechanical stimulation, meaning weight bearing and gross motor activity. One of the challenges in orthotic prescription for children with CP is to balance the need to provide some external stability yet not limit the opportunity for neuromechanical stimulation. Orthoses do provide opportunity for bearing weight and gross motor activity, but this is often done with the muscle in one fixed length versus allowing the muscle to work through its full range of motion. Although it has not been specifically studied or quantified, disuse atrophy of the gastrocnemius and soleus is a common side effect of long-term use of AFOs that block PF. The development of newer materials (plastics) that allow more dynamic orthoses may be one solution to this dilemma. Another solution may be that the theoretical framework for why we use orthoses needs to change to recognize the important role of muscle growth. Ultimately, this may lead to changes in design and dosage (hours of wear). The recent emphasis on the need to stimulate muscle growth may also be part of the explanation for why the evidence for night splints is insufficient and conflicting as noted earlier.[11] Newer evidence suggests that muscle (sarcomere) length is not the key problem in the development of contracture.[30] Although a low load prolonged stretch may be helpful for the connective tissue components, the muscle fibers themselves do not need to be lengthened.

MYELOMENINGOCELE

Of the diagnostic groups covered in this chapter, myelomeningocele has the fewest number of studies published regarding orthotic efficacy. Perhaps it is because this group may be the least controversial in regard to orthotic prescription. The studies of orthotic efficacy for myelomeningocele typically categorize the children into 2 groups: high-level lesions (upper lumber and thoracic level) and low-level lesions (lower lumber and sacral level). One systematic review by Mazur and Kyle[32] has been written, and only a few studies[33-35] have come out since that review was done. The systematic review by Mazur and Kyle[32] included 33 articles published between 1974 and 2003 with 20 of those studies focused on high-level lesions and 13 articles focused on lower-level lesions. The outcome of interest was how orthoses affected ambulation, with velocity and energy expenditure noted as the most common measures used.

For the high-level myelomeningocele category, Mazur and Kyle[32] concluded that there was little change in velocity or energy expenditure when walking with a parapodium, reciprocal gait orthosis, or HKAFO. The overall conclusion of Mazur and Kyle[32] was that ambulation training with orthoses for upper-level lesions was controversial because the data did not support that this was effective. However, none of the studies reviewed investigated the other possible benefits of orthotic use for this population, including prevention of secondary impairments or the benefits of standing (vs walking). The benefits of standing may include improved pulmonary and gastrointestinal function, better bone health, and even just the psychosocial benefits of being at eye level with peers who are standing.

Regardless of focus of past studies with the high-level myelomeningocele group, the current philosophy seems to be that orthoses may facilitate standing and that this may indeed be valuable during childhood. Ambulation with orthoses is often viewed as a form of exercise versus a means to acquire or improve ambulation ability. Often this is abandoned once children hit their adolescent growth spurt and their body size and weight become more challenging to manage.

Children with lower-level myelomeningocele often have a much better prognosis for achieving independent ambulation with orthoses and/or assistive devices. The Mazur and Kyle[32] systematic review concluded that ambulation training with orthoses that blocked PF (ie, AFOs) for this group was indeed effective. Their conclusions were that AFOs could decrease the excessive DF in stance phase (ie, crouch gait), decrease double support time, and increase velocity.[32] Although not explicitly stated, a decrease in double support time also means an increase in single limb support time and that may be interpreted as improved stability in stance. One final point from this systematic review was that AFOs may possibly increase the rotational forces in the transverse plane at the knee and that this must be carefully monitored.[32]

Since that review was published, a few additional studies have been published.[33-35] For the higher-level category, Arazpour et al[33] investigated isocentric reciprocal gait orthoses for 5 children with T12 to L3 lesions. The children did gait training, standing, and balance activities for 2 hours per day for 8 weeks. At the end of 8 weeks, the children showed improved hip range of motion in gait, increased velocity, increased step length, and decreased compensatory movements. An interesting note here is the intensity (frequency and duration) of the intervention in this study.[33] In the Mazur and Kyle[32] systematic review, most of the 20 studies involving high-level lesions did their data collection all in 1 day. The results of the Arazpour et al[33] study contradict what was stated by Mazur and Kyle,[32] and the intensity of the intervention in the Arazpour et al[33] study is one striking difference.

For the lower-level category, the studies that have been published since the systematic review have very small sample sizes and compare 2 types of AFOs.[34,35] The Kane and Barden[34] case report noted that a GRAFO gave the best results, even in the presence of significant unilateral tibial torsion. In a pilot study with 5 children, Wolf et al[35] found that a carbon fiber spring AFO offered a small increase in velocity, cadence, and step length when compared to a hinged AFO.

Overall, the state of the science for children with myelomeningocele is that there is not a large literature base but what is available is consistently supportive of the use of orthoses to improve ambulation for those with lower-level lesions, but the evidence is less clear for higher-level lesions. One study by Arazpour et al[33] with increased intensity of intervention showed the benefit of using reciprocating gait orthoses as exercise equipment, but the one systematic review noted no benefit with orthoses for ambulation training for children with higher-level lesions.[33] The benefits of standing have not been investigated.

HYPOTONIA AND DOWN SYNDROME

The population of children with hypotonia is very heterogeneous and often poorly defined as a result of the lack of a quantitative measure for hypotonia. Children with hypotonia should not be confused with children with flexible flat foot because these are 2 different conditions. The specific condition most often associated with hypotonia is Down syndrome (DS), and many studies on orthotic efficacy for this group focus on children with DS. Whether or not the results of these studies with children with DS can be generalized to children with hypotonia but without DS is a matter of debate, but there really is not much else to assist decision-making except for these studies.

One systematic review by Weber and Martin[36] has been published in regard to orthotic efficacy for children with hypotonia. Ten studies were reviewed, all of which had been published since 2001. The reviewed studies were too varied to perform a meta-analysis and the overall quality of the evidence was generally weak, but the primary conclusion of this systematic review was that both SMOs and FOs appear to improve body structure and activity level measures. One study by Looper and Martin[37] with participation level outcomes has been published after this systematic review.

Selby-Silverstein et al[38] used in-shoe pressure mapping sensors to evaluate the effect of custom-made FOs on foot function and gait in 16 children with DS (mean age ~5 years old). Selby-Silverstein et al[38] found immediate decrease in calcaneal eversion in standing and a decrease in variability in foot function during gait, meaning a more consistent pattern of movement was shown by the pressure mapping. Hashimoto et al[39] also documented the effects of shoes plus custom molded insoles (FOs) and found increased walking speed, step length, and single leg stance time compared to barefoot. Three case reports with children with hypotonia and varied conditions also provided evidence that FOs improve activity level measures through the use of portions of the Peabody Developmental Motor Scales before and after orthotic intervention.[40-42]

Ross and Shore[43] also studied the effects of FOs, but they used an off-the-shelf version. The study by Ross and Shore[43] was a randomized controlled trial comparing the effect of the FO alone to the FO in combination with "gross motor therapy" with children with developmental delay and flexible flat foot (mean age ~3 years old) who were ambulating independently. The specifics of the gross motor therapy were not well described in this article. Ross and Shore[43] study outcomes measures were the arch index and spatial-temporal gait data using the GAITRite mat.[44] The results showed significantly greater improvement in the arch index for the orthotic group and improvements toward age-appropriate normative values for the spatial-temporal data for both groups.[43] Although the arch index improved in the children using the FOs, this body structure measure has not been specifically correlated with function, and the authors did not report their reliability with this measure. Since the control group of children with DS also showed improved gait with just gross motor therapy, the benefit of using FOs may not be as important as the data seem to imply.[43]

Pitetti and Wondra[45] conducted a study with 25 children with developmental delay and hypotonia with a mean age of approximately 4 years old. The intervention was an off-the-shelf FO, and the outcome measure was the locomotion section of the Peabody Developmental Motor Scales, Second Edition. The participants were a very heterogeneous group, but overall, the authors reported significantly higher raw scores after 2 months of FO use. However, Pitetti and Wondra[45] made an interesting

observation about their data by stating that although the group showed significant improvements overall, the children with DS did not improve as much as the children with hypotonia from other conditions. Based on this observation, Pitetti and Wondra[45] recommended that although children with DS may benefit from an FO, an SMO would likely be more effective, and they proposed that children with DS need more support than the FO provided.

Multiple studies have examined the effect of SMOs with children with DS. Martin[46] found that children with DS who were walking independently (mean age ~6 years old) showed significant improvement in Gross Motor Function Measure (GMFM) scores immediately after fitting of the SureStep SMO[6] and then even more improvement in GMFM scores 7 weeks later. The balance subtest of the Bruininks-Oseretsky Test of Motor Proficiency was also used. The participants showed significant improvement on this measure after 7 weeks of SMO use. Martin[46] also looked at the impact of degree of joint laxity on the results, and although the children with greater laxity had fewer overall skills, their response to the orthotic intervention was similar to the children with less overall laxity. A single-system design study by Tamminga et al[47] compared 2 styles of SMOs, one more flexible and wraparound than the other. The study by Tamminga et al[47] only included 2 participants, so the results must be viewed with caution; however, the data appeared to indicate that the more flexible type of SMO was more effective and preferred over the more rigid style. Looper and Martin[37] did the only study to date that included participation level measures in 20 children with DS who had been walking for at least a year and had not used any orthoses for at least 1 month. After 4 weeks of using the SureStep SMO, improvements were seen in both activity level measures (GMFM Walking, Running, and Jumping scale) and parent-identified participation goals as determined by Goal Attainment Scaling. Parent-identified goals that were met with the use of orthoses included greater walking endurance and increased play time outside.[37]

The effectiveness of SMOs with children with DS has been the focus of several studies by Looper and colleagues.[37,48,49] Looper and Ulrich[48] followed up on the classic treadmill training study with infants with DS by adding SureStep SMOs to the protocol. This randomized controlled trial compared treadmill training with and without SMOs. The findings were mixed in that although the group with the SMOs achieved independent ambulation sooner (moderate treatment effect) than the control group, the control group had better overall GMFM scores at 1 month after onset of independent walking. Looper and Ulrich[48] suggested that although the SMOs appeared to speed up the acquisition of independent walking, they may have constrained the ankle too much and limited exploration of ankle control. The recommendation of Looper and Ulrich,[48] based on motor learning principles, was to wait until after the onset of independent walking to begin orthotic intervention.

The study by Looper and Ulrich[48] was the first to question when to initiate intervention. Common standard of care has always been to introduce orthoses when a child is interested in being on their feet and beginning to pull to stand. Although the randomized controlled design was strong, the sample sizes were small (experimental, n = 10; control, n = 7), and several children dropped out of the control group in order to initiate orthotic intervention. Thus, this recommendation to wait until after onset of independent walking to begin orthotic intervention remains controversial.

Because studies have shown beneficial effects of both FOs and SMOs for children with DS, an obvious question is how to choose between the 2 options. Looper et al[49] conducted a pilot study with 6 children with DS between the ages of 4 and 7 years to determine which data points might predict which style of orthosis (FO vs SMO) led to the best outcome. The results from the Looper et al[49] study were a bit surprising in that anthropomorphic data (height, weight, leg length, and joint hypermobility) may be better predictors than biomechanical data, such as calcaneal eversion in standing and navicular drop test. Looper et al[49] also acknowledged that biomechanical data were harder to get with this population and the sample size was quite small.[49] Thus, there is still no conclusive evidence to help with the FO versus SMO decision.

QUALITY OF THE EVIDENCE

For all 3 of diagnostic categories discussed, the evidence for orthotic efficacy suffers from small sample sizes, variability in the study designs and orthotic devices studied, use of barefoot as the control condition, and short-term intervention periods. The variability in design and orthoses studied prevents systematic reviews with meta-analysis. Even understanding the exact nature of the intervention is challenging as many orthoses are not completely described or different terms for similar devices are used across studies.[13] The barefoot condition is not a meaningful control condition because it overestimates the contribution of the shoe.[25,50,51] About half of all of the orthotic studies completed data collection all in 1 day; thus, these studies cannot provide insight into the long-term use of orthoses. Most children wear orthoses for months if not years, yet none of the studies provide data on the effects of orthoses for more than a few months at most.

Overall, the peer-reviewed literature provides preliminary evidence for the effects of orthoses on body structure and activity level measures. However, many gaps in our evidence exist, and current practice is still dictated by clinician experience and preference. The effect on participation outcomes and ideal dosing (length of time orthoses are worn) are 2 key questions that have not been addressed at all in the peer-reviewed literature. In addition, emerging understanding of muscle growth in CP and the application of motor learning principles to orthotic intervention may be changing the framework used to make decisions. Clearly the evidence is not sufficient, and many questions remained unanswered.

■ EVALUATION STRATEGIES

Evaluation of a child for orthoses should include a static standing postural assessment, gait analysis, and assessment of possible body structure impairments, such as limited range of motion, muscle length, and muscle strength. These assessments need to be done in a developmentally appropriate manner and thus may look quite different depending on the developmental status of the child. Gait analysis may be either visual or in a lab with motion capture and EMG data. Body structure impairments may be visually estimated or specifically measured and quantified, depending on the child's ability to participate. Ideally the evaluation will be as precise as possible, but this may not be possible for every child.

STATIC STANDING ALIGNMENT

A consistent and systematic approach to static standing postural assessment helps to ensure that all components are assessed. Working either from head to toe or toe to head is one good strategy. Key elements to note are ability to hold all body segments in midline and symmetry in both the frontal and sagittal planes.

Starting at the head, look for whether or not the head and trunk are in midline. View or palpate the spinal curves to look for appropriate kyphosis and lordosis. Check the pelvis to see if it is level and symmetrical. Although many trunk and head alignment issues may not be affected by a lower extremity orthosis, noting the position of the trunk and head prior to orthoses can assist with evaluation of the effect of an orthosis on posture up the kinetic chain. Any lower extremity orthosis that moves trunk and head alignment further away from ideal is likely not the right solution for that child.

All lower extremity joints should be assessed for static position in quiet standing, with specific care to note if the joint is near neutral in quiet standing or if the joint remains at end range while standing. For example, at the hips, is the child standing with the hip in neutral rotation and flexion/extension, or does the child "hang on their ligaments" by standing in hip extension? Does the child use excessive external rotation to widen the base of support or excessive internal rotation to gain stability from a closed-packed position? The knee should be assessed for excessive flexion or genu recurvatum in static stance. Genu valgum or varum beyond age-appropriate values should also be noted.

Impairment level measures that can be used to assess a child's need for orthoses include joint range of motion and muscle length (flexibility) testing. All lower extremity joints and muscles should be assessed, with particular emphasis on those that will be directly affected by the orthoses. Ankle motions, especially DF, and length of the gastrocnemius and soleus are critical for any orthosis that constrains the ankle joint. As noted earlier in the chapter, hamstring and hip flexor length needs to be assessed for consideration of a solid AFO for any child with crouch gait.

At the foot and ankle, alignment in all planes should be evaluated. Can the child maintain a foot flat position? Is there excessive DF or PF? The medial longitudinal arch should be visualized along with the position of the navicular bone. For children who are old enough to understand verbal cues, asking them to actively pronate and supinate while standing can be helpful to identify their ability to voluntarily change their foot posture. Measuring the amount of standing calcaneal valgus can also be quite helpful for young children. The

Valmassy criteria are based on this measurement of standing calcaneal valgus and propose that age-appropriate standing calcaneal eversion is derived from the formula of 7 minus a child's age in years.[52] The challenges with this test for young children are centered around the child's understanding of the directions and ability to stand quietly for the measurement. Finally, symmetry of foot posture between the 2 lower extremities should be noted.

GAIT ANALYSIS

A critical part of the evaluation for orthotic needs is gait analysis. Typically, the primary goal of orthotic intervention is to improve gait, so gait must be evaluated in order to identify the specific parts of the gait cycle that are problematic. The child should be observed walking at their self-selected pace and on a variety of surfaces and stairs as appropriate. The subjective history should help identify what environments are relevant for this part of the evaluation.

The child should be observed walking barefoot as well as with shoes. Walking barefoot allows better visualization of how the foot is functioning in gait, particularly calcaneal position in stance, presence or absence of the arch, and how much the navicular drops during stance phase. However, children in the United States rarely go barefoot outside the home, and sometimes not even in the home. Thus, evaluation of gait in their usual footwear is also important. Shoes do provide some added stability by splinting joints within the foot and reducing intrinsic foot motion.[50] Observing only barefoot gait fails to answer the question of whether or not a good supportive shoe would be enough to achieve the goals for improved gait.

Observational gait analysis is common because more sophisticated gait assessment systems, such as 3D video capture, EMG, and force plate data, are expensive and often challenging to get with children. However, capturing a simple cell phone video of the child walking can be very helpful, assuming appropriate security measures are in place to protect the child's privacy. Having video allows the use of slow motion or frame-by-frame advancement in order to see some of the nuances of the child's gait. When capturing video or just observing in real time, both the frontal and sagittal planes should be observed. The frontal plane provides visualization of trunk sway, abduction/adduction and internal/external rotation at the hip, genu valgum/varum at the knee, and pronation/supination at the foot. The sagittal plane provides information about flexion and extension of the trunk and all lower extremity joints.

Observational or video gait analysis should be conducted systematically to prevent missing important details. Focus on one part of gait at a time, such as stance phase or swing phase. It may be helpful to consider the big picture first and decide which phase of gait (stance or swing) is the most challenging for the child. This will help determine the goals of orthotic intervention. Does the child need more stability in stance phase, better foot clearance in swing phase, or both? When observing each of the 2 main phases of gait, either work from head to toe or toe to head. Observe one body segment at a time before moving up or down to the next one. Once all body segments have been

observed in one phase of gait, then repeat the same sequence for the other phase. This is why video can be helpful—it can be watched multiple times to facilitate this systematic approach without fatiguing the child.

MAT TABLE EVALUATION

After observing gait, an impairment level examination with the child in a non–weight-bearing position (sitting or lying) should come next. The gait analysis should have led to some hypotheses about the cause of the gait deviations. The impairment level examination should either confirm or refute these hypotheses. The key things to examine are joint range of motion, muscle length, and muscle strength.

The active and passive range of motion of all lower extremity joints should be examined. The key thing to note is if the range of motion at each joint is functional for gait and stairs (if appropriate). If the range of motion is limited, and the limitation is fixed (ie, contracture or bony end feel), then the orthosis will need to accommodate the deformity. If the malalignment or joint can be passively corrected, then an orthosis may be able to correct the deformity.

Muscle length is closely related to range of motion as a joint's movement may be limited either because of joint capsule/ligamentous tightness or by muscle length. Although all lower extremity muscles are relevant to gait, the key muscles to examine in regard to orthotic needs include the gastrocnemius, soleus, hamstrings, and the Thomas test (iliopsoas, rectus femoris, and iliotibial band). The length of these muscles should be sufficient to allow the functional ranges of motion.

Muscle strength is also important to consider, but formal testing of it (with manual muscle testing or hand-held dynamometry) is often challenging with children. Typically, a child must be at least 6 or 7 years old (and with age-appropriate cognition) in order to understand and comply with the directions for manual muscle testing. For younger children or children with cognitive impairment, observation of functional tasks, such as sit to stand, floor to stand transfers, and stairs, will have to serve as an assessment of strength. The child's voluntary control of each muscle group should also be considered. Better voluntary control may indicate better potential for strengthening and thus may allow a more dynamic or less restrictive orthosis.

Many practitioners also evaluate the hindfoot (calcaneal position) and forefoot alignment in an unweighted position, usually prone. The foot is passively moved into subtalar neutral, and then the alignment (to vertical/horizontal) of the hindfoot and forefoot are visualized. The value of examining the subtalar neutral alignment of the foot is debatable. Lee et al[53] believe this position is critical for molding an orthosis so that the foot is in its neutral position in the orthosis. The hindfoot and forefoot positions when the ankle/foot is in subtalar neutral may help to decide how much external posting to put on the orthosis in order to keep the foot in neutral when weight bearing. However, the validity of this perspective has never been proven, and some practitioners question the importance of subtalar neutral. The argument is that when a person without gait dysfunction walks, the foot and ankle pass through subtalar neutral but never stay there, and the foot and ankle are in the subtalar neutral position for less than 10% of the gait cycle. Because this is the way a typical foot and ankle function in gait, some question the need to have an orthosis keep the foot and ankle statically in the subtalar neutral position throughout the gait cycle. To date, there are no published data to help clarify this issue.

■ CONSIDERATION FOR CHOOSING AN ORTHOSIS

Obviously, the primary criterion for choosing an orthosis should be matching the indications for each specific device with the child's unique needs and abilities. However, there are additional factors to consider. The family's goals as well as the child's goals (when appropriate) should always be considered. Cosmesis of the orthosis and the family and child's acceptance of it must also be considered. An orthosis can only benefit a child when it is worn, so if the family and/or child dislike the orthosis and refuse to use it, then it will be a waste of time and money. A compromise may be necessary. This may mean choosing a less effective orthosis, but if it is one that will be worn, there will at least be some benefit versus no benefit from an ideal orthosis that is never worn.

Additional factors may include the geographical region where the family lives and the usual climate for that area. For children who live in areas with very high heat, their orthotic needs may require different considerations than children who live in colder climates. The materials for both the orthosis and the socks/garments worn under the orthosis may be different. Cultural influences (eg, style of shoes, how much shoes are worn) may also influence a family's acceptance and use of an orthosis. These issues need to be explored with the family prior to deciding upon a specific orthosis.

■ WHEN TO INTRODUCE AN ORTHOSIS

The current standard of care is often to provide the first orthoses when a child is interested in being on their feet. This is typically when a child is beginning to pull to stand or when the child can remain standing when placed in that position. The rationale for this is that the orthosis may provide improved stability and alignment so that the child will be more successful in attempting this new skill. As noted earlier though, Looper and Ulrich[48] were the first to question this standard of care, and they have suggested waiting until after the onset of independent ambulation. Looper and Ulrich's recommendation was specifically based on a study with young children with DS, but the motor learning theory they used to support their recommendation could apply to any population.[48] Their recommendation came from a very small sample size, and it has not been affirmed by any other study to date.[48] For this reason, the ideal time to introduce a first orthosis remains controversial.

For children who do not have the potential to stand or ambulate, the decision to provide orthoses is less clear. The primary goals for this group are often to prevent deformity or to prevent injury. Orthoses may be helpful in keeping a child's feet securely on the footplates of a wheelchair or to assist with positioning in a stander. The timing of providing orthoses to meet these goals will vary with each child and may depend on when the adaptive equipment is introduced or when concern about potential deformity rises to the level that the child's family is willing to add the orthoses to their daily routine.

■ HOW TO OBTAIN AN ORTHOSIS

Best practice for obtaining an orthosis involves a team approach between the family, the child's physician, the physical therapist, and the orthotist. Nearly all payment sources (insurance) require a physician's prescription before they will pay for an orthotic device. The physical therapist likely has the best understanding of the child's motor control, gross motor developmental status, and temperament with physical activities. The orthotist has the best understanding of materials and fabrication but very little time to get to know the child and family. Ideally, the physical therapist should accompany the family to the orthotic appointment and collaborate in person with the orthotist. The physical therapist should describe the child's motor function and propose how an orthosis may be used to meet the goals of the child and family. The orthotist needs this information to fabricate an appropriate device.

Some types of orthoses are available through mail order. These include many off-the-shelf orthoses (ordered by child's shoe size) and, most notably, orthoses made by Cascade DAFO.[7] Physical therapists can take cast molds of a child's foot and mail them directly to Cascade DAFO. The fabricated orthoses are mailed back to the physical therapist, and the physical therapist fits the orthoses to the child. Although the Cascade DAFO company has many excellent products to offer, the element of teamwork may be lost. Orthotists employed by Cascade DAFO can review videotapes of children and consult with the physical therapists by phone, but the opportunity to work with a child together is lost. In addition, if adjustments need to be made to orthoses obtained by mail, then the orthoses must be mailed back to the company, adjustments are made without seeing the orthoses on the child, and the orthoses are then mailed back to the family. This means that the child is without the braces for at least several days, and there is a chance that the adjustments will not be as accurate as needed because the orthotist was unable to see the orthoses on the child. When working with a local orthotist, the adjustments can be made while the child and family wait, and thus, the child is only without the orthoses for a brief amount of time.

In addition to the physician's prescription, most third-party payers require a letter of medical necessity before approving payment for orthoses. The letter of medical necessity must be explicit in identifying the child's specific needs and how and why an orthosis will improve function and prevent further injury and in providing specific details about the orthosis that is required. A key part of any letter of medical necessity is to provide insight on how this device will decrease future costs, such as improved safety with ambulation and decreased risk of injury from falling, prevention of deformity, and need for later intervention (eg, surgery). Most orthotists have templates for these letters that can be used as a starting point. Ideally, the orthotist and physical therapist should collaborate when developing this document.

ORTHOTIC FITTING AND CHECKOUT

The physical therapist's role in fitting orthoses will vary depending on whether they were obtained by mail order or through a local orthotist. When a local orthotist is not involved, clearly the physical therapist will have to do the initial fitting in addition to the ongoing evaluation, as described below. The initial fitting includes assessing the fit of the orthoses, the child's acceptance of them, and family education. The caregivers (and child as appropriate) must be taught how to don and doff the orthoses, how snug to pull the straps, and how to care for and clean the orthoses. Other safety considerations, such as providing assistance to the child with stairs and transitions until the child becomes used to the orthoses, and avoidance of activities that may damage the orthoses (eg, jumping, squatting) should be discussed. Another key part of the initial education includes teaching the family and child about how to assess the child's skin for excessive rubbing or pressure. A common guideline is usually that any area of redness that does not go away within 30 minutes of removing the orthoses is a potential problem and needs to be watched closely. Obviously, complaints of pain or discomfort from the child should also be taken seriously. Prolonged redness after removal and complaints from the child should trigger at least a phone call to the orthotist and likely an office visit so that the orthotist can more fully evaluate the fit.

Most orthotists recommend a break-in period with new orthoses that may last up to a week. The guideline is often to have the child wear the orthoses for 1 to 2 hours the first day and increase that wear time by approximately 1 or 2 hours each day until the child is able to wear the orthoses for most waking hours. Although there is no peer-reviewed evidence to help guide dosage decisions, the most common recommendation is that a child wear the orthoses 8 to 10 hours a day and definitely wear them for all gross motor activity. Only a few orthotic studies have reported how long the participant wore the orthoses each day, and this current standard of care of wearing orthoses for 8 to 10 hours a day is grounded in clinician experience and preference versus evidence.

Once the orthoses have been provided, reevaluating gait with the orthoses compared to shoes only can be a very useful activity. As previously noted, video in both the frontal and sagittal planes can be very helpful. Gait analysis can help confirm that the orthoses are meeting their intended purpose, can help the family see the value of the orthoses, and can perhaps help with payment from the third-party payer. Gait analysis may also reveal unintended consequences of orthotic use, such as new compensations in gait. This information can help both the physical therapist and the orthotist tweak their interventions to maximize the benefit of the orthoses.

The orthotist should be contacted for reevaluation of the orthoses if the child complains of discomfort, there is skin breakdown, there is redness lasting for more than 30 minutes after removal of the orthoses, or the identified goals of using the orthoses are not being met (eg, new and unacceptable compensations). In addition, the child must be monitored for growth. Most orthoses will accommodate 1 to 1½ shoes sizes of growth. Once a child has gone up one whole size in shoes, the fit of the orthoses needs to be closely monitored. This includes checking to see if the length of the footplate is still appropriate and if the molded arch in the orthosis still lines up with the arch of the foot and closely monitoring skin for redness and pressure areas.

ORTHOSES AND THE OVERALL PHYSICAL THERAPY PLAN OF CARE

Orthoses should be considered the same as any other intervention—it is one component of a plan of care and not something to be used in isolation. Orthoses should also not just be applied and forgotten. Like all other interventions used by physical therapists, the effect of orthoses must be continually assessed and the physical therapist must determine if the child's goals are being met. If the child is not making appropriate progress toward their goals, then the orthoses may need to be reevaluated or changed.

One key concept to remember is that strengthening will need to be a part of the overall plan of care, especially for those muscles constrained by an orthosis. As noted earlier in the review of evidence for CP, emerging evidence indicates that a key problem in CP is the failure of muscle to grow, and muscle requires neuromechanical stimulation to grow.[29] Neuromechanical stimulation means weight bearing and active contraction. Long-term use of rigid orthoses may limit the neuromechanical stimulation of key muscles needed for gait and thus lead to decreased muscle growth or even atrophy. Evidence conducted with athletes without disabilities seems to confirm the possibility of orthotic-induced atrophy. Morita et al[54] and Otsuka et al[55] concluded that toe flexor strength is significantly correlated with lower limb performance in tasks such as running and jumping. Yamauchi and Koyama[56] compared elastic ankle supports to a rigid ankle splint with healthy young adults and concluded that the rigid style of brace impaired the force produced by the plantar flexors and toe flexors and thus impaired physical performance. Although these studies were conducted with healthy athletes, the findings should make us pause and think about the long-term effects of rigid orthoses.[54-56] If more rigid styles of orthoses are used, then strengthening of the constrained musculature must also be a component of the plan of care, assuming the child has some voluntary control or ability to bear weight without the orthoses.

DISCONTINUING ORTHOSES

The decision of when to discontinue use of orthoses, or perhaps switch to a less supportive orthosis, should be based on outcome measures and progress toward the child's goals as much as possible. Helpful outcome measures will be discussed in the next section. Some children may need orthoses long term (eg, GMFCS level IV and V, children with ligamentous laxity or permanent deformity), but others may only need the orthoses for a shorter period of time. The child should be reassessed without the orthoses every few months to determine if the child is ready to function well without them. Orthotists are often available to help with these decisions by offering to collaborate on gait and task analysis without the orthoses or by offering a noncustom orthosis for a short trial to see if the child is ready to switch to a different style. The decision should also be made in collaboration with the child when appropriate and, of course, with the parents.

Some children and parents are eager to discontinue orthoses based on the "hassle factor" of daily use and the desire to not appear different from typically developing peers. The challenge for physical therapists is to predict future function if the child stops using the orthoses. Will the child be at risk for later orthopedic dysfunction and pain as a result of poor biomechanics when not using orthoses? As noted earlier, the peer-reviewed research does not offer much help in answering this question because most studies involved single-day data collection and the long-term effects of wearing (or not wearing) orthoses have not been documented. We should educate the child and family based on what is known and our clinical experience, but ultimately, this decision is still theirs. Older children and teens can go back into orthoses at a later time if pain or decreased function becomes an issue, but there is a likelihood that they may now have more of a fixed deformity and their options may be limited to orthoses that accommodate versus correct alignment.

■ OUTCOME MEASURES FOR ORTHOTIC EFFICACY

IMPAIRMENT LEVEL MEASURES

Common impairment level measures were discussed earlier in the chapter in the Evaluation Strategies section. These same measures may be helpful in documenting the effect of the orthoses over time, especially if improving range of motion was one of the identified goals. These measures include joint range of motion and muscle length (flexibility).

ACTIVITY LEVEL MEASURES

Gait analysis was discussed earlier in the chapter in the Evaluation Strategies section, and like impairment level measures, it can be helpful for both initial decision-making as well as for documenting improvement over time. For the majority of kids, improvement in gait is a key goal of orthotic intervention; therefore, gait analysis will be a key outcome measure. However, observational gait analysis is fairly subjective, and it should be supplemented with more objective tools. Oeffinger et al[57,58] have published 2 papers regarding outcome tools for ambulatory children with CP, including the minimally clinical important difference (MCID) when available. Other activity level outcome measures include the 1-Minute Walk Test,[59] 6-Minute Walk Test,[60,61] the Timed Up and Go (TUG) test,[62,63] and the Timed Up and Down Stairs (TUDS) test.[64] The Berg Balance Scale has also been validated for use with children and may be helpful, in addition to simply timing single leg stance for those children capable of doing this.[65]

The GMFM is a criterion-referenced outcome measure that has been validated with several groups of children, including those with CP and DS.[66] Two dimensions of this test, D (Standing) and E (Walking, Running, and Jumping) have particular relevance as they assess the skills most likely to be affected by orthotic use. Several norm-referenced tests also have components that included skills that will be affected by orthotic use,

including the Bruininks-Oseretsky Test of Motor Proficiency, Second Edition (BOT-2),[67] and the Peabody Developmental Motor Scales, Second Edition (PDMS-2).[68] This is not an exhaustive list of possible activity level outcome measures, and the key point is that objective, valid, and reliable measures should be used to document orthotic efficacy.

PARTICIPATION LEVEL MEASURES

Participation is arguably the most challenging area to objectively document. This may be because the meaning of participation is unique to each child and family. There are currently no studies that report on changes in participation levels with orthotic intervention. However, several popular outcome measures do exist that may help the clinician track progress for a child in this area. The Pediatric Evaluation of Disability Inventory (PEDI),[69] the Pediatric Quality of Life Inventory (PedsQL),[70] and Goal Attainment Scaling[71] are just a few of the more common ways to assess participation level changes. As with impairment and activity level measures, the important point is to find a tool that is as objective as possible while also being reliable and valid.

■ SUMMARY

Orthotic intervention for children with disabilities is common and part of the standard of care. However, the peer-reviewed evidence provides only a partial guide for decision-making, and often decisions are based on clinician preference and experience. To improve the success of orthotic interventions, physical therapists should collaborate with their local orthotist as much as possible. Valid and reliable measures should be used to help establish both the child's baseline status (before orthotic intervention) and to document the results of using orthoses. Impairment and activity level measures are common, but participation measures are also important.

Many professional doctor of physical therapy programs have limited time in their curricula for pediatrics and even less time devoted to pediatric orthoses. Therefore, the new graduate may find this area overwhelming and confusing, especially with the abundance of options that are available for children. Partnering with an experienced pediatric physical therapist and a pediatric orthotist can help build knowledge and competence.

Case 1

Cerebral Palsy, GMFCS Level III

Tommy is a 32-month-old who was born prematurely at 30 weeks' postconception age. He is the youngest child living in a 2-story home with his biological parents, 4-year-old sister, and 6-year-old brother. Currently Tommy has been identified as having global developmental delays, and he is taking oral baclofen for spasticity management, albuterol for reactive airway disease, and lansoprazole (Prevacid) for gastroesophageal reflux.

His past medical history includes a 12-week stay in the neonatal intensive care unit with mechanical ventilation for the first 5 weeks of life; then, he was weaned to Vapotherm for 3 weeks, and finally nasal cannula for 2 more weeks. He had a grade III intraventricular hemorrhage in the first week of life and subsequently underwent surgery to place a ventriculoperitoneal shunt. He had laser surgery on both eyes at 10 weeks of age for retinopathy of prematurity.

Tommy has been referred to physical therapy for gross motor delay. Review of systems is as follows:

- Cardiopulmonary: Reactive airway disease; bronchopulmonary dysplasia/chronic lung disease.
- Integumentary: Unremarkable.
- Musculoskeletal: Increased thoracic kyphosis and forward head posture—correctable with handling; mild tightness in adductors, hamstrings, gastrocnemius-soleus bilaterally; moderate tightness in biceps, wrist and finger flexors, and pectoralis major and minor.
- Neuromuscular: Spastic quadriplegic CP with spasticity in all 4 extremities; hypotonia in the trunk.
- Cognitive: Mild to moderate delays; expressive language more delayed than receptive. He has 20 to 25 words he can use consistently.

Currently, Tommy can roll over in both directions, but he initiates it with an extensor pattern. He is able to sit independently for up to 1 minute if placed in sitting, but he is unable to get into sitting on his own. He can get into quadruped and "bunny hops" for mobility, meaning that he advances both lower extremities together and can only creep reciprocally with moderate assistance. Tommy will stand at a support when placed but stands with genu recurvatum, maximal pronation, and anterior pelvic tilt, and he must lean on the support and prop with both upper extremities. He is unable to take steps, feed himself, or assist with activities of daily living in an age-appropriate way. He is unable to play with toys requiring fine motor control.

Tommy's movement system diagnoses include movement pattern coordination deficit, force production deficit, and fragmentation of movement deficit. He has been classified as GMFCS level III and is currently receiving physical therapy through his state's Part C early intervention program. His parents' goals on his Individualized Family Service Plan are for Tommy to be more independent in playing with his siblings and to be able walk with assistance. Tommy has been wearing solid ankle AFOs for the past year but has outgrown them recently.

Discussion Questions

1. What factors will be important to consider in determining what Tommy's orthotic needs are at this time?
2. What style of orthosis would you recommend for Tommy and why?
3. How does the GMFCS classification of level III impact your decision-making?

Case 2

Myelomeningocele, L5-S1

Mary is a 24-month-old only child, living with her parents in a 2-bedroom apartment. She was born full term after an uneventful pregnancy and underwent surgical closure of her spine and placement of a ventriculoperitoneal shunt for hydrocephalus when she was 1 day old. She has had her shunt replaced twice in the first year due to blockage but has otherwise been healthy. She is not taking any prescription medications currently but is on a bowel management program with enemas 1 time daily. Her parents do intermittent catheterization for bladder management.

She was referred to physical therapy for gross motor delays. A review of systems for her includes the following:

- Cardiopulmonary: Small ventricular septal defect that spontaneously closed in the first month of life; otherwise unremarkable.
- Integumentary: Appears that sensation to light touch and hot/cold is not intact in both feet and ankles.
- Musculoskeletal: Increased anterior pelvic tilt in supported standing, vertebrae defect L5-S1.
- Neuromuscular: Absent hip extension, ankle plantar flexion and eversion, toe flexion and extension; hip abduction, knee flexion, and ankle dorsiflexion weak (unable to move through full range of motion against gravity); knee extension strength fair (able to move through full range against gravity).
- Cognitive: Appears to be age appropriate with minor delays in expressive language.

Mary is currently able to roll in both directions, get into sitting from prone or supine through side sit, and reach up to 10 inches outside her base of support while sitting. She can transition from the floor into standing if she can pull herself up with her upper extremities. She is able to stand at a support independently but with increased pronation, knee flexion and genu valgum, and hip flexion. Mary's primary means of mobility is creeping on her hands and knees or scooting on her bottom in a sitting position. Mary has recently begun taking steps if she has upper extremity and trunk support from an adult.

Mary's movement system diagnoses are force production deficit and sensory detection deficit. She has been receiving Part C early intervention services since she was 6 weeks old, and her parents' goals for her include walking independently and being able to get up from the floor by herself. She has not yet had any orthoses, but her physical therapist has mentioned to the parents that it is time to pursue this.

Discussion Questions

1. What factors will be important to consider in determining what Mary's orthotic needs are at this time?
2. What style of orthosis would you recommend for Mary and why?

Case 3

Down Syndrome

Abby is a 40-month-old female child who was born full term after an uncomplicated pregnancy. Down syndrome was not identified during the pregnancy but was suspected immediately upon her birth and confirmed during the first week of life. She lives with her parents, 4 older siblings (ages 12, 10, 7, and 5 years) and 1 younger sibling (4 months old). Dad works full time as an accountant, and Mom was employed part time in a retail setting prior to the birth of her sixth child. She has not yet returned to work but needs to soon for financial reasons. Abby attends developmental preschool at a nearby public elementary school 5 days a week, 8:30 am to 11:30 am. The family lives in a ranch home with a finished basement that serves as the kids' play area.

Abby's past medical history includes open heart surgery at 5 months of age to repair an atrioventricular (AV) canal defect and ear tubes placed at 8 months due to recurrent ear infections. She has had cervical radiographs (at 30 months of age), which did not show any atlantoaxial instability, and her thyroid function (thyroid-stimulating hormone) is in the low-normal range. She is currently taking digoxin and ramipril and is monitored every 6 months by her cardiologist.

Abby has been referred to physical therapy for gross motor delay. Review of systems is as follows:

- Cardiopulmonary: History of open-heart surgery for AV canal repair; poor overall endurance and exercise tolerance.
- Integumentary: Unremarkable.
- Musculoskeletal: Global moderate hypotonia and ligamentous laxity.
- Neuromuscular: Decreased coordination and postural control.
- Cognitive: Moderate cognitive disability; severe expressive language delay with 3 or 4 words; communicates with gestures; can follow 1-step commands.

Abby has excessive range of motion and ligamentous laxity in all joints; however, it is most pronounced in her hips (~90 degrees of abduction) and knees (~20 degrees of hyperextension), and ankles (>30 degrees of DF). Abby rolls easily both ways and can prop on extended arms in prone but with high cervical extension and frogged lower extremities (abduction, external rotation). She sits independently both on the floor and in a child-sized chair. She can reach approximately 3 to 4 inches outside her base of support without loss of balance. She can transition in and out of sitting independently but will go from prone directly into sitting by pushing back and using excessive hip abduction (does the splits). Abby can stand independently for more than 5 minutes at a time. She prefers to pull to stand at a support (through half kneel, right leg up first) but can come to stand in the middle of the floor through plantigrade. Abby walks independently with a wide base of support, knee hyperextension in stance, increased pronation, and increased foot progression angle (toe out). She tires quickly and will walk only about 3 to 5 minutes before sitting down and refusing to continue. She goes up and down stairs using 2-hand support (handrail or hands held) and using a step-to (marking time) pattern. When she does not have support, she crawls up the steps. She is unable to jump and attempts to run, but it is really just fast walking.

Abby's movement system diagnoses are force production deficit and postural control deficit. Abby is receiving 20 minutes of physical therapy per week at a local developmental preschool under Individuals With Disabilities Education Act Part B services, but her parents have decided to pursue additional outpatient physical therapy for her at this time. Their goals for her include to be able to go up and down stairs safely (with supervision) so that she can play in the basement with her siblings, to improve her walking endurance for family outings, and to be able to access the playground at school (fewer falls).

Discussion Questions

1. Abby has never worn orthoses. Would this be an appropriate intervention for her at this time?
2. What orthoses would you consider for Abby and why?

STUDY QUESTIONS

1. What does the peer-reviewed evidence show in regard to orthotic efficacy?
2. What are the important gaps in the peer-reviewed evidence in regard to orthotic efficacy?
3. How does an orthosis fit into the overall intervention plan for a child with movement dysfunction?
4. What are important considerations for determining the optimal orthosis for a child?
5. What are some common outcome measures that could be used to document the effect of an orthotic intervention?
6. What is the role of the orthotist in determining the optimal orthosis for a child?
7. How often and for how long should a child wear orthoses?

References

1. World Health Organization. *International Classification of Functioning, Disability and Health (ICF)*. World Health Organization; 2001.
2. Morris C, Bowers R, Ross K, Stevens P, Phillips D. Orthotic management of cerebral palsy: recommendations from a consensus conference. *Neurorehabilitation*. 2011;28:37-46.
3. Rogozinski BM, Davids JR, Davis RB, Jameson GG, Blackhurst DW. The efficacy of the floor-reaction ankle-foot orthosis in children with cerebral palsy. *J Bone Joint Surg*. 2009;91:2440-2447.
4. Owen E. Segmental kinematic approach to orthotic management: ankle-foot orthosis/footwear combination. In: M. Rahlin, ed. *Physical Therapy for Children with Cerebral Palsy*. Slack; 2016: 341-370.
5. Allard USA. Kiddie Gait AFO. Rockaway, NJ. Accessed November 20, 2023. https://www.allardusa.com/products/foot-drop-afos/pediatric/kiddiegait-r-2-p35545.
6. Midwest Orthotic and Technology Center. SureStep® SMO. South Bend, IN. Accessed November 20, 2023. https://surestep.net/products/surestep-smo/.
7. Cascade DAFO. Our history. Ferndale, WA. Accessed November 20, 2023. https://cascadedafo.com/about/our-history.
8. Midwest Orthotic and Technology Center. *SureStep Parents Guide*. South Bend, IN. Accessed November 20, 2023. https://surestep.net/blog/ultimate-guide-find-shoes-for-afos-smos/.
9. Crawford L. The mighty. April 18, 2017. Accessed November 20, 2023. https://themighty.com/topic/disability/guide-to-finding-shoes-that-fit-over-braces.
10. Katalinic OM, Harvey LA, Herbert RD, Moseley AM, Lannin NA, Schurr K. Stretch for the treatment and prevention of contracture (Review). *Cochrane Database Syst Rev*. 2010;9:CD007455.
11. Craig J, Hilderman C, Wilson G, Misovic R. Effectiveness of stretch interventions for children with neuromuscular disabilities:

evidence-based recommendations. *Pediatr Phys Ther.* 2016; 28:262-75.

12. Morris C. Orthotic management of children with cerebral palsy. *J Prosthet Orthot.* 2002;14:150-158.

13. Figueiredo EM, Ferreira GB, Moreira RCM, Kirkwood RN, Fetters L. Efficacy of ankle-foot orthoses on gait of children with cerebral palsy: systematic review of literature. *Pediatr Phys Ther.* 2008;20:207-223.

14. Betancourt JP, Eleeh P, Stark S, Jain NB. Impact of ankle-foot orthosis on gait efficiency in ambulatory children with cerebral palsy: a systematic review and meta-analysis. *Am J Phys Med Rehabil.* 2019;98:759-770.

15. Brehm M, Harlaar J, Schwartz M. Effect of ankle-foot orthoses on walking efficiency and gait in children with cerebral palsy. *J Rehabil Med.* 2008;40:529-534.

16. Kerkum YL, Brehm M, van Hutten K, et al. Acclimatization of the gait pattern to wearing an ankle-foot orthosis in children with spastic cerebral palsy. *Clin Biomech.* 2015;30:617-622.

17. Lam WK, Leong JCY, Li YH, Hu Y, Lu WW. Biomechanical and electromyographic evaluation of ankle foot orthosis and dynamic ankle foot orthosis in spastic cerebral palsy. *Gait Posture.* 2004;22:189-197.

18. Rosenburg M, Steele KM. Simulated impacts of ankle foot orthoses on muscle demand and recruitment in typically-developing children and children with cerebral palsy and crouch gait. *PloS One.* 2017;12(7):e0180219.

19. Leonard R, Sweeney J, Damiano D, Bjornson K, Ries J. Effects of orthoses on standing postural control and muscle activity in children with cerebral palsy. *Pediatr Phys Ther.* 2021;33:129-135.

20. Lindskov L, Huse A, Johansson M, Nygard S. Muscle activity in children with spastic unilateral cerebral palsy when walking with ankle-foot orthoses: an exploratory study. *Gait Posture.* 2020;80:31-36.

21. Desloovere K, Molenaers G, van Gestel L, et al. How can push-off be preserved during use of an ankle foot orthosis in children with hemiplegia? A prospective controlled study. *Gait Posture.* 2006;24:142-151.

22. Limpaninlachat S, Prasertsukdee S, Palisano R, Burns J, Kaewkungwal J, Inthachom R. Multidimensional effects of solid and hinged ankle-foot-orthosis in children with cerebral palsy. *Pediatr Phys Ther.* 2021;33:227-235.

23. Lohman M, Goldstein H. Alternative strategies in tone-reducing AFO design. *J Prosthet Orthot.* 1993;5:21-24.

24. Kabayashi T, Leung AKL, Hutchins SW. Design and effect of ankle-foot orthoses proposed to influence muscle tone: a review. *J Prosthet Orthot.* 2011;23(2):52-59.

25. Autti-Rämö I, Soranta J, Anttila H, Malmivaara A, Mäkelä M. Effectiveness of upper and lower limb casting and orthoses in children with cerebral palsy. *Am J Phys Med Rehabil.* 2006;85:89-103.

26. Westberry DE, Davids JR, Shaver JC, Tanner SL, Blackhurst DW, Davis RB. Impact of ankle-foot orthoses on static foot alignment in children with cerebral palsy. *J Bone Joint Surg.* 2007;89:806-813.

27. Ricks NR, Eilert RE. Effects of inhibitory casts and orthoses on bony alignment of foot and ankle during weight-bearing in children with spasticity. *Dev Med Child Neurol.* 1993;35:11-16.

28. Jarvis HL, Nester CJ, Bowden PD, Jones RK. Challenging the foundations of the clinical model of foot function: further evidence that the Root model assessments fail to appropriately classify foot function. *J Foot Ankle Res.* 2017;10:7-17.

29. Herskind A, Ritterband-Rosenbaum A, Willerslev-Olsen M, et al. Muscle growth is reduced in 15-month-old children with cerebral palsy. *Dev Med Child Neurol.* 2016;58:485-491.

30. Willerslev-Olsen M, Lorentzen J, Sinkjaer T, Nielsen JB. Passive muscle properties are altered in children with cerebral palsy before the age of 3 years and are difficult to distinguish clinically from spasticity. *Dev Med Child Neurol.* 2013;55:617-623.

31. Willerslev-Olsen M, Lund MC, Lorentzen J, Barber L, Kofoed-Hansen M, Nielsen JB. Impaired muscle growth precedes development of increased stiffness of the triceps surae musculotendinous unit in children with cerebral palsy. *Dev Med Child Neurol.* 2018;60:672-679.

32. Mazur JM, Kyle S. Efficacy of bracing the lower limbs and ambulation training in children with myelomeningocele. *Dev Med Child Neurol.* 2004;46:352-356.

33. Arazpour M, Soleimani F, Sajedi F, et al. Effect of orthotic gait training with isocentric reciprocating gait orthosis on walking in children with myelomeningocele. *Top Spinal Cord Inj Rehabil.* 2015;23:147-54.

34. Kane D, Barden J. Comparison of ground reaction and articulated ankle-foot orthoses in a child with lumbosacral myelomeningocele and tibial torsion. *J Prosthet Orthot.* 2010;22(4):222-229.

35. Wolf SI, Alimusaj M, Rettig O, Döderlein L. Dynamic assist by carbon fiber spring AFOs for patients with myelomeningocele. *Gait Posture.* 2008;28:175-177.

36. Weber A, Martin K. Efficacy of orthoses for children with hypotonia: a systematic review. *Pediatr Phys Ther.* 2014;26:38-47.

37. Looper J, Martin K. The effect of supramalleolar orthotic use on activity and participation skills in children with Down syndrome. *J Prosthet Orthot.* 2020;32:222-228.

38. Selby-Silverstein L, Hillstrom HJ, Palisano RJ. The effect of foot orthoses on standing foot posture and gait of young children with Down syndrome. *Neurorehabilitation.* 2001;16:183-193.

39. Hashimoto K, Aoki S, Miyamura K, Kamide A, Honda M. Clinical efficacy of shoes and custom-modeled insoles in treating Down syndrome children with flatfoot. *Phys Med Rehabil Int.* 2015;2:1061-1063.

40. Buccieri KM. Use of orthoses and early intervention physical therapy to minimize hyperpronation and promote functional skills in a child with gross motor delays: a case report. *Phys Occup Ther Pediatr.* 2003;23(1):5-20.

41. George DA, Elchert L. The influence of foot orthoses on the function of a child with developmental delay. *Pediatr Phys Ther.* 2007;19:332-336.

42. Parent-Nichols J, Nervik D. Using orthoses to advance motor skills in a child with Noonan syndrome: a case report. *J Prosthet Orthot.* 2014;26:61-67.

43. Ross CG, Shore S. The effect of gross motor therapy and orthotic intervention in children with hypotonia and flexible flatfeet. *J Prosthet Orthot.* 2011;23:149-154.

44. CIR Systems. GAITRite Mat. Franklin, NJ. Accessed November 20, 2023. https://www.gaitrite.com/.

45. Pitetti KH, Wondra VC. Dynamic foot orthosis and motor skills of delayed children. *J Prosthet Orthot.* 2005;17:21-26.

46. Martin K. Effect of supramalleolar orthoses on postural stability in children with Down syndrome. *Dev Med Child Neurol.* 2004;46:406-411.

47. Tamminga JS, Martin KS, Miller EW. Single-subject design study of 2 types of supramalleolar orthoses for young children with Down syndrome. *Pediatr Phys Ther.* 2012;24:278-284.

48. Looper J, Ulrich DA. Effect of treadmill training and supramalleolar orthosis use on motor skill development in infants with Down syndrome: a randomized clinical trial. *Phys Ther.* 2010;90:382-390.

49. Looper J, Benjamin D, Nolan M, Schumm L. What to measure when determining orthotic needs in children with Down syndrome: a pilot study. *Pediatr Phys Ther*. 2012;24:313-319.

50. Wegener C, Hunt A, Vanwanseele B, Burns J, Smith RM. Effect of children's shoes on gait: a systematic review and meta-analysis. *J Foot Ankle Res*. 2011;4:3-16.

51. Churchill AJG, Halligan PW, Wade DT. Relative contribution of footwear to the efficacy of ankle-foot orthoses. *Clin Rehabil*. 2003;17:553-557.

52. Valmassy RL. Biomechanical evaluation of the child. In: *Clinical Biomechanics of the Lower Extremities*. Mosby; 1996:243-277.

53. Lee WC, Lee CK, Leung AK, Hutchins SW. Is it important to position foot in subtalar joint neutral position during non-weight bearing molding for foot orthoses? *J Rehabil Res Dev*. 2012;49:459-466.

54. Morita N, Yamauchi J, Kurihara T, et al. Toe flexor strength and foot arch height in children. *Med Sci Sports Exerc*. 2015;47:350-356.

55. Otsuka M, Yamauchi J, Kurihara T, Morita N, Isaka T. Toe flexor strength and lower-limb physical performance in adolescent. *Gazetta Med Ital*. 2015;174:307-313.

56. Yamauchi J, Koyama K. Influence of ankle braces on the maximum strength of plantar and toe flexor muscles. *Int J Sports Med*. 2015;36:592-595.

57. Oeffinger D, Bagley A, Rogers S, et al. Outcome tools used for children who are ambulatory with cerebral palsy: responsiveness and minimal clinically important differences. *Dev Med Child Neurol*. 2008;50:918-925.

58. Oeffinger DJ, Rogers SP, Bagley A, Gorton G, Tylkowski CM. Clinical applications of outcome tools in ambulatory children with cerebral palsy. *Phys Med Rehabil Clin North Am*. 2009; 20: 549-565.

59. McDowell BC, Kerr C, Parkes J, Cosgrove A. Validity of a 1-minute walk test for children with cerebral palsy. *Dev Med Child Neurol*. 2005;47:744-748.

60. Maher CA, Williams MT, Olds TS. The six-minute walk test for children with cerebral palsy. *Int J Rehabil Res*. 2008;31:185-188.

61. Vis JC, Thoonsen H, Duffels MG, et al. Six-minute walk test in patients with Down syndrome: validity and reproducibility. *Arch Phys Med Rehabil*. 2009;90:1423-1427.

62. Carey H, Martin K, Combs-Miller S, Heathcock JC. Reliability and responsiveness of the timed up and go test in children with cerebral palsy. *Pediatr Phys Ther*. 2016;28:401-408.

63. Williams EN, Carroll SG, Reddihough DS, Phillips BA, Galea MP. Investigation of the timed "up & go" test in children. *Dev Med Child Neurol*. 2005;47:518-524.

64. Zaino CA, Gocha Marchese V, Westcott SL. Timed up and down stairs test: preliminary reliability and validity of a new measure of functional mobility. *Pediatr Phys Ther*. 2004;16:90-98.

65. Franjoine MR, Gunther JS, Taylor MJ. Pediatric balance scale: a modified version of the Berg balance scale for the school-age child with mild to moderate motor impairment. *Pediatr Phys Ther*. 2003;15:114-128.

66. Russell DJ, Rosenbaum PL, Avery LM, Lane M. *Gross Motor Function Measure (GMFM-66 & GMFM-88) User's Manual*. Mac Keith Press; 2002.

67. Bruininks RH, Bruininks BD. *Bruininks-Oseretsky Test of Motor Proficiency Manual*. 2nd ed. NCS Pearson; 2005.

68. Folio MR, Fewell RR. *Peabody Developmental Motor Scales Examiner's Manual*. 2nd ed. Pro-Ed; 2000.

69. Haley SM, Coster WJ, Ludlow LH, Haltiwanger JT, Andrellos PJ. *Pediatric Evaluation of Disability Inventory*. PEDI Research Group; 1992.

70. Varni JW, Seid M, Rode CA. The PedsQL: measurement model for the pediatric quality of life inventory. *Med Care*. 1999;37:126-139.

71. Turner-Stokes L. Goal attainment scaling (GAS) in rehabilitation: a practical guide. *Clin Rehabil*. 2009;23:362-370.

The Role of the Physical Therapist in Assistive Technology Service Delivery

Michelle Schladant, PhD, ATP, Sadie Vega-Velasquez, MS, CCC-SLP, Cristina Pujol, MS, CCC-SLP, and Ana Nevares, MA

LEARNING OBJECTIVES

Upon completion of this chapter, the reader will be able to:

- Define assistive technology (AT) devices and services in pediatric populations.
- Describe a range of AT from low tech to digital tech.

- Discuss legislative issues affecting funding and delivery of AT services.
- Discuss principles of AT assessment and service delivery, including the role of the physical therapist as part of an interdisciplinary team.

■ INTRODUCTION

Children with disabilities often need and can benefit from the use of assistive technology (AT) devices and services. These services and supports can increase children's participation in everyday activities at home, school, and in the community. Unfortunately, AT is highly underused,[1] and too few service providers know how to implement AT in the services they provide.[2] Physical therapists have long been involved in the practice of providing adaptive equipment for positioning and mobility.[3] However, the role of the physical therapist in AT services delivery is much more than that. Physical therapists, along with other service providers, also need to know how to consider a range of ATs to optimize the overall functioning of children with disabilities[1] and support their participation in everyday activities.[4] Physical therapists also need to know about laws and legislations to support the acquisition of AT devices and services and how to access additional AT training and resources to support children's use and maintenance of AT. Physical therapists are in an ideal position to consider, recommend, and in many cases implement AT services because they are often one of the first service providers to provide interventions to children with disabilities.[2] Unfortunately, physical therapists and other service providers often feel inadequately prepared in obtaining and using AT.[2,5] Therefore, the purpose of this chapter is to provide a broad overview of AT for pediatric populations, including how to identify funding sources and AT resources. We will also discuss the role of the physical therapist as a member of an interdisciplinary team and describe principles of AT assessment and service delivery.

■ OVERVIEW OF ASSISTIVE TECHNOLOGY

In the past 40 years, there has been an explosion of AT devices from low tech to high tech, including digital tech.[3] This section will focus on the definition of AT and highlight different types of AT devices for pediatric populations.

WHAT IS ASSISTIVE TECHNOLOGY?

A formal definition of AT and AT services, outlined in **Table 20-1**, comes from the Technology-Related Assistance for Individuals with Disabilities Act (29 USC §2202, 1999) and the Individuals with Disabilities Education Act (20 USC §1400, 2004). In simplified terms, AT is *any* tool to help a person with a disability to do *something* they have trouble doing. AT can range from low-tech options such as pencil grips to more high-tech options such as computerized communication devices. AT also includes adaptive equipment such as wheelchairs, walkers, reachers, and positioning equipment (Technology-Related Assistance for Individuals with Disabilities Act, 29 USC §2202, 1999), as well as digital technologies such as tablets with learning applications. AT is a broad umbrella term that includes equipment, devices, technologies, services, systems, and processes that people with disabilities use to support their independence and full participation in society.[6] When do technology, environmental modifications, and services become AT? How does one

TABLE 20-1 • Definitions of Assistive Technology and Assistive Technology Services

Assistive technology: Any item, piece of equipment, or product system, whether acquired commercially off the shelf, modified, or customized, that is used to increase, maintain, or improve functional capabilities of individuals with disabilities.

Assistive technology services: The evaluation of the needs of the child; purchasing, leasing, or otherwise acquiring a specific device; selecting, designing, fitting, customizing, adapting, applying, maintaining, repairing, or replacing specific devices; coordinating and using other services such as therapy, education, rehabilitation, and vocational training or technical assistance or training for professionals or others who provide services to the child.

differentiate AT from other technologies? Technology, environmental modifications, and services become *assistive* when these adaptations are individualized and follow the user.[7] As shown in **Figure 20-1**, AT optimizes functioning by (1) enhancing residual capacities (eg, an orthotic splint); (2) replacing missing parts (eg, a prosthetic limb); (3) providing an alternative means of function (eg, an augmentative or alternative communication device); and (4) minimizing environmental barriers (eg, the use of wheelchair ramps).

CATEGORIES OF ASSISTIVE TECHNOLOGY

AT devices are often categorized as low tech, mid-tech, high tech, or digital tech. Low-tech devices are simple to make and easy to obtain. These types of AT do not require a battery or

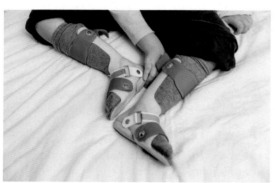

A

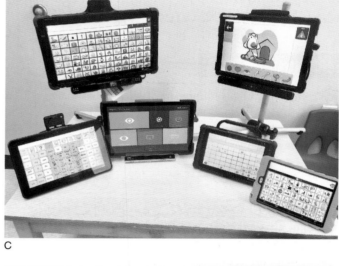

C

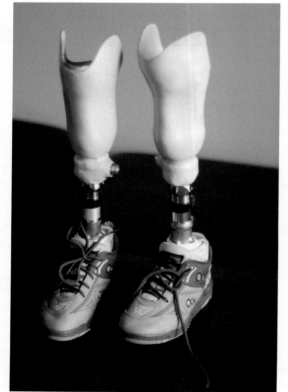

B

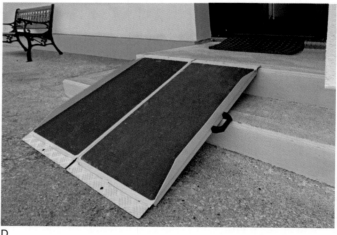

D

FIGURE 20-1 **(A) Splint.** (Used with permission with Jordi Mora/Shutterstock.) **(B) Prosthetic limb.** (Used with permission with Ryan Rodrick Beiler/Alamy Stock Photo.) **(C) Augmentative and alternative communication devices. Top row from left to right: PRC Accent 1400 with eye gaze and head tracker and Forbes AAC Winslate for Kids with eye gaze. Bottom row from left to right: Satillo Chat Fusion, TobiiDynavox, PRC Accent 800, and iPad with Proloqou2Go vocabulary system. (D) Wheelchair ramp.** (Used with permission with Ballygally View Images/Shutterstock.)

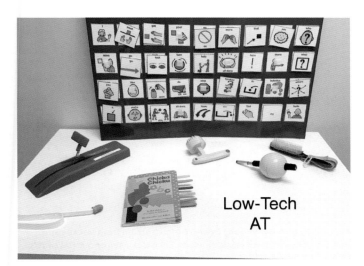

FIGURE 20-2 **Low-tech assistive technology. Top to bottom from left to right: Low-tech communication board, adaptive tabletop scissor, universal knob handle, adaptive hairbrush, adaptive page turner, adaptive book with sticks, and Arthwriter Hand Aid.**

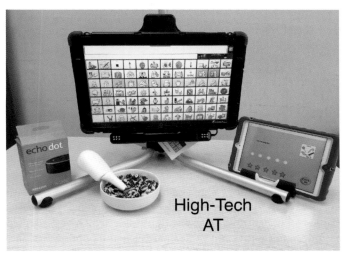

FIGURE 20-4 **High-tech assistive technology. Top to bottom from left to right: Amazon Echo Dot environmental control unit, PRC Accent 1400 with eye gaze and head tracker, iPad mini with Working 4 Application (token economy), and Google Liftware spoon.**

much training, may have a lower cost, and do not have mechanical features or complex functions. As shown in **Figure 20-2**, examples include pencil grips, adaptive equipment, picture boards, and magnifiers.

Mid-tech devices may have more complex features, are more expensive, may be electric or battery operated, and may require some training to learn how to use. As shown in **Figure 20-3**, examples are manual wheelchairs, switches, alternative mouse or keyboards for the computer, and 1-message voice-output device.

High-tech devices are the most complex devices or equipment. They may have digital or electric features, are more customizable to suit the needs of the user, and usually require training. Overall, high-tech devices are expensive and

sometimes harder to obtain. As shown in **Figure 20-4**, examples are speech-generating devices, computers, educational software, electronic aids for daily living, and powered mobility.

In recent years, there has been an explosion of digital technologies and mobile devices. It is essential for persons with disabilities to have the same access to these technologies (eg, smart devices, websites, social media, video games, computers, and electronic books) as their peers.[7] Different platforms for computer and smart devices include as part of their operational settings accessibility features that offer support for vision, hearing, or physical interactions. As shown in **Figure 20-5**, these options can include screen readers, text-to-speech, speech-to-text, magnification, hearing aid compatibility, and an array of access controls that incorporate direct touch, switches, head trackers, or eye gaze systems.

EXAMPLES OF ASSISTIVE TECHNOLOGY

There is a large body of research to support the effectiveness of AT to support children with disabilities across all ages and

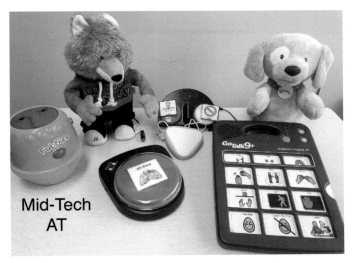

FIGURE 20-3 **Mid-tech assistive technology. Top to bottom left to right: Fubbles switch activated bubble machine, AbleNet plush switch-activated toy, AbleNet AbleLink connectable 2-button message-output device, AbleNet plush switch-activated toy, Big Mack communicator 1-message device, AlbeNet Big Candy Corn proximity senor switch, and Enablemart Go Talk 9+.**

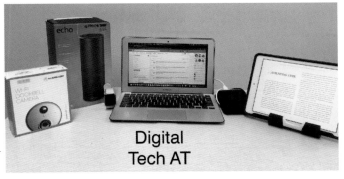

FIGURE 20-5 **Digital-tech assistive technology. Top to bottom from left to right: Alarm.com Wifi doorbell camera, Amazon Echo environmental control unit, Apple Watch, laptop, hard drive, and iPad with Amazon Kindle application.**

in many aspects of daily life such as learning, communication, and social interactions.[8] AT for pediatric populations can be categorized as (1) adapted toys; (2) aids for daily living; (3) AT for mobility, seating, and positioning; (4); hearing and vision devices; (5) augmentative and alternative communication (AAC); (6) electronic aids for daily living (EADLs); and (7) learning aids.

Adapted Toys

Play is an integral part of a child's development. Children with disabilities may face challenges playing and interacting with others. There is well-documented evidence that AT devices such as adapted toys can benefit infants and toddlers with special needs.[9] As seen in **Figure 20-6**, adapted toys such as battery-operated toys for use with a single switch and adapted nonmechanical toys and game boards expand opportunities for young children with disabilities to interact with their environment, exert some control, and engage with others. Many typical toys can be adapted for a child with a disability through the use of switches. Switches provide a way to operate battery-operated toys, radios, televisions, tape players, and games. Switches can be activated by many parts of the body, including hand, foot, head movement, eyebrow wiggle, tongue pressure, and eye glance. Nonmechanical toys can be adapted with big buttons, large handles, bright lights and colors, sounds, textures, and vibrations depending on the child's particular needs. The PACER Center (https://www.pacer.org/stc/tikes/) offers AT training and resources for parents and providers of young children from birth to 5 years old.

Pediatric Aids for Daily Living

Aids for daily living include tools that provide functional solutions for children to accomplish everyday tasks that otherwise they would not be able to do on their own. These tasks include daily activities such as dressing, eating, and personal care. Some examples of dressing aids, as shown in **Figure 20-7**, include zipper pulls, aids for putting on socks, and adapted button hooks for single-hand use. For eating, a spoon/fork combination, cups

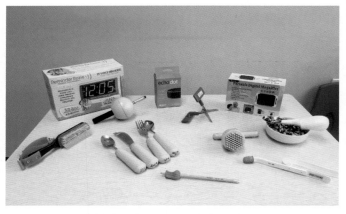

FIGURE 20-7 **Aids for daily living. Top to bottom from left to right: Reminder Rosie alarm clock, Amazon Echo dot environmental control, digital magnifier, adaptive hairbrush, Arthwriter Hand Aid, adaptive scissors, Google Liftware spoon, weighted utensils, universal knob handle, pencil grip, and page turner.**

with snorkel lids to suck fluid, plates and bowls with suction cups for stability while eating or enlarged rims for scooping, and modified handles can offer extra support. Aids for daily living can also assist with grooming, oral hygiene, and bathing tasks. Such tools can include longer or extra grip handles for a hairbrush or toothbrush and adaptive bathroom equipment, such as shower chairs, adaptive seating, or lifts.

Assistive Technology for Mobility, Seating, and Positioning

Providing proper seating, positioning, and mobility for young children is especially important because it enhances the visual information that children receive, heightens sensitivity to objects and events beyond the arm's reach, promotes goal-oriented behavior, and increases control over the environment.[7] As shown in **Figure 20-8**, seating, positioning, and mobility adaptations help to improve stability and seating posture, provide trunk or head support, and reduce pressure on the skin surface.

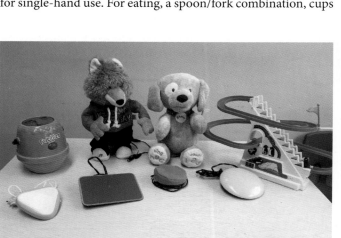

FIGURE 20-6 **Adapted toys. Top to bottom from left to right: Fubbles switch-activated toy, AlbeNet plush switch-activated toys, Penguin Race switch-activated toy, AbleNet Big Candy Corn proximity sensor switch, Adaptivation Pal Pad switch, AbleNet Pillow switch, and Smoothie switch.**

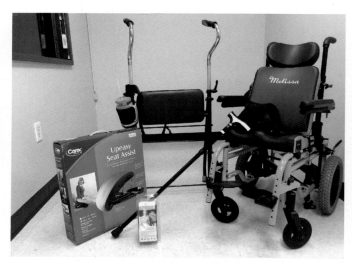

FIGURE 20-8 **Seating, positioning, and mobility options. Left to right: Carex Upeasy Seat Assist, walker, Stander Bed Caddie, cane, and manual wheelchair.**

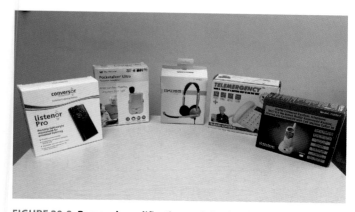

FIGURE 20-9 Personal amplification and alerting devices. Left to right: Conversor Listenor Pro, Pockettalker Ultra, Koss Headset, Telemergency, and Digital Enhanced Cordless Telephone.

Proper seating systems provide external support for a child to support musculoskeletal alignment, postural control, muscle tone, and strength.

Hearing and Vision Devices

AT for individuals with hearing impairments can generally be classified as personal amplification devices or alerting devices, using sound, light, or vibration. Personal amplification devices help individuals with hearing loss hear better. These types of AT devices can range in price and can be purchased with a prescription or a hearing evaluation. Children who have hearing aids or cochlear implants may still benefit from personal amplification devices (**Figure 20-9**). Alerting devices are defined as reactions to alarm situations and are used to inform persons who are deaf or hard of hearing that some condition is occurring. As shown in Figure 20-9, examples of alerting devices include tactile alarm clocks on the bed or pillow, flashing lights for doorbells and smoke alarms, and silent alarms that transmit to a wrist receiver.

Aids for individuals with visual impairments include devices for all degrees of vision loss that affect the individual's ability to perform the usual tasks of daily life. Products for individuals who are blind or visually impaired are designed to provide access to information, ensure safe travel, and assist with activities of daily living. Vision devices can be optical and nonoptical aids and electronic devices. Optical magnification aids are instruments for improving vision and range in cost. As shown in **Figure 20-10**, examples include handheld magnifiers, standing magnifiers, spectacles, contact lenses, and magnifying glasses. Nonoptical aids are instruments that can be used in combination with magnifiers and other optical devices. These devices can assist an individual with reading and other tasks. Nonoptical aids include enlarged print books and computer screens, high-contrast colors, and illumination controls (Figure 20-10). Electronic vision aids are available in several different options, including different sizes, depending on the task or activity. Examples of electronic vision aids (**Figure 20-11**) include closed-circuit devices (eg, closed-circuit television, which increase image size), automatic reading of text

(eg, text-to-speech or text-to-Braille, talking books, newspapers, magazines on MP3s), and synthetic speech output reading machines.

Augmentative and Alternative Communication Aids

AAC is a form of AT focused on communication. These devices provide a means for expressive and receptive communication for persons with limited or no speech. There are 2 types of AAC systems: aided and unaided. An aided AAC system is when an individual uses a tool or device. As shown in **Figure 20-12**, there are a variety of aided AAC options for individuals, including low-tech communication boards, mid-tech 1-message switches, and high-tech or digital-tech speech-generating devices. An unaided AAC system does not require anything other than the person's body to communicate (eg, sign language). Despite the growing empirical evidence that early AAC implementation can aid in the development of natural speech and language,[10] AAC myths persist (**Table 20-2**).

Aids for Computer Use, Including Electronic Aids for Daily Living

Individuals with complex physical difficulties may require AT to meet their needs. Depending on their physical abilities and specific needs, it is possible for a person to navigate, control, and activate a computer, touchscreen device, communication aid, or environmental control unit using a slight movement of their hand or foot, an eye blink, or head movement (**Table 20-3**). These various methods of controlling devices are considered access methods. Direct methods of access include pressing, touching, pointing, eye tracking, or head tracking. Some individuals may have the ability to use their fingers to point at pictures or touch a screen to make a selection or type a message, whereas others may be able to point or type using a different part of their bodies.

If pointing with any part of the body is still challenging, relying on head tracking or eye gaze could be a more suitable option, offering a quick and efficient access method. Head tracking enables a software or application to recognize a person's head movements using a basic front-facing camera on a computer or touch screen device. By moving the head and dwelling on specific options on the screen, a person can make a selection on the device without moving any other part of their body except their head. Similarly, with an eye gaze system mounted to a computer or touch screen device, a person can look and hold their gaze for a preset length of time to make a selection on the screen using their eyes.

Indirect access allows a person to use switches to operate a computer or touch screen device. There are many different types of switches of different sizes and colors. The individual needs to be able to activate either a single switch or a number of switches connected to the computer or touch screen device to make a selection as long as the computer or device is compatible with switch input. Some switches require a light touch to activate or provide visual and auditory feedback (eg, a light flashing or a beeping sound), whereas others can control scanning.

Simple switches require the person to press a button using their hands or any other part of their body (eg, elbow or foot). To offer the user an alternative option, switch scanning is a

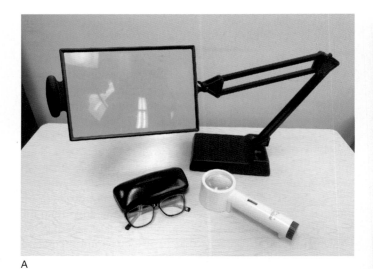

A

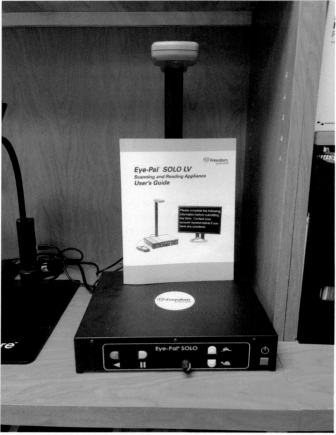

B

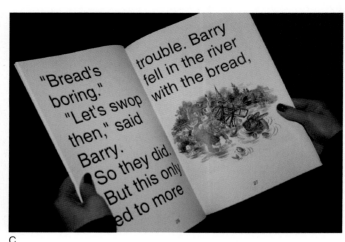

C

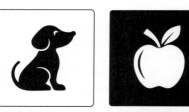

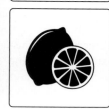

D

FIGURE 20-10 **(A, B) Optical aids and (C, D) nonoptical aids. (A) Left to right: Glasses, table magnifier, and handheld magnifier. (B) Eye-Pal SOLO LV. (C) Large-print books. (Image courtesy of Google.) (D) High-contrast images.** (Used with permission with Chamopcs/Shutterstock.)

setting available in certain software that enables a scan box to move across a series of on-screen items, highlighting or providing an auditory prompt for each item. The person can then activate a switch to select the desired item. There are different levels of switch scanning options. Single-switch scanning is when only one switch is used for automatic scanning. The device automatically controls the scanner, and the person presses a switch to select the desired item. In 2-switch scanning, 2 switches are used to control the scanning. Switch 1 is used to move from one option to the next, and switch 2 is used to

select the desired item or options when reached. More specialized control sites that use head or forehead pointers, eye blink switches, muscle movement detectors, and sip/puff switches by mouth or chin are also available for people who cannot activate a button switch reliably using their hand, fingers, elbow, knee, or foot. Selecting the most reliable access site will offer greater access to communication and increase their efficiency in selecting messages. Regardless of switch type, switches need to be secured and mounted in the ideal position to facilitate the individual's successful use of the device.

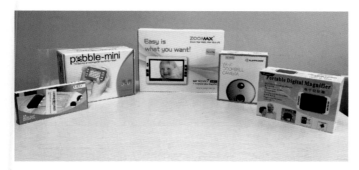

FIGURE 20-11   Electronic vision aids. Left to right: Handheld magnifier, pebble mini magnifier, ZoomMax magnifier, Alarm.com Wifi doorbell camera, and portable digital magnifier.

Learning Aids to Enhance Education

Different types of AT for students with disabilities can enhance their learning. Ranging from low tech to high tech, some AT options include computers and tablets, reading and writing aids, and adaptive learning tools. Different computer and laptop platforms (eg, Windows, MacOS, and Google Chrome) have embedded features for reading and writing such as screen readers, dictation, word prediction, and proofreading options. Text-to-speech offers students the option to see and hear text read aloud at the same time from a computer screen, either by word or by paragraphs. Audio and digital books allow students to hear books read aloud, typically recorded by a human voice. Optical character recognition (OCR) programs allow students to take a photo of a worksheet or scanned document and have the text read aloud.

Writing supports, such as graphic organizers, serve as visual representations, such as diagrams and maps to help students organize ideas and concepts. Students can use these tools to

TABLE 20-2 • Myth and Facts Regarding Augmentative and Alternative Communication (AAC)

Myth	Fact
AAC is a "last resort" in speech-language intervention.	The use of AAC interventions should not be contingent on failure to develop speech skills or considered a last resort because AAC can play many roles in communication development.[11,12] In fact, it is critical that AAC be introduced before communication failure occurs.
AAC hinders or stops further speech development.	Many parents and practitioners fear AAC will become the child's primary communication mode and take away the child's motivation to speak. This is not supported by the available empirical data. The literature actually suggests the opposite outcome: improvement in speech skills after AAC intervention.[13]
Children must have a certain skill set, age, or cognitive level to benefit from AAC use.	There is no evidence suggesting that children must be a certain age or posses a certain skill set to optimally benefit from AAC interventions. In fact, newer AAC tools, especially those offered via smart devices or dynamic displays, are more intuitive and require less training than in the past.

take notes while reading and they can help with comprehension. When speech is clear, students can write or type by using their voice as the words they speak appear on the screen using dictation or speech-to-text programs. Word prediction programs help students by suggesting correct spellings of words after only a few letters are typed, or they may include a word bank of the most commonly used words. Adaptive learning tools are simple tools that support the learning experience of children with physical impairment. Items such as book holders, slant boards, page turners, modified desks, and seating/standing equipment facilitate daily classroom activities.

■ ASSISTIVE TECHNOLOGY LEGISLATION AND FUNDING OVERVIEW

With the passage of federal laws, the consideration of AT to ensure equal access to school, community, and ultimately work for children with disabilities is a mandated practice.[14] Below are brief summaries of 4 main federal legislations that affect AT service delivery: (1) the Americans with Disabilities Act (1990) (ADA) (PL 101-336); (2) the Technology-Related Assistance for Individuals with Disabilities Act (1999) (Tech Act) (PL 100-407); (3) the Individuals with Disabilities Education Act (2004) (IDEA) (PL 105-17); and (4) the Rehabilitation Act of 1973 (1993).

THE AMERICANS WITH DISABILITIES ACT (ADA) (PL 101-336 [42 USC 12101])

The ADA (1990) is one of the first landmark laws prohibiting discrimination based on disability in employment, state

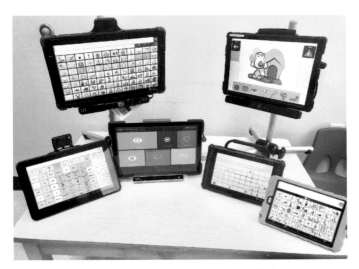

FIGURE 20-12   Photos of different augmentative and alternative communication options. Top row from left to right: PRC Accent 1400 with eye gaze and head tracker and Forbes AAC Winslate for Kids with eye gaze. Bottom row from left to right: Saltillo Chat Fusion, TobiiDynavox, PRC Accent 800, and iPad with Proloqou2Go vocabulary system.

TABLE 20-3 • Different Types of Adaptive Equipment

Type of Assistive Technology	Definition
Alternative keyboard	Keyboards that have larger, more widely spaced keys or one-handed, color-coded, or on-screen keyboard options. Some include keyguards, which are plastic or metal plates that sit above the keys on a standard keyboard. Keyguards isolate the keyboard's keys to help stabilize and position fingers or pointers.
Alternative mouse	Allows the user to move the computer cursor more easily with his or her hand or by not using hands at all. May include trackballs, joysticks, touch screens, head pointers, or touch pads.
Head pointers	Allow the movement of the mouse pointer to be controlled by voluntary head movements. A special camera sits on a monitor or laptop screen. The person controls the pointer on the screen by tracking a removable, reflective dot placed on a person's forehead, glasses, or finger.
Speech input software	An alternate way to type text and also control the computer. The person can speak commands and dictation to a word processing application to directly control computer and browser options.
Accessibility features	Designed to help people with disabilities use computers and smart devices more easily. Although some accessibility features require special software downloads, many are built into the computer or mobile device operating system. Common features include display controls to change the font or contrast on the screen, increase the size of icons such as the cursor, magnification options, screen readers, and keyboard shortcuts.

and local government, public accommodations, commercial facilities, transportation, and telecommunications. ADA has 4 main titles, all of which include AT provisions. Title I requires employers to make reasonable accommodations, including AT for people with disabilities. Titles II and III require that public transportation and public accommodations be accessible for people with disabilities, respectively. Title IV addresses telephone and television access such as text telephones (TTYs) and closed captioning. The following website provides more information about AT and ADA: https://www.ada.gov/law-andregs/ada/.

TECHNOLOGY-RELATED ASSISTANCE FOR INDIVIDUALS WITH DISABILITIES ACT

The Tech Act was passed in 1988 and amended in 1994, 1998, and 2004 and was passed to help states increase awareness, access, and acquisition of AT. This important legislation includes several provisions that positively impact the lives of persons with disabilities through monetary assistance to every state and territory in the United States. Throughout all authorizations, state AT programs are required to serve all people with all types of disabilities, of all ages, in all environments (early intervention, kindergarten through grade 12, postsecondary, vocational rehabilitation, community living, and aging services) and include all types of AT. These state AT programs funded by the Tech Act are a great source of information for physical therapists and other service providers. Each state AT program provides the following services:

- Device reutilization program: Provides for the exchange, repair, and recycling of AT devices
- Device loan program: Provides short-term device loans to individuals, employers, public agencies, or others seeking to meet the needs of people with disabilities
- Device demonstration program: Demonstrates a variety of AT devices

For a list of state AT programs, visit https://www.at3center.net/stateprogram.

INDIVIDUALS WITH DISABILITIES EDUCATION ACT (IDEA)

IDEA (2004) was initially passed in 1975 as Public Law 94-142. That law, known as the Education for All Handicapped Children Act, or the EHA, guaranteed that eligible children and youth with disabilities were entitled to a free and appropriate public education (FAPE), designed to meet their unique educational needs. Public Law 94-142 has been amended many times since passing in 1975 and, most recently, in 2004 as the Individuals with Disabilities Education Improvement Act (IDEIA). According to IDEIA (2004), public schools must ensure that AT devices and services are available for children receiving special education services. School teams must consider a continuum of AT devices as part of the child's Individualized Education Program (IEP). Once school teams identify the need for AT on the child's IEP, they must provide the device at no cost to parents.[14] For example, a school team might suggest a laptop and word-processing software such as Read & Write (www.texthelp.com) as a tool to help a student with grammar, reading aloud text, spelling, and word prediction.[15] AT services include AT evaluations; purchasing, selecting, designing, and customizing devices; and training and technical assistance for the child, teachers, parents, and other professionals involved in providing AT services. Lack of funding or local services is not sufficient reason to deny AT devices justified in the IEP.[7] Additionally, the law includes provisions that clearly state that AT provided by the school may be made available in the child's home or in other settings if the IEP team determines that the child requires the AT to receive FAPE.[16] Visit http://idea.ed.gov/ for more information.

THE REHABILITATION ACT OF 1973 (AMENDED IN 1993)

The Rehabilitation Act of 1973 (amended in 1993) is a civil rights law that prohibits discrimination and mandates reasonable accommodations in all federally funded programs. Section 504 provides reasonable accommodations to children with disabilities who do not qualify for special education services under the IDEA. A 504 plan is a formal document that schools use to provide students with disabilities the proper supports; this includes AT. If the school team determines that a child needs AT to access their education, the school must provide the AT to the child at no cost to the parents. The law also requires that AT be included in state vocational rehabilitation services plans and Individualized Plans for Employment. Section 508 of the law mandates that all electronic and information technology developed, maintained, or used by the federal government be accessible to people with disabilities. More information can be found at https://www.hhs.gov/web/section-508/what-is-section-504/index.html.

FUNDING

Public, private, and alternative programs are available for the purchase of devices. Medicaid is the largest funding source of AT for recipients who qualify. Medicaid is an income-based program for individuals who need medical and rehabilitative services. Medicare is another major funding source for AT for individuals who are 65 years or older and for individuals of all ages who meet the standards of disability under the Social Security Act.[7] State-funded Medicaid/Medicare programs and private managed care are the primary sources of funding for AT that is considered durable medical equipment, prosthetics, or specialized equipment such as speech-generating devices.[3] Other funding sources include private health insurance and alternative funding programs such as low-interest loans offered by many state AT programs and private foundations and charitable organizations.

Justifying funding for AT services and devices through public and private funding sources requires adequate documentation and proof of need. The essential question that funding sources want answered is how this technology will improve the individual's functioning. Whether it is medical, vocational, or an educational need, there are essential components that should be included in any written justification: an AT assessment, documentation of a trial period, and the physician's prescription for an equipment considered to be "medically necessary." Medical necessity refers to a medical diagnosis or condition that is specifically coupled to the functional impairment being addressed by the device.[17] The letter of medical necessity written by the physician needs to include the person's disability and prognosis.

Every funding agency has an appeals process for funding denial. Almost all funding programs will provide an explanation for the denial in writing. By knowing the reason for the denial, an appeal plan can be developed. In short, an appeal plan allows for the development of a specific statement of why the denial is wrong and why it should be reversed.

Justifying funding for AT for a child who attends the public school system through IDEA must be documented on an Individualized Family Service Plan (IFSP) for children birth to age 3 or the IEP for children age 3 to 21 years. If AT is identified as necessary for FAPE, it must be included in the IFSP/IEP and the device and service must be provided. The caveat is that the device is the property of the school but can transition to home, work, and community settings if the child needs the AT to access their education (IDEA, 2004).

OVERVIEW OF THE INTERDISCIPLINARY ASSISTIVE TECHNOLOGY SERVICE DELIVERY PROCESS

Although considering AT to support the needs of children with disabilities is a mandated practice in community, educational, and vocational settings, physical therapists and other service providers are faced with the challenge of how to actually implement AT service delivery practices.[2,14,18] AT service delivery is integral to pediatric physical therapy because it helps children with disabilities navigate through barriers to participate more fully in daily activities. AT service delivery has a critical role in determining whether individuals will successfully use and benefit from AT.[19] This process can be complex and involve multiple steps and stakeholders.[20]

AT services are most effective when provided by an interdisciplinary team, which may include AT professionals (ATPs), physical therapists, occupational therapists (OTs), speech-language pathologists (SLPs), educators, vendors, medical professionals, the child, and family members.[21,22] When forming an interdisciplinary team, all stakeholders involved in the care of the child should be aware of protocols for AT service delivery.[15] Central to the team are the family and child. A family- and person-centered approach provides a process for identifying family resources and ensures shared goals and decision-making for AT use.[23] Responsibilities of an interdisciplinary team include obtaining necessary referrals, setting goals in collaboration with the family, conducting evaluations and trials, selecting devices and vendors, identifying funding sources, determining training needs, following up on how the AT is working, and modifying goals when necessary.[14] Team members work together to gather and synthesize information and collaborate to develop coordinated recommendations for the child. The configuration of the AT team will vary depending on the needs of the child and family and the setting. Effective communication and coordination of AT service among team members are essential to ensure the appropriate selection of AT and reduce the risk of device abandonment.[3,21]

Other members of the AT team may include the child's doctor or medical professional and a designated AT specialist/professional. The medical professional provides important information such as how the child's disability or diagnosis affects participation in daily activities and what medications the child takes. When obtaining funding for the AT devices, physicians may also be required to provide a prescription for the AT assessment and a letter of medical necessity for the AT devices and services. The ATP or AT specialist can be any member of the team from any discipline (eg, OT, physical therapist, SLP, educator) who has specialized training and expertise in AT service delivery. These individuals may also be Rehabilitation Engineering and Assistive Technology Society of North America (RESNA)-certified ATPs, although this designation is not necessary. RESNA is an interdisciplinary professional association established in 1995 whose activities focus on ATs. Its members come from many disciplines and a variety of settings, and their activities involve the full scope of AT applications. RESNA offers a professional certification program that is based on standards of practice for ATPs and

AT suppliers. The credentialed ATP means that the professional has specialized training and experience in AT and promotes a standard of safety and effective AT service delivery.[3] For a list of ATPs in your area and for more information on RESNA, visit www.RESNA.org.

Additional resources to consider when forming the interdisciplinary team include access to your state AT Tech Act program and AT vendor or manufacturer. State AT programs can provide additional support to the AT team by providing device demonstrations and short-term device loans during the AT assessment and trial periods.[24] During the acquisition phase, state AT programs can also provide device training and technical support on various types of AT such as AAC, mobility devices, and electronic aids for daily living for members of the AT team and caregivers. State AT programs can also be an initial point of contact to provide referrals to AT specialists and professionals and/or agencies that provide AT assessment services. For a list of state AT programs, visit https://www.at3center.net/stateprogram. Similar to state AT programs, an AT vendor or manufacturer can provide device demonstrations and equipment rentals during the AT assessment and trial phases. AT vendors can also assist with acquiring funding from the documentation provided by the AT team and help with the funding process.[24]

ROLE OF THE PHYSICAL THERAPIST IN ASSISTIVE TECHNOLOGY

According to Long and Perry[2] and the Commission on Accreditation in Physical Therapy Education, physical therapists should have knowledge and skills to examine an individual in the area of assistive and adaptive devices (criterion number CC-5.30d) and provide intervention including prescribing, applying, and, as appropriate, fabricating devices and equipment (criterion number CC-5.39e). Physical therapists are one of the most common collaborators on the interdisciplinary team and typically assist with seating, positioning, and device access; however, physical therapists may assist with other aspects of the AT service delivery as deemed necessary by the interdisciplinary team.[2] Unfortunately, most physical therapists in general have limited knowledge of AT service delivery, which may inadvertently restrict a child's access to AT.[19]

Therefore, it is important that physical therapists gain their own competence in AT service delivery so that families have access to practitioners with the knowledge and skill to support children who need and use AT. One way for physical therapists to improve their AT competence is to join interdisciplinary professional organizations such as RESNA (www.RESNA.org), the Assistive Technology Industry Association (www.atia.org),

and the International Society for Augmentative and Alternative Communication (www.isaac-online.org). These organizations offer membership to professionals from many disciplines interested in AT.

Another consideration for physical therapists is to become a certified ATP through RESNA. There is an increasing need for physical therapists to be credentialed. According to RESNA, 647 physical therapists are credentialed ATPs, which is 7.7% of all credentialed ATPs.[25] Physical therapists and other service providers who often provide AT services to children should consider obtaining credentialing.[3]

■ ASSISTIVE TECHNOLOGY SERVICE DELIVERY

When considering AT for a child with a disability, merely providing the child access to the device is not enough.[26] Systematic approaches and evidenced informed decisions are necessary to identify the most appropriate technology for the user and to provide the necessary training and support for all stakeholders. **Figure 20-13** shows a 6-step process for how to assess a child for AT.[24]

During the referral and intake process, the AT team must collect background information on the child and family. Background information should include relevant medical information, diagnosis, educational setting, therapies (current and past), AT needs, and AT experience. It is also important to gather the child's IEP or the IFSP and any previous evaluations or progress notes related to the therapies that the child is currently receiving (eg, speech and language, occupational, physical).[24]

After gathering information from the intake process, the AT team conducts the initial evaluation to consider the child's need for AT, assess the child's skills, and determine the device characteristics. Numerous frameworks exist[27] to guide decision-making and include the following elements: (1) child factors to support AT use; (2) participation in activities or tasks; and (3) context and environment in which AT is needed. **Table 20-4** provides a brief summary of some of the more common frameworks. This chapter will focus on 2 of these frameworks: the International Classification of Functioning, Disability, and Health (ICF; most familiar to physical therapists) and the Human Activity Assistive Technology Model.

THE INTERNATIONAL CLASSIFICATION OF FUNCTIONING, DISABILITY, AND HEALTH

The ICF is a familiar and useful model to help guide physical therapists in the initial evaluation of AT needs.[3] The ICF

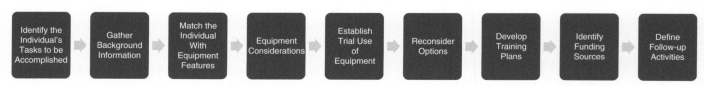

FIGURE 20-13 **Steps in the assistive technology service delivery process.** (Source: https://ndassistive.org/wp-content/uploads/2013/04/assistive-technology-assessment-process-2011.pdf)

TABLE 20-4 • Models and Frameworks for the Consideration of Assistive Technology	
Model	**Key Considerations**
The International Classification of Functioning, Disability, and Health[28]	The ICF framework focuses on the child's ability to participate in desired activities with an emphasis on what the child can do in important contexts.
HAAT[7]	The Human Activity Assistive Technology (HAAT) Model focuses on the interaction of the human skills to perform an activity within a context in which the assistive technology enables the human to perform the activity.
MPT[36] http://www.matchingpersonandtechnology.com	The Matching Person with Technology (MPT) Model focuses attention on the needs of the user, the aspects of the environments in which it will be used, and the functions and features of the technology.
SETT[37,38] http://www.joyzabala.com/	The Student, Environments, Tasks, Tools (SETT) Model provides a framework to evaluate systematically the student, the environment, the tasks, and the technology to be used.

Source: Wissick CA and Gardner JE. Conducting assessments in technology needs: From assessment to implementation. (33(2): 78-93, Copyright © 2008 by SAGE publication). Reprinted by permission of SAGE publications.

framework is an ideal framework because it focuses on the child's ability to participate in desired activities with an emphasis on what the child can do in important contexts. As shown in **Figure 20-14**, the ICF framework is a hierarchical scheme for the child's health condition based on 2 main parts: (1) functioning and disability and (2) contextual factors. The ICF framework is well suited to guide AT service delivery because it includes the contextual factors (personal and environmental) that may support or inhibit participation in daily activities and how AT can be used to augment body functions and structures. The physical therapist, family, and other team members work collaboratively to analyze factors that are impacting the child's functioning and participation in daily activities and how AT can be beneficial.

Steel et al[19] offer a guide for how to use the ICF framework.

1. Identify strengths and challenges in body functions and identify goals to improve activities and participation.

2. Determine environmental and personal factors that are barriers and facilitators and identify AT based on those needs.
3. Seek out databases through state-funded AT programs to explore and compare options. These programs often offer short-term loans to trial different devices.
4. Collect data in collaboration with family to evaluate the selected AT's suitability for the child. This includes gaining feedback on the preferences of the child and family. The ICF framework is also a useful tool to compare the child's functioning with and without AT.[29]

THE HUMAN ACTIVITY ASSISTIVE TECHNOLOGY MODEL

One of the most widely known and comprehensive frameworks in AT service delivery is the Human Activity Assistive Technology (HAAT) Model.[3,20,30] HAAT is an ecological and

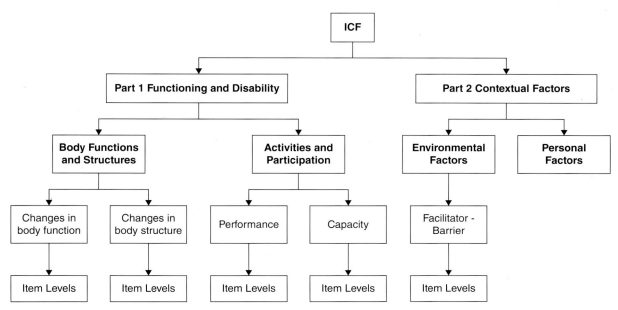

FIGURE 20-14 **International Classification of Functioning, Disability, and Health (ICF) framework.**[6] (Reprinted from On modelling assistive technology systems—Part I: Modelling framework, 20, Hersh MA & Johnson MA. *Technology and disability*, 193-215, 2008, with permission from IOS press. The publication is available at IOS Press through http://dx.doi.org/[10.3233/TAD-2008-20303])

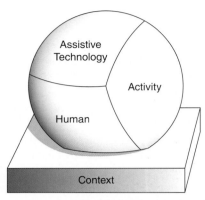

FIGURE 20-15 Visual representation of Human Activity Assistive Technology (HAAT) Model.[7] (Reproduced with permission from Cook AM, & Polgar JM. Assistive technologies: *Principles and Practice*, 4th ed: Elsevier; 2015.)

transactional construct. The 4 contextual components include (1) someone (human) doing (2) something (activity) in a (3) specific context using (4) technology as an enabler. As seen in **Figure 20-15**, the human, activity, and AT are interlocked in a sphere. Holding all these parts as depicted in a shallow box is the context in which AT is used. The components in the HAAT Model are comparable to those of the ICF framework: human (person), activity (occupation or performance of a task or activity), and the context (environment). According to Wissick and Gardner,[15] the activity is the goal to be achieved, and the human has the skills available to meet the goal. The context brings these skills and goals together and defines constraints on achieving goals. The AT therefore provides an external way for the human to perform the activity. While there are many models that can be used and adapted for individuals of any age or ability, what differentiates the HAAT Model from other models is that the focus is not only on the human's performance. In the HAAT Model, the context is broader to include social and cultural aspects as well as environments and physical conditions (eg, temperature, noise level, lighting) that may impact AT use.

When using the HAAT Model, the AT team conducts an assessment of the child's intrinsic enablers, the activities where AT is needed, and contextual factors that may facilitate or inhibit AT use and a trial of AT options. Let us consider the case of Mary who is a 17-year-old high school student with spina bifida. She will be attending a local community college for a degree in business in the fall. She is interested in AT to help her take notes during class.

Human Component (Intrinsic Enablers)

The first step in the HAAT Model is the human component and includes the user's intrinsic enablers or abilities in motor, sensory, cognitive, and affective areas. It also includes the user's roles in life and experience with technology (eg, motivation). In this stage of the HAAT Model, Mary's team considers what abilities (ie, intrinsic enablers) she will bring to the task of writing. With regard to sensory input, her team considers her ability to hear (auditory) the teacher and see (vision) the lecture

notes on the white board and paper. Once the sensory input has been determined, the team considers her cognitive abilities (ie, central processing). The team considers whether Mary is able to understand and interpret what the instructor is saying (language) and what the instructor writes on the white board (perception). They must also consider whether Mary is able to determine which information is pertinent (decision-making) and retain that information long enough to write it down (short-term memory) in her notes. Lastly, the team considers Mary's motor output. They consider her fine motor abilities to write. Other factors that may affect the effectiveness of motor output include automatic movements (eg, primitive reflexes, righting reactions, equilibrium reactions), muscle tone (flaccidity/hypotonicity and spasticity/hypertonicity), posture, strength, endurance, range of motion, and pain.

The Activities

The next component of the HAAT Model is to consider the activities (ie, purposeful tasks) that the user needs to perform throughout the day in the areas of self-care, learning, work, and leisure. At this stage, it is important for her team to consider Mary's various roles. A person may have multiple roles, and the roles may change with time. For example, Mary will not always be a student. When she graduates from college, her role may change to that of a business owner, or she may pick up additional roles.

Initially, when Mary was younger and began using a wheelchair, she needed her AT team to instruct her in manual tasks such as grooming, dressing, and bathing. As Mary grew older and started school, her AT team helped her develop skills to conserve her energy during daily manual tasks and reduce stress on her body. Currently, she is seeking AT to learn how to use technology to help her take notes in her role as a student. In the future, she may also need AT to drive, write term papers, and help her run a home-based Internet business.

When determining the activities, a task analysis should be completed to break the activity down into its individual components. For example, if the task for Mary is taking notes in class, some of the tasks may include pulling out a piece of paper, picking up and positioning the writing implement in the hand ready to write, hearing the teacher and processing what the teacher is saying, and writing down the pertinent points. The task analysis will enable the team to see whether Mary has the intrinsic skills or abilities—what she brings to the task, what parts of her body move, how fast her reaction time is, and what her proficiency level is to complete the task of writing and if an alternative approach will be needed. For example, as a student, Mary may need to use a computer or typing aid to take notes; however, she may require practice.

The Context

The third component of the HAAT Model is the context, also known as the environment. The context includes physical context (physical environments that support or hinder participation), social context (the individuals who interact in the user's environment), cultural context (beliefs, rituals, and values that are important to the user), and institutional context (eg, legislation, policy, funding). According to Cook and Polgar,[7] the contexts in which the human carries out the activity are frequently forgotten when AT applications are considered. However, the context is often the determining factor in the success or failure of the AT system. In Mary's case, she has a strong family and social support network. Her team must also consider whether she will need to perform writing tasks at school, at home, or in other setting.

The Assistive Technology (ie, Human-Technology Interface)

The fourth component is the human-technology interface (HTI). The HTI is the interaction between the human and the AT, which leads to an activity output in the areas of communication, mobility, manipulation, or cognitive processing. The purpose of these outputs is to link a human interaction (pressing a switch) to an activity (moving or speaking) in an assistive or augmentative way. Mary's team considers a range of AT from low-tech to high-tech devices. In the note-writing example, depending on Mary's deficits, some of her no-tech to high-tech alternatives include the following:

- Having a classmate take notes for her and give her a copy
- Using an adapted pencil/pen grip (**Figure 20-16**)
- Audio recording the notes
- Using note-taking applications: AudioNote, Notability, Inspiration Maps
- Typing up the notes using a laptop with a word processing program such as Read&Write for Google (https://chrome.google.com/webstore/detail/readwrite-for-google-chro/inoeonmfapjbbkmdafoankkfajkcphgd?hl=en-US)
- Using voice dictation software such as Dragon Speak
- Using the Livescribe Smart Pen (https://www.livescribe.com/en-us/smartpen/) to audio record notes while writing notes

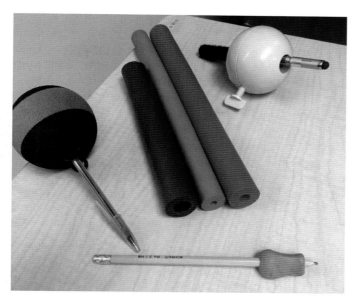

FIGURE 20-16 Adapted pencil grip. Top to bottom from left to right: Ball grip, grips, Arthwriter Hand Aid, and pencil grip.

The team will need to trial different AT options to determine which will be most beneficial. The AT system chosen must be tried out in the different contexts in which it will be used under varying circumstances (eg, various classrooms, teachers, and subjects). When an AT is not successful, use the activity analysis to assess at which component the AT system was successful, and then make corrections as needed. Input from the user and family is important throughout the whole process. There are times when the team feels an AT system is the best solution but the user (or caregiver) is not interested in it, and if this is the case, the AT system may fail.

After the initial evaluation, the team will make recommendations on the most appropriate AT device and write a report detailing the results of the initial evaluation. Once the report is written, the AT team must submit the report and any other documentation to the funding source to acquire the device. Other documents may include a prescription, a certificate of medical necessity, release of information for AT vendor, device selection form, and/or plan of care.

Once the device is received, caregivers (including service providers) should be trained on how to use, program, and maintain the device. Once again, the state AT program can assist caregivers and team members with device programming and training. As described in step 5 of the AT service delivery process, the follow-up will involve additional training to maintain use and identifying successes and problems with the AT device that have occurred since implementation. Lastly, in step 6, the follow along, the individuals with disabilities who are using AT devices should be assessed periodically to determine the need for changes.

The Assistive Technology Outcomes Measures Project (ATOMS Project), funded in part by the National Institute on Disability and Rehabilitation Research (NIDRR) under the Disability and Rehabilitation Research Projects (DRRP) program, provides access to an information database of AT assessment data collection tools.[31] This online database contains information on 43 different AT assessment tools. The tools are divided into 5 categories: AAC, seating and positioning, computer access, school and education, and other. Physical therapists and other practitioners can search the database for assessment tools that seem appropriate to meet the child's needs.[15] For more information on the database, visit http:www.r2d2.uwm.edu/atoms. **Table 20-5** provides information on specific AT centers and organizations that provide free downloads and assessment protocols.

■ TELE-AAC SERVICE DELIVERY MODEL

The coronavirus disease 2019 (COVID-19) global pandemic affected the disability community across the world[32] and affected access to education and essential rehabilitation therapies worldwide. Educators and service providers from all disciplines were required to swiftly shift and adapt traditional face-to-face service delivery to telehealth services to ensure the safety of their students and clients.[24] Telehealth, also known as telepractice, is defined by the American Speech-Language-Hearing

TABLE 20-5 • Assistive Technology Resources

Assistive technology Assessment	Web Site	Resources
ATOMS	http://www.r2d2.uwm.edu/atoms	Assistive Technology Outcomes: Informational database of AT assessments; graphic model of the IMPACT2 model
ATTO	http://atto.buffalo.edu	Assistive Technology Training Online: Handouts and tutorials on software use; AT process guide and forms based on SETT model
Boston Access Center	http://boston.k12.ma.us/teach/technology/access.asp	Student Access Map (SAM) model planning form to consider standards, student, barriers, and tools
GPAT	http://www.gpat.org	Georgia Project for Assistive Technology: Videos, handouts, and charts with definitions on types of devices
UKAT	http://serc.gws.uky.edu/www/ukatii	University of Kentucky Assistive Technology Toolkit: Complete manual for assistive technology
NATRI	http://natri.uky.edu	National Assistive Technology Research Institute: Information on the AT Planner Implementation Guide
TATN	http://www.texasat.net	Texas Assistive Technology Network: Complete implementation training module with training guide and forms based on the SETT framework
Tools for Life	http://www.gatfl.org/ldguide/default.htm	Specific information on tools for students with learning disabilities
RESNA	http://www.resna.org	Rehabilitation Engineering and Assistive Technology Society of North America: List of Tech Act Funded AT centers
SETT Framework	http://sweb.uky.edu/~jszaba0SETT2.html	Setting the Stage for Success: Detailed information on the SETT framework and on the quality indicators for assistive technology implementation (QIAT)
TAM	http://www.tamcec.org	Technology and Media Division of Council for Exceptional Children: Resource for AT Planner and monographs on AT implementation
WATI	http://www.wati.org	Wisconsin Assistive Technology Initiative Free download of "Hey Can I Try That?" and information on Education Tech Points

Source: Wissick CA, and Gardner JE. Conducting assessments in technology needs: From assessment to implementation. (33(2) 78-93, Copyright © 2008 by SAGE publication). Reprinted by permission of SAGE publications.

Association (ASHA) as "the application of telecommunications technology to the delivery of speech-language pathology and audiology professional services at a distance by linking clinician to client/patient or clinician to clinician for assessment, intervention, and/or consultation."[22] Research from multiple disciplines confirms that telehealth services empower both the client and the provider in determining the best approach to care while considering demographics, location, and diagnosis. Telehealth services reduce health disparities by providing access to high-quality, cost-effective care, especially for families in rural areas.[33] Tele-AAC, a specialized and unique type of service delivery, requires a provider to have technical expertise in both telepractice and AAC systems.[34]

Using Health Insurance Portability and Accountability Act–compliant video conferencing platforms, direct and indirect services can be provided to the AAC user. Direct services include the AAC user receiving real-time feedback on their device from an experienced provider, and indirect services include family members or caregivers receiving training and feedback on how to support the AAC users' communication.[35] Tele-AAC practices provide access to skilled AAC clinicians that may not be otherwise available in the AAC users' community due to geographic, travel (eg, access to a converted van), and time constraints. Additionally, tele-AAC services reduce barriers to obtaining ongoing services at home and promote collaboration with the AAC users' treating home health providers. **Table 20-6** demonstrates one example of how to implement an interdisciplinary tele-AAC assessment.[24]

Although tele-AAC practices have shown promising results, this practice is not a one-size-fits-all approach, and its appropriateness and use should be carefully considered for each child. Some families may prefer or require face-to-face support and intervention. Therefore, a hybrid approach that incorporates both telehealth practices and face-to-face services should be considered based on the family's preference and specific needs.[24,35] It is important for clinicians to become familiar with telehealth practices as the introduction of the Expanded Telehealth Access Act of 2021 will enable outpatient therapy providers, such as physical therapists, physical therapy assistants, OTs and their assistants, and SLPs, to continue using telehealth as a service delivery option for Medicare- and Medicaid-insured patients beyond the COVID-19 pandemic.

TABLE 20-6 • Interdisciplinary Tele-AAC Process and Communication Methods

Key Components	Tele-AAC Steps	Communication Methods/ Technology Needs
Conduct a technology-based assessment to prepare the family for the tele-AAC assessment.	1. Caregiver emails, completed questionnaire forms, previous evaluations, and video to ATP 2. ATP schedules call or Zoom with caregiver to discuss: • Tele-AAC assessment process • HIPAA-compliant technology to be used during the tele-sessions • Review consent forms (FERPA, video consent) 3. ATP and SLP conduct an initial video consultation to determine the caregiver's technology needs and computer equipment needed for the AAC assessment: • Computer/tablet, Zoom for video conferencing • Smartphone/tablet with mount for viewing AAC screen • Bluetooth headphones to communicate with caregiver • Preprogrammed AAC device(s) to use with person with CCNs 4. ATP and SLP assess the home environment to determine: • Where the assessment will take place • Where to position the camera • What activities to prepare in advance 5. ATP and SLP discuss with caregiver the possibility of inviting person's service providers (SLP, OT, PT) to the tele-AAC assessment 6. SLP borrows AAC, and additional technology needed (tablet with mount, Bluetooth headphones, mount) from state AT Tech Act program, preprograms the AAC device, and ships to caregiver 7. Caregiver receives preprogrammed AAC devices and technology for the AAC assessment from state AT Tech Act program	Phone, email, computer/tablet, video conferencing platform, US Postal Service, FedEx, UPS
Conduct tele-AAC assessment guided by the interdisciplinary team and facilitated by the caregiver.	8. SLP conducts tele-AAC assessment via video conferencing platform by coaching the caregiver 9. Other members of AAC team (eg, ATP, OT, PT) join video conferencing platform to assist SLP in determining the device access method 10. The person's service providers join via video conferencing platform or at person's home 11. The SLP uses screen mirroring app and screen sharing to program the device on the spot 12. AAC team, caregiver, and service providers determine AAC to trial	Computer/tablet, video conferencing platform, smartphone/tablet, mount, Bluetooth headphones, preprogrammed AAC device(s), screen mirroring app, screen sharing
Coach caregiver during tele-AAC device trial.	13. ATP coordinates a device loan from local AAC vendor or state AT Tech Act program to use during device trial 14. AAC vendor and SLP meet with caregiver and person to provide training and technical support on how to use the AAC device during the trial. Vendor or SLP uses the following technology: • Screen share • Remote into AAC device • Screen mirroring app 15. SLP conducts trial sessions via video conferencing platform, coaches caregiver to facilitate the communication interactions, and gathers data to determine appropriate AAC system • May include OT for access and/or ATP for caregiver device training • May include the person's service providers	Computer/tablet, video conferencing platform, preprogrammed AAC device, Bluetooth headphones, screen mirroring app, screen sharing
Provide ongoing support to the AAC user and caregiver(s) during acquisition, programming, and maintenance of the AAC device.	16. ATP works with family via phone or video conferencing platform to apply for AAC funding 17. ATP and SLP provide AAC resources from state AT Tech Act program for device training and continued support	Phone or computer/tablet, video conferencing platform

Abbreviations: AT, assistive technology; ATP, assistive technology professional; AAC, augmentative and alternative communication; CCN, complex communication need; FERPA, Family Educational Rights and Privacy Act; HIPAA, Health Insurance Portability and Accountability Act; OT, occupational therapy; PT, physical therapy; SLP, speech-language pathologist.

■ SUMMARY

Children with disabilities often need and can benefit from the use of AT devices and services. These services and supports can increase children's participation in everyday activities at home, at school, and in the community. Physical therapists, along with other service providers, need to know how to consider a range of ATs to optimize the overall functioning of children with disabilities and support their participation in everyday activities. Physical therapists are in an ideal position to consider, recommend, and in many cases implement AT devices and services because they are often one of the first service providers to provide interventions to children with disabilities.

AT is a broad umbrella term that includes equipment, devices, technologies, services, systems, and processes that people with disabilities use to support their independence and full participation in society. AT ranges from low tech to high tech and digital technology and includes adapted toys; aids for daily living; AT for mobility, including seating and position; hearing and vision devices; AAC devices; EADLs; and learning aids. Mandated laws such as IDEA, ADA, Tech Act, and Section 508 provide provisions for AT service delivery to ensure children with disabilities have equal access to school, community, and ultimately work. Public and private funding sources are available to help children with disabilities and their families acquire AT devices and services.

AT service delivery is integral to pediatric physical therapy because it helps children with disabilities navigate through barriers to participate more fully in daily activities. Physical therapists are one of the most common collaborators on the interdisciplinary team, typically assisting with seating, positioning, and device access; however, physical therapists may assist with other aspects of the AT service delivery as deemed necessary by the interdisciplinary team. As a member of the AT team, it is important that physical therapists gain their own competence in AT service delivery so that families have access to practitioners with the knowledge and skills to support children who need and use AT through membership in interdisciplinary professional organizations and/or certification in AT through RESNA.

AT assessment is a complex, collaborative, and evolving decision-making process undertaken by a team of professionals, individuals with disabilities, and their day-to-day contacts, including families, teachers, and school support staff. Other members of the team may include an AT specialist/professional, representatives from state AT programs, and/or AT vendors. When considering AT for a child with a disability, merely providing the child access to the device is not enough. Systematic approaches such as the ICF framework and HAAT Model are necessary to make informed decisions and identify the most appropriate technology for the user and to provide the necessary training and support for all stakeholders. Free resources such as state AT Tech Act programs are also available to provide physical therapists and other service providers with additional AT information and training.

Case 1

Alex is a 31-month-old child with cerebral palsy. Alex has severe spasticity in the extremities with hypotonia in the trunk. He has a severe motor impairment with high cognitive abilities. Alex communicates by vocalizations, facial expressions, body movements, and looking at desired objects in his environment. Alex receives occupational, physical, and speech therapies. The family would like Alex to be able to communicate with siblings and parents.

Questions

1. What recommendations would you make for curriculum adaptations and access to materials?
2. What recommendations would you make for access to toys, computers, and appliances?
3. What recommendations would you make for communications?

Case 2

Joanna, age 5, was involved in a near-drowning accident approximately 2 years ago. Prior to her near-drowning, her family indicated that she had been developing like a typical child her age, and they described her as being affectionate, sociable, and verbal. Joanna was found floating in a lake. She had been immersed for approximately 8 to 10 minutes and required cardiopulmonary resuscitation at the scene. She suffered anoxic encephalopathy. She was hospitalized for 2 weeks (in a coma) and then was transferred to an inpatient rehabilitation unit, where she spent 3.5 months. Upon admission, she exhibited extensor posturing, and no purposeful movement was observed. In addition, she exhibited flexion to painful stimuli on the left side, extension to painful stimuli on the right upper extremity, and minimal response to painful stimuli in the right lower extremity. No response to visual or auditory stimuli was elicited. She exhibited crying but no verbalization. At the time of discharge from inpatient rehabilitation, Joanna had made considerable progress. She was described as attentive and interactive, was using toys appropriately, and was activating switches. Fine and gross motor skills were estimated to be at an 8-month level, receptive language was at the 9- to 11-month level, and expressive language at the 3- to 4-month level. She had progressed from tube feeding to oral feeding of pureed textures and thickened liquids. She was dependent in all activities of daily living. Subsequent to discharge, she was enrolled in a preschool program where she received occupational therapy, physical therapy, and speech-language therapies.

Now, 2 years after injury, Joanna is eligible to begin kindergarten. She has made considerable progress in all areas, with cognitive skills clustering at the 3.5-year-old level. She is ambulatory, but continues to exhibit ataxia. Both gross and fine motor skills are below her age level due to her difficulty with motor control. Expressive language continues to be the area of greatest impairment. She has begun to show initiation of communication, using vocalization (but no words), gestures, and a picture exchange communication system. However, she is beginning to demonstrate significant frustration when unable to communicate her needs. Her family and school personnel believe that her current communication system is not maximizing her ability to communicate and would like to investigate other alternative communication systems. Joanna is becoming more independent but continues to need considerable assistance in activities of daily living. Her family and teachers have described Joanna as having considerable difficulty in switching from one activity to the next, tending to display perseverative behavior at times. Her teachers have also described her as being easily distracted.

Questions

1. Joanna is participating in an inclusive kindergarten program and is developing friendships with several girls in her class. All the girls like to play with Barbie dolls, but Joanna has great difficulty with manipulation. Using the 4 components of the HAAT Model, what recommendations and/or accommodations would you suggest to facilitate her play?

Case 3

Darian is an 11-year-old boy with a diagnosis of congenital spastic quadriparesis secondary to cerebral palsy. Darian has a gastrostomy tube and is nonverbal. Estimates of his intelligence are based on checklists since a consistent method of response to testing has not been found. Darian's mental age has been judged to be at the 18-month level. His teacher, however, feels that this is a gross underestimate of his ability. His teacher states that "he understands everything, but just can't talk." Darian gets around with a manual wheelchair that his caregivers must push since his motoric capabilities are limited. Visual and auditory acuity appear to be within normal limits. His parents and teachers are seeking recommendations.

Questions

1. Describe the entire assessment process for Darian.
2. What team members will be involved in his case?
3. What will their responsibilities be?
4. What low-tech and high-tech AT recommendations would you make?
5. Why does Darian need low-tech devices if he is able to use a high-tech communication device?

STUDY QUESTIONS

1. What differentiates AT from other types of technologies?
2. Where can you find information about any of the Tech Act projects?
3. Describe each component of the HAAT Model and give an example of each.
4. From your experience, name the disciplines that represent the members of the AT team and describe their roles.
5. From your personal experience, describe the following parts of the AT service delivery process: (a) assessment, (b) follow-up, and (c) follow along.

References

1. Desideri L, Hoogerwerf EJ, Roentgen U, et al. Recommending assistive technology (AT) for children with multiple disabilities: a systematic review and qualitative synthesis of models and instruments for AT professionals. *Technol Disabil.* 2013;25(1):3-13.
2. Long TM, Perry DF. Pediatric physical therapists' perceptions of their training in assistive technology. *Phys Ther.* 2008;88(5):629-639.
3. O'Shea RK, Bonfiglio BS. Assistive technology [supplemental material]. In: Campbell SK, Palisano RJ, Orlin MN, eds. *Physical Therapy for Children.* Elsevier Saunders; 2012.
4. Adya M, Samant D, Scherer MJ, et al. Assistive/rehabilitation technology, disability, and service delivery models. *Cogn Process.* 2012;13(1):75-78.
5. Weintraub Moore H, Wilcox MJ. Characteristics of early intervention practitioners and their confidence in the use of assistive technology. *Top Early Childhood Special Educ.* 2006;26(1):15-23.
6. Hersh MA, Johnson MA. On modelling assistive technology systems–part I: modelling framework. *Technol Disabil.* 2008; 20(3):193-215.
7. Cook AM, Polgar JM. *Assistive Technologies: Principles and Practice.* Elsevier Health Sciences; 2015.
8. Alper S, Raharinirina S. Assistive technology for individuals with disabilities: a review and synthesis of the literature. *J Special Educ Technol.* 2006;21(2):47-64.
9. Mistrett S. Assistive technology helps young children with disabilities participate in daily activities. *Technol Action.* 2004;1(4):1-8.
10. Romski MA, Sevcik RA, Barton-Hulsey A, Whitmore AS. Early Intervention and AAC: What a Difference 30 Years Makes. Augment Altern Commun. 2015;31(3):181-202. doi: 10.3109/07434618.2015.1064163
11. Cress CJ, Marvin CA. Common questions about AAC services in early intervention. *Augment Altern Commun.* 2003;19:254-272.
12. Reichle J, Beukelman D, Light J, eds. *Implementing an Augmentative Communication System: Exemplary Strategies for Beginning Communicators.* Paul H. Brookes; 2002.
13. Romski MA, Sevcik RA. *Breaking the Speech Barrier: Language Development Through Augmented Means.* Brookes; 1996.
14. Lee H, Templeton R. Ensuring equal access to technology: providing assistive technology for students with disabilities. *Theory Pract.* 2008;47(3):212-219.
15. Wissick CA, Gardner JE. Conducting assessments in technology needs: from assessment to implementation. *Assess Effect Interv.* 2008;33(2):78-93.
16. Georgia Project for Assistive Technology. Legal mandates for assistive technology. 2007. Accessed June 19, 2019. http://www.gpat.org/Georgia-Project-for-Assistive-Technology/Pages/Legal-Mandates-for-Assistive-Technology.aspx#prov.
17. Golinker L, Mistrett SG. Funding assistive technology. *Rehabil Ther.* 1997:211-233.
18. Dusing SC, Skinner AC, Mayer ML. Unmet need for therapy services, assistive devices, and related services: data from the national survey of children with special health care needs. *Ambul Pediatr.* 2004;4(5):448-454.
19. Steel EJ, Gelderblom GJ, de Witte LP. The role of the International Classification of Functioning, Disability, and Health and quality criteria for improving assistive technology service delivery in Europe. *Am J Phys Med Rehabil.* 2012;91(13):S55-S61.
20. Friederich A, Bernd T, De Witte L. Methods for the selection of assistive technology in neurological rehabilitation practice. *Scand J Occup Ther.* 2010;17(4):308-318.

21. Jackson D, Schladant M. Interdisciplinary assessment and intervention for aided augmentative and alternative communication. Paper presented at the Assistive Technology Industry Association, Orlando, FL; January 2017.

22. American Speech-Language-Hearing Association. Telepractice. Accessed November 21, 2023. https://www.asha.org/Practice-Portal/Professional-Issues/Telepractice/.

23. Mandak K, O'Neill T, Light J, & Fosco GM. Bridging the gap from values to actions: A family systems framework for family-centered AAC services. *Augmentative and Alternative Communication.* 2017;33(1):32-41.

24. Pujol CL, Nevares A, Schladant M. Increasing access to augmentative and alternative communication services for people with complex communication needs during COVID-19 and beyond. *Dev Disabil Netw J.* 2021;1(2):15.

25. Binger C, Ball L, Dietz A, et al. Personnel roles in the AAC assessment process. *Augment Altern Commun.* 2012;28(4):278-288.

26. RESNA. Member directory. Retrieved November 5, 2008. https://www.resna.org/member-directory/individual.

27. Schladant M, Dowling M. Parent perspectives on augmentative and alternative communication in children with fragile x syndrome: it starts in the home. *Intellect Dev Disabil.* 2020;58(5): 409-421.

28. Schiariti, V., Longo, E., Shoshmin, A., (2018). Implementation of the International Classification of Functioning, Disability, and Health (ICF) core sets for children and youth with cerebral palsy: global initiatives promoting optimal functioning. *Int J Environ Res Public Health.* (2018);15(9):1899.

29. Edyburn DL. 2003 in review: a synthesis of the special education technology literature. *J Special Educ Technol.* 2004;19(4):57-80.

30. Bernd TD, Der Pijl V, De Witte LP. Existing models and instruments for the selection of assistive technology in rehabilitation practice. *Scand J Occup Ther.* 2009;16(3):146-158.

31. Giesbrecht E. Application of the Human Activity Assistive Technology model for occupational therapy research. *Aust Occup Ther J.* 2013;60(4):230-240.

32. Edyburn DL, Smith RO. Creating an assistive technology outcomes measurement system: validating the components. *Assist Technol Outcomes Benefits.* 2004;1(1):8-15.

33. World Health Organization. Disability considerations during the COVID-19 outbreak. March 26, 2020. https://www.who.int/publications/i/item/WHO-2019-nCoV-Disability-2020-1.

34. American Physical Therapy Association. Position paper: Expanded Telehealth Access Act of 2021. Updated November 2021. Accessed July 28, 2022. https://www.apta.org/advocacy/issues/telehealth/expanded-telehealth-access-act-of-2021.

35. Anderson K, Boisvert MK, Doneski-Nicol J, et al. Tele-AAC resolution. *Int J Telerehabil.* 2012;4:2.

36. Hall N, Boisvert M. Clinical aspects related to tele-AAC: a technical report. *Perspect Augment Altern Commun.* 2014;23(1): 18-33.

37. Scherer M, Jutai J, Fuhrer M, Demers L, & Deruyter F. A framework for modelling the selection of assistive technology devices (ATDs). *Disabil Rehabilitation Assist.* 2007;2(1), 1-8.

38. Zabala J. The SETT Framework: Critical Areas To Consider When Making Informed *Assistive Technology Decisions.* 1995.

21

Physical Therapy Practice in Parts C and B of the Individuals With Disabilities Education Act

Tricia Catalino, PT, DSc, Kendra Gagnon, PT, PhD, Priscilla Weaver, PT, DPT, PhD, Susan W. Cecere, PT, MHS, and Denise Swensen, PT, DPT

LEARNING OBJECTIVES

Upon completion of this chapter, the reader will be able to:

- Appraise the current federal laws that govern early intervention and school-based practice and how they impact physical therapy decision-making.
- Analyze the philosophies of early intervention and school-based practice.
- Describe evaluation and eligibility determination for Parts C and Part B of the Individuals With Disabilities Education Improvement Act.

- Describe how physical therapy interventions may be embedded into natural environments and daily routines for children in early intervention and school settings.
- Discuss the physical therapist's role as a member of a multidisciplinary team in early intervention and school-based settings.
- Explain the physical therapist's role in planning and documentation in early intervention and school-based environments.

■ INTRODUCTION

The purpose of this chapter is to describe physical therapist practice in early intervention (EI) and school-based settings under Parts C and B of the Individuals With Disabilities Education Improvement Act (IDEA) of 2004. The law mandates family-centered and educationally relevant services and supports for children with or at risk for disabilities from ages birth through 21 years. Providing services through IDEA can be a rewarding yet challenging endeavor. Physical therapists who provide EI and school-based services have the opportunity to influence child and family outcomes in the places where children spend their days— in their homes, schools, and communities. However, providing physical therapy in these settings can be demanding as therapists navigate federal and state laws and regulations, strive to implement evidence-based practices, collaborate on multidisciplinary teams, and advocate for families and children. In this chapter, we will describe the context of EI and school-based physical therapy; outline the laws, philosophies, and evidence that guide best practice in these settings; and provide examples of what physical therapy looks like in these settings.

To understand the context of EI and school-based practice, therapists must consider the intersection of health/medical models of care and the developmental/educational framework of IDEA. Although IDEA is an education law, it includes direct or related services from health professionals to support children and families. As part of a multidisciplinary team, physical therapists are asked to apply their knowledge, skills, and expertise about health conditions and disabilities to individual service plans focused on participation for children in the context of their home, community, or school environment. Physical therapists are expected to engage in collaborative and team-based decision-making by considering all the factors that contribute to a child's level of function including family needs and priorities and/or educational priorities. Decision-making is also influenced by mandates outlined in IDEA for determining eligibility and providing services that require therapists to integrate the physical therapy patient management model into the EI and school-based environments.

As a foundation for the scope of this chapter, the authors acknowledge the unique factors that influence practice for providers in EI and school-based settings. Physical therapists must adhere to their state practice act regarding their jurisdictional scope of practice and requirements for patient/client evaluation and examination, documentation, levels of supervision, and direct access/physician referral while also providing services under the federal laws of Section 504 of the Rehabilitation Act of 1973,[1] the Americans With Disabilities Act of 1990,[2] and the IDEA of 2004.[3] Physical therapists should reference the *Guide to Physical Therapist Practice 3.0*[4] and the International Classification of Functioning, Disability, and Health (ICF)[5] during the process of examination, evaluation, and treatment planning. Finally, therapists must adhere to the American Physical Therapy Association (APTA) Code of Ethics[6] and strive to achieve published competencies[7,8] related to practice under either Part C or B of IDEA.

■ INDIVIDUALS WITH DISABILITIES EDUCATION IMPROVEMENT ACT

What is now known as IDEA, the Education of All Handicapped Children Act became law in 1975 requiring all states that received funding from the federal government to provide equal access to public education for children with disabilities. In 1986, the law was amended to include services for infants and toddlers with disabilities and subsequently reauthorized and amended to include Parts C and B of IDEA in 1997. The law was reauthorized in 2004 as the Individuals With Disabilities Education Improvement Act and, as of the time of this writing, is overdue for reauthorization.[3]

The IDEA statute is made up of 4 provisions. Part A contains *General Provisions* of the statute; Part B, *Assistance for All Children With Disabilities*, provides the framework for free appropriate public education services for children with disabilities ages 3 through 21 years; Part C, *Infant and Toddlers With Disabilities*, is the framework for EI services for children birth to age 3 years and their families; and Part D, *National Activities to Improve Education of Children with Disabilities*, provides grants for a variety of training and technical assistance. In this chapter, we will focus on Parts C and B of IDEA.

TEAMING AND COLLABORATION IN PARTS C AND B OF IDEA

Teaming and collaboration, while not unique to EI and school-based practice, are essential components of these practice settings. Physical therapists regularly partner, consult, co-treat, and collaborate with professionals from a range of disciplines and backgrounds. IDEA Parts C and B provide guidance on the composition of the team in both school-based and EI settings, respectively, and this will be described in more detail later in the chapter. However, it can be broadly stated that, under IDEA, the team consists of the child and family, any educators or providers working directly or indirectly with the child or family, the individual or agency that coordinates the service plan, and other individuals invited by the family to participate on the team.

There are 3 primary models of team interaction that the physical therapist may encounter in EI and school-based practice: multidisciplinary, interdisciplinary, and transdisciplinary.[9] The discussion surrounding teaming models has been highly dynamic in recent years, and there continues to be gaps in evidence and implementation of teaming practices varies.[10] However, teaming models are generally defined as presented in **Table 21-1**. It should be noted that the term *multidisciplinary* is used here to describe a model of team interaction that differs from the IDEA definition of *multidisciplinary*, which simply refers to the involvement of 2 or more professions/disciplines.

■ IDEA PART C

Part C of IDEA is a federal grant program that assists states in operating a comprehensive statewide program of EI services for infants and toddlers with developmental delays or disabilities, ages birth to 3 years, and their families. Congress originally established the Education of the Handicapped Act Amendments of 1986 in recognition of "an urgent and substantial need" to:

TABLE 21-1 • Teaming and Collaboration Models		
Model	**Definition**	**What It Looks Like**
Multidisciplinary	Providers work on discipline-specific goals. They may communicate with and value input from other team members but generally stay within clear professional boundaries with limited interactions between disciplines. Roles are clearly defined.	The physical therapist (PT) implements the plan of care, including discipline-specific goals. Services are provided one-on-one, directly with the child.
Interdisciplinary	Providers may work on skills and goals within their own discipline but do work with other professionals on evaluation, planning, and implementation of services. Roles are defined but may be relaxed.	The PT implements a plan of care with collaboration/input from the team. However, PT goals and interventions are discipline specific. PT services are provided to and on behalf of the child. The PT may share a nonskilled "home exercise program" and/or general strategies with the team (including teachers and family members) on environmental modifications to support participation. However, the PT generally does not share discipline-specific expertise.
Transdisciplinary	Providers work across disciplines and share information. Role release, in which a team member implements strategies of other disciplines, may occur. Goals and interventions are not discipline specific. All providers work together on all goals.	The PT plan of care is developed in collaboration with the team and embedded within non–discipline-specific educationally relevant or family-centered goal areas such as self-care, community living, and recreation/play. Discipline-specific expertise is shared among all team members so that suggested strategies may be implemented during daily routines.

1. enhance the development of infants and toddlers with disabilities and to minimize their potential for developmental delay, and to recognize the significant brain development that occurs during a child's first 3 years of life;
2. reduce the educational costs to our society, including our Nation's schools, by minimizing the need for special education and related services after infants and toddlers with disabilities reach school age;
3. maximize the potential for their independently living in society;
4. enhance the capacity of families to meet the special needs of their infants and toddlers with disabilities; and
5. enhance the capacity of state and local agencies and service providers to identify, evaluate, and meet the needs of all children, particularly minority, low-income, inner-city, and rural children and infants and toddlers in foster care.[11]

To participate in Part C, a state must guarantee that EI services are available to every eligible child and their family. In addition, states must meet the conditions outlined in IDEA that include components of service delivery to receive federal funding. For example, the governor must designate a lead agency to administer the program and appoint an Interagency Coordinating Council (ICC), including parents of young children with disabilities, to advise and assist the lead agency. The full list of components is included in **Table 21-2**. States must also assure that EI services meet the intent of Part C related to family-centered care, providing services in natural environments, service coordination, and implementing the Individualized Family Service Plan (IFSP)–the legal written document of Part C.

FAMILY-CENTERED CARE AND NATURAL ENVIRONMENTS

Family-centered care and providing services in natural environments are based on the philosophy that the best way to meet a child's needs is within their families and in the context of the naturally occurring routines that take place in the child's home and community. The agreed-upon mission of family-centered care in EI states: "Part 6C early intervention builds upon and provides supports and resources to assist family members and caregivers to enhance children's learning and development

TABLE 21-2 • Components of Part C Early Intervention

- Early intervention services for all infants and toddlers with disabilities (from birth to age 3) and their families
- Child Find: A system to identify, locate, and evaluate children with disabilities
- Comprehensive, multidisciplinary evaluation (MDE)
- Individualized Family Service Plan (IFSP)
- Procedural safeguards
- Public awareness program
- Central directory
- Comprehensive system of personnel development
- Administration by a lead agency
- State interagency coordinating council

TABLE 21-3 • Key Components of Family-Centered Care[13]

- Engaging with family members to understand their lives, goals, strengths, and challenges and developing a relationship between family and practitioner.
- Working with the family to set goals, strengthen capacity, and make decisions.
- Providing individualized, culturally responsive, and evidence-based interventions for each family.

through everyday learning opportunities."[*,12] Family-centered care emphasizes collaboration between the family and service providers and supports the view that families have the capacity to make informed decisions and act on them. **Table 21-3** lists key components of family-centered care.[13]

By definition, a natural environment means "settings that are natural or normal for the child's age peers who have no disabilities."[14] However, natural environments are more than just a physical location. In addition to the physical environment (eg, space, materials, climate), natural environments encompass the social environment (eg, relationships and interactions with caregivers, siblings, peers) and the temporal environment (eg, sequence and length of routines and activities).[15] In 2008, a multidisciplinary group of EI researchers, leaders, and EI providers published key principles for providing services in the natural environment.[12] The key principles are as follows:

1. Infants and toddlers learn best through everyday experiences and interactions with familiar people in familiar contexts.
2. All families, with the necessary supports and resources, can enhance their children's learning and development.
3. The primary role of a service provider in EI is to work with and support family members and caregivers in children's lives.
4. The EI process, from initial contacts through transition, must be dynamic and individualized to reflect the child's and family members' preferences, learning styles, and cultural beliefs.
5. IFSP outcomes must be functional and based on children's and families' needs and family-identified priorities.
6. The family's priorities, needs, and interests are addressed most appropriately by a primary provider who represents and receives team and community support.
7. Interventions with young children and family members must be based on explicit principles, validated practices, best available research, and relevant laws and regulations.[*,12]

Part C of IDEA requires that EI services for infants and toddlers with disabilities are provided "to the maximum extent appropriate, in natural environments."[16] Providing EI services in settings other than a natural environment is an option only if the team, including the parents, can justify that child and family outcomes cannot be achieved in the natural environment. This option is meant to be temporary, and the team must have a plan to return services to the natural environment.

*Reproduced with permission from Workgroup on Principles and Practices in Natural Environments, OSEP TA Community of Practice: Part C Settings. (2008, March). Agreed upon mission and key principles for providing early intervention services in natural environments. Retrieved from http://ectacenter.org/~pdfs/topics/families/Finalmissionandprinciples3_11_08.pdf

Family-centered care and providing services in natural environments aligns with a relationship-based approach to service provision. Relationship-based practices are grounded in research that confirms the critical influence that relationships have on child health and development.[17,18] In EI, relationship-based practices support the parent-child relationship while acknowledging the influence of other important relationships to the parent and child such as siblings, neighbors, and the EI team of service providers.[17,18] Implementing relationship-based practices requires a number of skills that may stretch a physical therapist beyond their technical skill base. Pilkington and Malinowski[18] identified relationship-based practice skills for service providers that apply to relationships with families and team members. These skills include "the capacity to: (1) listen carefully; (2) demonstrate concern and empathy; (3) promote reflection; (4) observe and highlight the parent/child relationship; (5) respect role boundaries; (6) respond thoughtfully in emotionally intense interactions; and (7) understand, regulate, and use one's own feelings."[19] Case 1a illustrates relationship-based practices in the context of family-centered care and natural environments.

Case 1a

Example of Relationship-Based Practices in the Context of Family-Centered Care and Natural Environments for Elijah
Relationship-based practices include fostering connections between all members of the child's team by listening, observing, validating, and communicating. Relationships between the caregiver and infant, caregiver and therapist, and infant and therapist are important for learning in the natural environment. Using a routines-based interview, the physical therapist considered all the dimensions of Elijah's and his mother's environment and began building a respectful and trusting relationship with the family. Their experience during the first 2 years of Elijah's life revolved around doctors and specialists in a hospital setting. We noticed the many-faceted interactions between Elijah, his mother, and his nurse. We connected with Elijah's mother, listened to her concerns as a young, single mother with no family support in the area, and explained our role and that of the program using coaching strategies with the family's needs at the center.
- Building a good relationship between the caregivers (mother and nurse) and the therapist helped support Elijah's functioning and development by empowering the caregivers to play a crucial role in his progress in all areas.
- We were sensitive to the relationship between Elijah and his mother and the stress they both experienced in the first 2 years of his life. Visits were scheduled around the family's routines and incorporated positioning and play. Adjustments were made when either one seemed overwhelmed with therapy interventions. Collaboration between multiple service providers included joint visits, phone and email conversations regarding treatment strategies, equipment management, and upcoming meetings and appointments with specialists.
- The providers developed a secure and trusting relationship with Elijah over time. He became comfortable with handling and positioning, enjoyed interactions during play, and engaged for a variety of learning opportunities.

Source: Academy of Pediatric Physical Therapy. *Resource/Fact Sheet. Weaving Relationship-based Practices into Intervention: A Guide for Pediatric Physical Therapists.* Academy of Pediatric Physical Therapy; 2018).

SERVICE COORDINATION

In Part C EI, each child and their family are assigned a service coordinator who is responsible for coordinating the provision of EI services. Service coordination includes responsibilities such as (1) assisting families in obtaining access to EI services and other services in the IFSP; (2) coordinating EI services or other services; (3) coordinating evaluations and assessments and IFSP meetings; (4) monitoring the delivery of EI services; (5) informing families of their rights and procedural safeguards; (6) coordinating funding sources for services; (7) and facilitation of the transition plan.[20] Each state defines the role of a service coordinator and who is qualified for this position. It is possible in some states for a physical therapist to serve as a service coordinator. For instance, at the time of this writing, Illinois allows a physical therapist to be employed as a service coordinator in a geographic area where they are not providing EI services as a physical therapist. The physical therapist must meet the qualifications for both services set forth by the program.[21]

EVALUATION, ASSESSMENT, AND ELIGIBILITY

Evaluation and assessment are distinctly defined in Part C of IDEA. Evaluation is the process of determining initial and ongoing eligibility for Part C services. According to Part C regulations, procedures that must take place during an evaluation include:

1. Administering an evaluation instrument;
2. Taking the child's history (including interviewing the parent);
3. Identifying the child's level of functioning in each of the developmental areas;
4. Gathering information from other sources, such as family members, other caregivers, medical providers, social workers, and educators, if necessary, to understand the full scope of the child's unique strengths and needs; and
5. Reviewing medical, educational, or other records."[22]

For children who are eligible for Part C EI, assessment is the process of identifying the child's and family's strengths and needs to determine appropriate EI services to meet those needs.[23] The assessment of the child must be conducted by qualified personnel and include a review of the results of the initial or subsequent evaluation, personal observations of the child, and identification of the child's needs in each of the 5 developmental areas. As part of the assessment process, caregivers may also voluntarily participate in a "family-directed assessment of the resources, priorities, and concerns of the family and the identification of the supports and services necessary to enhance the family's capacity to meet the developmental needs of the child."[24]

All evaluations and assessments must be conducted by a multi-disciplinary team in the family's preferred language and in a non-discriminatory manner. According to IDEA, a multidisciplinary team is made up of individuals representing 2 or more separate disciplines or professions and may include one individual who is qualified in one or more disciplines or professions. Each state determines who may conduct evaluations to determine initial eligibility for Part C services. For example, some states have dedicated evaluation teams based on geographic regions where providers may only perform eligibility evaluations outside the region where they provide direct services. Other states allow EI providers to participate on evaluation teams and provide services in the same geographic region without restriction.

Beyond the required components of evaluation and assessment under Part C of IDEA, physical therapists should consider additional practices and methods to gather information to determine eligibility for services and to help team-based decision-making as part of the IFSP process. For example, a state may provide a list of approved standardized tests and measures to determine eligibility for all children. This list may not include an approved tool that is appropriate for a specific child's diagnosis or level of functioning. Physical therapists may need to administer other tests and measures to gather data to support the IFSP. Further, many researchers recognize that traditional testing procedures and types of standardized assessments may not be developmentally appropriate for young children in EI.[25-30]

EI providers are encouraged to include authentic and functional assessment as part of a holistic assessment approach. Bagnato and Ho[30] define *authentic assessment* as "the systematic recording of developmental observations over time about the naturally occurring behaviors and functional competencies of young children in daily routines by familiar and knowledgeable caregivers in the child's life." *Functional assessment* is inclusive of authentic assessment and is defined as "a continuous, collaborative process that combines observing, asking meaningful questions, listening to family stories, and analyzing individual child skills and behaviors within naturally occurring everyday routines and activities across multiple situations and settings."[31] To support implementation of functional assessment as part of EI practice, the Virginia EI Program identified 8 high-quality assessment practices that make up functional assessment as illustrated in **Figure 21-1**.

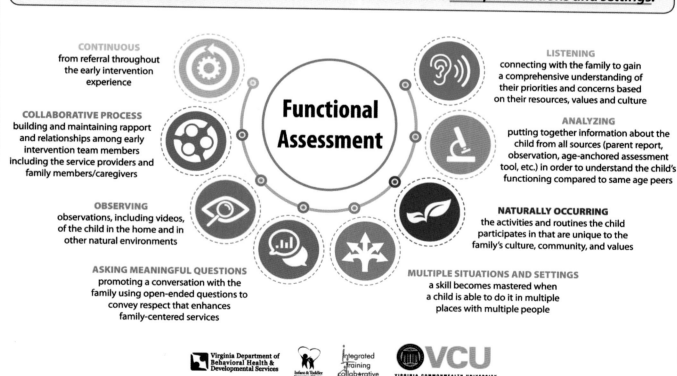

FIGURE 21-1 Definition of functional assessment. (Reproduced with permission from VCU, Virginia Department of Behavioral Health and Developmental Services.)

According to Part C of IDEA, infants and toddlers are eligible for EI services if there is an identified developmental delay or disability (or diagnosed physical or mental condition with a high probability of resulting in developmental delay) in any one or more of the following 5 areas: physical development, cognitive development, communication development, social or emotional development, and adaptive development.[32] The exact eligibility criteria for EI varies from state to state. Physical therapists who provide services under Part C must be familiar with their state's eligibility requirements. Case 1b provides an example of an initial eligibility evaluation and application of the functional assessment approach.

Case 1b

Example of an Initial Eligibility Evaluation and Application of the Functional Assessment Approach for Elijah

Elijah has a complex neonatal history including hypoplastic left heart syndrome (HLHS); cortical visual impairment (CVI); moderate bilateral hearing loss; lung, liver, and kidney dysfunction; and diffuse cerebral atrophy. He was born at 34 weeks' gestation and spent his first 25 months of life in various hospitals. During that time, he had 18 surgeries for the correction of various congenital anomalies. He currently has a tracheostomy, gastrojejunostomy tube, and pressure equalization (PE) tubes, and is ventilator-dependent with supplemental oxygen. He has a large team of doctors at the local children's hospital and has specialized equipment to assist with his complex needs.

A multidisciplinary team was assembled for the initial assessment and evaluation in his home when Elijah was 31 months of age. This was the family's first exposure to the IDEA process. The team included his mother, his private-duty nurse, and his Medicaid case manager, as well as the EI team from the local school system, which consisted of a special educator, an occupational therapist, a physical therapist, an educational audiologist, a teacher of the visually impaired, a speech-language pathologist, and a school nurse. At the assessment and evaluation, a routines-based interview was conducted with his mother for the purpose of gathering information about Elijah and his family's ecology. Standardized testing and clinical observations were also used to determine eligibility for services according to state guidelines.

The functional assessment was conducted during a discussion with his mother and private duty nurse in the home about Elijah's functional abilities during naturally occurring routines and activities. The team observed Elijah who was awake and alert during the assessment and interacted with various members of the team by smiling and moving his arms and legs while he was held by his mother and nurse. The team listened to his mother's concerns, priorities, and needs for her son, which included her desire for Elijah to sit up on his own and develop as normally as possible. His mother shared that Elijah expresses himself through crying, body movements, and facial expressions/smiling. Her concerns included managing his multiple medical needs, difficulty with bathing routines, and transporting him outside of the home. The team gathered information about Elijah by observation, use of assessment tools, and asking open-ended questions to understand his level of functioning compared to same-aged peers. Elijah had needs in all areas of development as well as concerns with hearing and vision.

Because children's functional abilities overlap domains of development, a summary was reviewed that combined all Elijah's functional abilities, strengths, and needs into 3 functional outcome areas: Developing Positive Social-Emotional Skills and Relationships, Acquiring and Using Knowledge and Skills, and Using Appropriate Behaviors to Meet Needs (Child Outcome Summary).

After analyzing all available data and collaborating with the family, Elijah was determined to be eligible for Part C services based on a diagnosed condition with a high probability of developmental delays in all areas of development as well as concerns with hearing and vision. An Initial IFSP was developed by the team and family that addressed concerns with Elijah's development in the areas of cognitive ability, gross and fine motor skills, communication, and social-emotional skills. Because of his age and complex profile, the meeting also included a discussion of Elijah's eligibility for Part B services after the age of 3. The team concluded the assessment by stating that there will be continuous monitoring of Elijah's progress and ongoing collaboration with his family to determine his needs in the home and other natural environments where he may spend time.

INDIVIDUALIZED FAMILY SERVICE PLAN

The IFSP is the written plan for providing EI services to eligible infants and toddlers with developmental delays or disabilities and their families. The plan is developed at an IFSP meeting involving the multidisciplinary team who performed the evaluation, the parents, service coordinator, providers involved in delivering EI services (as appropriate), and other family members or advocates requested by the parents. The meetings are conducted in settings and at times that are accessible and convenient to the family. The communication with the family must be in their native language or by other means of communication unless clearly not feasible. Family participation and team collaboration are critical when developing and implementing the IFSP. Prior to initiating EI services prescribed in the IFSP, the parents must fully understand and accept the IFSP through written consent. Detailed information on the IFSP is in IDEA Sec. 303.340-346.[33] The IFSP must include the following content:

- Child's present levels of physical development, communication development, social or emotional development, and adaptive development
- Family's resources, priorities, and concerns related to enhancing the development of the child
- Measurable outcomes expected to be achieved for the child and family
- Specific EI services, explanation of services in natural environment or otherwise, and payment arrangements
- Other services the child is receiving or is recommended to receive outside of EI
- Name of service coordinator
- Steps for transition process from Part C

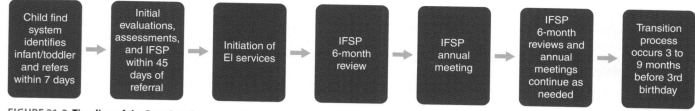

FIGURE 21-2 Timeline of the Part C early intervention process. IFSP, Individualized Family Service Plan.

The state comprehensive child find system must refer infants and toddlers to the lead agency or EI service provider no more than 7 days after identifying a potential need for EI services. The initial evaluations, initial assessments, and IFSP meeting and written plan must be completed within 45 days of receiving the referral by the lead agency or provider. A review of the IFSP occurs every 6 months or more often to determine progress toward achieving outcomes and whether modification of the plan is necessary. An annual IFSP meeting is conducted to reevaluate and revise the IFSP based on current assessments of the child and family. The transition process from Part C services occurs 3 to 9 months prior to a child's third birthday. **Figure 21-2** portrays the timeline of the EI process.

The Role of the Physical Therapist on the IFSP Team
A physical therapist plays a significant role on the IFSP team to assist in developing a plan that meets the individualized needs of each child and family. The physical therapist must demonstrate effective interpersonal and communication skills to promote team collaboration and family participation. All initial and ongoing evaluations and assessments conducted by the physical therapist are documented and the findings clearly communicated to the IFSP team. A key responsibility of the physical therapist is contribution to the development of IFSP outcomes at the initial and ongoing meetings that support the child's participation in everyday routines and activities and the family's capacity to meet those needs. Family outcomes also promote access to community resources to support the child's development. Outcomes reflect the family's priorities and needs relating to their child's development based on evaluations and assessments of both child and family. The child and family outcomes and strategies are first developed, and then the team discusses the services and supports that are necessary to achieve the outcomes. An IFSP may include physical therapy services based on the assessed needs of the child and family and identification of services appropriate to meet those needs. Physical therapists' expertise in the movement system offers a unique contribution to the IFSP team to support family and child outcomes.

Developing the IFSP: Outcomes, Strategies, and Services
The development of IFSP outcomes is a collaborative process by the IFSP team at the initial and ongoing meetings. Initial and ongoing evaluations and assessments provide the team with the family's priorities and concerns and a child's strengths and developmental needs. This information is a guide for the team to develop family and child outcomes. The family outcomes place the parents in an active role of promoting the participation of their child in daily activities and routines that are meaningful to the child and family within their natural environment. The child outcomes promote a variety of functional skill development across developmental domains and through participation in everyday activities. IFSP outcome statements must be meaningful to and easily understood by the family, be measurable, and be written in a discipline-free manner. It is not appropriate to identify "PT goals" on an IFSP. Instead, the team might identify a child outcome involving a family routine where the child needs to move from place to place in their home. After the outcomes are developed, the team decides on services, strategies, and supports to include in the IFSP. The ECTA Center provides resources and training materials for EI providers on developing high-quality, participation-based functional IFSP outcome statements. Case 1c describes a case with examples of IFSP outcomes and strategies.

Case 1c

Examples of IFSP Outcomes and Strategies for Elijah
The ECTA Center provides the following guidance on developing high-quality, participation-based functional outcomes:
- The outcome is necessary and functional for the child's and family's life.
- The outcome reflects real-life contextualized settings.
- The outcome integrates developmental domains and is discipline free.
- The outcome is jargon free, clear, and simple.
- The outcome emphasizes the positive, not the negative.
- The outcome uses active words rather than passive words.

Below is an example of a functional outcome addressing the family's priorities for Elijah:

What would we like to see happen within our daily activity/routine?

Elijah will sit in his high chair to look at or touch pictures in a book with his mother or other caregivers.

What are some initial strategies to begin/continue with?

Physical support, including the use of towels, pool noodles, or household items will be used while Elijah is seated in his high chair to improve his posture to enable him to maintain his head erect and use his hands more effectively during a book routine. The provider and parent will collaborate on strategies, toy suggestions, and activities to increase the mobility of Elijah's arms and fingers during periods of stability in the high chair such as popping bubbles, container play to facilitate voluntary grasp and release patterns, block activities, and the use of an ice cube tray for finger isolation. The provider will model and coach the caregiver to create a routine of reading and use strategies such as hand-over-hand assistance and tactile cueing to help facilitate isolated finger movements to point to pictures in a book. The caregiver will give Elijah a choice between 2 books, use books that have simple pictures and textures, model simple actions and sounds for him to imitate, and focus on the pictures to tell his own "story."

How will we know we've achieved this? By when?

We will know this has been achieved when Elijah reaches and touches the pictures in a book held by his mother or caregiver 3 or more times during a 2- to 5-minute book routine for 5 consecutive days when positioned in his high chair or adapted chair with support at the upper trunk with his head erect.

Source: Early Childhood Technical Assistance Center. Enhancing recognition of high quality, functional IFSP outcomes. Accessed November 25, 2023. https://ectacenter.org/~pdfs/pubs/rating-ifsp.pdf.

During the initial and subsequent IFSP meetings, the team decides on the EI services that will best meet the unique needs of the child and the family to achieve the IFSP outcomes. The child and family may receive any combination of the services listed in **Table 21-4** to support achieving the IFSP outcomes. The type and amount of services documented in the IFSP are (1) length of time the service is provided during each session; (2) duration of time to meet IFSP outcomes; (3) frequency of service (number of days or sessions) and intensity; (4) individual or group session; (5) and method of how the service is provided.

Teaming and Collaboration in Early Intervention

As a member of a multidisciplinary IFSP team, the physical therapist will participate in teaming and collaboration with one or more individuals from different professions. The model of team interaction for EI service delivery is decided by the IFSP team and should be based on the priority needs and preferences of the child and family. Federal and state laws and regulations do not specify models of team collaboration; however, some states describe specific team collaboration models in their EI policies. The 3 primary models of team interaction have been discussed previously in this chapter. In EI, the interdisciplinary and transdisciplinary models are most reflective of the philosophies of teaming and collaboration in this setting. The emphasis for both interdisciplinary and transdisciplinary models is communication among the team during evaluations and assessments, IFSP development, and implementation of the IFSP.

IFSP teams using an interdisciplinary approach to teaming and collaboration select one or more service providers to support the established IFSP outcomes pertinent to the providers' knowledge, skills, abilities, and scope of practice for their discipline. Each provider schedules individual reevaluations and treatment sessions with the child and family. Regular communication occurs between providers, and co-visits are an option to support progress toward outcomes in areas outside of one's area of expertise.

In one transdisciplinary approach to teaming and collaboration, the IFSP team selects one member of the team to be the primary service provider (PSP),[34] identified as the "primary coach" in some EI programs. The PSP is selected based on the match between the needs and priorities of the child and family and the knowledge and skills of the provider. If possible, the PSP remains consistent throughout the family's participation in the program; however, a change in PSP may occur over time based on ongoing evaluations and assessments to continually meet the changing needs of the child and family. The PSP schedules individual treatment sessions regularly with the child and family. To address child and family needs and priorities beyond the provider's individual area of expertise, the other team members may coach the PSP and family through joint visits, video or tele-conference sessions, and planned consultative time. Utilizing coaching practices builds the capacity of the family in promoting child learning and development.[35]

The implementation of each model of team interaction, especially transdisciplinary approaches, is highly variable across and even within a state; thus, physical therapists must ensure compliance with state practice acts and payor sources. The decision on team approach should reflect the individual needs and preferences of the child and family being served in the program and reviewed on a continual basis to ensure progress toward outcomes.

PHYSICAL THERAPY SERVICE DELIVERY IN EARLY INTERVENTION

Physical therapists and other team members are charged with applying EI philosophies, key principles, and agreed-upon practices for providing services in the natural environment when working with families and young children.[12,36] EI services and specific physical therapy interventions are highly individualized to the child and family and guided by the IFSP. When planning an intervention, the ICF framework[5] can help direct physical therapists in clinical reasoning and decision-making when implementing strategies that promote child and family participation in their natural environment. Physical therapists implement strategies that facilitate all areas of development by applying principles of motor learning[37] and promoting perceptual-motor experiences.[38] Supports may be recommended by the team to enhance a child's ability to learn and play such as mobility devices, adaptive toys, and positioning supports. An example of a physical therapist implementing intervention strategies in the natural environment is provided in Case 1c.

TABLE 21-4 • Part C Early Intervention Services

- Family training, counseling, home visits
- Special instruction
- Speech-language pathology and audiology services and sign language and cued language services
- Occupational therapy
- Physical therapy
- Psychological services
- Service coordination
- Medical services only for diagnostic or evaluation purposes
- Early identification, screening, and assessment services
- Health services necessary to enable the infant or toddler to benefit from the other early intervention services
- Social work services
- Vision services
- Assistive technology devices and services
- Transportation and related costs necessary to receive early intervention services

Case 1c

Example of a Physical Therapist Implementing Intervention Strategies in the Natural Environment

A variety of equipment was provided to give Elijah head and trunk support for upright positioning to allow him to use his hands for play. Establishing head control was a main priority. Neither his travel chair seating system nor high chair provided adequate support to enable him to use both his hands simultaneously. A corner chair, modified with a pommel, pool noodles, Velcro straps, and a neoprene trunk binder allowed him to sit upright without distress and enabled his caregiver to sit in front of him to engage him in an activity. The addition of a floor desk with a large surface area allowed the introduction of switches and electronic musical devices for him to activate and explore.

Engaging in coaching strategies is another important aspect of service delivery in EI. A physical therapist may serve as a coach or receive coaching depending on the agreed-upon roles of the team, areas of expertise, and family concerns and priorities. While any provider may use coaching strategies across a myriad of settings and contexts, coaching in EI is defined by Rush and Shelden[39] as "an adult learning strategy in which the coach promotes the learner's (coachee's) ability to reflect on his or her actions as a means to determine the effectiveness of an action or practice and develop a plan for refinement and use of the action in immediate and future situations."

It is important to acknowledge that coaching is intentional and meant to enhance confidence and competence in the person who is the recipient of coaching. Coaching on its own is not an intervention. However, coaching may be used to co-construct meaningful and evidence-informed intervention strategies with the family or other service providers. For example, a physical therapist may notice a parent already implementing effective strategies to help their child sit without support. In a coaching relationship, the physical therapist would provide affirmation to the parent and build upon this strength by engaging in a constructive discussion about why the parent chose the specific sitting strategy. The physical therapist might also begin to discuss other options for supporting transition to and from sitting and start by asking the parent for their ideas first.

THE PHYSICAL THERAPIST'S ROLE IN DOCUMENTATION IN EARLY INTERVENTION

Physical therapists providing services under EI must comply with documentation requirements of both state Part C laws and regulations and physical therapy state practice acts. Documentation in EI is written in family-friendly language. It may be necessary for a physical therapist to maintain supplementary documentation separate from the IFSP with more technical language to further detail the physical therapy examination, plan of care, and intervention strategies as required by a state practice act or other entities such as payor sources. The physical therapist will document evaluations and assessments used to determine eligibility or, in some cases, to assess a child already in the program due to additional developmental concerns by the IFSP team. The content in the IFSP is specified in the federal law, but the format of the IFSP varies by state.

Once services are initiated, physical therapists will document each visit to capture interventions, progress toward achievement of outcomes, communication with the family, and the provider plan. The physical therapist may need to conduct more frequent reevaluations than what is required by Part C depending on their state practice act. Federal IDEA legislation does not require a discharge summary; however, state Part C regulations and state practice acts may have additional requirements for a physical therapy discharge summary. Regardless, physical therapists should document when a child is exiting EI or transitioning to Part B or other services. Physical therapists working in EI will likely contribute to their state's performance plan or annual performance report, which evaluates the state's compliance with implementing the IDEA requirements.[40]

TRANSITION FROM PART C

Transition is described by the Division for Early Childhood[15] as "the events, activities, and processes associated with key changes between environments or programs during the early childhood years and the practices that support the adjustment of the child and family to the new setting." For children receiving Part C EI services, the transition process begins 3 to 9 months prior to the child's third birthday when the child is referred to the state education agency to determine eligibility for Part B services. The IFSP must include a transition plan that supports a smooth transition of the child from the Part C program. State policies and procedures mandate the steps required to guide the transition to preschool services under Part B of IDEA, to other appropriate services for toddlers, or to exit the EI program with no other services recommended.[41] A state may elect the option to continue EI services for toddlers eligible for preschool services under Part C until the child enters into preschool, kindergarten, or elementary school.[42] Physical therapists should be aware of the resources that are available for families from their state EI program to help guide the transition process.

The transition process can be a challenging time for the child and family with changes in team members, the environment, and service delivery. A physical therapist may assume an active role throughout the transition process from Part C EI to Part B school-based services. Physical therapists should participate in evaluations, transition meetings, and communications (with parental consent) with the school-based physical therapist. A transition fact sheet was developed by the APTA Academy of Pediatric Physical Therapy[43] to promote information sharing between physical therapists in EI and the school on child and family personal factors, participation, environmental factors, activities, body structures and functions, and intervention strategies that were successful while in EI.

■ IDEA PART B

Part B of IDEA is the current law that governs public education for students with disabilities, ages 3 through 21 years.[44] IDEA Part B ensures that all children with disabilities have access to free and appropriate public education in an environment with children who are not disabled to the maximum extent possible. Key elements of IDEA Part B are listed in **Table 21-5** and are described below.

TABLE 21-5 • Key Elements of IDEA Part B
• Free and appropriate public education (FAPE) for eligible students, age 3-21, with disabilities • Least restrictive environment (LRE) • Appropriate evaluation, with reevaluation at least once every 3 years • Determination of eligibility; eligibility categories • Individualized Education Program (IEP) • Parental consent and participation • Procedural safeguards • Administration by a local educational agency • State monitoring and enforcement

TABLE 21-6 • Part B Categories of Disabilities
To be eligible for special education and related services, a child must be identified as a "child with a disability" as evaluated in accordance with the following categories: • Intellectual disability • Hearing impairment (including deafness) • Speech or language impairment • Visual impairment (including blindness) • Serious emotional disturbance • Orthopedic impairment • Autism • Traumatic brain injury • Other health impairment • Specific learning disability • Deaf-blindness • Multiple disabilities

PHYSICAL THERAPY AS A RELATED SERVICE

Physical therapy is considered a related service under IDEA Part B. Section 300.34 of IDEA defines related services as "transportation and such developmental, corrective, and other supportive services as are required to assist a child with a disability to benefit from special education." The related service of physical therapy, as defined by the law, means "services provided by a qualified physical therapist."[45] In most states, physical therapy as a related service means that physical therapy services may only be provided if the student is eligible for special education and related services following the evaluation process. This requires physical therapy services be only as "special as necessary" and "educationally relevant." "Special as necessary" means only the expertise of a physical therapist can support the access and/or participation of the student. Educationally relevant means the activity or routine being supported is aligned with an activity and/or routine of a student's day that are necessary and expected. It is critical for the physical therapist to understand their role as a related service provider in evaluation, collaboration with the educational team, Individualized Education Program (IEP) development, and decision-making related to service delivery.

EVALUATION AND ELIGIBILITY

According to IDEA Part B, a student age 3 through 21 years must go through the child find process of referral, special education evaluation, and review of all pertinent assessments as part of the complete evaluation process. The initial evaluation is conducted by a team of professionals, which may include physical therapy, to determine (1) if a child is a child with a disability and (2) the educational needs of the child.[44] A physical therapist may be part of the evaluation team if there are concerns related to the movement system, functional mobility, and/or gross motor skills ability that impact the student's ability to benefit from their educational program. To be eligible for Part B services, the child must be evaluated as having a disability in 1 of 13 categories (**Table 21-6**).[46] Once the evaluation team has determined the child is eligible for Part B services, they will determine the student's educational needs and compose the IEP.

INDIVIDUALIZED EDUCATION PROGRAM

The IEP is a document developed by the educational team that is used to guide special education and related services for preschool-age and school-aged children. According to IDEA 2004, the IEP must include the following:

- A statement of the child's present level of academic achievement and functional performance (PLAAFP)
- A statement of measurable annual goals, including academic and functional goals
- A description of how the student's progress toward meeting the annual goals will be measured
- A statement of special education and related services and supplementary aids and services to be provided to the child
- An explanation of the extent to which the child will not participate with nondisabled children
- A statement of any individual appropriate accommodations that are necessary to measure the academic achievement and functional performance of the child on state and district-wide assessments
- The projected date for the beginning of the services and modifications, and the anticipated frequency, location, and duration of those services and modifications
- Beginning not later than the first IEP to be in effect when the child is 16, a transition plan including measurable postsecondary goals and transition services needed to assist the child in reaching those goals

Once a child is determined to be eligible for special education and related services, the team considers all pertinent data, including the physical therapy assessment, to develop the IEP. The IEP serves as a collaborative tool, and all IEP team members contribute to the document.

The IEP team should include members whose expertise is needed to ensure that free and appropriate public education is met through the IEP. At a minimum, the team must include the parents of the child with a disability, one regular education teacher of the child, one special education teacher of the child, a representative of the local educational agency, an individual who can interpret instructional implications of evaluation results, other individuals who have knowledge expertise regarding the child, including related services personnel, and whenever appropriate, the child with a disability.[47] The IEP team works closely throughout evaluation, reevaluation, and IEP development processes and collaboratively makes decisions regarding eligibility and services.

The IEP team is required to meet at least annually to review and revise the IEP and may meet more frequently if needed. Any member of the IEP team can call for a meeting, including the physical therapist, at any time. Reevaluation is required every 3 years but can be done more frequently if necessary.

Educational Placement and Least Restrictive Environment

Least restrictive environment (LRE) is a tenet of Part B IDEA 2004 and is defined as follows: "to the maximum extent appropriate, children with disabilities, including children in public or private institutions or other care facilities, are educated with children who are non-disabled." As part of the IEP process, a determination of educational placement is made. This is a team decision to determine the educational environment that best supports the needs of the student and offers the greatest opportunity for goal achievement as well as the integration with typical peers to the "maximum extent possible."[48] Physical therapists play a key role in the support of student success in the LRE and must have the expertise to provide services in any and all educational environments based on student needs and the expectations and requirements for that particular environment.

The Role of the Physical Therapist on the IEP Team

As a member of the team, the physical therapist should attend all IEP meetings and participate in all aspects of the teaming process. According to IDEA 2004, members of the IEP team may use alternative means of participation, such as phone or video conference, if agreed upon by the parent of a child with a disability and the local educational agency. Team members, including the physical therapist, may be excused from attending an IEP meeting if the parent and local educational agency consent to the excusal and the physical therapist submits their input in writing to both the parent and the IEP team. In the event that the related services provided by the physical therapist are not being modified or discussed, the parent and local educational agency may agree that the physical therapist's attendance is not necessary. As a member of the IEP team, the physical therapist must effectively communicate and form partnerships with team members to provide coordinated care. According to Effgen et al,[8] competencies are necessary for physical therapists on the IEP team in the following areas: collaboration, consultation, education, supervision, and advocacy.

If part of the IEP team, the physical therapist may contribute to the following:

1. Determining eligibility for special education and related services
2. Interpreting and communicating examination findings
3. Discussing student performance within school activities and routines
4. Discussing and prioritizing educationally relevant goals, objectives, supplementary aids, and services related to the child's educational needs
5. Assisting the IEP team in determining the need for physical therapy as a related service to support student access and participation in the general education curriculum; this includes dosing decisions as well as the method(s) of service delivery
6. Contributing to student placement decisions
7. Developing mechanism for ongoing coordination and communication[8]

> ### TABLE 21-7 • Elements of the Present Level of Academic Achievement and Functional Performance (PLAAFP)
>
> Consider the following elements for the PLAAFP:
> - Student grade, educational environment, and type of physical therapy supports over the past Individualized Education Program (IEP) cycle
> - Progress toward goals and objectives
> - Participation in educationally relevant activities and routines, such as arrival, dismissal, and lunchtime
> - Description of student strengths
> - Clear description of student needs
> - Clear description of the impact of the student needs on participation and progress

The Physical Therapist's Role in Documentation in the IEP

Before the physical therapist develops or contributes to the student's IEP goals, they contribute to the PLAAFP. The PLAAFP is a snapshot of student performance and should include the following: (1) data-based information about the student's current academic achievement and functional performance; (2) strengths of the student; (3) needs resulting from the disability; and (4) impact of the disability on involvement and progress in the general education curriculum.[49] The PLAAFP is the baseline in which educational benefit is measured and should be written collaboratively with the IEP team and based on educationally relevant data. Physical therapist considerations for contributing to the PLAAFP may be found in **Table 21-7**. See Case 2a for an example of a PLAAFP for Thom, a fourth grader with Down syndrome.

Case 2a

Case Application of PLAAFP for Thom, a Fourth Grader With Down Syndrome

Thom is fourth grade student with Down syndrome in an inclusive program at Johnny Appleseed Elementary School and has received physical therapy services to support his active participation in school activities and routines.

Thom rides the bus to school, ascending and descending the bus steps using both railings. He transitions to the classroom with his peers, but his pace of walking is slower and a concern of the classroom staff. He requires cues to keep pace and focused in order to arrive at any location at the same time as his peers. Using a 2-minute walk test, Thom was able to walk 330 ft, which is significantly less than the distance walked by other students his age, where the range is 401.84 to 681.30 ft within 2 minutes. During hallway transitions, he needs cues to avoid others, maintain his space, and change speed as the situation indicates.

In the classroom, sitting and remaining awake remain challenging; a low bench and ball chair are available for use to assist with his alertness level. He requires verbal prompts to use the ball chair appropriately at times. He transitions independently, although getting up from a low position is difficult and slow. A 5 times sit to stand test was used to assess Thom's strength and balance and demonstrated significant challenges: he took 43.25 seconds to do 5 repetitions due to difficulty following the directions, pace, and poor lower extremity strength (typical for his age would be up to 18 seconds). Thom navigates the classroom without difficulty, entering and exiting doorways without assistance.

Per classroom staff report, Thom has challenges with his self-care routines; he does not complete his toileting routine without adult assistance for clothing management, reminders (to go and sit long enough), and prompts to complete a handwashing/drying skill.

Thom participates in lunch with his classmates and requires supports for food selection and the setting up of some food items at the table, although his ability to open containers and packages has improved according to his classroom staff. He safely gets on and off the cafeteria bench. He has occasional spillage from his tray as holding the tray with both hands steady without it dropping forward is challenging for him. In physical education class, observed locomotor skills are not age appropriate due to gross motor delays and his weight. He tends to mark time when ascending and descending a short flight of steps to the school stage unless prompted not to do so. Thom participates in music and art with assistance to stay engaged and enjoys playing on the school's playground and can transit all surfaces. On community-based instruction trips, he has difficulty keeping pace with his classmates per teacher report.

Supports to Participation (Strengths)
- Can move on his own throughout the school building and classroom with verbal prompts only
- Has good static and dynamic sitting and standing balance
- Can sit on a variety of surfaces and transition independently
- Able to negotiate curbs, ramps, and stairs without physical assistance
- Enjoys adapted physical education (APE) and other movement-oriented activities
- Will follow simple directions

Participation/Activity Restrictions (Needs)
- Needs adult assistance for clothing management
- Needs adult supervision for cafeteria participation in order to select items, set up items, and occasionally assist with the tray
- Requires adult supervision and verbal cues to travel within the school building with his peers due to speed and distractibility
- Thom's weight impacts his skills in APE and his speed and endurance for activities and timely transitions within the school building

Instructional Implications for Child's/Student's Participation in General Curriculum/Learning Environment
Thom's lack of speed, decreased endurance, distractibility, and weight are factors that impact his participation. He requires adult supervision, occasional adult assistance, and verbal prompting/redirection to actively participate in all of his school activities.

As part of the IEP team, the physical therapist contributes to the IEP goals. Development of IEP goals is a complex process and requires an understanding of the student, collaboration with the IEP team, focusing on relevant and meaningful tasks, and embracing recommended practices.[50] Physical and occupational therapy experts have reached consensus on several key characteristics of IEP goals: measurability, educational relevance, and content that is specific, jargon-free, meaningful, and child-focused.[51] IEP goals should be written to support participation

in the child's educational environment, be discipline-free, and use positive language describing what the child can and will do. In addition, IEP goals should be SMART (specific, measurable, achievable, relevant, and time limited). An example of a school-based SMART goal for Thom is provided in Case 2b.

Case 2b

School-Based Example of SMART Goal for Thom
SMART goals describe the following: Who? Will do what? By when? Under what conditions? How well?

Make the goal SMART:

Specific: Describes "who" and the conditions of the goal, such as "when given adult support at the elbow when ambulating."

Measurable: Clear objective data point to be gathered, such as time, distance, or number of prompts.

Achievable: Based on prognosis and clinical reasoning, can the student meet the identified goal?

Relevant: Appropriate to the school environment and connected to school program.

Time limited: Can be achieved in a set period of time; generally, the length of the IEP cycle.

Example: Thom will walk from the bus into his homeroom and take a seat at his desk within 2 minutes of his peers in 4 out of 5 observed trials within a 4-week period.

The physical therapist will also collaborate with the team to determine the special education and related services, including supplementary aids and services, that will be provided for the child to meet their IEP goals. The physical therapist may include supplemental supports, instructional supports, behavioral supports, and personnel/staff supports. Case 2c includes examples of supplementary aids and services for Thom.

Case 2c

Supplementary Aids and Services for Thom
- Adult assistance for food setup
- Consultation with physical education to support the development of endurance and speed
- Adaptive seating for engagement
- Adult supervision for pacing and focus while transitioning
- Consultation with classroom staff and speech pathologist to develop strategies and verbal cues to assist with focus while transitioning

In addition to the IEP documentation developed collaboratively in accordance with federal law, the physical therapist may be required to maintain supplemental documentation to support the practice of physical therapy, including a physical therapy plan of care that is separate from the IEP and student encounter documentation in alignment with their state practice act.

PROGRESS MONITORING
IDEA 2004 requires regular progress reporting. However, there are no specific federal guidelines outlining how progress must be

TABLE 21-8 • Service Delivery Models in School-Based Practice

Service Delivery Model	Definition	What It Looks Like
Direct	The direct model of service delivery is the traditional model of service delivery in which the physical therapist provides 1-on-1 services with the child. This model of service delivery should be used infrequently in school-based and early intervention environments. When utilized, the physical therapist should implement direct services in natural environments and daily routines, rather than providing these services in a restrictive environment such as a private therapy room.	The physical therapist works 1-on-1 with the student at a set duration and frequency to develop a skill such as the ability to transfer. This service is delivered in the location where the challenge is, such as in the bathroom or classroom.
Integrated	In the integrated model of service delivery, the therapist provides direct services to the child alongside the child's family and/or teacher. Integrated services are typically carried out in natural environments and may involve extensive instruction of the child's family and/or teacher/aide and may involve coaching them to implement strategies between therapy visits.	The physical therapist is working 1-on-1 with the student on ambulation skills during a naturally occurring opportunity such as transitioning; the student's assigned adult assistant accompanies the physical therapist and student during the session to be coached on the proper hand support to facilitate skill development in order for the student to have practice opportunities.
Consultative	When providing consultative services, the physical therapist is primarily in contact with the child's family, teacher, or aide/paraprofessional. This indirect model of service delivery involves meeting with the child's family and/or team and providing recommendations/demonstration so that these individuals may carry out strategies to meet the child's outcomes.	The physical therapist works with the Individualized Education Program (IEP) team to design and/or discuss ways for the student to have practice opportunities for improved participation. Data may be reviewed as part of consultative services.
Monitoring	Monitoring is a model of indirect service that may be used as part of the child's transition to discharge from physical therapy. In a monitoring model, the physical therapist periodically checks on the child and meets with the child's family and/or teachers/aides to ensure the child is successful in the family and/or educational environment and to make recommendations for environmental modifications as needed.	The physical therapist feels as though a student has plateaued in the skill development. With a set frequency, the physical therapist will observe the student to ensure continued use of a skill (maintenance), consult with other providers, and/or review data to ensure the student continues to have practice opportunities to generalize the skill.

monitored. The progress monitoring plan should be developed collaboratively, with the specifics discussed by the team at the IEP meeting, and should include the method and criterion for data collection, including the frequency of data collection and by whom. Case 2d includes an example of a Thom's progress monitoring plan.

Case 2d

Progress Monitoring Plan for Thom
- Timed walking from bus to classroom: baseline time at start of IEP cycle.
- Paraprofessional will time Thom 3 days per week.
- Data will be collected over 1 month.
- Physical therapist will review data with classroom staff monthly.
- Adjustments may be made to strategies following data review.
- Progress will be reported quarterly based on report card cycle.

PHYSICAL THERAPY SERVICE DELIVERY IN SCHOOL-BASED PRACTICE

In a school-based setting, physical therapy services may be provided directly to the child or on behalf of the child to support the child in benefitting from their special education. Physical therapy services and specific physical therapy interventions are highly individualized, should be decided collaboratively by the

team, and should be guided by the IEP. Regardless of the individual or setting, the physical therapist must define the following parameters when making intervention decisions: service delivery method/model, intensity, frequency and duration, and progression. Definitions and examples of service delivery models frequently used in a school-based setting are outlined in **Table 21-8**.

Determining the amount and type of services based on the educational and functional needs of students is a complex process. Surveys of school-based physical therapists in the United States reveal a wide range in the type and duration of services provided to students with disabilities.[52] There is little evidence to support these decisions in pediatric populations, and this issue has emerged as a key focus for pediatric rehabilitation research.[53,54] When making service delivery recommendations, the physical therapist must consider best available evidence, as well as the ICF framework, *The Guide to Physical Therapist Practice 3.0*, federal law including IDEA, special education laws and physical therapist practice acts of their respective states, and policies and procedures of their local school district.[55] Dosage considerations for school-based physical therapy services, including examples, are described for Thom in **Table 21-9**. When considering dosing, the Academy of Pediatric Physical Therapy describes 4 intensity levels: intermittent (low dose provided irregularly), periodic (low dose provided at regularly scheduled intervals, such as quarterly),

TABLE 21-9 • School-Based Physical Therapy Dosage Considerations for Thom

Consideration	Example for Thom
Participation restrictions. Student demonstrates restrictions of functional or foundational skills that limit participation within the educational program.	Thom is limited in his speed and endurance, which impacts his participation in transitions in the school building and on field trips and making progress on his physical education benchmarks. He is continually late for class, impacting his instructional time.
Chronologic age/readiness for skill acquisition. The dosage of services must reflect the potential for skill acquisition during a critical period of development and the child's intrinsic desire to participate in the educational program.	Thom is a 9-year-old boy with Down syndrome. The physical therapist (PT) must consider Thom's age as well as his rate and stage of learning and level of engagement in the proposed strategies when determining the dose of school-based physical therapy service that may produce the speed and endurance changes desired. (See PT Now, Down Syndrome Clinical Summary, at https://www.ptnow.org/clinical-summaries-detail/down-syndrome.)
Impact of therapeutic intervention. The PT uses evidenced-based practice and considers the student's health condition/medical diagnosis, participation restrictions, personal factors, and gross motor prognosis when determining the effectiveness of interventions and making decisions regarding the student's potential to benefit from physical therapy	The PT should review previous interventions and outcomes if aligned with speed and endurance in order to make a decision regarding Thom's potential for change. If interventions for speed and endurance have not been applied previously, baseline data must be collected using appropriate tools (https://www.ptnow.org/clinical-summaries-detail/down-syndrome). Given his underlying diagnosis and complicating comorbidities, the PT must determine how often data should be gathered in order to track change and determine if changes in interventions are warranted. Age and engagement are key factors to consider.
Support available at the school. Considers the expertise/competency of other school-based providers who may support the student's participation in the educational program.	Thom is in a self-contained classroom where the adult-to-student ratio is 3:1. He receives adapted physical education twice a week due to his educational placement. This allows for him to have the adult support for cueing and frequent opportunities to work on speed and endurance with another service provider. The PT will work with the classroom and other staff to develop strategies in which Thom will work on speed and endurance as well as classroom seating to help with focus. Once these strategies are in place, consistent intervention from the PT in a 1:1 way will not be necessary,
Transitions. Considers student's transition to and present level of performance in a new program, placement, or environment, as well as available supports.	Thom will be transitioning to middle school, where the physical demands of the environment are greater than in elementary school. Distances between classes, including to and from the cafeteria, will impact his access and participation and timely availability for instruction.
Expertise and amount of clinical decision-making and problem solving needed from a PT. PTs are movement specialists who assist in optimizing movement for participation within the educational program.	The PT will work with the classroom to embed speed and endurance strategies and where to embed them. It will be up to the classroom staff to communicate with the PT on a preset basis to determine impact and need for regular PT support. The PT will also work with the physical education (PE) teacher to embed speed and endurance strategies into PE class. The PE teacher will work with Thom twice a week as part of his regular school program. The PT will review progress toward goals with the PE teacher and modify or revise strategies based on progress toward goals.
Previous therapy intervention. Uses the principles of evidence-based practice and considers the extent of and response to previous physical therapy interventions.	Thom received physical therapy services in the infant and toddler program to support his family and his global developmental delays; he received preschool services to monitor his continued gross motor skills development. He has not received services to support speed and endurance development to date.
Health condition. A student who experiences a change in medical status may require modifications to school-based physical therapy services.	Thom's medical diagnosis of Down syndrome is complicated by his obesity, hypotonia, sleep apnea, and intellectual disability. His caregiver reports he is medically stable and is aware of his sleep apnea. The Individualized Education Program (IEP) team has discussed the issue of obesity and its impact on school participation and has provided resources to support (see https://www.cdc.gov/healthyweight/assessing/bmi/children_bmi/about_childrens_bmi.html).
Assistive technology (AT). AT is any item, piece of equipment, or product that is used to increase, maintain, or improve a student's participation within and access to the educational program.	Thom has challenges staying awake in class due to his sleep apnea. A ball chair has been selected in order to keep him engaged during instruction. The classroom teacher ensures it is used for all tabletop, stationary activities. His fine motor challenges with producing written work are being addressed using adapted paper and pencil and supported by occupational therapy.

frequent (moderate dose provided consistently, such as weekly or biweekly), or intensive (highly concentrated dose provided frequently, such as twice weekly).[55] An example of Thom's service delivery plan is described in Case 2e.

Case 2e

Method of Service Delivery for Thom Based on His PLAAFP, Supplementary Aids and Services, Goals and Objectives, and Factors Considered as Part of Dosing Decision
- Service to the student (1:1)
- Objective measurement of speed (2-minute walk) and strength (5 times sit to stand)
- Once baseline data are gathered, reassessment by the physical therapist once per quarter using the same tools to monitor progress
- Services on behalf of the student: Monthly
- Adaptive seating monitoring
- Consultation with classroom staff on transitioning performance
- Consultation with physical education (PE) to develop strategies embedded into PE class
- Discuss Thom's engagement during transitions with verbal cues developed by the speech-language pathologist and team

TRANSITION

Services provided under IDEA Part B, including specialized instruction and related services, end on the student's 22nd birthday. According to IDEA, a transition plan must be in place beginning no later than the first IEP to be in effect when the student turns 16 years. The transition plan must include measurable postsecondary goals related to training, employment, and independent living, as well as transition services necessary to meet those goals. When postsecondary goals and transition services are under consideration, the child must be invited to attend their IEP meeting and participate as part of the team. The physical therapist can play a crucial role in the IEP team by providing supports and services to help the student, family, and IEP team reach postsecondary goals and create a vision for transition to adult life.

■ THE RELATIONSHIP BETWEEN IDEA, SECTION 504 OF THE REHABILITATION ACT, AND THE AMERICANS WITH DISABILITIES ACT

IDEA is not the only disability rights law that governs special education and related services in public schools. Section 504 of the Rehabilitation Act of 1973 was the first disability civil rights law to be enacted in the United States.[56] It prohibits discrimination against individuals with disabilities in programs that receive federal financial assistance, including public schools. Even if a child with a disability does not qualify for special education services under IDEA, they may be entitled to supports and services under Section 504 to ensure that they are receiving the same access to education as their peers. Supports such as accommodations or related services

may be documented in a 504 plan. For example, a student with an amputation or with diabetes could have a 504 plan that includes physical therapy if their health condition impacts a major life activity, even if the student does not qualify for special education services.

The Rehabilitation Act of 1973 set the stage for enactment of the Americans With Disabilities Act (ADA). This civil rights law, signed in 1990, protects the millions of Americans with disabilities as it relates to "virtually all aspects of public life."[2] Applied to a school setting, this means students should have physical access to any and all parts of the school environment, including bathrooms, stadiums, study halls, playgrounds, and classrooms. Under ADA, physical therapists may be called upon to assist school systems in the design of spaces used by students with disabilities and or to make recommendations to make a space accessible to students. Examples include adding bars to a bathroom stall, helping to design an accessible playground, or recommending an evacuation device for safe egress for a student who is unable to descend stairs.

As recipients of federal funding, public schools must adhere to Section 504 of the Rehabilitation Act and the ADA.[57] Section 504, ADA, and IDEA work together to protect children and adults with disabilities from exclusion and unequal treatment in schools, jobs, and the community.

■ COMPARISON OF PARTS C AND B OF IDEA

EI and school-based practice under Parts C and B of IDEA share similarities such as individualized service plans; evaluation, assessment, and service delivery by qualified multidisciplinary teams; participation-based outcomes, goals, strategies, and interventions; and consideration of federal and state law for documentation, direct access, and supervision. These practice settings are also quite distinct with a focus on family-centered care in EI and educationally relevant services in the school-based setting. **Table 21-10** compares several elements of Parts C and B of IDEA.

■ PROFESSIONAL DEVELOPMENT

All graduates of entry-level physical therapist education programs are expected to be competent in the knowledge, skills, and abilities essential for pediatric practice.[58] Physical therapists who decide to practice under IDEA will benefit from ongoing mentorship and professional development specific to EI[59,60] and school-based physical therapy.[61] EI and school-based competencies outline specific knowledge and skills for physical therapists to effectively serve children in these environments.[7,8] A physical therapist should self-assess and develop an ongoing professional development plan using resources available through the APTA Academy of Pediatric Physical Therapy.[60,61]

■ CONCLUSION

EI and school-based practice offers the physical therapist opportunities to work as part of a team to enhance child participation in the naturally occurring activities that are

TABLE 21-10 • Comparison of Elements of Parts C and B of IDEA

IDEA Elements	Part C	Part B
Eligibility criteria	Varies by state. Automatic eligibility for specific medical diagnoses or determined eligible by standardized testing criteria showing delay in one or more areas of development. May also determine eligibility by clinical opinion in some cases.	Based on the need for specialized instruction and related services
Categories of disabilities	Not applicable	13 educational disabilities, plus an option for a state to include developmental delay as an educational disability
Type of service	Physical therapy can be a stand-alone direct service.	Physical therapy is a related service, in general, not a stand-alone service.
Team structure and function (note: IDEA only identifies team structure)	Member of a multidisciplinary team. (Team function emphasizes transdisciplinary teaming; primary service provider/primary coach approach.)	Member of a multidisciplinary team. (Team function emphasizes interdisciplinary or transdisciplinary teaming.)
Service plan	Individual Family Service Plan (IFSP)	Individualized Education Program (IEP)
Frequency of evaluation and service plan review	At minimum, initial eligibility, 6-month review, and annual review	At minimum, initial IEP, annual review, and reevaluation every 3 years
Outcomes/goals/objectives	Family and child outcomes	Student goals and objectives
Environment of intervention	Natural environment	Least restrictive environment
Practice philosophy	Family-centered care	Educationally relevant

important for children to grow, develop, and thrive in their homes, schools, and communities. These practice settings require deep understanding of the laws and philosophies that guide practice while also implementing evidence-based assessment and intervention practices. Physical therapists must strive to achieve published competencies for EI and school-based practice and advocate for the role of the physical therapist on these multidisciplinary teams. Physical therapists may also be challenged by some of the demands of these practice settings but may ultimately find satisfaction in supporting children and families to achieve meaningful goals, objectives, and outcomes.

STUDY QUESTIONS

1. Compare and contrast the role of the physical therapist in Part C as a direct service provider and in Part B as a related service provider.

2. Think about the different models of service delivery. How do they align with the concepts of the natural environment in Part C and least restrictive environment (LRE) in Part B?

3. Compare and contrast assessment and eligibility determination under Part C and Part B of Individuals With Disabilities Education Act.

4. As a physical therapist in the early intervention setting, how do you work with the Individualized Family Service Plan (IFSP) team to determine when physical therapy services should be included in the IFSP? As a school-based physical therapist, how do you work with the Individualized Education Program (IEP) team to determine when physical therapy services are necessary and educationally relevant?

5. Explain the importance of family-centered care in the context of providing services in the natural environment in Part C early intervention.

6. In the school setting, is it possible that a physical therapy service could be medically necessary but not educationally relevant (or vice versa)? Why or why not? Provide an example.

7. What are some of the potential challenges a physical therapist may face when providing services that "push in" to the regular classroom environments, activities, and routines?

8. Provide examples of interventions that can be provided in the natural environment or school environment for the cases presented in this chapter (Elijah and Thom).

References

1. Office for Civil Rights (OCR). Discrimination on the basis of disability. HHS.gov. Published May 31, 2019. Accessed June 15, 2019. https://www.hhs.gov/civil-rights/for-individuals/disability/index.html.
2. 2010 ADA regulations. Information and Technical Assistance on the Americans with Disabilities Act. Accessed June 11, 2019. https://www.ada.gov/2010_regs.htm.
3. IDEA 2004 Summary, LD Topics, LD OnLine. Accessed May 31, 2019. http://www.ldonline.org/article/IDEA_2004_Summary.
4. American Physical Therapy Association. *Guide to Physical Therapist Practice 3.0*. American Physical Therapy Association; 2014. http://guidetoptpractice.apta.org/.
5. World Health Organization. International Classification of Functioning, Disability and Health (ICF). Published March 2, 2018. Accessed June 15, 2019. https://www.who.int/classifications/icf/en/.
6. American Physical Therapy Association. Code of ethics for the physical therapist. Accessed June 11, 2019. https://www.apta.org/uploadedFiles/APTAorg/About_Us/Policies/Ethics/CodeofEthics.pdf.
7. Chiarello L, Effgen SK. Updated competencies for physical therapists working in early intervention. *Pediatr Phys Ther*. 2006;18(2):148-158.
8. Effgen SK, Chiarello L, Milbourne SA. Updated competencies for physical therapists working in schools. *Pediatr Phys Ther*. 2007;19(4):266-274.
9. Section on Pediatrics of the American Physical Therapy Association. Team-based service delivery approaches in pediatric practice. Published 2010. https://pediatricapta.org/includes/fact-sheets/pdfs/Service%20Delivery.pdf.
10. King G, Strachan D, Tucker M, Duwyn B, Desserud S, Shillington M. The application of a transdisciplinary model for early intervention services. *Infants Young Child*. 2009;22(3):211.
11. Section 1431 (a), Individuals with Disabilities Education Act. Accessed June 8, 2019. https://sites.ed.gov/idea/statute-chapter-33/subchapter-III/1431/a.
12. Workgroup on Principles and Practices in Natural Environments. Agreed upon mission and key principles for providing early intervention services in natural environments. Accessed November 26, 2023. http://ectacenter.org/~pdfs/topics/families/Finalmissionandprinciples3_11_08.pdf.
13. National Resource Center For Family Centered Practice. What is family centered practice? Accessed May 31, 2019. https://clas.uiowa.edu/nrcfcp/what-family-centered-practice.
14. Sec. 303.26 Natural environments, Individuals with Disabilities Education Act. Individuals with Disabilities Education Act. Accessed June 8, 2019. https://sites.ed.gov/idea/regs/c/a/303.26.
15. Division for Early Childhood. DEC recommended practices in early intervention/early childhood special education. Published 2014. Accessed November 26, 2023. http://www.dec-sped.org/recommendedpractices.
16. Sec. 303.126 Early intervention services in natural environments, Individuals with Disabilities Education Act. Accessed June 8, 2019. https://sites.ed.gov/idea/regs/c/b/303.126.
17. National Research Council (US) and Institute of Medicine (US) Committee on Integrating the Science of Early Childhood Development. Shonkoff JP, Phillips DA, eds. *From Neurons to Neighborhoods: The Science of Early Childhood Development*. National Academies Press; 2014.
18. Pilkington KO, Malinowski M. The natural environment II: uncovering deeper responsibilities within relationship-based services. *Infants Young Child*. 2002;15(2):78.
19. Gilkerson L, Taylor Ritzler T. The role of reflective process in infusing relationship-based practice into an early intervention system. In: Finello KM, ed. *The Handbook of Training and Practice in Infant and Preschool Mental Health*. Jossey Bass; 2005:427-452.
20. Sec. 303.34 Service coordination services (case management), Individuals with Disabilities Education Act. Accessed June 15, 2019. https://sites.ed.gov/idea/regs/c/a/303.34.
21. Illinois Department of Human Services Division of Family and Community Services Bureau of Early Intervention. *Illinois Early Intervention Provider Handbook*. Published December 2016. Accessed June 15, 2019. http://www.wiu.edu/ProviderConnections/pdf/Illinois%20Early%20Intervention%20Provider%20Handbook%20-%20R12-2016.pdf.
22. Sec. 303.321 (b), Individuals with Disabilities Education Act. Accessed June 8, 2019. https://sites.ed.gov/idea/regs/c/d/303.321/b.
23. Sec. 303.321 (c) (1), Individuals with Disabilities Education Act. Accessed June 8, 2019. https://sites.ed.gov/idea/regs/c/d/303.321/c/1.
24. Sec. 303.321 (c) (2), Individuals with Disabilities Education Act. Accessed June 8, 2019. https://sites.ed.gov/idea/regs/c/d/303.321/c/2.
25. Bagnato SJ. The authentic alternative for assessment in early intervention: an emerging evidence-based practice. *J Early Interv*. 2005;28(1):17-22.
26. Bagnato SJ, Goins DD, Pretti-Frontczak K, Neisworth JT. Authentic assessment as "best practice" for early childhood intervention. *Top Early Child Special Educ*. 2014;34(2):116-127.
27. Bagnato SJ, McLean M, Macy M, Neisworth JT. Identifying instructional targets for early childhood via authentic assessment: alignment of professional standards and practice-based evidence. *J Early Interv*. 2011;33(4):243-253.
28. Neisworth JT, Bagnato SJ. The mismeasure of young children: the authentic assessment alternative. *Infants Young Child*. 2004;17(3):198.
29. Macy M, Bagnato SJ, Gallen R. Authentic assessment: a venerable idea whose time is now. *Zero Three*. 2016;37(1):37-43.
30. Bagnato SJ, Ho HY. High-stakes testing with preschool children: violation of professional standards for evidence-based practice in early childhood intervention. *KEDI J Educ Policy*. 2006;3:1. http://search.proquest.com/openview/f340c4a901ed9fe46a-8b76e1f5e0fdf5/1?pq-origsite=gscholar&cbl=946348.
31. Virginia's child outcomes booklet: team engagement in the child outcomes summary process. Published 2018. http://www.infantva.org/documents/va_child_outcomes_booklet%20-%20Final.pdf.
32. Sec. 303.321 Evaluation of the child and assessment of the child and family, Individuals with Disabilities Education Act. Accessed June 8, 2019. https://sites.ed.gov/idea/regs/c/d/303.321.
33. eCFR—Code of Federal Regulations. Electronic Code of Federal Regulations. Published June 13, 2019. Accessed June 15, 2019. https://www.ecfr.gov/cgi-bin/text-idx?SID=ac1a16592105fa1aaab3d6f-95f330c6f&mc=true&node=sg34.2.303_1322.sg15&rgn=div7.
34. Shelden ML, Rush DD. *The Early Intervention Teaming Handbook: The Primary Service Provider Approach*. Brookes Publishing Company; 2013.
35. Rush DD, Shelden ML, Hanft BE. Coaching families and colleagues: a process for collaboration in natural settings. *Infants Young Child*. 2003;16(1):33.
36. Workgroup on Principles and Practices in Natural Environments. OSEP TA Community of Practice: Part C Settings. Agreed upon practices for providing early intervention services in natural environments. February 2008. Accessed November 26, 2023. http://www.ectacenter.org/~pdfs/topics/families/AgreedUponPractices_FinalDraft2_01_08.pdf.

37. Valvano J. Activity-focused motor interventions for children with neurological conditions. *Phys Occup Ther Pediatr.* 2004; 24(1-2):79-107.

38. Lobo MA, Harbourne RT, Dusing SC, McCoy SW. Grounding early intervention: physical therapy cannot just be about motor skills anymore. *Phys Ther.* 2013;93(1):94-103.

39. Rush DD, Shelden ML. *The Early Childhood Coaching Handbook.* Brookes Publishing Company; 2011.

40. State Performance Plans/Annual Performance Reports (SPP/APR), Individuals with Disabilities Education Act. Accessed June 15, 2019. https://sites.ed.gov/idea/spp-apr/.

41. Sec. 303.209 Transition to preschool and other programs, Individuals with Disabilities Education Act. Accessed June 15, 2019. https://sites.ed.gov/idea/regs/c/c/303.209.

42. Sec. 303.211 State option to make services under this part available to children ages three and older, Individuals with Disabilities Education Act. Accessed June 16, 2019. https://sites.ed.gov/idea/regs/c/c/303.211.

43. American Physical Therapy Association, Academy of Pediatric Physical Therapy. Fact sheet: gross motor considerations for a successful transition from Part C to Part B. Published 2020. Accessed November 26, 2023. https://pediatricapta.org/includes/fact-sheets/pdfs/Gross%20Motor%20Considerations%20for%20Part%20C%20to%20B%20Transition.pdf.

44. Individuals with Disabilities Education Act, Subchapter II; 2004. Accessed June 11, 2019. https://sites.ed.gov/idea/statute-chapter-33/subchapter-II.

45. Individuals with Disabilities Education Act, Sec. 300.34 Related services. Accessed June 12, 2019. https://sites.ed.gov/idea/regs/b/a/300.34.

46. Individuals with Disabilities Education Act. Sec. 300.8 Child with a disability. Accessed June 12, 2019. https://sites.ed.gov/idea/regs/b/a/300.8.

47. Individuals with Disabilities Education Act. Sec. 300.321 IEP team. Accessed June 12, 2019. https://sites.ed.gov/idea/regs/b/d/300.321.

48. Individuals with Disabilities Education Act. Section 1412 (a) (5). Accessed June 17, 2019. https://sites.ed.gov/idea/statute-chapter-33/subchapter-II/1412/a/5.

49. SeekFreaks. IEP 4.0, Creating an intentional plan of care. Accessed June 12, 2019. https://www.seekfreaks.com/index.php/2016/05/04/iep-4-0-creating-an-intentional-plan-of-care/.

50. Wynarczuk KD, Chiarello L, Fisher K, Effgen S, Palisano RJ, Gracely E. Development of student goals in school-based practice: physical therapists' experiences and perceptions. *Disabil Rehabil.* 2020;42(25):3591-3605.

51. Dole RL, Arvidson K, Byrne E, Robbins J, Schasberger B. Consensus among experts in pediatric occupational and physical therapy on elements of individualized education programs. *Pediatr Phys Ther.* 2003;15(3):159-166.

52. Jeffries LM, McCoy SW, Effgen SK, Chiarello LA, Villasante Tezanos AG. Description of the services, activities, and interventions within school-based physical therapist practices across the United States. *Phys Ther.* 2019;99(1):98-108.

53. Dumas HM, Fragala-Pinkham MA, Rosen EL, Folmar E. Physical therapy dosing: frequency and type of intervention in pediatric postacute hospital care. *Pediatr Phys Ther.* 2017;29(1):47-53.

54. Kolobe THA, Christy JB, Gannotti ME, et al. Research summit III proceedings on dosing in children with an injured brain or cerebral palsy: executive summary. *Phys Ther.* 2014;94(7):907-920.

55. Antosyk S, Kaminker MK, Devenport G, et al. *Dosage Considerations: Recommending School-Based Physical Therapy Interventions under IDEA Resource Manual.* American Physical Therapy Association; 2014. https://pediatricapta.org/includes/fact-sheets/pdfs/15%20Dosage%20Consideration%20Resource%20Manual.pdf?v=1.

56. Rehabilitation Act. 1973. Accessed November 26, 2023. https://www.govinfo.gov/content/pkg/STATUTE-87/pdf/STATUTE-87-Pg355.pdf.

57. US Department of Justice Civil Rights Division Disability Rights Section. A guide to disability rights laws. Published July 2009. Accessed June 11, 2019. https://www.ada.gov/cguide.htm.

58. Rapport MJ, Furze J, Martin K, et al. Essential competencies in entry-level pediatric physical therapy education. *Pediatr Phys Ther.* 2014;26(1):7-18.

59. Catalino T, Chiarello LA, Long T, Weaver P. Promoting professional development for physical therapists in early intervention. *Infants Young Child.* 2015;28(2):133.

60. Academy of Pediatric Physical Therapy. Early intervention competencies for physical therapists: personal professional development plan. Published 2017. Accessed November 26, 2023. https://pediatricapta.org/includes/fact-sheets/pdfs/17%20EI%20Competencies%20Prof%20Dev%20Plan.pdf.

61. Academy of Pediatric Physical Therapy. Professional development plan for school-based physical therapists. Published 2018. Accessed November 26, 2023. https://pediatricapta.org/includes/fact-sheets/pdfs/18-SBPTProf-Dev-Plan.pdf.

22

Promoting Successful Transition to Adulthood: The Role of Physical Therapy

Melissa Moran Tovin, PT, MA, PhD, Rania Massad, PT, DPT, and
Martha H. Bloyer, PT, DPT

LEARNING OBJECTIVES

Upon completion of this chapter, the reader will be able to:

- Discuss the state of transition of health care services in adolescents and young adults with special health care needs.
- Describe the various pathways for transition to adult living (independent or supported), postsecondary education, employment, and community participation.

- Recognize that there are multiple models for transition.
- Identify facilitators, challenges, and barriers to successful transition to adulthood.
- Describe the role of the physical therapist in transitions through the life course.
- Recognize the numerous resources available for all stakeholders in the transition of youth with special health care needs.

INTRODUCTION

The longevity of children and youth with special health care needs (CYSHCN) has resulted in an increase in adolescents with disabilities attending nonpediatric traditional settings. Improving the transition from pediatric to adult care providers is a national priority that has been addressed by the Health Resources and Services Administration (HRSA),[1] an agency of the US Department of Health and Human Services, the American Academy of Pediatrics,[2] the American Physical Therapy Association (APTA) Academy of Pediatric Physical Therapy,[3] the Association of Maternal and Child Health Programs,[4,5] and many other stakeholders. Title V (of the Social Security Act) funds support programs for children with special health needs to facilitate the development of family-centered, community-based, coordinated systems of care, which include transition of care.[6]

There is a need to educate pediatric physical therapists and physical therapist assistants on their role in transition of care. In addition, adult care physical therapists and physical therapist assistants require knowledge on adolescent development, chronic childhood neurodevelopmental disabilities,

and techniques to guide adolescent and young adult patients through the transition process.

The purpose of this chapter is to describe the various paths and strategies for successful transition from adolescence to adulthood. The authors of this chapter acknowledge that *transition* occurs during various critical time frames in the lives of families and children with special health care needs; such as from early intervention to school-based services, from elementary to middle school, or from middle school to high school. However, the focus and objectives of this chapter are to describe and assist with the transition of adolescents with health care needs to an adult model of health care, community participation, and adult living (independent and supported).

CHILDREN AND YOUTH WITH SPECIAL HEALTH CARE NEEDS

Children and youth with special health care needs (CYSCHN) is a broad umbrella term that covers a range of children and youth with chronic health conditions and disabilities. The term CYSHCN includes children with chronic conditions (eg, cystic fibrosis, type 1 diabetes mellitus), children with

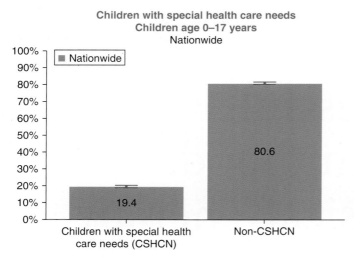

FIGURE 22-1 **Nationwide children with special health care needs.**[9]

neurodevelopmental disabilities (eg, autism, cerebral palsy, spina bifida), children with more medically complex health issues (eg, cancer), and children with behavioral or emotional conditions (eg, attention-deficit disorder). CYSHCN are defined by the federal Maternal and Child Health Bureau as "those who have or are at increased risk for a chronic physical, developmental, behavioral, or emotional condition and who also require health and related services of a type or amount beyond that required by children generally."[7,8] According to the 2019/2020 National Survey of Children with Special Health Care Needs, approximately 14.1 million children ages 0 to 17 years in the United States, or nearly 19.4%, meet this definition of CYSHCN (**Figure 22-1**).[9] This estimate has increased from the 2016/2018 survey when approximately 13.7 million children had been identified as meeting the criteria for the definition of CYSHCN.[9]

The National Alliance to Advance Adolescent Health estimates that chronic health conditions affect approximately 25% of the 18 million US young adults age 18 to 21 who should be transitioning to adult-centered health care. It is reported that, each year, approximately 750,000 young people in the United States with special health care needs transition to adult care. CYSHCN account for as much as 70% of child health care expenditures, and most of these individuals will survive into adulthood as the life expectancy of children with chronic illness continues to increase.[10] It is also reported that only 1 in 5 CYSHCN receive care in a well-functioning system with the most opportunity for improvement in the medical home and adolescent transition to adult health care.[11,12]

LIFE EXPECTANCY IN CHILDREN AND YOUTH WITH SPECIAL HEALTH CARE NEEDS

Life expectancy, or the statistical expectation of remaining years of life starting from birth, is the mean survival time remaining for any cohort.[13] The life expectancy of children and youth with disabilities continues to improve due to advances in medical care in the United States.[12] According to the National Institute of Neurological Disorders and Strokes, children with

spina bifida can lead full active lives. Their prognosis, activity, and participation are dependent on the type of spina bifida, but also on the care they receive throughout their life span.[14] The life expectancy for individuals with Down syndrome has increased dramatically in recent decades, from 25 years in 1983 to 60 years today.[15] It is also reported that the life expectancy for persons with mild cerebral palsy may be similar to that of the general population in the United States, 78.7 years.[16] Refer to additional chapters in this book for greater detail regarding specific diagnoses.

■ THE STATE OF TRANSITION OF CARE FROM ADOLESCENT TO ADULT CARE

Adolescents are defined as persons from ages 10 to 19, and young adults are persons from ages 20 to 24. Together, they make up 22% of the population of the United States.[17] Adolescence is recognized as a critical developmental period of transition from childhood to adulthood that includes biological changes of puberty and the need to negotiate key developmental tasks, such as increasing independence and normative experimentation, particularly being sensitive to environmental—that is, contextual or surrounding—influences. Public health and social problems either peak or start during adolescent years. Some examples of these problems include homicide; suicide; motor vehicle crashes, including those caused by drinking and driving; substance use and abuse; smoking; sexually transmitted infections; teen and unplanned pregnancies; and homelessness.[18] These adolescent experiences and social situations can be similar to or no different from those experienced by adolescents with special health care needs.[17]

According to the July 2021 US Census Bureau annual estimate of the population, 43 million youth in the United States are between the ages of 10 and 19, and 5 million people in this age range have a special health care need.[19] Furthermore, a 2019 report revealed that nearly 3 million (6.1%) of transition-aged youth and young adults (ie, age 14-24 years) in the United States have a documented disability as defined by the US Census.[20] It is reported that older adolescents and young adults, including those with chronic health conditions, may face challenges as they transition from the child to the adult health care system. Some of the challenges include changes in their insurance coverage and legal status, and there may be a decreased attention to their developmental and behavioral needs.[21] Compared to individuals without disabilities, individuals with disabilities are more likely to experience challenges finding a job, being included in regular educational classrooms, attending college, receiving preventive health care services, using fitness facilities, using health information technology, and obtaining sufficient social-emotional support.[21]

The Disability and Health (DH) topic of Healthy People 2020 further describes goals and delineates objectives related to transition of care. The Barriers to Health Objective DH-4 states, "Reduce the proportion of adults with disabilities aged 18 years and older who experience delays in receiving primary and periodic preventive care due to specific barriers," and DH-5 states, "Increase the proportion of youth with special health care needs whose health care provider has discussed transition planning from pediatric to adult health care."[22] In addition, the Environmental Objective DH-8 states, "Reduce the proportion of adults with disabilities aged 18 and older who experience physical or program barriers that limit or prevent them from using available local health and wellness programs."[22] These goals and objectives further solidify that health professional organizations and public health agencies continue to articulate the importance of health care transition from adolescent to adult health care environments.

FEDERAL EFFORTS FOR TRANSITION OF CARE

National reports, initiatives, and research have described or called for frameworks, standards, and various measures to advance a comprehensive system of care for CYSHCN and their families. Title V (included in the Social Security Act of 1935) is a partnership between the State Maternal and Child Health and Children with Special Health Care Needs programs and gives individual states flexibility with accountability for systemic approaches to improve health access and outcomes for all women, children, youth, and families.[6,23] Efforts in creating a comprehensive system of care for CYSHCN, including transition of care, had been taking place for more than three decades (since the 1980s).[24] These efforts had not resulted in an agreed-on national set of standards that could be used and applied within all health care and public health systems and other child-serving systems to improve health care quality and health outcomes for CYSHCN. In March 2014, the central purpose of the National Consensus Framework for Improving Quality Systems of Care for CYSHCN Project developed a core set of structure and process standards for systems of care, called the National Standards Version 1.0.[25] These standards are based on the research and national consensus among a diverse group of stakeholders with expertise in various professions. The standards in the document are intended for use by a range of national, state, and local stakeholder groups including state Title V CYSHCN programs, health plans, state Medicaid and Children's Health Insurance Program (CHIP) agencies, pediatric provider organizations, children's hospitals, insurers, health services researchers, families/consumers, and others.[25] The standards are grounded in 6 core outcomes for systems of care for CYSHCN (**Figure 22-2**).[25]

Building on the National Standards Version 1.0 Core Domains, in June 2017, the Standards for Systems of Care for Children and Youth With Special Health Care Needs Version 2.0 (**Table 22-1**) was released in order increase the readability and ease of use of the standards, while also maintaining their integrity and essential content.[25]

ADDITIONAL EFFORTS FOR TRANSITION OF CARE

The American Academy of Pediatrics has recognized the need for an earlier and more coordinated approach to transition for youth with special health care needs from pediatric to adult health care settings. In November 2018, the academy released the "Clinical Report Guidance for the Clinician in Rendering Pediatric Care: Supporting the Health Care Transition From Adolescence to Adulthood in the Medical Home."[2]

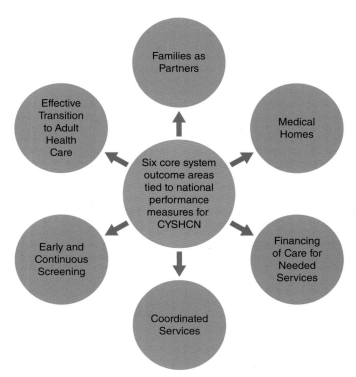

FIGURE 22-2 Six core system outcome areas tied to national performance measures for children and youth with special health care needs (CYSHCN).[25]

In 2005, the APTA House of Delegates identified the need for improving transition from pediatric to adult health care in physical therapy by passing RC34–05, and the Continuum of Care for People With Lifelong Disabilities (COCLLD) TASK FORCE was developed.[26]

The goals set forth by RC34–05 include the following:

1. Explore the magnitude of the issues.
2. Improve the content of entry-level education within the context of a doctoring profession.

TABLE 22-1 • National Standards, Version 2.0[25]
Core Domains for System Standards of Care for Children and Youth With Special Health Care Needs
1. Identification, Screening, Assessment, and Referral
2. Eligibility and Enrollment in Health Coverage
3. Access to Care
4. Medical Home, including: • Pediatric Preventive and Primary Care   • Medical Home Management   • Care Coordination   • Pediatric Specialty Care
5. Community-Based Services and Supports, including: • Respite Care   • Palliative and Hospice Care   • Home-Based Services
6. Transition to Adulthood
7. Health Information Technology
8. Quality Assurance and Improvement

3. Educate members to create an environment of autonomous practice for physical therapists working with people who have lifelong disabilities.
4. Explore and promote the role of physical therapists in a variety of practice settings to the membership and the public.[26]

Since its inception, the task force has developed continuing education courses and technical assistance documents addressing transitioning individuals with lifelong disabilities to adult-oriented health care.[26] In addition, the Academy of Pediatric Physical Therapy created the Adolescents and Adults With Developmental Disabilities Special Interest Group, whose purpose is "to foster the development of education, research, and practice in physical therapy that focus on the improving service satisfaction, health, quality of life, participation, and activity of adolescents and adults with developmental disabilities, or any chronic childhood disabling condition."[27]

■ HEALTH CARE TRANSITION: GUIDANCE FOR MEDICAL TRANSITION OF CARE

Health care transition (HCT) occurs across the life span of children, youth, and adolescents. Within the context of CYSHCN, the definition used by Blum et al[28] is "the purposeful, planned movement of adolescents and young adults with chronic physical and medical conditions from child or family-centered to adult-oriented health care systems" and is the definition applied in this chapter.[28] It is important to note that HCT differs from a single event, such as transfer to another *new* health care provider, but encompasses a process of planning, transferring, and integrating CYSHCN from parent- or caregiver-centered and supervised health care to patient-centered adult health care. HCT transition has evolved from a focus of transition from pediatric providers to adult providers to a *shared responsibility* of both pediatric and adult providers.

The goal of transition in health care for young adults with special health care needs is to *maximize lifelong functioning* and potential through the provision of high-quality, *developmentally appropriate* health care services that *continue uninterrupted* as the individual moves from adolescence to adulthood.[29]

As previously mentioned, due to technologic advances in health care, an increased number of adolescents with disabilities are transitioning from pediatric services to adult-focused care. However, adult services have not been able to respond to the specialized needs of these patients, and few models for transition of care have been developed. This gap has resulted in individuals with disabilities experiencing gaps in continuity of care.[30] In an effort to ameliorate these gaps, additional frameworks have been developed to assist with the medical transition of care.

EXISTING NATIONAL PRINCIPLES AND/OR FRAMEWORKS IN THE HEALTH CARE TRANSITION

A program of the National Alliance to Advance Adolescent Health, Got Transition, is funded through a cooperative agreement from the federal Maternal and Child Health Bureau and the HRSA. The aim of Got Transition is to improve transition from pediatric to adult health care through the use of innovative

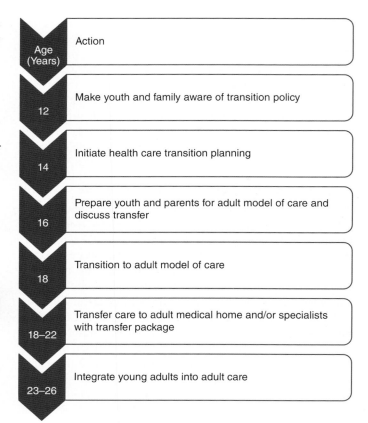

Age (Years)	Action
	Action
12	Make youth and family aware of transition policy
14	Initiate health care transition planning
16	Prepare youth and parents for adult model of care and discuss transfer
18	Transition to adult model of care
18–22	Transfer care to adult medical home and/or specialists with transfer package
23–26	Integrate young adults into adult care

FIGURE 22-3 Recommended health care transition timeline.[31]

strategies for health care professionals, youth, families, and caregivers. Got Transition developed a toolkit for families to use during pediatric-to-adult HCT and includes resources for both parents/caregivers and youth/young adults in pediatric, family medicine, and internal medicine practices. The toolkit includes a recommended timeline (**Figure 22-3**), starting at age 12, to prepare for transition and provides sample tools to implement and evaluate the readiness for transition.[31]

In alignment with the American Academy of Pediatrics (AAP), American Academy of Family Physicians, and American College of Physicians, the Six Core Elements of Health Care Transition 2.0 were identified.[31-34] These Six Core Elements include establishing a transition policy, tracking progress, administering transition readiness assessments, planning for adult care, transferring, and integrating into an adult practice. The Six Core Elements (**Table 22-2**) are intended for use in primary and specialty settings.[32-34]

Key themes that can be summarized in the literature to assist health care providers in assisting families navigate the transition process include (1) developing a written transition plan with the patient and their parents or guardians, (2) updating the plan throughout the transition process, (3) conducting readiness assessments, and (4) completing the transition. In addition, pediatric and adult providers should have open communication *prior to, during, and after* the transition with guidance using the 4 Best Practice Principles of HCT (**Figure 22-4**).[30]

In a summary review by Feinstein et al,[35] the HCT transition of patients with 4 specific illnesses (cystic fibrosis, sickle

TABLE 22-2 • Six Core Elements of Health Care Transition (Version 2.0)[32]	
The Six Core Elements of Health Care Transition[32-34]	
1. Transition Policy/Guide	Health care systems, along with input from families and youth, should develop a policy addressing the system's approach to the transition process. Health system staff should be educated on the policy and their roles in transition.
2. Transition Tracking and Monitoring	Health care systems should develop a process for identifying patients ready to begin at age 12 and follow them through the transition process. A systematic transition registry should be created to track transition progress. Integration with the electronic medical record (EMR) is preferable.
3. Transition Readiness	The provider should conduct regular transition readiness assessments of patients beginning at age 14. Patients and providers should communicate about readiness and jointly develop transition goals that promote self-advocacy and self-care.
4. Transition Planning	Patients and providers should develop and regularly update the patient's transition plan of care. Providers should prepare patients for an adult approach to care at age 18. Patients, caregivers, and providers should discuss the need for decision-making supports for youth with intellectual disabilities, optimal time of transfer, and the identification of adult providers. Linkages to insurance and other resources should be provided.
5. Transfer of Care	Pediatric providers should confirm the first adult provider appointment, transfer the patient when they are stable, and prepare a transfer package, including the final transition readiness assessment, plan of care, medical summary, and emergency care plan. The package should be sent to the identified adult provider.
6. Transfer Completion	Pediatric providers should follow up with patients and caregivers 3-6 months after the last pediatric visit to confirm transfer of care. Pediatric and adult primary and specialty care doctors should continue to build collaborative partnerships.

cell disease, congenital heart disease, and cancer) revealed that despite the challenges involved in designing and implementing randomized controlled trials, it is imperative that research be funded to decrease the challenges associated with the transition so as to improve the quality of life of youth with special health care needs.

CARE COORDINATION IN HEALTH CARE TRANSITION

Decentralization of health care from receiving services in a hospital setting to a more decentralized community-based model increased opportunities for medical, educational, social, and emotional needs of children and their families and increased their ability to receive services in their own communities. However, decentralization of services also made it difficult for all the providers who serve CYSHCN to coordinate care. Coordination of care in a decentralized model can often be fragmented, lack a universal electronic health record or other consistent means for providers and agencies to communicate, and result in the added burden of care coordination and facilitating communication

among providers falling onto the families.[36] In an effort to ameliorate some of these challenges, the most common model of care coordination is the medical home model.

The AAP characterizes the medical home as "not a building, house, or hospital, but rather an approach to providing continuous and comprehensive primary pediatric care from infancy through young adulthood, with availability 24 hours a day, 7 days a week, from a pediatrician or physician whom families trust."[37,38] In most medical home models, care coordination is traditionally centered around the primary care physician as the primary "home" or person who coordinates care.[38] However, the Agency for Health Research and Quality describes a patient-centered medical home in which the coordinator role is filled by the most appropriate provider within each patient's care team. Therefore, one potential role for physical therapists is to take the lead in care coordination or assume certain parts of the care coordinator's role when they are the primary, most frequent service provider for CYSHCN. Another potential role for physical therapists is as a member of an interprofessional team within a physician-centered medical home model. Ultimately, the physical therapist's role may vary as medical home team member, primary care coordinator, researcher, or advocate, and the role may change as care coordination models and direct access continue to develop.[36]

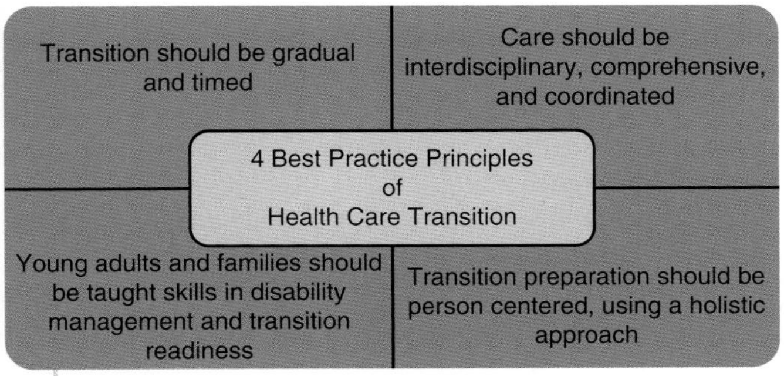

NAVIGATING FROM PEDIATRIC OR CHILD-CENTERED CARE TO ADULT-CENTERED CARE

In a study by Cheak-Zamora and Teti,[39] key themes emerged from focus group discussions with youth with autism spectrum disorder (ASD) and their caregivers regarding HCT. From the parent's discussions, the key themes identified were as follows:

1. Loss of relationship with providers and lack of support transitioning from pediatric to adult care

FIGURE 22-4 **Four best practice principles of health care transition (HCT).**

2. Lack of education and sensitivity about ASD among providers
3. Concerns about losing guardianship

The key themes that youth emphasized their confusion and anxiety around were as follows:

1. Medical providers' role, especially in the transition to adulthood
2. Managing their medical lives independently

One overarching key theme across the groups was related to independence with managing health-related medical decisions and readiness for the transition regardless of the individual having reached age 18, the age of maturity, as the medical decisions involve many factors, not just turning 18. From this study, the authors emphasize the need to help youth with ASD and their caregivers through a step-by-step process by defining their goals, developing action plans to achieve them, teaching specific health-related skills, and orienting the patients and caregivers to available services.[39]

Regarding health care professionals and their views on HCT, it is reported that pediatric or child-centered health care professionals have a hard time "letting go" of the children they have served for many years. They may also feel a distrust of the adult-centered health care environment. Adult providers have reported they feel unprepared to work with individuals with lifelong disabilities. Therefore, for HCT to be successful, both pediatric providers and adult providers must understand their role in working with individuals with lifelong disabilities.[26,40] Pediatric physical therapists should take an active role in discussing HCT with patients and families, assess readiness for transition, and assist with the transition process into the adult health care environment. Physical therapists providing care in adult practices should understand and recognize that although their patient or client has a medical diagnosis given to them when they were a child, their reason for seeking services as an adult are for adult-related concerns and needs. Many of these concerns and needs are a result of secondary impairments experienced over the course of time. Therefore, the adult provider's role and interventions may include treatment of chronic overuse conditions (eg, arthritic changes, pain, tendonitis); preventing additional secondary impairments; promoting community, leisure, and health-related fitness activities; determining and providing appropriate supports, adaptations, and accommodations; and advocating for routine health care screenings and tests.[26] Transition toolkits are available for physicians and may be adapted for use by other health care professions. Examples of disease-specific toolkits can be found at the American College of Physicians: Pediatric to Adult Care Transitions Initiative website.[41]

THE FUTURE OF HEALTH CARE TRANSITION FROM PEDIATRIC TO ADULT MEDICAL CARE

Despite the rising number of CYSHCN entering adulthood each year, recent literature demonstrates that the majority of these children are not receiving transition planning from pediatric to adult medical care providers.[42-44] This outcome can be partly attributed to variability in HCT training and preparation in pediatric, internal medicine, and combined internal medicine and pediatrics (med-peds) residency programs, as well as a lack of research on clinical and health systems barriers to effective HCT. Additional barriers include gaps in HCT knowledge and lack of research about HCT educational models and clinical outcomes of transition care strategies and models.[45,46]

Even with the unfavorable outcomes and ongoing barriers described above, there is evidence of an increased focus on medical transition care, including the development of HCT research frameworks, curricula, and collaboration within medical residency training programs.[45] In 2018, the HCT Residency Curriculum Collaborative Improvement Network was established to facilitate collaboration of med-peds residency program directors to improve educational methods and program evaluation for transition care training.[47]

While the body of literature on HCT training, models, and program evaluation continues to grow, physical therapists play a role in helping children and families access and navigate transitional care clinics and resources for specific diagnoses/medical needs such as juvenile diabetes, organ transplant, sickle cell disease, cystic fibrosis, spina bifida, epilepsy, and autism. Referring clients to clinics or pediatric hospital departments designed to effectively transition youth can lead to successful HCT outcomes, such as improved medication adherence, increased appointment attendance, decreased hospital admissions, and improved self-advocacy and patient-initiated communication.[48]

■ SCAFFOLDING FOR SUCCESS: USING A CONCEPTUAL APPROACH TO BUILDING SKILLS FOR ADULT TRANSITIONS

Transitioning to adulthood is complex and multifaceted. There are many paths one can take to reaching their full potential as an adult. The choices along the way, and the ultimate endpoint, will depend on many contextual and disability-related factors. That said, the physical therapist and other members of the health care team can support families and children in developing and scaffolding skills for success across all areas and levels of transition. Applying the psychosocial concepts of *self-efficacy, self-determination, self-advocacy,* and *empowerment* to transition planning and implementation throughout the life course, team members can facilitate capacity building for success into adulthood and beyond. *Capacity building* refers to the process of providing knowledge, skills, competence, strategies, and resources to meet current and future needs. These terms are interrelated and integral to successful transitions for children and families, regardless of the path they choose (**Figure 22-5**).

The concept of *self-efficacy* was initially proposed by psychologist Albert Bandura in 1977, and self-efficacy theory has since been applied to research, education, and clinical practice in psychology across disciplines, including health psychology.[49,50] Self-efficacy refers to an individual's confidence in their ability to meet challenges and complete tasks successfully. Self-efficacy beliefs greatly influence human

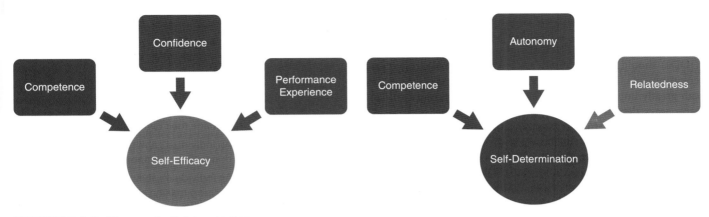

FIGURE 22-5 Self-efficacy and self-determination.

behaviors including goal setting, effort toward goal achievement, and the likelihood of achieving goals.[49] The construct of self-efficacy has been applied to a range of health topics including management of chronic disease, smoking cessation, human immunodeficiency virus (HIV) prevention, exercise, and pain management.[49]

Another concept from the field of psychology that is related to health management and behavior is *self-determination*. Self-determination is closely linked to motivation and behavior. It refers to one's ability to make choices and manage their own life. According to self-determination theory, motivation (both intrinsic and extrinsic) is driven by 3 psychological needs: autonomy (a sense of being in control of one's actions and goals), relatedness (a sense of belonging and connection to others), and competence (confidence in one's mastery of skills).[51] Refer to Figure 22-5. According to the theory, addressing and facilitating each of these 3 needs will result in motivation and, ultimately, the desired health behavior.[52] Self-determination theory has been applied to research and clinical practice for health management and disability independence.

Distinguishing between these 2 terms can seem confusing, as both concepts are applied in seemingly similar ways for the purpose of improving and studying health-related behaviors such as exercise, self-care, and independent living. Self-efficacy is dependent on self-perceived beliefs in one's skill level (and performance experience) and ability to accomplish a behavior, whereas self-determination relates to motivation for engaging in a behavior and is guided by a need for competence, autonomy, and relatedness[53] (**Figures** 22-5 and **22-6**). Moreover, experiences of autonomy and competence are essential to meaningful behavior changes.[52] Health providers can play an important role in supporting autonomy and improving competence by building knowledge and skills and providing guided experience for contextual learning. Pediatric physical therapists are well situated to promote self-determination and self-efficacy in patients throughout childhood and into adulthood. "Promoting self-determination and self-efficacy of individuals with neuromotor disabilities and their families" was recently established as a research priority at the Academy of Pediatric Physical Therapy Research Summit V.[54]

Promoting self-efficacy and self-determination for individuals with disabilities should begin in early childhood and include parents and/or primary caregivers. There is evidence that increased self-efficacy in parents leads to increased self-efficacy and improved long-term outcomes in young adults.[55] Likewise, parental modeling of self-advocacy and adaptation results in development of self-determination in children and can improve treatment outcomes.[56,57] *Empowerment* that results from increased self-efficacy and self-determination can alleviate stress and anxiety in caregivers. Caregiver anxiety can lead to behaviors such as overprotectiveness, which can limit development of independent skills in children.[57] Parent training and skill building to help them deal with challenges of caregiving for a child with a disability can lead to greater self-efficacy and thereby benefit both the parent and the child.[57-59] For example, a parent who feels confident in their knowledge, skills, and ability to handle behavioral, social, and physical challenges in their child will be able to more effectively support their child's emotional, physical, and social needs and support therapeutic goals.

Self-determination is positively related to improved outcomes in postsecondary employment, independence, and quality of life for young adults with disabilities.[60] According to a recent meta-analysis by Burke et al,[61] interventions that promote self-determination can be effective for students with disabilities

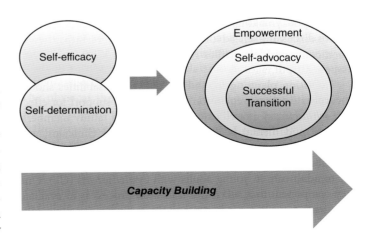

FIGURE 22-6 Scaffolding for successful transition to adulthood.

FIGURE 22-7 Success in postsecondary education requires a balance across 3 domains.

the student, student advocate (parent or other), and community support coordinators (eg, vocational rehabilitation case coordinator, Home and Community-Based Services Medicaid across grade levels (including transition-aged students), disabil-

waiver support coordinator) should be an integral part of the transition process before, during, and following successful transition. Refer to Appendix 22-1 for a postsecondary education transition checklist.

There are several tools for evaluating function, participation, and satisfaction across domains in postsecondary settings. Some examples include the Children's Assessment of Participation and Enjoyment (CAPE) and its companion Preferences for Activities of Children (PAC), Vineland Adaptive Behavior Scales Third Edition, Quality of Life Scale (QOLS), World Health Organization Quality of Life Assessment Abbreviated Version (WHOQoL-BREF), and goal attainment scaling (GAS). Using a family- and student-centered approach, GAS is an individualized outcomes measure used to calculate the level at which goals are attained. It is an effective and reliable method of measuring and tracking the student's progress toward achieving student goals in all areas of postsecondary transition and function. Collaborative goal setting and tracking through GAS, when used in pretransition planning, empowers the student by including them in the process of setting goals, identifying potential barriers, identifying resources, and determining how goal achievement will be measured. This process builds self-determination and self-efficacy, which improves long-term outcomes in adulthood. In a study by Cussen et al,[80] adolescents with CP age 14 to 16 years old shared their future aspirations during a series of interviews. Like their neurotypical peers, these teens identified their desire to maintain close relationships with family and friends, choose their own future, and partake in leisure activities in the coming years. Leisure activities they aspired to were mostly in a social context, such as going to the gym, camping, and socializing with friends. They also expressed their goals related to education, work, leisure, and living situations.[80] Unlike their peers, however, young adults with CP are less likely to achieve the same adult milestones (eg, marriage, independent living, employment). Depending on the severity of their disability, most require focused support and/or assistance. These findings support the importance of collaborative goals setting throughout the transition process and the value of including and encouraging individuals with CP and other disabilities to identify their priorities and aspirations and participate in the planning process. GAS enables these collaborative discussions and planning. See Chapter 3 for more information on GAS and other assessment tools.

EMPLOYMENT

The individual and societal benefits of employment are well-documented. Employment is linked with financial security, as well as psychological and health benefits. Employment also has a positive impact on the local community and society at large. This is no different for individuals with disabilities. For the individual with a disability, employment can result in economic self-sufficiency, access to health care, opportunity to use skills, more meaningful participation in the community, and improved perceived quality of life.[81-83] Individuals with cognitive disabilities who are unemployed score significantly lower in independent living and self-advocacy skills.[81] Employment can also reduce the incidence of mental health issues and need

for services.[82,83] Furthermore, lost wages and government subsidies for unemployed persons with disabilities have a significant economic impact on society.[84] Increasing employment for individuals with disabilities "saves the federal and state government money by reducing dependency on cash and medical and disability benefits."[85] Employing people with disabilities can specifically benefit businesses in a number of ways including a reduction in employee turnover rate, increased productivity, access to a broader pool of people with desired talents and skills, a stronger connection with the local community, and tax incentives such as the work opportunity tax credit.[86-88]

Despite the known benefits to individuals, employers/businesses, and society, individuals with disabilities are much less likely to be employed than individuals without a disability. According to 2021 data released by the US Bureau of Labor Statistics, only 19.1% of persons with a disability were employed, compared to 63.7% of persons without a disability.[89] Moreover, individuals with disabilities between the ages of 16 and 19 years (ie, transition age) are employed at nearly half the rate of nondisabled peers.[90] Individuals with disabilities face a range of barriers to obtaining and maintaining employment.[91] Some of these barriers are listed in **Table 22-4**. Furthermore, low limits on assets and income cause individuals with disabilities to limit self-employment and/or the number of work hours for fear of losing public benefits such as Medicaid and Supplemental Security Income (SSI).[92] SSI is a program administered by Social Security that provides monthly cash benefits

TABLE 22-4 • Barriers to Obtaining and Maintaining Employment	
Preemployment Barriers	**Barriers Once Employed**
Little or no postsecondary education despite cognitive capacity	Poor job matching regarding skills versus job requirements
Little to no community-based vocational experience or work-based learning	Low expectations and job discrimination
Little or no employability training	• Less opportunity for advancement or to try new positions
Little or no formal transitioning planning (from school to work)	• Negative attitudes of managers/coworkers
Overutilization of "prevocational" programs and "disability-only" workshops with pay below minimum wage and little expectation of moving into competitive jobs	Employer's concerns
	• Safety
	• Behavior issues
	Transportation challenges
Impaired social skills	Lack of assistive technology
Fear of losing public benefits limits number of hours available to work	Lack of awareness/understanding among coworkers and direct supervisors
	Limited work hours for fear of losing public benefits
	Lack of support or communication
	• From school or agency
	• Lack of resources or training for employer/staff

to individuals with limited income and resources who are disabled, blind, or age 65 or older.[92]

Individuals with disabilities who are transitioning from school-based services with a goal for employment can begin preemployment services and training during high school. The State Vocational Rehabilitation Program is a federal program that provides grants to assist states in operating statewide vocational rehabilitation (VR) programs to assist individuals with physical or intellectual disabilities achieve employment goals.[93] Moreover, each state's VR program provides preemployment transition services (PTSs) to eligible high school students with disabilities. PTSs enable students to explore career options, obtain job skills training, pursue postsecondary education, and support successful transition to employment. PTSs include career counseling, work readiness training, work-based learning experiences, supported employment, on-the-job coaching, employer training and support, independent living skills training, and peer mentoring. Opportunities for dual enrollment in postsecondary education (eg, technical, vocational, or community college programs) programs can also better position students for employment after high school.[87] Initiating these services during high school, particularly work-based experiences and paid employment, can facilitate successful transition to postsecondary education, employment, and independent living.

Work-based learning programs aim to provide work experiences and employability training to high school students with disabilities. Experiences include job shadowing, work aptitude assessments, resumé building, interview skill building, paid and unpaid internships, summer employment, and more. These experiences, both paid and unpaid, are strong predictors of employment after high school.[94,95] Work-based programs are often developed as partnerships between Exceptional Student Education programs at high schools, partnering businesses, and state agencies such as VR agencies. Riesen and Oertle indicated that employers have positive views of work-based training and believe it has social benefits for both the students with IDDs and the employees at the business.[86] Riesen and Oertle[86] also view it as a way to train and build their work force, as often these young adults are hired by the work sites after completing the program. Employers are open to offering work-based job training opportunities, as long as the training is provided through an established work-based program.[86]

Many individuals and families are concerned about the individual's ability to earn income that will allow them to be self-sufficient for independent living and relinquish public benefits. For this reason, many choose to seek part-time employment only, which limits employment opportunities. Programs such as the Social Security Ticket to Work Program is a federally funded employment program designed to support individuals entering the workforce and maintain employment with the goal of becoming economically self-supporting over time and less reliant on public benefits.[96] The program enables workers with disabilities to transition to full-time work without losing SSI benefits.

As with all transition episodes, a family-centered and interprofessional team approach is important for successful transition to employment. Families often continue to be very involved in the lives of young adults with disabilities and can positively influence employment success.[97-99] Family members may also have expectations, perspectives, and opinions regarding their loved one's abilities and preferences that can positively or negatively influence vocational choices.[100] For example, a parent's employment goals and priorities for their adult child with a disability may conflict with the adult child's goals and preferences. Preemployment assessment (eg, job skills and aptitude), as well as open communication before and during transition to employment, can promote a positive and successful process.[101] Employment transition is more likely to be effective when individuals and family members are engaged in the process in a way that encourages self-determination, by respecting and encouraging them to share their opinions, and when planning is focused on early intervention to address transition issues as they arise.[87,101] Strategies include incorporating interests in career decisions yet providing honest information for realistic expectations, a style of management that supports autonomy by maintaining open and explicit communication with the employee, and providing opportunity for social connection in the workplace (eg, peer mentors, staff disability awareness training).

The ICF framework can facilitate identification of participant needs and goals related to employment. Several contextual (ie, personal and environmental) factors and strategies that promote successful employment for individuals with disabilities have been identified. Some factors relate to the individual, and some relate to the employer and work environment. In addition to job-related training and skills, *job matching* (ie, matching skills strengths and interests to the job) is seen as a key factor for successful employment.[86,102] Factors related to the employer and work environment that promote successful employment for individuals with disabilities include a supportive work culture that promotes inclusion and diversity, employer knowledge and awareness of needs and limitations of workers with disabilities, awareness training for nondisabled employees, and open communication between employers and employees.[101-104]

Some individuals present with both strengths and challenges that result from disability-specific impairments, and employers can anticipate these challenges and implement strategies to maximize strengths and minimize challenges to promote successful employment. For example, Dreaver et al[102] identified strategies and supports across domains that facilitate successful employment for individuals with ASD. (Refer to **Figure 22-8** and **Table 22-5**).

External supports for employers can greatly influence employment outcomes for employees with disabilities.[101] These supports include disability-specific awareness training to promote positive attitudes for a supportive and understanding work environment, external employment support services, and expert consultation and assistance during challenging situations.[103] This aligns with the ICF and underscores the role of the environment in supporting function and participation of individuals with a disability across contexts.[104-106] The importance of providing knowledge and training to employers and employees to promote positive attitudes and an understanding environment is also consistent with Fishbein and Ajzen's Theory of Reasoned Action, which supports the impact of beliefs and attitudes on behavior and the potential for new information to change beliefs and attitudes and, ultimately, behavior.[107,108]

Strategies and Supports that Facilitate Successful Employment of persons with ASD				
Social Support	**Adaptive Strategies**	**Cognitive Supports**	**Employment Support Services**	**Vocational Training Supports**
"Additional supervision" for employee with ASD	*"Written step by step procedures"*	*"Reinforce positive behavior"*	Job matching support Initial support and leadership training for line manager	Personal care training and education
"Open, honest conversations"	*"Written job description"*	Co-workers model expected behavior	Ongoing *"general autism training"* for line manager and co-workers	Transport training
Supportive work team,	Introducing routine and structure into the workplace	*"Reassurance" "Encouragement"*	*"Regular catch-ups"* for line managers and employees with ASD	*"Formulating realistic goals"*
Low number of immediate team members	Restructuring job role to avoid unsuitable tasks	*"Problem solving strategies"* Preparation for new tasks or disruptions	Open communication between line manager and external support worker	Education about appropriate physical boundaries
Line managers and co-workers with an *"open door policy"*	Established and defined lines of communication	*"Regular feedback"* and *"informal evaluations"*	*"Expert"* available to assist with *"unexpected"* or *"difficult situations"*	*"Business writing skills"* training *"Integrity training"*
"Open minded line managers and co-workers"	Alternative to interview process	*"Strategies to overcome stress"*	*"External support"* for employee with ASD	Education about *"workplace basics"* (i.e. shared workspaces)
Co-worker to mentor and support employee with ASD	Alternative transport options		*"One-on-one support within the workplace"* for employee with ASD, if necessary	
Regular communication and support between line manager and employee with ASD	Accommodations to sensory demands of the environment (i.e., dimming lights, blinds, headphones, reducing ambient noise)			
Employee with ASD is aware of line manager's expectations				

FIGURE 22-8 Categories of strategies and supports that facilitate successful employment of persons with autism spectrum disease, as reported by participants. (Reproduced with permission from Dreaver J, Thompson C, Girdler S, Adolfsson M, Black MH, Falkmer M. Success factors enabling employment for adults on the autism spectrum from employers' perspective. *J Autism Dev Disord.* 2020;50[5]:1657-1667.

TABLE 22-5 • Absolute and Relative Frequencies of Abilities and Skills of Persons With Autism Spectrum Disorder as Reported by Participants (n = 20)

Abilities and Skills	No. (%)
Attention to detail	8 (40%)
Goal-directed behavior	8 (40%)
Passion	8 (40%)
Task focus	8 (40%)
Intellectual functions	7 (35%)
Loyalty	7 (35%)
Trustworthiness and dependability	7 (35%)
Ability to adhere to routine	7 (35%)
Expertise in a certain area	6 (30%)
Good memory	6 (30%)
Ability to tolerate monotonous tasks	6 (30%)
Honesty	6 (30%)
Technical abilities (eg, computer skills and knowledge)	5 (25%)

Note. No. indicates number of participants.
Source: Reproduced with permission from Dreaver J, Thompson C, Girdler S, Adolfsson M, Black MH, Falkmer M. Success factors enabling employment for adults on the autism spectrum from employers' perspective. J Autism Dev Disord. 2020;50(5):1657-1667.

INDEPENDENT LIVING AND OTHER LIVING OPTIONS

The concept of independent living is a philosophy and a model that today emphasizes consumer control—the idea that individuals with disabilities are the best experts on their own needs, having a crucial and valuable perspective to contribute and deserving of equal opportunity to decide how to live, work, and take part in their communities, particularly in reference to services that affect their day-to-day lives and access to independence.[109] Centers for independent living (CILs) are community-based, cross-disability, nonprofit organizations that are designed and operated by people with disabilities. CILs offer support, advocacy, and information on empowerment in the attainment of independence. The independent living model sees the problem not as a disability needing a "cure" but understands disability as a construct of society. In this model, the problem lies in the environment, not the individual.[110] When addressing transition from dependence to independence of young adults, this also includes determining independent living or other living options. These living arrangements can range from independent living to supported housing options that match the developmental and physical readiness of the individual.

For youth with disabilities whose families are involved in the transition process for living options, acknowledging parent expectations can serve as a contributing factor, and the expectations can also act as mediators to outcomes via the decision-making processes, which can be a central part to the successful dynamic transition-to-adulthood period.[111] By applying this concept, practitioners and researchers can better understand, account for, and address parent expectations, without allowing these expectations to become a barrier or challenge for the transition. In addition, when determining independence, families and caregivers should understand that independence does not mean ability to do things without assistance, but that the young adult can take responsibility for the direction of their care, which may include directing an attendant to assist with specific activities. It is crucial to encourage the continuous support and encouragement from the family for the young adult to attain autonomy and achieve the self-perception from being "disabled" to being "competent."[29] Not all youth need support related to their living arrangements, but many youth and adolescents may lack the natural support networks (ie, family support network) for successful decisions and living options.[112] Therefore, having the family as support has been identified as critical in the success to independent or other living options.

As previously discussed, youth with disabilities present with a range of medical, physical, cognitive, and/or emotional limitations. These limitations, as well as individual characteristics and contextual factors, should be considered when determining appropriate living options. According to some studies, in individuals with emotional and behavioral needs, although independent, noncongregate housing is generally preferable, supported housing can be critical and an important step to the success of transition-age youth who are learning to live on-their-own.[113] Dreaver et al[102] suggested that individuals with ASD had less residential independence and more often live with their parents or in other supported living options as compared to adults with Down syndrome and youth with other educational classifications including intellectual disabilities, traumatic brain injury, learning disabilities, speech-language impairments, sensory impairments, or emotional disturbances.[102] A study by Reiss et al[113] addressed factors that affect transition and found that young adults with impaired cognitive ability but sufficient skills for independent living could transition successfully, provided that they received additional supports to address cognitive deficits.[113]

In adults with amyoplasia, the most common form of arthrogryposis, living an independent active life with physical challenges requires individualized adapted solutions but is an achievable option with the use of compensatory techniques, adaptations to the environment, and assistive devices required to perform activities of daily living.[114] (Refer to Case 2: Norah.) Ultimately, for individuals with any special health care needs, just having a health care provider ask questions about the youth's future can prompt caregivers to teach youth independent living skills and lead to increased youth independence and a successful transition.

Alongside occupational therapists, physical therapists have the professional skills to participate in evaluating and addressing areas of independent living skills, community participation, and vocational skills.[115] As part of the evaluation for independent living, therapists should use transition readiness assessment tools. The Enderle-Severson Transition Rating Scale (ESTR-S), a criterion-referenced tool readiness scale designed for learners with mild to moderate disabilities from 14 to 21 years of age, can be used in addressing the needs,

preferences, and interests of learners with disabilities who prepare to transition and become successful adults in community environments. The ESTR-S assesses students' performance in each of the following 5 categories: (1) jobs and job training, (2) recreation and leisure, (3) home living, (4) community participation, and (5) postsecondary training and learning opportunities.[115] The ESTR-S can be found at ESTR Publications.[116]

Using the ICF can provide the conceptual framework in identifying both personal and environmental factors that may affect the participation of individuals with disabilities in activities that are important and meaningful to them, and this includes addressing residential independence and living options. Physical therapists can identify changes in body structure and function, analyze how these changes may affect participation in independent or other living options, and address the multiple unique contextual factors that can impact the individual's experience. In addition, physical therapists play an important role in educating individuals with disabilities and their caregivers of the importance of allowing individuals with disabilities to fully participate in activities of independent or assisted living in order to prevent further changes to body structure and function over their life course.[26,117] As part of the team, physical therapists can address independent living or other living options by assessing and teaching independent living skills; providing recommendations for supportive technology, mobility options, and environmental adaptations; and being a part of the individual's development process for a successful transition.[26,118] Successful transition to independent living requires skills in self-determination, self-efficacy, empowerment, and self-advocacy. Physical therapists can incorporate activities and opportunities for growth and skill development to build capacity for independence regardless of living option.

HEALTH BEHAVIORS AND HEALTHY LIFESTYLE

The ability to make healthy choices and practice healthy behaviors is an important aspect of adulthood and greatly impacts personal safety, relationships, overall health and well-being, and quality of life. Development and maintenance of healthy behaviors throughout the life course and especially into adulthood are particularly important for individuals with developmental disabilities regardless of their transition path.[119] Whether the young adult attends postsecondary education, seeks employment, lives independently, or lives with assistance or supervision, transition planning should include realistic and appropriate goals for healthy behaviors based on the individual's needs, interests, level of function and participation, available resources, and environmental factors.

Health behaviors, or *health-related behaviors*, are intentional or unintentional actions that can promote or detract from the individual's (or others') health,[120] and include behaviors in many areas of life. Some examples of health-related behaviors include smoking, substance or alcohol use, diet and nutrition, relationships, sexual behaviors, sleep, and physical activity. Additionally, taking actions to seek health and preventive care and adhere to health recommendations and medication schedules are health-related behaviors.

The term *social determinants of health* refers to the social and physical experiences and conditions within environments and settings that affect health, functioning, and quality of life.[120,121] In other words, a combination of many factors impact health and health-related behaviors. These include individual characteristics (eg, education, income, health beliefs, disability) and social and physical contexts (eg, families, schools, workplaces, community, sociopolitical environment), some of which contribute to health disparities faced by some populations. While health providers cannot control some of these factors, they can improve others through strategies such as education, support, and capacity building. As stated earlier, *capacity building* refers to the process of providing knowledge, skills, competence, strategies, and resources to meet current and future needs, and in this case, for the individual to engage in positive health-related behaviors and healthy lifestyle into adulthood. The ability to engage in positive health behaviors is also dependent on an individual's self-determination and self-efficacy, which are integral to building capacity. The process of building capacity for positive health behaviors should begin in childhood, and progress can be monitored using a tool such as the TRANSITION-Q. The TRANSITION-Q can be used in transition programs with adolescents starting at 12 years of age to measure and track the development of skills they need to acquire to manage their health and health care.[122]

As "movement experts who improve quality of life through prescribed exercise, hands-on care, and patient education,"[123] physical therapists are well positioned to support individuals, including those with disabilities, develop positive health behaviors and build capacity for a healthy lifestyle throughout the life course. The physical therapist scope of practice includes prevention, health promotion, wellness, fitness, and screening activities with the broad intervention goal of minimizing impairments and activity limitations, reducing health costs, and promoting optimal function and participation.[123] Furthermore, the goal of pediatric physical therapists is for the family, as well as the child, to "adopt fitness as an important activity and to carry the fitness program forward," and this includes transition ages of 16 to 22.[124] Once physical therapy goals are reached, the physical therapist should refer individuals to community-based fitness professionals for continued health promotion, long-term fitness, and wellness programs. Effective hand-off is important, and prior to referral, the physical therapist must be sure that the community-based professionals understand the disability and specific needs of the individual and family. Follow-up training and consultation may be indicated to ensure and maintain positive outcomes.

It is well established that regular participation in leisure and physical activity has positive effects on physical and mental health and improves perceived quality of life. Some pediatric disability populations, however, have lower levels of leisure and physical activity than their nondisabled peers and often do not meet the minimum levels of physical activity recommended by the Centers for Disease Control and Prevention (CDC). This places them at risk for secondary physical and mental health issues and poor long-term outcomes. Moreover, adults with disabilities are more likely to be sedentary than those without disabilities.[125] While it is beyond the scope of this chapter to specifically address physical activity limitations and related issues for adult transitions for each childhood disorder, those most frequently seen by physical therapists are discussed below.

Research findings indicate that children, adolescents, and adults with IDDs are less physically active than nondisabled peers and are not sufficiently physically active to achieve health benefits.[126-130] According to findings from a study by Rimmer et al,[131] adolescents with autism and Down syndrome are 2 to 3 times more likely to be obese than same-age peers in the general population. Additionally, obese adolescents with IDDs had a higher rate of secondary health conditions including high blood pressure, high blood cholesterol, diabetes, depression, fatigue, liver or gallbladder problems, low self-esteem, preoccupation with weight, early maturation, and pressure sores.[131] This pattern of low physical activity and sedentary behavior for individuals with IDDs persists in adulthood, leading to increased risk with age for overweight and obesity, as well as other serious health ramifications.[132-136]

The benefits of leisure and physical activity are well documented, and these benefits also apply to individuals with disabilities. In fact, the social and physical benefits are particularly important for individuals with disabilities to maintain functional capacity for participation across life domains to the greatest extent, both physically and socially, and to prevent health consequences that result from sedentary behavior. Research findings suggest that moderate physical activity contributes to improved physical functioning and performance, as well as physical fitness, balance, self-efficacy, and self-confidence in persons with developmental and intellectual disabilities.[137-143] Exercise has also been shown to reduce challenging behaviors in individuals with developmental and intellectual disability and emotional disorders.[144] Furthermore, leisure time physical activity can provide mortality benefits in adults with intellectual disabilities.[145]

For individuals with ASD and intellectual disabilities, vigorous-intensity aerobic and individually focused exercise can reduce repetitive and stereotypical behaviors, self-injurious behaviors, and hyperactivity that can interfere with task performance, function, and participation.[146,147] Furthermore, exercise has been shown to improve academic performance and executive function in individuals with ASD.[148-150]

Adolescents and adults with CP are less physically active than nondisabled peers and do not meet the CDC recommended guidelines for physical activity.[128,129] As adults, individuals with CP demonstrate a decrease in gross motor function, and of those who are ambulatory, 10% stop walking before the age of 35 years because of increasing levels of fatigue, pain, balance impairments, and environmental barriers.[151,152] Moreover, adults with CP demonstrate a decline in long-term health outcomes, including perceived health and functional level.[153] Pain and severe fatigue are among the most common health-related issues for adults in this population,[153-155] which along with reduced gross motor function contributes to reduced physical activity.[152,156,157] Poor coordination of services during transition to adulthood can result in loss of physical therapy services, which may contribute to reduced functional mobility, participation, and physical activity in adults with CP.[158] In addition to demonstrated health benefits seen in the general population, physical activity can reduce fatigue and pain and improve mental health in adolescents and adults with CP.[154,155,159]

Another patient population commonly seen by pediatric physical therapists is patients with CF. The benefits of physical activity for individuals with CF are well documented and include improved pulmonary function, functional capacity, quality of life, and life span. Physical activity has also been shown to reduce fatigue.[160-162] Moreover, regular engagement in physical activity could facilitate a healthy identity and a sense of "fitting in" with same-aged peers.[158] There is evidence to support the need for "regular, appropriate habitual physical activity, exercise and sports for all patients with CF," throughout their life course.[160] Nevertheless, children with CF do not achieve the recommended level of physical activity.[163] However, there is some evidence to support considerations for improving physical activity in this population. It is important that providers consider the impact of the social environment from the perspective of the individual with CF.[161,164] In a study by Street et al,[161] perceptions of the social environment facilitated participation in exercise for some individuals with CF, while it appeared to hinder physical activity levels for others.[161] For some participants, physical activity facilitated a stronger sense of self and positive outlook that improved exercise adherence. For others, physical activity "emphasized differences and left them 'exposed' and feeling vulnerable as they focused more attention on the CF."[161] These findings reinforce the importance of determining individual needs and goals when planning physical activities and building capacity for healthy lifestyle.

Some individuals with disabilities are physically unable to perform moderate to vigorous aerobic exercise or exercise in weight-bearing positions or require some adaptations or assistance to engage in physical activity. Some may also face other barriers to physical activity such as environmental access and transportation issues. For these persons, alternative delivery models and modes of physical activity can effectively provide physical, social, and/or emotional benefits. For example, aquatic exercise can be effective in improving aerobic capacity, lower extremity strength, mobility, endurance, and functional ability and can also positively impact anthropometric parameters (eg, body weight) in individuals with Down syndrome[165,166] and individuals with mild to moderate intellectual disability.[138] Yoga is another example of an alternative to impact physical activity that can be adapted to an individual's level and need (eg, can be performed in a wheelchair). Yoga has been shown to improve physical functioning and psychosocial well-being among adults with IDD.[167] There are many adaptive and inclusive community-based physical activity programs that can increase fitness parameters, provide psychosocial benefits, and offer opportunity for engagement. Examples include adaptive surfing, dance, martial arts, Pilates, bowling, and more. Remote videoconference and telefitness technologies can provide alternative opportunities for individuals to access guided support for physical activity. According to Ptomey et al,[168] group-based physical activities delivered via videoconference may be a feasible approach to physical activity promotion in adolescents with IDDs.[168]

For the general population, there are a broad range of factors that contribute to diminished physical activity levels, both intrinsic and extrinsic, such as age, educational level, socioeconomic status, self-determined motivation, and time constraints. Children, adolescents, and adults with developmental disabilities face additional barriers to participation in physical activities that are directly and indirectly related to their disability. Severity of intellectual disability, lower gross motor function, diminished physical performance, and social-communication impairments greatly impact participation in physical activities for children and adults with disabilities.[127,137,146,152,155,169] There are also social and environmental barriers to physical activity. For example, in children with intellectual disability, social and environmental barriers include competing family responsibilities, parental overprotection, and lack of opportunities or accessible programs,[127,169,170] whereas for adults, these include lack of support, lack of interest and motivation, and other medical factors.[171] For individuals with CP, social and environmental barriers include physical inaccessibility, lack of knowledgeable program staff, competitive attitude and environment, and a lack of understanding for personal and environmental factors.[157] Finally, perceived social environment can be a barrier to physical activity engagement in individuals with CF.[172] Early, collaborative, and well-coordinated transition planning may help individuals and families identify resources and strategies to overcome many of these barriers.

While barriers to physical activity exist, the literature also support several facilitators to leisure and physical activity engagement for individuals with disabilities. In a qualitative study, Mahy et al[171] explored perceived barriers and facilitators to physical activity for adults with Down syndrome.[171] Findings revealed that support from others, engaging in physical activity that was fun or interesting, and maintaining routine and familiarity all facilitated physical activity.[171] These findings are consistent with those from other studies and expert advice that emphasize the importance of including people who are part of the individual's support system or social circle (eg, family members, caretakers, friends) to facilitate a healthy lifestyle.[146,164,173-175] Select activities that are interesting, fun, and enjoyable for the individual.[164,176] Additional strategies to optimize outcomes of interventions to improve physical activity and healthy behaviors in individuals with disabilities across the life course are listed below:

- Develop goal-directed interventions.[175]
- Use mentors or peer-to-peer support.[177,178]
- Promote self-determination, self-efficacy, and self-advocacy through education, creating opportunity to express preferences and make choices, and planning real-life situations to develop social and communication skills needed for participation,[176,178] as well as using a life-coach model for capacity building[179] and promoting mastery of skills.[180]
- Ensure activity adaptation and modification for accessibility.[176]
- Collaborate with and train community providers (eg, personal trainers, coaches) and program staff.[176]
- Plan structured leisure or physical activity programs for easier integration into daily routines improved long-term adherence.[140,181,182]
- Telehealth is a feasible and acceptable option for delivery of interventions for adults with developmental disabilities.

As with other areas of transition to adulthood, the literature points toward initiating planning and interventions to promote a healthy lifestyle during childhood and continuing to support the development of healthy behaviors through the life course.[119] As previously discussed, physical activity levels often decline in adolescence and adulthood. Transition efforts should focus on promoting physical activity engagement, particularly during adolescence. Physical activity during adolescence contributes to a more physically active lifestyle during adulthood.[152,183]

■ CONCLUSION: ROLE OF PHYSICAL THERAPY ACROSS ADULT TRANSITION

Among transition-aged youth and young adults with disabilities, nearly 13% present with impaired self-care, over 34% present with impaired independent living skills, nearly 15% have impaired ambulation, and 69.5% are cognitively impaired.[20] These youth are less likely than their nondisabled peers to finish high school, obtain postsecondary education, and/or gain employment.[20] Less than one-half of youth with special needs receive adequate supports and services to successfully transition to adult life to their fullest potential.[184] Early, collaborative, and coordinated transition planning and support are essential to long-term success for the individual and family. Effective transition planning should include the individual and family throughout the process, which aims to (1) identify unique strengths, needs, and goals of the individual; (2) identify resources, barriers, and strategies for success; (3) facilitate communication between pediatric and adult agencies, providers, and programs; (4) identify service providers; and (5) ensure a seamless transition for continued support as needed throughout the life course. Successful transition planning focuses on career/vocational exploration and development, postsecondary education or training opportunities, supporting independent

life skills, building social skills and community engagement, HCT, and enhancing health and well-being (**Figure 22-9**).

In this chapter, the importance of building capacity for individuals and families as a key component of successful transition in all domains and regardless of living option was addressed. Several concepts important to building capacity, including self-efficacy, self-determination, self-advocacy, and empowerment, were described. Self-efficacy and self-determination are essential to empowerment and to enable individuals to self-advocate and successfully navigate challenging transition episodes on the road to adulthood and beyond. Scaffolding skills for success begins in childhood, for both child and family, by building confidence, competence, and self-awareness through opportunity for experience, opportunities for choice-making, positive role modeling, guidance, and support. Over time, support should fade to allow individuals and families to realize their potential for independence, yet they should have the understanding, knowledge, and resources to get support or assistance when needed.

Pediatric physical therapists are an integral part of the health care team for children and youth with disabilities and play a significant role in preparing individuals and families for transitioning to adulthood and beyond. As movement experts and patient advocates, physical therapists can assist individuals in achieving and maintaining mobility for participation at all points along the path to adulthood, and they can also promote health, wellness, and prevention through consultation, education, training, episodic care, capacity building, and empowerment for self-advocacy and independence throughout the life course.

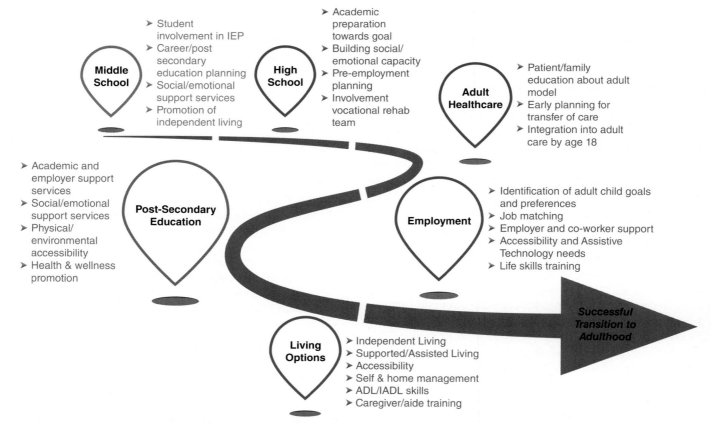

FIGURE 22-9 Considerations for transition episodes on the path from adolescence to adulthood.

Case 1

Luis

History

Luis is a 19-year-old boy with a diagnosis of spina bifida. He has been receiving physical therapy services throughout his life-time in various settings including school, home, and episodes of care at an outpatient (OP) clinic. Luis had a recent ventric-uloperitoneal shunt malfunction resulting in a revision and a 2-week hospital stay. Upon discharge from the pediatric hospital, he was referred for outpatient physical therapy services to address recent changes in his functional status. He returned to the OP clinic where he had been receiving services since his childhood. Although Luis has been attending the same OP clinic for many years and is well known by the staff, he is starting to feel uncomfortable entering a clinic that is primarily for pediatric clients.

Clinical Presentation

Let's look at Luis using the ICF framework at the time of HCT:

Impairments	Activity Limitations	Participation Restrictions
• Paraplegia • Contractures of lower extremities • Impaired sensation of lower extremities • Impaired dynamic sitting balance • Impaired cardiovascular endurance	• Independent with manual wheelchair mobility at home and in community • Independent with bed mobility • Minimal assistance with transfers • Minimal assistance for activities of daily living, dressing, and bathing • Independent with feeding	• Accessing classrooms and school buildings • Participating in social activities and school-related organizations • Ability to self-manage studying and school work • Participation in exercises/wellness program

Facilitators	Barriers
• Parental support and advocacy • Had a physical therapist well versed in HCT	• Patient's sense of discomfort in primarily pediatric clinical setting • Upcoming changes in Medicaid benefits when he turns age 21

Key Transition Periods and Role of Physical Therapist

The transition to an adult-based physical therapy clinic was discussed with Luis and his mother at the age of 14. However, at that time, he and his mother felt they were not "ready" for a change or to discuss a change in providers. At this time, he informs the therapist he feels he is ready to attend an adult clinic the next time he needs therapy but expresses he is still nervous about the change. Now at age 19, Luis currently has Medicaid as his primary insurance and the coverage for therapy services will end in almost 15 months, when he turns 21.

Strategies	Transition to Adult Health Care

Use of health care transition toolkit	• Date and summary when transition discussed/shared with youth and parent
	  ◦ Physical therapist started conversations with Luis and his mother at 14 years old to allow sufficient time for Luis and his mother to prepare for the transition and to be able to discuss concerns on an ongoing basis.
	• Date and summary after any transition readiness assessment conducted
	  ◦ Reviewing and assessing Luis's knowledge of his medical condition, ability to express his medical surgical history to others, knowledge of his medications and allergies
	  ◦ Information and resources provided to apply for health care coverage for individuals with lifelong disabilities
	    • As a result of that conversation, Luis's mother had registered with their state's Medicaid waiver programs for individuals with lifelong disabilities.
	• Date and information of the adult therapy provider selected, including provider name and contact information
	  ◦ Care coordination and discussions had been taking place with the case manager at local adult care OP hospital-based clinic.
	• Transfer of care
	  ◦ Comprehensive transfer package, including the following, sent to the adult care provider at the OP hospital-based clinic
	    • Transfer letter, including effective date of transfer of care to adult provider
	    • Final transition readiness assessment
	    • Plan of care, including goals and actions
	    • Updated medical summary and emergency care plan
	    • Legal documents, if needed
	    • Condition fact sheet, if needed
	    • Additional provider records, if needed
	  ◦ Date and summary of communication with adult provider about transfer
	• Elicit feedback from young adult after transfer from pediatric care
	  ◦ The therapist followed up with Luis after he was transferred to the adult provider to obtain feedback regarding the transfer.

Outcomes

The OP clinic Luis attends has had a transition policy in place and Luis's physical therapist is knowledgeable regarding her role in HCT. She had been using concepts and resources from existing models and available toolkits for HCT. As part of his medical record, the therapist documented the initiation of a transition process and has been completing a checklist that has been updated during subsequent visits during the past several years. The above transition steps incorporates The Six Core Elements of Health Care Transition as modified from the Transition Checklist for Young Adults With Neurological Disorders.[185]

Case 2 ....

Norah

History

Norah is a 28-year-old woman born with arthrogryposis multiplex congenita. She has an extensive complex medical and surgical history, including prolonged ventilator support, severe scoliosis, more than 30 corrective orthopedic surgeries on her spine and lower extremities by age 17, and reliance on a gastrostomy tube for feeding up until age 20. Norah received pediatric physical, occupational, and speech therapy since birth in a variety of settings to maximize her strength, functional potential, and independence.

Clinical Presentation

Let's look at Norah using the ICF framework at the start her post-secondary education career:

Impairments	Activity Limitations	Participation Restrictions
• Quadriplegia • Contractures in upper and lower extremities • Absent upper extremity function for manipulation • Impaired sitting balance	• Independent with power mobility • Able to use adaptive equipment for phone and computer use • Total dependence for bed mobility and transfers • Total dependence for feeding, grooming, bathing, dressing, and toileting	• Accessing classrooms and campus buildings • Managing entrance/exit of dorm room without upper extremity function • Participating in student organizations • Ability to self-manage school and work responsibilities • Attend social and professional student activities

Facilitators	Barriers
• Parental support and advocacy • Familiarity with government programs/resources • Access to adaptive van for transportation • History of adaptive sports participation • Prior experiences of autonomy and competence • Financial resources	• Lack of reliability with contracted personal aides through insurance • Complete dependence on personal care services/aide for daily routine and toileting needs • Family no longer lives geographically nearby • Lack of familiarity with/transition of medical care with moves out of state

Key Transition Periods and Role of Physical Therapist

As mentioned, Norah began building her independence very early on. Norah began managing a wheelchair by kindergarten and learned to use a mouth stick for manipulation tasks. A rigorous daily to weekly routine of standing and physiologic walking remained part of her plan of care through age 17 with the use of standers and orthoses for spine and lower extremities. Norah's parents and family also played a pivotal role in supporting therapy goals at home through exercises and activity adherence, using available governmental resources, and advocating for her with respect to her health, education, and participation in the home and community.

Below is a chart outlining the role of physical therapy in preparing Norah to succeed in her postsecondary education career.

Strategies	Transitions to College and Graduate School
Early Planning for Adulthood	• Patient/family education on accommodations for education • Patient/family education on screening educational institutions for accessibility, support, and transportation options, including personal care needs ◦ Able to find unique program that included aides for meals, classroom, homework, and personal care • Referral to vocational rehabilitation for future employment plans • Collaboration between rehab and medical care to prepare for transitions to elementary, middle, and high school
Promoting self-efficacy and self-determination	• Identifying assistive technology needs in current and future home and educational settings • Trained on how to self-direct care for activities of daily living and instrumental activities of daily living • Confidence building through rigorous exercise routine and self-care as well as adaptive sports participation • Parental encouragement of summer as receptionist at age 16 • Education on communicating accessibility needs to teachers, peers, and administrators in all education settings. • Referral to Self-Advocacy Leadership Training program

Outcomes

After graduating high school on time at 17, Norah went on to complete a bachelor's in psychology and master's in clinical mental health counseling at a university in her home state. Additionally, as part of her master's program, she was awarded a graduate assistantship in a campus dormitory and was successful in managing a residential housing facility. Immediately following, Norah partnered with vocational rehabilitation to become successfully employed as an intake coordinator in a drug and alcohol rehabilitation program. After 4 years of employment, Norah has now enrolled in a clinical psychology doctorate program; this did entail moving much further away from her family, but Norah has been successful in self-managing and advocating for all her personal and occupation needs. Interestingly, although she had received intensive physical therapy services up through high school, she did not have physical therapy again for nearly 10 years, until she recently chose to establish an exercise routine and revisit the idea of physiologic walking as part of improving her overall wellness and health.

Case-Related Items for Norah

YouTube videos from her channel
Assistive technology and arthrogryposis[186]
Norah's daily routine[187]

Case 3

Phoebe

History

Phoebe is a 30-year-old woman with a history of hemiplegic cerebral palsy. She underwent extensive outpatient rehabilitation starting at a young age, including physical therapy, occupational therapy, speech therapy, and vision therapy with a goal of attaining independence with activities of daily living, functional mobility including walking recovery, and speech fluency and vestibular interventions. Her physical therapy providers always involved her parents in the care plans in clinic and in school; Phoebe's parents were overly involved and at times hindered her independence with tasks and felt a need to protect her from challenging situations in both academic and social arenas. Her mother had a tendency to overly assist her with activities of daily living, whereas her father discouraged participation in adaptive sports for fear that she would feel less capable or get injured.

Clinical Presentation

Let's look at Phoebe using the ICF framework at the start her postsecondary education career:

Impairments	Activity Limitations	Participation Restrictions
• Left hemiparesis • Impaired static and dynamic balance • Double vision (diplopia), nystagmus, and saccades • Impaired coordination • Impaired proprioception • Mild dysarthria • Impaired hearing • Decreased standing and walking endurance • Decreased gait speed • Seizures	• Use of weighted rolling walker for all mobility • Transfers from low seat heights • Picking up objects from floor • Household and community ambulation • Walking with changes in direction, over uneven and outdoor surfaces, motor and cognitive dual-tasking • Walking in crowded areas • Stair negotiation • Unable to drive	• Accessing classrooms and common student areas • Attending on-campus and off-campus social events • Participating in student organizations • Going to social event and outings with friends • Using wellness/fitness centers safely where adaptive equipment was not available

Facilitators	Barriers
• Access to university-based health care clinics, including physical therapy and vision therapy • Ability to live on campus for undergraduate education	• Decreased self-efficacy due to history of parents being overly involved and protective • Limited decision-making during educational planning • Lack of transportation and heavy reliance on friends due to parents working full time • Depression and anxiety • Fear of falling

Key Transition Periods and Role of Physical Therapist

Phoebe's ability to self-advocate and build self-efficacy were not well developed during her middle and high school years, and she displayed signs of depression and anxiety during her transition to high school. Although her physical therapists took a family-centered approach to her care, her parents did not consistently promote maximal independence and self-management skills for their daughter. Phoebe expressed interest in attending college after high school graduation; however, her parents were not initially supportive due to concerns of safety and the chance of being unsuccessful.

After a long hiatus from school and PT clinic settings, Phoebe enrolled in college at age 25 to pursue a bachelor's degree in education. Upon college graduation, she took additional prerequisite courses to meeting the requirements for entrance to a master's in speech-language pathology program.

Below is chart outlining the active role of physical therapy to facilitate Phoebe maximizing her independence and participation in her postsecondary education career.

Strategies	Transition to College	Transition to Graduate School
Increase access to physical environment	• Training for getting on/off campus shuttle with rolling walker • Gait training on outdoor and uneven surfaces, elevator transitions with crowds, and negotiating stationary and moving obstacles • Endurance training for walking longer distances when shuttle unavailable	• Floor mobility training for management of pediatric clients during clinical education experiences • Balance training for safe classroom negotiation when RW did not fit • Referral to county transportation service for disabled persons
Maximize social and leisure participation	• Gait training over sandy/dirt surfaces to attend beach event • Transfers training and education on fitness equipment at campus wellness center (include group yoga classes)	• Education on hotel and air travel accommodations for professional student conferences • Referral to on-campus counseling services for self-management, adjustment to living back at home with parents
Promote independent living and self-advocacy	• Referral to on-campus counseling services for stress management and coping related to disability • Referral to residential housing for safe dormitory access • Referral to Self-Advocacy Leadership Training program	• Collaboration with disability office for physical environment accommodations during education experiences for pediatric client safety • Referral to neurologist for new onset of seizures associated with increased stress

Outcomes

Over the course of her undergraduate education, Phoebe was not only successful in completing all her required coursework but was also able to be employed at a poster-printing shop as well as volunteer at an on-campus radio station. Throughout her postsecondary education, she has multiple episodes of physical therapy care at a campus-based outpatient clinic to address endurance and balance deficits, orthopedic injuries due to frequent falls, and exercises and wellness training. All physical therapy goals were directly related to her educational participation across the domain of academics, leisure and recreation, and independent living.

STUDY QUESTIONS

1. Discuss the state of transition of health care services in adolescents and young adults with special healthcare needs. What challenges do they face? What systems, programs and/or frameworks are in place to support healthcare transition?

2. In what ways, and at what key transition points, can a pediatric physical therapist prepare families for successful transition to adult healthcare? Complete the following table as a guide:

Key Transition Point	Strategies to Prepare Families
1.	a.
	b.
	c.
2.	a.
	b.
	c.
3.	a.
	b.
	c.
4.	a.
	b.
	c.
5.	a.
	b.
	c.

3. Poor job-matching is a barrier to both obtaining and maintaining employment for individuals with disabilities. What are some ways the transition planning team can address this throughout the high school years. What role can PT specifically play in the planning process to facilitate successful employment after high school.

4. *Capacity building* is central to a family centered approach to care during childhood and throughout the lifecourse. Identify and define five key concepts that contribute to capacity building, and provide specific examples for building capacity during infancy, childhood, adolescence, and adulthood.

5. Compare and contrast the ways different members of the healthcare team, including PT, can collaborate to promote positive health-related behaviors in transitioning adults for each the following:

- Smoking
- Substance or alcohol use
- Diet and nutrition
- Relationships,
- Sexual behaviors,
- Sleep,
- Physical activity.
- Seek health and preventive care
- Adhere to health recommendations and medication schedules

References

1. Health Resources and Services Administration. Children and Youth With Special Health Care Needs (CYSHCN). June 2022. Accessed October 1, 2022. https://mchb.hrsa.gov/programs-impact/focus-areas/children-youth-special-health-care-needs-cyshcn.

2. American Academy of Pediatrics; American Academy of Family Physicians; American College of Physicians; Transitions Clinical Report Authoring Group; Cooley EC, Sagerman PJ. Supporting the health care transition from adolescence to adulthood in the medical home. *Pediatrics.* 2011;128(1):182-200.

3. American Physical Therapy Association (APTA) Academy of Pediatric Physical Therapy. *Fact Sheet Transition to Adulthood: Guidelines for Patients with Neuromuscular Disorders.* Accessed on October 1, 2022. https://pediatricapta.org/includes/fact-sheets/pdfs/FactSheet_TransitiontoAdulthoodPatientsNeuromuscular Disorders_2022.pdf.

4. Association of Maternal and Child Health Programs (AMCHP). *CYSHCN Overview.* Accessed October 1, 2022. https://amchp.org/cyshcn/.

5. National Standards for CYSHCN. Standards for systems of care for children and youth with special health care needs. Accessed October 1, 2022. http://cyshcnstandards.amchp.org/app-national-standards/#/.

6. Health Resources and Services Administration. Title V Maternal and Child Health Services Block Grant Program. Accessed October 1, 2022. https://mchb.hrsa.gov/maternal-child-health-initiatives/title-v-maternal-and-child-health-services-block-grant-program.

7. McPherson M, Arango P, Fox H, et al. A new definition of children with special health care needs. *Pediatrics.* 1998;102(1 Pt 1): 137-140.

8. National Disability Navigator Resource Collaborative. American Association on Health and Disability. Population Specific Fact Sheet. 2015. Accessed October 1, 2022. https://

nationaldisabilitynavigator.org/wp-content/uploads/Materials/Population-Specific-Fact-Sheet-CYSHCN.pdf.

9. Child and Adolescent Health Measurement Initiative. 2019-2020 National Survey of Children's Health (NSCH) Data Query. Data Resource Center for Child and Adolescent Health supported by Cooperative Agreement U59MC27866 from the US Department of Health and Human Services, Health Resources and Services Administration's Maternal and Child Health Bureau (HRSA MCHB). Accessed October 1, 2022. www.childhealthdata.org.

10. National Alliance to Advance Adolescent Health. Promote effective transition from pediatric to adult health care. Accessed October 1, 2022. https://www.thenationalalliance.org/transition.

11. Ghandour RM, Hirai AH, Kenney MK. Children and youth with special health care needs: a profile. *Pediatrics.* 2022;149(Suppl 7): e2021056150D.

12. McLellan SE, Mann MY, Scott JA, Brown TW. A blueprint for change: guiding principles for a system of services for children and youth with special health care needs and their families. *Pediatrics.* 2022;149(Suppl 7):e2021056150C.

13. US Department of Health and Human Services. Centers for Disease Control and Prevention. National Center for Health Statistics. *National Vital Statistics System Report 2014.* Accessed October 1, 2022. https://www.cdc.gov/nchs/data/nvsr/nvsr62/nvsr62_07.pdf.

14. National Institute of Neurological Disorders and Stroke. Spina bifida fact sheet. Accessed October 1, 2022. https://www.ninds.nih.gov/Disorders/Patient-Caregiver-Education/Fact-Sheets/Spina-Bifida-Fact-Sheet.

15. National Down Syndrome Society. Down syndrome facts. Accessed October 1, 2022. https://www.ndss.org/about-down-syndrome/down-syndrome-facts/.

16. Day SM, Reynolds RJ, Kush SJ. Extrapolating published survival curves to obtain evidence-based estimates of life expectancy in cerebral palsy. *Dev Med Child Neurol.* 2015;57(12):1105-1118.

17. US Department of Health and Human Services. Adolescent Health. Healthy People.Gov 2020. Accessed October 1, 2022. https://www.healthypeople.gov/2020/topics-objectives/topic/Adolescent-Health.

18. US Department of Health and Human Services. Healthy People 2030 Adolescents. Accessed October 1, 2022. https://health.gov/healthypeople/objectives-and-data/browse-objectives/adolescents.

19. US Census Bureau. National Population by Characteristics: 2020-2021. Annual Estimates of the Resident Population by Single Year of Age and Sex for the United States: April 1, 2020 to July 1, 2021. (2022, April 5). Accessed October 1, 2022. census.gov/data/datasets/time-series/demo/popest/2020s-national-detail.html.

20. Institute for Educational Leadership. *The 2019 Youth Transition Report: Outcomes for Youth and Young Adults with Disabilities.* Institute for Educational Leadership; 2019. Accessed October 1, 2022. https://iel.org/2019-youth-transition-report-outcomes-youth-and-young-adults-disabilities/.

21. University of New Hampshire, Institute on Disability. *2016 Disability Statistics Compendium.* University of New Hampshire, Institute on Disability; 2016. Accessed October 1, 2022. https://disabilitycompendium.org/sites/default/files/user-uploads/2016_AnnualReport.pdf.

22. Department of Health and Human Services. Healthy People.Gov 2020: disability and health: objectives. Accessed October 1, 2022. https://wayback.archive-it.org/5774/20220414161601/https://www.healthypeople.gov/2020/topics-objectives/topic/disability-and-health/objectives.

23. US Department of Health and Human Services, Health Resources and Services Administration, Maternal and Child Health Bureau.

The National Survey of Children with Special Health Care Needs Chartbook: 2005–2006. US Department of Health and Human Services; 2008. Accessed October 1, 2022. https://www.cahmi.org/docs/default-source/resources/the-national-survey-of-children-with-special-health-care-needs-chartbook-2005-2006-(2007).pdf?sfvrsn=1dbd8f83_0.

24. Magrab P, Millar HEC. *Surgeon General's Conference: Growing up and Getting Medical Care: Youth With Special Health Care Needs: A Summary of Conference Proceedings.* Georgetown University Child Development Center; March 1989. Accessed October 1, 2022. https://profiles.nlm.nih.gov/spotlight/nn/catalog/nlm:nlmuid-101584932X870-doc.

25. Association of Maternal and Child Health Programs. National Standards for Systems of Care for Children and Youth With Special Health Care Needs. Accessed October 1, 2022. https://www.nashp.org/wp-content/uploads/2019/10/Standards-for-Systems-of-Care-for-Children-and-Youth-with-Special-Health-Care-Needs-Version-2.0.pdf.

26. Orlin MN, Cicirello NA, O'Donnell AE, Doty AK. The continuum of care for individuals with lifelong disabilities: role of the physical therapist. *Phys Ther.* 2014;94(7):1043-1053.

27. Academy of Pediatric Physical Therapy. Adolescents and Adults with Developmental Disabilities Special Interest Group. Accessed October 1, 2022. https://pediatricapta.org/special-interest-groups/sigs.cfm?sig=ADD.

28. Blum RW, Garell D, Hodgman CH, et al. Transition from child-centered to adult health-care systems for adolescents with chronic conditions. A position paper of the Society for Adolescent Medicine. *J Adolesc Health.* 1993;14(7):570-576.

29. Binks JA, Barden WS, Burke TA, Young NL. What do we really know about the transition to adult-centered health care? A focus on cerebral palsy and spina bifida. *Arch Phys Med Rehabil.* 2007;88(8):1064-1073.

30. Kingsnorth S, Lindsay S, Maxwell J, et al. Implementation of the LIFEspan model of transition care across pediatric and adult rehabilitation providers. *Int J Child Adolesc Health.* 2011;3: 547-560.

31. Got Transition. *A Family Toolkit: Pediatric to Adult Healthcare Transition.* Accessed July 31, 2022. https://www.gottransition.org/news/index.cfm.

32. Got Transition. *The Six Core Elements of Health Care Transition.* Accessed July 31, 2022. https://www.gottransition.org/six-core-elements/.

33. Gabriel P, McManus M, Rogers K, White P. Outcome evidence for structured pediatric to adult health care transition interventions: a systematic review. *J Pediatrics.* 2017;188:263-9.e15.

34. CHOP. *Transition to Adult Care: Supporting Youth with Special Healthcare Needs.* Policy Lab: Evidence to Action Brief. Spring 2017. Accessed October 1, 2022. https://policylab.chop.edu/evidence-action-brief/transitioning-adult-care-supporting-youth-special-health-care-needs.

35. Feinstein R, Rabey C, Pilapil M. Evidence supporting the effectiveness of transition programs for youth with special health care needs. *Curr Probl Pediatr Adolesc Health Care.* 2017;47(8): 208-211.

36. McSpadden C, Therrien M, McEwen IR. Care coordination for children with special health care needs and roles for physical therapists. *Pediatr Phys Ther.* 2012;24(1):70-77.

37. Medical Home Initiatives for Children With Special Needs Project Advisory Committee, American Academy of Pediatrics. The medical home. *Pediatrics.* 2002;110:184-186.

38. Strickland B, Mcpherson M, Weissman G, van Dyck P, Huang ZJ, Newacheck P. Access to the medical home: results of the national

survey of children with special health care needs. *Pediatrics.* 2004;113(5 Suppl):1485-1492.

39. Cheak-Zamora NC, Teti M. "You think it's hard now … It gets much harder for our children": youth with autism and their caregiver's perspectives of health care transition services. *Autism.* 2015;19(8):992-1001.

40. Lindsay S, Cruickshank H, McPherson AC, Maxwell J. Implementation of an inter-agency transition model for youth with spina bifida. *Child Care Health Dev.* 2016;42(2):203-212.

41. American College of Physicians. Pediatric to Adult Care Transitions Initiative. Accessed October 1, 2022. https://www.acponline.org/clinical-information/high-value-care/resources-for-clinicians/pediatric-to-adult-care-transitions-initiative.

42. Fernandes P, Timmerman J, Hotez E, et al. A residency program curriculum to improve health care transitions for autistic individuals. *Pediatrics.* 2022;149(Suppl 4):e2020049437U.

43. Lebrun-Harris LA, McManus MA, Ilango SM, et al. Transition planning among US youth with and without special health care needs. *Pediatrics.* 2018;142(4):e20180194.

44. Goodman DM, Hall M, Levin A, et al. Adults with chronic health conditions originating in childhood: inpatient experience in children's hospitals. *Pediatrics.* 2011;128(1):5-13.

45. Sadun RE, Chung RJ, Pollock MD, Maslow GR. Lost in transition: resident and fellow training and experience caring for young adults with chronic conditions in a large United States' academic medical center. *Med Educ Online.* 2019;24(1):1605783.

46. Betz CL, O'Kane LS, Nehring WM, Lobo ML. Systematic review: health care transition practice service models. *Nurs Outlook.* 2016;64(3):229-243.

47. Feeney C, Hotez E, Wan L, et al. A multi-institutional collaborative to assess the knowledge and skills of medicine-pediatrics residents in health care transition. *Cureus.* 2021;13(12):e20327.

48. Davis AM, Brown RF, Taylor JL, Epstein RA, McPheeters ML. Transition care for children with special health care needs. *Pediatrics.* 2014;134(5):900-908.

49. Carey MP, Forsyth AD. *Teaching Tip Sheet: Self Efficacy.* American Psychological Association; 2019. Accessed October 1, 2022. https://www.apa.org/pi/aids/resources/education/self-efficacy.

50. Bandura A. Self-efficacy: Toward a unifying theory of behavioral change. *Psychol Rev.* 1977;84(2):191-215.

51. Ryan RM, Deci EL. *Self-Determination Theory: Basic Psychological Needs in Motivation, Development, and Wellness.* Guilford Publishing; 2017.

52. Center for Self-Determination Theory. Self-determination theory: healthcare. Available at https://selfdeterminationtheory.org/. Accessed October 1, 2022

53. Garrin JM. Self-efficacy, self-determination, and self-regulation: the role of the fitness professional in social change agency. *J Soc Change.* 2014;6(1):41-54.

54. Sargent B, Harbourne R, Moreau NG, et al. Research summit V: optimizing transitions from infancy to early adulthood in children with neuromotor conditions. *Pediatr Phys Ther.* 2022;34(3):411-417.

55. Ivey JK. What do parents expect? A study of likelihood and importance issues for children with autism spectrum disorders. *Focus Autism Other Dev Disabil.* 2004;19(1):27-33.

56. Field S, Hoffman A. The importance of family involvement for promoting self-determination in adolescents with autism and other developmental disabilities. *Focus Autism Other Dev Disabil.* 1999;14(1):36-41.

57. Karst JS, Van Hecke AV. Parent and family impact of autism spectrum disorders: a review and proposed model for intervention evaluation. *Clin Child Fam Psychol Rev.* 2012;15(3):247-277.

58. Leef J. A clinical intervention program for children with Asperger syndrome and their parents: promoting children's social skills and parents' self-confidence. *Autism NewsLink.* 2005:14-15.

59. Whittingham K, Sofronoff K, Sheffield J, Sanders MR. Stepping stones triple p: an RCT of a parenting program with parents of a child diagnosed with an autism spectrum disorder. *J Abnorm Child Psychol.* 2009;37(4):469-480.

60. White K, Flanagan TD, Nadig A. Examining the relationship between self-determination and quality of life in young adults with autism spectrum disorder. *J Dev Phys Disabil.* 2018;30(6):735-754.

61. Burke KM, Raley SK, Shogren KA, et al. A meta-analysis of interventions to promote self-determination for students with disabilities. *Remedial Spec Educ.* 2020;41(3):176-188.

62. Shogren KA. A social-ecological analysis of the self-determination literature. *Intellect Dev Disabil.* 2013;51(6):496-511.

63. Taylor WD, Cobigo V, Ouellette KH. A family systems perspective on supporting self-determination in young adults with intellectual and developmental disabilities. *J Appl Res Intellect Disabil.* 2019;32(5):1116-1128.

64. SelfAdvocateNet. What is self advocacy? Accessed October 1, 2022. https://selfadvocatenet.com/what-is-self-advocacy/.

65. Miller RJ, La Follette M, Green K. Development and field test of a transition planning procedure 1985-1988. *Career Dev Except Individ.* 1990;13(1):45-55.

66. Martin JE, Huber Marshall L, Maxson LL. Transition policy: infusing self-determination and self-advocacy into transition programs. *Career Dev Except Individ.* 1993;16(1):53-61.

67. National Rehabilitation Information Center. Advocacy, self-advocacy, and self-determination for individuals with disabilities. 2017;12(1). Accessed October 1, 2022. https://www.naric.com/sites/default/files/reSearch%20Vol.%2012%2C%20Issue%201.pdf.

68. Okumura MJ, Ong T, Dawson D, et al. Improving transition from paediatric to adult cystic fibrosis care: programme implementation and evaluation. *BMJ Qual Saf.* 2014;23(1):i64-72.

69. Sawicki GS, Lukens-Bull K, Yin X, et al. Measuring the transition readiness of youth with special healthcare needs: validation of the TRAQ—Transition Readiness Assessment Questionnaire. *J Pediatr Psychol.* 2011;36(2):160-171.

70. Department of Pediatrics, East Tennessee State University. Transition Readiness Assessment Questionnaire. Accessed October 1, 2022. https://www.etsu.edu/com/pediatrics/traq/.

71. Jeannis H, Goldberg M, Seelman K, Schmeler M, Cooper RA. Barriers and facilitators to students with physical disabilities' participation in academic laboratory spaces. *Disabil Rehabil Assist Technol.* 2020;15(2):225-237.

72. White SW, Elias R, Salina CE, et al. Students with autism spectrum disorder in college: results from a preliminary mixed methods needs analysis. *Res Dev Disabil.* 2016;56:29-40.

73. Gelbar N, Smith I, Reichow B. Systematic review of articles describing experience and supports of individuals with autism enrolled in college and university programs. *J Autism Dev Disord.* 2014;44(10):2593-2601.

74. Cai R, Richdale AL. Educational experiences and needs of higher education students with autism spectrum disorder. *J Autism Dev Disord.* 2016;46(1):31-41.

75. Bencini GML, Garofolo I, Arenghi A. Implementing universal design and the ICF in higher education: towards a model that achieves quality higher education for all. *Stud Health Technol Inform.* 2018;256:464-472.

76. Van Hees V, Moyson T, Roeyers H. Higher education experiences of students with autism spectrum disorder: challenges, benefits and support needs. *J Autism Dev Disord.* 2015;45(6):1673-1688.

77. College Living Experience. Accessed October 1, 2022. https://experiencecele.com/our-work-2/.

78. McPherson AC, Rudzik A, Kingsnorth S, King G, Gorter JW, Morrison A. "Ready to take on the world": experiences and understandings of independence after attending residential immersive life skills programs for youth with physical disabilities. *Dev Neurorehabil.* 2018;21(2):73-82.

79. Ho D. Optimizing movement to improve the college experience. *Pediatr Phys Ther.* 2015;27(4):E8.

80. Cussen A, Howie L, Imms C. Looking to the future: adolescents with cerebral palsy talk about their aspirations—a narrative study. *Disabil Rehabil.* 2012;34(24):2103-2110.

81. Sharma RN, Singh S, Kutty AT. Employment leads to independent living and self-advocacy: a comparative study of employed and unemployed persons with cognitive disabilities. *Asia Pacific Disabil Rehabil J.* 2006;17(1):50-60.

82. Shogren KA, Mayumi Hagiwara, Wehmeyer ML, Dean EE. How does employment influence health outcomes? A systematic review of the intellectual disability literature. *J Vocational Rehabil.* 2018;49(1):1-13.

83. Robertson J, Beyer S, Emerson E, Baines S, Hatton C. The association between employment and the health of people with intellectual disabilities: a systematic review. *J Appl Res Intellect Disabil.* 2019;32(6):1335-1348.

84. Ganz ML. The lifetime distribution of the incremental societal costs of autism. *Arch Pediatr Adolesc Med.* 2007;161(4):343-349.

85. Employer Assistance and Resource Network on Disability Inclusion (EARN). Employer Assistance and Resource Network Report. 2013. Accessed October 1, 2022. https://askearn.org/.

86. Riesen T, Oertle KM. Developing work-based learning experiences for students with intellectual and developmental disabilities: a preliminary study of employers' perspectives. *J Rehabil.* 2019;85(2):27-36.

87. Sansosti FJ, Merchant D, Koch L, Rumrill P, Herrer A. Providing supportive transition services to individuals with autism spectrum disorder: Considerations for vocational rehabilitation professionals. *J Vocat Rehabil.* 2017;47(2):207-222.

88. Internal Revenue Service. Tax benefits for businesses who have employees with disabilities. June 13, 2022. Accessed October 1, 2022. https://www.irs.gov/businesses/small-businesses-self-employed/tax-benefits-for-businesses-who-have-employees-with-disabilities.

89. US Bureau of Labor Statistics. Employment Status of the Civilian Noninstitutional Population by Disability Status and Selected Characteristics, 2021 Annual Averages. Economic News Release. February 22, 2022. Accessed October 1, 2022. https://www.bls.gov/news.release/disabl.t01.htm.

90. US Bureau of Labor Statistics. Persons with a disability: labor force characteristics summary. February 24, 2002. Accessed October 1, 2022. https://www.bls.gov/news.release/disabl.nr0.htm.

91. The ARC. Employment, training and wages. Accessed October 1, 2022. https://thearc.org/policy-advocacy/employment-training-and-wages/.

92. Social Security Administration. What is Social Security income? Accessed July 31, 2022. https://www.ssa.gov/ssi/.

93. US Department of Education. Vocational rehabilitation state grants. Accessed July 31, 2022. https://www2.ed.gov/programs/rsabvrs/index.html.

94. Siperstein GN, Heyman M, Stokes JE. Pathways to employment: a national survey of adults with intellectual disabilities. *J Vocat Rehabil.* 2014;41(3):165-178.

95. Wehman P, Sima AP, Ketchum J, West MD, Chan F, Luecking R. Predictors of successful transition from school to employment for youth with disabilities. *J Occup Rehabil.* 2015;25(2):323-334.

96. Ticket to Work. About Ticket to Work. Accessed October 1, 2022. https://yourtickettowork.ssa.gov/about/index.html.

97. Nicholas DB, Mitchell W, Dudley C, Clarke M, Zulla R. An ecosystem approach to employment and autism spectrum disorder. *J Autism Dev Disord.* 2018;48(1):264-275.

98. Taylor JL, Seltzer MM. Employment and post-secondary educational activities for young adults with autism spectrum disorders during the transition to adulthood. *J Autism Dev Disord.* 2011;41(5):566-574.

99. Cadman T, Eklund H, Howley D, et al. Caregiver burden as people with autism spectrum disorder and attention-deficit/hyperactivity disorder transition into adolescence and adulthood in the United Kingdom. *J Am Acad Child Adolesc Psychiatry.* 2012;51(9):879-888.

100. Van Hees V, Roeyers H, De Mol J. Students with autism spectrum disorder and their parents in the transition into higher education: impact on dynamics in the parent–child relationship. *J Autism Dev Disord.* 2018;48(10):3296-3310.

101. Goldfarb Y, Gal E, Golan O. A conflict of interests: a motivational perspective on special interests and employment success of adults with ASD. *J Autism Dev Disord.* 2019;49(9):3915-3923.

102. Dreaver J, Thompson C, Girdler S, Adolfsson M, Black MH, Falkmer M. Success factors enabling employment for adults on the autism spectrum from employers' perspective. *J Autism Dev Disord.* 2020;50(5):1657-1667.

103. Walsh L, Lydon S, Healy O. Employment and vocational skills among individuals with autism spectrum disorder: predictors, impact, and interventions. *Rev J Autism Dev Disord.* 2014;1(4):266-275.

104. Pfeiffer B, Brusilovskiy E, Davidson A, Persch A. Impact of person-environment fit on job satisfaction for working adults with autism spectrum disorders. *J Vocat Rehabil.* 2018;48(1):49-57.

105. de Schipper E, Mahdi S, de Vries P, et al. Functioning and disability in autism spectrum disorder: a worldwide survey of experts. *Autism Res.* 2016;9(9):959-969.

106. World Health Organization. International Classification of Functioning, Disability and Health: Children and Youth Version: ICF-CY. 2007. Accessed October 1, 2022. http://apps.who.int/iris/bitstream/handle/10665/43737/9789241547321_eng.pdf;jsessionid=9A68CA3A170B91FE820A42E689E3FBB1?sequence=1.

107. Fishbein M, Ajzen I. *Belief, Attitude, Intention and Behavior: An Introduction to Theory and Research.* Addison-Wesley; 1975.

108. Ajzen I, Fishbein M. *Understanding Attitudes and Predicting Social Behavior.* Prentice-Hall; 1980.

109. Disability Community Resource Center. What is independent living? Accessed October 1, 2022. https://www.dcrc.co/independent-living/#:~:text=Independent%20living%2C%20as%20seen%20by,determination%2C%20and%20self%2Drespect.

110. National Council on Independent Living. Accessed October 1, 2022. https://ncil.org/.

111. Kirby AV. Parent expectations mediate outcomes for young adults with autism spectrum disorder. *J Autism Dev Disord.* 2016;46(5):1643-1655.

112. Woolsey L, Katz-Leavy J. *Transitioning Youth With Mental Health Needs to Meaningful Employment and Independent Living.* National Collaborative on Workforce and Disability for Youth, Institute for Educational Leadership. 2008. Accessed October 1, 2022. https://nccollaborative.org/wp-content/uploads/2017/01/Transitioning-Youth-with-Mental-Health-Needs-to-Meaningful-Employment-and-Independent-Living-2.pdf.

113. Reiss JG, Gibson RW, Walker LR. Health care transition: youth, family, and provider perspectives. *Pediatrics.* 2005;115(1):112-120.

114. Steen U, Wekre LL, Vøllestad NK. Physical functioning and activities of daily living in adults with amyoplasia, the most common

form of arthrogryposis. a cross-sectional study. *Disabil Rehabil.* 2018;40(23):2767-2779.

115. Kardos MR, White BP. Evaluation options for secondary transition planning. *Am J Occup Ther.* 2006;60(3):333-339.

116. ESTR Publications. *Transition Rating Scales for Learners With Disabilities, TSR 1.0, TSR 2.0, TSR 3.0.* Accessed July 31, 2022. https://estr.net/index.cfm.

117. Roush S, Sharby N. Disability reconsidered: the paradox of physical therapy. *Phys Ther.* 2011;91(12):1715-1727.

118. Kohler PD, Gothberg JE, Fowler C, Coyle J. *Taxonomy for Transition Programming 2.0: A Model for Planning, Organizing, and Evaluating Transition Education, Services, and Programs.* Western Michigan University; 2016. Accessed September 30, 2022. https://floridadcdt.org/uploads/3/5/7/1/35718381/taxonomy_for_transition_prog._2.0.pdf.

119. Palisano RJ, Di Rezze B, Stewart D, et al. Promoting capacities for future adult roles and healthy living using a lifecourse health development approach. *Disabil Rehabil.* 2020;42(14):2002-2011.

120. Short SE, Mollborn S. Social determinants and health behaviors: conceptual frames and empirical advances. *Curr Opin Psychol.* 2015;5:78-84.

121. Office of Disease Prevention and Health Promotion. Social Determinants of Health. Healthy People 2020. Accessed September 30, 2022. https://wayback.archive-it.org/5774/20220413203948/https://www.healthypeople.gov/2020/topics-objectives/topic/social-determinants-of-health.

122. CanChild. TRANSITION-Q: What Is It? Accessed September 30, 2022. https://canchild.ca/en/shop/6-transition-q.

123. American Physical Therapy Association (APTA). What physical therapists do. Alexandria, VA. Accessed September 30, 2022. https://www.apta.org/your-career/careers-in-physical-therapy/becoming-a-pt.

124. Academy of Pediatric Physical Therapy (APPT). The Role and Scope of Pediatric Physical Therapy in Fitness, Wellness, Health Promotion, and Prevention. Fact Sheet, 2012. Accessed September 30, 2022. https://pediatricapta.org/includes/fact-sheets/pdfs/12%20Role%20and%20Scope%20in%20Fitness%20Health%20Promo.pdf.

125. Chiu C-Y, Ruopeng A. Physical activity patterns among U.S. adults with disabilities. *Rehabil Res Policy Educ.* 2016:30(1):77-88.

126. Pan CY, Frey GC. Physical activity patterns in youth with autism spectrum disorders. *J Autism Dev Disord.* 2006;36(5):597-606.

127. Downs SJ, Fairclough SJ, Knowles ZR, Boddy LM. Physical activity patterns in youth with intellectual disabilities. *Adapt Phys Activ Q.* 2016;33(4):374-390.

128. Usuba K, Oddson B, Gauthier A, Young NL. Leisure time physical activity in adults with cerebral palsy. *Disabil Health J.* 2015;8(4):611-618.

129. Carlon SL, Taylor NF, Dodd KJ, Shields N. Differences in habitual physical activity levels of young people with cerebral palsy and their typically developing peers: a systematic review. *Disabil Rehabil.* 2013;35(8):647-655.

130. Sundahl L, Zetterberg M, Wester A, Blomqvist S. Physical activity levels among adolescent and young adult women and men with and without intellectual disability. *J Appl Res Intellect Disabil.* 2016;29(1):93-98.

131. Rimmer JH, Yamaki K, Lowry BM, Wang E, Vogel LC. Obesity and obesity-related secondary conditions in adolescents with intellectual/developmental disabilities. *J Intellect Disabil Res.* 2010;54(9):787-794.

132. Maïano C. Prevalence and risk factors of overweight and obesity among children and adolescents with intellectual disabilities. *Obes Rev.* 2011;12(3):189-197.

133. Pierce M, Ramsey K, Pinter J. Trends in obesity and overweight in Oregon children with down syndrome. *Glob Pediatr Health.* 2019;6:2333794X19835640.

134. Pitchford EA, Adkins C, Hasson RE, Hornyak JE, Ulrich DA. Association between physical activity and adiposity in adolescents with Down syndrome. *Med Sci Sports Exerc.* 2018;50(4):667-674.

135. Curtin C, Anderson SE, Must A, Bandini L. The prevalence of obesity in children with autism: a secondary data analysis using nationally representative data from the National Survey of Children's Health. *BMC Pediatr.* 2010;10:11.

136. Tyler CV, Schramm SC, Karafa M, Tang AS, Jain AK. Chronic disease risks in young adults with autism spectrum disorder: forewarned is forearmed. *Am J Intellect Dev Disabil.* 2011;116(5): 371-380.

137. Xu J, Choi P, Motl RW, Agiovlasitis S. Is physical activity associated with physical performance in adults with intellectual disability? *Adapt Phys Activ Q.* 2020;37(3):289-303.

138. Hakim RM, Ross MD, Runco W, Kane MT. A community-based aquatic exercise program to improve endurance and mobility in adults with mild to moderate intellectual disability. *J Exerc Rehabil.* 2017;13(1):89-94.

139. Pan C-C, Mcnamara S. The impact of adapted physical education on physical fitness of students with intellectual disabilities: a three-year study. *Int J Disabil Dev Educ.* 2020;69(4):1257-1272.

140. Collins K, Staples K. The role of physical activity in improving physical fitness in children with intellectual and developmental disabilities. *Res Dev Disabil.* 2017;69:49-60.

141. Bartlo P, Klein PJ. Physical activity benefits and needs in adults with intellectual disabilities: systematic review of the literature. *Am J Intellect Dev Disabil.* 2011;116(3):220-232.

142. Heller T, McCubbin JA, Drum C, Peterson J. Physical activity and nutrition health promotion interventions: what is working for people with intellectual disabilities? *Intellect Dev Disabil.* 2011;49(1): 26-36.

143. Kapsal NJ, Dicke TD, Morin AJS, et al. Effects of physical activity on the physical and psychosocial health of youth with intellectual disabilities: a systematic review and meta-analyses. *J Phys Act Health.* 2019;16(12):1187-1195.

144. Cannella-Malone HI, Tullis CA, Kazee AR. Using antecedent exercise to decrease challenging behavior in boys with developmental disabilities and an emotional disorder. *J Posit Behav Interv.* 2011;13(4):230-239.

145. Diaz KM. Leisure-time physical activity and all-cause mortality among adults with intellectual disability: the National Health Interview Survey. *J Intellect Disabil Res.* 2020;64(2):180-184.

146. Srinivasan SM, Pescatello LS, Bhat AN. Current perspectives on physical activity and exercise recommendations for children and adolescents with autism spectrum disorders. *Phys Ther.* 2014;94(6):875-889.

147. Ali SH, Azar NR, Sutherland CA, Horton S. Understanding repetitive behaviors and the use of exercise as an intervention for adults with autism spectrum disorder and an intellectual disability. *Critical Rev Phys Rehabil Med.* 2018;30(2):151-179.

148. Anderson-Hanley C, Tureck K, Schneiderman RL. Autism and exergaming: effects on repetitive behaviors and cognition. *Psychol Res Behav Manag.* 2011;4:129-137.

149. Oriel KN, George CL, Peckus R, Semon A. The effects of aerobic exercise on academic engagement in young children with autism spectrum disorder. *Pediatr Phys Ther.* 2011;23(2):187-193.

150. Nicholson H, Kehle TJ, Bray MA, Heest JV. The effects of antecedent physical activity on the academic engagement of children with autism spectrum disorder. *Psychol Sch.* 2011;48(2):198-213.

151. Palisano RJ, Shimmell LJ, Stewart D, Lawless JJ, Rosenbaum PL, Russell DJ. Mobility experiences of adolescents with cerebral palsy. *Phys Occup Ther Pediatr.* 2009;29(2):133-153.

152. Waltersson L, Rodby-Bousquet E. Physical activity in adolescents and young adults with cerebral palsy. *Biomed Res Int.* 2017;2017:8080473.

153. Benner JL, Hilberink SR, Veenis T, Stam HJ, van der Slot WM, Roebroeck ME. Long-term deterioration of perceived health and functioning in adults with cerebral palsy. *Arch Phys Med Rehabil.* 2017;98(11):2196-205.e1.

154. Jacobson DNO, Löwing K, Tedroff K, Jacobson DN. Health-related quality of life, pain, and fatigue in young adults with cerebral palsy. *Dev Med Child Neurol.* 2020;62(3):372-378.

155. McPhee PG, Brunton LK, Timmons BW, Bentley T, Gorter JW. Fatigue and its relationship with physical activity, age, and body composition in adults with cerebral palsy. *Dev Med Child Neurol.* 2017;59(4):367-373.

156. Orlin MN, Palisano RJ, Chiarello LA, et al. Participation in home, extracurricular, and community activities among children and young people with cerebral palsy. *Dev Med Child Neurol.* 2010;52(2):160-166.

157. Koldoff EA, Holtzclaw BJ. Physical activity among adolescents with cerebral palsy: an integrative review. *J Pediatr Nurs.* 2015;30(5):e105-117.

158. Liljenquist K, O'Neil ME, Bjornson KF. Utilization of physical therapy services during transition for young people with cerebral palsy: a call for improved care into adulthood. *Phys Ther.* 2018;98(9):796-803.

159. Slaman J, van den Berg-Emons HJ, van Meeteren J, et al. A lifestyle intervention improves fatigue, mental health and social support among adolescents and young adults with cerebral palsy: focus on mediating effects. *Clin Rehabil.* 2015;29(7):717-727.

160. Orava C, Fitzgerald J, Figliomeni S, et al. Relationship between physical activity and fatigue in adults with cystic fibrosis. *Physiother Can.* 2018;70(1):42-48.

161. Street R, Mercer J, Mills-Bennett R, O LC, Thirlaway K. Experiences of physical activity: a phenomenological study of individuals with cystic fibrosis. *J Health Psychol.* 2016;21(2):261-270.

162. Swisher AK, Hebestreit H, Mejia-Downs A, et al. Exercise and habitual physical activity for people with cystic fibrosis: expert consensus, evidence-based guide for advising patients. *Cardiopulm Phys Ther J.* 2015;26(4):85-98.

163. Guthold R, Stevens GA, Riley LM, et al. Worldwide trends in insufficient physical activity from 2001 to 2016: a pooled analysis of 358 population-based surveys with 1·9 million participants. *Lancet Glob Health.* 2018;6(10):e1077-1086.

164. Denford S, van Beurden S, O'Halloran P, Williams CA. Barriers and facilitators to physical activity among children, adolescents, and young adults with cystic fibrosis: a systematic review and thematic synthesis of qualitative research. *BMJ Open.* 2020;10(2):e035261.

165. Boer P, Beer Z. The effect of aquatic exercises on the physical and functional fitness of adults with Down syndrome: a non-randomised controlled trial. *J Intellect Disabil Res.* 2019;63(12):1453-1463.

166. Boer PH, Moss S. Effects of continuous aerobic vs interval training on selected anthropometrical, physiological and functional parameters of adults with Down syndrome. *J Intellect Disabil Res.* 2016;60(4):322-334.

167. Crowe BM, Allison CK, Van Puymbroeck M, Adams EV, Schmid AA. Exploring the physical and psychosocial benefits of yoga for adults with intellectual and developmental disabilities. *Am J Rec Ther.* 2019;18(4):38-48.

168. Ptomey LT, Willis EA, Greene JL, et al. The feasibility of group video conferencing for promotion of physical activity in adolescents with intellectual and developmental disabilities. *Am J Intellect Dev Disabil.* 2017;122(6):525-538.

169. Bhat AN, Landa RJ, Galloway JC. Current perspectives on motor functioning in infants, children, and adults with autism spectrum disorders. *Phys Ther.* 2011;91(7):1116-1129.

170. Barr M, Shields N. Identifying the barriers and facilitators to participation in physical activity for children with Down syndrome. *J Intellect Disabil Res.* 2011;55(11):1020-1033.

171. Mahy J, Shields N, Taylor NF, Dodd K J. Identifying facilitators and barriers to physical activity for adults with Down syndrome. *J Intellect Disabil Res.* 2010;54(9):795-805.

172. McGarty AM, Melville CA. Parental perceptions of facilitators and barriers to physical activity for children with intellectual disabilities: a mixed methods systematic review. *Res Dev Disabil.* 2018;73:40-57.

173. Nguyen T, Henderson D, Stewart D, Hlyva O, Punthakee Z, Gorter JW. You never transition alone! Exploring the experiences of youth with chronic health conditions, parents and healthcare providers on self-management. *Child Care Health Dev.* 2016;42(4):464-472.

174. Burk BN, Sharaievska I. Health and recreation perceptions of adults with developmental disabilities. *Ther Recreat J.* 2017;51(3):179-192.

175. Willis C, Nyquist A, Jahnsen R, Elliott C, Ullenhag A. Enabling physical activity participation for children and youth with disabilities following a goal-directed, family-centred intervention. *Res Dev Disabil.* 2018;77:30-39.

176. Palisano RJ. Physical activity of children with cerebral palsy: what are the considerations? *Dev Med Child Neurol.* 2012;54(5):390-391.

177. Marks B, Sisirak J, Magallanes R, Krok K, Donohue-Chase D. Effectiveness of a peer-to-peer program for people with intellectual and developmental disabilities. *Intellect Dev Disabil.* 2019;57(3):242-258.

178. Kunstler R, Thompson A, Croke E. Inclusive recreation for transition-age youth: promoting self-sufficiency, community inclusion, and experiential learning. *Ther Recreat J.* 2013;47(2):122-136.

179. Shpigelman C-N. A proposed framework for using the life-coaching process to enhance the quality of life of individuals with intellectual and developmental disabilities: a case study. *J Policy Pract Intellect Disabil.* 2019;16(3):150-159.

180. Michalsen H, Wangberg SC, Anke A, Hartvigsen G, Jaccheri L, Arntzen C. Family members and health care workers' perspectives on motivational factors of participation in physical activity for people with intellectual disability: a qualitative study. *J Intellect Disabil Res.* 2020;64(4):259-270.

181. Hassan NM, Landorf KB, Shields N, Munteanu SE. Effectiveness of interventions to increase physical activity in individuals with intellectual disabilities: a systematic review of randomised controlled trials. *J Intellect Disabil Res.* 2019;63(2):168-191.

182. Melville CA, Mitchell F, Stalker K, et al. Effectiveness of a walking programme to support adults with intellectual disabilities to increase physical activity: walk well cluster-randomised controlled trial. *Int J Behav Nutr Phys Act.* 2015;12:125.

183. Hallal PC, Victora CG, Azevedo MR, Wells JC. Adolescent physical activity and health: a systematic review. *Sports Med.* 2006; 36(12):1019-1030.

184. Manus MA, Pollack LR, Cooley WC, et al. Current status of transition preparation among youth with special needs in the United States. *Pediatrics.* 2013;131(6):1090-1097.

185. Child Neurology Foundation. Transition Checklist. Accessed September 28, 2022. https://www.childneurologyfoundation.org/wp-content/uploads/2017/08/B_TransitionChecklist.pdf.

186. YouTube. Assistive technology and arthrogryposis. Accessed September 28, 2022. https://youtu.be/nI-lbFCIXMw.

187. YouTube. Quadriplegic morning routine. Arthrogryposis woman morning routine/GRWM. Accessed September 28, 2022. https://www.youtube.com/watch?v=mxjqFfrSSNw.

23

Legal Foundations

Ron Scott, PT, JD, EdD, MA (Spanish), MSBA, MSPT

LEARNING OBJECTIVES

Upon completion of this chapter, the reader will be able to:

- Determine the scope of professional activities that may give rise to a pediatric physical therapy malpractice claim or lawsuit.
- Document pediatric patient/client care and related activities effectively and in compliance with accepted ethicolegal standards.
- Analyze ethicolegal practice-related problems associated with contracting and education, employment, and regulatory law compliance.

- Practice effective clinical liability risk management in any pediatric physical therapy practice setting.
- Develop and implement a comprehensive clinic-specific liability risk management checklist.
- Synthesize legal and ethical principles learned into pediatric physical therapy practice in clinical, education, research, and all other settings.

INTRODUCTION

Pediatric physical therapists (PTs) and their assistants, like all health professionals, are charged with having at least a basic understanding of an ever-more-complex legal practice environment. From allegations of malpractice brought by patients or their representatives to employment contracting pitfalls to intellectual property issues, among a myriad of other considerations, pediatric PTs must stay abreast of legal standards and developments, and devise and execute optimally effective practice and personal risk management strategies and tactics in order to survive and thrive in a highly and ever-expanding litigious business world.

Several considerations complicate the legal landscape. First, legal obligations incumbent on every health care provider exist in many forms at both federal and state levels—constitutional mandates, statutory requirements, judge-made case law pronouncements, and a seemingly endless and ever-expanding set of administrative rules and regulations. Local city and/or county legal standards also apply to health professional practices. Second, these voluminous mandates are subject to constant change by courts, legislatures, executive agencies, and regulatory entities at all levels. Third, association ethical standards and even private accreditation guidelines often blend with legal mandates, creating additional potential bases for financial or liability exposure incident to practice.

Perhaps the most efficacious way to stay abreast of the legal environment and what is expected of pediatric PT professionals is to consult proactively and on a regularly recurring basis with personal attorneys of choice. That kind of relationship is customized, largely privileged from outside disclosure, and relatively low cost, and offers a high level of benefits, namely probable liability minimization in practice.

THE LEGAL MILIEU OF PEDIATRIC PHYSICAL THERAPY PRACTICE

Although health care malpractice civil cases brought by patients or their representatives against pediatric PTs are relatively few in number, the consequences of being claimed against and/or sued—irrespective of whether the PT-defendant wins or loses—are devastating in terms of personal stress, injury to professional and personal reputation, legal costs, and possible financial loss incident to a money judgment. Although the direct adverse effects of financial outlays may be dampened or eliminated through professional liability insurance, the other named adverse consequences still loom large. Therefore, the truism that the best way to avoid a lawsuit is to prevent it applies with full force to pediatric physical therapy practitioners.

The American Physical Therapy Association's *Physical Therapy Professional Liability Exposure: 2016 Claim Report Update* and the *Risk Control Self-Assessment Checklist*[1,2] (available for free online at http://www.hpso.com) are among the many available resources that spell out straightforward, practical strategies and tactics to minimize liability exposure in pediatric physical therapy practice. Certain basic methods for patients' protection from unreasonable harm incident to care are self-evident:

- Clutter-free or clutter-reduced physical pediatric clinical practice environments to minimize risks of falls or related injuries

- Secure storage of hazardous chemicals and compliance with the US Department of Labor, Occupational Safety and Health Administration's Safety Data Sheets' content, display, and reporting requirements
- Appointing every staff member in the clinic as a primary safety officer, charged with the critical job function of maintaining constant due diligence over the premises
- Evidence-based clinical practice
- Acquiring patient and parental/guardian informed consent prior to examination and intervention
- Systematic calibration of therapeutic equipment and modalities
- Practicing only within your scope of practice and personal competence

All of these are common-sense ways to minimize the risks of avoidable patient harm and liability exposure.

Practicing defensively, so called "defensive medicine," is not efficacious. Sanger-Katz[3] cited studies showing increased costs of care with such practices, although they neither improved outcomes nor caused more litigation. Researchers cited suggest practices such as shielding primary health care providers from personal liability if they adhere to "common standards of care," nonfault payment systems, or having health care malpractice cases adjudicated by administrative courts instead of juries, whose members often inflate verdicts based on sympathy or other considerations.

Every pediatric physical therapy professional should form and foster an ongoing professional relationship with an attorney-advisor before or at the start of their career, or as soon as is feasible, if not currently in place, in order to effectively navigate the legal milieu that they operate within. Perhaps the best 2 ways to engage a personal attorney are through positive recommendations from peers who have employed and been satisfied with a particular attorney or by telephoning the city, county, or state bar (professional) association and asking for the names of, and contact information for, attorney-specialists who represent pediatric PTs.

Another acceptable and commonly employed way to meet and establish a long-term professional relationship with an attorney is to contact the city, county, or state bar association's lawyer referral service (LRS) and set up a meeting with one of their attorneys. Be sure to ask the receptionist for exactly what you need—for example, an attorney-specialist who represents pediatric PTs (and, if applicable, describe the precise legal issue, eg, "to help me to interpret an employment contract's covenant not to compete").

Also, remember to ask for an attorney who offers a free, or low-cost, initial consultation. In every state in the United States, actively licensed attorneys are expected to provide at least 50 hours of pro bono legal services to the public. Some states, including my home state, Texas, require attorneys to input their pro bono hours annually as part of the relicensing process.

I carry out the bulk of my 50 to 100 hours of pro bono legal work as a volunteer attorney-mediator at the Bexar County Justice Center in San Antonio, Texas. (More information about mediation and other forms of alternative dispute resolution is provided later in this chapter.) Many attorneys in every state carry out their pro bono obligations by volunteering for LRS.

After meeting with an LRS-recommended attorney, decide whether to ask for their business card so that you can call on them for legal advice (at regular fees) in the future. It is an efficient and facile way to promote peace of mind.

It is important to consider engaging a personal attorney for the long term when first entering specialty practice. Finding an attorney through any of the 3 methods previously discussed can eliminate potential legal problems for the pediatric PT, including those arising from managing complex legal issues such as the formation of a partnership or another legal form of business, contracting for staff, writing and managing restrictive contractual covenants (eg, covenants not to compete and nondisclosure agreements), resolving zoning issues with local municipalities, business tax payment compliance, and many others.

A personal attorney can also assist the pediatric PT in deciding which types of liability, premises, and umbrella insurance coverage to carry. Relative to professional liability insurance, there are 2 basic types: claims-made and occurrence. Claims-made professional liability insurance coverage protects the insured for covered liability claims made during a finite start and end period, usually the period of employment for an employee or the period of coverage for an ongoing business. An expired claims-made policy cannot be used to pay prior or follow-on claims made by patients, families, or others, unless the insured has purchased (expensive) extended reporting period coverage (including prior acts and tail coverage).

Occurrence professional liability insurance potentially protects employees and employers from liability that occurred when the insurance policy was in effect, irrespective of whether it is still effective. For that reason, occurrence liability insurance is superior to claims-made in every respect except (for pediatric and other insured PTs) a minor differential in cost.

PEDIATRIC PATIENT AUTONOMY ISSUES

Only since 1972, in the seminal federal court case, *Canterbury v. Spence*,[4] has it been universally recognized and accepted that it is patients who control the treatment decisional process, not their physicians or other health care providers. *Canterbury* identified respect by health care professionals for patient autonomy over care-related decision-making as the preeminent biomedical ethical principle undergirding patient rights. Patients therefore have the fundamental right to receive disclosure of relevant medical information about their care that enables them to give informed consent or to refuse their providers' recommended interventions.

Autonomy, or self-determination, over medical decision-making therefore reigns supreme over the other biomedical ethical principles governing our health care practices. The subordinate, but also critically important, remaining cornerstone ethical principles include beneficence (acting always in patients' best interests), justice (striving to ensure equality in health care delivery at societal and individual levels), and nonmaleficence (vowing to never commit and, in practice, never committing intentional malicious harm to patients under care).

Informed consent, epitomizing respect for patient self-determination, consists of a rigid litany of disclosure elements, imparted to patients or their surrogate decision makers prior to examination or treatment, in the patient's language and at the patient's level of understanding. These include the following:

- Explanation of a patient's diagnosis
- Details about recommended interventions
- Delineation of the expected benefits and any material risks of possible harm associated with recommended interventions
- Summarization of feasible alternatives to the proposed interventions, if any, and their respective benefits and risks
- Soliciting and satisfactorily answering patient or surrogate decision-maker questions

Can a patient refuse care delivery altogether or tailor the dimensions of their health care delivery? Yes, within the bounds of patient safety and the safety of relevant others. It is the patient, not the health care provider, team, institution, or governmental entity, who sets the parameters and limits of care. Everything recommended (even pursuant to a physician order) is just that—a recommendation, which the patient can choose to approve or reject. As pediatric PTs, we use our best clinical judgment and skills to attempt to communicate to patients that the treatment options we recommend are in their best interests. The Centers for Medicare and Medicaid Services provides guidelines that include a provision describing the probable consequences of declining recommended or alternative therapies (informed refusal).

Landro[5] noted that the concept of informed consent may be the "biggest misnomer in medicine." In his article, Landro highlighted the Joint Commission's "teach back" approach to informed consent, which includes the feedback step of having patients repeat what they hear during informed consent disclosure. The Veterans Administration's iMedConsent approach is also mentioned. It contains electronic pictorial and simple word consent forms written at the sixth-grade level. A University of California–San Francisco study is mentioned in Landro's article,[5] which concluded that patients in general understand informed consent disclosure from 28% to 98% better if the forms are written at the sixth-grade level.

In the case of pediatric patients, autonomy rights are treated differently as a matter of customary practice and societal and judicial tolerance. For the most part, parents or guardians make decisions on behalf of their children; the children do not make their own decisions. Although statutes, regulations, and judge-made case law may afford children fewer rights than adults, it is noteworthy that the federal Constitution—the supreme law of the land—does not distinguish between children and adults in its personal rights protections.

There are several recognized exceptions to the requirement to obtain informed consent from patients. Minors are generally considered by law to lack the legal capacity to make their own decisions about health care; so instead, parents or guardians are charged with the authority to make such decisions for them. An exception to this exception is that statutory laws in a few jurisdictions permit minors to retain their autonomy and make their own choices concerning treatment of alcohol or other drug abuse and sexually transmitted diseases, as well as to make decisions about their sexual health and pregnancy.

In some instances, judge-made case law decisions grant minors the right to make their own medical decisions. Courts rarely may serve as substitute decision makers for parents, when it is deemed that parents might not act in the child's best interests. Incarcerated teens may also be considered emancipated and allowed to make their own medical decisions without parental involvement or veto.

Other exceptions to informed disclosure and consent include surrogate decision makers for patients who lack mental capacity, the emergency doctrine, and therapeutic privilege, all of which may affect pediatric patients and clients. Under the emergency doctrine, it is generally presumed that a patient in a comatose state or in cardiorespiratory arrest consents to life-saving medical interventions. There are, however, exceptions to this exception, including the existence and knowledge of patient advance directives, living wills, and durable powers of attorney for health care decision-making.

Therapeutic privilege involves a gag order imposed by a physician-head of an interdisciplinary team on team members not to discuss with a patient their diagnosis or prognosis. This unilateral transfer of power from the patient to the physician, and usurpation of power from the team to one member, is based on a physician's belief that the patient cannot effectively process a terminal diagnosis or prognosis. Therapeutic privilege is rarely invoked by physicians, and even more rarely permitted by the courts in the face of a challenge, because it derogates from respect for patient autonomy over medical decision-making, enunciated by the 1972 court in *Canterbury*.

If a pediatric PT disagrees with a physician's invocation of therapeutic privilege, they can take one or more of the following steps. The PT can speak with the physician and ask that the therapeutic privilege order be rescinded. The PT may call for advice from the health care system's institutional ethics committee on the issue. If these measures fail, the PT may need to recuse themself from the care team, if a suitable substitute provider is available to take over. These kinds of issues and options require that a PT consult first with their attorney for specific advice before acting.

In an interesting *New York Times* article, Hoffman[6] explored the issue of adolescents facing the end of life secondary to cancer, cardiac disease, and congenital abnormalities (accounting for 11% of adolescent deaths annually [1700 deaths]). These "near-adults," although legally limited from making their own medical decisions because they are minors, usually possess the capacity to at least contribute their individual end-of-life preferences, according to Hoffman. A monograph titled *Voicing My Choices*[7] is cited as a unique end-of-life guidebook for adolescents and young adult patients.

Hester,[8] in *Guidance for Healthcare Ethics Committees*, also addressed societal norms regarding pediatric and adolescent patient informed consent. He opined that, as teens mature, they possess a "developing capacity" to participate in, and even make outright, their own treatment-related decisions.

The federal Health Insurance Portability and Accountability Act of 1996 (HIPAA),[9] in its Privacy Rule, states that parents or legal guardians of children are their personal representatives for purposes of protected health information (PHI) privacy.

Parents have the right of direct access to their children's medical records unless either the parent agrees that the minor and health care professional may have a confidential relationship; the state does not require the parent's consent and the minor manages their own care; or the child obtains care at the direction of a court. Once a minor becomes emancipated, the parent or legal guardian no longer has access to the minor's medical records.

A provision in HIPAA's Privacy Rule, Section 164.502(g)(5)(ii), states:

Notwithstanding a State law or any requirement of this paragraph to the contrary, a covered entity may elect not to treat a person as the personal representative of an individual if the covered entity (i.e. provider), in the exercise of professional judgment, decides that it is not in the best interest of the individual to treat the person as the individual's personal representative.

The American Physical Therapy Association's Code of Ethics for the Physical Therapist,[10] Section 3A (2020), states:

Physical therapists shall demonstrate independent and objective professional judgment in the patient's or client's best interest in all practice settings.

Pediatric PTs should not assume that this ethics provision empowers them to withhold pediatric patients' PHI from their parents. If a legitimate basis exists for possibly withholding such information (eg, child abuse, neglect, or abandonment), then it should be communicated to relevant authorities and to institutional attorneys for action—most likely, a court order appointing a guardian.

■ LIABILITY FOR PATIENT OR CLIENT CLAIMS OF INJURY

Pediatric PTs, like all PTs and other health care co-professionals, face liability exposure for patient injury incident to care delivery. Health care malpractice is defined as physical and/or mental injury to a patient-plaintiff by a health care professional–defendant during the course of care delivery, coupled with a legal basis for imposition of liability.

Professional liability for patient injury, in the form of a money judgment, can arise in any practice setting. It requires more than just patient injury, however. Liability must be based on one or more of the following 5 legal principles:

- Professional negligence
- Intentional misconduct
- Actionable breach of a therapeutic promise
- Patient injury from dangerously defective care-related products or equipment
- Patient injury from abnormally dangerous clinical activities

Professional negligence equates to substandard care delivery. It is conduct, incident to patient care, that falls below minimally acceptable practice standards and directly or indirectly injures a patient. It is usually proven by a preponderance, or greater weight, of evidence through the introduction of in-court expert witness testimony. (Preponderance of evidence is also the standard of proof in licensing board and most other administrative proceedings.) What the legal standard of care is for members of a defendant's professional discipline or specialty can also be supported in a malpractice trial by reference to textbooks, peer-reviewed journals, and official documents, such as the American Physical Therapy Association Code of Ethics.

Intentional misconduct involves malicious intended acts or omissions, or reckless conduct, that injures a patient under care. Conduct such as the intentional infliction of emotional distress and sexual assault and battery fall under this category.

Pediatric PTs in all 50 states and the US territories—like all licensed health professionals—have the legal duty to report observed or reasonably suspected child abuse or neglect to appropriate authorities, such as child protective services. It is intentional misconduct and, in most cases, criminal not to report child abuse or neglect.

Child abuse may be grossly underreported by health professionals. Reasons it may not be reported include, among others, a health provider's perception of insufficient evidence to report, a fear of litigation, and a desire to maintain professional relations with a pediatric patient and their family. One Canadian study reported that health professionals report the lowest number of child abuse cases to authorities (10% in Canada and 8% in the United States).[11]

After reading this chapter, I invite readers to investigate their individual state's specific reporting statutes, regulations, and case law. They are then encouraged to create or amend their clinic policy and procedure manuals, as necessary, to ensure compliance with legal child abuse standards by staff, in consultation with their practice attorneys. Researchers can easily access these laws through the free online resource, Mandatory Reporting Laws by State 2023 (https://worldpopulationreview.com/state-rankings/mandatory-reporting-laws-by-state).

Actionable breach of a therapeutic contractual promise made to a patient is rarely a basis for malpractice liability and is further limited by administrative and judicial hurdles in jurisdictions where it may be recognized. The most straightforward risk management tactic for pediatric PTs to avoid breach of contract malpractice liability exposure may be to not make therapeutic promises to pediatric patients or their parents or guardians.

Whereas professional negligence, intentional wrongdoing, and breach of therapeutic promises are all fault-based categories of malpractice liability, liability for patient injury from dangerously or defectively designed or manufactured care-related products or equipment and from abnormally dangerous clinical activities (eg cervical manipulation) are non–fault based. These 2 bases of malpractice liability—also much less common than professional negligence and intentional misconduct—require only that a patient suffer injury incident to care by one of these 2 means.

To better understand the distinction between fault and non-fault bases of malpractice liability, consider the analogous concepts of primary and secondary, or vicarious, liability. Primary liability is generally fault based. Vicarious liability, such as the indirect financial responsibility for the conduct of employees and volunteers within the scope of their duties, is non–fault based. A pediatric physical therapy practice owner who renders substandard care and directly causes a patient injury from therapeutic exercise is primarily liable for professional negligence. Alternatively, they might be free of culpability but vicariously liable for the same injury caused by a PT assistant working in the clinic.

Many factors—both internal to health care disciplines and specialties and external—have contributed to an increase in clinical health professionals' liability exposure in recent times. Internal factors include an ever-expanding scope of practice, resulting in greater legal responsibility; greater accountability for practice and outcomes pursuant to evidence-based practice; and higher entry-level graduate education requirements. External factors include a consistently high level of litigiousness in society; expansive governmental and nongovernmental regulation and oversight; and the changing nature of health care delivery, with its greater focus on costs, revenue, and volume of patients. Consider Case 1.

Case 1

When Does the Legal Duty of Care Commence?

As with all other licensed health care (and other) professionals, the law holds pediatric PTs to a special duty of due care that is higher than that incumbent upon the general public. When is that special, high legal duty of care owed to patients?

A. When the patient calls for an appointment
B. When the patient arrives at your clinic and is greeted by the receptionist
C. At the start of the initial clinical examination
D. When the physical therapist accepts the patient for appropriate intervention

The answer is choice D. At the commencement of the initial clinical examination, the physical therapist owes a special duty to impart informed disclosure about the examination; to obtain the patient (or parent's) informed consent to proceed; and to carry out the clinical examination competently, within the legal standard of care. The full-blown special legal duty of care arises when the physical therapist completes the clinical examination; determines that the patient's problem is within the scope of physical therapy practice and the provider's scope of clinical competence; and accepts the patient for appropriate intervention.

At the commencement of the initial clinical examination, the PT owes a special duty to impart informed disclosure about the examination, obtain the patient (or parent's) informed consent to proceed, and carry out the clinical examination competently within the legal standard of care. The full-blown special legal duty of care arises when the PT completes the clinical examination, determines that the patient's problem is within the scope of physical therapy practice and the provider's scope of clinical competence, and accepts the patient for appropriate intervention.

Pediatric PTs owe a special duty not only to patients under their care but also sometimes to others. Under the 1976 Tarasoff Rule, based on the seminal legal case *Tarasoff v. Regents of the University of California*,[12] clinical health professionals have the legal duty to protect individuals who are being threatened with

bodily harm by a patient. According to case holding, that duty may be discharged in one of several ways, including notifying law enforcement, warning the intended victim, or taking other reasonable steps to protect a threatened individual, possibly including involving hospital security and social work services.

Consider the hypothetical exemplar in Case 2.

Case 2

Reporting Requirements: Suicide Threat

Sue is a clinical pediatric PT working at a large urban children's medical center. Her adolescent cancer patient, Toni, confidentially informs Sue during a PT session that she plans to take her own life at home the next weekend. Reflect on what Sue's legal and ethical responsibilities are.

Sue has a duty to act reasonably to safeguard her patient's life, including, at a minimum, immediate consultation with the patient's referring or attending physician. What are other possible actions? What if Sue were in private practice?

The National Practitioner Data Bank (NPDB) is part of the Health Care Quality Improvement Act of 1986. Besides recording physician and dentist malpractice payments, the NPDB collects and records any negative action or finding by state licensing agencies, peer review organizations, and private accreditation organizations against all health care practitioners, including PTs. For medical doctors, dentists, and other licensed health professionals, once liability in a malpractice claim or lawsuit is established and either a civil court judgment is rendered or a settlement is reached and paid by a defendant's insurer, employer, or other third party, the responsible licensed health professional's name must be reported, and their name is entered permanently into the NPDB, which is administered by the US Department of Health and Human Services.

Who can access adverse provider information stored in the NPDB? There is no public access to the NPDB, nor may information be released to defense attorneys or medical malpractice insurers. It is mandatory for employing hospitals to query the NPDB about new privileged providers, and every 2 years thereafter. Permissive queries are allowed by state licensing agencies and law enforcement officials. Plaintiffs' attorneys and pro se plaintiffs (those self-representing) in malpractice cases may, under limited circumstances, query the NPDB for information about a defendant-provider. Providers may always self-query the NPDB and should consider systematically doing so as a matter of prudent liability risk management. Details on how to do so are found at https://www.npdb.hrsa.gov.

Alternative dispute resolution includes 3 extrajudicial processes, within which parties in administrative, civil, or criminal disputes can resolve their legal issues. *Conciliation* involves resolution by the parties themselves, without attorney or other representative intervention. *Mediation* entails appointing a neutral third party (usually an attorney) to assist the parties in civilly and cooperatively resolving their dispute. *Arbitration* is similar to mediation, in that a neutral third party is appointed or hired to hear evidence from both sides and render a binding decision that the parties agree in advance to abide by. Both mediation and arbitration are characterized by confidentiality, relative low cost, and streamlined resolution of disputes. In many or most cases, no written record needs to be generated.

Jenkins et al[13] reported a high degree of efficacy for court-ordered mediation for health care malpractice disputes. Legal expenses decreased by 87%, and over an 8-year period (2008–2015) in Florida, the average time from receipt of the case to resolution was 6 months.

■ LEGAL ISSUES IN SCHOOL-BASED PRACTICE SETTINGS

Pediatric PTs must be cognizant of legal issues in school law, especially if they work in education environments. This section overviews the key federal constitutional concepts and statutory and regulatory school laws affecting providers in these settings.

The Individuals With Disabilities Education Act (IDEA)[14] is the national special education statute that entitles all children ages 3 to 21 with disabilities to a free and appropriate public education in the least restrictive environment. IDEA also vests specific rights and protections in disabled students' parents or guardians, known as procedural safeguards.

Originally authorized as the Education for All Handicapped Children Act in 1975, the statute was reauthorized by Congress in 1990 and its name changed to IDEA. The law was reauthorized again in 2004 as the Individuals With Disabilities Education Improvement Act.

In 1985, the US Supreme Court in *Irving Independent School District v. Tatro*[15] interpreted the Education for All Handicapped Children Act for the first time to include medical services provided by primary care providers other than physicians. The high court ruled that simple related medical services such as catheterization were required to comply with the statute in order to support special education students. (Amber Tatro, who was at the center of this case, went on to graduate and become a productive member of the workforce, serving disabled children. She died on August 8, 2018, at age 42.)

Since *Tatro*, in order to help enable disabled students to achieve their educational goals and needs, rehabilitation professionals—including physical, occupational, and speech therapists—work with students, families, and teachers to reach the zenith of their educational potential within Individualized Education Programs (IEPs). As part of a multifactored evaluation, therapists initially conduct individualized school functional assessments, focusing on barriers to learning and to participation by disabled students. The service delivery models for these health professional services include direct (hands-on intervention), indirect (through extenders), and consultative.

To qualify for special education under IDEA, a student's disability must fall within 1 or more of the following 13 enumerated disability categories under the statute:

- Autism spectrum disorder
- Blindness
- Deafness
- Emotional disturbances
- Hearing impairment
- Intellectual disability
- Multiple disabilities
- Orthopedic impairment

- Other health impairment (including attention-deficit/hyperactivity disorder)
- Specific learning disabilities
- Speech or language impairment
- Traumatic brain injury
- Visual impairment

The presence of a disability that falls within 1 of the 13 categories triggers applicability of IDEA. However, having 1 of the 13 disabilities does not automatically qualify a child for services under IDEA. To be eligible, a student must have a disability and, as a result of that disability, require special education in order to make reasonable progress in school.

Because schools generally are public, they are required by the US Constitution to afford due process of law to students and their parents and to public employees, visitors, and relevant others within these institutions. *Due process* is a federal constitutional protection that applies to conduct by the federal government (under the 5th Amendment of the Bill of Rights) and to the states (under the post–Civil War 14th Amendment to the Constitution). It has 2 components: procedural due process and substantive due process.

Procedural due process requires public entities to give reasonable notice of a pending adverse action and a reasonable opportunity to challenge the impending adverse action. *Substantive due process* can be thought of as fundamental fairness.

A student's IEP is a public contract, subject to procedural and substantive due process. Like any contract, it requires active participation, negotiation, and approval by a student's parent(s) or guardian(s). An established IEP is a binding legal document on the school and team and is subject to at least annual review. Students and parents or guardians have legal rights to constitutional due process, mediation of disputes, and access to the courts for judicial redress for denial of necessary services, after exhaustion of their internal administrative remedies.

A landmark IDEA legal case, *Endrew F. v. Douglas County School District*,[16] came before the US Supreme Court in 2017. The facts of that case were that the parents of a child with autism were unsatisfied with their child's progress in public school. They transferred their child to a private school and then sought reimbursement from the school district for the fees associated with attending the private school. The issue before the court was: Did the school district comply with IDEA's mandate that disabled children are entitled to a fair and appropriate public education that meets their individual needs? The 10th Circuit Court of Appeals ruled that school districts are not liable for private educational costs if they provide "more than *de minimis*" education services themselves. Endrew's parents appealed that decision to the US Supreme Court. The 10th Circuit's opinion was based on its perception of a high-cost burden for school districts.

The US Supreme Court decision on March 22, 2017, affecting some 6.7 million students with disabilities covered by IDEA, rejected the state's de minimis standard but did not specify what is required, ruling that students' individual circumstances will determine that. Chief Justice Roberts, writing the 8–0 opinion, stated:

[A disabled child's] educational program must be appropriately ambitious in light of his circumstances.... [E]very child should have the chance to meet challenging objectives.... When all is said and done, a student offered an educational program providing 'merely more than de minimis' progress from year to year can hardly be said to have been offered an education at all.... For children with disabilities, receiving instruction that aims so low would be tantamount to sitting idly, awaiting the time when they were old enough to "drop out."[17]

Two related laws complement IDEA. They are Section 504 of the Rehabilitation Act of 1973[18] and the Americans With Disabilities Act of 1990 (ADA).[19] All 3 are federal statutes that require accommodation of individuals' physical and mental disabilities. Three characteristics differentiate IDEA from Section 504 and the ADA. Whereas the ADA and Section 504 are nearly global in their scope of coverage (commercial, educational, employment, and most other settings), IDEA addresses only education services. Both ADA and Section 504 are broader in their scope of disability coverage, in that a covered disability is defined as follows: "An individual with a disability means any person who: (i) has a mental or physical impairment that substantially limits one or more major life activity; (ii) has a record of such an impairment; or (iii) is regarded as having such an impairment." Finally, only IDEA requires the creation of an enforceable public contract for services—a special education student's IEP.

The Family Educational Rights and Privacy Act of 1974 (FERPA)[20] affords parents and students the privacy right to protect student education records from being released to third parties. For purposes of the statute, education records are those records that directly relate to a student and are maintained by an educational agency or institution or by a party acting for the agency or institution. The issue of when and which medical records of special education students are covered under FERPA and HIPAA is unnecessarily complex.[21]

Students age 18 years or older who are not dependents of their parents or guardians can shield their education records from their parents or guardians. Also under FERPA, graduate school applicants have the right of access to their letters of recommendation, unless they waive that right.

Analyze and discuss with colleagues Case 3.

Case 3

Reporting Misconduct in Education Settings

During a parent-teacher conference, a teacher solicits a date with his student's legally separated mother and shortly thereafter moves in with her and the student.

What ethical, legal, and practical problems does this scenario engender? What is a school-based PT's responsibility, if any, if the student brings this issue to the PT's attention, saying that it severely disturbs her?

The teacher is a fiduciary, just as a parent or PT is. This conduct by the teacher and parent on its face seems to violate the high duty owed to the dependent child. The suggested approach to the mandatory reporting issue is to analyze this

fact scenario under your state's unique governing child abuse/neglect reporting statutes and regulations. Share results and opinions. At a minimum, reporting to school administration seemingly is required.

CONTRACTING ISSUES IN PEDIATRIC PHYSICAL THERAPY

As a preliminary point, recognize that every therapeutic encounter between a pediatric PT and a patient (or pediatric patient's parent[s] or guardian) involves an implied (implicit) business contract. This "implied-in-fact" nonspecific contractual relationship may be embellished with explicit details, converting it into an express contract, which may or may not be in writing.

A contract is a promise or set of promises enforceable as binding legal obligations by the parties. By making a contract, individuals are allowed to create their own "private law," provided that what they agree to does not violate administrative, civil, or criminal laws, or public policy.

Under the PT-patient therapeutic contract, the therapist promises to use their best clinical judgment and skills to achieve an optimal therapeutic result for the patient. The patient promises, normally through a third-party payer (insurer), to pay reasonable fees for therapy services. Consider also asking patients under your care to make an express promise to actively cooperate with, and participate in, their care plan, to the maximum degree possible.

There are 5 fundamental elements to a business contract:

1. Who are the parties to the agreement?
2. Does the contract clearly show agreement by the parties (ie, "mutuality of assent")?
3. Does the contract evidence legal "consideration," that is, a mutual exchange of something of value? "Value" need not include one party paying for services, just something of value given in exchange for the other person's contractual promise.
4. Do all of the parties have legal capacity, that is, the legal ability to enter into a binding contract? Capacity excludes minors (except for absolute necessities) and incapacitated persons.
5. Does the contract comply with the law and with public policy?

A business contract does not normally need to be in writing to be enforceable. Practically, however, most business lawsuits are over oral contracts. It is always good business practice and liability risk management to reduce business agreements to writing and to have them reviewed by both parties' attorneys before signature.

Certain contracts must be in writing in order to be enforceable, under a medieval law called the Statute of Frauds (having nothing to do with fraud). These include cosigning for another person's loan, prenuptial and postnuptial marital agreements, long-term land leases, and business contracts that cannot be fulfilled within 1 year from the time they are signed (the "1-year rule").

There are 3 basic types of money damage remedies for another party's breach (violation) of a contract. They are restitution damages (restoring the parties to their precontractual positions, or "status quo ante"); reliance damages (reimbursing the aggrieved party's reasonable out-of-pocket losses); and expectancy (awarding the aggrieved party the full benefit of the bargain, including incidental [direct] and consequential [indirect] expenses, and provable lost profits caused by the breach).

Quasi-contract involves a situation where there is no contractual agreement between 2 parties; however, a contract-like remedy is required to prevent an unfair gain by one party over the other. Consider the example in Case 4.

Case 4

Quasi-Contractual Equitable Remedy (When Is a Noncontract a Contract?)

Henrietta, a rehab aide, commences to work in Indira's pediatric clinic, believing that she has been hired, a mistake of fact. After 3 days, Indira informs Henrietta of her mistake and dismisses her without compensation for her services.

A court might impose a quasi-contractual "implied-in-law" remedy in this situation to prevent unjust enrichment by Indira.

Pediatric PTs frequently are asked by new or existing employers to sign *covenants not to compete*. Covenants not to compete have become pervasive in the United States over the past 20 years, encumbering over a quarter of the workforce.

There is absolutely no consideration given by an employer for an employee to sign one of these documents. They are exclusively "one-way" contractual obligations, binding only the employee. Awarding the employee a job position is not consideration for the employee agreeing to be bound under a covenant not to compete.

A covenant not to compete can severely restrict a pediatric PT's ability to work after terminating employment. Although courts initially did not recognize them as legal (and California, North Dakota, Oklahoma and the District of Columbia still do not generally recognize them), recently, courts and legislatures in the vast majority of states have taken a business-friendly "caveat emptor" approach and have come to tolerate them, especially when signed by highly educated employees such as PTs and physicians. Still, a covenant not to compete must be declared by any court in a legal dispute to be reasonable in terms of the scope and breadth of employment activities that are restricted, the geographic scope of its coverage, and its effective time period. Pediatric PTs are strongly urged to consult with their personal or practice legal counsel before ever signing one of these burdensome legal instruments.

Consider the exemplar described in Case 5.

Case 5

Covenant Not to Compete Case Exemplar

Ron Scott, PT, PCS, an employee of Hypothetical Children's Medical Center, voluntarily agrees to the following: Upon termination of employment for any reason, at any time, I will not work as a clinical physical therapist anywhere in the southwest United States (Arizona, California, Nevada, New Mexico, Texas, or Utah), nor within 1 mile of any ABC facility anywhere in the United States, for a period of 3 years.

Identify what might be unreasonable about these conditions. A redacted (lined out and corrected) agreement might be crafted that would meet both the professional employee's and employer's needs. Any changes should limit to reasonable parameters what activities are proscribed, for what time period, and for how long. Arguably, all of the terms of this covenant are unreasonable.

Other restrictive employment-related covenants, or contractual promises, include nondisclosure agreements, non-moonlighting agreements, and "no poaching" and wage-fixing agreements among employers. Before ever signing one of these agreements, please consult with legal counsel for advice on how to proceed.

■ CONCLUSION

The legal environment that pediatric PTs work in is obviously complex. This chapter provides an introduction to select basic ethicolegal practice issues. It strives to enable therapists, assistants, and other extenders to meet their high fiduciary duty owed to pediatric patients under care, while at the same time protecting themselves from avoidable liability exposure.

As fiduciaries, or professionals in special trust relationships with their patients, pediatric PTs are charged by law and ethical and moral standards to place patient interests above all others, including financial considerations. This is a particularly difficult task in the cost containment–focused world of managed health care.

Therapists and patients automatically form a business contractual relationship when they agree to professional service delivery. PTs' contractual promise to patients is to use their best clinical judgment to help patients reach the zenith of their rehabilitation potential. Pediatric patients (through parents or guardians) agree to pay the reasonable costs of services and to cooperate with plans of care established for and with them. It is critically important for pediatric and other PTs not to appear too business-focused with their patients because this approach derogates from the close bond normally established between them. As a result, patients and families may be more inclined to file claims or lawsuits for alleged or actual injuries.

Pediatric PTs face ever-increasing malpractice liability exposure in practice because of factors as diverse as consumer greed, doctoral entry-level education, expanding scopes of practice, noncompliance with clinical practice guidelines and evidence-based practice, and increasing governmental regulation and oversight. Most malpractice cases brought against PTs involve allegations of professional negligence or substandard care. To minimize their liability exposure, pediatric PTs must stay abreast of, and practice according to, state-of-the-art developments in evidence-based practice and clinical research.

As employees, pediatric PTs should form legally privileged (confidential) relationships with personal attorneys in order to safeguard their professional well-being. This includes consulting with attorneys before becoming bound by potentially onerous restrictive employment provisions, such as covenants not to compete with current or former employers. Like erroneous patient care documentation, offensive provisions in such covenants can be stricken, initialed, and refused by employees, yet professional employees continue to sign them in record numbers.

The best legal advice is to continue to care for your patients as you always have—with compassion and dedication, never defensively. Patients can readily sense defensive health practice and will be more inclined to treat such providers also in a business-like manner in the event of care-related disputes. Fine-tune your practices, as needed, in consultation with your personal or practice attorneys, and consult with them—not just reactively after an adverse event, but proactively and systematically as well.

Best wishes for ongoing practice success!

STUDY QUESTIONS

1. What specific safety measures do you employ in clinical practice to minimize patient, staff, and visitor injuries?

2. What specific communicative and clinical practice strategies and tactics do you employ in clinical practice to minimize malpractice liability exposure?

3. Should a pediatric PT form a professional relationship with a health law attorney before one is even needed? Support your answer.

4. How should a health professional find an appropriate attorney to represent them after receiving a formal legal complaint from a former patient?

5. Why isn't every patient injury legally actionable as malpractice?

6. Justify why a clinical practice should include a health law attorney for annual continuing education.

7. What constitutional protections prevent school districts from making major, unilateral modifications to disabled students' IEPs without parental consultation or approval? What roles do pediatric PTs working in school districts play to protect the rights of disabled students under IDEA?

8. Delineate the similarities and differences among the ADA, IDEA, and Section 504 of the Rehabilitation Act of 1973.

9. Should you, as a clinical pediatric PT, ask patients (or their parents or guardian) to sign written contracts of care? What are the relative advantages and disadvantages of reducing care contracts to writing?

10. What risk management measures do you or will you employ to attempt to limit the scope and duration of employment-related covenants not to compete?

References

1. American Physical Therapy Association. Physical Therapy Professional Liability Exposure: 2016 Claim Report Update. Accessed November 26, 2023. https://www.hpso.com/getmedia/5e41bb-f5-8b7e-4f5f-a932-460629bb4770/CNA_PT_CS_020116_CF_PROD_ASIZE_ONLINE_040417_SEC_1.pdf.

2. American Physical Therapy Association. Risk Control Self-Assessment Checklist. 2016. Accessed July 17, 2018. https://www.hpso.com.

3. Sanger-Katz M. Doctors' fears of liability may hit patients in the wallet, study hints. *New York Times*, July 24, 2018, B4.

4. *Canterbury v. Spence*, 409 U.S. 1064, 93 S. Ct. 560, 34 L. Ed. 2d 518 (U.S,. November 1, 1972).

5. Landro L. Consent forms patients can understand. *Wall Street Journal*, February 6, 2008, D1, 3.

6. Hoffman J. Teenagers face early death, on their terms. *New York Times*, March 29, 2015, A1, A20.

7. Department of Health and Human Services. *Voicing My Choices: A Planning Guide for Adolescents and Young Adults.* Department of Health and Human Services; 2015.

8. Hester DM. Ethical issues in pediatrics. In Hester DM, Schonfeld T, eds. *Guidance for Healthcare Ethics Committees.* Cambridge University Press; 2012:114-121.

9. Health Insurance Portability and Accountability Act of 1996, 42 USC 1320d *et seq.*

10. American Physical Therapy Association. *Code of Ethics for the Physical Therapist.* Section 3A. American Physical Therapy Association; 2020.

11. Tonmyr L, Li Y, Williams G, Scott D, Jack S. Patterns of reporting by health care and non-health care professionals to child protection services in Canada. *Paediatr Child Health.* 2010;15(8):e25-e32.

12. *Tarasoff v. Regents of the University of California*, 17 Cal. 3d 425, 551 P.2d 334, 131 Cal. Rptr. 14 (Cal. 1976).

13. Jenkins R, Firestone G, Aasheim K, Boelens B. Mandatory presuit mediation for medical malpractice: eight-year results and future innovations. *Conflict Res Q.* 2017;35(1):73-88.

14. Individuals with Disabilities Education Act. Accessed August 14, 2018. https://sites.ed.gov/idea/.

15. *Irving Independent School District v. Tatro*, 468 U.S. 883 (1984).

16. *Endrew F. v. Douglas County School District*, 137 S. Ct. 988 (2017).

17. *Endrew F. v. Douglas County School District*, RE-1, 580 U.S. (2017).

18. Section 504 of the Rehabilitation Act of 1973, Section 504, 29 U.S.C. § 701 et seq.

19. American With Disabilities Act of 1990, 42 U.S.C. 12101 et seq.

20. Family Educational Rights and Privacy Act of 1974, 20 U.S.C. 1232g.

21. Department of Health and Human Services. Does FERPA or HIPAA apply to elementary or secondary school student health records maintained by a health care provider that is not employed by a school? Accessed August 16, 2018. https://www.hhs.gov/hipaa/for-professionals/faq/514/does-hipaa-apply-to-school-student-health-records/index.html.

This chapter provides legal information only and not specific legal advice. Such advice can only be rendered by one's personal attorney, acting on fact-specific law.

Emergency Response of Physical Therapy During a Crisis or Pandemic

Roberta Bertie Gatlin, PT, DScPT, Jonathan Greenwood, PT, MS, MBA, DPT, and Mary Devine, MPH

LEARNING OBJECTIVES

Upon completion of this chapter, the reader will be able to:

- Recognize the incident command system response model and the role that physical therapy has in this process during a crisis.
- Identify ways that a crisis may affect the operations of physical therapy and determine ways to minimize the impact of a crisis.

- Distinguish methods to expand services during the midst of a crisis.
- Understand the importance of supporting the impact that working through a crisis has on mental health.

DEFINING A CRISIS: NATURAL DISASTER (eg, HURRICANE, TORNADO, WILDFIRES) AND PANDEMIC (eg, CORONAVIRUS [COVID-19])

The emergency response of physical therapy during a crisis is something we as a profession do not often think about. Physical therapists (PTs) and physical therapist assistants (PTAs) may play a role in the emergency department of a hospital or as a first responder on the athletic field in response to an athletic injury. However, what happens when a natural disaster strikes a region or a pandemic is experienced by a nation? The professional roles and responsibilities are tested, patient care access may be altered, and creativity in the delivery of care is needed.

Crisis is defined as a time of intense difficulty, trouble, or danger. A crisis situation may encompass a series of events of a situation or disease that may take a turn for the worse. Many events across the United States and across the globe have qualified as regional, national, or global crises, such as wildfires, hurricanes, tornados, and pandemics. In the health care environment, there can be many different types of crisis. This can include global events such as pandemics or natural disasters or more targeted events, such as

information technology (IT) outages or a pipe bursting in a clinic. A crisis impacts all individuals, but there are additional considerations needed when considering vulnerable populations such as pediatric patients, individuals with disabilities, and those with special health care needs. Children are more vulnerable during disasters due to several factors, such as the following:

- Structural differences are present in the anatomy of children; for example, children inhale more air than adults and therefore may absorb airborne materials more easily than adults.
- When receiving medical treatment, there is a need for specialized equipment, supplies, and pharmaceuticals that may be extremely limited during a disaster. This could lead to greater morbidity and mortality of this population based on the lack of resources.
- Based on their age, children may not be capable of communicating their symptoms or their needs during a disaster.
- Children depend on others for almost all needs, including safety. If a child does not have an advocate, not only does this impact their medical needs but it also affects their safety and can lead to serious safety issues, such as child abduction.

Both national and more local emergencies may impact physical therapy in similar ways. These include the following:

- Destruction of property and infrastructure necessary to provide care (clinic buildings/hospitals)
- Disruption to technology and methods of communication including access to the electronic health record or ability to access cell phones
- Staffing shortages, as staff may be affected by the event or need to attend to family members impacted by the event. This is particularly challenging if child care is impacted.
- An increase in the need for PT services due to injuries caused by the crisis

Working on a comprehensive emergency response plan can address how to cope with these issues, increase resilience, and minimize the impact on a physical therapy department. Being prepared to respond to the impact of a crisis can help a department maintain operations during a crisis.

During the coronavirus disease 2019 (COVID-19) pandemic crisis in 2020, the American Physical Therapy Association (APTA) board of directors stated that PTs and PTAs should "use their professional judgment to determine when, where, and how to provide care, with the understanding this is not the optimal environment for care, for anyone involved."[1] This statement holds true for any crisis situation. During the coronavirus pandemic, PTs were treated as essential health care providers by federal, state, and local agencies. The APTA encourages PTs and PTAs to review the Centers for Disease Control and Prevention (CDC) guidelines and use their professional judgment in providing services to their clients.[2] The APTA board of directors' statement on patient care and practice management during COVID-19 was to build communities that continue to assist in advancing the profession of physical therapy to improve the health of our society.[1] This statement holds true during any crisis situation, and emergency preparedness is essential to the response of our profession in times of crises.[3]

■ THE PHYSICAL THERAPIST'S ROLE IN EMERGENCY PREPAREDNESS AND RESPONSE

PTs must identify a new culture of emergency preparedness. Emergency preparedness is not a new concept. Individuals are reminded every year to prepare. Prepare for routine safety measures such as changing the batteries in smoke detectors and prepare for annual storms (eg, hurricanes, snow, tornados) with enough food, water, and supplies to meet a shelter in place or know evacuation routes should evacuation be needed. With the recent national and global disasters, such as wildfires, hurricanes, tornadoes, and pandemics, our health care community has heightened the awareness of the ancillary health care professionals in preparing for when, not if, a national disaster occurs. Pediatric PTs and PTAs will need to identify the role emergency management plays in their unique specialty across all settings.

Regulatory agencies of health care systems require emergency preparedness. The Joint Commission, a state organization responsible for accrediting health care organizations and programs, requires several planning activities as part of hospital accreditation. This includes developing response plans and maintaining an emergency drill program.[3] All emergency preparedness should be structured within an emergency management program. An emergency management program is responsible for the planning and implementation of response policies during an emergency.

One major aspect of a hospital's emergency management program is the implementation of a hospital incident command system (HICS).[3] This is an incident management system used to approach the coordination of an emergency response by adopting a standardized organizational structure.[4,5] It is a way an organization can quickly and effectively collaborate across departments and structures to coordinate an effective response after a crisis. Large organizations, like hospitals, are required to use this model to structure an emergency response. The group of individuals within HICS will be sending out pertinent information about the emergency and be developing the response plan for that specific crisis. HICS is organized around the following 5 categories:

- **Command,** which defines the incident command goals and operational objectives
- **Operations,** which establishes strategy and tactics to operationalize the objectives set by the command group
- **Logistics,** which facilitates the equipment, supplies, and staff needed to act out the operational objectives
- **Planning,** which coordinates and plans for the implementation of the response as well as compiles pertinent information about the response
- **Administration/finance,** which coordinates the administrative and finance needs of the response

PTs may play a role in this structure. They may need to attend meetings to help plan for and respond to an emergency. They may receive important updates about the situation through regularly scheduled briefings. The role of the PT within the HICS might be to answer questions about the impact of the emergency or act as a conduit of information to others in the physical therapy department. It is important for all to know who is designing the emergency response and what role the department and the PT and PTA will play within that response.

Another emergency preparedness setting in which PTs play a role is assisting with school disaster planning for students with disabilities. Title II of the Americans With Disabilities Act (ADA) addresses "discrimination on the basis of disability in the activities of places of public accommodation such as restaurants, movies, and schools."[6] Most schools have an evacuation procedure that calls for a person with a disability to shelter in place on the landing of the stairwell and wait for emergency medical services (EMS) rescue. That may not be enough of a response given today's current climate. Many schools in the United States have policies for disaster preparedness, and the PT may play an intricate role in this planning for students with disabilities. "In 2020–21, the number of students ages 3–21 who received special education services under the Individuals with Disabilities Education Act (IDEA) was 7.2 million, or 15 percent of all public school students. Among students receiving special education services, the most common category of disability was specific learning disabilities (33%)."[7] In this era of threats, it is paramount that school systems offer an effective emergency evacuation plan for students with disabilities.

Planning is the key to successful school evacuations. Schools must design plans for all students who have disabilities, such as those with sensory disabilities, those who lack the understanding of the situation, and those who are unable to act quickly in an emergency or are nonmobile. The PT may offer suggested evacuation needs for specialized routes and equipment needs for students utilizing adaptive equipment such as crutches and/or wheelchairs and assign specific personnel to student(s). Evacuation routes are often compounded by the nature of the emergency route designs. PTs can offer guidance and training for school system personnel to assist in the use of proper emergency equipment and strategic locations throughout the facility to safely evacuate students with disabilities. Information regarding the emergency evacuation of school students with disabilities is provided by IDEA Part B services, the National Fire Protection Association (NFPA), and the US Department of Transportation Federal Highway Administration.[8-10] These organizations offer planning and preparation for evacuating populations with special needs. Suggested requirements of transporting students with disabilities include the following:

1. Need to coordinate the identification of individuals with special needs, their locations, and their requirements for transportation assistance. This will be listed on the student's individualized education program (IEP).
2. Need to coordinate roles, responsibilities, and dispatching of personnel for transit services to evacuate individuals requiring transportation.
3. Need to coordinate resumption of critical health care functions once evacuated to a safe environment.
4. Need to coordinate postevent efforts and manage students within a safe environment.

Evidence-based information provides a guide to school authorities in adapting and mitigating school environmental changes. The PT is an integral part of this evacuation plan.

During the recent COVID-19 pandemic, physical therapy professionals were advised to follow the information provided by the CDC. The CDC provides information regarding the short- and long-term health effects associated with the COVID-19.[2] A recent Delphi study by Magnusson et al[10] set out to gather competencies for educating the physical therapy student regarding their roles in population health, prevention, health promotion, and wellness. The authors identified competencies for population health as well as health systems and polity categories. The authors indicate the discrepancy identified in Commission on Accreditation for Physical Therapy Education (CAPTE) standards due to the recent shift in population health focus: Research has continued to promote the need for physical therapists and physical therapy educational models to reinforce population health and health promotion into practice. The World Confederation for Physical Therapy (WCPT) Summit on Global Health has been developing mechanisms for integrating health-focused physical therapy professions."[10]

The fact that the physical therapy profession is working toward competencies in public health and public wellness (PHPW) at the profession's entry educational level will assist in changing the culture around our role as health care practitioners in public health, as well as in emergency preparedness.[10] The vision of the APTA is to transform society by optimizing movement to improve the human experience.[11] The mission statement is to build a community that advances the profession of physical therapy to improve the health of society.[11] These 2 statements recognize the role of the PT in PHPW. Achieving PHPW competencies at the entry level begins the cultural transition to ensure that PTs and PTAs encompass their role in emergency preparedness.[12]

The role of the PT and PTA in disaster management is an important component of emergency preparedness, disaster response, and recovery. The profession of physical therapy is well positioned to assist other health care providers in understanding mechanisms of injuries and other health-related conditions that might result from disaster. The PT and PTA may assist in the area of triage, providing interventions for acute injuries such as traumatic brain injury, fractures, and burns. The PT is able to assess a patient's mobility, address their need for accessibility, and provide interventions in an intensive care unit (ICU) environment to help mobilize patients for improved recovery and transition out of ICU to a regular floor. This assists in freeing up ventilators and/or ICU beds for more critically ill patients.

In 2018, the APTA House of Delegates (HOD) recognized the importance of roles the PT and PTA can have in disaster management. The HOD charged the association with the following: "That the APTA engage and collaborate with disaster management agencies to identify the professional roles of the PT and PTs assistant in disaster preparation, response, relief, and recovery. Further, the APTA promotes the role of the PT and PTA to members, and to agencies that study and manage disasters so that the expertise of PTs and PTAs can be utilized appropriately."[12] PTs and PTAs are poised to define the essential scopes of practice in which to participate during a crisis. We should also define a triage process for patients requiring the skills of a PT or PTA for care delivery during a crisis. This triage process will vary based on the practice setting, type of crisis, and length of the emergency response. For example, PTs working in an acute care setting during the COVID-19 pandemic may have needed to define a triage process for patient care elevating direct patient care for those in pulmonary distress as a part of the proning team, whereas those deconditioned following a noninjurious fall may not elevate to a high level of care in the triage process (**Table 24-1**). Additionally, it is important to understand that the staffing of PTs or PTAs during a crisis may also impact the availability of physical therapy services for patient care or emergency response, thus creating a need to prioritize those with a greater need for receiving physical therapy. PTs and PTAs might also be required to respond to a crisis with more nontraditional roles and responsibilities.

APTA recommends using the World Health Organization (WHO) Minimal Technical Standards and Recommendations

TABLE 24-2 • US Department of Education's 5 Mission Areas	
Prevention	Means the capabilities to secure schools against acts of violence and man-made or natural disasters
Protection	Focuses on ongoing actions that protect students, teachers, staff, visitors, networks, and property from a threat or hazard
Mitigation	Means the capabilities necessary to eliminate or reduce the loss of life and property damage by lessening the impact of an event or emergency
Response	Means the capabilities necessary to stabilize an emergency once it has already happened or is certain to happen in an unpreventable way; establish a safe and secure environment; save lives and property; and facilitate the transition to recovery
Recovery	Means the capabilities necessary to assist schools affected by an event or emergency in restoring the learning environment

TABLE 24-3 • Categories of Hazards		
Type of Hazard	**Definition**	**Example**
Natural	These are events caused by forces of nature within the natural environment. These events happen within our environment and are only an issue when they come into contact with the built environment.	Wildfire: Wildfires frequently occur in nature. These naturally occurring fires are ecologically beneficial for the environment. If uncontrolled, they cause significant damage to businesses and housing developments in the path of the fire.
Technological	These hazards are emergencies that impact man-made materials and have a great impact on how business is conducted and how we communicate with the public.	Network downtime: If health care institutions are not able to access the network, this means that providers will not be able to access critical information about patients (health records) or communicate through email/portal, significantly impacting patient care.
Adversarial (human caused)	These are emergencies caused by human beings, either intentionally or unintentionally.	Cyberattack: Malware rendering a computer unusable unless a ransom is paid has been a significant threat in the business community over the past few years. This can cost an organization both time and money and result in system vulnerability.

Developing an emergency response plan should be done prior to an emergency. There are a few steps to developing a comprehensive emergency response plan, including:

- Completing a risk assessment
- Determining the response objectives and strategies
- Developing a comprehensive training plan to ensure all roles know what to do during a response

A basic risk assessment for a department does not have to be formal. Hosting a departmental meeting and brainstorming what hazards the department may have dealt with in the past year can help structure a conversation around preparedness. Was there a day when staff could not access the electronic health record? What happened in this scenario? What were the roadblocks, and what ideas do staff have to make that an easier situation? There may have been a bad storm or a time when a pipe burst, impacting the way the department could function. Discussing these scenarios is how you start thinking about your plan. This exercise can lead you to determine what the response objectives are and what strategies should be implemented during a crisis. If there is not a safe space to see patients, will the clinic need to close operations for that day? If so, how will the patients and staff be notified of this change? Writing out a process to respond to these crises will help while experiencing the crisis.

When trying to understand the impact of an emergency, it is important to think about the different types of threats that may impact physical therapy. There are different types of emergencies that may require different responses based on the type of emergency. A severe technological disruption such as an Internet outage may require a vastly different response than a hurricane or other natural disaster. Both will have a large impact on patient care, but the needs may be different. Within the emergency management field, there are different categories of hazards that help to assess the risk an organization has of being impacted (**Table 24-3**).

After a risk assessment, it is important to document what steps would need to be taken during an emergency. When compiling a plan (**Table 24-4**), it is important to consider the following:

- What are the operational objectives to this plan?
  - What is the overall goal and purpose of the plan- be specific.
- How will these objectives be met?
  - Who specifically (what roles) will be carrying out these objectives?
- What is needed for the response?
  - Are there specific supplies or equipment that is needed?
- How will you recover from this emergency?
  - When and how will the services revert to normal operations?

Understanding the needs of an emergency before an organization is impacted by that crisis can help streamline a response and quickly address the needs of that organization. By taking

Type of Plan	Explanation	Example
Strategic	The strategic planning focuses on the overall objectives of the response. This outlines the strategy of the response.	During a hurricane, the objective might be to ensure safety of patients and staff through evacuation of a building.
Operational	Operational planning focuses on the roles, responsibilities, and tasks that need to be completed to ensure the objective of the response is accomplished.	During a hospital evacuation, planning is needed to understand which roles will evacuate patients and how they will evacuate patients.
Tactical	A tactical plan focuses on what is needed to physically execute the objectives of the response and what types of staff, equipment, and supplies will be used in the response.	During a snowstorm, 5 extra staff members may need to be advised to deliver food to inpatients to supplement for staff who are unable to come into the hospital.

TABLE 24-4 • The Different Types of Organizational Response Plans

time to understand what the overall goals are in a response, what is needed during that response, and how to get resources for that response, the impact of that response on departmental operations can be greatly reduced.

After a plan has been developed, the last and most important part of the planning phase is to ensure all staff understand what the plan is in case of emergency. There is a need to train all staff on their role during an emergency. This should consist of both didactic training and a simulation. The didactic training should involve discussion-based instruction allowing for staff members to understand aspects of the plan. After a basic comprehension, some plans may require a simulation for staff to fully understand their roles during an emergency. A response to an active shooter may require a PT or PTA to work in an unfamiliar area or under more stress than during their usual workday. Simulations can help create realistic situations during which an individual can practice their response to an emergency.

RESPONSE DURING A CRISIS

Response to a crisis can look very different based on the type of hazard. An earthquake may require the PT and PTA to help assess multiple crush injuries that victims coming into an emergency room might have. A hurricane response may require the PT and PTA to help evacuate hospitals, offices, or residences of people with access and functional needs. Response to a pandemic may require the PT and PTA to don proper personal protective equipment (PPE) in order to prevent the spread of infectious disease. These different types of responses all require the PT and PTA to be flexible within their role and open to learning new processes. Before responding to any of these scenarios, the PT and PTA should understand their role, the risks involved, and ways to

protect themselves while delivering care. During an emergency, a designated safety representative from the organization should be able to instruct a PT or PTA about these issues. Emergency response can be time consuming, hectic, stressful, and at times dangerous. As a crisis responder, it is important to determine what your needs are during a response and how to communicate those needs. A responder needs to prioritize their physical needs during a response because those who are exhausted, mentally or physically, are prone to make errors and add to the victims of the response. When responding to a crisis, the following can be done to help be prepared to respond:

- Know how to communicate with your team members and your supervisors in case of an emergency.
- Understand when breaks will be allowed and how to access food and bathroom breaks.
- Communicate your plans with your family/friends/support network to ensure they know you are safe while responding to a crisis.
- If working a long shift, take frequent breaks and listen to your body.

A successful emergency response requires a large amount of support from individuals and the organization. Large-scale emergency response often requires long hours under stressful conditions. Ensuring that all responders' needs are met while responding can increase the success of that response and lessen the casualties from a response.

DELIVERY OF CARE DURING A RESPONSE

When a crisis occurs, daily functions change and the standard delivery of care changes. There are both clinical and nonclinical activities that require attention to support the delivery of care. The PT or PTA may be directly impacted by the crisis geographically or serve in a local community spared by the crisis and needing to offer support to those impacted. Safety and emergency response is often the first line of support in a crisis. As with the need for evacuation of patients or employees to follow local, state, or federal mandates, PTs or PTAs may take on a supporting role. This may be true in the prioritization of need for the population impacted, from ensuring proper nutrition by delivering food trays, to assisting triage in the emergency department, to assisting to contact parents of children attending schools and coordinating reunions. All of these nonclinical roles are important in the emergency response of your specified area of clinical practice. There are also clinical roles the PT or PTA may take on during a crisis, including the delivery of care based on setting and what phase the crisis is in.

Because PTs and PTAs have a particular area of expertise in the safe movement of nonambulatory patients, there may be a particular role for PTs and PTAs to help evacuate buildings during a crisis in which the elevators are not functional. For example, in the school setting, the PT and PTA may play an integral role in evacuation of nonambulatory students. The same can be true during a hospital evacuation during a natural disaster, such as responding to a hurricane or earthquake. During these scenarios, there may be multiple roles a PT or PTA can play during the response. The PT or PTA should help the care team understand safe lifting techniques to minimize injury to the care team and the patient. The PT or PTA may also be asked to come up with overall best practices in order to develop training for nonclinicians to understand safe ways to transport nonambulatory patients from adverse environments.

There are many other ways that the delivery of care for the PT or PTA could change during an emergency response. After a mass casualty incident such as a large explosion, an active shooter event, or building collapse, there may be an increased need for PT services as large amounts of people will be evacuating an area. During these events, there will be an increase in injuries not only from the cause of the event but also from individuals fleeing the scene. For example, there may be 30 people injured from an explosion, but the explosion may have occurred during a parade, causing many people to flee the area. While running from the area, sprained ankles and other injuries from trips and falls may occur. These types of injuries can result in an increased need for PT or PTA treatment. There may also be an increase in the need for PT postoperative services and rehabilitation in the days and months after a mass casualty incident.

The PT or PTA also may need to augment the way that they care for a patient during an emergency. During a pandemic, there may be a need to implement different infection control standards to ensure safety to both patients and staff members. This may require that PTs and PTAs don PPE such as facemasks, respirators, gloves, or face shields. This equipment allows for a safe way to see patients during an infectious disease outbreak. There may be other requirements based on the mode of infection, such as the need to leave a room vacant between patients for a certain amount of time to minimize transmission. The CDC or your local department of public health will issue instructions on how to treat patients in a safe environment during an infectious disease emergency.

Based on the recommendations from public health authorities, there may be a need to determine alternative ways to treat patients. During the COVID-19 pandemic of 2020, the emergency response varied across the country from clinic and school closures limiting access to physical therapy services to fully operational hospitals and clinics offering business as usual. These operations varied based on the virus exposure risk and governmental declarations regarding who could remain operational in their state. PTs needed to assess the clinical acuity of patient needs and resolve how to deliver care to those patients deemed essential for ongoing care, which patients could pause their clinical care without loss of function or decline in status, and which patients might need a hybrid model of care, including virtual service delivery. For example, a postoperative patient in the early phases of recovery may require direct in-person clinical care to progress from their surgery, whereas that same patient 12 weeks after the operation may have PT needs that are not clinically urgent.

The delivery of patient care during a crisis involves ensuring the environment is safe to deliver care for you and your patients. Whether in a hospital, school, clinic, or home, a determination needs to be made whether it is safe for the PT or PTA and the patient or student to deliver direct patient care. This is also true when delivering virtual care. The PT or PTA needs to ensure that the patient or student is safe within their environment and

that the equipment needed to deliver care is available. This may require creativity in using a different environment and different tools to achieve the therapeutic effects needed to deliver care.

■ MODELS OF SERVICE DELIVERY

DIRECT PATIENT CARE

Therapists may find it safe and essential to deliver care in person to their patient or student. The delivery of care during an emergency may be directed to include only essential treatments needed to progress postoperative patients, prevent loss of function in particular patients, and ensure rehabilitation needs are met at the functional level.

CONSULTATIVE MODEL OF CARE

Therapists may provide consultative models of service delivery in order to support those interacting with patients or students including parents, teachers, and other medical professionals. This model may be used to enable or support ongoing care, assist in decision-making by other medical professionals, or answer questions during a difficult and time-sensitive transition of care during a crisis.

VIRTUAL PATIENT CARE

Virtual patient care (or telehealth) may involve several modes of care including video and/or audio delivery of care. The APTA defines this model of health care delivery as follows: "Telehealth is a well-defined and established method of health services delivery. PTs provide services using telehealth as part of their scope of practice, incorporating elements of patient and client management as needed, to enhance patient and client interactions. The APTA supports: Inclusion of PT services in telehealth policy and regulation on the national and state levels to help society address the growing cost of health services, the disparity in accessibility of health services, and the potential impact of health workforce shortages."[25]

APTA offers information regarding guidelines and strategies to improve telehealth in various physical therapy settings or environments.[25] One link on the APTA website offers "telehealth modalities PTs and PTAs can use during the public health emergency and beyond."[25] APTA also provides information regarding the use of electronic information and telecommunication technologies to remotely provide health care in this new virtual world.[26]

Case 1

Care Delivery During a Crisis

In December 2019, severe acute respiratory syndrome coronavirus 2 (SARS-CoV-2), a novel coronavirus, was identified in Wuhan, China. SARS-CoV-2 is the virus that causes the disease COVID-19, a new virus in humans causing respiratory illness that can be spread through droplet transmission from person to person. The disease gained global attention after an outbreak was reported in Wuhan, China, in January 2020. In March, many states issued formal state of emergency declarations, giving the state administration more flexibility to respond to the coronavirus outbreak. By early

March 2020, after transmission was recorded throughout most of the world, the WHO designated COVID-19 as a global pandemic. The designation of a pandemic led to widespread restrictions across the world, including in the United States.

In mid-March, governors ordered that all businesses and organizations that do not provide "COVID-19 essential services" to close their physical workplaces and continue operations remotely where possible, which included schools. A stay-at-home order was also issued advising residents to stay home and avoid unnecessary travel. Travel restrictions, stay-at-home orders, and work-from-home mandates continued with varying degrees throughout 2020 and into 2021. On May 1, 2020, universal masking became required in all public places where social distancing was not feasible. By May 2020, 20 adult hospitals in Massachusetts reported that they were operating above capacity and using medical surge space to meet patient needs. Field hospitals were established in early spring 2020 due to increases in hospitalizations and overall hospital capacity concerns. Hospitals canceled elective procedures and postponed nonemergent appointments to address capacity issues.

During this time, clinics were asked to immediately decrease volume and implement stringent infection prevention strategies. This meant that only emergent cases were able to be treated. Clinicians were asked to don PPE, including masks, face shields, N95 respirators, gowns, and gloves, to ensure they were protected against the virus. Waiting rooms were augmented to ensure proper physical distancing, and a time frame was implemented in between patients to allow for safe patient care. All were expected to be masked in patient care areas, posing a greater risk for those treating individuals who were unable to wear masks.

■ MANAGING THROUGH A CRISIS

The ability to manage through a crisis is a challenge. Whether an independent clinician managing your individual caseload or a director of a large urban hospital or a team leader of a school district, many considerations and decisions need to be made to ensure safe and effective care is delivered to patients and students. First and foremost is the need to ensure employee and patient/student safety. Management of care delivery requires that those delivering care and those receiving care are all safe within the model of care delivery. Second, the management of care delivery requires a proper analysis that clinical needs within models of care delivery systems are proportional to the crisis and relative risk of accessing that care. This may involve the need for a clinical triage system to prioritize care delivery to those most in need. Finally, the management of care delivery needs to account for the well-being and mental health of care providers, patients, students, and caregivers.

When considering safety for employees, patients, students, and caregivers, the management includes the accessibility of brick-and-mortar locations versus virtual care delivery. In-person care delivery needs to account for resource allocation (ie, availability of clinicians and availability of PPE) to match these resources with the patient in need of in-person care delivery. If appropriate safety measures are in place and all parties are able to maintain the safety measures needed to deliver care,

then the efficacy of care can be determined. Considerations of blended models of care (in person and virtual) may be considered if service delivery is deemed to be effective in both models.

As we consider the appropriateness of various models of care and modes of patient care, certain patients may benefit more from one model over the other and some may only benefit from one model due to their unique clinical presentations. For example, a patient requiring manual assistance and the skills of a therapist to progress with their balance activities may not benefit from virtual visits. This same patient may progress with in-person therapy over several weeks and, after demonstrating improved balance, may be able to then benefit from virtual visits with the assistance of their caregivers. It is important to constantly assess the clinical needs of the patient and align them with the current crisis situation. As a crisis continues and time passes, a patient's or student's condition may also become more urgent to address. This is where a uniform decision tree or patient/student triage system may benefit an organization. This will allow multiple therapists to make similar decisions based on the clinical presentations of their patients. This triage system may assist in prioritization of patient care and will be unique to setting and the situation of the crisis.

Responding to an emergency can be emotionally, mentally, and physically exhausting. Working long hours in intense situations different from everyday environments can increase the stress levels of any individual. Depending on the emergency, the response and the individual responding to an emergency may cause trauma to the emergency responder in multiple ways. During a prolonged response with constantly changing guidance, there may be an increase in burnout as practitioners are asked to augment their practice for months at a time. During an intense immediate response where responders are exposed to multiple traumatic images (eg, an active shooter incident), a responder may experience traumatic event stress responses. These types of reactions may vary from person to person. The US Department of Health and Human Services' Substance Abuse and Mental Health Services Administration (SAMHSA) states that "Disasters have the potential to cause emotional distress."[27] They outline the following warning signs of distress after responding to a disaster:

- Sleeping too much or too little
- Stomachaches or headaches
- Anger, feeling edgy, or lashing out at others
- Worrying a lot of the time; feeling guilty but not sure why
- Overwhelming sadness
- Feeling like you have to keep busy
- Lack of energy or always feeling tired
- Drinking alcohol, smoking, or using tobacco more than usual; using illegal drugs more
- Eating too much or too little
- Not connecting with others
- Feeling like you won't ever be happy again

Many tactics can help minimize stress after a particularly stressful response, including the following:

- Undergoing a critical incident stress debriefing
- Taking time off away from work

- Ensuring a strong social support network following an event
- Acknowledging situations that may be more stressful after experiencing trauma
- Getting enough sleep and establishing healthy habits

Furthermore, as a crisis brings about constant change and ongoing analysis of the situation, this leads to uncertainty and increased stress of health care providers. APTA reported in August 2020 that 72% of PT practice owners reported a revenue loss of greater than 50% during early months of pandemic.[3] During this same time period, 36% of PTs had experienced a reduction in employed hours compared with before the pandemic.[3] The pandemic was reported to have a negative impact on the stress levels of both the medical and physical therapy students.[28-30] Gallagher and Schleyer[31] and Husky et al[32] reported that stress can be related to both personal life situations and professional sense of duty. Cao et al[33] reported in May 2020 that 7143 students from Changzhi Medical College in China completed the 7-item Generalized Anxiety Disorder Scale, with 21.3% reporting mild anxiety, 2.7% moderate anxiety, and 0.9% severe anxiety. Economic effects, effects on daily life, and delays in academic activities were positively correlated with anxiety symptoms, and social support was negatively correlated with anxiety levels. In July of 2020, Nakhostin-Ansari et al[34] reported medical clerks and interns at Tehron University of Medical Science in Iran had a 38.1% mild to severe anxiety level and 27.6% reported mild to severe depression. As a crisis continues and ongoing changes occur, stress and mental health conditions change. Employees wonder about job security for their own well-being and the security of their families personally. Therapists also maintain the responsibility of patient care management during the pandemic.[35]

An additional consideration as one manages through a crisis is the impact of finances on the individual therapist, the organization, and the patients/caregivers. The impact of the crisis on all of these aspects may lead an organization to make a decision for possible temporary staff reduction. This decision may allow the organization to close during the crisis with hopes to reopen when it is safe to do so. These decisions are difficult for management, and many financial considerations need to be made. Other organizations may creatively move therapists into other roles within the organization, such as patient triage or administrative roles in admissions. PTs must ensure that they are aware of their role and what their scope of practice allows in their state if functioning as a care provider. Even still, some organizations may be physically or financially compromised and may not be able to continue to provide care during or following a crisis. This is tragic for the therapist and the organization and even more so for the patients or students and caregivers. There is a duty to assist families in the coordination of services to other providers if appropriate in the region either during or after the pandemic.[36,37]

■ RESOURCES

During the outbreak of COVID-19, social media platforms and news outlets were important for disseminating information to the public and reporting on events around the globe. The CDC, the WHO, numerous journals, and other health care organizations regularly posted guidance across a host of platforms.[2,36,37] The need to receive and evaluate reliable information is critical to the success of the management of any crisis. It is important to find primary and trusted information sources when making decisions concerning for your profession, community, and patient care.

Primary sources of information include local, national, and global professional organizations; governmental organizations (eg, CDC, WHO, FEMA); and primary research and evidence sources.[2,21,36] Considerations must also be given to the organization within which the therapist works to ensure compliance with policies and procedures set forth to ensure adherence with regulatory agencies and safety for all employees, patients or students, and caregivers. It is important to maintain a questioning attitude during any crisis so that, as a medical professional, you are continually assessing the situation and asking questions regarding safety and efficacy of care delivery.

Communication is a key element during a crisis:

1. Communication from government agencies to the public
2. Communication between the organization and their employees
3. Communication between the organization or therapist and their patients or students
4. Communication at the department level on local implications of care delivery
5. Communication among peers within the organization

Transparent communication founded in evidence and fact is important so that everyone is educated and informed on the situation, impact to care delivery, impact to the organization, and the direction the organization is taking to navigate through the crisis. There are many forms of communication, and a multimodal approach is best. Written communication followed by verbal support and dialogue is needed to ensure questions are answered in a timely manner to address any situations that arise due to the new processes. Especially during a crisis, communication needs to be delivered consistently and repeatedly so that the message is clear. As a medical professional, it is also important to maintain an inquisitive mind and questioning attitude so that the information delivered is interpreted and applied to the patient care needs of the employee's unique situation. Any anomalies or safety concerns should be escalated to leadership or management using the proper channels of communication to ensure employee, patient or student, and caregiver safety and efficacy of care delivery.

There are many resources to increase your awareness of emergency preparedness. The following agencies provide a number of tools and training that would be helpful to explore for both personal and professional preparedness.

- FEMA (www.Ready.gov)
- CDC: Public health preparedness resources (www.cdc.gov)
- Department of Public Health (state-based resources)
- American Red Cross (www.redcross.org)
- Occupational Safety and Health Administration (OSHA): Emergency preparedness and response (www.osha.gov)

Many communities also offer ways for PTs and PTAs to be involved in response through medical volunteer corps or community emergency response teams.

SUMMARY[38,39]

Natural disasters and pandemic events are chaotic. Crucial decisions made by health care facilities can result in inconsistent action that is potentially adverse to patient and public interests. It is important to ensure organizational emergency plans are in alignment with public health and emergency management agency protocols to ensure capacity and guide crucial decisions in a disaster. The secretary of Health and Human Services should consider issuing early public health emergency declarations to reduce legal concerns and regulatory constraints in the delivery of health care.[40] National professional organizations and local professional organizations should align in solidarity to ensure that safe and effective care is provided to patients in need.

STUDY QUESTIONS

1. What are ways that a PT or PTA can be integrated into an emergency response?
2. What is the hospital incident command system?
3. How can an emergency plan be structured?
4. What are the different models of service that can be implemented in an emergency?
5. What are 3 ways a child may be impacted uniquely by a disaster?
6. What are the warning signs of distress that a clinician might experience after an emergency?
7. What are some tactics that clinicians can use to minimize stress after responding to an emergency?
8. Where can you find resources about emergency preparedness?

References

1. American Physical Therapy Association. Statement from the APTA Board of Directors on patient care and practice management during COVID-19 outbreak. APTA Professional Pulse APTA Leading the Way. *PTinMotionmag.org.* 2020;May:49-51.
2. Centers for Disease Control and Prevention. Coronavirus disease 2019 (COVID-19). CDC's response. Accessed November 29, 2023. https://www.cdc.gov/coronavirus/2019-ncov/cdcresponse/index.html.
3. Emergency management and the incident command system. https://www.hhs.gov/
4. American Physical Therapy Association. Impact of COVID-19 on the physical therapy profession. A report from the American Physical Therapy Association. 2020. Accessed October 7, 2020. https://www.apta.org/apta-and-you/news-publications/2020/impact-of-covid-19-on-the-physical-therapy-profession.
5. The Joint Commission (2020). Emergency management. Accessed January 13, 2021. https://www.jointcommission.org/resources/patient-safety-topics/emergency-management/.
6. National Center for Education Statistics. Resources. Accessed November 29, 2023. https://nces.ed.gov/programs/coe/indicator/cgg/

students-with-disabilities#:~:text=In%202020%E2%80%9321%2C%20the%20number,of%20all%20public%20school%20students.
7. National Center for Education Statistics. (2023). Students With Disabilities. Condition of Education. U.S. Department of Education, Institute of Education Sciences. Retrieved [date], from https://nces.ed.gov/programs/coe/indicator/cgg.
8. National Fire Protection Association. DARAC: Emergency Evacuation Planning Guide for People with Disabilities. June 2016. Accessed November 29, 2023. https://www.nfpa.org/downloadable-resources/guides-and-manuals/evacuation-guide-pdf?l=0.
9. US Department of Transportation. DOT emergency preparedness, response, and recovery information. Accessed November 29, 2023. https://www.transportation.gov/emergency.
10. Dean E, de Andrade AD, O'Donoghue G, et al. The Second Physical Therapy Summit on Global Health: developing an action plan to promote health in daily practice and reduce the burden of non-communicable diseases. *Physiother Theory Pract.* 2014;30(4):261-275.
11. American Physical Therapy Association. Vision, mission, and strategic plan. 2020. Accessed January 13, 2021. https://www.apta.org/apta-and-you/leadership-and-governance/vision-mission-and-strategic-plan.
12. American Physical Therapy Association. The role of the PT and PTA in disaster management. 2020. Accessed November 29, 2023. https://www.apta.org/patient-care/public-health-population-care/emergency-preparedness/role-of-pt-disaster-management.
13. Mosely J. Creating a culture of emergency preparedness. *Health Progress.* 2019;Nov-Dec:30-34.
14. Mills JA, Gosney J, Stephenson F, et al. Development and implementation of the World Health Organization Emergency Medical Teams: minimum technical standards and recommendations for rehabilitation. *PLOS Curr.* 2018;10:ecurrents.dis.76fd9ebfd8689469452cc8c0c0d7cdce.
15. Wiggermann N, Zhow J, Kumper D, et al. Proning patients with COVID-19: a review of equipment and methods. *Human Factors.* 2020;62(7):1069-1076.
16. Federal Emergency Management Agency. Developing and Maintaining Emergency Operations Plans. Comprehensive Preparedness Guide (CPG) 101. Version 2.0. November 2010. Accessed November 29, 2023. https://www.ready.gov/sites/default/files/2019-06/comprehensive_preparedness_guide_developing_and_maintaining_emergency_operations_plans.pdf.
17. Wilson MJ, Aw TG, Sherchan S, et al. The environmental health and emergency preparedness impacts of Hurricane Katrina. *Am J Public Health.* 2020;110(10):1476-1478.
18. American Physical Therapy Association. Coronavirus (COVID-19) resources for the physical therapy profession. 2020. Accessed January 13, 2021. https://www.apta.org/patient-care/public-health-population-care/coronavirus.
19. American Physical Therapy Association. Emergency preparedness. 2020. Accessed January 13, 2021. https://www.apta.org/patient-care/public-health-population-care/emergency-preparedness.
20. Institute of Medicine. *Crisis Standards of Care: A Systems Framework for Catastrophic Disaster Response.* National Academies Press; 2012.
21. US Department of Health and Human Services. Emergency management and the incident command system. 2020. Accessed January 13, 2021. https://www.phe.gov/Preparedness/planning/mscc/handbook/chapter1/Pages/emergency-management.aspx.
22. Federal Emergency Management Agency. Accessed November 29, 2023. https://www.fema.gov/.

23. US Department of Health and Human Services. Presidential Policy Directive 8: National Preparedness. August 14, 2018. Accessed January 13, 2021. https://www.dhs.gov/presidential-policy-directive-8-national-preparedness#:~:text=Presidential%20Policy%20Directive%20%2F%20PPD%2D8%20is%20aimed%20at%20strengthening%20the,pandemics%2C%20and%20catastrophic%20natural%20disasters.

24. US Department of Education. Creating emergency management plans. Emergency Response and Crisis Management TA Center. *ERCMExpress.* 2006;2:1-12. https://rems.ed.gov/docs/Creating-Plans.pdf.

25. American Physical Therapy Association. Position on telehealth. September 20, 2019. Accessed January 13, 2021. https://www.apta.org/apta-and-you/leadership-and-governance/policies/telehealth.

26. American Physical Therapy Association. Telehealth modalities PTs and PTAs can use during the public health emergency. December 16, 2020. Accessed January 13, 2021. https://www.apta.org/your-practice/practice-models-and-settings/telehealth-practice/telehealth-modalities-that-pts-and-ptas-can-use-during-the-public-health-emergency.

27. Substance Abuse and Mental Health Services Administration. Accessed June 2022. https://www.samhsa.gov/.

28. Rose S. Medical student education in the time of COVID-19. *JAMA.* 2020;323(21):2131-2132.

29. Schwartz AM, Wilson JM, Boden SD, et al. Managing resident workforce and education during the COVID-19 pandemic. *JB JS Open Access.* 2020;5(2):e0045.

30. Pappa S, Ntella V, Giannakas T, et al. Prevalence of depression, anxiety, and insomnia among healthcare workers during the COVID-19 pandemic: a systematic review and meta analysis. *Brain Behav Immun.* 2020;88:901-907.

31. Gallagher TH, Schleyer AM. We signed up for this! Student and trainee responses to COVID-19 Pandemic. *N Engl J Med.* 2020;25:382.

32. Husky MM, Kovess-Masfety V, Swendsen J. Stress and anxiety among university students in France during COVID-19 mandatory confinement. *Comp Psychol.* 2020;201:152191.

33. Cao W, Fang Z, Hou G, et al. The psychological impact of the COVID-19 epidemic on college students in China. *Psychiatry Res.* 2020;287:112934.

34. Nakhostin-Ansari A, Sherafati A, Aghajani F, et al. Depression and anxiety among Iranian medical students during COVID-19 pandemic. *Iran J Psychiatry.* 2020;15(30):228-235.

35. American Physical Therapy Association. Code of ethics for the physical therapist. 2020. Accessed November 29, 2023. https://www.apta.org/apta-and-you/leadership-and-governance/policies/code-of-ethics-for-the-physical-therapist.

36. World, H. O. (Ed.). (2023). World Health Organization (WHO). World Health Organization. https://www.who.int/.

37. Merchant RM, Lurie N. Social media and emergency preparedness in response to novel coronavirus. *JAMA.* 2020;323(20):2011-2012.

38. Pedersini P, Corbellini C, Villafañe JH. Italian physical therapists' response to the novel COVID-19 emergency, *Phys Ther.* 2020;100:1049-1051.

39. Berge-Poppe P, Hilfman C, Talja-Binoya MD, et al. Impact of physical therapist training, experience, and role certainty on confidence when responding to a public health event crisis. *Phys Ther J Policy Admin Leader.* 2019;19:1.

40. Powell T, Hanfling D, Gostin LO. Emergency preparedness and public health: the lessons of Hurricane Sandy. *JAMA.* 2012;308(24):2569-2570.

41. United Nations Office for Disaster Risk Reduction. Terminology. 2020. Accessed January 13, 2021. https://www.undrr.org/terminology.

25

The Role of Telehealth in Pediatric Physical Therapy

Jonathan Greenwood, PT, MS, MBA, DPT

LEARNING OBJECTIVES

Upon completion of this chapter, the reader will be able to:

- Understand the elements of synchronous and asynchronous telehealth.
- Identify 3 benefits of telehealth to the patient, provider, and society.

- Cite 5 elements of technology that contribute to the success of telehealth.
- Identify special considerations for pediatric telehealth service delivery.

INTRODUCTION

Telehealth in pediatric physical therapy has been gaining traction over the past few years. Although, 96% of surveyed pediatric physical therapists had never practiced using telehealth services prior to the coronavirus disease 2019 (COVID-19) pandemic, there has been a rapid increase in utilization of telehealth services with good clinical success.[1] With the advancement of technology in rehabilitation, the delivery of physical therapy to advance clinical care is adopting digital practice.[2] This includes the use of telehealth to provide evaluation, assessment, intervention, monitoring, and discharge to our patients.

American Physical Therapy Association Position

According to the American Physical Therapy Association, "Telehealth is a well defined and established method of health service delivery. Physical therapists provide services using telehealth as part of their scope of practice, incorporating elements of patient and client management as needed, to enhance patient and client interactions."[3]

Physical therapists (PTs) are advocates for and users of telehealth. Telehealth in physical therapy, often called telerehabilitation, refers to the delivery of rehabilitation and habilitation services via information and communication technologies. Telerehabilitation is primarily applied to physical therapy and occupational therapy services via telehealth, whereas *telepractice* is the term used for telehealth in speech-language pathology services.[1] PTs can use telephone, video, and synchronous and asynchronous modes of communication to deliver telehealth services in accordance with state practice, licensure, and regulatory bodies.

THE HISTORY OF TELEHEALTH IN HEALTH CARE AND PHYSICAL THERAPY

In the United States, telemedicine began in the 1950s with a collaborative project between NASA, Lockheed, and the US Public Health Service. A mobile van was connected via microwave television and phone to a fixed hospital that provided health care on the Papago Indian Reservation in Arizona. This project spanned 20 years. In 1968, Massachusetts General Hospital linked in microwave television with a medical station at Boston Logan Airport into the Bedford, Massachusetts, Veterans Affairs (VA) hospital. This later expanded to include local schools, courts, and prisons. During the same time, Dartmouth Medical School developed the Interact System servicing 8 communities in Vermont and New Hampshire plus the local VA hospital. Dartmouth medical school also supported an extensive continuing medical education program for physicians, nurses, and ancillary staff. Both of these programs spanned a period of 10 years. In the 1980s, telemedicine moved to television tape satellites linking the main campus of major medical centers.[4] Advancements in the delivery of telemedicine progressed over the decades as technology continued to advance. In the 1990s and 2000s, telehealth progressed to monitoring patients within their homes. In 2001, the US Department of Veteran Affairs was the first health care system to implement telehealth services.[5]

In 2014, 38 states in the United States did not have any telehealth laws and regulations for physical therapy services.[6] By 2018, only 8 states in the country had no telehealth laws or regulations for physical therapy services.[7] Some of these states with telehealth laws or regulations limited telehealth to use of live videos during treatments for the purpose of supervising physical therapist assistants (PTAs). The Physical Therapy Licensure Compact allows therapists licensed within a compact state to practice physical therapy in any other compact state, including providing services through telehealth.[7,8]

This brings us to modern-day telehealth services whereby PTs are delivering direct patient care through e-visits, virtual visits, telecommunications, and wearable technologies. Physical therapy may be considered a manual and hands-on service delivery model; however, the clinical decision-making and communication strategies needed to ensure safe and effective clinical care do not require hands-on service. PTs can use their skills of observation, analysis, critical thinking, coaching, patient instruction, intervention implementation, patient education, goal setting, and discharge planning to leverage the delivery of care remotely, both synchronously or asynchronously.

■ DEFINITIONS (EG, DIGITAL PRACTICE, TELEHEALTH, TELEREHABILITATION, VIRTUAL VISITS)

Two-way, real-time interactive communications, e-visits, virtual check-ins, remote evaluation of visual recordings, and telephone assessment and management services are telehealth services covered under Medicare when furnished by PTs in response to the COVID-19 public health emergency.[9] The use of any of these digital services to deliver physical therapy can be referred to as digital practice (**Table 25-1**).

TABLE 25-1 • Models of Telehealth in Physical Therapy[10-13]

Synchronous telehealth occurs when a physical therapist (PT) provides **live, real-time settings where the patient interacts with a provider** through discussion or communication over the telephone or combined video and audio.

Two-way, real-time interactive communications entail interaction between patient and caregiver using audio and visual technology.

Virtual check-ins are brief, real-time remote communication services for an already established patient.

Telephone assessment and management services are initiated by the patient or, for a child, the parent or guardian and involve a real-time discussion with the PT over the telephone.

Synchronous telehealth may result in a diagnosis, prognosis, treatment plan, intervention, or exercise prescription.

An **asynchronous visit** occurs when a PT collects information from an established patient and provides communication **not in real time** via texting, email, or a patient portal. Providers and patients can communicate online using digital formats or previously recorded information. This information is then reviewed at a later time by the PT. Asynchronous telehealth is also known as "store and forward."
- An **e-visit** is a patient-initiated online assessment and management service for an established patient that is furnished using an online patient portal, not in real time. This is an example of asynchronous, or store-and-forward, technology.
- **Remote evaluation of recorded video or images** is when a PT reviews a prerecorded video or image that an established patient has submitted not in real time via texting, email, or patient portal.

■ THE ADVANTAGES OF TELEHEALTH[2]

Physical therapy telehealth practice offers a number of advantages for patients, caregivers, service providers, and society.

The benefits of telehealth to patients and caregivers include the following:
- Expanded access to physical therapy providers and/or clinical specialists without regard to geographical proximity
- Decreased cost associated with travel and parking
- Increased patient/caregiver independence and control in managing their own health-related concerns by using wearable technology, online self-monitoring, and self-management resources
- Opportunities for flexibility in scheduling for patients and their caregivers, improving time lost on other activities including school, employment, and caring for others

There are also limits patients and families may experience in the delivery of telehealth physical therapy including limited access to technology or access to connectivity, limits to access of specific therapy equipment, and decreased effectiveness if evaluations or interventions require manual interventions or therapeutic touch.

The role of telehealth in pediatric physical therapy can provide many of the benefits noted earlier. Additional pediatric-specific benefits realized include the ability to observe the child and their caregivers in several of their natural environments. This includes problem solving within these environments in real time. Additional benefits for pediatric populations include decreasing the demands on the family unit for travel and time out of the home for scheduled medical appointments. Telehealth also shifts the responsibility of patient management to the caregivers, thus empowering them to carry over therapeutic intervention with the guidance of the PT and therefore improving home practice and repetition.

The benefits of telehealth to service providers include the following:
- Increasing workforce efficiencies such as reduction in travel between care settings
- Ability of the PT to monitor the delivery of care and patient outcomes with greater access to patients regardless of attendance of in-person visits
- Enhanced creativity when leveraging the advantages of new technology options (eg, connected accelerometers, pedometers, heart monitors) and software platforms
- New business opportunities, automation, and time savings with store and forward

Limitations and risks also exist for service providers, including limited payer practices for equitable reimbursement as compared to in-person visits, variable technology and connectivity during telehealth sessions, the need to ensure Health Insurance Portability and Accountability Act (HIPAA) compliance, and any potential safety risks posed to the patient during the session with a safety plan in place.

The benefits of telehealth to society include the following:
- Efficient use of physical therapy resources to deliver care
- Benefits to employers of patients or patient families, including fewer work or school absences

- Developing a better informed and autonomous public with regard to personal health
- Supports individuals wishing to leverage technology and engage in health care digitally
- Creates equity to access physical therapy services independent of geography
- Decreases environmental impact due to reduced travel, resulting in reduced demands on fuel, transportation services, and roadways

There are also limits to society, including varied practice acts from state to state creating artificial barriers to care delivery and payer limitations in their coverage of telehealth benefits for their customers. In addition, communities may also have areas of Internet inaccessibility, typically in lower socioeconomic areas or more rural areas of the country, thus creating health disparities due to lack of technology.[2]

■ WHAT BROUGHT ABOUT THE RAPID CHANGE IN TELEHEALTH PHYSICAL THERAPY?

During the COVID-19 pandemic of 2020, the health care system was challenged and disrupted due to the global pandemic. This pandemic was uncertain in how it was unfolding in the United States and worldwide. PTs were required to socially distance by maintaining a distance of 6 ft from others and use enhanced safety precautions in health care institutions. Patients were encouraged to stay at home or "shelter in place" by state governors' emergency executive orders, thus limiting the ability of patients to access necessary physical therapy services. This created an environment where the profession of physical therapy was required to embrace and expand its implementation and utilization of digital PT practice including telehealth (telerehabilitation) services. Building off an already robust platform, the American Physical Therapy Association (APTA) and PTs across the country quickly advocated for and implemented telehealth services to deliver the needed care for their patients. This included advocacy for legislative changes through state and federal support of regulatory guidelines and laws allowing telehealth practice by PTs where otherwise there were none or restricted practice. Changes in state law to relax licensure requirements varied across the country to allow for cross-border clinical telehealth practice. Many states also mandated that third-party payers and government payers reimburse telehealth practice at the same rate as in-person visits. This allowed PTs and their employers to continue to deliver physical therapy care with adequate reimbursement during this challenging time.

Not only was the delivery of telehealth physical therapy effective in providing direct care to patients, but Lee[14] notes that a transformation in PT practice took place. Telehealth allowed the preservation of scarce resources, including personal protective equipment, which was in high demand but difficult to access during the pandemic. Telehealth services allowed patients already involved in their course of care to continue with virtual visits so they could continue to benefit from physical therapy and work toward their functional recovery. COVID-19 was a catalyst of sorts for moving physical therapy practice toward embracing virtual digital care, through

telehealth, by PTs out of necessity. Our profession could not abandon our patients in need and thus needed to embrace the clinical practice, regulation, legislation, reimbursement, and scope of telehealth practice.

■ LIMITATIONS IN TELEHEALTH

There are limitations in the delivery of physical therapy using digital technology in the format of telehealth. These include patient and provider lack of access to secure technology, public and professional acceptance of practice, inability to deliver aspects of clinical care, licensure, regulatory guidelines, HIPAA compliance, and reimbursement regulations. See **Table 25-2**.

■ HOW TO DELIVER TELEHEALTH IN VARIOUS SETTINGS

EARLY INTERVENTION

Early intervention providers are already well versed in a coaching model of care. PTs in this setting are focused on the entire family and deliver care in a transdisciplinary model.[16] Early intervention providers and families report both benefits and barriers to the telehealth platform of service delivery.[17]

Benefits to telehealth in early intervention include the following:

- Improved scheduling flexibility
- Improved provider access to rural areas
- Improved caregiver engagement using the coaching method of care
- Ability to continue to provide care despite the restrictions of the COVID-19 pandemic

Limitations to telehealth in early intervention include the following:

- Caregiver access to technology
- Caregiver comfort and knowledge of technology
- Caregiver and practitioner perception that in-person visits are more personal and may be more effective
- Technology fatigue due to ongoing use of screens to deliver care

Emerging evidence on the use of telehealth in early intervention, however, suggests that telehealth may be as equally effective as in-person visits and that the coaching model for intervention is, indeed, considered to be best practice in this service delivery model.[17] Perhaps the forced exposure of clinicians and families to telehealth during the COVID-19 pandemic will help to shift attitudes regarding efficacy and efficiency toward supporting this platform in the future.

SCHOOL BASED

School-based PTs are accustomed to delivering care in a variety of models ranging from direct student care to consultative and collaborative models of care. Through the delivery of telehealth physical therapy, therapists provide virtual visits to individual children or small groups of children to increase their participation in school or, during the COVID-19 pandemic, when they return to school. Ideally, activities should be conducted collaboratively with a teacher if the child is in

TABLE 25-2 • Principles and Limitations to Consider Regarding Telehealth for Physical Therapy Practice[15]	
Technology	• **Connectivity:** Communities with inadequate Internet connectivity may have limited access to telehealth services. Physical therapists (PTs) must ensure equity in access to digital services. • **Technology:** Patients without technology may have limited access to telehealth services. PTs must leverage more cost-effective technology to deliver care. • **Utility:** Therapists and patient may be unable to use the technology. PTs must educate themselves and support the education of their patients on how to use telehealth technology. • **Security and integrity:** Lack of secure HIPAA-compliant technologies. *It is crucial for the practitioner to use secure, HIPAA-compliant technology and have Business Associates Agreements in place with their telehealth vendor and any other related business associates.* • **Quality:** Lack of video quality (eg, lighting, camera resolution, camera height, audio quality, background). PTs need to consider their background to limit distractions or interruptions as well as the child's video quality to achieve the assessment and interventions needed.
Reimbursement and compliance	• **Insurance:** Telehealth may not be recognized for reimbursement by insurance and third-party payers. Ensure codes used for billing are recognized by the payer and advocate/contract for equal reimbursement for services rendered noting that the clinical skills needed are equitable and costs are comparable to face-to-face visits given additional technologies, training, and possibly space. • **Regulation:** PT must ensure compliance with all state practice act and billing/documentation requirements (APTA.org).
Education	• **Training:** PTs need to have the understanding, knowledge, and skills to practice digitally. Each facility should have a policy on what trainings and competencies are needed for successful and safe delivery of telehealth services.
Research	• **Evidence:** PTs must be aware of the telehealth evidence related to digital practice (both positive and lacking evidence). • **Application of current practice:** PTs must apply sound clinical reasoning and follow standards of practice and codes of conduct.
Outcomes	• PTs must routinely assess telehealth service delivery to ensure expected patient outcomes are achieved. This may require intervals of face-to-face visits if manual assessment is needed. • PTs should determine what outcomes can be measured via telehealth and what outcomes may require a face-to-face visit ahead of establishing a plan of care in order to set expectations on service delivery models with the patient or caregivers.
Regulation	• **Laws and regulations:** States differ in their governance over telehealth for physical therapy. It is the responsibility of the PT to be aware of the laws and regulations that govern their practice. • **Compliance:** It is critical for PTs to review their state's laws and regulations, physical therapy practice act, and Medicaid/private payer coverage policies to determine any limitations to using telehealth in the state or district in which they practice. • **PT Compact:** There are several states that belong to the PT Compact. Among those states, if a PT has compact privileges in another of those states, they could deliver telehealth services in accordance with that state's regulations.

school or a parent or caregiver if the child is at home. One example of telehealth services in the school setting would be a video meeting during a preschool motor group with 3 to 4 children. The therapists would collaborate with the teacher ahead of time to develop a list of activities. During the video session, the therapist would consult with the teacher on ways to promote optimal student participation. Another example of telehealth services would be during a video meeting with a parent or caregiver and child who is at home and needs assistance for positioning at home while participating in school activities. For children and families who have limited access to Internet and technology, therapists may provide consultation via telephone calls to discuss and collaborate on home activities. The goals of telehealth services are to maintain or increase a child's access to education and curriculum so that they can fully participate in school activities at home and when they return to the school setting.[18]

Benefits to telehealth in schools include the following:

• Improved provider access to rural schools or across various school districts
• Improved caregiver or teacher engagement when implementing telehealth in small groups, classrooms for observations and instructions, and carryover interventions with families during home-schooling activities

Limitations to Telehealth in Schools include the following:

• School access and comfort with technology
• Teacher and practitioner perception that in-person visits are more personal and may be more effective
• Ensuring service delivery models including telehealth within the child's Individualized Education Program (IEP)
• Time available for a teacher or aide to provide the assistance to deliver physical therapy using telehealth during the school day

OUTPATIENT

Outpatient-based providers traditionally deliver physical therapy services in a clinic setting face to face with their patients. In a telehealth model of outpatient service delivery, PTs use their observational skills during virtual visits to evaluate patients' motor skills and movement patterns in order to make recommendations about positioning, how to use adaptive equipment, or ways to move in the home setting to prevent impairments and facilitate movement activities and participation. Therapists may consult with parents and other caregivers about how they can provide safe hands-on assistance to children who cannot move safely on their own. They may also provide recommendations using verbal feedback on ways to adapt the environment or activity to improve participation in motor activities. Overall, the PT can deliver high-quality therapeutic interventions not requiring manual skills for assessment or treatment to patients through telehealth modalities.

Benefits of telehealth for outpatient physical therapy include the following:

- Improved scheduling flexibility
- Improved provider access for specialty services and when geographically challenged
- Provide in-home (in-community) assessment for improved understanding of natural home environments and how therapy services can enhance function within that environment
- Utilization of technology for health monitoring

Limitations of telehealth for outpatient physical therapy include the following:

- Caregiver access to and comfort with technology
- Caregiver and patient need for manual hands-on interventions to meet outcomes
- Overutilization of telehealth platforms and visits. leading to decreased motivation during session or preference for in-person visits
- Limited equipment access in the home location, leading to failure to meet therapeutic benefit needed
- Limited reimbursement for telehealth services
- Limitations in service delivery as determined by state licensure or governing agencies and across jurisdictions (state to state)

INPATIENT

Inpatient-based providers are usually seeing patients at the bedside in an acute care or acute rehabilitation facility. During the COVID-19 pandemic, there was a demand for increased use of personal protective equipment (PPE) for all patient encounters. This created a shortage globally with a need to conserve PPE. In an effort to decrease utilization of personal protective equipment and limit contact with patients presenting with COVID 19, therapists needed to think of new models of delivery in an acute care setting. Telehealth was a model of direct patient care delivery to enhance caregiver education and even participate remotely in bedside or team rounding on patients without the need to don & use new PPE. Inpatient PTs could leverage use of remote technology for telehealth

visits without the need to enter the patient's room and deliver care with instruction to caregivers, nurses, and other medical providers.

Benefits of telehealth for inpatient physical therapy include the following:

- Access to patients on isolation restrictions within the acute care setting
- Access to specialty services beyond the hospital walls for clinical consultation

Limitations of telehealth for inpatient physical therapy include the following:

- Caregiver and patient need for manual hands-on interventions to meet outcomes, enhance discharge, and ensure safe patient handling and education
- Interactions in rounds when multiple clinicians are attending via telehealth and need to contribute to the rounding process

■ SPECIAL CONSIDERATIONS FOR PEDIATRIC TELEHEALTH SERVICE DELIVERY

The World Confederation of Physiotherapy notes special considerations for the delivery of telehealth, including considerations needed when using digital modalities to engage with vulnerable individuals or groups such as children.[2] Specific consent and participation may be needed by caregivers for the pediatric population. The PT must consider in what circumstances the parent, caregiver, or advocate needs to be present. This relates to patient safety during a telehealth visit, the need for collecting information for evaluation and assessment, and overall performance throughout the telehealth visit.

The PT needs to know their ability to deliver care between state lines and internationally. In some countries, a proliferation of digital service options could result in patients shopping around more for services, leading to discontinuity of care. This can be managed or mitigated in the PT practice setting by having policies regarding patients seeking care with multiple providers for physical therapy. This standard should also apply to telehealth services. Culturally specific considerations may need to be observed when using telehealth services. In some cultures, eye contact is not considered respectful. This may impact a telehealth session when looking at a screen is required. In other cultures, image recording or image capture may be considered inappropriate. The PT/PTA should ask for permission prior to recording or capturing the image of the patient in all situations. The therapist's gender must be considered where disrobing may be required. If the PT does not speak the same language as the patient or family, ancillary services may be required (eg, medical interpreter). Considerations must be made to ensure that the interpreter is familiar with telehealth practice. There needs to be a safety plan in place if a parent is not in the room so that the parent can safely supervise or assist the child or communication can be had with the parent in the event of an emergency or clinical need.

INFORMED CONSENT

Obtaining informed consent is part of a process that ensures compliance with all rules, regulations, and ethical responsibilities and ensures the patient is informed, understands, and is comfortable with treatment via telehealth. The PT should ensure that the consent process meets all state practice act, state law, and payer policies. This may include consideration of written versus oral consent, consent for each visit or one-time consent for the episode of care, consent for specific treatments, and the use of a standardized form for the patient's consent. For pediatric patients, practitioners must verify whether the caregiver, parent, or guardian is required to be present in accordance with state law, malpractice insurance, and/or payer policy. The practitioner must also make sure that informed consent is obtained from the parent or guardian if the patient is a minor.[9,10] Specific to telehealth, it is important to explain to the patient that they are encouraged to ask questions before, during, and after the session and can also stop the session at any time. Patients also have the right to refuse a telehealth session and request an in-person visit at any time. It may also be important to explain that there is the possibility for technical difficulties during the session due to the nature of the online platform.[10]

DOCUMENTATION

Clinical documentation of telehealth visits must adhere to the same rigor as in-person clinical documentation, with several additional components to consider:

- Documentation of start and stop time
- Location of the patient and provider
- Reason patient/caregiver initiated the request for the PT virtual visit
- Consent of patient/caregiver to PT virtual visit
- Documentation of clinical decision-making because this is critical to justify that the visit is necessary and requires the skills of a PT

EQUIPMENT

It is important to establish the need for appropriate equipment related to technology and the therapeutic devices the patient and caregiver will need at home in order to be successful in the implementation and progression of therapy activities. This may include sending a patient home with the progression of therapy bands with instruction to use the lessor of the resistance until the virtual visit when the PT can then progress to greater resistance over time during the virtual visits.

COACHING MODELS OF CARE

According to Rush et al,[16] "Coaching in early childhood is an interactive process of observation and reflection in which the coach promotes a parent's or other care provider's ability to support a child's participation in everyday experiences and interactions with family members and peers across settings. Focusing on collaborative relationships, coaching provides a supportive structure for promoting conversations between family members, childcare providers, and early interventionists to select and implement meaningful strategies to achieve functional

outcomes that focus on the child's participation in natural settings." This model of service delivery is helpful to guide the clinician in the telehealth platform. The clinician observes, reflects, and evaluates the patient in their natural environment and makes recommendations to the patient or caregiver on what to do in order to address impairments, activity limitations, and participation restrictions in order to progress the plan of care.

■ EVALUATIONS VERSUS ESTABLISHED PATIENTS

There are some restrictions in the delivery of telehealth by state licensure and practice acts including the delivery of telehealth with new patients versus patients with established relationships. This may impact the ability to legally perform evaluations via telehealth. Additional considerations for completing evaluations via telehealth are the abilities to obtain the patient/client history and perform tests and measures in order to make the movement system diagnosis and determine the needs of the patient.[19] There may be assessments, tests, and measures that are unable to be completed without an in-person visit such as manual muscle testing, tone and spasticity assessments, and several standardized tests and measures. That considered, there are many assessments that can be completed via telehealth, including formal and informal observational movement assessments.

Case 1

Durable Medical Equipment Delivery

John is an 8-year-old boy with spastic quadriplegic cerebral palsy. He was seen in the outpatient physical therapy clinic for an equipment evaluation prior to the COVID-19 pandemic with his parents, his PT, and his equipment vendor. The team agreed on and measured John for a supine stander, adapted stroller, and bath chair. A letter of medical necessity was generated, and the request was sent to John's insurance company for approval. John's PT received notification from the equipment vendor that John's equipment was approved and that the order had been placed. Three months later, at the beginning of the COVID-19 pandemic, John's PT received notification that the equipment had been delivered to the vendor and was ready for fitting with John and his family. Typically, this visit would take place in the outpatient clinic with the patient, his family, the PT, and the vendor working collaboratively to assure that John was fitting comfortably and safely in his new equipment and that the family felt comfortable with management. However, the outpatient clinic, during this time, had restricted in-person visits to only those patients considered to be urgent. This was established to ensure the safety of the caregivers and the staff. It was determined that equipment follow-up visits of this nature did not fall within that category.

The PT and vendor discussed telehealth as a possible solution to this novel barrier. The family was contacted to discuss the possibility of a telehealth visit in which the vendor would deliver the equipment to the patient's home face to face and the PT would join this visit via a secure, HIPAA-compliant audiovisual platform. The family consented to this visit. On the date of service, the PT successfully joined the visit remotely and provided the vendor and the family guidance and recommendations throughout the visit. John was safely and effectively fitted in his new equipment. The family worked actively with the vendor and under the guidance and coaching of the PT to position John and manage the new equipment. The family felt empowered as an active part of the team and felt supported by the PT who was confident that the family was independent and safe with John's new equipment. This telehealth visit allowed the family to remain safely in their home, eliminating a trip to the hospital and needing to transport equipment back to their home. It is possible that this form of equipment follow-up could be used outside of the pandemic environment to improve efficiencies and decrease unnecessary burden of travel on families while still supporting an effective outcome for the patient and family.

Case 2

A Baby With Congenital Muscular Torticollis

During the COVID-19 pandemic, normal operations in the outpatient clinic were halted for patients who were not considered to be urgent in nature due to safety concerns. This left baby Luke in the care of his parents and without skilled intervention. Luke had been seen in the clinic prior to the pandemic to address a left head tilt and developmental asymmetry associated with congenital muscular torticollis. The parents were proficient in their home exercise program but had noted some development of atypical creeping and were unsuccessful in fully resolving Luke's head tilt. They contacted the physical therapy department and were scheduled for a virtual follow-up with a new provider because their previous provider was unavailable.

Upon initiation of the virtual visit, the clinician introduced herself and offered her credentials as well as cautiously preparing the parents for the visit and its potential barriers from a technology and intervention perspective as this was a new relationship and a new platform for the therapist, family, and patient. All consented to the visit and agreed to proceed. Luke was encouraged to interact and move in his natural environment with his parents while the therapist observed. Dialogue between the therapist and family progressed, and it was quickly identified that Luke was now moving around on the floor on his bottom with an asymmetrical pattern that was driven by his residual head tilt. More observation with the coaching of the therapist revealed mild weakness on the right side of his neck as observed by the Muscle Function Scale that was administered by the parents under the guidance of the PT. After careful consideration, the therapist decided that the family would be able to administer some simple handling in order to mediate the asymmetrical patterns.

Both parents were eager to learn and demonstrated proficiency in a short time with coaching from the PT. It was agreed that the parents would implement these strategies over the next week and reschedule a virtual follow-up visit to reassess and progress the plan of care. During this next visit, Luke had made significant gains in symmetry under the parents' care. The therapist was able to repeat the observation, assessment, and intervention cycle, discussing the parents' concerns regarding asymmetry in the high chair and making recommendations for

intervention accordingly. Each subsequent visit followed a similar pattern, assessing the patient and evaluating parent concerns with appropriate recommendations and follow-through. The patient had full resolution of asymmetry in mobility and posture within 6 visits and was discharged to the parents' care without the need for an in-person visit. The parents had become skilled observers of Luke's movements and had the tools to intervene on their own, having been empowered to do so throughout this virtual plan of care. Telehealth proved to be not only effective in this case but also extremely efficient because the parents had truly learned to be the interventionists and developed the confidence and skill to take over in the home. The parents were thrilled with the results and all remained safe in their homes.

STUDY QUESTIONS

1. What are the similarities and differences between Synchronous and Asynchronous methods of telehealth?

2. Discuss what advantages physical therapy telehealth practice offers to patients, caregivers, service providers, and society?

3. Consider the limitations of telehealth and discuss how they may limit patient access to physical therapy services?

4. Provide benefits and limitations to tehelealth practices in the following treatment settings: School? Outpatient? Acute Care? Early Intervention?

5. How does a coaching model of care impact the delivery of PT services via telehealth in pediatrics?

References

1. Exum E, Hull BL, Lee AC, Gumieny A, Villarreal C, Longnecker D. Applying telehealth technologies and strategies to provide acute care consultation and treatment of patients with confirmed or possible COVID-19. *J Acute Care Phys Ther.* 2020;11(3):103-112.

2. World Confederation of Physiotherapy/International Network of Physiotherapy Regulatory Authorities. Report of the WCPT/INPTRA Digital Physical Therapy Practice Task Force. World Confederation of Physiotherapy/International Network of Physiotherapy Regulatory Authorities. Published March 2020. Accessed August 20, 2022. https://world.physio/sites/default/files/2020-06/WCPT-INPTRA-Digital-Physical-Therapy-Practice-Task-force-March2020.pdf.

3. American Physical Therapy Association. Telehealth HODP06-19-15-09. Published September 20, 2019. Accessed August 19, 2022. https://www.apta.org/apta-and-you/leadership-and-governance/policies/telehealth.

4. Jerant AF, Epperly TD. Fundamentals of telemedicine. *Mil Med.* 1997;162(4):304-309.

5. Lee AC, Harada N. Telehealth as a means of health care delivery for physical therapist practice. *Phys Ther.* 2012;92(3):463-468.

6. Calouro C, Kwong MW, Gutierrez M. An analysis of state telehealth laws and regulations for occupational therapy and physical therapy. *Int J Telerehabil.* 2014;6(1):17-23.

7. Bierman RT, Kwong MW, Calouro C. State occupational and physical therapy telehealth laws and regulations: a 50-state survey. *Int J Telerehabil.* 2018;10(2):3-54.

8. Federation of State Boards of Physical Therapy. General information about interstate compacts. Published 2022. Accessed August 19, 2022. https://www.fsbpt.org/Free-Resources/Physical-Therapy-Licensure-Compact/General-Information.

9. American Physical Therapy Association. Telehealth. Published September 20, 2019. Accessed August 19, 2022. https://www.apta.org/apta-and-you/leadership-and-governance/policies/telehealth.

10. American Physical Therapy Association. Telehealth state and federal regulations and legislation. Published December 22, 2020. Accessed August 19, 2022. https://www.apta.org/your-practice/practice-models-and-settings/telehealth-practice/state-regulations.

11. US Department of Health and Human Services. Health It Playbook. HealthIT.gov. March 11, 2020. Accessed August 19, 2022. https://www.healthit.gov/playbook/patient-engagement/#section-5-3. Published

12. American Physical Therapy Association. Telehealth modalities PTs and PTAs can use during the public health emergency. Published December 16, 2020. Accessed August 19, 2022. https://www.apta.org/your-practice/practice-models-and-settings/telehealth-practice/telehealth-modalities-that-pts-and-ptas-can-use-during-the-public-health-emergency.

13. US Department of Health and Human Services. Asynchronous direct-to-consumer telehealth. Telehealth.HHS.gov. Published February 9, 2021. Accessed August 19, 2022. https://telehealth.hhs.gov/providers/direct-to-consumer/asynchronous-direct-to-consumer-telehealth/.

14. Lee AC. Covid-19 and the advancement of digital physical therapist practice and telehealth. *Phys Ther*. 2020;100(7):1054-1057.

15. American Physical Therapy Association. Telehealth state and federal regulations and legislation. Published December 22, 2020. Accessed August 19, 2022. https://www.apta.org/your-practice/practice-models-and-settings/telehealth-practice/state-regulations.

16. Rush DD, Shelden MLL, Hanft BE. Coaching families and colleagues. *Infants Young Child*. 2003;16(1):33-47.

17. Cole B, Pickard K, Stredler-Brown A. Report on the use of telehealth in early intervention in Colorado: strengths and challenges with telehealth as a service delivery method. *Int J Telerehabil*. 2019;11(1):33-40.

18. Hall JB, Luechtefeld JT, Woods ML. Adoption of telehealth by pediatric physical therapists during COVID-19: a survey study. *Pediatr Phys Ther*. 2021;33(4):237-244.

19. American Physical Therapy Association. Guide to Physical Therapist Practice. Second Edition. American Physical Therapy Association. *Phys Ther*. 2001;81(1):9-746.

Appendices

Appendix 1-1

Applying Developmental Theories to a Play Activity

Apply the discussed development theories in this chapter to tasks including swinging a bat and walking. Use the information in Chapter 1 as a guide for your answer.

EXAMPLE: KICKING A SOCCER BALL

Dynamical systems theory	A developing child's body will grow and develop. This growth and development occur because of a combined interaction of:
	• The internal body systems (eg, cardiorespiratory system, musculoskeletal system, and neuromuscular system)
	• The external environmental systems (eg, amount of play area to explore, toys, other children to observe play)
	• The tasks that are given to the child (those activities that motivate the child's behavior)
	If the child is given the opportunity (affordances) to participate in learning to manipulate a ball, and the child's constraints work in favor of the child learning about foot and ball manipulation, then motor patterns will emerge in which the child learns to play and kick a ball.
Neuronal group selection theory	When a child is developing in utero they will begin to show movement. This initial movement originates in the activation of specific cortical structures that cause movement of the developing fetus (primary variability). As the fetus develops sensory organs that interact with the brain, it begins to learn from these movements, which furthers the development of a feedback mechanism. As this feedback mechanism advances in the infant and child, they learn from the interaction of the body and its environment. This progressive learning evolves into more and more mature movement activities, with greater expression of variation in movements. This continued development of movement is an ongoing interaction of neural control, gene expression, and environmental influences that eventually lead to learning the skill of kicking a ball.
Schema and motor programming theory	Children learn to move their body by performing tasks that build on previously learned tasks.
	Learning to kick a ball is a specific skill that, when practiced, will progressively lead to refined coordination of the activity of kicking a ball. Practice is very important for this skill to be achieved at a proficient level. The motor memory advances as this skill is worked on. Initial kicking practice will result in immature kicking patterns. There will most likely be invariant features of the movement; however, as the skill improves, the parameters of the task, including the force and speed, will change, leading to an improved kicking pattern.

AMERICAN SPINAL INJURY ASSOCIATION

INTERNATIONAL STANDARDS FOR NEUROLOGICAL CLASSIFICATION OF SPINAL CORD INJURY (ISNCSCI)

ISCoS INTERNATIONAL SPINAL CORD SOCIETY

Patient Name _____   Date/Time of Exam _____

Examiner Name _____   Signature _____

RIGHT

LEFT

MOTOR KEY MUSCLES

SENSORY KEY SENSORY POINTS

MOTOR KEY MUSCLES

Light Touch (LTR) Pin Prick (PPR)

Light Touch (LTL) Pin Prick (PPL)

C2
C3
C4

UER (Upper Extremity Right)
Elbow flexors C5
Wrist extensors C6
Elbow extensors C7
Finger flexors C8
Finger abductors (little finger) T1

UEL (Upper Extremity Left)
C5 Elbow flexors
C6 Wrist extensors
C7 Elbow extensors
C8 Finger flexors
T1 Finger abductors (little finger)

T2
T3
T4
T5
T6
T7
T8
T9
T10
T11
T12
L1

Comments (Non-key Muscle? Reason for NT? Pain? Non-SCI condition?):

MOTOR (SCORING ON REVERSE SIDE)
0 = Total paralysis
1 = Palpable or visible contraction
2 = Active movement, gravity eliminated
3 = Active movement, against gravity
4 = Active movement, against some resistance
5 = Active movement, against full resistance
NT = Not testable
0*, 1*, 2*, 3*, 4*, NT* = Non-SCI condition present

SENSORY (SCORING ON REVERSE SIDE)
0 = Absent   NT = Not testable
1 = Altered   0*, 1*, NT* = Non-SCI
2 = Normal   condition present

LER (Lower Extremity Right)
Hip flexors L2
Knee extensors L3
Ankle dorsiflexors L4
Long toe extensors L5
Ankle plantar flexors S1

LEL (Lower Extremity Left)
L2 Hip flexors
L3 Knee extensors
L4 Ankle dorsiflexors
L5 Long toe extensors
S1 Ankle plantar flexors

S2
S3
S4-5

(VAC) Voluntary Anal Contraction (Yes/No)

RIGHT TOTALS (MAXIMUM)   (50)

(56)   (56)

(56)   (56)

LEFT TOTALS (MAXIMUM)   (50)

(DAP) Deep Anal Pressure (Yes/No)

• Key Sensory Points

Palm   C6
C5
T1
T2
C6
Dorsum

C2
C3
C4
C2
C3
C4
T3
T4
T5
T6
T7
T8
T9
T10
T11
T12
L1
L2
L3
L4
L5
S3
S4-5
S2
L2
L3
L4
L5
S1

MOTOR SUBSCORES

UER [ ] + UEL [ ] = UEMS TOTAL [ ]
MAX (25)   (25)   (50)

LER [ ] + LEL [ ] = LEMS TOTAL [ ]
MAX (25)   (25)   (50)

SENSORY SUBSCORES

LTR [ ] + LTL [ ] = LT TOTAL [ ]
MAX (56)   (56)   (112)

PPR [ ] + PPL [ ] = PP TOTAL [ ]
MAX (56) (56)   (112)

NEUROLOGICAL LEVELS
Steps 1 - 6 for classification as on reverse

	R	L
1. SENSORY		
2. MOTOR		

3. **NEUROLOGICAL LEVEL OF INJURY** (NLI) [ ]

4. **COMPLETE OR INCOMPLETE?**
Incomplete = Any sensory or motor function in S4-5 [ ]

5. **ASIA IMPAIRMENT SCALE (AIS)** [ ]

6. **ZONE OF PARTIAL PRESERVATION**
Most caudal levels with any innervation

	R	L
SENSORY		
MOTOR		

(In injuries with absent motor OR sensory function in S4-5 only)

This form may be copied freely but should not be altered without permission from the American Spinal Injury Association.

Page 1/2   REV 04/19

Muscle Function Grading

0 = Total paralysis

1 = Palpable or visible contraction

2 = Active movement, full range of motion (ROM) with gravity eliminated

3 = Active movement, full ROM against gravity

4 = Active movement, full ROM against gravity and moderate resistance in a muscle specific position

5 = (Normal) active movement, full ROM against gravity and full resistance in a functional muscle position expected from an otherwise unimpaired person

NT = Not testable (i.e. due to immobilization, severe pain such that the patient cannot be graded, amputation of limb, or contracture of > 50% of the normal ROM)

0*, 1*, 2*, 3*, 4*, NT* = Non-SCI condition present[a]

Sensory Grading

0 = Absent **1** = Altered, either decreased/impaired sensation or hypersensitivity

2 = Normal **NT** = Not testable

0*, 1*, NT* = Non-SCI condition present[a]

[a] Note: Abnormal motor and sensory scores should be tagged with a '*' to indicate an impairment due to a non-SCI condition. The non-SCI condition should be explained in the comments box together with information about how the score is rated for classification purposes (at least normal / not normal for classification).

When to Test Non-Key Muscles:

In a patient with an apparent AIS B classification, non-key muscle functions more than 3 levels below the motor level on each side should be tested to most accurately classify the injury (differentiate between AIS B and C).

Movement	Root level
Shoulder: Flexion, extension, abduction, adduction, internal and external rotation **Elbow:** Supination	C5
Elbow: Pronation **Wrist:** Flexion	C6
Finger: Flexion at proximal joint, extension **Thumb:** Flexion, extension and abduction in plane of thumb	C7
Finger: Flexion at MCP joint **Thumb:** Opposition, adduction and abduction perpendicular to palm	C8
Finger: Abduction of the index finger	T1
Hip: Adduction	L2
Hip: External rotation	L3
Hip: Extension, abduction, internal rotation **Knee:** Flexion **Ankle:** Inversion and eversion **Toe:** MP and IP extension	L4
Hallux and Toe: DIP and PIP flexion and abduction	L5
Hallux: Adduction	S1

ASIA Impairment Scale (AIS)

A = Complete. No sensory or motor function is preserved in the sacral segments S4-5.

B = Sensory Incomplete. Sensory but not motor function is preserved below the neurological level and includes the sacral segments S4-5 (light touch or pin prick at S4-5 or deep anal pressure) AND no motor function is preserved more than three levels below the motor level on either side of the body.

C = Motor Incomplete. Motor function is preserved at the most caudal sacral segments for voluntary anal contraction (VAC) OR the patient meets the criteria for sensory incomplete status (sensory function preserved at the most caudal sacral segments S4-5 by LT, PP or DAP), and has some sparing of motor function more than three levels below the ipsilateral motor level on either side of the body. (This includes key or non-key muscle functions to determine motor incomplete status.) For AIS C – less than half of key muscle functions below the single NLI have a muscle grade ≥ 3.

D = Motor Incomplete. Motor incomplete status as defined above, with at least half (half or more) of key muscle functions below the single NLI having a muscle grade ≥ 3.

E = Normal. If sensation and motor function as tested with the ISNCSCI are graded as normal in all segments, and the patient had prior deficits, then the AIS grade is E. Someone without an initial SCI does not receive an AIS grade.

Using ND: To document the sensory, motor and NLI levels, the ASIA Impairment Scale grade, and/or the zone of partial preservation (ZPP) when they are unable to be determined based on the examination results.

Steps in Classification

The following order is recommended for determining the classification of individuals with SCI.

1. Determine sensory levels for right and left sides.
The sensory level is the most caudal, intact dermatome for both pin prick and light touch sensation.

2. Determine motor levels for right and left sides.
Defined by the lowest key muscle function that has a grade of at least 3 (on supine testing), providing the key muscle functions represented by segments above that level are judged to be intact (graded as a 5).
Note: in regions where there is no myotome to test, the motor level is presumed to be the same as the sensory level, if testable motor function above that level is also normal.

3. Determine the neurological level of injury (NLI).
This refers to the most caudal segment of the cord with intact sensation and antigravity (3 or more) muscle function strength, provided that there is normal (intact) sensory and motor function rostrally respectively.
The NLI is the most cephalad of the sensory and motor levels determined in steps 1 and 2.

4. Determine whether the injury is Complete or Incomplete.
(i.e. absence or presence of sacral sparing)
*If voluntary anal contraction = No AND all S4-5 sensory scores = 0 AND deep anal pressure = No, then injury is **Complete**. Otherwise, injury is **Incomplete**.*

5. Determine ASIA Impairment Scale (AIS) Grade.

Is injury Complete? If YES, AIS=A

NO ↓

Is injury Motor Complete? If YES, AIS=B

NO ↓
(No=voluntary anal contraction OR motor function more than three levels below the motor level on a given side, if the patient has sensory incomplete classification)

Are at least half (half or more) of the key muscles below the neurological level of injury graded 3 or better?

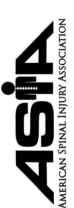

NO ↓ YES ↓

AIS=C   AIS=D

If sensation and motor function is normal in all segments, AIS=E
Note: AIS E is used in follow-up testing when an individual with a documented SCI has recovered normal function. If at initial testing no deficits are found, the individual is neurologically intact and the ASIA Impairment Scale does not apply.

6. Determine the zone of partial preservation (ZPP).
The ZPP is used only in injuries with absent motor (no VAC) OR sensory function (no DAP, no LT and no PP sensation) in the lowest sacral segments S4-5, and refers to those dermatomes and myotomes caudal to the sensory and motor levels that remain partially innervated. With sacral sparing of sensory function, the sensory ZPP is not applicable and therefore "NA" is recorded in the block of the worksheet. Accordingly, if VAC is present, the motor ZPP is not applicable and is noted as "NA".

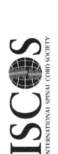

AMERICAN SPINAL INJURY ASSOCIATION

ISCOS
INTERNATIONAL SPINAL CORD SOCIETY

INTERNATIONAL STANDARDS FOR NEUROLOGICAL CLASSIFICATION OF SPINAL CORD INJURY

Page 2/2

Appendix 11-1

Resources for Autism Spectrum Disorder

■ ONLINE RESOURCES

Centers for Disease Control and Prevention (CDC) Act Early Campaign and Milestone Tracker app:

- https://www.cdc.gov/ncbddd/actearly/index.html
- https://www.cdc.gov/ncbddd/actearly/milestones-app.html

American Academy of Pediatrics, Developmental Screening Technical Assistance and Resource Center (STAR)

- https://www.aap.org/en/patient-care/screening-technical-assistance-and-resource-center/

CDC Screening and Diagnosis of Autism Spectrum Disorder for Healthcare Providers

- https://www.cdc.gov/autism/hcp/diagnosis/screening.html

American Physical Therapy Association Fact Sheet: Autism: Current Practice Resources for Physical Therapists

- https://pediatricapta.org/includes/fact-sheets/pdfs/14%20Autism%20Current%20Practice%20Resources.pdf

AUTISM SPEAKS

- Autism Speaks toolkits (resource guides by life stage and audience): https://www.autismspeaks.org/resource-guide
- ABA family toolkit: https://www.autismspeaks.org/toolkit/atnair-p-parents-guide-applied-behavior-analysis

AUTISM SPECTRUM AUSTRALIA (ASPECT)

- http://www.autismspectrum.org.au/
- A variety of autism fact sheets available related to topics (eg, siblings, positive behavior support, mental health and wellbeing, coping with death)
- https://www.facebook.com/AutismSpectrumAustralia/
- Writing social stories

CANCHILD

- Autism spectrum disorder: https://canchild.ca/en/diagnoses/autism-spectrum-disorder
- Offers a variety of resources including ACSF:SC (Autism Classification System of Functioning: Social Communication)
  - https://canchild.ca/en/resources/254-autism-classification-system-of-functioning-social-communication-acsf-sc

SOCIAL STORIES AND OTHER COMMUNICATION RESOURCES

- https://www.autism.org.uk/advice-and-guidance/topics/communication/communication-tools
- https://carolgraysocialstories.com/

Appendix 22-1

Sample Post-Secondary Education Transition Checklist

Today's Date:
Student Name:
DOB:
Anticipated Graduation (month/year):
Name and role* of individual(s) involved in transition planning:
1.
2.
3.
4.
5.
6.
*(teacher, guidance counselor, ESE coordinator, college admissions counselor, vocational rehab case coordinator, advocate, waiver support coordinator, occupational/physical therapist, speech language pathologist, mental health counselor)

Student's Transition Goals:
• Personal/leisure/community participation:
  ◦ Resources needed:
  ◦ Essential transition team members/support personnel:
  ◦ Supplemental programs/supports available:
• Education/training (may include academic, vocational, independent living training):
  ◦ Resources needed:
  ◦ Essential transition team members/support personnel:
  ◦ Supplemental programs/supports available:
• Career/employment:
  ◦ Resources needed:
  ◦ Essential transition team members/support personnel:
  ◦ Supplemental programs/supports available:

	YES/NO	Comments/Plans for follow-up	Team member initials	Student initials
Personal/leisure/community participation goal(s) discussed				
Education/training goal discussed				
Career/employment goal discussed				
Legal decision-making status (eg, independence, guardianship, health surrogate) discussed, information, and resources provided				
Transition to adult healthcare/primary care physician discussed, information, and resources provided				
Waiver programs discussed (eligibility and availability), information, and resources provided				
Post-secondary living options discussed, information, and resources provided				
Transportation options discussed/ training initiated: 1. Para-transport 2. Public transportation 3. Driving	1. 2. 3.			
Vocational rehabilitation services/options discussed. Evaluation initiated if appropriate				
Healthy habits discussed, information, and resources provided (physical activity and fitness adult groups and organizations)				
Social supports and resources discussed, initiated (adult support groups, special interest groups, community clubs)				
Other:				
Other:				

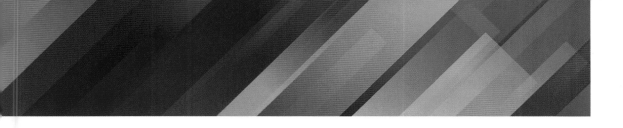

Glossary

6-Minute Walk Test (6MWT): Functional assessment of endurance that measures how far an individual can walk in 6 minutes.

Activities of daily living (ADLs): Activities related to independent living such as dressing, preparing meals, bathing, and mobility.

Adapted toys: Toys that are adapted with special features for children with disabilities.

AGA: Appropriate for gestational age.

Aids for daily living: Any product, device, or equipment used in everyday, functional activities such as feeding, dressing, and attending to personal hygiene.

Alerting devices: Devices designed to alert a person with a hearing impairment that some condition is occurring, such as a smoke alarm or a doorbell ring.

Americans with Disabilities Education Act (ADA): A civil rights law that prohibits discrimination against individuals with disabilities in all areas of public life, including jobs, schools, transportations, and all public and private places open to the general public.

Ankle-foot-orthosis (AFO): An orthotic device that provides functional support, positioning, or restriction of undesired movement at the ankle joint and foot.

Apgar: 8^1 9^5 indicates a score of 8 at 1 minute, and a score of 9 at 5 minutes.

Applied behavior analysis (ABA): A form of therapy based on the science of learning and behavior, that aims to increase desired behaviors to facilitate learning, and reduce behaviors that negatively impact learning.

ART: Artificial reproductive technology.

ASD: Atrial septal defect.

Asphyxia: A condition in which there is a deficiency of oxygen and an increase in carbon dioxide in the blood and tissues. Perinatal asphyxia is lack of oxygen just prior to, during, or shortly after birth.

Aspiration: Breathing a foreign substance such as meconium, formula, or stomach contents into the lungs.

Assistive technology (AT): Any item, piece of equipment, or product system, whether acquired commercially off the shelf, modified, or customized, that is used to increase, maintain, or improve functional capabilities of individuals with disabilities.

Assistive technology professional (ATP): A certification process that demonstrates that a person has met competence in analyzing the needs of consumers with disabilities in the selection of appropriate AT and providing training in the use of the selected devices.

Assistive technology services: The evaluation of the needs of a consumer in the purchasing, leasing, or acquisition of specific AT. Also includes selecting, designing, fitting, customizing, adapting, applying, maintaining, repairing, or replacing specific devices and coordinating and using other services such as therapy, education, rehabilitation, and vocational training or technical assistance or training for professionals or others who provide services to the child.

Atelectasis: Collapse of the air sacs in the lungs.

Augmentative alternative communication (AAC): A set of devices, tools, and strategies that an individual uses to solve everyday communication challenges.

Augmentative and alternative communication (AAC): Ways to communicate without talking. AAC can be unaided (eg, gestures, sign language) or aided (eg, picture boards, computer technology).

BAER: Brainstem auditory evoked response test; a method for early detection of hearing loss in neonates in which brain wave response to a variety of sound levels is assessed.

Betamethasone: A steroid given to a mother before a threatened preterm birth to help the baby's lungs mature.

Bilirubin: A yellowish substance produced when red blood cells break down; may cause jaundice, and in large amounts, kernicterus, with resultant basal ganglia damage and possible athetoid-type cerebral palsy.

Biological hazard: A hazard of organic origin or conveyed by biological vectors, including pathogenic microorganisms, toxins, and bioactive substances. Examples are bacteria, viruses (eg, SARS-CoV-2, which was responsible for the COVID-19 pandemic), parasites, venomous wildlife and insects, poisonous plants, and mosquitoes carrying disease-causing agents.

Blood gas: A sample of blood that measures the amount of oxygen, carbon dioxide, and acid it contains; ABG—arterial blood gas; CBG—capillary blood gas; VBG—venous blood gas.

Bottom-up approach: Approach to treat the underlying deficit with the goal of positively affecting function.

Bronchopulmonary dysplasia: An iatrogenic condition characterized by changes and alterations of the normal development of the air passages of the lungs and lung tissues. Generally occurs following prolonged treatment with a respirator.

Capacity building: The process of providing knowledge, skills, competence, strategies, and resources to meet current and future needs.

CDH: Congenital diaphragmatic hernia.

Chalasia: Relaxation or immaturity of the sphincter between the esophagus and the stomach, resulting in vomiting; may be referred to as gastroesophageal reflux disease.

CHARGE association: Coloboma of the eye, heart defects, atresia of the nasal choanae, delay of growth development, genital hypoplasia, ear anomalies, and deafness.

CHD: Congenital hip dislocation.

Children's Hospital of Philadelphia Infant Test for Neuromuscular Disorder scale (CHOP INTEND): 16-item scale designed specifically to capture motor function in infants with spinal muscular atrophy (SMA) type I.

CLD: Chronic lung disease.

Clinical practice guideline: Evidence-based statement that includes recommendations for patient care.

CMV: Conventional mechanical ventilation.

CMV infection: Cytomegalovirus (CMV) infection.

Complementary and alternative medicine (CAM): Medical treatments and practices that are not part of standard care and while some are supported by research, some may lack scientific evidence for effectiveness and/or safety.

Congenital myopathies (CMs): Genetic muscle disorders that involve abnormal myofiber structure and/or abnormal protein accumulation in the sarcoplasm and that present with hypotonia, slowly progressing or nonprogressing weakness, reduced endurance, and pain.

Consultation: The formal act of discussion. In a therapeutic setting, team members come together to discuss expectations and problem solve.

Coordination: The organization of components of a motor activity to allow for accurate completion of that task.

CPAP: Continuous positive airway pressure; the constant flow of high pressure being blown into the lungs.

CVL: Central venous line.

C-X or C-SECT: Cesarean section.

Developmental coordination disorder (DCD): A neurodevelopmental diagnosis resulting in challenges with acquisition and refinement of motor skills. For individuals with DCD, completion of activities of daily ADLs living is challenging.

Developmental domains: The five areas of child development—motor (gross motor and fine motor), language (expressive and receptive), cognitive, adaptive (self-help), and social.

Disaster: A serious disruption of the functioning of a community or a society at any scale due to hazardous events interacting with conditions of exposure, vulnerability, and capacity, leading to one or more of the following: human, material, economic, and environmental losses and impacts.

Disaster management: The organization, planning, and application of measures preparing for, responding to, and recovering from disasters.

Disseminated intravascular coagulation: A condition in which the platelets and other clotting factors of the blood are consumed because of infection, hypoxia, acidosis, or other diseases or injuries; this results in excessive bleeding and often requires transfusions.

Duchenne muscular dystrophy (DMD): The most common of the childhood muscular dystrophies, characterized by mutations that result in no functional dystrophin production.

Ductus arteriosus: A fetal blood vessel extending from the pulmonary artery to the aorta.

Dystrophin: A protein naturally present in skeletal and cardiac muscle, but also in other tissues such the brain and in the retina. In muscle, it plays a role in stabilization of the sarcolemma during muscle contraction and for appropriate force transmission and is also important in cell signaling, calcium homeostasis, and the nitric oxide pathways.

Dystrophinopathies: Diseases caused by some type of mutation in the *DMD* gene located in the short arm of the X chromosome.

Eclampsia: Toxemia of pregnancy, accompanied by high blood pressure, albuminuria, oliguria, tonic and clonic convulsions, and coma; may occur before, during, or after childbirth.

ECMO: Extracorporeal membrane oxygenation

EDC: Expectant date of confinement.

Egen Klassifikation (EK) scale: Functional scale focused on activities of daily life for use with children who are not ambulatory, which also includes coughing ability.

ELBW: Extremely low birth weight (<1000 g).

Electronic aids to daily living (EADLs); also known as environmental control units (ECUs): Voice activation, switch access, or computer interface devices that interact and manipulate electronic appliances such as televisions, radios, phones, lights, or fans using voice activation, switch access, or a computer interface.

Emergency: Sometimes used interchangeably with the term *disaster*, as, for example, in the context of biological and technological hazards or health emergencies. However, emergencies can also relate to hazardous events that do not result in the serious disruption of the functioning of a community or society.

Empowerment: An individual's ability to have control over decision-making about their present and future life.

Endotracheal intubation: Passage of a small plastic tube through the trachea, past the vocal cords, and into the bronchial tree for assisted ventilation.

Environmental hazard: A hazard that may include chemical, natural, and biological activity. They can be created by environmental degradation or physical or chemical pollution in the air, water, and soil. However, many of the processes and phenomena that fall into this category may be termed drivers of hazard and risk rather than hazards in themselves, such as soil degradation, deforestation, loss of biodiversity, salinization, and sea-level rise.

Erythroblastosis fetalis: Blood type incompatibility between the mother and baby, causing maternal antibodies to attack neonatal blood cells and causing severe anemia and jaundice in the newborn.

Eteplirsen: A drug that promotes dystrophin production by excision of exon 51 and is used in patients with Duchenne muscular dystrophy.

Executive function: Higher-level cognitive skills that allow for organization of resources to complete a task.

FAS: Fetal alcohol syndrome.

Free and appropriate public education (FAPE): One of the primary purposes of Individuals with Disabilities Education Act (IDEA), which provides a FAPE to children with disabilities.

FTT: Failure to thrive.

GA: Gestational age.

Gavage feeding: Feedings given through a tube passed through the nose or mouth and into the stomach in babies who may be too immature to bottle feed, who are medically unable to bottle or breastfeed, or who are unable to feed orally.

GBS: Group B streptococci.

Generalization of skill: The ability to use a skill developed in one setting and apply it to a novel setting or situation.

Geological or geophysical hazard: A hazard that originates from internal earth processes. Examples are earthquakes, volcanic activity and emissions, and related geophysical processes such as mass movements, landslides, rockslides, surface collapses, and debris or mud flows. Hydrometeorological factors are important contributors to some of these processes. Tsunamis are difficult to categorize; although they are triggered by undersea earthquakes and other geological events, they essentially become an oceanic process that is manifested as a coastal water-related hazard.

GERD: Gastroesophageal reflux disease.

Glucocorticoids: A class of corticosteroids that are well established in the treatment of the child with Duchenne muscular dystrophy. Long-term use of glucocorticoids results in slower progression of muscle degeneration and damage, with prolonged functional use of lower extremities, upper extremities, and respiratory muscles.

Goal Attainment Scale: A 5-point rating scale that allows for measurement of criterion-referenced, functional goals.

Gower sign: A clinical sign of proximal lower extremity muscle weakness that consists of using the upper extremities to "walk" up the body during a floor to stand transfer.

Hammersmith Functional Motor Scale–Expanded (HFMSE): Key outcome measure in SMA clinical trials; gives objective information on motor ability and clinical progression for individuals with type II and type III SMA.

Hazard: A process, phenomenon, or human activity that may cause loss of life, injury, or other health impacts; property damage; social and economic disruption; or environmental degradation.

HBF: Fetal hemoglobin.

Healthcare transition: The purposeful, planned movement of adolescents and young adults with chronic physical and medical conditions from child- or family-centered to adult-oriented health care systems.

HELLP: Hemolysis, elevated liver enzymes, low platelets count.

HFJV: High-frequency jet ventilation.

HFNC: High-flow nasal cannula.

HFOV: High-frequency oscillation ventilation.

HIE: Hypoxic-ischemia encephalopathy.

High-tech devices: Devices that are the most complex. They may have digital or electric features, are more customizable to suit the needs of the user, and require training.

Hip-knee-ankle-foot orthosis (HKAFO): An orthotic device that provides functional support, positioning, or restriction of undesired movement at the hip joint, knee joint, ankle joint, and foot.

HMD: Hyaline membrane disease, respiratory disease that affects preterm babies; it is caused by a lack of surfactant, a substance that prevents collapse of the alveoli.

HSV: Herpes simplex virus

Human Activity Assistive Technology (HAAT) Model: Exemplifies AT usability by describing the interaction of a user with an AT (device) to accomplish an activity in a given context.

Human-technology interface (HTI): The interaction between humans and technology.

Hydrometeorological hazard: A hazard of atmospheric, hydrological, or oceanographic origin. Examples are tropical cyclones (also known as typhoons and hurricanes); floods, including flash floods; drought; heatwaves and cold spells; and coastal storm surges. Hydrometeorological conditions may also be a factor in other hazards such as landslides, wildland fires, locust plagues, epidemics, and in the transport and dispersal of toxic substances and volcanic eruption material.

Hyperalimentation: Intravenous administration of glucose, protein, minerals, and vitamins; used when oral feedings cannot be initiated; this is also called total parenteral nutrition.

IDM: Infant of diabetic mother.

IGG: Immunoglobulin indicative transfer from mom to baby.

IGM: Immunologic indicative of baby (viral test).

Individualized Education Plan (IEP): Mandated by IDEA; a written plan for children and adults age 3 to 21 who attend public schools and are eligible for special education.

Individualized Family Service Plan (IFSP): Mandated by IDEA; a written plan for children age 0 to 3 years that describes a child's current needs and prescribes the services needed to support the family and child's development.

Individuals with Disabilities Education Act (IDEA): A federal law that ensures students with disabilities are provided with free and appropriate public education (FAPE) that is tailored to their individual needs.

Indomethacin: A drug used to close the patent ductus arteriosus.

Interdisciplinary team: A group of providers from different fields who work together or toward the same goal to provide the best care or outcome for patients.

International Classification of Functioning, Disability and Health (ICF): A framework for organizing information on functioning and disability. It provides a standard language and a conceptual basis for the definition and measurement of health and disability.

Intrinsic enablers: Part of the HAAT Model that describes the user's abilities in motor, sensory, cognitive, and affective areas and includes the user's roles and AT experience.

IUGR: Intrauterine growth retardation.

IVH: Intraventricular hemorrhage.

Knee-ankle-foot orthosis (KAFO): An orthotic device that provides functional support, positioning, or restriction of undesired movement at the knee joint, ankle joint, and foot.

Learning aids: Any equipment, tools, and devices that aid in the learning and development process of an individual.

LBW: Low birth weight (between 1501 and 2500 g).

LGA: Large for gestational age (>4000 g).

LMP: Last menstrual period.

Loading dose: Sufficient amount of medication to obtain a therapeutic blood level.

Lordotic stance: Biomechanical postural changes that occur in DMD over time that include a progressive increase in lumbar lordosis, posterior weight shift to promote antigravity control of the hip, and increased anterior pelvic tilt due to hip flexor tightness.

Low-tech devices: Devices that are simple to make and easy to obtain. These types of AT do not require a battery or much training, may have a lower cost, and do not have mechanical features or complex functions.

LPI: Late preterm infant.

LS ratio: A ratio between two factors in surfactant (lecithin and sphingomyelin) in the amniotic fluid; this ratio is used as an indicator of lung maturity in the fetus.

MAP: Mean arterial pressure

MAS: Meconium aspiration syndrome.

Medicaid: A state and federal program that provides health coverage for low-income individuals.

Medicare: A federal program that provides health coverage for individuals over 65 years old, or less than 65 if they have a disability, regardless of income.

Mid-tech devices: AT devices that have more complex features, are more expensive, may be electric or battery operated, and may require some training to learn how to use.

Motor function measure (MFM): Functional assessment of motor skills with 32 items in three subsections—standing and transfers, axial and proximal motor capacity, and distal motor capacity.

Muscular dystrophies: A diverse collection of inherited disorders that affect the muscle component of the motor unit and can be classified in several ways including age of onset, rate of progression, genotype, and other factors. The hallmark of muscular dystrophies is insidious weakness accompanied by secondary impairments such as contractures, postural changes, pathologic biomechanics, decreased endurance, difficulties with functional tasks, and impaired motor development when the onset occurs during childhood or infancy.

NAS: Neonatal abstinence syndrome.

NCPAP: Variable flow nasal continuous positive airway pressure.

NEC: Necrotizing enterocolitis.

Neonate: A baby less than 4 weeks of age.

Neuromuscular diseases: Diseases that affect any of the components of the motor unit, including the motor neuron, peripheral nerves, neuromuscular junction, and muscle. In these diseases, dysfunction of the motor unit results in loss of strength, range of motion, and functional abilities.

NICU: Neonatal intensive care unit.

NIDCAP: Newborn individualized developmental care assessment program.

NIICU: Neonatal intermediate intensive care unit or step-down neonatal unit.

NO: Nitric oxide.

Nonnutritive sucking: Sucking on finger or pacifier, purpose is not for oral intake.

Nonoptical aids: Assist a person with a visual impairment through more low-tech tools such as high contrast, large print publication, and text reading software.

North Star Ambulatory Assessment (NSAA): Functional assessment for preclinical or ambulatory assessment of DMD.

NPO: Nothing by mouth.

Nusinersen: An antisense oligonucleotide that targets *SMN2*, resulting in an increase in functional production of survival motor neuron (SMN) protein. It is administered by intrathecal injection and results in improvement of motor function for pediatric patients with type II and type III SMA and improved survival in pediatric patients with type I SMA.

OFC: Occipital frontal circumference head size measurement.

Oligohydramnios: A greatly reduced amount of amniotic fluid.

OOP: Osteopenia of prematurity.

Optical magnification aids: Assist a person with a visual impairment by magnifying text or pictures to read more easily.

PaCO$_2$: Partial pressure of carbon dioxide in arterial blood.

Pancuronium bromide (Pavulon): A drug that acts on the myoneural junction and produces temporary paralysis; often used to prevent a baby from "fighting" the respirator.

PaO$_2$: Partial pressure of oxygen in arterial blood.

Patent ductus arteriosus: A condition in which this vessel fails to close after birth, which results in poor oxygenation and generally requires either medical or surgical intervention for closure.

PCA: Postconception age.

Pediatric evaluation of disability inventory (PEDI): A global clinical assessment that evaluates key functional capabilities and performance in children between the functional ages of 6 months and 7½ years.

Pediatric quality of life inventory (PedsQL): A measure of health-related quality of life in children and adolescents.

Periodic breathing: Breathing interrupted by pauses of 10 or more seconds; common in preterm babies.

Persistent fetal circulation: A condition in which the blood continues to flow through the ductus arteriosus and bypass the lungs; this usually occurs in term and postterm infants following hypoxia.

Personal amplification devices: Wearable, electronic products that are intended to amplify sound.

Physical environment: The physical space, toys, and opportunities for play afforded a child. Physical environment includes the child's home, extended family's homes, and the childcare environments where the child spends their days and nights.

Postural control: The ability to assume, maintain, or reestablish upright posture during an activity.

PIH: Pregnancy-induced hypertension.

PIV: Peripheral intravenous line.

Placenta abruptio: Premature separation of the placenta from the uterus with resultant bleeding and neonatal asphyxia.

Placenta previa: A condition in which the placenta is abnormally positioned over the cervix, thereby preventing a normal vaginal delivery.

Pneumogram: Monitoring a baby's heart rate and respiratory patterns for several hours to detect any abnormalities either during waking or sleeping.

PO: Feeding by mouth.

Polycythemia: Abnormally high number of red blood cells, causing "sluggish" circulation; this is also called hyperviscosity.

Polyhydramnios: Excessive amount of amniotic fluid.

Positive end-expiratory pressure: A constant amount of pressure exerted by the respiratory system to keep the lungs expanded.

PPHN: Persistent pulmonary hypertension of the newborn.

Premature rupture of membranes: The breaking of the membrane surrounding the fetus before the beginning of labor; this results in an increased possibility of infection.

Preparedness: The knowledge and capacities developed by governments, response and recovery organizations, communities, and individuals to effectively anticipate, respond to, and recover from the impacts of likely, imminent, or current disasters. Preparedness action is carried out within the context of disaster risk management and aims to build the capacities needed to efficiently manage all types of emergencies and achieve orderly transitions from response to sustained recovery.

Primary impairments: Problems arising directly from the identified health concerns.

Proprioception: The sense of the relative position of body parts in space in static positions and during dynamic movement.

Pseudohypertrophy: Appearance of increased muscle bulk that is caused by fat infiltration and loss of muscle tissue in muscular dystrophies.

PT: Prothrombin time or preterm infant.

PTT: Partial thromboplastin time.

PVL: Periventricular leukomalacia.

Quality of life: An individual standard of health and happiness.

RA: Room air.

Reciprocating gait orthosis (RGO): An orthotic device that encompasses both lower extremities along with a trunk support component and that controls or facilitates reciprocal motion of the lower extremities for therapeutic or functional gait.

Red flags: Developmental milestones a child should be doing at a certain age but is not. Reasons for future evaluation or referral to a pediatrician.

Rehabilitation Act of 1973: A federal law that prohibits discrimination based on disability in programs conducted by federal agencies, in programs receiving federal financial assistance, and in federal employment and the employment practices of federal contractors.

Rehabilitation Engineering and Assistive Technology Society of North America (RESNA): A professional organization dedicated to promoting the health and well-being of people with disabilities through increasing access to technology solutions.

Respiratory distress syndrome: Term used interchangeably with hyaline membrane disease.

Retinopathy of prematurity: A condition of the eyes related to prematurity, oxygen concentration, and possibly other factors that affects the blood vessels of the eyes and can result in blindness; previously called retrolental fibroplasia.

Revised Upper Limb Scale (RULM): Twenty-item instrument to assess activities of daily living (ADLs) in patients with SMA through items involving shoulder, elbow, wrist, and hand function such as bringing hands from lap to table, picking up small items, pushing buttons, and bringing hands above shoulders.

School Function Assessment (SFA): An assessment of performance of functional tasks related to academic and social aspects of school participation.

Secondary impairments: Problems arising from a health concern that become apparent as time passes.

Self-advocacy: An individual's ability to speak up for the things that are important to them.

Self-determination: An individual's ability to make choices and manage their own life.

Self-efficacy: An individual's confidence in their ability to meet challenges and complete tasks successfully.

Sensory processing disorder: A disorder that arises when sensory processing impairments lead to a variety of sensory modulation difficulties, atypical activity levels, behavioral and emotional problems, and developmental delays.

Sensory-motor loop: The coupling of the sensory and motor systems. Coordination of these 2two systems drives accurate movement.

Sepsis: Generalized infection characterized by proliferation of bacteria in the bloodstream, due to the fact the newborn has little capacity to localize or encapsulate infections.

Septal defects: Congenital defects in the heart muscle. Ventricular septal defect (VSD) is an opening between the right and left ventricles. Atrial septal defect (ASD) is between the right and left atria. These defects generally require surgical repair.

Serial casting: A procedure that helps reduce contractures and increase available range of motion by applying a cast in a stretched position and doing subsequent applications at increased ranges.

Sexually transmitted disease: Infection passed prenatally or perinatally to the infant whose mother is infected; examples include syphilis, herpes, and gonorrhea.

SIMV: Synchronized intermittent mandatory ventilation.

Small for gestational age: Newborn whose growth parameters (weight, length, and head circumference) are less than the fifth percentile for gestational age; also called intrauterine growth restriction (IUGR).

SMN-dependent pharmacologic therapies: Medications that try to increase the available amount of functional SMN protein by either modifying the splicing of *SMN2* RNA (with the goal of producing functional SMN protein) or replacing the faulty *SMN1* gene (using viral vector–based gene therapy).

SMN-independent pharmacologic therapies: Medications that try to ameliorate symptoms of SMA by enhancing muscle activation.

Social story: A form of social narrative intervention that aims to explain confusing or difficult social concepts, interactions, or situations in a meaningful way for the individual.

Spinal muscular atrophy (SMA): A disease in which degeneration of α-motor neurons in the lower spinal cord leads to progressive muscle weakness and atrophy. The death of these motor neurons is related to lack of SMN.

Spinal muscular atrophy classification by types: A classification approach for SMA based on age of onset and expected function that divides patients with SMA into type I (Werdnig-Hoffmann), type II, or type III (Kugelberg-Welander). Types I to III are ordered from younger to older age of onset and from lower to higher expected functional ability. Other types exist, including type IV and type X-linked, but they are not as common.

Spinal muscular atrophy functional classification: A classification approach for SMA based on functional ability that divides patients with SMA into nonsitters, sitters, and walkers.

Surfactant: A substance manufactured by the lungs to prevent alveolar collapse.

Survival motor neuron (SMN): A protein encoded by the *SMN1* and *SMN2* genes that is involved in cellular homeostatic pathways, mRNA trafficking and local translation, cytoskeletal dynamics, endocytosis, and bioenergetic pathways.

Task analysis: The breakdown of a more complex skill into its component parts.

Technological hazard: A hazard that originates from technological or industrial conditions, dangerous procedures, infrastructure failures, or specific human activities. Examples include industrial pollution, nuclear radiation, toxic wastes, dam failures, transport accidents, factory explosions, fires, and chemical spills. Technological hazards also may arise directly as a result of the impacts of a natural hazard.

Technology-Related Assistance for Individuals with Disabilities Act: Provides federal funding from the US Department of Education to each state and territory to support "state efforts to improve the provision of AT to individuals with disabilities of all ages through comprehensive statewide programs of technology-related assistance."

TEF: Tracheoesophageal fistula.

Theophylline: A stimulant drug used in the treatment of apnea; caffeine citrate is also used for this purpose.

Thoracolumbosacral orthosis: An orthotic device used for trunk positioning and control.

Timed functional tests: Tests that require the child to perform a specific functional task and can serve as predictors of expected functional changes based on the time taken to complete the task. Examples include 10-m walk test, supine to stand, climb 4four stairs, Timed Up and Go (TUG), and single limb stance.

Tocolytic drugs: Drugs used to stop premature labor (eg, ritodrine).

TOF: Tetralogy of Fallot.

Top-down approach: Uses cognition to drive motor output. Requires that the patient think about the task.

TORCH: Toxoplasmosis, rubella cytomegalovirus, herpes simplex, and HIV.

TORCH titers: A blood test to determine the presence of certain viral agents including toxoplasmosis, syphilis, rubella, cytomegalovirus, and herpes simplex.

Transcutaneous monitor: A device to monitor oxygen concentration in the blood by means of a skin electrode.

Twin-to-twin transfusion syndrome: Rapid respiratory rate generally seen in term infants born by cesarean or with precipitous deliveries, related to poorly absorbed lung fluid; may be referred to as wet lung.

UAC OR UA: Umbilical artery catheter.

UVC OR UV: Umbilical vein catheter.

Vernix: White fatty substance that protects the fetus skin in utero and serves as an antimicrobial barrier.

Visualization/imagery: The practice of imagining successful completion of all the components of a motor task from beginning to end.

Visual-spatial tasks: Tasks requiring the knowledge of items' arrangements and relationships in space.

VLBW: Very low birth weight (between 1001 and 1500 g)

VSD: Ventricular septal defect.

Woman's reproductive history:

Example: G4 P 2-1-1-3

G: gravida – total number of pregnancies.
P: para – pregnancy outcomes.

Numbers following P are:

First number: number of full-term deliveries.
Second number: number of preterm deliveries.
Third number: number of abortions (spontaneous or elective).
Fourth number: number of living children.

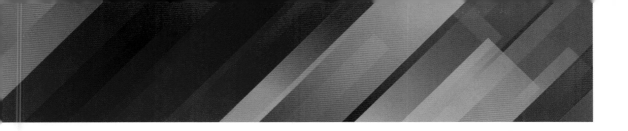

Index

Note: Page numbers followed by an "*f*" indicate figures; page numbers followed by a "*t*" indicate tables.